CLINICAL PRACTICE OF

TRANSFUSION
MEDICINE

THIRD EDITION

CLINICAL PRACTICE OF
TRANSFUSION
MEDICINE

THIRD EDITION

Edited by

LAWRENCE D. PETZ, M.D.
Professor of Pathology and Laboratory Medicine
Department of Pathology
University of California, Los Angeles
UCLA School of Medicine
Director of Transfusion Medicine
UCLA Medical Center
Los Angeles, California

SCOTT N. SWISHER, M.D.
Professor Emeritus
Department of Medicine
College of Human Medicine
Michigan State University
East Lansing, Michigan

STEVEN KLEINMAN, M.D.
Professor of Clinical Pathology
and Laboratory Medicine
Department of Pathology
University of California, Los Angeles
UCLA School of Medicine
Co-director of Transfusion Medicine
UCLA Medical Center
Los Angeles, California

RICHARD K. SPENCE, M.D.
Professor
Department of Surgery
University of Medicine and Dentistry
of New Jersey
Robert Wood Johnson Medical School
Head, Section of Vascular Surgery
Cooper Hospital/University Medical Center
Camden, New Jersey

RONALD G. STRAUSS, M.D.
Professor
Departments of Pathology and Pediatrics
University of Iowa College of Medicine
Medical Director
DeGowin Blood Center
University of Iowa Hospitals and Clinics
Iowa City, Iowa

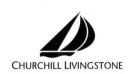

CHURCHILL LIVINGSTONE

New York, Edinburgh, London, Madrid, Melbourne, San Francisco, Tokyo

Library of Congress Cataloging-in-Publication Data

Clinical practice of transfusion medicine / edited by Lawrence D. Petz
   ... [et al.]. – 3rd ed.
     p.   cm.
  Includes bibliographical references and index.
  ISBN 0-443-08981-7
  1. Blood–Transfusion.   I. Petz, Lawrence D.
  [DNLM: 1. Blood Transfusion. WB 356 C6415 1995]
  RM171.C524 1995
  615'.39–dc20
  DNLM/DLC
  for Library of Congress   95-32421
                                    CIP

Distributed in the United Kingdom by Churchill Livingstone, Robert Stevenson
House, 1–3 Baxter's Place, Leith Walk, Edinburgh EH1 3AF, and by associated companies, branches, and representatives throughout the world.

Accurate indications, adverse reactions, and dosage schedules for drugs are provided
in this book, but it is possible that they may change. The reader is urged to review
the package information data of the manufacturers of the medications mentioned.

The Publishers have made every effort to trace the copyright holders for borrowed
material. If they have inadvertently overlooked any, they will be pleased to make
the necessary arrangements at the first opportunity.

Acquisitions Editor: *Kerry Willis*
Assistant Editor: *Marc Strauss*
Copy Editor: *Elizabeth Bowman-Schulman*
Production Supervisor: *Laura Mosberg Cohen*
Cover Design: *Paul Moran*

Printed in the United States of America

First published in 1996   7 6 5 4 3 2

Contributors

Kenneth C. Anderson, M.D.
Associate Professor, Department of Medicine, Harvard Medical School; Medical Director, Blood Component Laboratory, Division of Hematologic Malignancies, Dana-Farber Cancer Institute, Boston, Massachusetts

Maureen Andrew, M.D.
Professor, Department of Paediatrics, McMaster University School of Medicine, and Hamilton Civic Hospitals Research Centre, Hamilton, Ontario; Staff, Department of Paediatrics, Children's Hospital, Chedoke-McMaster Hospitals, and The Hospital for Sick Children, Toronto, Ontario, Canada

Kaaron Benson, M.D., Ph.D.
Assistant Professor, Department of Pathology and Laboratory Medicine, University of South Florida College of Medicine; Director, Blood Bank, HLA/Immunogenetics Laboratory, Pathology Service, H. Lee Moffitt Cancer Center, Tampa, Florida

Mark E. Boyd, M.D.
Associate Professor, Department of Obstetrics and Gynecology, McGill University Faculty of Medicine; Director of Gynecology, Department of Obstetrics and Gynecology, Royal Victoria Hospital, Montreal, Quebec, Canada

Lu Ann Brooker, R.T.
Staff, McMaster University School of Medicine and Hamilton Civic Hospitals Research Centre, Hamilton, Ontario, Canada

Michael P. Busch, M.D., Ph.D.
Associate Professor, Department of Laboratory Medicine, University of California, San Francisco, School of Medicine; Vice President, Research and Scientific Services, Irwin Memorial Blood Centers, San Francisco, California

James B. Bussel, M.D.
Associate Professor, Department of Pediatric Hematology/Oncology, Cornell University Medical College; Associate Attending Pediatrician, Department of Pediatric Hematology/Oncology, New York Hospital, New York, New York

Mitchell S. Cairo, M.D.
Director, Hematology/Oncology Research and Bone Marrow Transplantation, Department of Hematology/Oncology, Children's Hospital of Orange County, Orange, California

Loni Calhoun, M.T.(A.S.C.P.)S.B.B.
Senior Technical Specialist, Education and Research, Division of Transfusion Medicine, UCLA Medical Center, Los Angeles, California

Jeffrey L. Carson, M.D.

Professor of Medicine and Chief, Division of General Internal Medicine, Department of Medicine, University of Medicine and Dentistry of New Jersey Robert Wood Johnson Medical School, New Brunswick, New Jersey

J. Michael Cecka, Ph.D.

Associate Professor, Department of Surgery, University of California, Los Angeles, UCLA School of Medicine; Staff, UCLA Tissue Typing Laboratory, and United Network for Organ Sharing, UCLA Medical Center, Los Angeles, California

Roger Y. Dodd, Ph.D.

Head, Transmissible Diseases Department, Jerome H. Holland Laboratory, American Red Cross Blood Services, Rockville, Maryland

Janice P. Dutcher, M.D.

Professor of Medicine, Departments of Oncology and Medicine, Albert Einstein Cancer Center, Bronx, New York

Walter H. Dzik, M.D.

Assistant Professor, Department of Internal Medicine, Harvard Medical School; Director, Transfusion Medicine, New England Deaconness Hospital, Boston, Massachusetts

Cherie S. Evans, M.D.

Assistant Clinical Professor, Department of Laboratory Medicine, University of California, San Francisco, School of Medicine, San Francisco, California; Medical Director, Blood Bank of the Alameda Contra Costa Medical Association, Oakland, California

Laura Gindy, M.T.(A.S.C.P.)S.B.B.

Senior Specialist, Division of Transfusion Medicine, UCLA Medical Center, Los Angeles, California

Jonathan C. Goldsmith, M.D.

Vice President of Clinical Research, and Medical Director, Alpha Therapeutic Corporation, Los Angeles, California

Paul V. Holland, M.D.

Clinical Professor, Division of Hematology/ Oncology, Department of Internal Medicine, University of California, Davis, School of Medicine; Medical Director and Chief Executive Officer, Sacramento Medical Foundation Blood Center, Sacramento, California

Heather Hume, M.D., F.R.C.P.C.

Assistant Professor, Department of Pediatrics, Université de Montréal; Pediatric Hematologist/ Onocologist, Department of Hematology/Oncology, Hôpital Ste-Justine, Montreal, Quebec, Canada

Paul W. Jenner, M.D.

Director, Medical Affairs, Blood Systems, Inc., Scottsdale, Arizona

Elaine Jeter, M.D.

Associate Professor and Medical Director of Transfusion Medicine, Department of Pathology and Laboratory Medicine, Medical University of South Carolina College of Medicine, Charleston, South Carolina

Anne Kessinger, M.D.

Professor, Section of Oncology/Hematology, Department of Internal Medicine, University of Nebraska Medical Center, Omaha, Nebraska

Sherwin V. Kevy, M.D.

Associate Professor, Department of Pediatrics, Harvard Medical School; Director, Transfusion Service, Department of Laboratory Medicine, Children's Hospital, Boston, Massachusetts

Harvey G. Klein, M.D.

Director, Department of Transfusion Medicine, Warren G. Magnuson Clinical Center, National Institutes of Health, Department of Health and Human Services, Bethesda, Maryland

Steven Kleinman, M.D.

Biomedical Consultant, Victoria, BC, Canada

Roger H. Kobayashi, M.D.

Clinical Associate Professor, Division of Immunology, Department of Pediatrics, University of California, Los Angeles, UCLA School of Medicine, Los Angeles, California; Partner, Allergy, Asthma and Immunology Associates, Omaha, Nebraska

Margot S. Kruskall, M.D.

Associate Professor, Departments of Pathology and Medicine, Harvard Medical School; Director, Division of Laboratory Medicine, Beth Israel Hospital, Boston, Massachusetts

Sanford R. Kurtz, M.D.

Chairman, Department of Laboratory Medicine, Director, Transfusion Medicine, Lahey Clinic, Burlington, Massachusetts

Karen Shoos Lipton, J.D.

Chief Executive Officer, American Association of Blood Banks, Bethesda, Maryland

Carma Lizza, M.T.(A.S.C.P.)S.B.B.

Manager, Division of Transfusion Medicine, UCLA Medical Center, Los Angeles, California

Jeffrey McCullough, M.D.

Professor, Department of Laboratory Medicine and Pathology, University of Minnesota Medical School—Minneapolis; Director, Blood Bank, Health Sciences Center of the University of Minnesota, Minneapolis, Minneapolis, Minnesota; Director, American Red Cross Regional Blood Program, St. Paul, Minnesota

Judith Myers, M.T.(A.S.C.P.)S.B.B.

Supervisor, Division of Transfusion Medicine, UCLA Medical Center, Los Angeles, California

Harold A. Oberman, M.D.

Professor, Department of Pathology, University of Michigan Medical School; Director, Blood Bank and Transfusion Service, University of Michigan Medical Center, Ann Arbor, Michigan

Lawrence D. Petz, M.D.

Professor of Pathology and Laboratory Medicine, University of California, Los Angeles, UCLA School of Medicine; Director of Transfusion Medicine, UCLA Medical Center, Los Angeles, California

Joseph Rosenthal, M.D.

Associate, Blood and Bone Marrow Transplantation, Children's Hospital of Orange County, Orange, California

Steven Ross, M.D.

Associate Professor, Department of Surgery, University of Medicine and Dentistry of New Jersey Robert Wood Johnson Medical School; Head, Division of Trauma Emergency Surgical Services, Cooper Hospital/University Medical Center, Camden, New Jersey

Merlyn H. Sayers, M.D., Ph.D.

Associate Professor, Department of Medicine, Division of Hematology, University of Washington Medical School; Director, Transfusion Surveillance, Puget Sound Blood Center, Seattle, Washington

Ramesh A. Shivdasani, M.D., Ph.D.

Assistant Professor, Department of Medicine, Harvard Medical School; Instructor, Department of Medicine, Dana-Farber Cancer Institute, Boston, Massachusetts

Ira A. Shulman, M.D.

Professor and Director of Transfusion Medicine, University of Southern California School of Medicine; Chief, Division of Transfusion Medicine, Immunology, and Microbiology, Los Angeles County/University of Southern California Medical Center; Medical Director, Blood Bank and Transfusion Services, USC Kenneth Norris Jr. Comprehensive Cancer Institute, Los Angeles, California

Arthur J. Silvergleid, M.D.

Associate Clinical Professor, Department of Medicine, University of California, Los Angeles, UCLA School of Medicine, Los Angeles, California; Medical and Executive Director, Blood Bank of San Bernardino and Riverside Counties, San Bernardino, California

Daniel W. Skupski, M.D.
Assistant Professor, Division of Maternal-Fetal Medicine, Department of Obstetrics and Gynecology, Cornell University Medical College, New York, New York

Richard K. Spence, M.D.
Professor, Department of Surgery, University of Medicine and Dentistry of New Jersey Robert Wood Johnson Medical School; Head, Section of Vascular Surgery, Cooper Hospital/University Medical Center, Camden, New Jersey

Linda Stehling, M.D.
Vice President, Medical and Regulatory Affairs, Blood Systems, Inc., Scottsdale, Arizona

E. Richard Stiehm, M.D.
Professor and Chief, Division of Immunology/ Allergy, Department of Pediatrics, University of California, Los Angeles, UCLA School of Medicine; Attending Pediatrician, UCLA Medical Center, Los Angeles, California

Ronald G. Strauss, M.D.
Professor, Departments of Pathology and Pediatrics, University of Iowa College of Medicine; Medical Director, DeGowin Blood Center, University of Iowa Hospitals and Clinics, Iowa City, Iowa

Scott N. Swisher, M.D.
Professor Emeritus, Department of Medicine, College of Human Medicine, Michigan State University, East Lansing, Michigan

Roger Vertrees, B.A., C.C.P.
Instructor and Perfusionist, Division of Cardiothoracic Surgery, The University of Texas Medical Branch University of Texas Medical School at Galveston, Galveston, Texas

Carl F.W. Wolf, M.D.
Professor of Clinical Pathology, Department of Pathology, Cornell University Medical College; Director, Blood Bank and Transfusion Service, The New York Hospital, New York, New York

Edward L. Wolf, M.D.
Senior Associate General Counsel, Office of General Counsel, American Red Cross, Washington, D.C.

Priscilla Yam, F.I.B.M.S.
Senior Research Associate in Gene Therapy Research, Division of Pediatrics, City of Hope Medical Center, Duarte, California

John A. Zaia, M.D.
Professor and Director of Virology and Infectious Diseases, Division of Pediatrics, City of Hope Medical Center, Duarte, California

Howard L. Zauder, M.D., Ph.D.
Professor Emeritus, Department of Anesthesiology, State University of New York Health Center at Syracuse College of Medicine, Syracuse, New York; Chief, Anesthesia Section, Carl T. Hayden Veterans Affairs Medical Center, Phoenix, Arizona

Preface to the Third Edition

Since the second edition of *Clinical Practice of Transfusion Medicine*, published in 1989, the field of transfusion medicine has continued to grow, develop, and respond to rapid changes in basic science, clinical practice, and health care organizations, as well as new forces in the economic, political, legal, and regulatory spheres. Many of these changes are shared with the entire health care system and are linked to profound movements within American society. This edition of the book responds to this dynamic environment. It has resulted in a major reorganization of the book and the addition of three new members, all recognized authorities in transfusion medicine, to the editorial group.

Surgically oriented topics have been drawn together by Richard Spence, who has studied many aspects of the requirement for transfusion secondary to blood loss in surgical and non-surgical settings. He has also contributed to the study of oxygen-carrying blood substitutes and to the still controversial topic of the "transfusion trigger." His experience in the surgical care of patients who refuse transfusion has provided an opportunity to investigate many of these issues. Ronald Strauss has done the same for those problems related to pediatric transfusion, including disorders of hemostasis and congenital anemias. With experience in pediatrics, transfusion medicine, and blood banking, he has greatly extended the range of topics covered in this area of the book. There is now increased emphasis on neonatal physiology of hematopoiesis and hemostasis as it relates to transfusion practice.

Steven Kleinman expanded coverage of infections transmissible by transfusion. This section now deals in more detail not only with the well-known infections transmissible by transfusion, but also with problems that may be emerging. His experience in blood center and hospital blood bank management has also contributed to focusing attention on issues of donor selection that minimize the threat of transmitted infection.

We have again tried to deal with some issues that may become clinically relevant in the near future: immune modulation caused by transfusion, ambulatory transfusion, issues associated with organ, marrow, and stem cell transplantation, and modification of the immune system by several therapeutic approaches. A completely new section on medicolegal aspects of transfusion deals with some of the recent pertinent decisions specific to this field, written by two attorneys with long experience in transfusion-related litigation. Chapters dealing with organizational, management, and regulatory matters have also been revised.

Finally, many new contributors have been recruited to the book, further to diversify the viewpoints expressed. We thank them for their participation and extend the same thanks to those authors who have contributed to the previous editions. We again express our gratitude to the editorial staff of Churchill Livingstone for their personal support and professional skills that have gone into this book in its past and present editions.

Lawrence D. Petz, M.D.
Scott N. Swisher, M.D.

Preface to the Second Edition

Since the publication of the first edition of this book in 1981, a sweeping change has occurred in the practice of transfusion medicine. Most of the material for that edition was prepared in late 1979 and early 1980. The problem of acquired immunodeficiency syndrome, now called AIDS, was just emerging at that time. There was no mention of it in the first edition.

Since then, progress in understanding the infectious nature of the disease and its epidemiology has occurred at an unprecedented rate. Although AIDS is spread primarily by sexual routes, it became apparent early on that the transfusion of blood or blood products derived from an infected donor usually transmits the infection to the recipient. Although there is still no effective therapy for infection with the human immunodeficiency virus, HIV, sensitive tests for antibodies to this agent have been developed that at least permit identification of blood donors who are probably infectious. It appears that once an individual is infected, the virus remains in the blood for the life of the patient and can be transmitted to a recipient by transfusion of blood or blood products that, as of yet, cannot be rendered noninfectious by in vitro treatment.

Although the risk of transmission of HIV by blood transfusion is low, and only a small proportion of the total number of patients with AIDS have been infected due to transfusion, the serious nature of the infection has produced major changes in the practice of blood banking and transfusion medicine. Screening of donors for evidence of infection, testing of all units for antibody to HIV, mechanisms for self–deferral of potential donors who are at high risk of the infection, and methods of sterilization of some of the plasma–derived therapeutic products are among the changes that have occurred as part of a major effort to control this route of transmission. Fortunately, these measure have been quite successful, although some risk for the patient remains.

The small residual risk of infection with HIV has produced a major change in the way transfusion therapy is viewed and utilized in clinical practice. More conservative risk/benefit evaluations of the need for transfusion are being made today. Thus, in the second edition, one will find evidence of a new awareness of the risks of transfusion and frequent suggestions of more conservative indications for administration of blood and blood products. This may be beneficial in several respects. In avoiding transfusion because of the risk of HIV infection, the other well known risks of transfusion are also avoided. For example, the problem of transfusion– related hepatitis is still with us, and its avoidance may be even more important in the epidemiological sense than is eliminating the small risk of transmission of HIV. That the use of marginally justified transfusion therapy should continue to decrease is a view strongly advocated by many specialists in transfusion medicine.

A lack of public awareness about how AIDS can be spread has had a major impact on transfusion medicine, one that is unfortunate as seen from the point of view of blood transfusion services. For example, at one time public opinion data indicated that many people thought transfusion was one of the major routes of transmission of HIV infection. Many people also felt that donating blood would put them at risk of acquiring this infection. The effect of this level of public apprehension was to reduce the blood supply at a time of continuing growth of demand. In turn, this has raised costs of providing blood, since recruitment of donors has had to be increased. The more conservative use of transfusion did not offset the decrease in supply. The blood supply of the United States is again in a marginal balance with utilization, a situation that is only slowly improving as this edition goes to print.

There are also a number of technical and scientific changes that have occurred since publication of the first edition. For example, additional screening tests for exclusion of potentially infectious donors with hepatitis have been introduced. This is further reducing the blood supply by deferring a larger number of donors. Again, this will increase the costs of providing blood at a time when there is a major emphasis on reducing the costs of health care. Thus far, blood services have been able to cope without having to implement major changes, but whether our present system can continue to accommodate the adverse economic changes remains to be seen. It would be paradoxical indeed if the generally excellent, safe, and effective blood supply that has evolved in the United States, Canada, and much of Western Europe were to be adversely affected by this unfortunate combination of social and economic factors.

A number of new contributors have been added to the present edition in order to introduce differing viewpoints of topics of interest and importance. We thank previous contributors whose material in some instances has been consolidated by the editors or new contributors into new chapters. Much of this has been done to make space for new material in the second edition. We acknowledge the continuing value of these previous contributions.

The target audiences and the purposes of the second edition remain unchanged, although we have changed the title of the book to emphasize that we focus on the clinical aspects of transfusion medicine while attempting to provide an understanding of it on a scientific and practical basis. This emphasis on clinical practice should not detract from the fact that we have tried to give appropriate weight to laboratory aspects of transfusion medicine, which included immunohematology as well as the collection of blood, and its processing, storage, and administration. This inclusion of both clinical and laboratory components of transfusion medicine arises from our strong commitment to the principle of improving communication between primary care physicians and laboratory workers about all aspects of transfusion medicine. In this regard, we feel that blood bank technologists have played an extraordinary role in that they are highly skilled and dedicated, have participated in extensive continuing education programs including national and international meetings, and have taken on an exceptional amount of responsibility in solving difficult immunohematologic problems. We hope communication between primary care physicians and laboratory workers will continue to improve and that this book will be a single source of information to facilitate such interaction. We intend for the book to be useful on a frequent basis, not merely to provide a repository of reference information.

Many people have been helpful in the preparation of the second edition, too many to cite individually. Our colleagues in our own institutions have been particularly helpful as critics. We also appreciate the tolerant help of our publisher, Churchill Livingstone, and our editor, Robert Hurley.

Lawrence D. Petz, M.D.
Scott N. Swisher, M.D.

Contents

Chapter 1

Overview and General Principles of Transfusion Medicine

Scott N. Swisher and Lawrence D. Petz

In spite of the major role transfusion therapy has in today's health care, only rough estimates of the extent of blood banking activity were available in the United States until about 1990. Efforts to document the scope of blood banking activities in this country by more systematic data gathering started with the work of Surgenor et al.[1] Their data covering the period from 1982 to 1988 and a later related publication of Wallace et al.[2] that reported on a survey of transfusion activities in 1989 provide the best estimates available of the available national blood resource and its utilization.

The 1982 to 1988 survey indicated a peak blood collection in 1986 of 13.4 million units, with essentially the same figure for the following 2 years. Autologous blood collections rose from 30,000 in 1982 to 397,000 in 1987. In this study, transfusions of red cells or whole blood, 12.2 million in 1986, declined more than 1 million units by 1987, and continued at about this level through 1988. It was noted in this report that there were 6.4 million units of platelets transfused in 1987. During the period 1980 to 1987, the proportion of platelets obtained from single donors rose from 11 to 25 percent. Plasma transfusion were relatively constant over this period at 2.1 to 2.3 million units.

The later study reported by Wallace et al.[2] of data about activity in 1989 utilized a different method in which the survey data were extended to a sample of hospitals and results were extended to the national level by statistical analysis. These data show a somewhat higher level of activity, as might be expected from the larger survey base, that is, 14.3 million units collected, somewhat more than 12 million red cell/whole blood transfusions to 3,159,000 recipients, for an average of 3.8 units/patient transfused. At this time, 655,000 units of preoperative autologous blood were drawn, a 65 percent increase since 1987, but 55 percent of these units were not transfused and were presumably discarded. Similar data on the utilization of autologous transfusion suggests that, with the present safety of allogeneic transfusion, the practice of autologous transfusion may have become cost-ineffective, in part because of the high rate of discard of such units.[3] Platelet transfusions were estimated at 7,258,000 units, an increase of 13.7 percent since 1987. A more limited study of blood collection and distribution provided data concordant with those cited when consideration is given to differing methods.[4,5] This report indicates that the growth in the U.S. blood supply has been slower since 1988. There is, however, no indication (as of early 1995) that the total U.S. supply is inadequate to meet real needs, even though there have been reported regional shortages that have been managed by resource-sharing programs.

The U.S. blood supply nevertheless may be in some jeopardy, based on economic forces developing in the health care program of this country, possible slow adverse shifts in public attitudes about dona-

1

tion, and the introduction of new technologies that require large amounts of donor blood. In this respect, better and more current data about blood service activity in the United States would be of great value in detecting impending shortages before they become severe. More comprehensive information would also be valuable in economic and organizational planning for blood resources in the U.S. health care system changes in which are now under consideration.

COMPONENT THERAPY

The introduction of component therapy during the 1960s, in which the donated unit of whole blood was broken down into sedimented red cells, platelets, cryoprecipitate, fresh frozen plasma, or other components, has had a major impact on the practice of blood transfusion. A much larger number of useful therapeutic units, from 2 to 2.5 per donation, are now derived from a single donation. There is no comprehensive historical information about the impact of component therapy on transfusion practice throughout the entire country. It has become widespread if not universal. The effective practice of component therapy still varies to some degree throughout the country, which seemingly is dependent on the level of organization, sophistication, and effectiveness of the available transfusion services in a region.

Component therapy has been of major significance in two ways. It has provided more specific replacement of the blood component(s) that the patient needs. As a corollary, it has also made unnecessary the administration of components that the patient does not require. This has improved both the safety and the efficacy of blood transfusion. Of almost equal importance has been the impact of component therapy on the national blood supply. It has permitted much more efficient utilization of available donor resources to meet a still-expanding need for transfusion.

NATIONAL BLOOD SUPPLY

If component therapy were used in a maximally useful way in the United States and if overuse of blood transfusion not well justified by clinical or scientific data were greatly reduced, the presently marginal blood supply of the United States would be in better balance with the real needs of our population. Further growth in the need for blood would, in effect, then depend largely on the introduction of new therapeutic procedures that require blood or one or more of its components. A relatively modest rate of future growth can be predicted on the basis of increasing population, an older population, and increasing participation of presently underserved segments of the U.S. population in the health care service system. Other potential changes in medical practice might also reduce the need for blood.

IMPACT OF NEW MEDICAL TECHNOLOGY

The introduction of a major new medical or surgical technique might increase the requirement for blood transfusions on a major scale even though such innovations are not presently a prospect. However, plans to develop an increased blood supply are rarely undertaken before the appearance of the increased need in a relatively acute form. In this respect, it is interesting to examine the past impact of the introduction of coronary artery bypass surgery and cardiac surgery in general on the national blood supply. These procedures depended very directly on the availability of blood transfusions for their development. This has been true of many surgical developments in this century and of a number of medical procedures, such as renal dialysis. With improvements in anesthesiology and physiologic understanding of the surgical patient, enormous advances in all areas of surgery have occurred since 1945. Until the introduction of cardiac surgery, with its requirement for cardiac bypass pump priming and substantial intraoperative and postoperative blood replacement during the developmental phase, the growth of the blood donor base in the United States kept up reasonably well with the need for blood.

The sudden, almost explosive rise in cardiac surgical procedures that occurred in the early 1970s seriously stressed the blood supply of the country. For example, it was found that more than one-third of the blood supply in Milwaukee at that time was directed to cardiac surgical patients. It was difficult for well organized, efficient blood banks to keep pace with the increased demand. Their carefully constructed volunteer donor base was threatened by calls from hospitals and surgeons for recruitment of professional donors. It was probably only the threat of the hepatitis hazard associated with professional blood donation that prevented re-emergence of substantial commercial blood banking activity in United States at that time. As new medical technologies dependent on blood transfusion are introduced, it would be wise to examine their possible impact on the blood supply. Plans could then be made for further development of the donor base, if this is necessary, or for more efficient utilization of blood resources already available.

Newer medial approaches to remaining serious health problems in some instances might have the opposite effect on the national blood supply. At the present time, for example, large numbers of blood platelets are administered to patients undergoing chemotherapy for malignant diseases, particularly acute leukemia. If a more effective treatment of these disorders were to be discovered or if ways to improve effectiveness of platelet transfusions or prevent refractoriness were found, the demand for platelets would immediately be affected. This in turn would have major economic effects on the national blood services and might cause a readjustment of pricing policies for other blood components to meet the costs of operating the system as a whole in the face of lost revenue from platelet production. At present, there is controversy over the use of platelet transfusions given prophylactically to prevent bleeding in severely thrombocytopenic patients undergoing intensive chemotherapy. Approaches using a lower transfusion trigger than usual have been suggested, and such policies might also have an effect on the blood supply and the economics of blood services. An even greater impact on platelet transfusion may result from the introduction of thrombopoietin (see Chapter 16). Even without new technology, changes in established practice that are based on better information will affect blood services in ways that are not easy to predict.

NEW PLASMA PRODUCTS

It is possible that a number of additional components of plasma may be isolated and found to be clinically useful. If this were to occur, additional products with economic value and unknown demand or need would then be available. Again, this might result in a restructuring of the needs, demands, and economics of plasma-derivative production. It is increasingly recognized that serum albumin is overutilized in the United States and in many Western European countries. Fresh frozen plasma has been substituted for the albumin to some degree resulting in an unstable market for serum albumin and albumin products.[1] This may indirectly affect the price and availability of antihemophilic factor, the other major economically important component of plasma for which there has been in the past a relative imbalance between need and supply. The availability of recombinant factor VIII now provides another economic force. The uses for plasma immunoglobulin have also changed suddenly and dramatically with the availability of safe products for intravenous administration (see Chapter 45). The impact of these changes on the operation of the total blood services system of the country and the Western world remains to be seen. The system is dynamic. Changing clinical guidelines and practice can also affect the blood economy.[6]

For these reasons and others, there appears to be a need for a more integrated management of the national blood resource than the present system, or nonsystem, provides. There is support for the opinion that this management should be developed outside the complete control of government, but the specific agencies or organizations that might implement it effectively are uncertain and unlikely to be defined in the present political climate. Some would argue for a return to a more or less completely free market situation as the most effective and efficient way of achieving the best relationship between costs, safety, and availability of blood and blood products. This is equally unlikely in view of the past experiences in the United States and the Western world. A market approach is incompatible with the widely accepted concept that the blood service complex is, in fact, a human service and not primarily a commercial enterprise. How these matters will be resolved ultimately in the United States and in other countries will be of great interest.

PROBLEMS OF MEDICAL EDUCATION AND PUBLIC EDUCATION

By any assessment, the systematic exposure of medical students and residents to even fundamental information about blood transfusion at the clinical level is still inadequate. Transfusion practice and related research have not experienced widespread acceptance in academic circles until recently. As a result, many medical students and residents learn what they do know about blood transfusion by the process of "chaining." Chief residents pass along what they have learned, which was gathered in an entirely unsystematic way, to the assistant residents who then in turn teach the interns and medical students as they rotate through the various clinical services. The teaching is usually unsystematic and largely in the context of the transfusion management of individual patients. Consequently, many physicians enter their definitive careers with a shallow and narrow understanding of the appropriate management of one of their most important therapeutic tools.

This is partly a reflection of the fact that, in many medical institutions, the blood transfusion service is still regarded as primarily a laboratory service. The laboratory aspects of blood transfusion services are, of course, of great importance. Without them, in their highly developed present state, little of modern transfusion practice could exist. Unfortunately, many clinical pathologists and laboratory directors have not been particularly well informed about the clinical management of blood transfusion. Many of the standard textbooks in medicine, surgery, pediatrics, obstetrics, and gynecology have, in the past, had little to say about blood transfusion at the clinical level, although they are slowly improving. One of the major goals of this book is to bring this clinical perspective to an audience of clinicians and laboratory personnel.

One of the major goals for the future should be to improve the education of medical students, all residents, and the senior staffs of all medical institutions in the proper management of blood transfusion in clinical practice. To accomplish this, these groups will have to be convinced of the favorable impact of such knowledge on the patient's welfare. Soumerai et al.[7] showed that changes in practice can be affected by educational interventions. Performance in this area should be subjected to the same scrutiny by peers as performance of surgical or medical procedures themselves. Informed transfusion committees play a vital role in this respect. A number of the now-outmoded concepts and some of the myths about blood transfusion therapy must be abandoned and replaced by what we know based on

a reasonably firm scientific basis. This will result not only in better patient care but also in a more intelligent, rational, and cost-effective use of this precious human resource. We should look for improvements in blood services in this country in the near future. The National Institutes of Health and the Heart, Lung, and Blood Institute provided leadership in this regard with the development of the Transfusion Medicine Academic Award Program, which was initiated in 1983, with the last 5-year grant being awarded in 1991. Also, the support of research by the National Blood Foundation of the American Association of Blood Banks plays a significant role in providing opportunities for improving the practice of what is now called transfusion medicine.

Not all changes in transfusion practice occur as the results of research, education, or organization and management. The discovery that the human immunodeficiency virus (HIV) is transmissible by transfusion and the transfusion acquired immunodeficiency syndrome scare that followed has changed the practice to transfusion medicine in a major way and very rapidly. Knowledge of transfusion-induced hepatitis had a similar but much smaller effect. Autologous transfusion, intraoperative blood salvage, hemodilution, and directed donations were among the responses generated by this knowledge. In addition, transfusion practice, particularly for red cells, became more conservative. Lower pre- and post-operative hematocrits were accepted, and efforts have been made to minimize transfusion of acutely and chronically anemic patients.

Many of these changes in practice have probably been beneficial to patients, by minimizing their exposure to known, if small, risks. Some, such as directed donations, probably serve primarily the psychological needs of patients but remain controversial in terms of risk reduction. There is now the concern that some patients are being undertransfused, to their detriment.[8] This risk is greatest when transfusion rates are guided primarily by laboratory measurements rather than by a clinical evaluation in which relevant laboratory data are a part.

COST-EFFECTIVENESS

Blood transfusions now enjoy a relatively well developed and mature technology that can meet most major demands on the system at the present time.

At least these needs can be met within the current biologically imposed limitations on the effectiveness of transfusion of red cells, platelets, leukocytes, and the currently available plasma derivatives. Present technologies still can be substantially improved. However, one must now examine the marginal value of these improvements. For example, improvement of the period of in vitro storage of red cells from the present 42-day limit to 50 days would probably have relatively little value. On the other hand, improvement of in vitro storage to beyond 60 days, if this could be accomplished with a greater than 90 percent viability of the transfused red cells, might have a substantial value. This value would also have to be judged in terms of the cost of the new system before it might be expected to replace the present technology. Almost any improvement in the in vitro preservation of function and storage life of platelets would be of some value, provided that this could be accomplished without an accompanying increase in the risk of bacterial infection. Practical and safe blood substitutes may become available. Other improvements in the technology of production, storage, and distribution of blood components must be similarly compared with the current methods, and the marginal value of the improvements must be estimated. With increasingly tight controls on all health care-related costs, future practice will probably require higher cost-benefit ratios; this will differ from the past tendency to introduce innovations that provided only a small improvement in efficacy without regard for cost.

ORGANIZATIONAL IMPROVEMENTS

Improved organization of blood services with better coordination between their various elements and improved professional utilization of the products of the blood transfusion services of the country still present major opportunities for better patient care. More effective approaches to donor recruitment, particularly, those that tend to level the blood supply around the calendar year, could be expected to contribute to resolution of nagging problems of periodic low blood availability. Resource sharing, by which supply and demand are adjusted over wide areas and nationally, has contributed to the security of the blood supply for individual institutions and the pa-

tients they serve. There is need for a clear, coherent, and unified message to blood donors of the country. Most of these changes are possible with little or no additional costs; they have the possibility of reducing costs by improving efficiency.

These reasonable and obviously needed changes are now being overshadowed by a process of imposed change by regulation. A brief review of some of the historical background of this development is helpful in understanding its impact.

Since World War II, three major events have serially transformed the nature of blood services in the United States and the developed world. These have been (1) the concept and discovery of effective methods of red cell preservation, which made blood banking, as we know it, possible; (2) the development of plastic transfusion equipment, which brought component therapy into practice; and (3) the discovery that HIV infection could be transmitted by blood transfusion and was indeed present in the U.S. blood supply. The effects of the first two developments led to the creation of a technically advanced transfusion service; these effects are still developing. The change wrought by the problem of HIV infection transmitted by transfusion has already revolutionized the organization and management of blood services in the United States and in many other developed countries; its final impact is still to be learned.

Three major related processes of change have been operating in this arena. First, transfusion practices have become more conservative as the issues raised by the HIV problem have been clarified. The public has reinforced these changes, and methods such as autologous transfusion have been developed to avoid many transfusions with donor blood in response to these pressures. Second, blood service organizations have examined their practices and have instituted changes designed to reduce the HIV hazard and the risk of hepatitis. Third, intensive research and development in both the public and private sectors has provided much of the technology and information that has made this possible.

Finally, there has been a major change in the regulatory environment under the authority of the Food and Drug Administration (FDA). This agency was in the process of reorganizing and reorienting its mechanisms for regulating biologic materials, including the many new products of biotechnology, when the need for change in blood services regulation became apparent. During intensified inspection programs by the FDA, it was recognized that many blood centers lacked standard operating procedures or did not follow adequately those that they had. Although there were few releases of dangerous units, this called for a regulatory response.

It seems clear that the agency did not have at that time the resources, financial and personnel, to carry out these changes with maximal efficiency and dispatch. Rather, the regulatory environment became a moving target with constantly increasing stringency of requirements on all aspects of the transfusion services of the country.

Present Regulatory Environment (1995)

The most recently imposed regulations involve the application of what is known as the Code of Good Manufacturing Practices (GMPs) on blood service organizations. These regulations have long controlled the manufacture and distribution of drugs, for which purpose they were specifically developed. Their applicability to biologic and blood products in general can be questioned. The environment of the pharmaceutical industry is different from that in which blood products are procured, processed, and distributed. GMPs now control essentially every aspect of providing blood and blood products at all levels of the system.

GMP regulations are oriented toward complete standardization and documentation of all aspects of the collection, processing, and distribution of blood and blood products. Qualifications, training, retraining, and documentation of proficiency are also under strong regulation. This has added greatly to the cost of blood and blood products, and these costs continue to increase. In some centers, it is said that an equal amount of time is being spent on documenting what is done as in actually carrying out the operation itself.

Critics of this situation maintain that this type of regulation actually derogates the safety of the products rather than ensures it. This question has not been put to a scientific evaluation, nor has the claim of the FDA that this level of regulation will improve safety. The fact is that the law under which the FDA operates in this field has no such requirement, nor are they required to consider costs or cost-benefit

relationships. The agency's decision, internally developed with or without attention to public comment, stands as law. The costs involved are yet unknown but are certainly high, with a predictable pattern of increase. These expenditures come at a time when the United States has found it difficult to finance even basic health care for millions of people in whom its need and efficacy are unquestioned.

As a governmental agency involved in many health-related issues, the FDA is particularly sensitively exposed to the political process. Because the political process, in this case, has been driven to a large extent by public and media hysteria about the HIV problem in transfusion, it is not unexpected that increased regulation would be proposed as a solution to the problem, even in the absence of evidence of efficacy. This approach leaves the impression that "something is being done" when that may not be the case.

The argument that the use of GMP regulations will not improve the safety of heterologous transfusion can be summarized as follows: Donor screening and testing have markedly reduced the risk of transfusion-transmitted disease already. The principal remaining risk is posed by the so-called window period, particularly for hepatitis C and HIV infection. Increased regulation, particularly that which focuses on the minutia of documentation, will not influence this risk at all. It must be recognized that the blood supply can never be made completely safe, given the present state of our knowledge. Rather, regulation appears to have the purpose of creating an enhanced trail of responsibility.

Without question, the ongoing regulatory process has uncovered and corrected a significant number of problems in the way that U.S. blood services have operated in the past. The regulatory agency, the FDA, should be given full credit for these accomplishments. Also, it must be said that, without these uncomfortable and disrupting regulatory interventions, some of these might not have been corrected. The question that remains in the minds of many is whether the current level of regulations create only a burden without improvement in safety. If the pendulum of regulation has swung too far in the direction of over-regulation, it is hard to see how this can be corrected in light of the history of governmental regulations in general. On the other hand, it is a sad fact that, even in a service-driven industry such as blood services, which under the best circumstances should be largely self-regulating, there are marginal operators who would take advantage of any relaxation of regulations if it were personally profitable or just more convenient, even if some element of safety were sacrificed. We again have the paradigm of the many suffering for the sins of the few.

A reasonable level of regulation focused on correctable problems is undoubtedly important and almost universally accepted. However, regulatory "overkill" tends to increase costs without reasonable benefit. Is there a middle road? Recently, attention has been given to the need for a regulatory code specifically designed for blood services. This concept includes participatory development of the new code of regulations by the FDA with the regulated community, U.S. blood services. This process, properly pursued, could develop a regulatory process that serves the causes of safety and efficacy while still facilitating the economic and management problems of the blood service organizations.

In this section on the regulatory environment in which blood services now operate, no attempt has been made to give any details of the requirements of the specific regulations themselves. Rather, the effort has been to provide a general understanding of the situation blood services face for those who use them. The specific requirements of these regulations if they are of interest to the reader should be sought in the official FDA publications themselves or in reliable guides to their interpretation, which should be available in all blood banks and hospital transfusion services.

These many changes have had a heavy impact on U.S. blood services. A de facto reorganization of these services is in progress. McCullough[9] summarized the situation circa 1993 in an important publication. The pace of change remains rapid, and the outcome configuration of U.S. blood services is unpredictable. Similar changes are occurring in many countries of the developed world. The best hope is for a structure that is based on and supports scientific findings while providing safe and affordable blood and blood products to patients in need. This is in accord with the long-standing traditions of the field.

GENERAL PRINCIPLES OF TRANSFUSION MEDICINE

Replacement

Transfusion therapy, in almost all instances, is based on replacing a blood component that is present in inadequate amounts in a patient with that component derived from the blood of a donor. For transfusion therapy to be rational and effective, the deficient component must be identifiable and preferably measurable so that therapy can be guided in part by objective quantification and by observation of the clinical effect of the replacement.

Amount of Replacement

It is important to recognize at the outset that complete replacement of a deficient blood component is almost never needed for an adequate therapeutic effect. Indeed, it may not even be possible to achieve complete replacement in a safe and cost-effective way. Thus, it is important to know the critical levels of deficiency that will probably be associated with adverse effects such as clinically significant anemic anoxia in the case of red blood cell deficiency or bleeding in the case of a deficiency of one or more of the components of the hemostatic system. Furthermore, there are variations between patients in the levels of deficiency that produce clinical adverse effects. Even within the same patient, clinical manifestations may occur at variable levels of deficiency of a blood component from time to time.

The reasons for the variability of critical levels of deficiency among patients and in one patient over time are not all known. Some of the factors that might play a role are the presence of other illnesses such as infections, cardiac insufficiency, trauma, and the like. This fact is essential in understanding transfusion therapy as a primarily clinical discipline based on careful and intelligent clinical patient evaluations. Laboratory measurements of the concentrations of the deficient component in the patient are of supplementary value in deciding on the amount and timing of replacement of components but do not provide the complete basis for most such decisions.

Role of the Laboratory

Laboratory measurements of the levels of a deficient component, such as hemoglobin, in certain patients with anemia permit a rough calculation of the amount of a blood component, in this case, red blood cells, that will be necessary to raise the level of the component to a safer or more effective level. This calculation is based on an estimate of the blood volume derived from body weight, the measured level of the component, the desired level, and the amount of the component in a therapeutic unit that contains that component. The period during which a transfused component will be effective depends on its natural half-life or the rate at which it is being lost, inactivated, or consumed and the rate at which the patient may be replacing the component. These are, in general, inaccurate calculations that serve only as a general guide or as a way of approximating the amount of a replacement transfusion. The clinical evaluation of effectiveness of replacement takes precedence over laboratory measurements in almost all instances.

Inadequate Response to Replacement

If a replacement transfusion has been given that should have corrected the abnormality but did not, one has an indication that there might be a complication that has not been evaluated adequately. This should prompt a detailed re-evaluation of the entire clinical picture in search of previously unrecognized pathologic processes.

Other reasons for inadequate responses to replacement transfusions are the use of a material that, for some reason, has become inactive, the presence in the patient of a mechanism that inactivates or destroys the transfused component, or the fact that the component replaced was not the deficiency that was actually responsible for the clinical abnormality, even though the laboratory measurement was in fact correct in indicating the presence of a deficiency. Mechanisms that inactivate or destroy transfused blood components are commonly of immunologic origin. The development of modern component transfusion therapy has closely paralleled the development of the science of immunology.

Replacement Only of Needed Components

Finally, the most general principle of modern component transfusion therapy is the administration of the component that the patient needs and, ideally, no others. Application of this principle has virtually eliminated the empiric transfusion of whole blood for indications other than rapid bleeding. The strategy of component therapy depends on recovering a maximal number of therapeutically valuable components from each blood donation. Some products are the result of manufacturing processes that concentrate a given component, such as antihemophilic factor for the treatment of hemophilia A. Others, such as concentrated red blood cells and blood platelet concentrates, are produced and distributed by blood centers to hospitals and clinics where they are transfused. To manage transfusion therapy properly, the physician should understand the logistic system that makes these products available and the economics of that system.

Infections Transmitted by Transfusion Therapy

Any blood component that cannot be sterilized in vitro can transmit infection from donor to recipient. Of the infections thus transmitted, hepatitis in its several forms is, by far, the most important numerically. In general, the only products that can be sterilized or rendered noninfectious are plasma derivatives that are produced by manufacturing processes. Thus, it is important to recognize that manufactured products such as factor VIII are derived from large pools of plasma. If the plasma of even one infected donor is present in the pool, the entire pool is contaminated and can only be made safe by sterilization, with inactivation of infectious agents in the final product. Fortunately, the technology for accomplishing this has improved greatly.

In contrast, it is still not possible to sterilize cellular products prepared in blood centers. Viable cells are destroyed by all known sterilization procedures. These products are rendered safer, but not absolutely safe, by careful screening of donors by multiple methods, including history and a number of relevant laboratory tests. Although this approach has rendered the blood supply of much of the Western World much safer, it must be recognized that the risk of transmission of infection by transfusion is still present (Chs. 36 to 40). This becomes one of the primary risks to be evaluated in making the decision to transfuse any potentially infectious product.

These comments have been provided to emphasize certain critical principles of transfusion medicine. More detailed discussions are to be found in appropriate chapters of this text.

MEDICOLEGAL CONCERNS

Incidents related to transfusion have long been a favorite target of malpractice litigation. Since the recognition that the human immunodeficiency virus (HIV) can be transmitted by blood and blood products, the filing of lawsuits alleging transfusion-related injury has increased greatly. Some of these cases have resulted in large awards. Kern and Croy analyzed the outcomes of 163 legal actions involving HIV infection in which adequate data were available.[10] In 14 cases, more than $75 million were awarded to plaintiffs. Most of these judgments were assessed against physicians and surgeons, particularly cardiothoracic surgeons. There may be a trend toward successful defense of such suits and a decrease in filings in some areas of the United States.

Other transfusion-related risks, including transmission of hepatitis, continue to pose threats of litigation. The most frequent claims are for malpractice, including unnecessary transfusions, and failure to obtain informed consent. In our experience, an inadequate medical record that fails to document the need for transfusion, the risks of not transfusing the patient, and details of the informed consent obtained frequently make a claim difficult or impossible to defend. A clear comprehensive clinical record is the key to the prevention of or successful defense against such litigation; transfusion review committees of hospitals should make this a requirement for all transfused patients.

This edition features a completely revised chapter (15) dealing with medicolegal issues of transfusion by two highly experienced lawyers working in this field. They have reviewed current trends in this area of legal practice and indicate that this is still evolving. Reading of this chapter is strongly recommended. Possible tort law reform will not eliminate this area of concern in the practice of transfusion medicine.

REFERENCES

1. Surgenor DM, Wallace EL, Hao SHS, Chapman RH: Collection and transfusion of blood in the United States, 1982–1988. N Engl J Med 322:1646, 1990
2. Wallace EL, Surgenor DM, Hao HS et al: Collection and transfusion of blood and blood components in the United States, 1989. Transfusion 33:139, 1993
3. Etchason J, Petz LD, Keeler E, et al: The cost effectiveness of preoperative autologous blood donations. N Engl J Med 332:719, 1995
4. Forbes JM, Laurie ML: Blood collections by community blood centers, 1988 through 1992. Transfusion 34:392, 1994
5. Devine P, Linden JV, Hoffstadter LK, et al: Blood donor-, apheresis-, and transfusion-related activities: results of the 1991 American Association of Blood Banks Institutional Membership Questionnaire. Transfusion 33:779, 1993
6. Lawrence VA, Birch S, Gafni A: The impact of new clinical guidelines on the North American blood economy. Transfusion Med Rev 4:232, 1994
7. Soumerai SB, Salem-Schatz S, Avorn J et al: A controlled trial of educational outreach to improve blood transfusion practice. JAMA 270:961, 1993
8. Dzik WH: Blood usage reviews. JAMA 272:896, 1994
9. McCullough J: The nation's changing blood supply system. JAMA 269:2239, 1993
10. Kern JM, Croy BB: A review of transfusion-associated AIDS litigation: 1984 through 1993. Transfustion 34:484, 1994

The History of Transfusion Medicine

Harold A. Oberman

The therapeutic benefits of blood have been recognized for centuries; however, blood transfusion as we know it today is of comparatively recent vintage. Not until the present century was there full appreciation of the scientific rationale for blood transfusion, or complete realization of its consequences.

The evolution of blood transfusion is a fascinating story, ranging from mysticism and pseudoscience to present-day rational therapy. It also reflects the parallel expansion of knowledge in bioengineering, physiology, immunology, mechanical engineering, biochemistry, and genetics. The history is enhanced by the role of a variety of personages who became famous in other areas, both medical and nonmedical, yet all of whom played a role in the dramatic story of transfusion.

EARLY BEGINNINGS

One of the first references to blood transfusion is contained in the seventh book of the *Metamorphoses* by Ovid.[1] Jason pleaded that Media restore the youth of his father, King Aeson. She complied as follows:

Medea took her unsheathed knife and cut the old man's throat, letting all of his old blood out of him. She filled his ancient veins with a rich elixir. Received it through his lips and wound, his beard and

hair no longer white with age, turned quickly to their natural vigor, dark and lustrous; and his wasted form renewed, appeared in all the vigor of bright youth.

Medea's remarkable success was achieved with an elixir brewed in a bronze cauldron containing

root herbs, seeds and flowers, strong juices, and pebbles from the farthest shores of oceans east and west, hoarfrost taken at the full of the moon, a hoot owl's wings and flesh, a werewolf's entrails, the fillet of a snake, the liver of a stag, and the eggs and head of a crow which had been alive for nine centuries.

Medea's practice as a transfusionist was not confined to this single event. Later, when she wished to kill Pelias, she pretended to perform a similar miracle on him. Before killing Pelias, Medea gained his confidence by changing an aged sheep into a lamb.

There are several citations in the Old Testament indirectly bearing on blood transfusion that have had a social impact to the present day. Denial of blood transfusion on religious grounds has its foundation in passages such as the following:

For the life of the flesh is in the blood: and I have given it to you upon the altar to make atonement for your souls: for it is the blood that maketh atonement by reason of the life. Therefore, I said unto the children of Israel: No soul of you shall eat blood, neither shall any stranger that sojourneth among you eat blood.[2]

Only flesh with the life thereof, which is the blood thereof, shall ye not eat.[3]

Be steadfast in not eating the blood; for the blood is the life; and thou shalt not eat the life with the flesh. Thou shalt not eat it; thou shalt pour it out upon the earth as water.[4]

There are many ancient references to the use of blood. For example, Pliny described the drinking of the blood of dying gladiators "as if out of loving cups" as a cure of epilepsy and also noted the practice of Egyptian kings bathing in blood as a cure for elephantiasis. Galen advised the drinking of the blood of a weasel or of a dog for the cure of rabies. Similarly, ancient Norwegians drank the blood of seals and whales as a remedy for epilepsy and scurvy.[5] Whereas these references refer to the drinking of blood or the application of blood to the skin, an ancient reference to the possible transfusion of blood is contained in an ancient Hebrew manuscript:

Naam, leader of the armies of Ben-Adad, King of Syria, afflicted with leprosy, consulted physicians, who, in order to kill him, drew out the blood from his veins and put in that of another.[6]

In the 13th century, Petro de Abano described the management of an adverse reaction occasioned by ingestion of blood:

He who drinks of menstrual blood or that of a leper will be seen to be distracted and lunatic, evil-minded and forgetful, and his cure is to drink of daisies powdered and mixed with water of honey, and to bathe in tepid water and to copulate with girls according to the law natural, and to play with pretty girls and young boys; and the antidote is to eat serpents whose heads and tails have been cut off with the edge of a palm frond.[5]

Aside from other significant events of 1492, did the first transfusion also occur in that year? In 1492, Pope Innocent VIII was terminally ill with what likely was chronic renal disease. According to legend, a mystic arrived in Rome and promised to cure the pope by exchanging his blood with that of three young boys.

Three 10-year-old boys were selected and paid one ducat apiece, and the procedure was instituted. Villary states that the blood of the dying pope was cast into the veins of the boys, who gave him their own in exchange.[7] Each boy died shortly after the procedure, and there was no modification of the pope's illness.

It seems probable that this presumed transfusion stems from an incorrect translation of an earlier account of the pope's illness. What most likely happened is that the blood of the three young boys was intended for use in preparation of a potion for the pope. However, when the pope heard of this, he condemned the practice, refused the potion, and ordered the mystic punished.[8]

TRANSFUSION IN THE 17TH CENTURY

The event that first kindled interest in blood transfusion was the description of the circulation of blood by William Harvey in 1613, which was subsequently published in his *De Motu Cordis* in 1628. This occasioned considerable speculation regarding the possibility of blood transfusion and also pertaining to the infusion of other medications. For example, in 1628, Giovanni Colle suggested transfusion as a means of prolonging life,[9] and a decade earlier, in 1615, Andreas Libavius, the renowned chemist, postulated the following in a satirical sense while defending his theories against his critics:

Let there by a young man, robust, full of spirituous blood, and also an old man, thin, emaciated, his strength exhausted, hardly able to retain his own soul. Let the performer of the operation have two silver tubes fitting into each other. Let him open the artery of the young man and put into it one the tubes, fastening it in. Let him immediately after open the artery of the old man, and put the female tube into it, and then the two tubes be joined together, the hot and spirituous blood of the young man will pour into the old one as if it were from a fountain of life, and all of his weaknesses will be dispelled. Now, in order that the young man may not suffer from weakness, to him is to be given good care and food, but to the doctor, hellebore.[5]

In the middle of the 17th century, several claimants presented themselves for the honor of being the first to transfuse blood. Based upon his reading of Ovid's story of Medea, Frances Potter may have been the first to conceive of transfusion on a practical basis. Potter was a recluse whose efforts were documented in the writings of his contemporary John Aubrey. Apparently, Potter originated the idea of transfusion as early as 1639 and devised quills and tubes for the purpose. In 1649 he reportedly attempted the procedure of transfusion on a pullet; however, probably because of the size of the bird, it proved unsuccessful.[10]

Sir Christopher Wren, who achieved lasting fame as an astronomer and architect, in 1656 first proposed the intravenous administration of medications into the veins of dogs.[11] For this purpose he devised an animal bladder attached to quills. Wren was assisted in this endeavor by his contemporary, Robert Boyle. Four years later Johannes Elsholtz, a physician in Brandenburg, began his experiments on the intravenous injection of wine and emetics into the veins of dogs. These were summarized in his book *Chlysmatica Nova*, published in 1667.[12] Other 17th century experiments in intravenous medication administration were performed by using nitric acid, sulfuric acid, beer, or water.

In a book published in 1660, Francesco Folli of Florence described techniques for transfusion using silver tubes inserted into the vein of the recipient that were connected with the artery of an animal. He also stated that he demonstrated this procedure in 1654, although there was never a public presentation.[5]

At a meeting of a learned society held in Paris in July 1658, Robert des Gabets, a Benedictine monk, enunciated the concept of transfusion and noted that 7 years earlier a friar, Pichot, had prepared an instrument consisting of two small silver cannulae connected by a small leather bag that could be used for this purpose.[13]

It seems most likely that the first public demonstration of transfusion was presented by the English physician Richard Lower, who began his experiments at Oxford in late February 1665 (Fig. 2-1).

Lower initially attempted to join the jugular veins of two dogs, but the blood promptly clotted in the tubing. He thereupon cannulated a cervical artery in one dog and attached it to the jugular vein of the recipient, thereupon exsanguinating the donor animal. Boyle invited Lower to demonstrate this before the Royal Society, and it was subsequently documented in its *Philosophical Transactions* in December 1666.[14]

It seems clear that Lower was the first to define the appropriateness of transfusional replacement of blood in severe hemorrhage since he was able to demonstrate that a dog could be exsanguinated to the point of death and then be completely restored by transfusion. It is interesting to note that a contemporary record of this experiment is contained in the diary of Samuel Pepys. His entry of November 14, 1666, notes that

> Dr. Croone told me that, at the meeting at Gresham College tonight there was a pretty experiment of the blood of one dog let out till he died, into the body of another on one side, while all his own run out on the other side. The first died upon the place, and the other very well and likely to do well. This did give occasion to many pretty wishes, as of the blood of a Quaker to be let into an Archbishop, and such like; but, as Dr. Croone says, may if it takes, be of mighty use to man's health, for the amendment of bad blood by borrowing from a better body.[15]

Lower's efforts were the stimulus for a series of experiments upon animals by a multitude of workers throughout Europe and eventually led to the transfusion of blood from an animal into a human. The priority for the latter procedure occasioned a rancorous debate across the English Channel.

On November 23, 1667, Lower, assisted by Dr. Edmund King, transfused a man named Author Coga, described by Pepys as "a man that is a little frantic, that hath been a kind of minister, that the College hath hired for twenty shillings" (Fig. 2-2A). Pepys observed that the members of the Royal College "differ in the opinion they have of the effects [of the transfusion]; some think it may have a good effect upon the man as a frantic man by cooling his blood, others that it will not have any effect at all." The experiment, using blood of a lamb, apparently

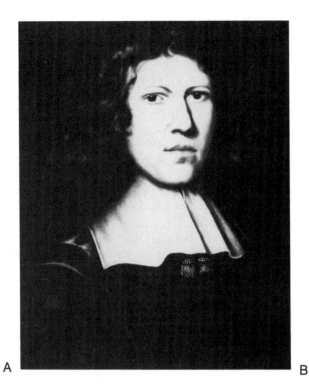

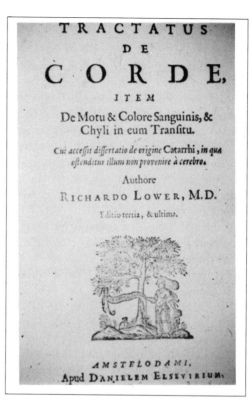

A   B

Fig. 2-1. **(A)** Portrait of Richard Lower. (From Wellcome Museum of History of Medicine, London.) **(B)** Title page of Lower's book, *Tractatus de Corde* (1969), in which transfusion of blood is described in detail.

proceeded without mishap, and afterward, Coga allowed that he felt better, although Pepys observed that "he is cracked a little in the head."[16]

A second and uneventful transfusion of Coga took place the following month; however, it was never recorded in the transactions because of events that transpired almost simultaneously in France.

Jean Denis, a young physician on the large staff attached to King Louis XIV, read of Lower's experiments in the *Journal des Savants* of January 31, 1667. In association with a surgeon, Paul Emmerez, Denis initiated his own trials approximately a month later and performed numerous dog-to-dog transfusion. Eventually, on June 15, 1667, Denis transfused a 15-year-old boy who had a febrile illness of unknown nature with associated extreme weakness, likely related to multiple bloodlettings. The youngster was relieved following the transfusion (Fig. 2-2B). Denis' second human transfusion was performed on a 45-

year-old man, apparently with little clinical indication. Denis reported that this individual felt stronger than before the transfusion. Shortly thereafter, the son of the minister of state to the king of Sweden became seriously ill while traveling in Paris and was transfused twice by Denis. Denis subsequently transfused a hemiplegic woman during the autumn of 1667.[17,18]

Denis submitted the report of his transfusion of the teenage boy to Henry Oldenburg, editor of the *Philosophical Transactions*, in July 1667, and the letter was published in the July 22, 1667, issue. However, because of Oldenburg's confinement in the Tower of London at that time, he did not formally recognize it until the issue of September 23, 1667.[19] Nevertheless, considering that Lower did not perform his first human transfusion until November of that year, there seems little question that Denis was the first to perform transfusion of a human being.

(489)   *Numb.*27.

A LETTER

Concerning a new way of curing sundry diseases by Transfusion of Blood, Written to Monsieur de MONTMOR, *Counseller to the* French King, *and Master of Requests.*

By J: DENIS *Professor of* Philosophy, *and the* Mathematicks.

Munday July 22. 1667.

SIR,

HE project of causing the Blood of a healthy animal to passe into the veins of one diseased, having been conceived a-bout ten years agoe, in the illustrious Society of *Virtuosi* which assembles at your house; and your goodness having received M. *Emmeriz,* & my self, very favorably at such times as we have presum'd to entertain you either with discourse concerning it, or the sight of some not inconsiderable effects of it : You will not think it strange that I now take the liberty of troubling you with this Letter, and design to inform you fully of what pursuances and successes we have made in this Operation; wherein you are justly intitled to a greater share than any other, considering that it was first spoken of in your *Academy,* & that the Publick

---

An Account
Of the Experiment of *Transfusion,* practised upon a Man in *London.*

This was perform'd, Novemb. 23. 1667. *upon one* Mr. Arthur Coga, *at* Arundel-*House, in the presence of many considerable and intelligent persons, by the management of those two Learned Physitians and dextrous Anatomists* Dr. Richard Lower, *and* Dr. Edmund King, *the latter of whom communicated the Relation of it, as followeth.*

THe Experiment of Transfusion of Blood into an *humane* Veine was made by Us in this manner. Having prepared

M m m   the

Fig. 2-2. (Top) Account of Denis and Emmerez's first human transfusion in *Philosophical Transactions.* **(Bottom)** Lower's report of human transfusion in *Philosophical Transactions* 4 months later.

Denis favored use of animal blood for his transfusion experiments because he believed it less likely to be rendered impure by passion or vice." In contrast to Lower, he favored use of a femoral artery in the donor animal rather than the cervical vessels used by Lower.[17]

Following transfusion of the four individuals described earlier, Denis and his associate performed a fifth transfusion later in 1667 that was to have far-reaching repercussions. A 34-year-old man, Antoine Mauroy, had had a severe "phrensy" for 7 or 8 years, ostensibly occasioned by an unfortunate love affair. His madness was manifested by his running naked through the streets of Paris. Denis's patron, Monsieur de Montmor, proposed transfusion because he believed it would allay the "heat of his blood." Following removal of 10 oz of blood from a vein in the man's right arm, 5 or 6 oz of blood from a calf was administered without event.[20]

Two days later a second transfusion of Mauroy took place, more plentiful than the first. This resulted in what we would now recognize as a hemolytic transfusion reaction. Denis' description can be considered a medical classic:

As soon as the blood began to enter into his veins, he felt the heat along his arm and under his armpits. His pulse rose and soon after we observed a plentiful sweat over all his face. His pulse varied extremely at this instant and he complained of great pains in his kidneys, and that he was not well in his stomach, and that he was ready to choke unless given his liberty. He was made to lie down and fell asleep, and slept all night without awakening until morning. When he awakened he made a great glass full of urine, of a color as black as if it had been mixed with the soot of chimneys.[21]

Denis recounted that the following morning the subject also manifested hemoglobinuria and had epistaxis. However, by the third day his urine cleared, and he improved his mental status and returned to his wife. Denis attributed the color of the urine to a "black choler" that had been retained in the body and had sent vapors to the brain that caused the subject's mental disturbance.[21] Several months later Mauroy again became violent and irrational, and his wife persuaded Denis and Emmerez to repeat the transfusion. Transfusion was attempted; however, mechanical difficulties precluded its performance. Mauroy died the following night.

Through their experiments of the previous year, Denis and Emmerez had acquired many enemies among the physicians of Paris. Three of these persuaded Mauroy's widow to accuse Denis and Emmerez of contributing to the death of her husband by the transfusion. Moreover, other physicians published pamphlets condemning the work of Denis and Emmerez. At one time the widow offered to withdraw the lawsuit provided she would receive payment from Denis; however, he responded "that those physicians, and herself, stood more in need of the transfusion than ever her husband had done."[20] Denis lodged a countercomplaint against the widow. At the subsequent trial he was exonerated, and the widow was subsequently shown to have poisoned her husband with arsenic.

Most important, the Faculty of Medicine of Paris issued a decree based on the results of the trial that stated that the procedure of transfusion was a criminal act unless given sanction by the Faculty of Medicine.[5] It must be recalled that the faculty was an extremely conservative body that had refused for many years to recognize Harvey's theory of circulation.

By 1678 an edict of the French parliament specifically forbade transfusion in France, and the procedure also was outlawed by the Royal Society in London. In 1679, the pope joined the outcry and banned the procedure. Therefore, interest in transfusion quickly waned.[22]

It is of interest that, aside from Lower's comments associated with his initial dog experiments, in the 17th century little consideration was given to the use of transfusion for replacement of blood loss. Most popular was the possibility of altering mental aberration through transfusion. Considerable importance was attached in contemporary writings to the possibility of restoring youth to the aged, and it was even suggested that marital discord might be settled by reciprocal transfusions of the blood of husband and wife. In line with the mysticism associated with transfusion, it was speculated that a dog transfused with sheep blood might grow wool, cloven hooves, and horns. There was even an account of a young girl who received blood from a cat and was quickly endowed with feline characteristics.[5]

Only sporadic efforts at transfusion were undertaken during the remainder of the 17th and throughout the 18th century, all representing instances of transfusion of animal blood to humans. Not until 1749 did a member of the Faculty of Medicine of Paris, Cantwell, state that transfusion was valuable and advocate its use as a procedure in extreme emergencies.[6]

TRANSFUSION IN THE 19TH CENTURY
James Blundell and the Rebirth of Transfusion

Blood transfusion lay dormant for a century and a half. The credit for rekindling interest in the procedure and providing it with a semblance of a rational approach must be given to James Blundell. Blundell, born in 1790, was a physician with far-reaching interests (Fig. 2-3). He was one of the outstanding obstetricians of his day, and between 1816 and 1834 he delivered lectures on midwifery at Guy's Hospital in London. These were printed in *Lancet* and subsequently were published in book form both in England and in the United States. Among the new operations that Blundell proposed were operative reduction of intussusception, sterilization by bilateral partial salpingectomy, bilateral oophorectomy for severe dysmenorrhea, a method for removal of the cancerous uterus either through the abdominal wall or the vagina, and cesarean hysterectomy.[24] It should be noted that, although he suggested these procedures, he did not actually perform all of them.

Blundell's interest in blood transfusion stemmed from his perception that this would be an appropriate treatment for postpartum hemorrhage. He initially experimented on dogs by exsanguinating them and subsequently reviving them by transfusion of arterial blood obtained from other dogs.[25] From his experiments he concluded that the blood of one animal could not be substituted for that of another with impunity, and he thereupon turned to use of human blood for human transfusion.

It should be appreciated that Blundell received his medical degree from the University of Edinburgh and undoubtedly was influenced in his early experiments by the experiments of John Leacock.[26] Although Leacock's manuscript on the subject was written while he was in Barbados, his experiments were performed during his tenure in Edinburgh where one of his contemporaries was Blundell. Utilizing a 6-in length of ox ureter with crow quills attached to each end, Leacock operated on dogs and resuscitated exsanguinated animals by transfusion. Although Leacock did not perform human transfusion, he argued against mixing blood of different species, and his experiments quite clearly pointed to the efficacy of such treatment.

Blundell initially advocated direct transfusions; however, he showed that blood was still satisfactory if allowed to remain in a container for only a few seconds and then injected by syringe. Blundell described transfusion by syringe in several papers and noted the necessity of removing air from the instrument before the transfusion.

Following his experiments with animals, Blundell turned to transfusing humans with human blood. On December 22, 1818, Blundell transfused a 35-year-old man with gastric carcinoma (Fig. 2-4). When first seen by Blundell, the patient was severely wasted and near death. Approximately 14 oz of blood was administered by syringe in small amounts at intervals of 5 to 6 minutes; however, despite temporary improvement, the patient died 56 hours later.[27]

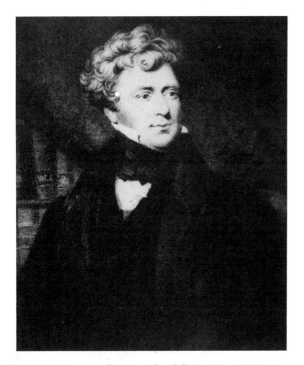

Fig. 2-3. Portrait of James Blundell (1790–1877). (From Jones et al.,[23] with permission.)

SOME ACCOUNT OF A CASE

OF

OBSTINATE VOMITING,

IN WHICH

AN ATTEMPT WAS MADE

TO PROLONG LIFE,

BY THE

INJECTION OF BLOOD INTO THE VEINS.

BY JAMES BLUNDELL, M.D.

LECTURER, IN CONJUNCTION WITH DR. HAIGHTON, ON PHYSIOLOGY
AND MIDWIFERY, AT GUY'S HOSPITAL.

Read Dec. 22, 1818.

Fig. 2-4. Report of Blundell's first transfusion. (From Blundell,[27] with permission.)

This transfusion is generally accepted as the first transfusion of a human with human blood. However, a footnote in an American journal along with a report of the transfusion in England notes that Dr. Philip Syng Physick performed the procedure "under precisely the same circumstances" in 1795.[28] It is impossible to verify this citation, for in contrast to Blundell's numerous publications, Physick never recorded this event. His biographer notes that Physick "maintained a most invincible repugnance to appear before the public in the shape of an author; and this feeling induced him to exact the promise that none of his manuscripts, lectures or letters should be published."[29]

Blundell subsequently transfused several women with postpartum hemorrhage and consulted in numerous other transfusions at that time. In 1828, defending the use of human rather than animal blood for transfusion, he noted the impracticality of animal blood because of the difficulty of finding the appropriate animal in an emergency:

What is to be done in an emergency? A dog might come when you whistled, but the animal is small; a calf might have appeared fitter for the purpose, but then it had not been taught to walk properly up the stairs.[30]

Blundell was also aware that the operation might be performed needlessly and emphasized that it should be reserved for desperately ill patients.

Blundell stimulated his contemporaries to practice transfusion. For the most part, these were obstetricians who utilized the procedure in cases of postpartum hemorrhage. Two of the most active transfusionists were Waller and Doubleday.[31,32] The medical writing of the time is remarkably descriptive, as exemplified by Doubleday's description of his transfusion of a woman with postpartum hemorrhage with her husband's blood. After 6 oz had been administered, the woman, previously semicomatose, suddenly exclaimed, "by Jesus, I feel strong as a bull."[32]

Similarly, Blundell, in 1829 describing a transfusion for postpartum hemorrhage, claimed that "the patient expresses herself very strongly on the benefits resulting from the injection of the blood; her observations are equivalent to this—that she felt as if life were infused into her body."[33] It is of interest that this report, in *Lancet*, is in apposition to the thorough documentation of the murder trial of the notorious resurrectionists Burke and Hare.

Blundell developed several different methods of transfusion. Following his demonstration of the effectiveness of a syringe, he devised an "impellor," an instrument in which the blood was collected in a metal cup surrounded by warm water and then in-jected into the vein of the recipient with the aid of an attached syringe (Fig. 2-5A). He also fabricated a piston-syringe-cup device, a tube for direct transfusion, and a gravitator (Fig. 2-5B). In the gravitator technique, blood from the donor dripped into a cup several feet above the arm of the recipient and flowed through tubing into the recipient vein.[34]

Apparently Blundell performed transfusions on 10 different occasions, 5 being successful. In three

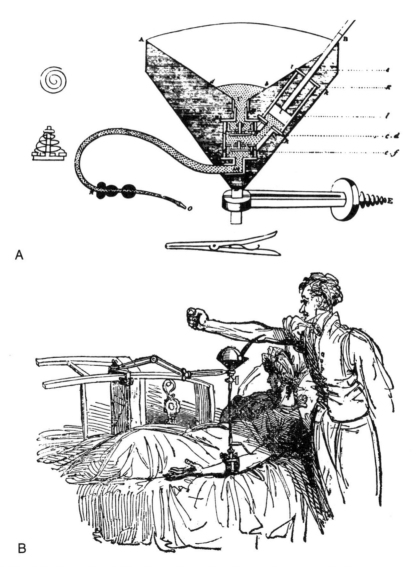

A

B

Fig. 2-5. **(A)** Blundell's "impellor." Blood is indicated by dots and is surrounded by warm water, indicated by horizontal lines. (From Jones et al.,[23] with permission.) **(B)** Sketch of Blundell's gravitator. (From Blundell,[34] with permission.)

of the unsuccessful cases, the patient was moribund when transfused. Blundell also served as a consultant in many other cases. One of these, in 1840, was most significant, for it was the first demonstration that a freshly drawn blood product could correct the bleeding tendency in hemophilia A.[35] In this situation, the patient was an 11-year-old boy who had persistent hemorrhage after operative correction of strabismus (Fig. 2-6).

Although Blundell was remarkably progressive in developing his techniques of transfusion, it should be noted that he commonly applied leeches to the skin of the donor and recipient in an effort to prevent inflammation of the veins.[36] After 1830, his interest in transfusion waned. He retired from medical practice in 1847, undoubtedly facilitated by a fortune of a half-million pounds sterling he had accumulated in practice and in bequests. Blundell lived in comparative obscurity until his death in 1878. He was a controversial figure, frequently at odds with the Medical Society of London and with the directors of Guy's Hospital. His retirement from Guy's, in 1838, was occasioned by the appointment of a successor as chairman of obstetrics during Blundell's temporary absence. A heated dispute ensued, which led to his severance of all relations with the hospital.[23]

Considerable debate occupied London during the mid-19th century regarding the use of transfusion, as evidenced by the minutes of the Medical Society. Many felt that the procedure was dangerous and that it may have hastened the death of some of the patients on whom it was used. Furthermore, it was claimed that most of the patients who benefited from the procedure would have recovered without its use.

Conversely, Blundell argued strenuously on its behalf, noting that the danger of hemorrhage in these patients far outweighed the possible danger resulting from transfusion.[30]

This debate was still raging in 1849 when Routh reviewed all of the transfusions published to that date.[37] He was only able to find 48 recorded cases, of which 18 had a fatal outcome. This gave a mortality rate "rather less than that of hernia, or about the same as the average amputation." Furthermore, he noted that the mortality rate was unjustly high, for in many of these patients death was due to causes other than the transfusion. Routh concluded that the greatest danger was transmission of air, and he suggested that the quantity of blood transfused should not be less than 6 oz nor more than 16 oz.

Among the indications for transfusion that were cited by Routh were severe hemorrhage, extreme exhaustion from dyspepsia, stricture of the esophagus, collapse following fever, and severe diarrhea or dysentery.

Early Transfusion In the United States

Aside from the unproven transfusion by Physick, it is doubtful that transfusion was practiced in the United States before 1830. The citations of transfusions in the early American literature most likely were culled from foreign journals, often without appropriate credit. As late as 1853, Benedict, in a review of the subject, stated that he had no knowledge of the procedure being performed in the United States.[38] The following year, an anonymous report of a transfusion in New Orleans was published.[39] The recipient was a patient with cholera who received 10 oz of human blood by syringe but died a few minutes later. Four years later, Benedict transfused a young woman with yellow fever.[40] Austin Flint reviewed the subject in 1874 and noted that his son had performed the procedure in New Orleans during the winter of 1860 to 1861.[41] However, during the entire Civil War, only four transfusions are recorded.[42] It is of interest that two of these took place within a 10-day interval in 1864, one in Louisville, Kentucky, and the other in Alexandria, Virginia.[43]

Although never published, George McClellan was said to have transfused a patient with cholera in 1832, and William Hammond, an army surgeon, transfused soldiers with cholera in New Mexico in

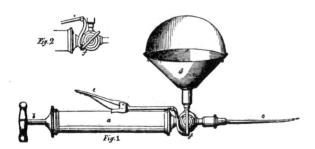

Fig. 2-6. Syringe used by Samuel Lane for transfusion in 1840. (From Lane,[35] with permission.)

1849.[42] Hammond subsequently became surgeon general of the Union Army during the Civil War. There is no record of the use of transfusion by the Confederate forces during the Civil War.

Anticoagulation—Early Efforts

It is obvious that one of the problems that had to be solved before blood transfusion could be placed on a practical basis was the prevention of coagulation. Attempts to achieve this took several forms in the 19th century. Blundell observed in his writings the need for rapid performance of transfusion to avoid coagulation and initiated the use of a syringe to overcome this problem. He also noted the impracticality of vein-to-vein direct transfusion and encouraged the use of direct transfusion by using the artery of the donor attached to the vein of the recipient.

In 1835 Bischoff proposed the use of defibrinated blood.[44] A variety of techniques were used for this purpose, the majority incorporating some form of a stirring process. One of the first to use an anticoagulant additive was Neudorfer, who in 1860 recommended the addition of sodium bicarbonate as an anticoagulant.[45] Two physicians who were to achieve fame in other areas actively sought an answer to the problem of blood coagulation. Braxton-Hicks utilized a solution of sodium phosphate as an anticoagulant in six unsuccessful transfusions,[46] while Brown-Sequard used defibrinated blood for his experiments performed in the early 1850s.[47] Nevertheless,

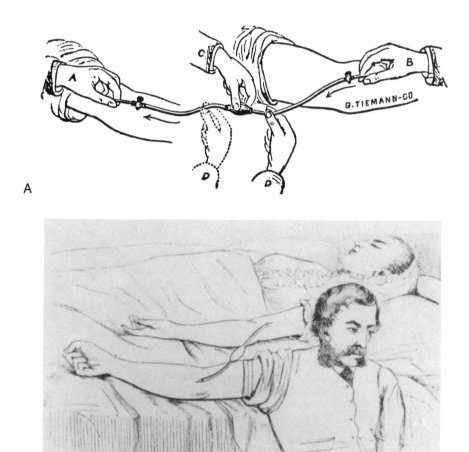

Fig. 2-7. **(A)** Direct transfusion as practiced by Aveling in 1872. **(B)** The donor artery was connected to the recipient vein, and pumping action was provided by a rubber bulb. (From Aveling,[48] with permission.)

half a century was to elapse before a practical means of anticoagulation was derived.

Late 19th Century Transfusion

During the remainder of the 19th century, efforts were directed toward improvement of devices for indirect transfusion or refinement of surgical techniques to facilitate direct transfusion (Figs. 2-7 to 2-9). Nevertheless, indiscriminate use of transfusion resulted in increasing numbers of untoward reactions in recipients so that the procedure fell into disfavor. Once again, transfusion of animal blood to humans was attempted; however, the experiments of Ponfick and Landois, in effect, put an end to heterologous blood transfusion.[9] Ponfick also was the first to note that the dark urine following an incompatible blood transfusion was hemoglobinuria, not hematuria, and resulted from destruction of the donor red cells and not those of the recipient.

During the final quarter of the 19th century, frustration and discouragement with blood as a transfusion product resulted in a brief wave of enthusiasm for transfusion of milk as a blood substitute.[51] This form of treatment achieved its greatest popularity in the United States between 1873 and 1880, with milk from cows, goats, and humans being used. The most outspoken advocate of milk transfusion was Thomas, who discouraged the use of blood transfusion be-cause of "the inherent difficulties and dangers of the operation, almost all of which arise from the tendency to coagulation."[52] Prout supported Thomas and even postulated a medical-legal use for milk transfusion in that it might prolong life for a sufficient time to permit "the victim of an assault to identify his assailant."[53]

By 1878 Brinton predicted that transfusion of milk would entirely supersede transfusion of blood.[54] However, by 1880 increasing numbers of adverse reactions associated with its administration led to its abandonment. This was hastened by the advent of saline infusion as a "blood substitute" in 1884.[55]

THE ADVENT OF MODERN BLOOD TRANSFUSION

At the end of the 19th century, blood transfusion was only slightly less primitive than at its inception 2½ centuries earlier. The principal accomplishment during this interval was the recognition of the inappropriateness of animal blood for human transfusion. Beyond that, solutions to such problems as anticoagulation, immune destruction of transfused red cells, long-term preservation of blood for transfusion, recognition of the serologic heterogeneity of

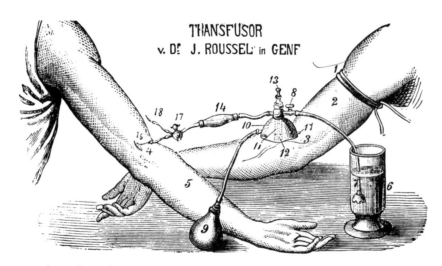

Fig. 2-8. Roussel's method of direct transfusion. In this technique, a lancet was inserted into the donor's vein, and a suction cup as well as an in-line rubber bulb was used to maintain adequate flow. (From Roussel,[49] with permission.)

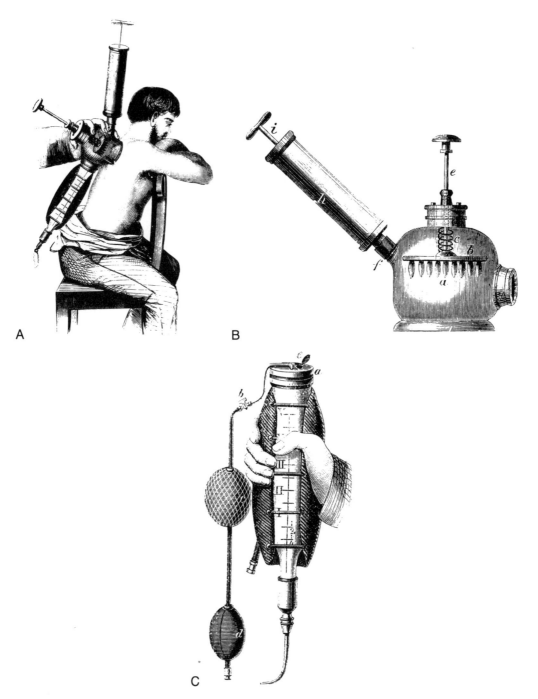

Fig. 2-9. **(A)** Collection and transfusion of capillary blood by the method of Gesellius. **(B)** An evacuated suction cup was placed over the back of the donor, and multiple lancets were plunged into the skin. **(C)** A graduated cylinder surrounded by warm water was disconnected from the donor apparatus and used for the transfusion. (From Gesselius,[50] with permission.)

red cells, and component preparation awaited developments of the 20th century.

The Discovery of Blood Groups

The modern era of blood transfusion was initiated with the epochal work of Landsteiner who demonstrated the presence of A, B, and O isoagglutinins in serum in 1900 and in the following year divided human blood into three groups on the basis of the serologic reactions of red cells with these agglutinins. Landsteiner's initial publication was in the form of a footnote to an article on bacterial fermentation.[56] In his 1901 article, Landsteiner indicated the importance of taking into account these blood differences for the successful outcome of transfusion.[57] Unfortunately, several years were to pass until such a practice was introduced. In 1902 the fourth blood group, AB, was described by DeCastello and Sturli.[58] Following these initial studies, Lansteiner abandoned his work on blood groups for over 20 years to pursue other interests.

In 1907 Richard Weil, a pathologist at German Hospital in New York, alerted his intern, Reuben Ottenberg, to the importance of Landsteiner's discovery.[59] Ottenberg was the first to perform ABO typing of patient and donor before blood transfusion and also was the first to use compatibility testing before transfusion. Furthermore, he first suggested inheritance of the ABO types and noted the relatively minor role of donor antibodies in transfusion therapy.

While the ABO blood types were defined in the first years of this century, considerable debate ensued relative to their appropriate terminology. In his original paper, Landsteiner identified the three groups as A, B, and C. Working independently, Jansky of Czechoslovakia in 1907 and Moss of the United States in 1910 described four blood groups by using Roman numeral designations. Unfortunately, Moss was unaware of Jansky's work and, in classifying the groups, transposed the order of the Roman numeral designations. In 1927 the American Association of Immunologists, in an effort to resolve the resultant terminologic confusion, sponsored a new classification, suggested by Landsteiner, which is the present one used for the ABO system.

Although Moss is remembered for his efforts in classifying the ABO group, his most important contribution may have been his demonstration that isohemolysis was parallel to isoagglutination. This permitted determination of blood groups by agglutination reactions rather than by the more laborious hemolysis tests.[60]

Blood Preservation and the Advent of the Blood Bank

The second major problem solved in the 20th century was that of anticoagulation and preservation of blood for transfusion. In the early years of the century, coagulation was prevented by improved methods of direct transfusion. Anastomosis of blood vessels for direct transfusion, first performed by Alexis Carrel, was refined and popularized in 1907 by George Crile who utilized a cannula through which the vein of the recipient and the artery of the donor were drawn (Fig. 2-10). Although other methods for direct transfusion were devised (Fig. 2-11), such procedures necessitated sacrifice of the two vessels; therefore, these operations did not have long-lasting popularity.

Various paraffin-coated tubes were employed for direct transfusion in an effort to forestall coagulation; however, of greater significance was the comparatively simple multiple-syringe method, proposed in 1913 by Edward Lindeman, representing a rediscovery of a method that had been described in 1892 by von Zeimssen.[63] The syringe procedures

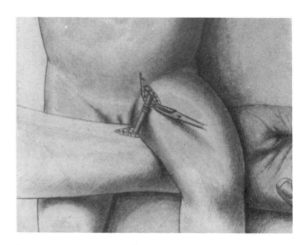

Fig. 2-10. Direct transfusion using artery-vein anastomosis by Crile's technique for hemorrhagic disease of the newborn. (From Lespinasse,[61] with permission.)

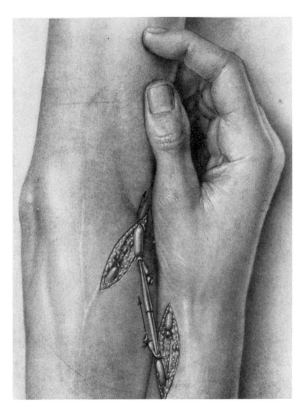

Fig. 2-11. Artery-vein anastomosis using paired tubes as devised by Bernheim. (From Bernheim,[62] with permission.)

effectively put an end to direct vessel anastomosis transfusion.

The principal advantage of the Lindeman technique was the elimination of the need for dissection of blood vessels in either the donor or the recipient.[64] The direct anastomosis procedure often proved more difficult than the operation it was intended to support. Furthermore, with the use of syringes the exact quantity of blood transfused was known; however, repeated filling and washing of syringes required several operators because rapid injection of the blood was essential to avoid coagulation. Two years later Unger devised a simple syringe method using a four-way stopcock that overcame many of the difficulties of the Lindeman procedure.[65] Dozens of variations of Unger's syringe technique appeared during the following 2 decades, as did mechanical devices for direct transfusion (Fig. 2-12).

In 1914 and 1915, the use of sodium citrate as an anticoagulant was proposed independently from four different sources. In March of 1914, Albert Hustin, a Belgian, apparently was the first to use citrate in a solution containing salt and glucose.[59] His solution rendered the red cells so dilute as to be impractical. In November of the same year, Luis Agote of Buenos Aires performed a transfusion in which citrate alone was used. As Agote noted, this had the potential of eliminating the need for arteriovenous anastomosis as a prelude to transfusion and the inability to determine the amount of blood being transfused. Rather than publishing his report in a medical journal, Agote gave the story to *La Prensa*, the leading newspaper of Buenos Aires, and it was also published in detail in the *New York Herald*.[68]

Two months later, two New York physicians independently provided the most significant impetus for the use of citrate as an anticoagulant. Richard Lewisohn, a surgeon at Mount Sinai Hospital, used citrate for human blood transfusion only after performing multiple studies of citrate toxicity in dogs (Fig. 2-13). He carefully demonstrated the optimal citrate dose for anticoagulation. Simultaneously, Richard Weil, the pathologist who had served as a stimulus for Ottenberg, noted that citrated blood could be stored in a refrigerator for several days before use.[70]

Based upon Weil's and Lewisohn's work, Rous and Turner prepared a solution of salt, isocitrate, and glucose to accomplish both anticoagulation and preservation of blood.[71] The addition of glucose to the anticoagulant was the seminal contribution that permitted delayed transfusion of blood. This was a most cumbersome method in that there was a tremendous excess of anticoagulant solution to blood volume that required removal of the anticoagulant before transfusion. However, it was the only such solution available for almost 25 years.

The availability of the Rous-Turner solution permitted an American physician attached to the British Army to perform the first transfusions with preserved blood during World War I. Oswald Robertson transfused 20 casualties on 22 occasions during the Battle of Cambrai in November 1917. The blood units had been preserved for 10 to 26 days before transfusion. Robertson used only group O blood.[72]

By March 1918, citrated blood had become the official method for combating shock in both the Brit-

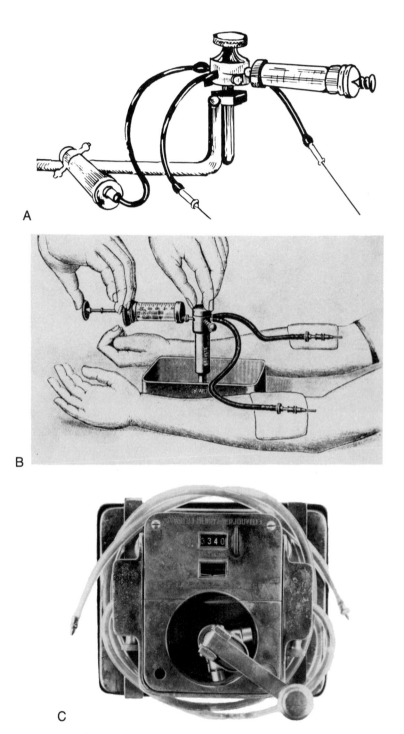

Fig. 2-12. **(A)** Unger's device for transfusion by syringe with a four-way stopcock. (From Killduffe et al.,[65] with permission.) **(B)** Tzanck's modification of the Unger technique. (From Tzanck,[67] with permission.) **(C)** Device of Henry and Jouvelet (1934) for direct transfusion that uses a manual roller pump. (From the author's collection.)

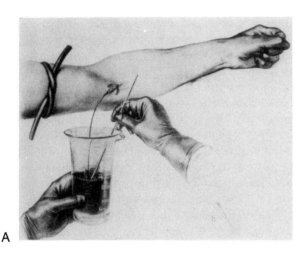

A

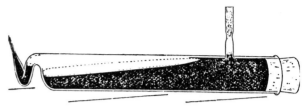

Fig. 2-14. Kimpton-Brown tube. Blood is drawn from the donor, and the tube is kept horizontal until transfusion. (From Kimpton and Brown,[74] with permission.)

ish and American armies.[73] Before that time, most transfusions in the war were by syringe or by related techniques such as the Kimpton-Brown tube (Fig. 2-14). The Kimpton-Brown tube, which was devised in 1913, is a paraffin-coated graduated glass cylinder with a horizontal side tube for suction. The bottom of the cylinder was drawn into an S-shaped cannula for use both in the donor and recipient veins.[74] A combination of the paraffin-coated cylinder with a syringe technique is shown in Fig. 2-15.

Blood preservation in the United States following World War I largely was through use of the Rous-Turner solution or subsequent minor modifications introduced in the early 1940s by DeGowin et al. and Alsever and Ainslee.[76,77] All of these solutions had the disadvantage of having a large volume of preservative solution in relation to the amount of blood. Blood preserved in this manner was used during most of World War II.

In December 1943, Loutit and Mollison intro-

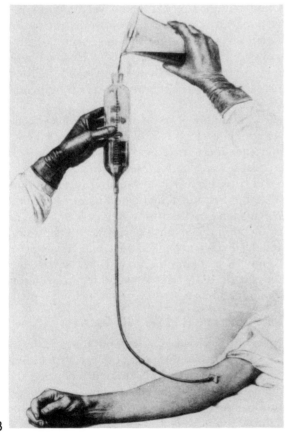

B

Fig. 2-13. Lewisohn's method of transfusion of citrated blood. **(A)** Blood is collected in a graduated flask and **(B)** is promptly transfused to the patient. (From Lewisohn,[69] with permission.)

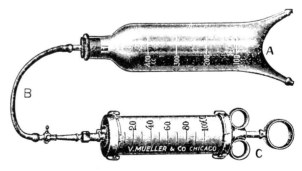

Fig. 2-15. Combination of syringe and paraffin-lined cylinder for transfusion as devised by Davis and Curtis. The cannula tips at A are attached to the recipient and donor veins. (From Davis and Curtis,[75] with permission.)

duced acid-citrate-dextros (ACD), wherein citric acid was added to the sodium citrate and dextrose, thereby mitigating the problem of caramelization in the sterilization process and reducing the volume of solution.[78] Before this development, the citrate and glucose solutions had to be autoclaved separately, with the glucose being added at the time the blood was collected, resulting in extra work and increasing the risk of contamination. Although the ratio of blood to preservative solution of Alsever's solution was 1:1, that of ACD, as initially formulated, was 4:1, and it was later reduced to 6:1. Moreover, ACD was simpler to prepare and to autoclave than Alsever's solution. However, because of the need for testing the new preservative as well as obtaining new bottles and transporting materials, ACD solution was not adopted by the United States Army until April 1945.[73]

Recognition of the so-called lesion of collection, and the need to prolong storage of blood beyond 21 days, led to the introduction of citrate-phosphate-dextrose (CPD) anticoagulant in 1957.[79] Shortly thereafter, the importance of maintaining 2, 3-diphosphoglyceric acid levels and of preserving adenine nucleotides was recognized, and this resulted in prolongation of storage by adding adenine to the preservative solution.

The discovery that glycerol could prevent damage to living sperm caused by freezing and thawing led to attempts to preserve other cells and ultimately resulted in the use of this method for long-term preservation of red cells. Initially it was demonstrated that red cells could be maintained for 3 months in plasma that contained glycerol, and this eventuated in the first transfusion of previously frozen red cells in 1951.[80]

Preserved blood originally was collected by using steel needles and glass bottles with rubber seals and tubing. All these products were reused after sterilization. Lack of removal of all of the blood or proteins from the apparatus as well as contamination by rinsing solutions often resulted in pyrogenic reactions in the recipients of subsequent units. Not until 1933 was the incidence of such reactions reduced through greater attention to bottle cleaning.[81] Moreover, evacuated blood collection bottles resulted in foaming of the collected blood with the attendant possibility of coagulation. Also, gravity-draw bottles carried

the risk of air embolism for the donor, while a similar risk existed for the recipient transfused with blood in glass bottles when air was pumped into the bottle to hasten transfusion.

A most significant expansion of the horizons of blood banking was the advent of plastic transfusion equipment. By 1949 trials of such equipment were conducted by the American National Red Cross and a few hospital blood banks; however, more than 10 years were to elapse before such equipment was incorporated into transfusion programs.[82] The use of plastic transfusion equipment facilitated the advent of blood component therapy, primarily a development of the 1950s and 1960s.

A major impetus for further development of blood component therapy was the revival of interest in the technique of plasmapheresis in the sixth and seventh decades of this century. This had been initially described in 1914 at Johns Hopkins Hospital by Abel et al., who proposed the technique as a method of increasing the yield of antitoxic sera from hyperimmune animals.[83]

The availability of perservative solutions along with the development of electrical refrigeration equipment permitted the development of organized programs for blood preservation. While the first blood bank likely was formulated in Leningrad in 1932, the first functional blood bank was instituted in Barcelona in 1936 in association with the need for blood in the Spanish Civil War.[84] Fantus organized the first blood bank in the United States at Cook County Hospital in Chicago in 1937. However, even in the early 1940s, direct or indirect transfusion of unmodified blood was favored in many hospitals.

Other Developments of the 20th Century

During the early years of the 20th century, the difficulty of direct transfusion and the relative impracticality of transfusion with citrated blood led to attempts to identify alternative sources of blood for transfusion. For example, in Moscow, Yudin initiated the use of cadaver blood for transfusion.[85] By 1938 he had accomplished 2,500 such transfusions. However, cadaver blood transfusion, even in Russia, never achieved significant popularity. Another alternative source of blood was placental blood, although there is no record that it ever achieved significant use in the United States.[86]

The development of blood banking in the third quarter of the 20th century has been phenomenal. Whereas only a handful of blood group systems had been identified by 1950, over 200 are now recognized. This expansion of knowledge of blood group serology has been reflected in enhancement of the safety of blood transfusion through pretransfusion testing.

One of the primary factors facilitating such testing was the advent of the antiglobulin reaction. Although originally described by Moreschi in 1908, current use of this test stems from the 1945 work of Coombs et al.[87] Not only has pretransfusion testing mitigated the risk of immune hemolysis of the transfused red cells, it also has optimized the survival of such cells through recognition of antibodies that occasion more protracted removal of the transfused erythrocytes.

The expansion of knowledge of blood group antigens is indicated by the fact that only the ABO system and the MN and P antigens were recognized by 1935. Landsteiner and Weiner coined the term Rh in 1940, although Levine had recognized Rh polymorphisms a year earlier.[88,89] Most significantly, in 1941, Levine and associates demonstrated that isoimmunization to the Rh antigen was the principal cause of hemolytic disease of the newborn.[90] Prior to that time, the latter disease often had been attributed to seronegative syphilis. The profusion of newly identified blood group systems was intimately related to the development of new methods of detection of IgG antibody. This included not only the antiglobulin test but also the use of high protein medium and enzyme techniques for serologic testing.[91]

As previously noted, Ottenberg initiated the use of compatibility testing in the form of a crossmatch to enhance the safety of transfusion.[92] He initially used a hemolysin technique, but Moss's observation that isoagglutination was comparable to isohemolysis opened the way for utilizing the more convenient agglutination tests for blood grouping as well as for the crossmatch.[60] The need for crossmatching was debated through the second decade of the 20th century. Although it was appreciated that the crossmatch complemented blood grouping, it was suggested as late as 1937 that, if selection of donors was restricted to individuals of the same blood group, no further test of compatibility was needed.[93]

In contrast, in 1939 Riddell concluded that performance of the crossmatch obviated the need for knowledge of the donor's and the recipient's blood groups.[94]

Subsequently, use of the antiglobulin procedure as well as incubation at 37°C allowed detection of IgG antibodies. Ottenberg, in his early publications, suggested that the minor crossmatch was unnecessary; however, not until 1968, with growing acceptance of pretransfusion antibody screening, was there a general concurrence that the minor crossmatch test lacked real significance.[95] During the 1970s the crossmatch procedure became unduly cumbersome with the use of various incubation temperatures as well as the use of high protein, antiglobulin, and enzyme reagents.[96] Recently, however, the crossmatch has been streamlined. This has come about by the introduction of some newer reagents such as low-ionic strength saline solution used as a suspension medium for red cells.[97] Even more important however, has been the careful reassessment of various compatibility test procedures, including the demonstration that the antiglobulin phase of the crossmatch does not contribute significantly to patient safety when the screening test for unexpected antibodies is negative[98] (see also Ch. 7). This re-emphasis on the importance of verification of ABO compatibility, coupled with the need to expedite issuance of blood and, simultaneously contain costs, led to adoption of the so-called electronic, or computer, crossmatch.[99]

Developments during the last decade have further enhanced the safe and effective utilization of blood as a therapeutic resource. For example, storage of blood has been prolonged by the development of newer blood preservative solutions. Moreover, through the use of automated and semiautomated equipment, the procurement of platelets and granulocytes for transfusion has been facilitated. The accumulation of clots and debris in blood containers led to realization of the need to filter blood before transfusion. In 1938 Fantus described a filter made from silk; glass bead and cotton mesh filters were introduced shortly thereafter.[100] Although difficult to clean, wire mesh filters were used in the 1940s; by the end of that decade, disposable cotton cloth filters with a pore size approximating 200 μm were utilized in all administration sets.

The demonstration of microaggregates composed of platelets, leukocytes, and fibrin led to the introduction in the early 1960s of microaggregate filters with a much smaller pore size. Initially these were screen filters with a pore size of 20 to 40 μm, but these soon were replaced by depth filters of varying composition and highly efficient adsorption filters, which not only removed microaggregates but also effectively reduced the volume of transfused leukocytes.

Improvement of methods for enhancement of agglutination in serologic testing has expedited provision of blood for transfusion. The safety of transfusion has been greatly enhanced through the advent of specific and surrogate serologic testing for hepatitis B, non-A, non-B hepatitis, and the human immunodeficiency virus; the recognition of the danger of blood obtained from commercial donors; the advent of quality control programs; and the promulgation of minimum performance standards with associated inspection programs. Automation also has greatly expanded the efficiency and accuracy of serologic testing in blood donor centers.

It is obvious that clinical acceptance of blood transfusion has been achieved only over the past several decades. The scope of transfusion medicine has now broadened to include numerous diagnostic and therapeutic implications. One can only wonder what the future holds in store for this rapidly changing field.

REFERENCES

1. Ovid's Metamorphoses. Vol. 2. Cornhill, Boston, 1941
2. Leviticus 17:11–12
3. Genesis 9:4
4. Deuteronomy 12:23–24
5. Brown HM: The beginnings of intravenous medication. Ann Med Hist 1:177, 1917
6. Dutton WF: Intravenous Therapy: Its Application in the Modern Practice of Medicine. FA Davis, Philadelphia, 1925
7. Villari P: The Life and Times of Giralamo Savonarola. T. Fisher Unwin, London, 1888
8. Lindeboom GA: The story of a blood transfusion to a pope. J Hist Med 9:455, 1954
9. Maluf MFR: History of blood transfusion. J Hist Med 9:59, 1954
10. Webster C: The origins of blood transfusion. Med Hist 15:387, 1971
11. Wren C: Philos Trans R Soc Lond [Biol] 1:128, 1665
12. Gladstone E: Johann Sigiss Elsholtz. Calif West Med 38:432; 39:45, 1933
13. Jennings CE: Transfusion. Leonard & Co, New York, 1883
14. Lower R: Philos Trans R Soc Lond [Biol] 1:353, 1666
15. Wheatley H (ed): The Diary of Samuel Pepys. Vol. 6. p. 14. G. Bell & Sons, London, 1896
16. Ibid. Vol. 7. p. 28
17. Brown H: Jean Denis and transfusion of blood, Paris, 1667–1668. Isis 39:15, 1948
18. Keynes G: Tercentenary of blood transfusion. BMJ 4:410, 1967
19. Denis J: Philos Trans R Soc Lond [Biol] 3:489, 1667
20. Denis J: Philos Trans R Soc Lond [Biol] 4:710, 1668
21. Denis J: Philos Trans R Soc Lond [Biol] 4:617, 1668
22. Hoff He, Guillemin R: The tercentenary of transfusion in man. Cardiovasc Res Cent Bull 6:47, 1967
23. Jones HW, Mackmull G: The influence of James Blundell on the development of blood transfusion. Ann Med Hist 10:242, 1928
24. Young JH: James Blundell (1790–1878): experimental physiologist and obstetrician. Med Hist 8:159, 1964
25. Blundell J: Experiments on the transfusion of blood by the syringe. Med Chir Trans 9:56, 1818
26. Leacock JH: On the transfusion of blood in extreme cases of hemorrhage. Med Chir J Rev 3:276, 1816
27. Blundell J: Some account of a case of obstinate vomiting in which an attempt was made to prolong life by the injection of blood into the veins. Med Chir Trans 10:296, 1819
28. Editorial: Transfusion of blood. Philadelphia J Med Phys Sci 9:205, 1825
29. Randolph J: Memoir of Dr. P.S. Physick. Am J Med Sci 24:93, 1839
30. Blundell J: The aftermanagement of floodings, and on transfusion. Lancet 13:673, 1828
31. Waller C: Successful transfusion. Lancet 11:457, 1827
32. Doubleday E: Another successful case of transfusion. Lancet 1:111, 1825
33. Blundell J: Successful case of transfusion. Lancet 1:431, 1829
34. Blundell J: Observations on transfusion of blood. Lancet 2:321, 1828
35. Lane S: Hemorrhagic diathesis. Successful transfusion of blood. Lancet 1:185, 1840
36. Blundell J: Lectures on the theory and practice of midwifery. Lancet 2:513, 1827
37. Routh C: Remarks statistical and general on transfusion of blood. Med Times 20:114, 1849
38. Benedict NB: On the operation of transfusion, being

the report of a committee. New Orleans Med Sci J 10:191, 1853

39. Charity Hospital Reports. New Orleans Med News Hosp Gaz 1:216, 1854

40. Benedict NB: Transfusion in yellow fever—successful case. New Orleans Med News Hosp Gaz 5:721, 1859

41. Flint A: Transfusion Med Rec 1:187, 1874

42. Schmidt PJ: Transfusion in America in the eighteenth and nineteenth centuries. N Engl J Med 279:1319, 1968

43. Kuhns WJ: Blood transfusion in the Civil War. Transfusion 5:92, 1965

44. Bischoff TLW: Beitrage zur Lehre von dem Blute und der Transfusion desselben. Arch Anat Physiol: p. 347, 1835

45. Neudorfer J: Uber Transfusionen bei Anaemischen. Oesterr Z Prakt Heild 6:124, 1860

46. Braxton-Hicks J: On transfusion and new mode of management. B M J 3:151, 1868

47. Brown-Sequard E: Experimental researches on the faculty possessed by certain elements of the blood of regenerating the vital properties. Med Times Gaz 11:492, 1855

48. Aveling JH: Immediate transfusion in England. Obstet J Gt Britain Ireland 5:289, 1873

49. Roussel J: Leçons sur la Transfusion Directe du Sang. Asselin et Houzeaw, Paris, 1885

50. Gesellius F: Die Transfusion des Blutes. E. Hoppe, Leipzig, 1873

51. Oberman HA: Early history of blood substitutes. Transfusion of milk. Transfusion 9:74, 1969

52. Thomas TG: The intravenous injection of milk as a substitute for the transfusion of blood. Illustrated by seven operations. N Y Med J 27:449, 1878

53. Prout JS: Intravenous injection of milk. Med Rec 13:378, 1878

54. Brinton JH: The transfusion of blood and the intravenous injection of milk. Med Rec 14:344, 1878

55. Bull WT: On the intravenous injection of saline solutions as a substitute for blood. Med Rec 25:6, 1884

56. Landsteiner K: Zur Kenntnis der antifermentativen, lytischen und agglutinierenden wirkungen des Blutserums und der Lymphe. Zentrabl Bakteriol 27:361, 1900

57. Landsteiner K: Uber Agglutinationserscheinungen normalen meuschlichen Blutes. Wien Klin Wochenschr 14:1132, 1901

58. DeCastello A, Sturli A: Uber die Isoagglutinine im Serum gesunder und kranker Menschen. Munch Med Wochenschr: p. 1090, 1902

59. Rosenfield R: Early twentieth century origins of modern blood transfusion therapy. Mt Sinai J Med 41:626, 1974

60. Moss WL: Studies on isoagglutinins and isohemolysins. Bull Johns Hopkins Hosp 21:63, 1910

61. Lespinasse VD: The treatment of hemorrhagic disease of the newborn by direct transfusion of blood. JAMA 62:1868, 1914

62. Bernheim BM: Blood Transfusion, Hemorrhage and the Anemias. JB Lippincott, Philadelphia, 1917

63. von Ziemssen H: Uber die subcutane Blutinjection und uber eine neue einfache Methode der intravenosen Transfusion. Munch Med Wochenschr 39:1, 1892

64. Lindeman E: Simple syringe transfusion with special cannulas. Am J Dis Child 6:28, 1913

65. Unger LJ: A new method of syringe transfusion. JAMA 64:582, 1915

66. Killduffe RA, DeBakey M: The Blood Bank and the Technique and Therapeutics of Transfusion. CV Mosby, St. Louis, 1942

67. Tzanck A: Techniques de transfusion sanguine. Paris Med 59:301, 1925

68. Kyle RA, Shampo MA: Louis Agote. JAMA 228:860, 1974

69. Lewisohn R: The citrate method of blood transfusion after ten years. Boston Med Surg J 190:733, 1924

70. Weil R: Sodium citrate in the transfusion of blood. JAMA 64:425, 1915

71. Rous P, Turner P: The preservation of living red blood cells in vitro. II. The transfusion of kept cells. J Exp Med 23:239, 1916

72. Robertson O: Transfusion with preserved red blood cells. BMJ 1:691, 1918

73. Kendrick DB (ed): Blood Programs in World War II. Department of the Army, Washington, DC, 1964

74. Kimpton AR, Brown JH: A new and simple method of transfusion. JAMA 61:117, 1913

75. Davis VC, Curtis AH: Recent experiences with blood transfusion. JAMA 62:775, 1914

76. De Gowin EL, Harris JE, Plass ED: Studies on preserved human blood. I. Various factors inducing hemolysis. JAMA 114:850, 1940

77. Alsever JB, Ainslee RB: A new method for the preparation of dilute plasma and the operation of a complete transfusion service. N Y State Med J 41:126, 1941

78. Loutit JF, Mollison PL: Advantages of a disodium-citrate-glucose mixture as a blood preservative. BMJ 2:744, 1943

79. Gibson JG, Rees SB, McManus TJ, Schleitlin WA: A citrate-phosphate-dextrose solution for the preservation of whole blood. Am J Clin Path 18:569, 1957

80. Mollison PL, Sloviter HA: Successful transfusion of previously frozen human red cells. Lancet 2:862, 1951

81. Lewisohn R, Rosenthal N: Prevention of chills following the transfusion of citrated blood. JAMA 100:467, 1933

82. Diamond LK: History of blood banking in the United States. JAMA 193:140, 1965

83. Abel JJ, Rowntree LG, Turner BB: Plasma removal with return of corpuscles. J Pharmacol Exp Ther 5:625, 1914

84. Jorda JD: The Barcelona blood transfusion service. Lancet 1:773, 1939

85. Swan H, Schechter DC: The transfusion of blood from cadavers: a historical review. Surgery 52:545, 1962

86. Hawkins J, Brewer H: Placental blood for transfusion. Lancet 1:132, 1939

87. Coombs RRA, Mourant AE, Race RR: A new test for the detection of weak and "incomplete" Rh agglutinins. Br J Exp Pathol 26:225, 1945

88. Levine P, Stetson RE: An unusual case of intra-group agglutination. JAMA 113:126, 1939

89. Rosenfield RE: Who discovered Rh? A personal glimpse of the Levine-Weiner argument. Transfusion 29:355, 1989

90. Levine P, Burnham L, Katzin EM, Vogel P: The role of isoimmunization in the pathogenesis of erythroblastosis fetalis. Am J Obstet Gynecol 42:925, 1941

91. Rosenfield RE: The past and future of immunohematology. Am J Clin Pathol 64:569, 1975

92. Ottenberg R: Transfusion and arterial anastomosis. Ann Surg 47:486, 1908

93. Hoxworth P, Ames A: Blood grouping and compatibility. JAMA 108:1234, 1937

94. Riddell VH: Blood Transfusion. Oxford University Press, London, 1939

95. Monroe CH, Jennings ER: The significance of the minor crossmatch—after ten years. In: A Seminar on Compatibility Testing. American Association of Blood Banks, Washington, DC, 1968

96. Oberman HA, Barnes BA, Steiner EA: Role of the crossmatch in testing for serologic incompatibility. Transfusion 22:12, 1982

97. Low B, Meseter L: Antiglobulin test in low-ionic strength salt solution for rapid antibody screening and cross-matching. Vox Sang 26:53, 1974

98. Oberman HA, Barnes BA, Friedman BA: The risk of abbreviating the major crossmatch in urgent or massive transfusion. Transfusion 18:137, 1978

99. Electronic verification of donor-recipient compatibility: The computer crossmatch. In Butch SH, Judd WJ, Steiner EA et al (eds): Transfusion 34:105, 1994

100. Fantus B: The therapy of the Cook County Hospital. Blood preservation technic. JAMA 111:317, 1938

Chapter 3

Immunology and Its Relation to Blood Transfusion

Lawrence D. Petz and Scott N. Swisher

The purpose of this chapter is to provide a review of selected aspects of immunology that have relevance to the practice of blood transfusion. A number of clinical applications of these immunologic principles are pointed out in this chapter. Although some of the basic immunology discussed does not yet have direct application to the practice of transfusion medicine, the information nevertheless allows the interested reader to develop greater depth of knowledge in these selected areas; it provides a basis for understanding some of the phenomenology of blood transfusion, enables the reader to cope with much of the modern medical literature, and points toward future developments in transfusion and transplantation biology.

IMMUNOLOGIC RECOGNITION OF ANTIGENS

Antigen-specific recognition of foreign antigens by the adaptive immune system is governed by three genetic systems as follows: (1) class I and II major histocompatibility complex (MHC) genes, (2) T-cell receptor genes, and (3) B-cell receptor (immunoglobulin) genes.[1] B cells, through their membrane immunoglobulin receptors, can interact directly with epitope conformations present on native, unmodified antigens. In contrast to B-cell receptors, antigen-specific T-cell receptors recognize a heterodimeric complex that consists of an antigen-derived peptide that is noncovalently bound to an HLA molecule. Antigen must be processed and appropriately presented by MHC molecules on the surface of antigen-presenting cells (APCs).

Engagement of the specific antigen receptors of B or T cells by the appropriate ligands during a primary response is insufficient to activate a B cell to produce antibody or a T cell to synthesize cytokines or acquire the function of cytotoxicity. Additional signals must be received by both cell types before activation can occur. In fact, there is abundant evidence that engagement of antigen receptors in the absence of critical costimulatory signals can deactivate cells and may prevent their activation by subsequent exposure to antigen (anergy). For B cells with receptors specific for protein antigens, the additional signals are provided primarily by T-helper cells. This response is referred to as a T-cell-dependent B-cell response. For T-cell responses, the signals are provided by APCs, which may be dendritic cells in a primary response and, in addition, by B cells or macrophages in a secondary response.[1]

Antigen-activated and memory T cells develop additional adhesion molecules that permit egress from capillaries and into sites of inflammation where they may then be retained by other specific adhesion molecules. Collectively, distribution of adhesion molecules on various T- and B-cell subpopulations defines precise and distinct homing routes. These molecules interact with complementary ligands present on endothelial cells and various extracellular matrices. Reviews of the role of leukocyte-endothelial adhesion molecules have been published,[2,3] including those related to altered expression of adhesion molecules in human disease.[4,5]

COMPONENTS OF THE IMMUNE SYSTEM

Stem Cells

The pluripotent stem cell gives rise to the production of all immune and blood cells.[6] At birth, the pluripotent stem cell has generated two populations of other stem cells, that is, hematopoietic stem cells and lymphopoietic stem cells. Hematopoietic stem cells differentiate into platelets, granulocytes, monocytes, and erythrocytes; lymphopoietic stem cells produce lymphocytes (Fig. 3-1). Both hematopoietic and lymphopoietic stem cells retain an important capacity, termed self-renewal, whereby some of their daughter cells remain as stem cells. Stem cells in adults are found in the bone marrow and look like small lymphocytes.

Antigen-Presenting Cells

The term APC refers to a set of functional attributes of different cell types that permit them to present peptides to T cells effectively.[1] During a primary immune response, the major cell type that can perform this function for naive, resting T cells is the dendritic cell. B lymphocytes and, to a lesser extent, macrophages can also present antigen to memory T cells previously exposed to the inducing antigen.

Effective activation of antigen-specific T cells by APCs involves the following four steps: (1) uptake and partial degradation of the antigen into peptides that bind to intracellular MHC molecules (processing), (2) re-expression of the peptide-MHC molecules on the cell membrane surface (presentation), (3) interaction of the T-cell antigen receptor with the peptide-MHC complex, and (4) interaction of accessory receptors with their ligands.

Dendritic Cells

Dendritic cells are derived from hematopoietic stem cells and, at some point during differentiation, develop into a specific lineage of cells distinct from

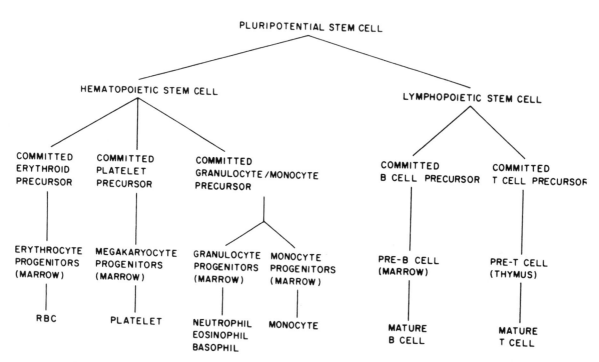

Fig. 3-1. Ontogeny and development of mononuclear cells. (From Dzik,[7] with permission.)

monocytes and macrophages. They are widely distributed in small numbers throughout most organs in the body. Although they constitute less than 0.1 percent of peripheral blood leukocytes, they are the major stimulator cell in mixed leukocyte cultures. In a primary humoral response, naive antigen-specific B cells are thought to interact with dendritic cell T-cell clusters, initiating B-cell activation and proliferation and immunoglobulin synthesis.

Additional interactions that occur between the T cell and APCs involve other accessory molecules and cytokines (see below) that are critical for effective T-cell activation. Presentation of antigen without this "second signal" may not only result in lack of proliferation but may also actually lead to a state of nonresponsiveness in the involved T cell (clonal anergy).

Cytokines

Lymphokines and cytokines are low-molecular-weight (10,000 to 60,000 D) glycoproteins primarily produced by lymphoid cells that act in a hormone-like fashion to regulate the immune system.[8] Lymphokines and cytokines have systemic and localized effects. These small glycoprotein molecules are grouped generally under the term *cytokine*. The more specific term *lymphokine* is commonly used to denote factors produced by lymphoid cells (lymphocytes) and monocytes or macrophages. Many of these cytokines have been extensively characterized, their genes have been cloned, and their production has been initiated in bacterial or mammalian engineered cellular systems (Table 3-1). Literally dozens of cytokines have been identified, including interleukin-1 (IL-1) through IL-11; α-interferon (INF-α) INF-β, and INF-γ; tumor necrosis factor-α (TNF-α) and TNF-β; a number of colony-stimulating factors (CSF), and numerous growth factors.

Cytokine production is required for the initiation and progression of a normal immune response. The lymphokines and cytokines work together in a complex interactive scheme, often in cascade fashion such that one factor induces another; no single factor is sufficient to promote an immune response by itself. Also, lymphokine regulation itself is a complex concept involving autocrine interactions, receptor up- and downregulation, and receptor affinity alterations. We are only beginning to appreciate the fine regulation of cytokine action and production.

Table 3-1. Cloned, Genetically Engineered Cytokines

Cytokine	Abbreviation
Interleukin-1 α, β	IL-1α, IL-1β
Interleukin-2	IL-2
Interleukin-3	IL-3
Interleukin-4	IL-4
Interleukin-5	IL-5
Interleukin-6	IL-6
Interleukin-7	IL-7
Interleukin-8	IL-8
α, β interferon	IFN-α, IFN-β
γ interferon	IFN-γ
Granulocyte colony-stimulating factor	G-CSF
Granulocyte-macrophage colony-stimulating factor	GM-CSF
Macrophage colony-stimulating factor	M-CSF
Tumor necrosis factor-α, β	TNF-α, TNF-β
Erythropoietin	EPO
Transforming growth factor-α, β	TGF-α, TGF-β

(From Rossio et al.,[8] with permission.)

Changes in the delicate equilibrium of the immune system are reflected by changes in lymphokine and cytokine levels in plasma or serum. Alterations or abnormalities in the production of lymphokines, or in the ability of target cells to respond appropriately to lymphokines, have been implicated in the pathogenesis of cancer, infectious disease, autoimmune diseases, and allergies.

Cytokines, especially those involving the immune system, are being increasingly used as immune stimulants in the clinical setting, particularly in the therapy of disorders such as cancer and acquired immunodeficiency syndrome. Clinical trials have involved many of the interleukins (IL-1α, IL-1β, IL-2, IL-3, and IL-4), granulocyte-macrophage CSF and granulocyte CSF, interferons (IFN-α, IFN-β, and IFN-γ), and others. Cytokine therapy is also being combined with standard types of therapy (i.e., radiation, surgery, and chemotherapy) in an effort to increase the effectiveness of the therapy.

B-Cell Development

One of the two major divisions of lymphocytes are B cells. These lymphocytes are so named because they were originally discovered in experiments on the chicken that showed that the cells developed from stem cells in an organ known as the bursa of Fabricius. In humans, B cells develop in the bone marrow. During this development, the most important activity of the cell is its commitment to produce a specific antibody should the cell later become activated.

All B cells arise in the bone marrow from pluripotent progenitor or stem cells that do not synthesize immunoglobulin molecules.[9] The next earliest cell that expresses B-lymphocyte markers is called the pre-B cell. This cell expresses cytoplasmic IgM only and no conventional light chains. Therefore, it is believed that pre-B cells do not respond to antigenic stimulation. The next stage of B-cell maturation involves the immature B cell, which expresses surface IgM. Once these immature cells leave the bone marrow, they continue to mature and start to express IgD in addition to IgM and are then called mature B cells. These mature B cells are likely to encounter antigen in the periphery and progress to become activated B cells. Activated B cells proliferate and differentiate into antibody-producing B cells. During this stage of B-cell differentiation, some B cells undergo heavy chain isotype switching. Others may not terminally differentiate into plasma cells and, instead, become memory B cells, the stimulation of which leads to secondary antibody responses.

After antigen binding to surface Ig on mature B cells, these cells have the potential to mount either a T-cell-dependent or an -independent response, depending on the nature and magnitude of the stimulus.

T-Cell-Independent B-Cell Responses

The T-cell-independent response can be initiated by bacterial products, such as lipopolysaccharide, that are potent polyclonal mitogens for mouse B lymphocytes. The interaction of multiple repeating determinants, such as those characteristic of many carbohydrate structures, cross-links the immunoglobulin receptor, which initiates steps of B-lymphocyte activation, resulting in the generation of a humoral response, usually restricted to the IgM subclass.

T-Cell-Dependent Activation of B Cells

T-cell-dependent antigens are proteins. After binding to the immunoglobulin receptor on B lymphocytes, they are endocytosed and processed as in other

APCs, such as macrophages. This sequence of events results in the generation of peptide fragments of the antigen, which are subsequently expressed on the surface of the B-cell surface, noncovalently bound to class II MHC molecules. These peptide-MHC class II complexes can now be recognized by antigen-specific helper T cells. After internalization and processing, the peptide fragments are presented in the context of MHC class II molecules to specific helper T cells. These antigen-specific helper T cells then secrete cytokines that stimulate the proliferation and differentiation of the antigen-specific B cells. Various cytokines play distinct roles during the different stages of B-cell differentiation and proliferation. The relative proportion of the different cytokines influences the nature and magnitude of an immune response because certain cytokines either synergize or inhibit one another's actions. The type of antigenic stimulus can also influence the degree of T-cell help and thus the production of the various cytokines.

T-Cell Development

The development of mature T cells from committed T-cell precursors follows a totally different path. Precursor cells leave the marrow and travel to the thymus gland (hence the term T cells). There, the pre-T cells come under the influence of local factors in the gland that cause these cells to develop into mature T cells. There are many different kinds of T cells, which are named according to their respective functions: helper T cells, suppressor T cells, killer T cells, and so forth. The process of thymic T-cell development involves not only a DNA commitment to respond to only one specific antigen (as in the case of the B cell) but also selection of a particular function among the variety of functions that T cells perform.

A great deal has been learned about the details of T-cell development in the thymus. As in the case of B cells, T-cell development follows a logical sequence, and the cells can be recognized at various stages of development by the different surface antigen phenotypes expressed. A systematic nomenclature has been developed for these cell surface molecules, the CD (cluster designation) system, in which the markers are numbered CD1, CD2, and so forth. Initially, CD defined the existence of a group of monoclonal antibodies with similar specificity, but it is now generally held that CD in fact designates a discrete antigen identified by two or more monoclonal antibodies. Monoclonal antibodies that identify CD antigens on the cell surface of hematopoietic cells have been essential in delineating the components of the immune system. CD molecules may serve as cell surface receptors for essential growth factors, cytokines, and serum proteins; may function as membrane enzymes; and may mediate cell adhesion to other cells and to extracellular matrix components. At a workshop in Vienna in 1989, 78 CDs were recognized.

Two general phenotypic categories of T cells, CD4-positive and CD8-positive types, have been well characterized. CD4 cells have the general property of helper/inducer cells, whereas CD8 cells have cytotoxic/suppressor properties, although these two populations are not always mutually exclusive. Both of these phenotypic cell types can be further subdivided into discrete functional categories according to the profile of lymphokines they secrete.

Th1 and Th2 Subsets

Th1 cells secrete predominantly IL-2 and IFN-γ. These cytokine profiles play a major role in the mediation of delayed-type sensitivity reactions. Th1 cells can activate B cells and cause their proliferation, but the cytokine profile secreted by these cells does not induce significant heavy chain class switching in B cells.

In contrast, a second type, referred to as Th2, secretes predominantly IL-4, IL-5, and IL-10. Cytokines produced by Th2 are essential for heavy chain switching in activated B cells to IgG, IgA, or IgE production. Th2 cells are the principal T-helper cells for B-cell maturation and antibody production. Th2 cells are also predominantly found in chronic inflammatory lesions in which IgE, mast cells, and eosinophils are major effector mechanisms, such as atopic allergic reactions and parasitic infestations.

Not all CD4-positive, T-helper cells show the distinctive cytokine profiles of Th1 and Th2 cells. In fact, a commonly observed profile in humans is T cells (called Th0) that produce most of the cytokines produced by both Th1 and Th2. Th0 cells may represent activated T cells not yet committed to a discrete pathway of cytokine synthesis. The various T-cell subsets may not be distinct lineages but, rather,

cells that have received different activating signals. Some evidence indicates that CD8-positive T cells similarly may be divided into populations with Th1- and Th2-like cytokine profiles.

HLA Molecules in Antigen Presentation

HLA molecules are two-chain, globular glycoproteins. Structurally, HLA molecules belong to the immunoglobulin superfamily of molecules. Six major types of HLA gene products have been identified: HLA-A, -B, -C, -DR, -DQ, and -DP. Based on physical characteristics, the gene products can be divided into two classes of molecules, termed class I and class II. (See Ch. 6 for a detailed discussion of the HLA system.)

The manner by which MHC gene products present peptides to T cells has been described. The α_1 and α_2 domains of the class I heavy chain each contain sequences of amino acids that assume an α-helical configuration (Fig. 3-2). These helices form the sides of a groove that can accommodate a peptide of approximately 8 to 20 amino acids. Virtually all of the amino acid differences that determine the defined polymorphism of the various HLA class I molecules occur in the sides of the floor of this so-called peptide groove. Thus, T cells, through their antigen

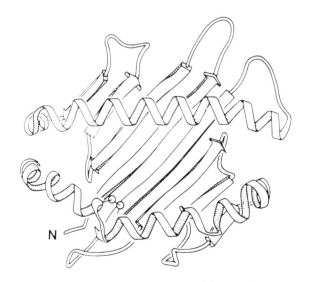

Fig. 3-2. Schematic representation of the peptide groove of an HLA class I molecule (see text). (From Bjorkman et al.,[10] with permission.)

receptors, recognize and bind to unique conformations that consist of an MHC molecule bearing a peptide of self or foreign origin. Analysis of the positions of amino acid sequence differences among class II molecules strongly suggests that these molecules have a similar peptide groove constructed from their α_1 and β_1 domains.

IMMUNE RESPONSE

B and T lymphocytes, the cells endowed with receptors to recognize specifically the subtle antigenic variations that distinguish self and nonself antigens, identify these differences through entirely separate mechanisms. B cells "see" foreign epitopes in the antigen's native conformation, whereas T cells "see" the antigen only after it has been processed into discrete peptides and presented on a histocompatibility molecule. T cells not only orchestrate T-cell responses but also are essential for most B-cell responses. If appropriate signals are not received in a timely fashion, T-cell activation may not occur; under these circumstances, T cells can develop anergy and not respond to a subsequent specific antigen challenge. Although T cells play a central role in immune responses, none of the responses will occur without an effective system of APCs.

Primary and Secondary Immune Responses

Primary and secondary immune responses refer to the generation of antigen-specific antibody populations during the first and subsequent exposures of an individual to exogenous antigens. The primary response is characterized by the appearance of antigen-specific IgM antibodies after 5 to 7 days, followed by IgG antibodies several days later; the titers of both antibodies usually diminish by 28 days.[9] However, on subsequent challenge with the same antigen, a rapid increase (within 48 hours) in predominantly IgG antibody ensues, which peaks at about 6 days after the challenge. This sequence of events explains the serologic and clinical manifestations that occur during a delayed hemolytic transfusion reaction (see Ch. 41).

STRUCTURE OF IMMUNE GLOBULINS

An understanding of antibody structure is essential to an understanding of immune recognition. There are eight chemically different types or classes of antibody: the four kinds of IgG plus IgM, IgE, IgA, and IgD. Their essential design is reasonably similar for all isotypes. Like many proteins, antibodies are multichain structures, that is, composed of linked subunits. IgG consists of two identical heavy chains and two identical light chains, hooked together by disulfide bonds. The molecule is entirely symmetrical, and the two portions that actually unite with antigen, the antibody-combining sites, are absolutely identical in a given molecule (Fig. 3-3).

DIVERSITY OF THE IMMUNE RESPONSE

The key puzzle is how the body, with a large but finite amount of genetic information, can create antibodies of enough different specificities to react against the amazing variety of antigens with which the immune system comes in contact. The essential element of such antibody diversity involves the principle of using combinatorial methods.[12] The heavy-chain V region is coded for by three separate genes: V, D, and J (Fig. 3-4) and the light chain V region, by two genes: V and J. There are 500 to 1,000 different V heavy-chain genes and about 10 D genes and 4 J genes. There are at least 200 different V light-chain genes, both κ and λ, and a total of 6 J genes. It should be immediately apparent that an antibody combining site that consists of randomly chosen gene products from no fewer than five genes, each of which permits multiple choices, can present enormous variability (i.e., $10^3 \times 10 \times 4 \times 200 \times 6$ or 5×10^7 to a first approximation) even before explanations such as somatic mutation or slightly imprecise joining at the D-J junction are proposed.

The diversity is provided by an extraordinary process of immunoglobulin gene somatic translocation (Fig. 3-4). During the differentiation of the B cell, a series of translocations takes place, which are different in every cell. First, one member of the set of D genes of the heavy chain translocates to join one of the available J genes, and then the intervening stretch of DNA is discarded from the cell. Next, one particular V gene moves next to the D gene, thus forming a VDJ set for the heavy chain. As indicated in Figure 3-3, this defines the particular messenger RNA for the variable portion of the heavy chain that this cell, and its progeny, can make. Then, a particular V gene for the light chain performs a similar

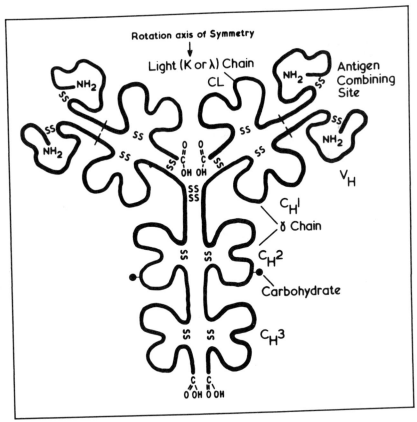

Fig. 3-3. Schematic diagram of a molecule of human IgG, showing the two light (κ or λ) chains and two heavy (γ) chains held together by disulfide bonds. The constant regions of the light (CL) and heavy (C_H1, C_H2, and C_H3 chains and the variable region of the heavy chain (V_H) are indicated. Loops in the peptide chain formed by intrachain disulfide bonds (C_H1, etc.) comprise separate functional domains. (From Nossal,[11] with permission.)

translocation to one J gene. As this random process of gene translocation occurs, uniquely for each different B-cell precursor, a whole repertoire of B cells is created, each of which has its own specificity. When a B cell is activated by antigen, it secretes large amounts of the antibody for which its translocated immunoglobulin genes code. Thus, the "one cell-one antibody" rule is an obligate consequence of the fact that each B cell has experienced its own series of gene translocations.

Nature still has another mechanism to produce a good antibody. Point mutation in DNA is a substitution of one nucleotide for another and is a rare error normally occurring only once in 10^8 or 10^9 times at a particular spot in the gene when a cell divides. As antigenically driven B cells divide, however, somatic

mutation occurs in immunoglobulin genes at about a 100,000-fold higher rate. This creates a tremendous opportunity for selection of variants with receptors of higher affinity for the antigen. Thus, an ongoing or repeated immune response includes affinity maturation, producing better and better antibodies over time. When activated B-cell clones revert to the resting state, they are known as memory cells.

The T-cell repertoire is based on a molecular system that has many similarities. The T-cell receptor is a heterodimer of two polypeptide chains, the α and β chains. These both have V regions with an N-terminal of 100 or so amino acids, and the genes coding for them are also broken into V, D, and J sets. During T lymphocyte differentiation, as in B-lymphocyte development, specific gene transloca-

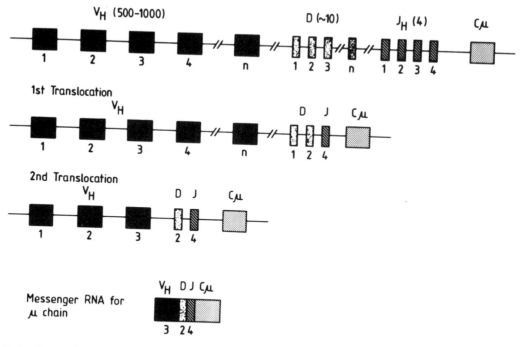

Fig. 3-4. Genetic basis for immune specificity. Gene translocations occur somatically, giving each lymphocyte its unique expression of immunoglobulin minigenes. For the heavy chain, a given D gene translocates to a given J gene. Then a given V gene translocates to the DJ combination. Transcription of the rearranged gene is followed by RNA processing to create a unique heavy-chain messenger RNA. Because a VJ translocation occurs for the light chain shortly thereafter, the combinational possibilities are enormous. $C\mu$ denotes the gene for the constant portion of the immunoglobulin μ heavy chain. (From Nossal,[11] with permission.)

tions occur that give each cell a unique specificity. The translocations and the whole process of T-cell genesis take place in the thymus.

Thus, for both T and B cells, germ-like repertoires are created through essentially antigen-independent differentiation of lymphoneogenesis. When antigen activates particular lymphocytes, then antigen-driven processes initiate a second cycle of multiplication and differentiation in which lymphocytes are turned into effector cells. Immunity therefore involves preantigenic and postantigenic components.

In summary, recognition in the immune system depends on random somatic translocations in immunocyte precursors that create diversified repertoires of B and T cells. Each cell has a single, unique combining specificity, and selective stimulation by antigen results in proliferation of clones of specific immunocytes.

Discrimination Between Self and Nonself

Immune responses to autologous antigens are kept within strict bounds. Although there is some formation of antibody to some bodily constituents, these minimal immune responses ordinarily are kept under adequate control and cause no disease. The spectrum of mechanisms that prevent autoimmune disorders is covered by the term *immunologic tolerance*.

Burnet's theory to explain immunologic tolerance stated that the potentially self-reactive cells are eliminated from the repertoire because contact between an immunocyte and an antigen reactive with it early in ontogeny, when the host is immature, leads to death of the cell. It is presently believed that, instead of being killed, B cells and probably T cells can be negatively signaled or downregulated by contact with antigen and rendered refractory to later triggering stimuli, a state termed clonal anergy.[13] This state is potentially reversible. Suppressor T lymphocytes play a role in some models of tolerance because there are T cells of the CD8 or T8 phenotype that, in ways still poorly understood, antagonize the helper function of CD4 lymphocytes or act directly to suppress B-cell activation.

Regulation of Immune Responses

There are many regulatory mechanisms of the immune system. Antigen itself is a key regulator. As it is catabolized or neutralized by antibody, only immunocytes with receptors of high affinity are able to compete effectively for the diminishing supply of antigen. Antibody is also a feedback regulator. It speeds antigen elimination, and soluble antigen-antibody complexes can downregulate individual immunocytes.

MHC genes and the antigens for which they code exercise a powerful regulatory function. If a given epitope from an antigen cannot make an effective union with any of the MHC antigens, the immune response cannot be initiated, and the host is considered a genetic nonresponder to that epitope. Also, antigen-specific helpers and suppressors exercise antagonistic controlling functions. Furthermore, lymphokines, which are released after specific activation, can have profound nonspecific effects, including the lowering of activation thresholds for nearby lymphocytes of different specificity and the recruitment of inflammatory cells that affect both antigen presentation and lymphocyte migration.

Finally, because every combining site is unique, it in itself is a unique antigen. The technical term for this unique property is its *idiotype*. Because the amount of any given idiotype in the body is small, immunologic tolerance may not be induced; thus, each idiotype is potentially an immunogen. If immunity is induced to an idiotype, the result is anti-idiotypic antibody or anti-idiotypic cytotoxic T cells. If tolerance is induced, the result could include a population of anti-idiotypic suppressor T cells. The potential exists for the immune system to constitute a network of idiotype-anti-idiotype interactions. The significance of such a network is a matter of intense investigational work.

IMMUNE RESPONSES TO RED CELL ANTIGENS

Classes of Immunoglobulin Produced

Although the primary immune response characteristically results initially in development of IgM antibodies, with a later switch to synthesis of IgG antibodies, it has been difficult to prove that this generalization applies to the production of red cell alloantibodies in humans.[14] It is not known with certainty whether IgM antibody is the first to be made in human subjects responding to the Rh antigen, but it is clear that, in most people, IgG anti-$Rh_o(D)$ antibody soon predominates and is often the only type that can be identified at any time. In a minority of challenged subjects, IgM anti-$Rh_o(D)$ is also produced in substantial amounts. In hyperimmunized donors with anti-Rh in their serum, "boosting" with small amounts of Rh-positive red cells is often followed by the production of IgM and IgG anti-Rh. In these hyperimmunized antibody donors, the anti-Rh is also often partly IgA. Responses to several other red cell antigens (e.g., K, Fy^a and Jk^a) appear to be similar to responses to Rh, that is, most antibodies are predominantly IgG, although in some subjects alloimmunized to these antigens a mixture of IgM and IgG antibodies is found.[15]

With the ABO system, perhaps all humans should be regarded as immunized. Moreover, ABO-incompatible pregnancies and injections of various animal products cause both quantitative and qualitative changes in anti-A and anti-B. Perhaps the most interesting fact about antibody production in the ABO system is that immune anti-A and anti-B are predominantly IgM in A or B subjects but may be largely IgG (and partly IgA) in group O subjects.

Relative Immunogenicity of Different Red Cell Alloantigens

An estimate of the relative immunogenicity of different red cell alloantigens can be obtained by comparing the actual frequency with which particular alloantibodies are encountered with the calculated frequency of the opportunity for immunization.[16] The relative opportunities for immunization to K and Fy^a can be estimated by simply comparing the frequency of the combination K-positive donor/k-negative recipient (i.e., $0.09 \times 0.91 = 0.08$), with the frequency of the combination Fy^a-positive donor/

Fy^a-negative recipient (i.e., $0.66 \times 0.34 = 0.22$). Thus, the opportunity for immunization to Fy^a is about 3.5 times greater than that for K (0.22 versus 0.08). Although opportunities for immunization to Fy^a are 3.5 times more frequent than those to K, anti-K is in fact found 2.5 times more commonly than anti-Fy^a; overall, K can be said to be nine times more potent than Fy^a. If a single transfusion of K-positive blood to a K-negative subject induces the formation of serologically detectable anti-K in 10 percent of cases, it can be predicted that the transfusion of a single unit of Fy(a+) blood to a Fy^a-negative subject would induce the formation of serologically detectable anti-Fy^a in about one percent of cases. Giblett[16] calculated that c and E of the Rh system were about one-third as immunogenic as K; Fy^a was calculated to be about one-twenty-fifth as potent, and Jk^a one-fiftieth to one-one-hundredth as potent as K.

Responders and Nonresponders

It has long been apparent that it is very difficult to elicit the formation of anti-D in some D-negative subjects; despite repeated injections of Rh-positive red cells, about 20 percent of Rh-negative subjects do not form anti-Rh.[14]

Krevans et al.[17] and Woodrow et al.[18] made an observation of great interest when they found that, within 6 weeks (sometimes longer) after a first injection of Rh-positive red cells, Rh-negative subjects could be divided into two classes: (1) those in whom the second and subsequent injections of ^{51}Cr-labeled Rh-positive red cells were rapidly eliminated and who formed anti-Rh after a few more injections and (2) those in whom the second and subsequent injections of Rh-positive red cells survived normally and who did not subsequently form anti-Rh. Although most Rh-negative responders produce serologically detectable anti-Rh after two injections of Rh-positive red cells given at an interval of 3 to 6 months, a few do not; such subjects can be classified as nonresponders only if the survival of Rh-positive red cells is measured or if several further injections of Rh-positive cells are given.

A few subjects produce trace amounts of anti-Rh after a few injections of Rh-positive cells, but increased antibody levels do not occur after further injections. The antibody may even become undetectable. Subjects who take a long time to produce anti-

Rh tend to produce low-titer antibody: of 116 subjects who produced anti-Rh within 9 months of the first immunization, the agglutination titer (in albumin) eventually reached 512 or more in all cases. In those in whom anti-Rh was first detected 12 months or more after the first injection, the titer reached a maximum of 128 or less in 8 of 18 cases.[14]

The genetic differences between individuals who are responders or nonresponders are generally not well understood. No consistent differences in HLA antigens have been identified. In a study of the association between responsiveness to Rh antigen and certain bacterial and other antigens, no relationship could be found.[19]

Effect of Rh$_o$(D) Alloimmunization on Formation of Other Red Cell Alloantibodies

Among Rh-negative volunteers deliberately injected with Rh-positive red cells, those who form anti-D also tend to form alloantibodies outside the Rh system, whereas those who do not form anti-D seldom form any red cell alloantibodies. In one series of 73 subjects who formed anti-D, 6 formed anti-Fy^a, 4 formed anti-Jk^a, and 4 formed other alloantibodies; by contrast, among 48 subjects who did not form anti-D, not 1 made any detectable alloantibodies.[20]

Several studies in which Rh-negative subjects have been deliberately immunized with Rh-positive red cells are available for analysis. The data indicate a tremendously increased response to antigens outside the Rh system in subjects responding to the D antigen. In subjects who formed anti-D and were also exposed to other potentially immunogenic antigens, 50 percent formed anti-K. The incidence rates of anti-Fy^a, anti-Jk^a, and anti-s in those who were challenged were about 20 percent in each instance.

COMPLEMENT

About 1 century ago, it was recognized that serum contained soluble and heat-labile proteins that could lyse bacterial cells in the wake of an antibody response to those cells. The term *alexin* or *complement* was used to describe these factors; over the years, complement has been used as a collective term to include the series of proteins required to mediate these biologic events.[21] The complement system is composed of a number of serum proteins that function in an orderly and integrated fashion. Activation of the complement system can either be beneficial to the host, as in resistance to invading microorganisms, or it can be detrimental to the host, as in a variety of immunopathologically mediated diseases. Activation can be accomplished by at least two different pathways: classic and alternative.

The rapid development of methodology in protein chemistry in the last several decades has led to a detailed understanding of the biochemistry and reaction mechanism of the components of the complement system. More recently, emphasis in complement research has been placed on the importance of complement activation in the production of inflammation, on the contribution of the components

to various aspects of host defense, and on the role of complement in human disease. Indeed, present-day investigative work utilizes molecular biology, genetics, biochemistry, immunology, and medicine.

Complement Activation

Two pathways of complement activation have been described (Fig. 3-5). These are called the classic pathway, which has been studied since the turn of the century, and the alternative pathway, which was discovered more recently.[22,23] Both function through the interaction of a series of proteins termed *components*. In general, the classic pathway is activated by antibody-coated targets or antigen-antibody complexes. The alternative pathway can be

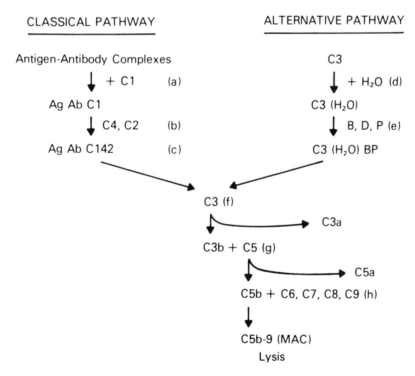

Fig. 3-5. Diagram showing the elements of the classic and alternative pathways, which converge to form a convertase that cleaves C3. In the classic pathway, antigen-antibody (Ag-Ab) complexes sequentially bind C1, C4, and C2. Binding is followed by activation. Cleavage fragments are not shown, except in the case of C3 and C5. In the alternative pathway, C3 undergoes hydrolysis of a high-energy thiol-ester bond, which induces a change in conformation. It now accepts factor B, which is cleaved by factor D to form a convertase, which in turn is stabilized by properdin (P). C3b, the cleavage product of C3, also has a cleaved thiol-ester bond and acts like hydrolyzed C3 to activate the alternative pathway. The convertase complex of the classic or alternative pathway with C3 continues sequential binding of each of the late-acting components until the reaction sequence is complete (see the text for details). MAC denotes membrane-attack complex. (From Frank,[22] with permission.)

activated by suitable targets in the absence of antibody. Both pathways proceed by means of sequential activation and assembly of a series of proteins, leading to the formation of a complex enzyme that can bind to and cleave a key protein, C3, which is common to both pathways. Thereafter, the two pathways proceed together through binding of the late-acting components to form a membrane attack complex (MAC), which ultimately causes cell lysis. The proteins of the classic pathway and the late-acting components are designated by numbers. Proteins of the alternative pathway are generally given letter designations, as are the proteins that induce complement component degradation.

C1 Activation Induced by Immune Complexes

C1 is activated by interaction with certain antigen-antibody complexes. Human IgG and IgM bind C1, but IgA, IgD, and IgE do not.[24] Furthermore, subclass specificity is a factor, with IgG3 being the most reactive and IgG4 the least reactive of the four subclasses of IgG.[24,25] Binding of antigen to antibody either induces a conformational change in the antibody's Fc portion, thereby facilitating C1 activation, or aggregates or clusters, Fcs, thereby enhancing the affinity for the multivalent C1q.[26]

Binding of C1q by Anti-Rh₀(D)

There is good evidence from a variety of sources that each C1q molecule must bind to two IgG molecules to bind C1 firmly enough for C1 activation to take place.[27] Thus, a single C1q molecule must bind to a pair of IgG molecules that are sufficiently close together to allow the C1q to span between them. The greater the density of antibody molecules is, the greater the chance of finding suitable pairs of binding sites. This requirement for dual binding of C1q has been offered as an explanation for the failure of certain antibodies to activate complement. The outstanding example of this is anti-Rh₀(D). However, many anti-K, anti-Jk^a, and anti-Fy^a antibodies activate complement, and there are far fewer K, Jk^a, and Fy^a sites on the red cell than D sites. Indeed, it has been shown that C1q can bind to anti-D-coated red cells provided that the density of anti-D on the surface is sufficiently great. Hughes-Jones and Ghosh[28] measured C1q binding on anti-D-sensitized erythrocytes using ^{125}I-labeled C1q. When red cells

were coated with about 10,000 anti-D molecules, 100 C1q binding sites were found on each cell. At higher anti-D densities, the number of C1q binding sites increased rapidly so that, with a doubling of the density to 20,000 anti-D molecules per cell, there was a five- to six-fold increase in C1q binding sites. Because it is probable that the D antigen is distributed at random on the red cell surface, the existence of this many binding sites indicates that some pairs of molecules will be present by chance within 30 nm of each other, the distance that can be spanned by a C1q molecule. Therefore, there must be a failure of bound C1 to activate because of unknown mechanisms.

Activation of C3

Figure 3-6 depicts the fragmentation sequence of C3 as it occurs under physiologic conditions. Native C3 consists of two nonidentical polypeptide chains held together by disulfide bonds and noncovalent forces. The α chain has a molecular weight of 110,000 D and the β chain, 70,000 D. During activation, the native molecule is cleaved, and two fragments are produced: C3a and C3b. The C3b fragment undergoes a rapid conformational change, which allows for its covalent binding with the complement-activating particle; however, many C3b fragments do not come in contact with the activating particle, hydrolyze, and become unreactive.

Regulation of C3b is effected by factors H and I. After binding of H to C3b, factor I cleaves the α chain of C3b twice and generates three unequal fragments of 67,000, 40,000, and 3,000 D. This cleavage gives rise to a new fragment, termed C3bi (or iC3b). Factor I cleaves a third bond in the 67,000-D α-chain fragment of C3bi and produces two fragments that are named C3dg and C3c.[30] As illustrated, C3dg is a single-chain molecule with a molecular weight of 43,000 D. C3c consists of three polypeptide chains and has a molecular weight of 150,000 D. The C3dg fragment remains associated with the activator (e.g., an antibody-coated erythrocyte); C3c is eluted. The most effective cofactor for this reaction is the complement receptor type 1 (CR1) (see Chemistry and Biology of Complement Receptors), although factor H at high concentrations or low ionic strength can substitute for CR1. The end products of C3 regula-

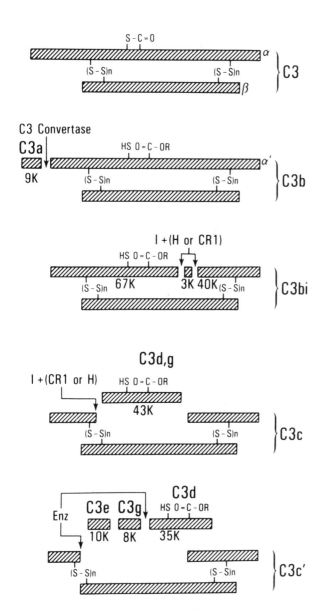

Fig. 3-6. Schematic description of the physiologic activation and control of C3. (From Schrieber,[29] with permission.)

tion are C3d and C3e; because C3c is a fluid-phase fragment, C3e exists only in solution.

Thus, red blood cells of patients with immune hemolytic anemias are coated with C3dg rather than with C3d. C3dg seems to be the final product of in vivo C3 activation in the fluid phase and on red cells.[31] However, conversion of C3bi or C3dg to C3d can be produced in vitro by certain enzymes.

Alternative Pathway of Complement Activation

The alternative pathway of complement activation provides the host with a humoral component of the natural defense mechanisms against infectious agents.[32] The six plasma proteins involved in recognition and activation perform a continuous surveillance function that does not require specific antibody to recognize potential pathogens. Discrimination between host and foreign particles occurs because activation of the system is under strict control by regulatory plasma and membrane proteins of the host. Full activation only occurs when the function of these regulators is dampened on the surface of foreign particles. Organisms sensitive to attack by the alternative pathway include bacteria, fungi, certain viruses, virus-infected cells, some tumor cell lines, a wide variety of naturally occurring polysaccharides and lipopolysaccharides, and human erythrocytes that lack the decay accelerating factor in their membrane.

Role of Antibody in Activation of the Alternative Pathway

It was recognized early that the alternative complement pathway can be activated in the absence of specific antibody. This occurs on the surface of certain cells and particles that provide a microenvironment in which the affinity of the regulatory protein H for surface-bound C3b is low. In addition, there is now abundant evidence that antibody can enhance activation.

The first demonstration that antibody led to the selective activation of complement by a mechanism that bypassed C1, C4, and C2 was reported by Sandberg et al.[33,34] These investigators worked with immune complexes and guinea pig complement. In addition, antibody has been found to play a role in augmenting the capacity of certain cells and particles to activate the alternative complement pathway, and the mechanism of augmentation may differ from that of insoluble immune complexes.

Winkelstein et al.[35] demonstrated this function of antibody by finding that C3 consumption in C4-deficient guinea pig serum by pneumococci that had been preincubated with guinea pig IgG was greater than that by unsensitized pneumococci. Furthermore, the augmenting capacity resided in the F(ab')$_2$ fragment, thereby excluding participation of C1q. The ability of antibody to enhance the endogenous capacity of a particle to activate the alternative pathway has implications not only for defense of the host against bacteria but also for defense against viral infection.

Also, in addition to augmenting the activating capacity of certain cells, antibody has been shown to confer the ability to activate on streptococci and sheep erythrocytes, which do not normally induce alternative pathway activation.

Finally, an autoantibody that activates the alternative pathway was discovered in the serum of some patients with membranoproliferative glomerulonephritis. This IgG autoantibody is called the C3 nephritic factor (C3NeF), and a similar factor has been found in the serum of patients with partial lipodystrophy, some of whom have hypocomplementemic glomerulonephritis. C3NeF is an autoantibody specific for the alternative pathway C3 convertase, and it creates a stable enzyme complex that escapes the regulatory mechanisms of the alternative pathway.[36]

Thus, different mechanisms of antibody-dependent alternative pathway activation are recognized from separate experimental conditions. The implication of these findings is that alternative pathway activation can use and regulate specific immunity under conditions that preclude activation of the classical pathway.

CHEMISTRY AND BIOLOGY OF COMPLEMENT RECEPTORS

Activation of the complement system gives rise to a number of molecular species that can interact with host-derived cells and regulate their function. This interaction is mediated through distinct cell surface CRs, and receptor engagement produces biologic responses that can either modulate host defense reactions or enhance inflammation (Table 3-2). By their interaction, with CR, small peptide fragments of

Table 3-2. Characteristics of Complement Receptors

Protein	Specificity	Size (kD)	Expression
CR1	C4b, C3b, iC3b	160–250	Erythrocytes, neutrophils, monocytes, glomerular podocytes, eosinophils, B and some T lymphocytes, follicular dendritic cells, macrophages
CR2	C3d, C3dg, iC3b, gp350	140	B lymphocytes, some B- and T-cell lines, follicular dendritic cells, some epithelial cells, thymocytes
CR3	iC3b, C3d	165 (α), 95 (β)	Monocytes, macrophages, neutrophils, natural killer cells, some cytotoxic T cells, follicular dendritic cells
CR4	iC3b, C3dg(?)	150 (α), 95 (β)	Neutrophils, monocytes, macrophages, natural killer cells, some cytotoxic T cells
DAF	C3b,Bb C4b, C2a	70	Leukocytes, erythrocytes, platelets, lymphocytes, epithelial cells
MCP	C3b, C4b, iC3b	45–70	Neutrophils, monocytes, platelets, reticulocytes, lymphocytes
C3a receptor	C3a, C4a	Unknown	Mast cells, neutrophils, monocytes, basophils, eosinophils, T lymphocytes
C3e receptor	C3e, C3dk	Unknown	Neutrophils, monocytes
Factor H receptor	Factor H	150	B lymphocytes, monocytes
Factor B receptor	Bb, Ba	Unknown	B lymphocytes
C5a receptor	C5a, C5a-des-arg	48	Mast cells, granulocytes, macrophages, neutrophils, monocytes
C1q receptor	C1q	70 (polymer)	Monocytes, neutrophils, macrophages, platelets, fibroblasts, lymphocytes

(Modified from Gaither and Frank,[37] with permission.)

complement components that are generated during complement activation may act as potent inflammatory mediators, and complement fragments that remain associated with activating particles may function as opsonins that aid in phagocytosis of the particles or as regulators of other aspects of the immune response.

Also, CR play a critical role in the regulation of the complement cascade at the cell surface. For example, the receptor for C3b/C4b, CR1, also acts as a cofactor to facilitate cleavage of bound C3b by the serum enzyme factor I. This cleavage results in the loss of hemolytic functional activity and the formation of an altered C3b molecule, referred to as C3bi. Furthermore, in the presence of CR1, factor I can proceed to degrade C3bi into a small membrane-bound fragment, C3dg, and a larger fragment, C3c, which is released from the membrane surface.

COMPLEMENT IN THE IMMUNE CLEARANCE OF BLOOD CELLS

As knowledge has accumulated concerning the proteins of the complement system and the specific receptors for complement proteins present on cell surfaces of erythrocytes and phagocytes, a more detailed understanding of immune cytolysis has developed. Thus, complement components or their fragments may serve as ligands between target cells and receptor cells. Receptor proteins on receptor-bearing cells express biologic activity toward complement fragments on target cells (e.g., erythrocytes), and these reactions determine the outcome of the interaction between the receptor-bearing and target cells. Such an interaction may be followed by phagocytosis or, in contrast, by rejection of the ligand by the receptor protein, which results in release of the adherent target cell from the phagocyte.

Deposition of Complement Proteins on Blood Cell Surfaces

Deposition of complement on blood cells usually occurs as a consequence of binding of specific antibody to the cell membrane, although it may apparently occur in the absence of antibody in a few clinical conditions. The potential for activation of the classic complement pathway is not a property unique to immunoglobulins because other proteins, carbohydrates, lipids, polyanions, and microbial material may bind and activate C1. However, IgG and IgM antibody-dependent complement activation is the prominent mechanism for complement deposition on blood cells in human disease. Although activation of the alternative pathway can proceed independently of the presence of immunoglobulins, specific antibody may enhance activation of this pathway. Deposition of complement on target cells enhances removal of IgG-sensitized cells through the reticulo-endothelial system and is absolutely required for clearance of IgM-sensitized target cells.[38]

Erythrocytes

Experimental and human studies have emphasized complement requirements together with the role of antibody class (i.e., IgG or IgM) and the number of antibody molecules bound per cell in the clearance of opsonized blood cells.[38] Thus, decreased survival of human erythrocytes coated with sufficient IgM antibody was found to be entirely dependent on complement; no acceleration of clearance of IgM-coated erythrocytes was seen in hypocomplementemic patients. Rapid sequestration of the cells occurred in the liver, whereas splenic clearance was inefficient, even for highly sensitized cells. Hepatic sequestration affected IgM- and C3b-coated cells in that a few of the cleared cells were phagocytized, whereas most cells returned to the circulation no longer bearing C3b but, instead, complement fragments recognized with anti-C3d antibody. Recirculating cells exhibited normal or greater than normal survival, which was attributed to a decreased capacity of the IgM-C3d (C3dg)-coated cells to bind additional C3b molecules.

In contrast to IgM-sensitized cells, increased clearance of IgG-coated erythrocytes occurs through splenic sequestration and is observed even in complement-deficient animals. Complement markedly enhances clearance of IgG-bearing cells through activation of the classic pathway without altering the exponential pattern of survival curves. Very few complement-fixing sites per cell are sufficient to accelerate clearance of IgG-sensitized autologous cells in guinea pigs. Splenic sequestration results in phagocytosis of IgG-coated target cells through interaction of the cells with Fc receptors of fixed phagocytes and probably through the enhancing effect of C3b receptor stimulation on IgG-dependent phagocytosis.

Whereas IgG-coated erythrocytes are cleared predominantly by the spleen, IgM-coated erythrocytes are mainly cleared through the liver with an absolute requirement for the complement system. Antierythrocyte antibodies express a variable capacity to activate complement on erythrocyte membranes through the classic or alternative pathways, depending on class, subclass, affinity for the antigen, and number of immunoglobulin molecules bound per erythrocyte.[38,39]

As mentioned previously, the role of complement in immunologically mediated clearance of blood cells is mainly to facilitate extravascular sequestration and interaction of complement-coated target cells with immunoglobulin and complement-receptor-bearing cells of the reticuloendothelial system. Complement activation at the surface of erythrocytes may, however, result in intravascular lysis (e.g., in alloimmune hemolytic anemias after certain incompatible blood transfusions, acute hemolytic episodes in cold agglutinin syndrome, some autoimmune hemolytic anemias, some drug-induced hemolytic anemias, and paroxysmal nocturnal hemoglobinuria).

Neutrophils

The sensitization of granulocytes by complement components may directly damage or transiently remove neutrophils from the circulating blood by causing their margination. C5a, C3b, Bb, and C5b,6,7 are chemotactic for neutrophils. The interaction between C5a and specific high-affinity receptors on neutrophils may explain the severe granulocytopenia that develops in patients during hemodialysis, nylon-fiber leukapheresis, and cardiopulmonary bypass procedures.

Complement activation is related to neutropenia and reversible intrapulmonary sequestration of neutrophils. Neutropenia can readily be induced by infusion of autologous plasma in which the alternative pathway has been activated by dialyzer cellophane membranes or by infusion of chemotactic factors. Also, binding of C5a to peripheral blood neutrophils induces increased adherence of granulocytes, lyso-somal enzyme release, and damage to endothelial cells.

Platelets

Immunologic alteration of human platelets with shortened platelet survival can result from the interaction of platelets with immune complexes, certain drug-induced antibodies, or antiplatelet antibodies. However, the role of complement in drug-induced thrombocytopenias and immune complex-mediated platelet clearance has not yet been fully investigated. A number of antibodies involved in drug-induced thrombocytopenias activate the complement system, resulting in assembly of the C5b-9 complex on the platelet membrane and in platelet lysis; elevated values for platelet-associated IgG and C3 have also been found in patients with drug-induced thrombocytopenia or systemic lupus erythematosus. The interaction of drug-induced immune complexes with the platelet membrane had been thought to be a result of the interaction of the IgG-Fc part of the complex with the platelet Fc receptor. However, more recent reports indicate that drug-antibody binding to platelets is mediated by the Fab domain and is not Fc dependent.[40,41]

Acquired alloantibodies secondary to transfusion or to contact with fetal platelets during pregnancy are responsible for rapid destruction of infused platelets, post-transfusion purpura, and alloimmune neonatal thrombocytopenia. Post-transfusion purpura and alloimmune neonatal thrombocytopenia usually occur as a result of immunization to the Pl^{A1} antigen as a result of transfusion or pregnancy.

Idiopathic thrombocytopenic purpura (ITP) is an immune-mediated disease that presents with abnormally high amounts of platelet-associated IgG. The role of complement in ITP is as yet ill defined. There is general agreement that free serum platelet autoantibodies have no complement-fixing properties, with only a few exceptions. It is, however, conceivable that minute quantities of complement are activated in vivo by platelet autoantibodies and bound to the platelet membrane. Indeed, there have been reports describing increased amounts of platelet-associated C3 in patients with ITP. On the other hand, platelet-associated C3 can also be elevated in presumed nonimmune thrombocytopenia.

COMPLEMENT SENSITIZATION IN DETECTING IMMUNE HEMOLYTIC ANEMIAS AND ALLOANTIBODIES

Evaluating the red cells of patients with acquired hemolytic anemias for the presence or absence of complement components by the direct antiglobulin test is valuable in developing a precise diagnosis.[42] In patients with the warm antibody type of autoimmune hemolytic anemia, the direct antiglobulin test reveals IgG and C3d in about 62 percent of patients, IgG only in 20 percent, and C3d only in 13 percent. The red cells of patients with cold agglutinin syndrome are sensitized with C3d but not with IgG. Patients with drug-induced immune hemolytic anemia caused by penicillin and methyldopa typically have red cells strongly sensitized by IgG but without fixation of complement. Other drug-induced immune hemolytic anemias are usually characterized by weak to moderate sensitization of red cells by complement components without detectable immune globulins. However, some such patients do have IgG on their red cells, more often in association with complement. Table 3-3 summarizes the characteristic antiglobulin test results in various hemolytic anemias.

A point that must be emphasized is that about 26 percent of patients with immune hemolytic anemias appear to have a negative direct antiglobulin test result unless the antiglobulin serum used contains antibodies against complement components (Table 3-4).

Although the results of the direct antiglobulin test provide valuable information if performed as described above,[43] they must be interpreted in conjunction with clinical and other laboratory data to avoid erroneous conclusions.[42,44,45] A positive direct antiglobulin test result occurs in situations other than immune hemolytic anemias. A positive direct antiglobulin test finding does not necessarily indicate the presence of autoantibody; furthermore, even if autoantibody is present, the patient may or may not have a hemolytic anemia. Thus, an independent clinical assessment must be made to determine the presence or absence of hemolytic anemia; the role of the direct antiglobulin test is to aid in the evaluation of the cause of hemolysis when present.

Table 3-3. Direct Antiglobulin Test Results in Immune Hemolytic Anemias Using Anti-IgG and Anti-C3 Antisera

	IgG	C3[a]
Warm antibody AIHA		
(67%)	+	+
(20%)	+	0
(13%)	0	+
Cold agglutinin syndrome	0	+
Paroxysmal cold hemoglobinuria	0	+
Penicillin or methyldopa induced[b]	+	0
Other drug-induced immune hemolytic anemias[c]	0	+
Warm antibody AIHA associated with systemic lupus erythematosus	+	+

Abbreviation: AIHA, autoimmune hemolytic anemia.

[a] Such cells are primarily sensitized with the C3d component of C3 (see text).

[b] Weakly positive reactions with anti-C3 may occur; invariably, reactions are strongly positive and anti-IgG.

[c] The most common pattern of red cell sensitization is indicated, but occasionally IgG may be detected with or without C3.

(From Petz and Garratty,[42] with permission.)

PATHOPHYSIOLOGY OF IMMUNE HEMOLYSIS

Lysis in vivo of red cells injured by immune mechanisms can result directly from the effects of complement on the red cell membrane or from the interaction of cells of the reticuloendothelial system with red cells sensitized with antibody and/or complement.[42] The former is often referred to as "intravas-

Table 3-4. Results of Direct Antiglobulin Test With Anti-IgG and Anti-C3 in 347 Patients With Autoimmune Hemolytic Anemia and Drug-Induced Immune Hemolytic Anemias

	Percent[a]	
IgG (no C3)	23	73% have IgG on RBC
IgG + C3	50	
C3 (no IgG)	26.4	76.4% have C3 on RBC

Abbreviation: RBC, red blood cells.

[a] Two patients (0.5%) had only IgA present on their red blood cells.

(From Petz and Garratty,[42] with permission.)

cular" hemolysis and the latter, as "extravascular" hemolysis. Clinical indications of intravascular hemolysis include increased plasma hemoglobin, methemalbuminemia, hemoglobinuria, and hemosiderinuria; even with only minimal intravascular hemolysis, the serum haptoglobin level is low or absent.[42,46,47] Prototype disorders that are primarily associated with intravascular hemolysis are ABO hemolytic transfusion reactions, mechanical hemolytic anemia, paroxysmal nocturnal hemoglobinuria, and paroxysmal cold hemoglobinuria. Extravascular hemolysis results in an increase in serum bilirubin concentration and in bilirubin degradation products in the urine and stool without causing evidence of release of free hemoglobin into the blood. Hemolysis in hereditary spherocytosis, or that induced by Rh antibodies or warm autoantibodies, is characteristically extravascular in nature.

It is useful to discuss intravascular and extravascular hemolysis separately, even though a sharp distinction between the two is not always justified, either on clinical grounds or in regard to the pathophysiologic process involved.[48] Indeed, with brisk hemolysis of any cause, some manifestations of intravascular hemolysis may be present. Also, complement may participate in red cell lysis by both mechanisms. Finally, it should be pointed out that, in many instances of immune hemolysis, the process of red cell destruction is multimodal, and it is currently impossible to separate and quantify the several processes going on simultaneously.

Intravascular Immune Red Cell Destruction

This type of immune red cell destruction is complement mediated. Not many alloantibodies are able to destroy red cells intravascularly; among the alloantibodies that do destroy red cells through this mechanism, anti-A and -B are the best examples; anti-Kidd, -Vel, -Tj^a and -Jk^a sometimes can also activate the complement cascade. Thus, on rare occasions, they can cause the intravascular lysis of donor red cells. Intravascular hemolysis is also uncommon in autoimmune hemolytic anemia. When it occurs, it is usually associated with paroxysmal cold hemoglobinuria, and, less commonly, with cold agglutinin syndrome and with cases of drug-induced hemolytic anemia caused by immune-complex formation. Intravascular hemolysis is less common in warm anti-

body autoimmune hemolytic anemia but does occur particularly in the hyperacute form of the disease.

Complement-mediated immune hemolysis occurs by way of the classic pathway of complement activation, which has been described in the preceding section. Theoretically, any of the many substances that can activate the alternative pathway could cause intravascular hemolysis, but there is at present no evidence to suggest that antibody-mediated red cell lysis occurs as a result of this pathway of complement activation. Indeed, studies by May et al.[49] on antibody-mediated cytolysis of erythrocytes and nucleated cells have indicated that the alternative pathway mediates cell lysis inefficiently or not at all.

Extravascular Immune Red Cell Destruction

The second major mode of in vivo erythrocyte destruction is mediated by a mechanism of temporary or permanent sequestration of erythrocytes within portions of the reticuloendothelial system, primarily in the liver and spleen. If red cells become sensitized with IgG or cells are sensitized with complement but do not proceed through the entire cascade to lysis, they may then be destroyed or damaged within the reticuloendothelial system.[50,51]

It is believed that red cells sensitized with antibody and/or complement are destroyed within the reticuloendothelial system by interaction with mononuclear phagocytes. The most important phagocyte that participates in immune red cell destruction is the macrophage, which arises primarily from bone marrow precursors, probably the promonocyte. After a short period of maturation in the bone marrow, monocytes are released into the blood. After spending a few days in the peripheral circulation, they migrate to the tissues, and there they mature functionally and morphologically to become typical histiocytic or exudative macrophages.[52] They are particularly prominent in the liver (Kupffer cells), lung (alveolar macrophages), spleen, and bone marrow. The survival time of mature tissue macrophages is thought to be several weeks or even months.[53]

Macrophage Receptors

Macrophages have receptors on their membranes that specifically recognize certain classes of immunoglobulins (either free or as part of an immune complex) and certain complement components.[50,51,54] One type of receptor can interact with the Fc portion of the IgG molecule, specifically with a portion of the molecule in the domain nearest to the carboxyl terminus of the heavy chain.[55] This site appears to be found on human IgG molecules of only the IgG1 and IgG3 subgroups.[56] It is not present on the IgM molecule.[57] Such receptor sites on the macrophages are relatively insensitive to digestion by proteolytic enzymes[58] and appear to be present on granulocytes and monocytes. Qualitatively similar sites are also demonstrable on certain lymphocytes.[59] Quantitative studies have indicated that there are approximately 1×10^6 IgG receptors on the membrane of each macrophage.[60] The number of receptor sites seems to increase during macrophage activation,[61] a finding that may have important clinical implications.

In addition, there appear to be receptors for a biologically active fragment of C3, C3b.[58,62] When C3b is enzymatically degraded by C3b inactivator, interaction with this receptor no longer occurs.[63] Other investigators have described receptors for C3c,[64] C4,[65,66] and C3d.[67,68]

MECHANISMS OF EXTRAVASCULAR IMMUNE HEMOLYSIS AND RED CELL FRAGMENTATION

Red cells sensitized by antibody and/or complement may fragment in vivo in several ways.[69] If two red cells approach each other closely enough to result in contact of their membranes, a small area of membrane fusion may result. When mechanical forces such as those found in the circulation force the cells apart, a long membrane thread may be drawn out and break off to form a small membrane fragment. This fragment was termed a myelin form by Ponder,[70] who first observed the phenomenon.[71] The process is enhanced by antibody and probably by complement components bound to the red cell membrane; it is easily observed in patients with autoimmune hemolytic anemia who are actively hemolyzing and who have spherocytes in their peripheral blood. Microspherocyte formation results from this loss of membrane material without loss of cell contents, thereby leading to a decrease in the ratio of surface area to volume. This causes the membrane

of the spherocytic cell to be rigid and results in its being unable to change its shape readily to traverse the fine channels of the spleen; the membrane is thus susceptible to early destruction by trapping.[72,74]

A second type of red cell fragmentation which may be induced by sensitization with antibody has been termed phagocytic fragmentation.[71] The attachment of appropriately sensitized red cells to macrophages can be visualized in vitro by so-called rosette formation; the macrophage becomes ringed by sensitized red cells, like petals on a flower (Fig. 3-7).[42] On attachment to the macrophage, the red cells usually undergo considerable distortion and deformity in the region of attachments.[75] Sensitized red cells may become completely engulfed by the macrophage and destroyed internally (Fig. 3-8).[76] However, in some instances, a red cell is only partially engulfed by a phagocytic cell (Figs. 3-9 and 3-10); it is then fragmented into two relatively large pieces, with the unengulfed fragment escaping into the circulation, possibly as a result of simple mechanical forces. This process results in small, variably shaped poikilocytic and spherocytic red cell fragments (Fig. 3-11),[77] which are presumably rapidly removed by subsequent phagocytosis or filtration in the spleen. Red cell-phagocyte interaction may also result in loss of small membrane fragments if the red cells are swept away by circulatory forces after they are attached but before phagocytic engulfment.

Although extravascular red cell destruction typically leads to the appearance in the plasma and urine of breakdown products of hemoglobin, such as bilirubin and urobilinogen, laboratory tests may show some results that are associated with intravascular lysis. For instance, hemoglobinemia and hemoglobinuria may occur after Rh-incompatible transfusions. The Rh antibodies in these cases have not been shown to fix complement, and it therefore seems likely that hemoglobin may be released into the blood after fragmentation of the red cells during macrophage-mediated cell damage, particularly when large amounts of blood are rapidly destroyed. Data also indicate that macrophages (and possibly lymphocytes) may destroy sensitized red cells by extracellular cytotoxicity[50,78] in addition to phagocytosis; this phenomenon may be an alternative explanation for hemoglobinemia and hemoglobinuria associated with extravascular lysis.

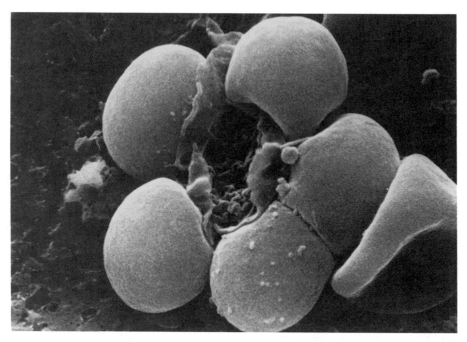

Fig. 3-7. Scanning electron micrograph illustrating the interaction of antibody-coated red cells and a phagocytic white cell. The white cell is surrounded by sensitized red cells, forming a rosette. (From Petz and Garratty,[42] with permission.)

Macrophage/Monocyte Cytotoxicity

Since the elucidation of macrophages as the major effector cell in immune red cell destruction, emphasis has been placed on the phagocytic properties of this cell. Recent studies suggest that an extracellular mechanism is operative, and perhaps the cytotoxic properties of the macrophage may be more important than first thought. Holm and Hammarstrom[79] showed that purified human monocytes were able to lyse red cells treated with hyperimmune anti-A. In fact, one monocyte was able to lyse two or three red cells within an 18-hour incubation period. Complement was not necessary for this reaction.

Kurlander et al.[80] demonstrated monocyte-mediated lysis in vitro of human red cells sensitized with IgG anti-Rh$_o$(D) and anti-A or -B. Cells sensitized only with human complement components (even up to 80,000 molecules per red cell) were not lysed, but C3b or C3d sensitization augmented IgG-mediated lysis and reduced the amount of IgG necessary to produce lysis.

Fleer et al.[81–83] suggested that cytotoxicity may play a more important role than phagocytosis in immune red cell destruction. Using ^{51}Cr-labeled human red cells sensitized with anti-D, they were able to demonstrate cytotoxicity by monocytes, independent of phagocytosis. Unlike other workers,[84–87] Fleer et al.[81–83] were not able to demonstrate lysis of Rh-sensitized cells by lymphocytes. Another important effect noted by Fleer et al.[88] was the development of an increased osmotic fragility of a considerable part of the nonlysed Rh-sensitized red cells. In fact, they found that the osmotically more fragile cells considerably outnumbered lysed and ingested red cells. A correlation with increased osmotic fragility and severity of autoimmune hemolytic anemia has been described previously.[89] The presence of spherocytes, for years, has been said to be a hallmark of autoimmune hemolytic anemia; the spherocytes are now thought to be formed through fragmentation of the sensitized red cells by macrophages. It has also been assumed that the increased osmotic fragility is due to the presence of spherocytes, but it may well be that the damage to the red cell membrane caused by cytotoxicity without fragmentation may also contribute to the increased fragility.

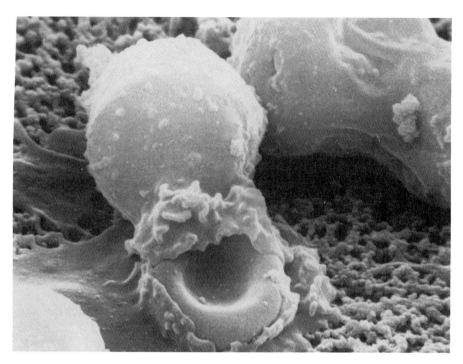

Fig. 3-8. Scanning electron micrograph illustrating the reaction of a phagocytic white cell with an antibody–coated red cell. Only a small exposed area remains of a nearly ingested red cell. (From Rosse and de Boisfleury,[76] with permission.)

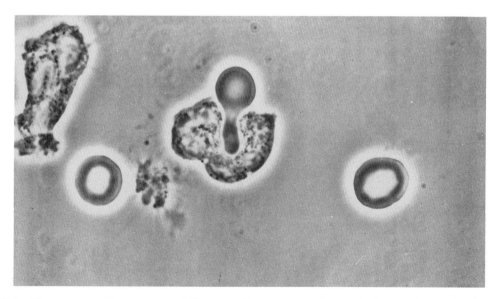

Fig. 3-9. Phase-contrast photomicrograph illustrating the interaction of an antibody-coated red cell and a phagocytic white cell. The red cell, having been taken by the metapod, is deformed as the metapod flows along its sides. (From Rosse et al.,[57] with permission.)

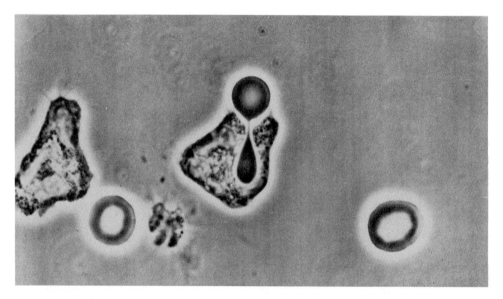

Fig. 3-10. Further interaction between the phagocytic white cell and the antibody-coated red cell results in internalization of a portion of red cell. (From Rosse et al.,[57] with permission.)

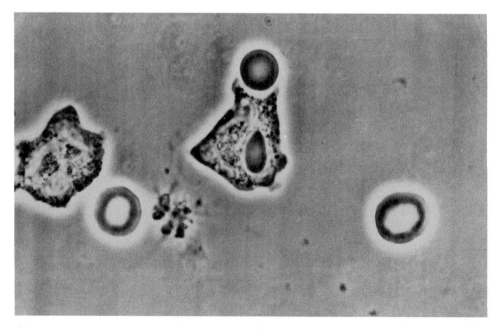

Fig. 3-11. The separation of the internal and external portions of the red cell is complete; the portion of the red cell outside the macrophage may escape and circulate as a spherocyte. (From Rosse et al.,[57] with permission.)

REFEREN

1. Rod
zat¹
an
B¹

2. (
°

3.

/

...ow JC, Finn R, Krevans JR: Rapid clearance of
...ositive blood during experimental Rh immuniza-
...Vox Sang 17:349, 1969

...Vit, CD and Borst-Eilers E: Lack of relationship
...ween the response to the D-antigen and to some
...er antigens. Vox Sang 16:222, 1969

...cher GT, Cooke BR, Mitchell K, Parry P: Hyperim-
...unisation des donneurs de sang pour la production
...es gammaglobulines anti-Rh(D). Rev Fr Transfusion
12:341, 1969

Petz LD: The role of complement in the immune response. In Tregellas WM, Keating LJ (eds): Immunology. p. 53. American Association of Blood Banks, Arlington, 1985

22. Frank MM: Current concepts: complement in the
pathophysiology of human disease. N Engl J Med 316:
1525, 1987

23. Morgan BP: Complement: Clinical Aspects and Relevance to Disease. Academic Press, New York, 1990

24. Augener W, Grey HM, Cooper NR, Muller-Eberhard
HJ: The reaction of monomeric and aggregated immunoglobulins with C1. Immunochemistry 8:1011,
1971

25. Schumaker VN, Calcott MA, Speigelberg HL, Muller-
Eberhard HJ: Ultracentrifuge studies of the binding
of IgG of different subclasses to the C1q subunit of
the first component of complement. Biochemistry 15:
5175, 1976

26. Metzger H: The effect of antigen on antibodies: recent
studies. Contemp Top Mol Immunol 7:119, 1978

27. Borsos T, Chapuis RM, Langone JJ: Distinction between fixation of C1 and the activation of complement
by natural IgM antihapten antibody: effect of cell surface hapten density. Mol Immunol 18:863, 1981

28. Hughes-Jones NC, Ghosh S: Anti-D coated Rh-positive
red cells will bind the first component of the complement pathway, C1q. FEBS Lett 128:318, 1981

29. Schrieber RD: The chemistry and biology of complement receptors. Springer Semin Immunopathol 7:
221, 1984

30. Lachmann PJ, Pangburn MK, Oldroyd RG: Breakdown of C3 after complement activation: identification
of a new fragment, C3g, using monoclonal antibodies.
J Exp Med 156:205, 1982

31. Lachmann PJ, Voak D, Oldroyd RG et al: Use of monoclonal anti-C3 antibodies to characterize the fragments
of C3 that are found on erythrocytes. Vox Sang 45:
367, 1983

32. Pangburn M, Muller-Eberhard HJ: The alternative
pathway of complement. Springer Semin Immunopathol 7:163, 1984

33. Sandberg AL, Osler AG, Shin HS, Oliveira B: The bio-

testing
De Macario EC, ...
Laboratory Immunology. A...
biology, Washington, DC, 1992

9. Silberstein LE: The antibody response to antigen. p.
25. In Nance SJ (ed): Alloimmunity: 1993 and Beyond.
American Association of Blood Banks, Bethesda, 1993

10. Bjorkman PJ, Saper MA, Samraoui B et al: Structure
of the human class I histocompatibility antigen, HLA-
A2. Nature 329:506, 1987

11. Nossal GJV: Current concepts: immunology. The basic
components of the immune system. N Engl J Med 316:
1320, 1987

12. Nossal GJV: Immunoregulation: the key to transplantation and autoimmunity. J Thorac Cardiovasc Surg
94:802, 1987

13. Nossal GJV: Cellular mechanisms of immunologic tolerance. Annu Rev Immunol 1:33, 1983

14. Mollison PL, Engelfriet CP, Contreras M: Blood
Transfusion in Clinical Medicine. Blackwell Scientific
Publications, Oxford, 1993

15. Polley MJ, Mollison PL, Soothill JF: The role of 19s
gammaglobulin blood group antibodies in the antiglobulin reaction. Br J Haematol 8:149, 1962

16. Giblett ER: A critique of the theoretical hazard of in-
ter- vs. intra-racial transfusion. Transfusion 1:233,
1961

17. Krevans JR, Woodrow JC, Nosenzo C, Finn R: Patterns
of Rh-immunization. 10th Congress of the International Society of Haematology, Stockholm, 1964

logic activities of guinea pig antibodies. II. Modes of complement interaction with gamma-1 and gamma-2 immunoglobulins. J Immunol 104:329, 1970

34. Sandberg AL, Oliveira B, Osler AG: Two complement interaction sites in guinea pig immunoglobulins. J Immunol 106:282, 1971

35. Winkelstein JA, Shin HS, Wood WB, Jr: Heat-labile opsonins to pneumococcus. III. The participation of immunoglobulin and of the alternative pathway of C3 activation. J Immunol 108:1681, 1972

36. Daha MR, Austen KF, Fearon DT: The incorporation of C3 nephritic factor (C3NeF) into a stabilized C3 convertase, C3b, Bb (C3Nef), and its release after decay of convertase function. J Immunol 119:812, 1977

37. Gaither TA, Frank MM: Complement receptors. p. 142. In Rose NR, De Macario EC, Fahey JL et al (eds): Manual of Clinical Laboratory Immunology. American Society for Microbiology, Washington, DC, 1992

38. Frank MM (moderator): NIH Conference: Pathophysiology of Immune Hemolytic Anemia. Ann Intern Med 87:210, 1977

39. Frank MM, Dourmashkin RR, Humphrey JJ: Observations on the mechanism of immune hemolysis: importance of immunoglobulin class and source of complement on the extent of damage. J Immunol 104:1502, 1970

40. Smith ME, Jordan JV, Jr, Reid DM et al: Drug antibody binding to platelets is mediated by the Fab domain and is not Fc-dependent. Blood, suppl. 64:91a, 1984

41. Christie DJ, Mullen PC, Aster RH: Fab-mediated binding of quinidine- and quinine-induced antibodies to platelets in drug-induced, immunologic thrombocytopenia. Blood, suppl. 1, 64:236a, 1984

42. Petz LD, Garratty G: Acquired Immune Hemolytic Anemias. Churchill Livingstone, New York, 1980

43. Engelfriet CP, Overbeeke MAM, Voak D: The antiglobulin test (Coombs test) and the red cell. p. 74. In Cash JD (ed): Progress in Transfusion Medicine. Vol. 2. Churchill Livingstone, Edinburgh, 1987

44. Petz LD, Branch DR: Serological tests for the diagnosis of immune hemolytic anemias. p. 9. In McMillan R (ed): Methods in Haematology: Immune Cytopenias. Churchill Livingstone, New York, 1983

45. Garratty G: The significance of IgG on the red cell surface. Transfusion Med Rev 1:47, 1987

46. Anderson MN, Gabrieli E, Zizzi JA: Chronic hemolysis in patients with ball-valve prosthesis. J Thorac Cardiovasc Surg 50:501, 1965

47. Brus I, Lewis SM: The haptoglobin content of serum in haemolytic anaemia. Br J Haematol 5:348, 1959

48. Petz LD: The diagnosis of hemolytic anemia. p. 1. In Bell CA (ed): A Seminar on Laboratory Management of Hemolysis. American Association of Blood Banks, Washington, DC, 1979

49. May JE, Green I, Frank MM: The alternate complement pathway in cell damage: antibody-mediated cytolysis of erythrocytes and nucleated cells. J Immunol 109:595, 1972

50. Engelfriet CP, Kr von dem Borne AEG, Beckers DO et al: Immune destruction of red cells. p. 93. In Bell CA (ed): A Seminar of Immune-Mediated Cell Destruction. American Association of Blood Banks, Arlington, 1981

51. Garratty G: Mechanisms of immune red cell destruction, and red cell compatibility testing. Hum Pathol 14:204, 1983

52. van Furth R, Cohn ZA, Hirsch JG et al: The mononuclear phagocyte system: a new classification of macrophages, monocytes and their precursor cells. Bull WHO 46:845, 1972

53. van Furth R: Origin and kinetics of monocytes and macrophages. Semin Hematol 7:125, 1970

54. Huber H, Fudenberg HH: Receptor sites of human monocytes for IgG. Int Arch Allergy Appl Immunol 34:18, 1968

55. Yasmeen E, Ellerson JR, Dorrington KJ, Painter RH: Location of the site of cytophilic activity toward guinea pig macrophages in the CH3 homology region of human immunoglobulin. J Immunol 110:1706, 1973

56. Huber H, Douglas SD, Nusbacher J et al: IgG subclass specificity of human monocyte receptor sites. Nature 229:419, 1970

57. Rosse WF, de Boisfleury A, Bessis M: The interaction of phagocytic cells and red cells modified by immune reactions. Comparison of antibody- and complement-coated red cells. Blood Cells 1:345, 1975

58. Lay WH, Nussenzweig V: Receptors for complement on leukocytes. J Exp Med 128:991, 1968

59. Dickler HB: Studies of the human lymphocyte receptor for heat-aggregated or antigen-complexed immunoglobulin. J Exp Med 140:508, 1974

60. Arend WP, Mannik M: Quantitative studies on IgG receptors on monocytes. In van Furth R (ed): Mononuclear Phagocytes in Immunity, Infection, and Pathology. Blackwell Scientific Publications, Oxford, 1975

61. Arend WP, Mannik M: The macrophage receptor for IgG: number and affinity of binding sites. J Immunol 110:1455, 1973

62. Huber H, Polley M, Linscott W et al: Human monocytes: distinct receptor sites for the third component of complement and for immunoglobulin. Science 162:1281, 1968

63. Logue GL, Rosse WF, Adams JP: Complement-depen-

dent immune adherence measured with human granulocytes: changes in the antigenic nature of red cell bound C3 produced by incubation in human serum. Clin Immunol Immunopathol 1:398, 1973

64. Polley MJ, Ross GD: Macrophage and lymphocyte receptor sites for complement (C3) and for immunoglobulin (IgG). Proceedings of an international symposium on The Nature of and Significances of Complement Activation. Ortho Diagnostics, Raritan, 1976

65. Iida K, Nussenzweig V: Functional properties of membrane-associated complement receptor CR1. J Immunol 130:1876, 1983

66. Ross GD, Polley MJ: Specificity of human lymphocyte complement receptors. J Exp Med 141:1163, 1975

67. Munn IR, Chaplin H, Jr: Rosette formation by sensitized human red cells—effects of source of peripheral leukocyte monolayers. Vox Sang 33:129, 1977

68. Atkinson JP, Frank MM: Role of complement in the pathophysiology of hemotologic diseases. Prog Hematol 10:211, 1977

69. Weed RI, Reed CF: Membrane alterations leading to red cell destruction. Am J Med 41:681, 1966

70. Ponder E: Hemolysis and Related Phenomena. Grune & Stratton, Orlando, 1971

71. Bessis M: Living Blood Cells and their Ultrastructure. Springer-Verlag, New York, 1973

72. Cooper RA: Loss of membrane components in the pathogenesis of antibody-induced spherocytosis. J Clin Invest 51:16, 1972

73. Mohandas N, de Boisfleury A: Antibody-induced spherocytic anemia. I. Changes in red cell deformity. Blood Cells 3:187, 1977

74. Weed RI: The importance of erythrocyte deformability. Am J Med 49:147, 1970

75. Lo Buglio AF, Cotran R, Jandl JH: Red cells coated with immunoglobulin G: binding and sphering by mononuclear cells in man. Science 158:1582, 1967

76. Rosse WF, deBoisfleury A: The interaction of phagocyctic cells and red cells following alteration of their form or deformability. Blood Cells 1:359, 1975

77. Brown DL, Nelson DA: Surface microfragmentation of red cells as a mechanism for complement-mediated immune spherocytosis. Br J Haematol 24:301, 1973

78. Urbaniak SJ: ADCC (K-cell) lysis of human erythrocytes sensitized with rhesus alloantibodies I. Investigation of in vivo culture variables. Br J Haematol 42:303, 1979

79. Holm G, Hammarstrom S: Haemolytic activity of human blood monocytes: lysis of human erythrocytes treated with anti-A serum. Clin Exp Immunol 13:29, 1973

80. Kurlander RJ, Rosse WF, Logue WL: Quantitative influence of antibody and complement coating of red cells on monocyte-mediated cell lysis. J Clin Invest 61:1309, 1978

81. Fleer A, van der Hart M, Kr von dem Borne AEG, Engelfriet CP: Mechanisms of antibody-dependent cytotoxicity by human blood monocytes towards IgG-sensitized erythrocytes. Euro J Clin Invest 6:333, 1976 (abstract)

82. Fleer A, van der Hart M, Kr von dem Borne AEG, Engelfriet CP: Monocyte-mediated lysis of human erythrocytes. p. 673. In Eijsvoogal VP, Roos D, Zeijlemaker WP (eds): Leucocyte Membrane Determinants Regulating Immune Reactivity. Academic Press, Orlando, 1976

83. Fleer A, Van Schaik MLJ, Kr von dem Borne AEG, Engelfriet CP: Destruction of sensitized erythrocytes by human monocytes in vitro. Effects of cytochalasin B, hydrocortisone and colchicine. Scand J Immunol 8:515, 1978

84. Handwerger BS, Kay NW, Douglas SD: Lymphocyte-mediated antibody-dependent cytolysis: role in immune hemolysis. Vox Sang 34:276, 1978

85. Hinz CF, Jr, Chickosky JF: Lymphocyte cytotoxicity for human erythrocytes. In Schwarz MR (ed): Leukocyte Culture Conference. University of Washington, Seattle, 1972

86. Northoff H, Kluge A, Resch K: Antibody-dependent cellular cytotoxicity (ADCC) against human erythrocytes, mediated by blood group alloantibodies: a model for the role of antigen density in target cell lysis. Z Immun Forsch 154:15, 1978

87. Urbaniak SJ: Lymphoid cell dependent (K-cell) lysis of human erythrocytes sensitized with rhesus alloantibodies. Br J Haematol 33:409, 1976

88. Fleer A, Koopman MG, Kr von dem Borne AEG, Engelfriet CP: Monocyte-induced increase in osmotic fragility of human red cells sensitized with anti-D alloantibodies. Br J Haematol 40:439, 1978

89. Kr von dem Borne AEG, Engelfriet CP, Beckers D, Van Loghem JJ: Autoimmune haemolytic anemias. Biochemical studies of red cells from patients with autoimmune haemolytic anemia with incomplete warm autoantibodies. Clin Exp Immunol 8:377, 1971

Immunomodulation Caused by Blood Transfusion

Harvey G. Klein

During the past decade, concerns about blood safety have focused on the highly publicized risks of transfusion-transmitted infection.[1,2] However, infusions of allogeneic cells and plasma proteins have many other potential drawbacks.[3] Transfusion has long been recognized as capable of eliciting immune responses from blood recipients. Acute immune-mediated hemolysis represents the most dramatic such response. Additional clinically important immune-mediated transfusion reactions range from urticaria and alloantibody formation to graft-versus-host disease to anaphylaxis (see Chs. 41 and 42). Laboratory and clinical evidence suggests that allogeneic transfusions may evoke other more subtle immunomodulatory effects, including immunosuppression and varying degrees of immune tolerance. If confirmed, these immune effects would have considerable consequences for the transfused patient.

Blood transfusions unquestionably cause a number of changes in the laboratory measurement of immune function. The reported findings in transfusion recipients include development of Fc receptor-blocking factors; lymphocyte activation, as measured by surface membrane antigens and functional studies; changes in lymphocyte subpopulations; and downregulation of antigen-presenting cells.[4] Reduced numbers of B lymphocytes and HLA-DR-positive cells and modified natural killer cell function may persist for years after the transfusion.[5] However,

the mechanisms for such changes, whether related to some aspect of the transfused component or to a special characteristic of the recipient, remain unclear. Neonates who receive washed and irradiated red blood cells, for example, do not exhibit many of the changes reported in adult transfusion recipients.[6] Furthermore, the clinical relevance of these findings remains uncertain.

Clinical evidence of the immunosuppressive effect of transfusion emerged from retrospective analyses of factors affecting renal cadaver allograft survival. Investigators noted the importance of graft match, organ quality, blood group, and previous organ transplant or pregnancy but further reported the unexpected and contradictory finding that blood transfusion before renal transplantation seemed to prolong allograft survival.[7] Furthermore, the transfusion effect appeared to be dose dependent (Fig. 4-1). These results confirmed previously reported observations in animals and were subsequently supported by similar findings for both living related renal grafts and for cardiac allografts.[8-11] More recent retrospective analyses indicate that the benefits of a "transfusion effect" for solid organ transplants is now difficult to discern because of the improved effectiveness of current potent immunosuppressive drug regimens. However, careful study of the HLA-DR status of donor and recipient indicate that transfusions matched for at least one DR

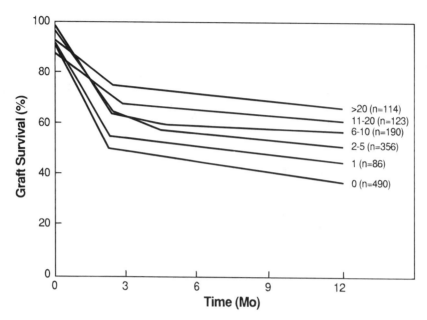

Fig. 4-1. Renal allograft survival in months as a function of prior allogeneic blood transfusion. Six groups have been defined based on the total number of transfusions, ranging from 0 to more than 20 units. Numbers in parentheses represent the number of patients in each group. (From Opelz and Terasaki,[8] with permission.)

antigen are still associated with improved survival of both cardiac and renal allografts.[11] Deliberate pre-transfusion protocols that use donor-specific transfusions are still in use in some centers. The immunologic complexities of tolerance and sensitization and their relationship to transfusion are still incompletely understood and do not explain the transfusion effect (see Chs. 6 and 35).

Several additional lines of evidence suggest that blood transfusions may have clinically important immunomodulatory effects. (Table 4-1). Among the po-

Table 4-1. Reported Clinical Outcomes From Immunomodulatory Effects of Blood Transfusion

Improved organ allograft survival[7–11]
Recurrence of malignancy[18–27]
Susceptibility to postoperative infection[25,31–36]
Prevention of recurrent abortion[13,47–49]
Suppression of inflammatory bowel disease[12,53–55]
Reactivation of latent viral infection[15,40,41,45,46]

tential benefits are the postulated amelioration of immune inflammatory illness such as Crohn's disease and the prevention of recurrent abortion.[12,13] Among the suspected adverse effects are the associations of transfusion with recurrence of malignancy, postoperative infections, and reactivation of latent viruses.[14,15] The latter effect may play a role in the reports of the rapid progression of acquired immunodeficiency syndrome (AIDS) in heavily transfused patients. Finally, one well recognized adverse effect of transfusion is graft-versus-host disease, a highly lethal disorder mediated by transfused immunocompetent lymphocytes that engraft and reject the transfused host (see Ch. 42).[16]

TRANSFUSION AND CANCER RECURRENCE

The role of blood transfusion in the recurrence rate and survival of patients with cancer has been disputed for more than a decade. Studies of various tumors in animal models yield conflicting results.[17] Some models suggest that transfusion stimulates tumor growth; others report suppression of growth.

Still others enumerate various modifications in the cellular immune responses of the animals tested. Because the tumors, the experimental animals, the transfusion component, and the experimental designs differ substantially, it is difficult to use these findings to construct a single unifying hypothesis and impossible to extrapolate these data to patients with cancer.

Studies concerning the role of transfusion in cancer recurrence and survival of patients undergoing cancer surgery are almost as contradictory and difficult to interpret as are the animal studies. Early retrospective reports of series of patients with colon cancer, matched for clinical stage, histologic characteristics, and various other factors such as tumor size, location, and adjuvant therapy, indicated that patients who received transfusions, and particularly those who were heavily transfused, fared less well in terms of recurrence, survival, and tumor-free survival than did the "control" group, generally patients from the same institution who received little or no transfusion (Fig. 4-2).[18–21] This observation has been confirmed in numerous subsequent retrospective studies, although other investigators did not detect a relationship between transfusion and clinical outcome.[22,23]

One large, multicenter, randomized, controlled study of surgery for patients with colorectal carcinoma found no relationship between allogeneic transfusion and prognosis; the control arm consisted of patients who received autologous transfusion.[24] However, transfused patients, those who received either allogeneic blood or autologous blood, showed a significantly increased risk of recurrence compared with that in the untransfused patients. The investigators explain the differences in this study compared with the effect of allogeneic blood alone reported in the retrospective studies as most likely related to patient selection factors. However, this prospective study limited patients to those who received two units or fewer and, using an intention-to-treat analysis, included in the control group a significant number of patients who received allogeneic blood (28 percent); in the allogeneic transfusion group, 44 percent of patients did not require transfusion. Furthermore, 14 of the centers re-

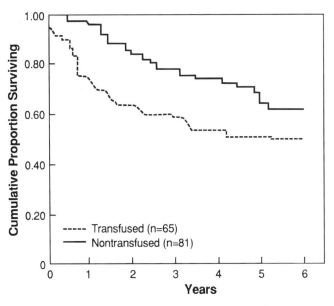

Fig. 4-2. Overall survival in colorectal cancer, Dukes stages A, B, and C by life-table analysis. Results are from a retrospective study comparing transfused and nontransfused patients. (Adapted from Foster et al.,[21] with permission)

moved the buffy coat from the red cell component.

A second randomized, controlled trial compared patients transfused with leukocyte-depleted blood (average leukocyte content $0.2 \times 10^6 \pm 0.3$) with those who received buffy coat-depleted blood (average leukocyte content 0.8×10^9).[25] No difference was found between the two groups in survival, disease-free survival, or cancer recurrence rate. In this series of 871 patients, those who received blood of any sort had a shorter 3-year survival than did those who received none, although the relationship is not necessarily a causal one. If the transfusion effect is more than selection of patients with more advanced disease, in this study, transfused patients derived no obvious benefit from the removal of most of the leukocytes from the blood components. The less favorable outcome in transfused patients may still be no more than a reflection of patient selection for disease severity.

A third randomized, controlled, prospective study of 120 patients undergoing colorectal surgery reported fewer recurrences in the autologous transfusion group than in the group that received allogeneic buffy coat-depleted blood.[26] Thus, two of the three prospective studies cast some doubt on the adverse effect of allogeneic transfusion on tumor growth and recurrence; none of the prospective studies disproves an adverse effect of transfusion on patient survival.

More than 40 studies of transfusion and cancer recurrence have now been published. Of the retrospective studies, those involving renal and lung cancer most often report a transfusion effect; however, some series of patients with soft tissue sarcoma or breast, head and neck, or prostate cancer have yielded similar findings. A prospective, but nonrandomized, study of radical retropubic prostatectomy for patients with prostatic malignancy did not find a relationship between transfusion and cancer recurrence or patient survival.[27] It is not yet possible to reconcile these findings. Any comprehensive analysis of the relationship of transfusion to cancer recurrence and patient survival has to account for such variables as study design, sample size, tumor type and stage, transfusion dose, component preparation and storage, patient selection, surgeon, and publica-

tion bias. Perhaps the two points to stress at this time are that (1) the prospective studies do not find an obvious immunosuppressive effect of blood transfusion, but neither is such an effect definitively excluded, and (2) none of the studies points to a prognostic benefit for the patient who receives a transfusion.

The most relevant clinical studies that evaluated the effect of perioperative allogeneic blood transfusion on the outcome in patients with colorectal carcinoma have been subjected to meta-analysis by two groups of investigators. One analysis indicates that the cumulative odds ratio of colorectal carcinoma recurrence, cancer-associated death, and death from any cause in allogeneically transfused patients are 1.80, 1.76, and 1.63, respectively.[28] These investigators concluded that their analysis supports the hypothesis that perioperative allogeneic blood transfusion is associated with an increased risk of colorectal carcinoma recurrence and death from this disease. Vamvakas and Moore[29] concluded that, if a deleterious effect of perioperative blood transfusion did exist, it would have to be small and could be reliably established only by means of a randomized controlled experiment. They thought that the extent of residual confounding in the data of the 11 observational studies pooled for their meta-analysis probably explained the full 37 percent excess risk calculated for the transfused patients. Thus, whether allogeneic blood transfusion affects tumor growth in humans is still an open issue,[30] and any radical alteration in perioperative transfusion practice aimed at thwarting a potential deleterious transfusion effect that leads to earlier cancer recurrence is presently premature.[29]

PERIOPERATIVE TRANSFUSION AND POSTOPERATIVE INFECTION

Similar controversy surrounds the relationship between perioperative transfusion and the risk of postoperative infection. As with tumor recurrence, animal studies suggest an adverse effect of allogeneic transfusion in experimental surgical models.[31] Retrospective analysis of records of orthopedic patients and of those undergoing open heart surgery and colorectal surgery indicate that perioperative (possibly excluding preoperative) allogeneic transfusion is associated with increased numbers of wound infections and increased numbers of distant infections, including pneumonitis and urinary tract infection.[14,32] The effect seems to be dose dependent, but unfortunately this variable is difficult to control with matched autologous blood recipients because of the limited amount of blood that most patients can predeposit.[33]

Retrospective chart analysis for study of postoperative infections presents numerous pitfalls. The definition of "infection" overestimates events if all febrile episodes are included and underestimates events if the inclusion criteria demand positive microbial cultures. Differences in surgical technique are extremely important variables, so that either a single surgeon or a randomized study is necessary to correct this potential bias. Furthermore, studies that use autologous blood recipients as matched controls often face the criticism that patients who are capable of donating their own blood may be healthier than those who cannot; this selection bias may account for the difference in infection rate. Finally, even if the difference in postoperative infection rates between patients who receive transfusions and those who do not is real, the difference may have nothing to do with the transfusion itself. Transfusion may be no more than a surrogate marker for some other factor, such as low hematocrit or chronic disease.

More than 20 retrospective studies of transfusion and postoperative infection have now been published. Almost all of these publications conclude that transfusion is a significant predictor of postoperative infection.[14] In most of these reports, transfusion was the single best predictor of infection.[34] Other factors that correlate with transfusion, such as hematocrit, blood loss, and duration of surgery, are generally not significant predictors in multivariate analysis models. Patients who receive comparable amounts of autologous transfusion still appear to have fewer infections than do those who receive allogeneic blood.

Four large, prospective, randomized studies of colorectal surgery have addressed the association between postoperative infection and perioperative transfusion.[24,25,35,36] One found no difference in infection rates between allogeneic and autologous transfusion recipients.[24] Two found a statistically significant increase in the number of postoperative infections in the cohort that receive allogeneic blood.[25,35] The fourth found no difference in the total number of infections, but there was a statistically significant increase in postoperative wound infections in patients who received whole blood compared with a cohort who received blood that was leukocyte depleted by filtration at the bedside.[36] Because of weaknesses in methodology and analysis, none of the studies is likely to be regarded as definitive. However, the great majority of both retrospective and prospective studies, when analyzed by multivariate analysis, find that perioperative blood transfusion is associated with postoperative infection as an independent variable.

Vamvakas and Moore[37] published a detailed review of evaluable accumulated clinical evidence that was performed to determine the validity of the reported association of transfusion with postoperative infection. They concluded that scientifically sound clinical studies unequivocally establishing the existence of an adverse effect (relating perioperative transfusion to septic complications of surgery) have not yet been published. Bordin et al[30] also reviewed published clinical studies and concluded that the relationship between allogeneic blood transfusion and bacterial infection has not been proved.

Vamvakas and Moore's[37] review of the methods used in published studies agreed with Alexander's[38] 1991 appraisal of the available evidence as "circumstantial." Nevertheless, there was a high degree of suspicion that some portion of the association under study truly exists, and it is certainly worthy of further investigation.

If an adverse effect is ultimately established, it would be prudent to consider the cost-effectiveness of remedial medical interventions (e.g., third-generation filters) before proposing modifications in standard transfusion practice.[37]

ALLOGENEIC TRANSFUSION AND HUMAN IMMUNODEFICIENCY VIRUS INFECTION

Another aspect of the relationship between allogeneic transfusion and infection involves patients infected with human immunodeficiency virus (HIV).

Several reports suggest that HIV-infected patients, and those with clinical AIDS, may experience more rapid disease progression, decreased survival, and increased frequency of cytomegalovirus (CMV) infection, bacterial infection, and wasting if exposed to allogeneic blood transfusion.[40–42] The effects appear to be dose dependent. An attractive explanation for these findings, and one that may have broader implications, involves the observation that allogeneic peripheral blood leukocytes stimulate replication and spread of HIV-1 in lymphocytes and monocytes in vitro.[15] Coculture of leukocytes with lymphocytes infected in vivo induced a dose-related activation of HIV-1 followed by dissemination of HIV to previously uninfected cells (Fig. 4-3). Partially purified red blood cells, platelets, and plasma from the same donors did not. Small numbers of leukocytes that are present in most blood components may thus play an important role in activation of latent viral infections.

Similarly, other transfusion-transmitted lymphotropic viruses such as CMV and Epstein-Barr virus (EBV) may play a role in HIV activation. Transfusion-related lymphocyte stimulation also likely affects other latent viral infections.[43,44] It has long been appreciated that transfusion may reactivate latent CMV infection and that the chance of reactivation correlates with the amount of blood transfused.[45] Furthermore, immediate-early proteins expressed by activated CMV have been demonstrated to inactivate the p53 gene, a tumor suppressor, the loss or inactivation of which may be associated with one-half of all human cancers.[46] These proteins are produced even in the absence of documented viral replication. Such activation of latent viral infections, HIV, CMV, EBV, or other oncogenic viruses, may be one mechanism by which allogeneic transfusions affect host immune defenses.

SPONTANEOUS ABORTION

Spontaneous abortion approximates a natural model of "allograft rejection" that provides further insight into the immunomodulatory effects of blood

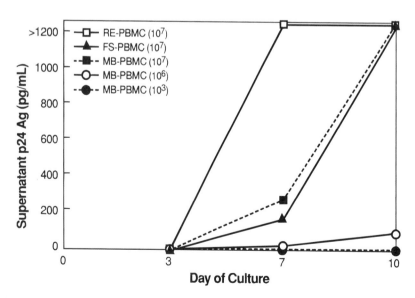

Fig. 4-3. Induction of HIV p24 antigen expression in the supernatant of cells from an HIV-infected patient cocultured with peripheral blood mononuclear cells (PBMC) from three normal donors (RE, FS, and MB). Antigen induction is dose dependent and absent at low numbers of PBMC. No p24 induction was observed with cocultures of red cells, platelets, or plasma. (Adapted from Busch et al.,[15] with permission.)

transfusion. In 1981, Taylor and Faulk[47] described three women, each of whom had a history of three or more spontaneous abortions, and each of whom shared one HLA haplotype with her husband. In an effort to desensitize the women, each was infused with pooled buffy coat-rich plasma from unrelated donors, and each subsequently delivered an infant at term. This report was sufficiently stimulating to prompt the design of a controlled trial. The value of transfusion for the prevention of recurrent spontaneous pregnancy losses is as yet incompletely evaluated because the results of only one controlled trial have been published. In 1985, Mowbray et al.[48] published a report of a controlled study of leukocyte infusions for women with at least three spontaneous abortions. One hundred five couples were randomized so that, at conception, the women received either autologous (control) white blood cells or allogeneic leukocytes from their spouses in a blinded, randomized fashion. The trial was halted when 17 live births occurred among 22 women who received paternal cells; 17 of 27 women who received autologous cells sustained another spontaneous abortion. Pregnancy rates were equal in both groups. The paternal leukocytes were superior to autologous cells in preventing spontaneous abortion, and 13 of 15 of these women carried subsequent pregnancies to term. The mechanism of the possible effect remains unknown, although the stimulation of HLA-DR antibodies or maternal blocking antibodies that cross-react with lymphocytes and trophoblast antigens have been postulated as potential mediators of tolerance.[49]

Mueller-Eckhardt's group[50,51] proposed that intravenous immune globulin should contain preformed antibodies of similar specificity, which might be as effective as allogeneic leukocyte therapy. The results of pilot studies demonstrated a successful outcome of pregnancy in approximately 80 percent of treated patients.[51] However, the evaluation and interpretation of such results has to take into account that the probability of a successful pregnancy in women with a history of three spontaneous abortions is about 60 percent without treatment. A specific therapeutic effect could not be verified in a German randomized, double-blind, multicenter trial in comparison with 5 percent human albumin, which was used as a placebo. The data for intravenous immune globulin and albumin show success rates in the range of results reported for allogeneic leukocyte treatment, and this might be interpreted to mean that these favorable results are due to a placebo effect. Indeed, Stray-Pedersen and Stray-Pedersen[52] demonstrated impressively the positive role of psychological influence on reproductive success in patients with recurrent spontaneous abortions. Women who received specific antenatal counseling and psychological support had a pregnancy success rate of 86 percent compared with a success rate of 33 percent observed in women who were given no specific antenatal care ($P < 0.001$).

CROHN'S DISEASE

Blood transfusion reportedly decreases the rate of recurrence in Crohn's disease, a chronic inflammatory bowel disease mediated in part by activated lymphocytes and treated routinely with combinations of antibiotics, immunosuppressive medication, and surgery. Williams and Hughes[12] reported a 5-year recurrence rate of only 19 percent in 28 patients who received between one and eight units of blood at the time of bowel resection. There was a 59 percent recurrence rate among the 32 patients who received no blood ($P = 0.006$). Although this analysis was retrospective, surgical indications for resection were similar for both groups, all operations were done by the same surgeon, and the transfused group had more severe disease, a finding that might predict a higher recurrence rate in this group. If transfusion has an immunosuppressive effect in this study, it must be an effect that persists for several years. Subsequent analyses of patients with Crohn's disease have yielded conflicting results.[53,54] A retrospective analysis of 197 patients with Crohn's disease has not confirmed a relationship between transfusion and recurrence.[55]

MECHANISMS OF THE TRANSFUSION EFFECT

If allogeneic blood has an immunomodulatory effect, the mechanism and pathogenesis of the effect remain unexplained (Table 4-2). Allogeneic transfusion may elicit a suppressor cell network or develop-

Table 4-2. Proposed Mechanisms of Immunomodulatory Effects of Blood Transfusion

Development of a suppressor-cell network
Anti-idiotype antibody formation
Clonal deletion
Transmission of infectious agents
Reactivation of latent viral infections
Effects of the preservative or storage process
Direct effects of minor cell populations or trace proteins
Combinations of the mechanisms above

ment of anti-idiotype antibodies. However, no evidence to support a clonal deletion mechanism has been provided. Cytokines accumulate in stored blood, and organic substances such as phthalate plasticizers leach from plastic storage containers during refrigerated storage. Anticoagulant preservative solutions may also affect lymphocyte function.[56] All of these may contribute to changes in immunologic responsiveness in the transfusion recipient.

Evidence is emerging that plasma, leukocytes, and latent transfusion-transmitted viruses may be involved in the immunomodulatory effects of transfusion. Blumberg and Heal[57] suggest that the plasma contained in whole blood may be related to immunosuppression and to recurrence of colorectal, cervical, and prostatic cancer. These investigators also analyzed several series of patients with AIDS and correlated progression of disease with volume of plasma received. They postulate further that the apparent decline in the tolerogenic effect of blood transfusion for renal allografts may relate to the increasing use of red blood cell concentrates that contain little plasma. Others have also implicated the plasma component as an important mediator of immunosuppression.[58,59] In patients with hemophilia, alterations of immune function develop that may result from repeated exposure to plasma protein and alloantigens contained in relatively impure concentrates of plasma-derived clotting factor concentrates.[60,61] HIV-seronegative hemophiliac patients treated with recombinant factor VIII, which contains only trace amounts of human plasma proteins other than albumin, show no evidence of such changes, and seropositive patients show no unexpected decline in CD4 cell count.[62] Comparisons of patients treated with plasma-derived high-purity concentrates and intermediate-purity concentrates report more rapid CD4 cell decline in the latter group.[63] Other studies show no effect of dose of low- or intermediate-purity concentrate on decline in CD4 cell count in either HIV-seronegative or HIV-seropositive hemophiliac patients.[64] Differences in study duration, treatment with anti-retroviral agents, and patient populations limit the significance of comparisons. Also, small changes in circulating CD4 cell counts may not be accurate as a surrogate marker of increasing clinical illness. It is also possible that, rather than an adverse effect of low-purity concentrates, high-purity concentrates either slow the HIV-mediated destruction of CD4 cells or alter their mobilization or traffic in the peripheral blood.

Experience with HIV suggests that one possible mechanism of transfusion-associated immunomodulation might be a direct effect of a transfusion-transmitted infectious agent. On the other hand, the studies of latent virus activation suggest that leukocytes may be the implicated component in these clinical circumstances. If so, one might expect leukocyte-poor components to have a reduced or unmeasurable effect. The current data are equivocal, and additional studies to investigate this possibility are being conducted.

The weight of evidence from basic science, preclinical, and clinical studies suggests that allogeneic transfusion exerts at least modest immunomodulatory effects on the recipient. The mechanisms of these effects, their clinical import, the specific components of blood transfusion involved, and the role of recipient-host factors are poorly understood. The possibilities of eliminating the transfusion effect or harnessing it for therapeutic use remain areas for further scientific inquiry. Until the implications of transfusion-associated alterations in the immune response are better understood, prudence dictates continued cautious use of allogeneic transfusion.

REFERENCES

1. Dodd RV: The risk of transfusion-transmitted infection. N Engl J Med 327:419, 1992
2. Blajchman MA, Ali AM: Bacteria in the blood supply: an overlooked issue in transfusion medicine. p. 213.

In Nance SJ (ed): Blood Safety: Current Challenges. American Association of Blood Banks, Bethesda, MD, 1992

3. Stehling LC, Cosgrove DM, Moss GS et al: Indications for the use of red blood cells, platelets, and fresh frozen plasma. Publication no. (NIH) 89-2974. U.S. Department of Health and Human Services, Bethesda, MD, 1989

4. Brunson ME, Alexander JW: Mechanisms of transfusion induced immunosuppression. Transfusion 30: 651, 1990

5. Mathiesen O, Lund L, Brodthagen U et al: The effect of previous blood transfusion on lymphocyte subsets and natural killer cell function in patients with colorectal cancer. Vox Sang 67:36, 1994

6. DePalma L, Duncan B, Chan MM et al: The neonatal response to washed and irradiated red cells: lack of evidence of lymphocyte activation. Transfusion 31: 737, 1991

7. Opelz G, Sengar DPS, Mickey MR et al: Effect of blood transfusion on subsequent kidney transplants. Transplant Proc 5:253, 1973

8. Opelz G, Terasaki PI: Improvement of kidney-graft survival with increased numbers of blood transfusions. N Engl J Med 299:799, 1978

9. Fabre JW, Morris PJ: The effect of donor strain blood pretreatment on renal allograft rejection in rats. Transplantation 14:608, 1972

10. Salvatierra O, Jr, Vincenti F, Amend W et al: Deliberate donor-specific blood transfusion prior to living related renal transplantation. Ann Surg 192:543, 1980

11. Lagaaij EL, Hennemann IPH, Ruigrok M et al: Effect of one-HLA-DR-antigen-matched and completely HLA-DR-mismatched blood transfusion on survival of heart and kidney allografts. N Engl J Med 321:701, 1989

12. Williams JG, Hughes LE: Effect of perioperative blood transfusion on recurrence of Crohn's disease. Lancet 2:131, 1989

13. Mowbray JF, Gibbings CR, Sidgwick AS et al: Effects of transfusion in women with recurrent spontaneous abortion. Transplant Proc 15:896, 1983

14. Blumberg N, Heal JM: Transfusion and host defenses against cancer recurrence and infection. Transfusion 29:236, 1988

15. Busch MP, Lee T-H, Heitman J: Allogeneic lymphocytes but not therapeutic blood elements induce reactivation and dissemination of latent HIV-1: implications for transfusion support of infected patients. Blood 83: 2128, 1992

16. Anderson KC, Weinstein H: Transfusion-associated graft-versus-host disease. N Engl J Med 323:315, 1990

17. Van Aken WG: Does perioperative blood transfusion promote tumor growth? Transfusion Med Rev 3:243, 1989

18. Burrows L, Tarrtar P: Effect of blood transfusions on colonic malignancy recurrence rate. Lancet 2:662, 1982

19. Blumberg N, Agarwal M, Chuang C: Relation between recurrence of cancer of the colon and blood transfusion. BMJ 290:1037, 1985

20. Creasy TS, Veitch PS, Bell PR: A relationship between perioperative blood transfusion and recurrence of carcinoma of the sigmoid colon following potentially curative surgery. Ann R Coll Surg Engl 69:100, 1987

21. Foster RS, Costanza MC, Foster JC et al: Adverse relationship between blood transfusions and survival after colectomy for colon cancer. Cancer 55:1195, 1985

22. Blair SD, Janvrin SB: Relation between cancer of the colon and blood transfusion. BMJ 290:1516, 1985

23. Frankish PD, McNee RK, Alley PG et al: Relation between cancer of the colon and blood transfusion. BMJ 290:1827, 1985

24. Busch ORC, Hop WCJ, Hoynck MAW et al: Blood transfusions and prognosis in colorectal cancer. N Engl J Med 328:1372, 1993

25. Houbiers JGA, Brand A, van de Watering LMG et al: Randomised controlled trial comparing transfusion of leucocyte-depleted or buffy-coat-depleted blood in surgery for colorectal cancer. Lancet 344:573, 1994

26. Heiss MM, Jauch K-W, Delanoff CH et al: Blood transfusion modulated tumor recurrence: a randomized study of autologous versus homologous blood transfusion in colorectal cancer surgery. Am J Clin Oncol 12: 1859, 1994

27. Ness PM, Walsh PC, Zahurak M et al: Prostate cancer recurrence in radical surgery patients receiving autologous or homologous blood. Transfusion 32:31, 1992

28. Chung M, Steinmetz OK, Gordon PH: Perioperative blood transfusion and outcome after resection for colorectal carcinoma. Br J Surg 80:427, 1993

29. Vamvakas E, Moore SB: Perioperative blood transfusion and colorectal cancer recurrence: a qualitative statistical overview and meta-analysis. Transfusion 33: 754, 1993

30. Bordin JO, Heddle NM, Blajchman MA: Biologic effects of leukocytes present in transfused cellular blood products. Blood 84:1703, 1994

31. Waymack JP, Warden GD, Alexander JW et al: Effect of blood transfusion and anesthesia on resistance to bacterial peritonitis. J Surg Res 42:528, 1987

32. Ottilo G, De Paulis R, Pansini S et al: Major sternal wound infection after open-heart surgery: a multivari-

ate analysis of risk factors in 2579 consecutive procedures. Ann Thorac Surg 44:173, 1987

33. Leikola J, Myllyla G: The clinical use of red blood cell components. p. 1. In Summers SH, Smith DM, Agraneklo VA (eds): Transfusion Therapy: Guidelines for Practice. American Association of Blood Banks, Arlington, VA, 1990

34. Murphy P, Heal JM, Blumberg N: Infection or suspected infection after hip replacement surgery with autologous or homologous blood transfusions. Transfusion 31:212, 1991

35. Heiss MM, Mempel W, Jauch K-W et al: Beneficial effect of autologous blood transfusion on infectious complications after colorectal cancer surgery. Lancet 344:573, 1994

36. Jensen LS, Andersen AJ, Christiansen PM et al: Postoperative infection and natural killer cell function following blood transfusion in patients undergoing elective colorectal surgery. Br J Surg 79:513, 1992

37. Vamvakas EC, Moore SB: Blood transfusion and postoperative septic complications. Transfusion 34:714, 1994

38. Alexander JW: Transfusion-induced immunomodulation and infection (editorial). Transfusion 31:195, 1991

39. Heiss MK, Mempel W, Jauch K-W et al: Beneficial effect of autologous blood transfusion on infectious complications after colorectal cancer surgery. Lancet 342: 1328, 1993

40. Ward JW, Bush TJ, Perkins HJ et al: The natural history of transfusion-associated infection with human immunodeficiency virus. Factors influencing the rate of progression to disease. N Engl J Med 321:947, 1989

41. Vamvakas E, Kaplan HS: Early transfusion and length of survival in acquired immune deficiency syndrome: experience with a population receiving medical care at a public hospital. Transfusion 33:111, 1993

42. Sloand E, Kumar P, Klein HG, Merritt S, Sacher R: Transfusion of blood products in HIV-1 infected persons: relationship to opportunistic infection. Transfusion 34:48, 1994

43. Margolick JB, Volkman DJ, Folks TM et al: Amplification of HTLV-III/LAV infection by antigen-induced activation of T cells and direct suppression by virus of lymphocyte blastogenic responses. J Immunol 138: 1719, 1987

44. Kenney S, Kamine J, Markovitz D et al: An Epstein-Barr virus immediate-early gene product trans-activates gene expression from the human immunodeficiency virus long terminal repeat. Proc Natl Acad Sci U S A 85:1652, 1992

45. Adler SP, McVoy MM: Cytomegalovirus infections in seropositive patients after transfusion: the effect of red cell storage and volume. Transfusion 29:667, 1989

46. Speir E, Modali R, Huang E-S et al: Potential role of human cytomegalovirus and p53 interaction in coronary restenosis. Science 265:391, 1994

47. Taylor C, Faulk WP: Prevention of recurrent abortion with leukocyte transfusions. Lancet 2:68, 1981

48. Mowbray JF, Lidell H, Underwood JL et al: Controlled trial of treatment of recurrent abortion with leukocyte transfusions. Lancet 2:941, 1985

49. Maternal blocking antibodies, the fetal allograft, and recurrent abortion (editorial). Lancet 2:1175, 1983

50. Mueller-Eckhardt G, Heine O, Neppert J et al: Prevention of recurrent spontaneous abortion by intravenous immunoglobulin. Vox Sang 51:122, 1989

51. Heine O, Mueller-Eckhardt G: Intravenous immune globulin in recurrent abortion. Clin Exp Immunol 97: 39, 1994

52. Stray-Pedersen B, Stray-Pedersen S: Etiologic factors and subsequent reproductive performance in 195 couples with prior history of habitual abortion. Am J Obstet Gynecol 148:140, 1984

53. Park RHR, Russell R: Effect of perioperative blood transfusion on recurrence of Crohn's disease. Lancet 2:631, 1989

54. Sutherland LR, Ramcharan S, Bryant H et al: Effect of perioperative blood transfusion on recurrence of Crohn's disease. Lancet 2:1048, 1989

55. Scott ADN, Ritchie JK, Phillips RKS: Blood transfusion and recurrent Crohn's disease. Br J Surg 78:455, 1991

56. Vliet WC, Dock NL, Davey FR: Factors in the liquid portion of stored blood inhibit the proliferative response in mixed lymphocyte cultures. Transfusion 29: 41, 1989

57. Blumberg N, Heal JM: Transfusion and recipient immune function. Arch Pathol Lab Med 113:246, 1989

58. Wobbes T, Joosen KHG, Kuypers HHC et al: The effect of packed cells and whole blood on survival after curative resection for colorectal carcinoma. Dis Colon Rectum 32:743, 1989

59. Marsh J, Donnan PT, Hamer-Hodges DW: Association between transfusion with plasma and the recurrence of colorectal carcinoma. Br J Surg 77:623, 1990

60. Teitel JM, Freedman JJ, Garvey MB, Kardish M: Two-year evaluation of clinical and laboratory variables of immune function in 117 hemophiliacs seropositive or seronegative for HIV-1. Am J Hematol 32:362, 1989

61. Cuthbert RJG, Ludlam CA, Steel CM et al: Immunological studies in HIV seronegative haemophiliacs: relationship to blood product therapy. Br J Haematol 80:364, 1992

62. Seremetis SV, Aledort LM, Bergman GE et al: Three-year randomized study of high-purity or intermediate purity factor VIII concentrates in symptom-free HIV seropositive hemophiliacs: effects on immune status. Lancet 342:700, 1993

63. Mannucci PM, Brettler DB, Aledort LM et al: Immune status of human immunodeficiency virus seropositive and seronegative hemophiliacs infused for 35 years with recombinant factor VIII. Blood 83:1958, 1994

64. Gjerset GF, Pike MC, Mosley JW et al: Effect of low- and intermediate-purity clotting factor therapy on progression of human immunodeficiency virus infection in congenital clotting disorders. Blood 84:1666, 1994

Blood Groups

Carma Lizza, Judith Myers, and Laura Gindy

Before 1901, agglutination of human red cells, when observed, was considered a phenomenon of disease and of no significance in transfusion. Karl Landsteiner's[1] correlation of visible clumping in mixtures of plasma and red cells from healthy individuals led to the discovery of the ABO system and one explanation for serious, hemolytic transfusion reactions. This single system is the primary basis for successful transfusion, even today.

Following the discovery of the ABO system, investigators searched for other naturally occurring antibodies to identify new systems, but were unsuccessful. Then, other blood systems were defined with antibodies produced by immunization of animals with human red blood cells. Development of new techniques and new reagents further expanded the list. By 1951, nine blood group systems were known. In order of discovery, they are ABO, MNSs, P, Rh, Lutheran, Kell, Lewis, Duffy, and Kidd. The number of red cell characteristics is now greater than 600 and continues to increase.[2] Some of the more recently detected antigens have been assigned to established blood group systems; others with recognizable relationships have been organized into new systems or placed in associated collections of antigens, and still others remain unclassified. A few of the previous classifications have been changed. The International Society of Blood Transfusion (ISBT)[3] currently lists 21 blood group systems, with an additional eight collections.

While the most important application of this knowledge is providing safe blood transfusion, the study of red cell polymorphism has made important contributions to anthropology, forensics, genetics, paternity testing, and immunology, among other areas. Blood groups appear to have some relationship to susceptibility to disease and play a role in successful transplantation. Research is intensifying in an effort to identify relationships, if any, with malignancy. Whatever the function, the existence of red cell polymorphism is genetically maintained.

ROLE OF THE BLOOD GROUP SYSTEMS

Theories on the biologic role of human blood groups have been postulated, but despite much speculation and discussion, their purpose remains unclear. Possible functions are recognition of self and nonself, the maintenance of cellular integrity, involvement in cell maturation, and susceptibility or resistance to disease. However, given the heterogeneity of human blood group systems, it is unlikely that a single function will be discovered. Our knowledge of the blood systems is continually evolving, but many conclusions, even those based on current knowledge, remain tentative.

Links with disease have been established, and anomalies of antigenic expression are found in many hematopoietic disorders. Changes in blood group antigens are observed with malignancies, but the causes or implications are not fully understood. Antibodies of the systems specific to hematopoietic tissue (Rh, Duffy, Kidd, and Kell) are directed primarily against the red cell. Human blood group systems with systemic antigens widely distributed throughout the body (ABH, Lewis, Ii, and P) can be obstacles in transplantation as well as in transfusion and pregnancy.[4] The Rh system and many high-incidence antigens are involved in autoimmune specificities. Investigations into the function of human blood groups may result in beneficial new prognostic and diagnostic information.

DEFINITION OF A BLOOD GROUP SYSTEM

A blood group system is composed of antigens inherited as a group. Each system is made up of antigens produced by alleles at a single genetic locus or at loci so closely linked that crossover does not occur. Red cell antigens that represent a single blood group are genetically controlled by allelic genes inherited independently of each other.

Within each system, groups of individuals may be distinguished from other groups by phenotype. A phenotype is the observed serologic red cell antigen type that may, in many instances, indicate the actual genotype. Until there are convenient laboratory test for blood group genes, a probable genotype may be deduced from phenotype but, generally, genotype must be substantiated by family studies.

Identification of a blood group system follows a natural sequence. An antibody detecting a specific new antigen is discovered, usually from a multiply-transfused patient or a multiparous woman. Once the corresponding antigen is found, the pattern of inheritance is studied and a search for the antithetical antigen begins. Later, more complex genetic relationships may be established when multiple alleles on a single chromosome are inherited as a set, such as in the MNSs blood group system, or several loci are involved as in the Lewis blood group system. Population studies are undertaken to calculate gene frequencies. Once a genetic relationship is confirmed, assignment to a blood group system can be made. If feasible, the biochemical structure of the antigen is determined, and the pathway of biosynthesis is formulated. Thus, blood groups are first de-fined immunologically, then genetically and biochemically.

Blood groups may be classified in the following ways: (1) by clinical significance (i.e., as a cause of hemolytic transfusion reactions [HTR] or hemolytic disease of the newborn [HDN]), (2) by the source of sensitization (i.e., exposure to similar antigens in the environment or immune stimulation by foreign antigens introduced by transfusion or pregnancy), or (3) biochemical relationships.

Nomenclature for blood groups is inconsistent. There are numerous conflicts with mendelian terminology, in which, traditionally, dominant traits are capitalized and recessive traits are designated by lower case letters. In the human blood groups, for example, the recessive amorph *O* is capitalized, while alleles *K* and *k* are co-dominant. In some systems, co-dominant alleles are assigned the same symbol distinguished by different superscript letters. Numbers are assigned to alleles in still other blood group systems. The use of as many as three different terminologies for the same system requires the ability to translate from one to another.[5] To eliminate confusion, the ISBT has formed a Working Party on Terminology for Red Cell Surface Antigens to recommend standard terminology and devise numerical designations for use with computers. Their definition of a blood group system remains essentially the same. Additionally, a blood group "collection" category has been added to gather together specificities that have a serologic, biochemical, or genetic connection. Specific guidelines are defined to establish new blood group systems or to include an antigen in a current blood group.[6]

IMMUNOLOGY

Antibodies defining blood group antigens are divided into three group: alloantibodies, autoantibodies, and heterologous antibodies.[7] Alloantibodies are either naturally occurring or immune antibodies, stimulated by transfusion or pregnancy, against antigens an individual lacks. Autoantibodies react with antigens of the same individual that formed the antibody and are generally directed against high-frequency antigens. Heterologous antibodies to human red cells are derived from other species.

An antigen induces formation of a specific antibody that is capable of combining with the antigen. The portion that binds strongly with antibody is the immunodominant determinant and is most often the terminal end. Antigenic determinants may be sequential, as with linear polypeptides and polysaccharides, or may involve structures that fold, as with proteins.

Specificity depends on chemical structure of the antigen, which permits stereochemical contact between antigen and antibody. The antigenic determinant is the accessible area that combines with antibody. The number and location of antigenic determinants vary widely from system to system and correlate with the strength with which different antigens react with their antibodies. Table 5-1 shows estimates of the numbers of antigen sites for selected antigens.[8-12] Wide variations help explain diversity of antigens' serologic behavior. Another contributing factor is the ability of some antigens to cluster together, increasing their accessibility, while others remain isolated from each other. ABO antigens cluster while Rh antigens do not.

Antibodies produced by a specific antigen may cross-react with other antigens. An antigen generally has more than one antigenic determinant that may also be found in unrelated antigens. Cross-reactivity occurs when the shared determinants are identical structures or when antigenic structures are similar, as in acquired B, where D-galactosamine residues react with the antibody specific for D-galactose.

The immunogenicity of an antigen is its ability to stimulate antibody formation. Not all antigens are equally immunogenic. Relative antigenicity can be estimated by calculating the number of transfused people negative for a specific antigen who develop the corresponding antibody, compared with the chances of receiving antigen-positive blood. Of the immune antibodies, Rh are the most common, followed by those of the Kell, Kidd, and Duffy blood group systems.[7] Formation of anti-D occurs in nearly 1 percent of total potential antigenic exposures, anti-K in approximately 0.1 percent, and anti-c and anti-E in about 0.04 percent.[4] Anti-Fya has been found to occur 25 times less frequently and anti-Jka 50 to 100 times less frequently than anti-K.[13]

Clinical importance is determined by whether the antibody destroys red cells in vivo, by whether the antibody can cross the placenta (and the antigen is well developed in the fetus), and by the relative frequency of the antigen. Using these criteria, ABO antibodies, which cause immediate intravascular destruction, are clearly the most important in transfusion, followed by Rh antibodies, which are readily formed by immune stimulation and may cause severe HDN or immune destruction of transfused red cells.

Table 5-1. Comparison of Estimated Antigen Sites on Individual Erythrocytes

Antigen	Phenotype	Average (No.) ($\times 10^3$)
A	A_1 adult	800
	newborn	300
	A_2 adult	240
	newborn	140
	A_1 B adult	660
	newborn	0.22
	A_2 B adult	140
	newborn	0.14
	A_3	<100
	A_x	<10
	A_m	<2
	A_{end}	$0-0.2^a$
	A_{el}	<1.4
B	B adult	750
	newborn	200
	A_1 B	430
I	I+	300
Le^a	Le(a + b −)	3
K	K + k −	6
	K + k +	3
D	CDe/CDe	17
	cDE/cDE	25
c	cde/cde	78
	Cde/cde	45
e	cde/cde	21
	cDE/cde	14
MN	M + N −, M − N +	1,000
S	S + s −	250
s	S − s +	170
Jk^a	Jk(a + b −)	14
Fy^a	Fy(a + b −)	17
	Fy(a − b +)	7
Fy^b	Fy(a − b +)	17

^{a} None on nonagglutinated cells; cells that agglutinate with anti-A have 200 antigen sites.

Naturally occurring antibodies describe those antibodies formed spontaneously without exposure to red cells. This does not mean there has been no antigenic stimulus, but rather that these develop as an immune response to substances with similar antigenic determinants found in the environment. "Naturally occurring" is a misnomer, but phrases that better describe the situation are inconvenient. In addition, some of the antibodies are to antigens that are unlikely to be found in the environment,[14] such as a few examples of anti-E, or antibodies to low-incidence antigens commonly found along with autoantibody in autoimmune hemolytic anemia.[15] The majority of naturally occurring antibodies are IgM and are primarily cold-reacting. An IgG fraction is present in a significant number, while a few may even be predominantly IgG. Anti-A, -B, -H, -PP_1P^k, and P^k are found in almost every individual who lacks the corresponding antigen. Anti-A_1, -Le^a, and -P_1 occur less frequently. Anti-Vw and -Wr^a are present in about 1 to 2 percent of all sera. Less common naturally occurring antibodies are anti-M, -S, -N, -Ge, -K, -Lu^a, -Di^a, and -Xg^a.[7]

Immune antibodies are typically IgG. Response to the first exposure to a foreign antigen tends to be slow, but upon second exposure to the same antigen, a large amount of antibody can be produced in a comparatively short time. The antibody formed initially in a primary response is IgM while IgG antibody occurs in the secondary response. Although IgM may be the first antibody formed, IgG is soon the predominant immunoglobulin in the human response to red cell antigens. Immune antibody, once formed, may persist over long periods of time or may disappear in relatively short periods, setting the stage for an anamnestic response upon subsequent exposure to the same antigen. Approximately 35 percent of clinically significant antibodies become undetectable in 1 year and nearly 50 percent are undetectable after 10 years.[16]

Individuals vary widely in response to different antigens, and this response may be determined by HLA-DR genes.[17] Genetic control also appears to be influenced by genes outside the HLA system. When exposed to an antigen, an individual may respond by producing antibody, and this antibody may be directed against different determinants on the antigen with varying affinities. Even when the antigen is relatively homogeneous, the response is heterogeneous. These polyclonal antibodies are developed by different cell lines of lymphocytes reacting to polymorphic determinants of the same antigenic structure. Clinically significant antibodies occur in about 1 to 2 percent of all transfused patients. Adults with sickle cell disease have the highest incidence, at approximately 25 percent. Other highly transfused hospital populations such as recipients of liver transplants run between 6 percent and 12 percent. Individuals with autoimmune antibodies tend to also have an increased frequency of alloantibodies. Individuals with complex, multiple alloantibody combinations are more likely to also have autoantibody.[16]

Monoclonal antibody (mAb) is produced by immunocytes cloned from a single cell. All molecules are identical and combine with identical sections of the antigen. Human mAbs are found in certain pathological conditions, such as cold hemagglutinin disease (CHD). The genome of a single human cell can be hybridized into a mouse cell to produce pure, well-defined monospecific antibodies against many human red cell determinants. These antibodies have great potential for biochemical and genetic research. Monoclonal antibodies have already made a significant contribution to the understanding of sialoglycoproteins and their relationship to red cell membranes.[18] Many commercial monoclonal antibodies are available for routine blood grouping and, inevitably, will replace other sources of reagents as availability and cost improve with refinement of production techniques. Mixtures of monoclonal antibodies to different epitopes of the same antigen may be blended to enhance affinity.

GENETICS

Each gene has a specific locus on a given chromosome and alternate genes that occupy a single locus are alleles that are responsible for specific antigens. Blood group genes are primarily located on the 22 paired autosomes. None have been found on the Y chromosome but sex-linked *Xg* and *Xk* genes are on the X chromosome. Table 5-2 lists known chromosome assignments.[19] In all autosomal gene pairs, an individual is homozygous if both alleles are the same, or heterozygous if the alleles are dissimilar. Most blood group alleles are co-dominant and, when pres-

Table 5-2. Chromosome Assignments

Chromosome	Blood Group	ISBT	Location
1	Rh	RH	p34–p36
	Scianna	SC	p32–p34
	Duffy	FY	q22–q23
	Cromer	CROMER	q32
	Ridley		p22.1–p34
	Dolton		
2	Gerbich	GE	q14–q21
4	MNSs	MNS	q28–q31
6	Chido/Rodgers	CH/RG	p21.3
7	Colton	CO	pter–p14
	Cartwright	YT	q22
	Kell	KEL	q33
9	ABO	ABO	q34
18	Kidd	JK	q11–q12
19	Lewis	LE	p--------
	LW	LW	p13–p11
	Lutheran	LU	q12–q13
	H	H	q-------
	Secretor		
22	P	P1	q11.2–qter
X	Xg^a	XG	p22–pter
	Kx	XK	p21

Abbreviations: p, short arm of chromosome; q, long arm of chromosome; ter, terminal end.

ent, the corresponding allele is expressed. A recessive trait is only demonstrated when an individual is homozygous, as with the Bombay phenotype. Some blood group genes may code for more than one antigen. For example, Fy^a and Fy^b genes produce not only their respective antigens but a common antigen Fy3 as well.

Genes located on the same chromosome are said to be syntenic, but all genes on a single chromosome are not necessarily transmitted as a unit, since crossover of material between paired chromosomes may occur during meiosis. Alleles positioned far apart tend to segregate independently. The closer together two loci are on a chromosome, the greater the linkage and the more likely the genes are inherited as a haplotype.[20]

Antigenic expression may be altered by gene interaction. Regulator or modifier genes not necessarily located at the same locus may modify a blood group. In addition, suppressor or modifier genes may affect expression of other genes through un-

known mechanisms. Interaction of gene products from three separate loci (*H, Le,* and *Se*) determine Lewis phenotypes. *In(Lu)* is a modifying gene that inhibits expression of Lutheran antigens along with P$_1$, i, Au^a, and others. Genetic interaction also explains weakened D expression when D is in transposition to the C allele.

When two silent or amorphic alleles are inherited, the result is a null or minus-minus phenotype.[21] There are null phenotypes in most of the major human blood group systems. The most common example is group O and, except for Fy(a−b−) and Le(a−b−) in the black population, the rest are rare. Two mechanisms have been proposed to explain null phenotypes. Both are based on the assumption that at least two genes are required: a regulator gene, which produces a precursor substance, and a structural gene, which acts on precursor to produce an antigen. If the regulator gene is absent, malfunctioning, or suppressed, no precursor substance is available, even when a normal structural gene is present. This explains the Bombay phenotype, some of the Rh nulls, and the McLeod phenotype. Absence of a functioning structural gene may explain Rh deletions. Other possibilities, such as an alternate allele coding for an antigen for which there is no antisera, or a relatively rare allele, remain viable explanations in some situations.

Percentages of different phenotypes vary widely according to race and geographic boundaries. Within a population, frequency of a particular gene is based on the number of homozygous and heterozygous individuals expressed as a percentage. This information may be helpful in estimating difficulty in locating compatible blood or probability of HDN, and in paternity or forensic investigations. Population and family studies are available for references.

Genetic Pathways

Proteins are direct products of gene action; therefore, blood group antigens that result from differences in amino acid sequence are direct gene products. The situation is more complicated when antigenic specificity is derived from carbohydrates. In this instance, the gene codes for a transferase that manufactures antigen by adding a sugar to a precursor structure.

Systems that appear to be direct gene products

need no explanation, but it may be that this simple approach is possible only because their complexity is not recognized. Blood group systems that are the result of gene interaction or modifying genes are explained by proposed genetic pathways, which suggest how genes interact to form specific antigens. Each new piece of information about a system challenges the explanation; a piece either fits or an alteration in the proposed pathway must be considered. As genes involved are cloned, many questions will be answered.

BIOCHEMISTRY

Blood group antigens are composed of glycoproteins secreted in biologic fluid and adsorbed onto cells or of glycoproteins and glycolipids synthesized by the red cell. Located on the external surface of the membrane are linear or branched carbohydrate structures attached by covalent bonds to membrane lipids or proteins. These peripheral structures are easily removed from the red cell membrane for study. Less easily obtained are transmembrane integral proteins that extend across the lipid bilayer. Proteins found only on the interior side of the red cell membrane have not been associated with blood group activity.[22]

Three types of structures on red cell membranes carry blood group determinants: glyco(sphingo)lipids, glycoproteins, and proteolipids. Glycolipids are either linear, branched structures of less than 20 carbohydrate units (ABH, P, P_1, P^k), or complex and hydrosoluble structures of 30 to 60 carbohydrates, called polyglycosylceramides (ABH, Ii).[23] Other blood group determinants have been identified as glycoproteins or proteolipids. Glycophorin A carries MN and En^a antigens. Glycophorin B is associated with Ss, 'N', and U antigens. Glycophorin C and D bear Gerbich specificities. The D polypeptide with a molecular weight of 30,000 daltons is associated with red cell skeletal structure and may be a proteolipid. A slightly larger polypeptide is associated with the C and E antigens. Kell antigens appear to be on a glycoprotein with a molecular weight of 93,000 daltons, while Duffy antigens are on a glycosylated protein of 35,500 to 90,000 daltons.[19]

Red cell antigens are distributed in soluble form in serum, saliva, urine, and other tissues. ABH, Lewis, Sd^a, and Ii are found in plasma, and, if a secretor, in all body secretions. Other antigens, such as P, Chido, Rodgers, and Bg antigens, are present in plasma, but not in secretions. Red cell antigens of ABO, Ii, P, and Lewis are also expressed on platelets, but the carbohydrate determinants appear to be passively acquired by incorporation of plasma glycolipids into the platelet membrane.

On glycoproteins and glycolipids, sequences of up to seven sugars combine to form antigenic determinants. Six sugars are responsible for specificity: D-galactose, N-acetyl-D-glucosamine, N-acetylneuraminic acid, D-mannose, L-fucose, and N-acetyl-D-galactosamine. Due to the difficulty of isolating antigens from erythrocyte membranes, most biochemical identification has been done on soluble counterparts. Several blood group antigens have the same immunodominant sugar, but specificity is dependent on the entire terminal structure of the oligosaccharide and the type of linkage. D-galactose is the chief determinant of B, P_1, and P^k. L-Fucose in different configurations is responsible for H, Le^a, and Le^b specificity. N-acetyl-D-galactosamine is the immunodominant sugar of A and P specificities.

Lectins are not true antibodies but instead are sugar-binding proteins that have been important in identifying composition of antigens composed of carbohydrates. Their specificity depends on configuration and amount of steric hindrance.[24] Many lectins have been reported but only a few have proved useful in routine blood banking: *Ulex europeaeous* (H specificity), *Dolichos biflorus* (A_1 specificity), and *Vicia graminea* (N specificity).

Biosynthesis of ABH, Ii, P, and Lewis Antigens

Glycolipid antigens of these four systems are essentially derived from the same precursor by sequential addition of sugars to similar oligosaccharide chains. There are many structural similarities, and a single molecule may have both ABH and Lewis specificities.[25] A simplified version of the biosynthetic pathway is shown in Figure 5-1. It is apparent that any influence on the precursor substance could affect expression of ABH, Ii, P, or Lewis, and this may, in part, be the explanation of observed inhibition of P_1 and i antigens by *In(Lu)*. P blood group antigens (double line) are related to the other antigens but are not located on the same structures. The *Ii* genes may code for an intermediate product that is the

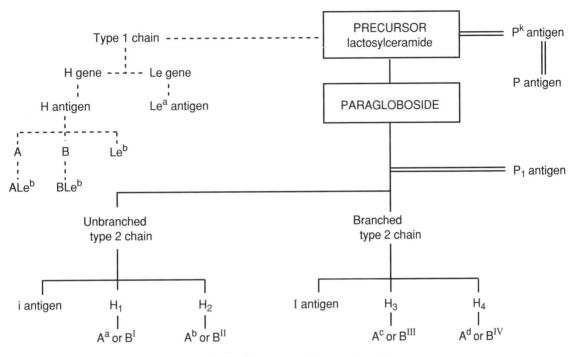

Fig. 5-1. Biosynthesis of antigens of ABO, Ii, P, and Lewis systems.

precursor of the H antigen, and therefore, of A and B antigens. The sequence, starting from the cell membrane, is P, I, H, AB, but branched glycosphingolipids are folded in their natural state, which narrows the distance in between.

Four H antigen structures have been identified: H_1 and H_2 are unbranched, whereas H_3 and H_4 are branched.[25] Since H is the substrate for A and B antigens, there are, in turn, four A and B structures. The ABH of the fetus and newborn is typically unbranched: A^a, A^b, B^I, B^{II}, H_1, H_2 with i antigen. Larger concentrations of branched ABH antigens are found on adult red cells: A^c, A^d, B^{III}, B^{IV}, H_3, H_4 with I antigen. This difference may be due to a maturation process.

Synthesis of plasma antigens (dotted line) only involves type 1 chain precursor. The level of A or B antigens in plasma is related to ABO type, secretor status, and Lewis phenotype. The secretor who is A_1, Le(a−b−) has a higher level of plasma antigens than one who is A_2 Le(a−b+). Secretors generally have greater amount of ABH substance than do nonsecretors of the same blood type.

Specificity of antibodies in these systems vary. Some (such as anti-A, anti-B, anti-H, anti-Le^a, and anti-P_1) react with the immunodominant sugar, or a complex containing this sugar, at or near the terminal end. Others, such as anti-i, react with both internal and repeating linear sequences. With branching of the structure, antibody recognition may become more complex, with some antibodies specific for different branches or reactive against all branches as seen with anti-I.

Given the close relationship of the structures, it is not surprising to find red cell specific antibodies that have a certain combination of antigens from the four systems. The most common of these is anti-IH, which requires the presence of both H and I antigens to react. Other antibodies, such as anti-IP or anti-A_1Le^b, also involve antigen combinations.

THE ABO BLOOD GROUP SYSTEM

ABO antigens are found not only on red cells but also on many other types of cells and as soluble substances in body fluids. Their biochemistry is well defined and synthesis of antigens well characterized. The reciprocal antibodies are expected when the antigen is not present. These naturally occurring antibodies are thought to be stimulated by antigens similar to A and B commonly found in nature. Unlike other blood group systems, ABO phenotypes are normally defined by both antigen on red cells and antibody in the serum.

Antigens

Four common phenotypes are encountered in routine testing: groups A, B, AB, and O. The antigens A and B are formed by addition of a group-specific sugar to H substance. Group O is a silent phenotype: nothing is added to the precursor H structure and there is no group O antigen. Reciprocal relationships exist between H antigen and ABO phenotype of the red cell. Although the original H antigen is still present, addition of A and B structures makes it less accessible. Reactivity of anti-H with red cells of different ABO groups tends to be $O > A_2 > B > A_2B > A_1 > A_1B$.

The frequency of ABO phenotypes varies in different populations and races. Overall, the white population in the United States is 44 percent group O, 44 percent group A, 9 percent group B, and 4 percent group AB. The black, Hispanic, and Oriental populations are 28 percent group A, while group B ranges from 15 to 25 percent.[26]

Antigens are not fully developed at birth and the number of antigen sites are considerably less than found on adult cells. Newborns that are genetically A_1 may appear to be type A_2 initially. It may be 6 to 18 months before the type changes to A_1. At the end of the first year, the number of antigenic sites has increased to nearly adult numbers, and by 2 to 4 years of age, adult numbers have been reached.[27]

ABH-Soluble Substances

About 80 percent of individuals secrete ABH substance in saliva. Presence of soluble A, B, and H in saliva is controlled by the *Se* locus independent of both *H* and *ABO* loci, and secretion does not require presence of an *H* gene. These glycoprotein substances are also detected in many other body secretions, including tears, urine, bile, milk, amniotic fluid, and some pathological fluids. In each individual, the amount of substance varies widely in differ-

ent secretions. A, B, and H antigens found in plasma as glycosphingolipids[28] are detectable regardless of secretor status, but plasma of a nonsecretor contains less ABH substance than plasma of a secretor.

ABO Subgroups

About 80 percent of A and AB phenotypes belong to subgroup A_1, with the remaining almost entirely A_2. Again, this varies with the population. A_2 is nearly absent in oriental populations while Lapps have an increased percentage of A_2 subgroups. The immunodominant sugar, N-acetyl-D-galactosamine, is identical for both A_1 and A_2. It appears that the distinction between the two is partly a quantitative difference in number and distribution of antigen sites on the erythrocyte. Some reagents recognize only a quantitative difference.[29] The argument of whether this difference is also qualitative has not been laid to rest; it is difficult to totally dismiss this idea given that anti-A_1 is formed by group A_2 individuals and the A_1 and A_2 transferases are different (Table 5-3).

Subgroups may be classified by their serological reactivity with anti-A, anti-B, anti-AB, anti-A_1, and anti-H. The amount of H detectable in weaker subgroups is inversely proportional to strength of reactivity with anti-A or anti-B. Often the only evidence that a subgroups may exist is a discrepancy between cell type and the expected reciprocal serum type. Definitive workups include saliva inhibition, adsorption and elution, transferase levels, and family studies. Commercial monoclonal ABO grouping reagents are superior to polyclonal human sera in that they detect weak subgroups more easily.

Subgroups of A are summarized in Table 5-4.[30,31] Group A intermediates (A_{int}) have some properties of both A_1 and A_2 antigens, and are relatively common in the black population. A_3 gives a characteristic mixed-field reactivity described as small agglutinates in a sea of unagglutinated cells while A_x is distinguished by stronger reactions with anti-A, B than with anti-A. In the weaker subgroups, specificity may only be demonstrable by adsorption and elution of anti-A. In addition to those included in the table, A_{bantu} and A_{finn} are considered to be variants of A_{end}. The unusual A_{pae} variant is thought to be a small piece of the normal A antigen.[32]

Although more variability is found with B antigen

Table 5-3. Comparison of A_1 and A_2 Red Blood Cells

Characteristics	A_1	A_2
Quantitative differences		
Anti-A	+ + + +	+ + +
Antigen sites adult	0.8×10^6	0.2×10^6
Qualitative differences		
A_1 lectin	+ + +	Negative
Anti-A_1 in serum	None	Sometimes
Antigenic structure	Type 1 and 2 chains	Type 2 chains only
Antigenic determinants	A^a, A^b, A^c, A^d	A^a, A^b only
Transferase activity	Active	Less active
	Optimal pH 6	Optimal pH 7
Transferase cofactor	Mn^{++} and Mg^{++}	Mg^{++} only
Isoelectric focus	pI 9–10	pI 6–7
Gene	A^1 gene	A^2 gene[a]

[a] Cloned gene differs by a single base substitution.

than with A antigen, there are no comparable B_1 or B_2 antigens. Rare subgroups of B do exist, but there has been little consistency in description and definition is complicated by apparent heterogeneity within the B group as a whole. Thermodynamic methods demonstrate a wide range of B-antigen agglutinability from one family to another, but this reactivity is consistent within a family.[33] Percentage of agglutination may be used to classify weak subgroups of B into B_{60}, B_{20}, and B_0. Others recommend use of terminology parallel to that used to describe A subgroups: B_3, B_x, B_{el}, and B_m (Table 5-5).[30,31] There is no proven equivalent to A_{end} or A_y, but a B variant similar to A_{pae} has been reported.

Classification of A and B subgroups provides a convenient method for discussion but actually may have limited meaning. Within each subgroup, there is a range of antigenic strength; this heterogeneity is inherited within a family. Although most subgroups fall into defined categories, many weakened expressions of A and B antigens may be unique and defy classification.

Antibodies

With the exception of group AB or newborns, agglutinins are normally present in plasma. The presence of anti-A is expected in the sera of individuals whose cells lack the A antigen and anti-B is expected in

Table 5-4. Characteristics of A Subgroups

Group	Anti-A	Anti-A,B	Anti-H	Saliva	Transferase	Remarks
A_1	+ + + +	+ + + +	Negative	A/H	A_1	A_1 lectin + + + +
A_2	+ + + +	+ + + +	+ +	A/H	A_2	A_1 lectin negative
A_{mt}	+ + + +	+ + + +	+ + +	A/H	Present	A_1 lectin + +
A_3	+ +^{mf}	+ +^{mf}	+ + +	A/H	Weak-to-none[a]	Anti-A_1 occ. in serum
A_x	+^{w}	+ +	+ + + +	(A_x)/H	Very weak	Anti-A_1 present
A_m[b]	0/+^{w}	0/+^{w}	+ + + +	A/H	A_1 most; few A_2	Anti-A_1 not found
A_y[b]	0/+^{w}	0/+^{w}	+ + + +	A/H	Present	Anti-A_1 not found
A_{end}[b]	+^{w} (1%)	+^{w} (1%)	+ + + +	H	None	Anti-A_1 occ. in serum
A_{el}[b]	0	0	+ + + +	H	None	Anti-A_1 usually present

Abbreviations: mf, mixed field; w, weak reactivity.
[a] Three different types are found: weak reactivity at pH 7, no reactivity, 50% normal activity at pH 6.
[b] Adsorption/elution may be necessary to demonstrate A specificity.

Table 5-5. Characteristics of B Subgroups

Group	Anti-B	Anti-A,B	Anti-H	Saliva	Tranferase	Remarks
B	+ + + +	+ + + +	+ +	B/H	Normal	
B_3	+ +^{mf}	+ +^{mf}	+ + +	B/H	Weak	
B_x	0/+^{w}	+/+ +	+ + +	H	None	Weak anti-B in serum
$B_m{}^a$	0	0	+ + +	B/H	Weak	
$B_{el}{}^a$	0	0	+ + +	H	None	Weak anti-B sometimes

Abbreviations: mf, mixed field; w, weak.
^{a} Adsorption and elution may be necessary to demonstrate B specificity.

those who lack the B antigen. Combinations of IgM and IgG are found; either immunoglobulin fixes complement and causes hemolysis. Concentration of antibody varies considerably but, in general, anti-A titers are higher than anti-B titers. In blacks, both anti-A and anti-B titers are consistently higher with anti-B levels equivalents to anti-A levels found in whites.[34]

Anti-A and anti-B not derived from mother have been detected in cord samples;[35] however, antibodies produced by infant are not readily demonstrable until 3 to 6 months. Maximum level is reached between 5 and 10 years, after which time the levels fall as the individual ages. IgG levels continue to persist, while IgM levels tend to disappear with aging. This observation is challenged by a recent study that concluded ABO antibodies were present in significant amounts in healthy elderly patients. If absent, a further explanation, other than age, may be found in most instances.[36]

Higher than normal antibody levels are found in autoimmune hemolytic anemia, alcoholic cirrhosis, and chronic active hepatitis. Antibody concentration is lower than normal in myeloma, Waldenström's disease, chronic lymphocytic leukemia, and other immunodeficiencies. Hypogammaglobulinemia is a common cause of decreased or absent antibody.[37]

Red cell stimulation and pregnancy may result in immune forms of antibodies with higher than normal titers that persist for long periods. The immune antibody produced in an A or B individual is primarily IgM but in group O is predominantly IgG. Because of exposure of antigens similar to A and B throughout life, an individual can develop high-titer, immune antibody without red cell stimulation. This is observed more often with anti-A than anti-B and the most commonly identified causes are vaccines and bacterial agents.

Anti-A,B found in group O sera is predominantly IgG capable of crossing the placenta. Although some have suggested that anti-A,B is a combination of anti-A and anti-B, it appears that the antibody reacts with a structure common to both antigens.[38] A and B antigens are structurally very similar and antibody formed by a group O person is developed against a shared portion, resulting in an antibody that is capable of reacting with either or both antigens.

Anti-A from a group B or group O person is a mixture of anti-A_1 and anti-A. This anti-A_1 is IgG, while anti-A_1 formed by a group A_2 individual is primarily IgM and does not react at 37°C. About 8 percent of group A_2 and 25 percent of A_2B have detectable anti-A_1. Anti-A_1 reactive at 37°C may develop in a small number of A_2 individuals after transfusion.[39] Although this antibody is characteristically biphasic and often only destroys a limited amount of A_1 red cells (leaving the majority with normal survival rates), a few hemolytic reactions have been reported. Passively infused anti-A_1 has been implicated in destruction of subsequently transfused A_1 cells.

Anti-H produced by A_1, B, or A_1B individuals is almost always a cold reactive autoantibody and not associated with significant red cell destruction. Allo-anti-H formed by the Bombay phenotype is a potent hemolysin reactive at 37°C and a cause of accelerated red cell destruction in vivo. Anti-IH reacts only with cells carrying both H and I specificities and is not uncommon during pregnancy. A more potent anti-IH is invariably found in the serum of H-deficient phenotypes.[31]

Anti-A and anti-B are occasionally found as harmless, cold autoantibodies, but intravascular hemolysis has been documented in a few instances. Anti-A$_1$ has been reported as an autoantibody.[40]

Genetics

The *A*, *B*, and *O* genes have been cloned. Both *O* and *B* mutated from the *A* gene. Near the N-terminus, a single deletion occurred, resulting in the *O* gene. The *B* gene differs from the *A* gene by a series of four single base substitutions. The *A^2* gene is a single base deletion from the *A^1* gene. It is probable that base substitutions account for other A and B subgroups.[7]

Four alleles (*A^1*, *A^2*, *B*, and *O*) are responsible for the majority of ABO blood groups, with 10 genotypes and six phenotypes. An individual's genotype is not always obvious. The phenotype A$_1$ could be *A^{1}A^1*, *A^{1}A^2*, or *A^{1}O* genetically, or even *A^1* combined with a weaker subgroup allele. *A* and *B* alleles are codominant and are expressed when present. Classically, *A^1* is considered dominant over the *A^2* allele but, even though an *A^{1}A^2* may appear to be A$_1$, both A$_1$ and A$_2$ enzymes are present in serum. Expression of A$_2$ antigen is hidden by A$_1$ antigen. Other A and B subgroups are masked unless paired with an *O* gene. Despite proposed models based on aberrant ABO phenotypes, it is generally accepted that alleles at the *ABO* locus are responsible.

Mosaicism has been reported in which two populations of red cells with different ABO phenotypes are inherited,[41] probably the result of rare alleles at the *ABO* locus. Chimerism or dispermy has been ruled out since this is an inherited characteristic.

There are well-documented cases in which *A* and *B* genes have been inherited on a single chromosome.[42,43] These may have arisen from an unequal crossover involving an *A* gene on one chromosome and a *B* gene on the other, or by mutation. The *AB$_{cis}$* allele is the predominant explanation for the occurrence of AB children from an *AB* × *O* mating.

Anomalies in ABO inheritance have been reported. The A$_y$ phenotype[44] appears to be the result of a recessive characteristic at another genetic locus, *Y*, independent of the *ABO* locus. Absence of a *Y* gene prevents normal expression of A antigens on the red cell. Dominant suppression of A and B has been described where red cells type group O, regardless of genotype.[45] A variety of situations result in unexpected phenotypes in family studies. A$_x$ has

been transmitted by an A$_2$B parent.[46] A$_x$ children have been born to group O parents.[23] No convincing explanations have been given for all of these contradictory inheritance patterns.

H Phenotypes

A functional *H* gene is necessary for formation of A and B antigens despite ABO genotype and presence of A or B transferases. The *H* gene has been cloned but the actual mechanism for regulation is as yet unknown. Without H substance there is little or no expression of A or B antigens on red cells. There are several H-deficient phenotypes known.[31]

The classic Bombay phenotype (O$_h$) is characterized by absence of A, B, or H antigens on red cells and in secretions, but anti-H is present in serum in addition to anti-A and anti-B. Synthesis of A and B antigens is blocked by the absence of precursor substance (H) necessary for their expression. These red cells react very strongly with anti-I, possibly because I receptors are more readily accessible. Absence of ABH antigens in this phenotype is not associated with membrane defect or changes in red cell survival but serum antibody makes transfusion difficult. All red cells except those from another Bombay phenotype are grossly incompatible. Frequency of the classic Bombay phenotype is about 1 in 13,000 in India but is rarely found in other populations.

Parabombay individuals demonstrate weak H antigens along with weak A or B antigens on red cells, but there is no H substance in saliva. Frequency of this phenotype in Thailand was about 1 in 5,000 normal donors. Mode of inheritance may be a rare allele at the *H* locus, which produces a limited amount of H antigen. Two other H-deficient phenotypes, Hz and Hm, have weak H antigens on cells with normal levels of H substance in saliva.[47,48] All H-deficient phenotypes are recessive characteristics with the exception of the H$_m$ Bombay.

Biochemistry

Gene products of the *ABO* locus are glycosyltransferases. The *A* gene produces *N*-acetylgalactosaminyl transferase which attaches *N*-acetylgalactosamine to the H determinant. The *B* gene produces D-galactosaminyl transferase that attaches D-galactosamine

Table 5-6. Biochemical Structure of Precursor and ABH Antigens

Chain/Antigen	Structure
Precursor chain[a]	CER-GALNAc-GAL-GLCNAc-GAL
H antigen	CER-GALNAc-GAL-GLCNAc-GAL $\vert$ FUC
A antigen	CER-GALNAc-GAL-GLCNAc-GAL-GALNAc $\vert$ FUC
B antigen	CER-GALNAc-GAL-GLCNAc-GAL-GAL $\vert$ FUC

[a] Precursor chains are type 1 or type 2 that differ in linkage of terminal galactose. Types 1 and 2 are found in secretions, body fluids, and tissues. Only type 2 chains are synthesized by the red cell; type 1 chains found on red cells are adsorbed from plasma.
Abbreviations: GAL, galactose; GALNAc, N-acetylgalactosamine; GLCNAc, N-acetylglucosamine; FUC, fucose; CER, ceramide.

to the H determinant (Table 5-6). The O gene product is a nonfunctional enzyme that adds nothing to the H structure. Determining transferases present in plasma may elucidate genotype in some cases since the transferase is present even when expression of antigen is masked.

Two A transferases have been isolated with different biochemical properties[49] (Table 5-3). The A_1 transferase is more efficient in adding the immunodominant sugar to H, and converts unbranched and branched H structures, forming four types of A antigens: A^a, A^b, A^c, and A^d. The A_2 enzyme only converts unbranched H structures into A^a and A^b antigens, leaving H_3 and H_4 antigens.[25] Red cells from newborns are deficient in branched H structures (H_3 and H_4); this is a possible explanation for the A_2 phenotype found in newborns that are genetically A^1. It is speculated that anti-A_1 might recognize A^c and A^d antigens present in an A_1 but not an A_2 individual. Others suggest that there is only a secondary modification rather than an actual difference between the two transferases, supporting the idea of a quantitative rather than a qualitative difference between A_1 and A_2 cells.

There are also two B enzymes with the same optimal pH and same cofactor. Four B antigens are formed from the four H structures: B^I, B^{II}, B^{III}, and B^{IV}. Results of transferase studies in B subgroups are comparable with those of A subgroups.[4,49]

Levels of transferases are decreased in pregnancy which corresponds with an observed weakening of red cell antigens.[50] Although transferase levels in newborns are higher than those found in the nonpregnant adult, there is a decrease in antigen sites that is most likely due to lack of substrate. Approximately 20 percent of blacks are known to have very strong B antigens with higher levels of B transferase.

At least 25 hematopoietic chimeras have been recognized in dizygotic twins, the result of a graft of hematopoietic tissue from one twin to the other in utero. Since this condition only affects red cells, the contribution of bone marrow cells to transferase levels can be estimated as the source of 20 to 30 percent of transferase, with the remainder contributed by other tissues.[51] This is confirmed by studies of A_m and B_m phenotypes, but the primary site of synthesis has not been identified.

Group AB Phenotypes

A and B enzymes vie for H substrate in the presence of each other. At least two factors affect synthesis of A and B antigens in group AB individuals. The B enzyme is more efficient than the A enzyme and there are indications that the B enzyme may have an inhibitory affect on the A enzyme. Weakened expression of A antigen is commonly observed in *trans*-AB phenotypes (A and B alleles on separate chromosomes). In the presence of a strong B-specified transferase, red cells may have the phenotype A_2B or possibly A_3B even with an A^1B genotype.[52] The genotype A^2B frequently appears to be A_3B or a weaker $A_{sub}B$ serologically. This leads to a relatively common error in determining blood group, since the weak A antigen may be overlooked. If an A^1 allele is paired with a weaker B allele, expression of the B antigen may be suppressed with a resulting A_1B_3 phenotype. Allelic enhancement has also been known to occur. In one case, an apparently normal A antigen in a group AB individual was expressed in the second generation as A_x when paired with an O gene.

The *cis*-AB phenotype results from a single allele

producing both the A and B antigen.[42,43] In most, the A and/or B antigens are weaker than expected. Two types of *cis*-AB phenotypes have been identified. The first produces a single abnormal enzyme caused by a structural mutation at the *ABO* locus. In the second, both A and B enzymes are present as the result of unequal crossover during meiosis. In most *cis*-AB, the B antigen is abnormal and alloanti-B is present in serum.

Acquired B phenotype has been described in numerous A_1 patients in relationship with gastrointestinal disorders. Anti-B is present but does not react with patient's own red cells. Two mechanisms are believed to be responsible for this: in one, a bacterial deacetylase[53] converts A antigen into galactosamine, which cross-reacts with anti-B, or, in the other, B-like substances[54] passively absorbs onto red cells of group A or group O individuals with *Proteus vulgaris* or *Escherichia coli* infections.

Acquired A antigen is associated with Tn polyagglutinability of group B or O red blood cells. The A-like antigen reacts with human and some monoclonal anti-A reagents but reactivity is destroyed by proteolytic enzymes.

In addition, there are reports of overlapping activity[55] with A and B transferases when tested with potent monoclonal antibodies. Under certain conditions or with an extremely active transferase, a small amount of the "wrong" antigen may be produced. In the presence of strong B transferases, a weak A antigen may be detected.[7] B determinants may be found in a group A individual with a strong H-transferase.

Clinical Significance

Transfusion with ABO-incompatible red cells is extremely serious; even small amounts may be fatal, especially in a debilitated recipient. Destruction of red cells is intravascular and immediate, and may trigger disseminated intravascular coagulation, renal failure, and death. The most common cause of mistransfusion is not technical error, but clerical mistakes.

ABO antibodies that cross the placenta are the most common cause of HDN. Fortunately, it is also the mildest form, rarely producing clinical disease. HDN is seen in group A or B offspring of group O mothers and may occur with the first pregnancy.

ABO incompatibility between mother and fetus offers protection against development of anti-D by removing fetal cells from maternal circulation before triggering an immune response.[56] If an Rh-negative mother of an Rh-positive child are ABO compatible, the mother is more likely to develop anti-D unless Rh immune globulin is administered. It is unclear whether this happens with other antibodies.

The importance of ABO in transplantation is variable.[57] Hyperacute rejection of an ABO-incompatible renal or heart transplant is initiated within minutes by recipient antibody while an ABO-incompatible liver may be successfully transplanted. However, successful renal transplants from A_2 donors into group O recipients have been documented. ABO-incompatible bone marrow requires additional manipulation for infusion but may successfully engraft since ABH antigens are not expressed on hematopoietic stem cells in any quantity. With the shift of ABO type to that of the marrow donor, ABO discrepancies due to bone marrow transplantation are becoming relatively common. A "pseudoautoantibody" of donor graft origin has been observed with ABO-minor mismatched transplants managed with cyclosporin. If viable donor lymphocytes of an organ from a group O donor transplanted to a group A recipient continues to produce anti-A and anti-B, there may be significant hemolysis of the recipient's group A red cells, even to the point of requiring exchange transfusion with group O red cells.

The role of ABH antigens[58] is difficult to define, but correlations with disease susceptibility and disease state do exist and may be prognostic. Acquisition of new antigens is associated with bacterial enzymes. There are quantitative variations of ABH antigens in neoplastic tissue and changes in phenotype are observed with hematopoietic disorders.

Numerous relationships between ABH antigens and widely diverse diseases ranging from infection to malignancy have been established both directly and indirectly. There is a 20 percent greater chance of cancer of the stomach in group A individuals compared with those of group O. Similar statistics are found in carcinomas of the colon, rectum, ovary, uterus, and cervix. An even higher (60 percent) incidence is seen with cancer of the salivary glands.[59]

Group O individuals are much more susceptible to bleeding duodenal and gastric ulcers. Duodenal ulceration occurs 50 percent more often in nonsecretors. Factor VIII levels are highest in group A, while group O has the lowest von Willebrand factor antigen levels. Thromboembolic disorders and acute myocardial infarcts occur more frequency in group A. Female group A and AB nonsecretors may be susceptible to recurring urinary tract infections and it is possible that those who lack anti-B may not be resistant to organisms with B-like antigens.[60]

Surface neoantigens or neoplastic cells, different from the antigens on normal cells derived from the same tissue, may be biochemically similar to the ABO system and may be accompanied by a decrease or absence of normal ABO antigen. A-like activity in adenocarcinoma is seen with group O and group B individuals. Acquired B phenotype is associated with gastrointestinal malignancies and alimentary infections. High levels of ABH and Lewis antigenic activity matching patient's own blood group have been detected in purified preparations of carcinoembryonic antigen (CEA) found in carcinoma of the colon. Disappearance of ABH antigens from epithelial tumor cells precedes development of metastases; continued presence of ABH antigens is considered a favorable sign.[61]

Hematopoietic disorders are known to alter the phenotypic expression of ABH antigens. Weakened expression of A and B are observed with leukemia, Hodgkin's disease, and aplastic anemia. Alterations may help predict outcome, classify leukemias, and determine type of malignancy. Loss or decrease in ABH antigenic expression indicates more aggressive malignancies with poorer prognoses. ABH anomalies are seen in myeloid rather than lymphoid disorders. Partial or complete loss of A or B antigens in patients with hypoplastic or sideroblastic anemia are very significant, since the patient frequently progresses to acute leukemia when this occurs.

In acute leukemia or preleukemia, mixed-field agglutination has been observed. Modification of ABH antigens may be related to reduction in levels of glycosyltransferase. Unlike A and B transferases, the source of H transferase is almost entirely hematopoietic and, with few exceptions, ABH antigenic alteration in hematopoietic disorders correlates with H-enzyme activity. A and B levels remain within normal limits while H-enzyme is markedly decreased. H-enzyme level rises again during clinical remission.[62]

THE I BLOOD GROUP COLLECTION

I and i are not antithetical: rather, the antigens are related structures. The i antigen is the precursor of I much the same as H is to A or B. There is also biochemical evidence that I and i are precursors of ABH antigens.[63] ISBT has designated Ii as an antigen collection rather than a blood group system.

Antigens

The two antigens, I and i, are high-frequency antigens with reactivity inversely proportional to each other. At birth, the newborn's red cells have a large amount of i antigen with almost undetectable I antigen. I increases as i decreases, until about 18 months, when red cells test I positive with little detectable i antigen. A few rare adults continue to have almost undetectable I antigen levels.

There are five classic phenotypes classified by reactivity with anti-I and anti-i: I, I intermediate, i_{cord}, i_2, and i_1. The normal adult phenotype is I; i_{cord} is the normal newborn phenotype. A very small percentage of adults react moderately with both anti-I and anti-i; they are designated I intermediate. The rarest phenotype, i_1, fails to react with anti-I and is found in less than 1 in 10,000 white adults. Another rare phenotype, i_2, reacts weakly with anti-I and is found in about 1 in 10,000 black adults.[4]

Other I specificities have been determined by reactivity on cord and adult cells. I^D (developed) is expressed on adult red cells, but not on i cord or i adult red cells. I^F (fetal) is expressed on both adult and cord cells, but not on i adult cells. I^T (transitional) is present during transformation of i to I, although "transitional" may not be an appropriate term, since fetal cells react more strongly with anti-I^T. I^S is secreted antigen, neutralized by saliva, human colostrum, and milk.[63]

Antigens of the I system are heterogeneous, and the amount of I antigen on red cells of different individuals varies. All I positive persons have some i and I^T antigen. The I antigen is poorly developed on cord red cells, but is usually present in trace amounts. It has been shown that i reactivity is increased in normal adults when bone marrow activity is increased by repeated phlebotomies[63] and that i reactivity becomes weaker as red cells age in circulation.[65]

I and i substances are found in many biologic fluids. In soluble form, they are present in serum, saliva, milk, amniotic fluid, urine, ovarian fluid, and hydatid cyst fluid. In contrast to red cell antigen activity the level of soluble I and i substances is the same in both adults and newborns. The level of I in secretions is greater among ABH secretors but this is not reflected in strength of expression on red cells.

Antibodies

Anti-I is found as a weak cold IgM autoantibody in the serum of most healthy individuals or as a potent cold IgM autoantibody implicated in acquired hemolytic anemia. Monoclonal antibody in cold hemagglutinin disease (CHD) commonly has anti-I specificity. Anti-I is also found as a weak alloantibody in the serum of most i adults but is not clinically significant, although increased clearance of normal I adult red cells was reported in one case.[66]

Anti-i was first described in the serum of a patient with reticulocytosis. It is common in the sera of patients with infectious mononucleosis and has been reported in myeloid leukemia and alcoholic cirrhosis.[67] Alloanti-i has not been reported.

It is difficult to classify strong cold autoagglutinins since their specificity ranges from entirely anti-I to entirely anti-i with combinations in between. Rarely, a sera will contain both anti-I and anti-i that is separable by adsorption.

A relatively potent anti-I^T possibly associated with parasitic infestation has been found in several populations, including the Melanesians and Yanomama Indians of Venezuela.[68] IgG anti-I^T has been detected in Hodgkin's patients with hemolytic anemia.

Genetics

It is unlikely that i and I result from alternate alleles. No single sugar has been identified with I or i specificity. A genetic pathway has not been defined, but the complex, repetitive glycosylation and branching needed to form the antigens suggest that a sequence is involved. Conversion of i to I may require at least 2 glycosylation steps to complete the branching process, and specific glycosylation steps are necessary for biosynthesis of i structure by assembling a linear sequence of repeating sugars.[69] The *I* gene may control the ability to convert i to I. Those that lack the gene would be adult i phenotypes. This is consistent

with several family pedigrees but too many adult i phenotypes have been found for this to be the only explanation.

Ii-deficient phenotypes with a dominant inheritance pattern have been described. The I-i- phenotype[70] is characterized by weak reactions with both anti-I and anti-i isand may be designated I-weak, i-weak, instead.

It has been suggested that presence of antigens on red cells and substance in secretions may be under separate genetic control, since levels of I and i substance do not correspond with levels on the red cell. The adult i phenotype has been shown to have the same level of I substance in milk and saliva as is found with I+ phenotypes.

Biochemistry

Even though the biochemistry of Ii has been partially clarified, specific glycosyltransferases have not been isolated. The i determinant is a straight oligosaccharide chain with repeating D-galactose-*N*-acetyl-D-glucosamine sequences attached to ceramide or protein. A branch of D-galactose-*N*-acetyl-D-galactosamine attached to the middle galactose of unbranched I determinant results in I specificity; up to five branches may be added per chain. The complexity and variety found in these structures suggest that heterogeneity of Ii antibodies is due not only to heterogeneity of carbohydrate sequences but also to the fact that antibodies are directed toward narrow domains within the antigenic determinant. Substitutions on terminal residues also appear to alter Ii specificity.

Clinical Significance

Anti-I and anti-i are generally not significant antibodies but anti-I and rarely anti-i may become significant in autoimmune hemolytic anemia with increased complement binding and thermal range of reactivity. The I system plays a very large role in CHD with very potent autoantibodies are capable of causing hemolysis. There are two forms of CHD seen: chronic with persistent production of monoclonal anti-I or acute following *Mycoplasma* or viral infections with transient product of polyclonal anti-I.[63] Leukopenia and thrombocytopenia occasionally seen in CHD may represent destruction by autoantibody since Ii antigens are present on white cells and platelets.

Anti-I has not been implicated in HDN, possibly because the newborn is I deficient. Rare cases of IgG anti-i that did cross the placenta have been reported, but these did not cause significant red cell destruction.

Anti-I[T] is found in Hodgkin's disease complicated by hemolytic anemia. Collected case reports of hemolytic anemias with cold autoagglutinins consistent with anti-I[T] specificity indicate that I[T] may be an important target for autoimmunity.[63]

Many variations in Ii strength are observed on cells of patients with various diseases, including hematologic malignancy. Both enhancement and depression of reactivity may occur. Reduction of I together with an increase in i reactivity on red cells has been reported in preleukemic and leukemic patients and in myeloproliferative diseases. Enhanced I antigen without changes in i reactivity has been reported in these same diseases. Increased i reactivity is seen in infectious mononucleosis, megaloblastic anemia, and HEMPAS.[60,71]

Even in the early stages of chronic lymphocytic leukemia, the amount of i antigen on lymphocytes is greatly reduced. Normal amounts are found on blasts of patients with acute lymphocytic leukemia and lymphosarcoma cell leukemia. Determining i antigen level may be helpful in diagnosis.[72]

The genes that code for i and autosomal congenital cataracts appear to be linked in Oriental populations, but not necessarily other populations.

Transient anti-I is found during infections with *Mycoplasma pneumoniae*. Hemolysis is usually self-limiting but can be dramatic and fatalities have occurred. Even though an I antigen cannot be demonstrated on the organism, it is possible that there are small amounts of I antigen present, or that an I cryptogen may be exposed by enzymatic activity. The antibody appears to be an immune response to the organism.

Transient, low-titer anti-i with a low thermal range is commonly found in the sera of patients with infectious mononucleosis. Rarely, autoimmune hemolysis occurs due to anti-i.

Drug-induced hemolysis involving I antigen has been reported, where binding of drug–antidrug complex is facilitated by the presence of I. This has been demonstrated with dexchlorpheniramine maleate, rifampicin, nomifensine, and nitrofurantoin.[63]

COLD-REACTING AUTOAGGLUTININS OTHER THAN Ii

The Pr series of antigens was first designated Sp for species, since it was thought that this specificity was common only to humans. The antigens were later found on red cells of nonhuman species and the name was changed to PR to reflect the fact that the antibody defines an antigen denatured by proteases. N-Acetyl-neuraminic acid (NeuNAc) appears to be the immunodominant carbohydrate and there is strong evidence that Pr antigenic determinants are carried on red cell glycophorins. Whereas reactivity of Ii is enhanced by all proteolytic enzymes, Pr activity is destroyed.

Gd, Sa, Fl, and Lud cold agglutinins also define a determinant with NeuNAc as the immunodominant sugar. Vo and Li cold agglutinins recognize sialic acid-dependent antigens expressed only on red cells of newborns.

These autoantibodies are included in the specificities of cold autoagglutinins associated with autoimmune hemolytic anemias. While the total incidence is low, most cold agglutinins not directed against Ii antigens have anti-Pr specificity. These antibodies are not found in healthy individuals; most follow a viral infection. Both low- and high-titer antibodies are observed and are oligoclonal or monoclonal. Low-titer cold agglutinins are probably of little significance, but high-titer anti-Pr has been found with chronic cold agglutinin disease and may be a symptom of benign gammopathy or B-cell lymphoma. A few have caused increased red cell destruction but there are also high-titer autoantibodies with Pr specificity that are clinically insignificant.[73]

THE LEWIS SYSTEM

Lewis is not primarily a blood group system but consists of soluble antigens in body fluids that are absorbed onto erythrocytes from plasma. Lewis also differs from other systems in that *Lele* interacts with *Hh* and *Sese* loci to produce Lewis antigens.

Antigens

Le^a antigen is found in about 22 percent of the population while 52 to 72 percent, depending on race, test positive for Le^b antigen. Approximately 6 percent of the white population and up to 28 percent of the black population are negative for both antigens. Testing with anti-Le^a and anti-Le^b identifies three common phenotypes: Le(a+b−), Le(a−b+), and Le(a−b−) Table 5-7.[2]

Many human cells are able to produce Lewis antigens, but the red cell is not one of them. In chimeras, observed Lewis type is indicative of true genotype, since red cells engrafted in utero do not contribute to Lewis phenotype.[74] In the presence of an *Le* gene, mucus cells, especially in the salivary gland, make and secrete a soluble glycoprotein with Le^a specificity. Interaction of genes at other loci is responsible for production of Le^b antigen. The glycoprotein antigen found in saliva is not adsorbed onto red cells, as is the glycosphingolipid secreted in plasma.[75] Even when Le^b antigen is formed, minute quantities of Le^a still remain in plasma and are adsorbed onto red cell, causing a trace amount of Le^a antigen to be detectable along with Le^b antigen.[76]

Other Lewis antigens have been described but these are not true antigens of the Lewis system, since the antibodies that define these antigens actually have other specificities. Most likely, Le^x is Le^a antigen. Le^c is unconverted type 1 chain and Le^d is type 1 H determinant.[4] Le^x and Le^y, specificities associated with malignancies, are type 2 chains.[60]

Rare examples of the unusual phenotype Le(a+b+) have been found in Southeast Asian countries. This occurs in Le(a−b+) individuals with an extremely efficient *Le* gene, or a defective *H/Se* gene-specified transferase that produces sufficient levels of both Le^a and Le^b, so that both are adsorbed onto red cells in detectable quantities.[77]

Development of Lewis Antigens After Birth

Lewis antigens are known to be synthesized by the fetus. Le^a and Le^b substance is detectable in the saliva of newborns, although there are no demonstrable Lewis antigens in plasma until about 10 days of life. Newborn infants do not have detectable Lewis antigens on red cells and typically type Le(a−b−). However, using an antiglobulin test system, 50 percent of infants typed at birth are Le(a+), while 80 percent type Le(a+) at 2 months, 45 percent at 1 year, and 22 percent at 2 to 3 years of age.[78] The increased number of Le(a+) may result from the use of antisera containing anti-Le^x.

It is thought that at about 2 months, the transferase coded for by the *Le* gene must be present in sufficient quantities to make Le^a, while H/Se-specified transferase production begins to reach adult levels at 1 year, as evidenced by a decrease in the number of Le(a+) persons. In the months in which production of Le^b is just the beginning, a child may type Le(a+b+) and this may continue until normal adult levels of Le^b substance are reached by 7 years of age.[78]

Lewis Antigens During Pregnancy

There is a decrease in expression of Lewis antigens on red cells during pregnancy. Some Le(a−b+) women (most often group A$_1$) may lose Le^b activity

Table 5-7. Interaction of Lewis, Secretor, and H Systems

Genes Present	Lewis Saliva Antigens	Lewis RBC Antigens	Lewis Phenotype	% Frequency White	% Frequency Black
Le, sese, H	Le^a	Le^a	Le(a+b−)		
Le, Se, hh	Le^a	Le^a	Le(a+b−)	22	20
Le, sese, hh	Le^a	Le^a	Le(a+b−)		
Le, Se, H	Le^a, Le^b	Le^b	Le(a − b +)	72	52
lele, Se, H	Type 1H	Type 1H	Le(a−b−c−d+)		
lele, sese, H	Type 1 chain	Type 1 chain	Le(a−b−c+d−)	6	28
lele, Se, hh	Type 1 chain	Type 1 chain	Le(a−b−c+d−)		
lele, sese, hh	Type 1 chain	Type 1 chain	Le(a−b−c+d−)		

altogether and type Le(a−b−) while pregnant. A greater fraction of Le[b] substance is bound by lipoproteins during pregnancy, leaving a much smaller quantity available for adsorption onto the red cell.[79] This may reach a level in which the quantity of Le[b] adsorbed is not detectable. Anti-Le[b] may form when red cell antigen level is decreased, but red cell phenotype usually reverts to original type after delivery and the antibody disappears.

Transfused Red Cells

Loss of Lewis antigens from transfused cells has been observed in vivo. Red cells with Le[a] or Le[b] antigens transfused into a Le(a−b−) recipient have been shown to lose Lewis specificity by the 7th day. Uptake of recipient's Lewis type has also been demonstrated on transfused cells after 5 days in circulation.[75] The continual exchange of glycolipids between red cell membrane and plasma is responsible for this conversion of phenotype.

Antibodies

Antibodies of the Lewis system are naturally occurring IgM antibodies that bind complement; a few may even cause in vitro hemolysis. Lewis antibodies are seen frequently during pregnancy. They often have an IgG fraction that crosses the placenta but does not cause HDN because of the Lewis status of newborns.[80]

Anti-Le[a] is a relatively common antibody found in up to 20 percent of people who are genetically *lele* and secrete H substance. It is detected more often in blacks because there is a higher incidence of Le(a−b−) in that population. Individuals with the Le(a−b+) phenotype do not form anti-Le[a], since it is not a foreign antigen; they have Le[a] substance in saliva and a trace amount of Le[a] antigen present on red cells. Secretor status may have an affect, since anti-Le[a] is most often made when the *Se* gene is present, but this observation has not been fully explained. Anti-Le[a] active at 37°C or causing hemolysis in vitro may cause an acute hemolytic reaction but delayed reactions are not seen.[7]

Anti-Le[b] is often seen as a weak antibody in the presence of a strong anti-Le[a] and is relatively common in individuals of the phenotype Le(a−b−) who are nonsecretors of ABH substance. Le(a−b−) secretors are possibly protected from forming anti-Le[b] because they have type 1 H (Le[d]) which is similar to Le[b].[2] Some examples of very strong anti-Le[a] with weak anti-Le[b] may be explained as very potent anti-Le[a] reacting with small amounts of Le[a] antigen adsorbed onto cells of a person who is phenotypically Le(a−b+). This also may be due to anti-Le[x].[2,4]

Two distinct variations of anti-Le[b] are encountered. Anti-Le[bL] reacts with all Le(b+) cells regardless of ABO group. Anti-Le[bH] is the more frequently identified antibody, reacting best with group O Le(b+) cells. This antibody is formed by people who have less H on their red cells (group A_1, B, AB) and both H and Le[b] antigens have to be present for agglutination. Anti-Le[b] does not characteristically cause hemolytic transfusion reactions, even though these antibodies occasionally cause hemolysis in vitro.[2,4,7]

Anti-Le[c] is directed against red cells from individuals who are genetically *lele, sese*, or *lele, hh*[81] and anti-Le[d] reacts with red cells of a person with the genotype *lele, Se, H*.[82] These antibodies are rarely found in humans but are produced by immunization of animals.[2]

Anti-Le[x] appears to react with Le[a] antigen, even in very small amounts, and detects anyone with a *Le* gene.[76] There is still unresolved controversy about the specificity of this antibody.

MAbs are available for routine Lewis typing. Other Lewis antibodies are produced in goats or rabbits. Pure Lewis substances obtained by chemical synthesis are available to immunize animals.[81] Using these better defined antibodies may help sort out the confusion created by human antibodies and antigens. mAbs also demonstrate heterogeneity of Lewis specificities.[4]

Genetics

The mode of inheritance, based on family studies of saliva phenotypes, indicates that *Lele, Sese, Hh*, and *ABO* genes all interact to determine Lewis phenotypes expressed on red cells. These are located at independent loci and segregate independently. Le(a+b−) individuals are secretors of Le[a] substance and nonsecretors of ABH. Lewis(a−b+) secrete Le[a] and Le[b] substance and are ABH secretors. Le(a−b−) are 80 percent secretors but will not have Le[a] or Le[b] substance in saliva.[82]

The first step of inheritance involves the *Le* locus. The dominant *Le* gene insures production of Le^a antigen. Both *Se* and *H* genes must be present in order to form Le^b antigen. If either is missing, only Le^a is produced. Also, Le^a is not formed when the genotype is *lele*; even with *Se* and *H* genes present, the phenotype remains Le(a−b−). *Le, Se,* and *H* genes need only be present in a single dose; amorphic genes *le, se,* and *h* must be present in a double dose to block the sequence. Refer to Table 5-7[7,31] for phenotypes formed by interaction of the three loci. Le^c, Le^d, and Le^x are not true Lewis antigens and have no alleles at the Lewis locus.

Biochemistry

The biochemistry as it unfolded confirmed inheritance patterns. Identification of biochemical structures further corroborated interaction of Lewis, Secretor, and ABH and delineated sequences of action. *Le* codes for a fucosyltransferase that adds fucose to the subterminal sugar of type 1 chains resulting in a structure with Le^a activity. When *H* and *Se* are both present, a fucose is added to the terminal sugar of type 1 chains forming type 1 H to which the transferase specified by the *Le* gene adds a fucose to the subterminal sugar to form Le^b. Interaction of *H* and *Se* cannot add a terminal sugar to chains that have already been changed into Le^a but it appears that the majority of chains are converted to type 1 H chains judging by the proportion of Le^a substance to Le^b substance found in saliva of secretors. Biochemical structures of the Lewis antigens are shown in Table 5-8.[31]

Clinical Significance

Most Lewis antibodies are not clinically significant, although some may cause hemolysis in vitro. It is known that IgG fractions do exist in the majority of anti-Le^a and there are a few reports of hemolytic reactions due to anti-Le^a. No problems are encountered when crossmatch compatible red cells are transfused. Antibodies that are demonstrable only below 37°C have no clinical significance in transfusion, and most should be ignored. There is little risk of HDN, since the newborn is Le(a−b−). However, IgG antibodies may cross the placenta and appear as an unexpected antibody in the serum of the newborn.[7]

Table 5-8. Lewis System Antigens

Antigen	Structure^a

Le^a	GAL-GLCNAc-GAL-
	          |
	         FUC

Le^b	GAL-GLCNAc-GAL-
	      | |
	    FUC FUC

Le^c (type 1 chain)
Le^d (type 1H)
	GAL-GLCNAc-GAL-
	GAL-GLCNAc-GAL
	           |
	         FUC

Le^x (subterminal Le^a and Le^b)	GLCNAc
	   |
	  FUC

^a Structures are attached to GLC-glycosphingolipid in plasma or GALNAc-glycoprotein in saliva.
Abbreviations: GAL, galactose; GLCNAc, N-acetylglucosamine; FUC, fucose; GALNAc, N-acetylgalactosamine.

The role of Lewis in transplantation is unclear. Survival rates of kidney transplants have been reported to be decreased in Le(a−b−) recipients. Recipients with HLA- and Lewis-matched kidneys had the best rates, while survival rates were the lowest when neither was matched. However, a more recent, prospective study of Lewis-matched and -mismatched pairs found no statistically significant difference in 1-year-graft survival.[83]

Lewis is of no significance in bone marrow transplantation. Plasma substance and antigen type of red cells and lymphocytes remain those of the recipient, confirming that antigens are adsorbed from plasma. Lewis substances are apparently not produced by red cell precursors.

There is a higher than expected incidence of Le(a−b−) individuals with Sjögren's syndrome.[56] The association has no known clinical significance. Association with malignancies exist. Glycolipids extracted from adenocarcinomas have Le^a and Le^b activity, regardless of Lewis blood type. Le^x and Le^y are major oncofetal antigens found in gastrointestinal, colorectal, and lung cancers. Le^x antigen is a marker for Reed-Sterling cells of Hodgkin's disease.[60]

P1 BLOOD GROUP SYSTEM AND THE GLOBOSIDE COLLECTION

In 1927, immunization experiments with rabbits resulted in discovery of anti-P_1. Later anti-Tj^a, a naturally occurring hemolysin, was found that defined antigens assigned to the P system. Recently, the system was renamed P1 with a single antigen, P_1, and other antigens have been reassigned to the globoside collection. For convenience, this section includes associated antigens.[5]

Antigens

Three antigens (P_1, P, and P^k) define five phenotypes. The majority of people have P antigen on their red cells and have either a P_1 or P_2 phenotype. The P_1 phenotype has P_1, P, and a trace of P^k on the red cells. Red cells lacking P_1 but possessing P are of the P_2 phenotype. In the white population, 80 percent are P_1 and 20 percent are P_2. The distribution in the black population is 95 percent P_1 and 5 percent P_2.

Only 1 in 100,000 is negative for P antigen. If these rare individuals have a P^k antigen, the phenotype is either P_1^k (P_1 and P^k) or P_2^k (P^k only). All three antigens are absent in the p phenotype, which is found only slightly more often than the P^k phenotype.[4,84]

Expression of P_1 antigen varies considerably from one individual to another, apparently a quantitative rather than a qualitative difference. There are no distinct categories. This variation may be a genetic trait or a variation due to homozygosity versus heterozygosity. All weak P_1 are heterozygous. Furthermore, red cells from P_1+ blacks characteristically have strong antigens. Since 95 percent of the black population is positive, more blacks are homozygous. P_1 antigen is not well developed at birth and does not reach full expression until 7 years of age.

Carbohydrate structures related to the P system are widely distributed in nature. P_1 and P^k are found in a variety of animal tissue,[85] including *Echinococcus* cyst fluid, bovine liver fluke, *Clonorchis sinensis*, *Lumbricus terrestis* (night crawler), pigeon, and turtle dove.

Luke, an antigen thought to demonstrate an association between P and ABO, adds even more complexity. There are three phenotypes: LKE−, LKEw, and LKE+. All p and P^k samples are LKE−. In addition, 1 to 2 percent of P_1 and P_2 subjects are negative for the Luke antigen.[86] More recent testing with other monoclonal antibodies has not entirely resolved questions about this antigen.[84]

Antibodies

Antibodies range from clinically insignificant to those capable of causing hemolysis. Individuals with unique phenotypes, P_1^k, P_2^k, and p, characteristically have naturally occurring hemolytic antibodies.

Anti-P_1 is possibly the most common naturally occurring antibody found outside the ABO system. It is a low titer IgM antibody in the sera of most P_2 individuals. More sensitive test methods increase the number of anti-P_1 detected. Anti-P_1 has been found in up to 90 percent of pregnant P_2 woman, but there is no strong evidence that this is a result of alloimmunization. Rare examples of anti-P_1 reactive at 37°C may cause in vivo hemolysis.[7]

Anti-P is found as an alloantibody in the sera of all P^k individuals[2] and reacts with all P_1 and P_2 cells. It is often a high titer antibody reactive at room temperature and 37°C with hemolytic activity.

Autoanti-P is the specificity attributed to the Donath-Landsteiner antibody responsible for paroxysmal cold hemaglobinuria (PCH), a type of autoimmune hemolytic anemia sometimes seen in children following a viral infection. This antibody is a potent biphasic IgG hemolysin that attaches to red cells in the cold and lyses them at warmer temperatures. Benign forms of autoanti-P have also been reported.[7]

Anti-PP_1P^k is found in the sera of all p phenotypes as a naturally occurring high titer IgM or IgG antibody reactive at 37°C. This is the antibody originally called anti-Tj^a. It is not present at birth but develops early without red cell stimulus. The antibody has been involved in hemolytic transfusion reactions and HDN.

Anti-P^k is not found as a single antibody in serum. An avid anti-P^k can be separated from some but not all anti-PP_1P^k sera by adsorption.

Anti-p has been reported. It appears that all cells have some p antigen: $P_1 < P_2 < p$. The "p antigen" is actually sialosylparagloboside but accumulates in those individuals who lack glycosyltransferases of the P system (p phenotype).

Genetics

Several genetic models have been proposed. The existence of at least two structural genes working sequentially is an implied minimum but the genetic pathway is currently unresolved. The biochemistry of the different antigens indicates that all originate from the common precursor lactosylceramide but that the process is not straightforward. Little is known about the genes involved or the actual gene products. The genetics will probably be worked out after the genes have been cloned. The gene responsible for LKE is dominant and segregates independently.[84]

Biochemistry

The original work identifying these antigens was done by inhibition studies using glycoproteins derived from hydatid cyst fluid. Later work used glycosphingolipids isolated from cell membrane. The antigenic determinants are immunodominant carbohydrates added to glycosphingolipids associated with the red cell membrane by transferases. Antigens are synthesized by red cells but are also found in plasma attached to glycoprotein. Red cell antigens are type 2 chains similar to those carrying ABO and Ii antigens (Table 5-9).

Ceramide dihexoside (CDH) is precursor to P^k and P. The addition of a terminal D-galactose converts CDH to ceramide trihexoside (CTH), which has P^k specificity. A terminal N-acetyl-D-galactosamine added to CTH forms globoside which has P specificity.

Paragloboside (CDH with N-acetyl-D-glucosamine attached) is the precursor of P_1 and p. A terminal D-galactose forms P_1, while p specificity results from addition of a terminal N-acetylneuraminic acid forming sialosylparagloboside.

A link between globoside (P antigen) and LKE has been established. Tippett[86] proposed the structure of galactose–galactose–globoside for LKE and that LKE + individuals possess a transferase acting in the pathway beyond globoside production.

Clinical Significance

Antibodies are naturally occurring. Anti-P_1 has been implicated as a rare cause of transfusion reactions and only when the antibody is active at 37°C. If compatibility testing is nonreactive, transfusion of P_1-positive red cells will not cause a reaction or shortening of the life span of donor cells. Anti-PP_1P^k (anti-Tj^a) and anti-P have caused both hemolytic transfusion reactions and HDN. Donath-Landsteiner antibody usually has anti-P specificity and is implicated in PCH.[7]

There is a high frequency of miscarriage and abortion in women who are phenotypically p and it is probable that anti-PP_1P^k is responsible.[88] Successful deliveries have been achieved when antibody titers were reduced by plasmapheresis. It is thought that only the IgG component of the antibody is responsible, but little is known about development of P antigens in the embryo. P antigen is present in the placenta.[60] A causal relationship between IgG subclass or cytotoxicity of antibody with early abortion has been suggested.[87,88]

Table 5-9. Structures with P Blood Group Antigenic Determinants

Red cell glycolipids	
CER-GLC-GAL	CDH (R^k, P precursor)
CER-GLC-GAL-GAL	P^k (CTH)
CER-GLC-GAL-GAL-GALNAc	P (globoside)
CER-GLC-GAL-GLCNAc-GAL	Paragloboside (P_1, p precursor)
CER-GLC-GAL-GLCNAc-GAL-GAL	P_1
Soluble glycoproteins	
GPC-GALNAc-GAL-GAL	Soluble P^k
GPC-GALNAc-GAL-GLCNAc-GAL-GAL	Soluble P_1
Associated structures	
CER-GLC-GAL-GLCNAc-GAL-NeuNAc	p (sialosylparagloboside)
GLOBOSIDE-GAL-GAL	LKE?
CER-GLC-GAL-GAL-GALNAc-GALNAc	Forssman

Abbreviations: CER, ceramide (N-acetylacylsphingosine); GAL, galactose; GALNAc, N-acetylgalactosamine; GLC, glucose; GLCNAc, N-acetylglucosamine; NeuNAc, N-acetylneuraminic acid; CDH, ceramide dihexoside; CTH, ceramide trihexoside; GPC, glycoprotein carrier.

Transient autoanti-PP_1P^k has been reported in approximately one-third of Australian women located near Perth who are threatened with a second abortion. This phenomenon has never been observed elsewhere. This antibody causes lysis of autologous cells in vitro, but there was no apparent destruction of red cells in vivo.[89]

"Illegitimate" P antigens appear on malignant cells. The first reported anti-Tj^a (anti-PP_1P^k) was in a patient with adenocarcinoma. An illegitimate (incompatible) P was present on malignant cells and it was thought that serum antibody caused inhibition of the tumor with long term survival. P^k antigen is expressed on tumor cells from Burkitt's lymphoma. Globoside (P antigen) is the precursor of Forssman antigen and illegitimate Forssman antigens are found in malignant tissues with a concurrent decrease of Forssman antibody in patients' sera.[60]

Parasitic infestations and anti-P_1 are often found together due to P_1 substance in various parasites. Potent anti-P_1 is reported in some cases of patients with hydatid cysts. The immune source is *Echinococcus* scolices found in cyst fluid. Extremely potent anti-P_1 has been detected in almost all cases of fascioliasis (bovine liver fluke).[90] In the populations of Kampuchea and Laos, where 80 percent are negative for P_1 antigen, approximately 50 percent have anti-P_1 which may reflect infestation with *Clonorchis*.[91]

Pyelonephritis has been associated with P antigens. Certain strains of *Escherichia coli* have receptors that preferentially attach to P receptors on uroepithelium of the bladder. Individuals of the p phenotype do not have these receptors on uroepithelial cells and are resistant to these strains.[60] Individuals who do not have the P antigen (P_1P^k, P_2P^k, and p phenotypes) are resistant to infection with parvovirus B19. The P antigen is the cellular receptor for the virus.[92]

MNSs BLOOD GROUP SYSTEM

Rabbit immunization experiments also resulted in identification of M and N in 1927. When S and s were discovered, family studies indicated, that although not alleles, these antigens were related to M and N. The U antigen was later placed in the MNSs system when it was shown that U− blood was S−s−

also. There are now 37 antigens assigned to this system.[93]

Antigens

M and N are antithetical: an individual is positive for one or both. Very rarely is one negative for both antigens. M negatives range from 22 percent of the white population to 30 percent of the black population, while about 27 percent of either population is N negative. A dosage effect is common with homozygosity. Cells that are negative for N antigen may react weakly when tested with anti-N. This specificity designated 'N' is part of the Ss antigenic structure.

S and s are antithetical. About 45 percent of whites and 69 percent of blacks are S negative. Those negative for s constitute 11 percent of whites and 3 percent of blacks. In the black population, about 1.5 percent of blood samples test S−s−, a null phenotype. Sixteen percent of these have the U antigen, while the rest are either U negative or have a variant of the U antigen. Only one S−s−U− white family has been reported.

There are many associated rare variants that, based on serologic reactivity and genetic associations, may be divided into quantitative variants, mosaics, qualitative variants, satellite antigens, or null phenotypes.[4]

Quantitative Variants

M_1 and M' are both associated with strong expression of the M antigen and may in fact be the same antigen. M_2 and N_2 are characterized by weak expression of M and N antigens, respectively.[23] M^r and M^z phenotypes have abnormal M and N levels and are sometimes accompanied by the St^a (Stones) antigen. S_2 is a weakened expression of the S antigen. U^z, and possibly U^x, may be a quantitative difference between S and s antigens.

Mosaics

M^A and N^A, proposed mosaics of M and N antigens, help explain antibodies that are not autoantibodies formed by antigen-positive people. U^A and U^B antigens are possible mosaics of the U antigen.

Qualitative Variants

M^g is an extremely rare antigen. M^o is an intermediate structure with similarities to both M and N antigens. Both are altered glycophorin A. M^v is a variant of glycophorin B.

Satellite Antigens

These are antigens, other than MNSs, genetically linked to the MNSs system. T^m (Sheerin) and Can (Canner) are relatively common. Hu (Hunter) is found in 7 percent and He (Henshaw) in 3 percent of the black population. Low-incidence antigens include: Vr^a (Verdegaal), Mt^a (Martin), St^a (Stones), Ri^a (Ridley), Cl^a (Caldwell), Ny^a (Nyberg), Sul (Sullivan), and Sj (Stenbar-James).

The Miltenberger subsystem with nine classes is a series of rare antigens within MNSs.[94] V^W(Verweyst) and Mi^a are antigens most often encountered in this subsystem. (Anti-Mi^a is a cross-reacting, polyspecific antibody and does not represent a single antigenic specificity.) The Mi antigens are associated with qualitative abnormalities of M, N, S, and s antigens along with membrane alterations.

Null Phenotypes

M^k expresses no M, N, S, or s antigens and has no detectable U, En^a, Wr^a, or Wr^b.[94] M^k is a silent gene complex that involves both the *MN* and *Ss* loci; both glycophorin A and glycophorin B are missing from the red cell membrane.

The rare En(a−) phenotype has no M, N, Wr^a, or Wr^b. Red cells lack glycophorin A and have a marked sialic acid deficiency with enhanced reactivity with saline anti-D.

The U− phenotype has no S, s, or U antigens. Red cells lack glycophorin B. While 0.2 percent of blacks are truly U negative, an additional 1 percent are weakly positive for the U antigen (U variants) and are thought to have a portion of the U antigen.[96]

Antibodies

Anti-M is a naturally occurring antibody reacting best at 4°C and weakly, if at all, at 37°C. Although generally considered to be IgM, up to 75 percent have an IgG fraction.[97] Anti-M may react better in albumin than saline media; some are only detectable at a reduced pH or when tested against M + N − cells. Anti-M that does not appear to be autoantibody has been detected in M + N + individuals,[98] apparently formed against an absent portion of M, the mosaic characteristic M^A. Autoanti-M-like antibody is rare but has been associated with hemolytic anemia.[99] Anti-M$_1$ occurs frequently in combination with anti-M. Anti-M$_1$ without the presence of anti-M has been described in an M + + individual.[100]

Anti-N, which is rarer than anti-M, is primarily a cold-reactive, naturally occurring IgM antibody reacting with both N and 'N' determinants. Clinically significant anti-N is almost only found in S − s − individuals.[101] Immune anti-N has been known to cause red cell destruction and has been implicated in mild HDN.[102] Anti-N has been detected in M + N + individuals, presumably directed against the mosaic antigen, N^A, and autoanti-N[103] has been implicated in autoimmune hemolytic anemia.

Glucose-dependent anti-M and anti-N have been described[104] and only react with antigen positive red cells incubated in a glucose solution. These specificities are designated M^D and N^D.

Anti-N may be found in sera of renal patients regardless of MN type who have undergone dialysis with equipment sterilized with formaldehyde.[105] Designated anti-N$_f$, the antibody reacts with any cell treated with formaldehyde. Titers decrease after exposure to formaldehyde is discontinued and almost always disappear after transplantation.

Murine monoclonal anti-M and anti-N are available commercially. There is no useful lectin for the M antigen but *Vicia graminea* has N specificity (N$_{vg}$). Both monoclonal anti-N and N selectin react with 'N' carried on the Ss glycophorin unless properly diluted.

Anti-S, anti-s, and anti-U differ from anti-M and anti-N in that they are generally clinically significant. Anti-S is found as a naturally occurring antibody but is more often seen as an immune antibody following red cell exposure. Anti-s is rarer and is also an immune antibody. Extremely rare, anti-U is immune and capable of causing red cell destruction and HDN. The anti-U developed in a U-negative individual will react with U variants, while U variants form many varieties of anti-U. All three antibodies (anti-S, -s, -U) may react best at temperatures lower than 37°C, even when using the indirect antiglobulin test.[106] In comparison, typical immune antibodies such as anti-D, anti-K, and anti-Fy^a, characteristically give strongest reactions at 37°C.

Autoanti-S has been reported.[107] Autoanti-U in combination with other autoantibodies is commonly found in autoimmune hemolytic anemias, especially if investigating antibodies that do not react with Rh$_{null}$ cells.[96]

Although there actually is no En^a antigen, En(a−) phenotypes form three different anti-En^a antibodies reacting with different portions of glycophorin A molecule. One example of naturally occurring anti-En^a has been reported.[108] Autoanti-En^a may be found in some warm autoimmune hemolytic anemias with reactivity against all cells except En(a−), although in most cases the specificity of an antibody is anti-Wr^b. (En(a−) cells are also negative for Wr^b.)

Antibodies to low incidence antigens in the MNSs system are not routinely detected because of relative scarcity of the antigens. Serologically similar to anti-M or anti-N, they most often are identified during investigations of mild HDN or unexpectedly incompatible crossmatches.

Genetics

Characterized by a growing number of genetic variants, the MNSs system is very complex. *MN* and *Ss* are pseudoalleles that combine to form four haplotypes. The loci for *MN* and *Ss* are so closely linked that crossover is not expected. An equal number of pairings between the alleles at the two loci would be expected, but the actual distribution is unequal. Of four possible haplotypes, *Ns* is the most common, followed by *Ms, MS,* and *NS,* in that order. There is no apparent advantage or explanation for the disequilibrium.

The actual genetics of the MNSs system is simpler than expected. Instead of one gene required for each specificity, a single gene codes for a polypeptide with multiple antigens. For example, the *N* gene codes for a structure that carries N, Tm, En^a, and Wr^b.

Genes responsible for MN and Ss specificity have been cloned, *GYPA* and *GYPB,* respectively. While investigating these genes, a third related gene, *GYPE,* was identified. Structural similarities suggest that *GYPB* and *GYPE* genes are derived by mutation from *GYPA. GYPB,* responsible for glycophorin B synthesis, arose by duplication and partial deletion of the *GYPA* gene, responsible for glycophorin A synthesis. Further mutations explain the variety of associated gene products. No corresponding cell structure has been identified for *GYPE,* but it most likely has M specificity and may correspond to a minor component on the cell membrane.[109]

Although it is rare, unequal crossover between the *GYPA* and *GYPB* genes produces hybrid molecules. *GYP(A-B)* recombinants have the N-terminal (outer) of glycophorin A and C-terminal (inner) of glycophorin B. *GYP(B-A)* recombinants have the outer portion of glycophorin B and inner portion of glycophorin A. GP(A-B) hybrids are larger than glycophorin B while GP(B-A) hybrids are smaller than glycophorin A. Miltenberger V and Mt^a are GP(A-B) hybrids; St^a and Dantu are GP(B-A) hybrids. There are even double crossovers designated GP(B-A-B) and GP(A-B-A).

Wr^a and Wr^b are not genetically controlled by the MNSs loci but it appears that Wr^b cannot be expressed unless the En^a structure is present.

Biochemistry

Two sialic acid rich glycoproteins with MN and Ss specificity have been identified; MN specificities are located on glycophorin A (GPA), also called MN-sialoglycoprotein, and Ss antigens are located on glycophorin B (GPB), also called Ss-sialoglycoprotein.[110]

GPA, composed of a sequence of 131 amino acids, has a C-terminal that extends through the red cell membrane into the red cell. The N-terminus outside the red cell membrane has 15 alkali-labile tetrasaccharides and a single alkali-stable oligiosaccharide. M and N specificity seem to lie in the first 5 amino acids (Table 5-10). The rest of the polysaccharide appears to be identical for both M and N. Normal GPA contains a sequence of several antigenic determinants: M or N, En^a, and Wr^b. The amino acid substitutions and glycosylation changes for many of the MN variants have been identified.

GPB is a shorter polypeptide than GPA with less than 100 amino acids and the C-terminal ending within the red cell membrane. The N-terminus has 11 alkali-labile tetrasaccharides that are probably the same tetrasaccharides present in GPA, but there is no alkali-stable oligiosaccharide. The first 25 amino acids have the same sequence as GPA. Of these, the terminal 5 amino acids and glycosylation of GPB are identical with the N antigen. This specificity is designated 'N' and, in contrast with N antigen, is trypsin-resistant. GPB at the C-terminal appears to be identical to GPA but the middle portion of GPB has no match on GPA. S-GPB differs from s-GPB at position

Table 5-10. Antigenic Determinants of Glycophorin A and Glycophorin B

Antigen	Structure	Amino Acid Position					
		1	2	3	4	5	29
M	GPA	SER-SER-THR-THR-GLY-R					
			TS	TS	TS		
N	GPA	LEU-SER-THR-THR-GLU-R					
			TS	TS	TS		
S and 'N'	GPB	LEU-SER-THR-THR-GLU-R-MET-R					
			TS	TS	TS		
s and 'N'	GPB	LEU-SER-THR-THR-GLU-R-THR-R					
			TS	TS	TS		

Abbreviations: SER, serine; LEU, leucine; THR, threonine; MET, methionine; GLY, glycine; GLU, glutamic acid; TS, alkali labile tetrasaccharide.

29; methionine is found in S specificity and threonine in s specificity. The GPB polypeptide is a sequence of several specificities: 'N' at the terminal end, S or s at position 29, and the U antigen. Other antigens found on GPB involve substitutions at different positions.

Recently, new terminology based on DNA analysis has been proposed to eliminate the Miltenberger subsystem and could be expanded to all phenotypes. Each specificity would be identified by GP. name of first propositus. Added to this would be the biochemical structure, when it is known. For example, Mi.III would be GP(B-A-B)Mur.[94]

Clinical Significance

Anti-M and anti-N are not clinically significant antibodies. Rarely has anti-M been implicated in hemolytic transfusion reactions or HDN and then only when antibody is active at 37°C. Most of the antibodies of this system do not appear to activate complement. Transient anti-M is sometimes associated with bacterial infection in children.

The anti-N formed by an individual with normal GPB is not capable of causing much harm because of the presence of 'N' antigen. However, anti-N developed by a recipient negative for both N and 'N' is significant. This occurs in the M + N − phenotype

with an abnormal GPB and has been documented in both U − and He + individuals.

Anti-S, -s, and -U do cause HDN and hemolytic transfusion reactions. Anti-U presents an unusual challenge in finding blood for transfusion or exchange because of rarity, multiple specificities of anti-U antibodies and variants of U antigen. Anti-En^a is also a problem for some of the same reasons.

Transfusion reactions and HDN due to antibodies against the low-frequency antigens of this system have been reported and are usually mild, although the first reported case of Far (Kamhuber) was severe.[111] When there is clinical evidence of HDN with no antibody detected, antigens in this system should be considered as a possible cause.

Autoantibodies of the MNSs system have been implicated in antibody-induced hemolytic anemia. Although benign examples of autoanti-En^a, autoanti-U, and autoanti-Wr^a have been described, these specificities are often seen in warm autoimmune hemolytic anemias.

Weakened expression of MN due to transferase deficiencies (possible the result of mutation of hematopoietic cells) along with Tn antigen exposure has been reported in preleukemia. Exposure of T antigen with weakened MN expression due to neuraminidase is found in bacterial infections.[60] For unknown reasons, weakened expression of Ss along with many other antigens occurs with stomatocytic hereditary elliptocytosis.[19]

The MNSs system has been useful in paternity testing. Antigens are well developed at birth; MN has been detected on fetal cells at 9 weeks gestation and Ss at 12 weeks. Direct exclusions are reliable. However, caution must be taken with indirect exclusions because of silent phenotypes and the number of low-incidence antigens.

Null phenotypes of this system have no disease association. There is no morphologic or functional abnormality of red cells, even though a large portion of normal red cell membrane structure is missing. This make it difficult to assign a function to these red cell sialoglycoproteins. When GPA or GPB is missing or abnormal, other proteins (possibly GPE) may take over necessary functions. Rh_{null} cells have decreased amount of GPB, and it is suggested that the Rh antigen complexes with GPB during biosynthesis, aiding its incorporation into the red cell membrane.[112] Glycophorin A and/or B appear to serve as a ligand for invasion by some strains of *Plasmodium falciparum*. Phenotypes with abnormal GPA or GPB are resistant.[60]

As detected in atomic bomb survivors, the gene cluster, *GYPA*, *GYPB*, and *GYPE*, is susceptible to somatic mutation. An increase in mutation rate is also seen in Bloom syndrome, suggesting a link with predisposition to cancer. Investigation of these situations might help in understanding the mechanisms of somatic mutation.[109]

THE Rh SYSTEM

The Rh system is the largest and most complex of the blood group systems. To date, at least 50 antigens (Table 5-11) have been defined by Rh specific antibodies. Rh antigens are only found on red cells and not on noncommitted precursor cells of the erythroid line or on other blood or tissue cells. The Rh antigens are embedded in the red cell membrane and are considered important to its integrity.

The Rh blood group system is second only to the ABO system in importance in transfusion medicine practice. Because certain Rh antigens are highly immunogenic in small doses,[7] Rh antibodies are the most common specificities stimulated through pregnancy and transfusion. They are responsible for the more severe forms of HDN, that is, those cases requiring treatment or causing fetal death,[113,114] as well as severe hemolytic transfusion reactions. Rh blood group specificities are frequently involved in warm autoimmune hemolytic anemia.

Table 5-11. Various Terms for Antigens of the Rh Blood Group System[a]

Numerical	CDE	Rh-Hr	Other	Numerical	CDE	Rh-Hr	Other
Rh1	D	Rh_0		Rh26	c-like		Deal
Rh2	C	rh′		Rh27	cE		
Rh3	E	rh″		Rh28		Hr^H	Hernandez
Rh4	c	hr′		Rh29			total Rh
Rh5	e	hr″		Rh30	D^{Cor}		Go^a
Rh6	ce	hr	f	Rh31		hr^B	
Rh7	Ce	rh_i		Rh32			Troll
Rh8	C^W	rh^{W1}		Rh33			
Rh9	C^X	rh^X		Rh34		Hr^B	Bastiaan
Rh10	ce^S	hr^V	V	Rh35			1114
Rh11	E^W	rh^{W2}		Rh36			Be^a
Rh12	G	rh^G		Rh37			Evans
Rh13		Rh^A		~~Rh38~~			Duclos
Rh14		Rh^B		Rh39	C-like		
Rh15		Rh^C		Rh40			Targett (Tar)
Rh16		Rh^D		Rh41	Ce-like		
Rh17		Hr_0		Rh42	Ce^S	rh^S	Thornton
Rh18		Hr		Rh43			Crawford
Rh19		hr^S		Rh44			Nou
Rh20	e^S		VS	Rh45			Riv
Rh21	C^G			Rh46			Sec
Rh22	CE		Jarvis	Rh47			Dav
Rh23	D^W		Weil	Rh48			JAL
Rh24	E^T			Rh49			STEM
~~Rh25~~			LW^a	Rh50			FPTT

[a] Terms: given in three nomenclatures (Fisher-Race, CDE; Wiener, Rh-hr; Rosenfield, numerical) and other known notations. Rh23 (LW^a) and Rh38 (Duclos) antigens no longer assigned to Rh system; now known to be products of genes independent of Rh.

There has been great interest in the Rh blood group system, followed by an immense amount of published studies for well over five decades. The extensive serologic observations that define the Rh antigens and antibodies lay a large foundation of understanding that is now being supported or refuted by the rapid accumulation of molecular and biochemical findings. This section will attempt to touch upon the more enduring theories and common characteristics of the Rh system, as well as some of the newer recognized biochemical features. Those interested in a more extensive look into the vast serologic, biochemical, and genetic complexities of the Rh system should refer to the cited references.

Early Milestones

In 1939, Levine and Stetson[115] described the first example of a human antibody as a disease causing mechanism for the previously unexplained HDN. A group O mother delivered a stillborn fetus and subsequently developed symptoms of a hemolytic transfusion reaction when transfused with her husband's blood. An antibody in the mother's serum was found to agglutinate her husband's group O cells and was found to be compatible with only 21 of 104 random group O donors. Levine and Stetson noted that the responsible antibody developed through an isoimmunizing property of an inherited factor from the fetus to the mother. They concluded that the antibody accounted for both the hemolytic transfusion reaction to the father's cells and the HDN. The antibody was not named at that time.

In 1940, Landsteiner and Wiener[116] reported on antibodies that were stimulated when Rhesus monkey cells were injected into rabbits and guinea pigs. They hoped that the Rhesus cells would be more immunogenic and produce an antibody that would react with red cell antigens in common with the similar human species. This work led to the discovery of the Rh system. The antibody, named anti-Rh, agglutinated approximately 85 percent of random human red cells tested. Its antigenic determinant was called the Rh factor. The Levine and Stetson antibody was subsequently reexamined and found to have the same pattern of reactivity as the anti-Rhesus antibody of Landsteiner and Wiener. Soon thereafter the scientific community began to realize the significance of the Rh factor.

In 1940, Wiener and Peters[117] demonstrated that anti-Rh was responsible for hemolytic transfusion reactions in patients transfused with ABO-compatible blood. Also in 1940, Levine and Katzin[118] reported additional associations between human antibodies formed in pregnancy and those of the animal anti-Rhesus sera. In 1941, Levine and associates[119] confirmed that Rh incompatibility between mother and fetus led to the pathogenesis of HDN.

Later, the animal anti-Rhesus of Landsteiner and Wiener was shown not to be the same as the human antibody. These antibodies indeed defined separate but related antigens.[120] The antibody causing human hemolytic disease of the newborn defined the Rh antigen and the name LW, in honor of Landsteiner and Wiener, was given to the human antigen defined by their original animal antisera.

Rh Genetics and Nomenclature

As other investigators began reporting on additional antibodies related to the Rh factor, it became apparent that there was not one simple Rh antigenic determinant, but a host of associated antigens defining an entire Rh blood group system. Various nomenclature systems and genetic models were developed to describe the system antigens and their mode of inheritance. Over the years, three primary concepts for the genetic control of Rh were postulated. During the early 1940s, the first two genetic models were formed along with their corresponding nomenclature systems. Later in 1986, a newer theory evolved based on more recent biochemical information at that time; this model has turned out to be true for the number of Rh genes or gene complexes responsible for Rh antigenic expression. As knowledge of the complexities of the Rh system advanced, difficulties in communicating about the Rh antigens in an easy and standard way has continued. This led to the development of a third numerical terminology as well as a notation system based on an international working group consensus.

To date, although at least 50 Rh antigens are defined, the first five common Rh antigens and their corresponding antibodies are responsible for most, perhaps more than 99 percent, of the serologic observations in the Rh system. The presence of the first known Rh specific red cell antigen, called Rh_o by Wiener, D by Fisher and later Rh:1, was used to define the commonly used term "Rh-positive." The $Rh_o(D)$ antigen occurs in approximately 85 percent of the population. Conversely, "Rh-negative" red cells, occuring in 15 percent of people, are defined by the absence of the Rh_o (D) antigen.

Rh Concept of Wiener

In 1943, using only three of the first four Rh antibodies, Wiener[121] suggested that a single gene at the *Rh* locus produces what he termed an *agglutinogen*, composed of several blood factors or antigenic determinants. The one *Rh* gene has multiple alleles. Each agglutinogen typically expressed the two or three common Rh antigens (factors); however, when rare antigenic variants were found, the *Rh* gene encodes for the production of a different agglutinogen expressing the rare variant alleles.

Wiener developed the Rh terminology to interpret his genetic theory (Table 5-12). Capital R is used as the gene encoding for the original Rh_o factor and Rh for the agglutinogen exhibiting this factor. Lower-case r and rh indicates that the original Rh factor is not encoded by the gene or included in the agglutinogen respectively.

The recent cloning of two *Rh* genes does not support the Wiener concept and his notations are nearly obsolete. Since his theory persisted and was debated over many years, it is included here for historic interest.

CDE Concept of Fisher and Race

In 1943, while Wiener was developing his theories, Fisher and Race,[122–125] working with the first four Rh antibodies, suggested that the Rh antigens were determined by three closely linked genes that encoded for three pairs of alleles, inherited as a unit. Fisher recognized the antithetical relationship of the Rh antibodies and called the first antigenic products of the allelic pairs of genes C and c, followed by D and E. Fisher predicted the future discovery of anti-d and anti-e. Mourant[126] confirmed this assumption with the discovery of anti-e two years later. Anti-d, however, has never been found and, as we now know, the *d* gene does not exist.

Fisher used the CDE terminology to show the eight possible combinations of the six genes (Table 5-12). The same letters were used to indicate the gene or the gene products. Fisher suggested that the sequence of the genes on the chromosome was probably *DCE* and that crossing over between the higher frequency gene complexes explained some of the rarer antigenic expressions. Later, the Fisher–Race theory was modified to include three subloci within a single genetic locus, since inheritance is always by an intact *Rh* gene complex contributed to the offspring.

The application of the two nomenclature systems has not been determined by the correctness of the genetic principles. CDE terminology has been adapted for everyday use, as it is easier to explain the written relationships between the antigens and antibodies. However, because CDE/cde combinations are cumbersome to communicate verbally, "shorthand R" symbols have been popularly adapted from Wiener's notations for ease in speaking to designate phenotypes (Table 5-13).

Rh Phenotypes and Genotypes

Red cells are tested with antisera to detect the five common Rh antigens D, C, c, E, e, in order to determine the Rh phenotype. It is now known that one *Rh* gene encodes for the C or c and E or e antigen of the antithetical pairs and a second *Rh* gene encodes for the presence or absence of D.[127] A person inherits one *Rh* haplotype from each parent, combining three or two common determinants of the two gene complexes. *Rh* genes are codominant, and thus the products of both haploid gene complexes inherited from each parent will be expressed on the red cells. If the haplotypes are identical, only one antigen of each of the genetic alleles will be detected on the red cells, the antigens will be present in dou-

Table 5-12. Comparison of Wiener and Fisher-Race Nomenclature

Rh-HR of Wiener			CDE of Fisher-Race	
Gene	Shorthand	Agglutinogen	Gene Complex	Antigens
Rh^0	R^0	Rh_0	*cDe*	c,D,e
Rh^1	R^1	Rh_1	*CDe*	C,D,e
Rh^2	R^2	Rh_2	*cDE*	c,D,E
Rh^Z	R^Z	Rh_Z	*CDE*	C,D,E
rh	*r*	rh	*cde*	c,e
rh′	*r′*	rh′	*Cde*	C,e
rh″	*r″*	rh″	*cdE*	c,E
rh^y	*r*^{y}	rh_y	*CdE*	C,E

Table 5-13. Frequencies of the Primary Rh Genes or Gene Complexes and Their RBC Phenotypes

Phenotype		Haplotype		Gene or Gene Complex—% Frequency in U.S.[a]			
CDE Term	Rh-Hr Shorthand	Rh-Hr	CDE	Whites	Blacks	Native Americans	Asians
cDE	R_0	R^0	cDe	4	44	2	3
CDe	R_1	R^1	CDe	42	17	44	70
cDE	R_2	R^2	cDE	14	11	34	21
CDE	R_Z	R^Z	CDE	Rare	Rare	6	1
cde	r	r	cde	37	26	11	3
Cde	r′	r′	Cde	2	2	2	2
cdE	r″	r″	cdE	1	Rare	1	Rare
CdE	r^y	r^y	CdE	Rare	Rare	Rare	Rare

[a] Rare denotes a frequency of less than 1% of population tested.
(Data from Walker.[5])

ble dose, and the person will be homozygous for those gene products. If, however, both antigenic products of the allelic pairs are present, the haplotypes will not be identical, and the person will be heterozygous for those gene products. In addition to the common Rh antigens, the products of rare variant alleles exist. Some *Rh* genes may encode for various amounts of antigens, or suppress, enhance, or influence the expression of other gene products. Examples of these are reviewed later in the section on Rh antigens and phenotypes.

Unless the haplotypes are homozygous, it is not known which antigens are inherited from which gene complex. Although the antigenic phenotype may be known, the genotype cannot be determined with certainty. The most probable genotype can be presumed on the basis of the known frequencies of genes and their products (Tables 5-13 and 5-14). The disequilibrium in the observed frequencies of the various gene complexes supports the theory that the *Rh* genes are so closely linked on the chromosome that crossing over is an extremely rare event. Otherwise, the gene complex frequencies would be expected to be similar. Racial origins need to be considered when interpreting the genotype, as significant differences in gene frequencies occur between ethnic groups. Determining the most probable *Rh* genotypes can be useful for population studies, paternity testing, and predicting the risk of HDN.

Differences in reactivity from the homozygous or heterozygous expression of some red cell antigens can be useful in predicting *Rh* genotypes. Dosage effect is sometimes observed with antibodies to the E or c antigens and occasionally to the C antigen. The D antigen, however, does not appear to show variation in strength of reactivity based on its homozygous or heterozygous state. The *D* gene zygosity is best predicted using gene frequency tables rather than quantitative red cell testing.

The quantitative expression of some antigens may also be influenced by gene interaction.[128] If there is increased or decreased antigen production due to the interaction between genes on the same chromosome, the result is called the "cis position effect." For example, the E antigen produced by *cDE* is weaker than the E produced by *cdE*. If the gene on one chromosome interacts with the production of an antigen from the gene on the opposite paired chromosome, the result is called the "*trans* position effect." The C and E antigens are weaker when produced by *Cde/cdE* than *Cde/cde* or *cdE/cde*. Antibodies to *cis* gene products may be helpful in differentiating between genotypes of the same phenotype.

Rosenfeld and ISBT Numerical Nomenclature

In 1962, Rosenfeld and coworkers[129] introduced a new numerical terminology to deal with the expanded complexities of the Rh system (Table 5-15). By then, 25 different antigens had been recognized, and neither the Fisher–Race nor Wiener nomencla-

Table 5-14. Common Rh Phenotypes and Estimation of Most Probable Genotype Based on Known Gene Frequencies[a]

Phenotype	% Frequency		Most Probable Genotype			
	Whites	Blacks	Whites		Blacks	
CcDee	35	26	CDe/cde	R^1r	CDe/cDe	R^1R^0
CCDee	19	3	CDe/CDe	R^1R^1	CDe/CDe	R^1R^1
ccee	15	7	cde/cde	rr	cde/cde	rr
CcDEe	13	4	CDe/cDE	R^1R^2	CDe/cDE	R^1R^2
ccDEe	12	16	cDE/cde	R^2r	cDE/cDe	R^2R^0
ccDEE	2	1	cDE/cDe	R^2R^2	cDE/cDE	R^2R^2
ccDee	2	42	cDe/cde	R^0r	cDe/cde	R^0r
					cDe/cDe	R^0R^0
Ccee	1	1	Cde/cde	$r'r$	Cde/cde	$r'r$
ccEe	1	Rare	cdE/cde	$r''r$	cdE/cde	$r''r$

[a] Using the five common Rh antisera, 18 phenotypes are possible. Phenotypes not listed occur with a frequency of less than 0.2%.

ture could satisfactorily accommodate this heterogeneity. The numerical system is not based on any genetic concept but is simply used to record serologic reactions. The advantage of a numerical terminology is its application for use with computers. Observations can be made more objectively, as genetic interpretations are not implied. Numbers are assigned to the antigens in chronologic order of their discovery. An antigen present on red cells is designated by the symbol Rh, followed by a colon and the number for that antigen. If red cells are tested with specific antisera and the antigen is not detected, that antigen would be written with a minus sign preceding its number. For example, the presence of the D antigen is indicated as Rh:1, whereas the absence of D is Rh:−1.

Table 5-15. Common Rh Antigens

Numerical	Nomenclatures		% Frequency in Whites
	Wiener	Fisher-Race	
Rh1	Rh^0	D	84
Rh2	rh′	C	70
Rh3	rh″	E	30
Rh4	hr′	c	80
Rh5	hr″	e	98
Rh6	hr	f	64
Rh12	rh^G	G	85

The international scientific community determined that there was a need for a universal terminology to interpret serologic reactions that was not linked to genetic concepts. The ISBT formed the working Party on Terminology for Red Cell Surface Antigens. Each blood group specificity verified as unique by the ISBT working party is given a six digit number. The first three numbers represent the blood group system (004 for Rh system) and the last three numbers represent the differing antigens assigned to the system. The recording of individual antigen phenotypes, genes, genetic alleles, and haplotypes follows a system similar to that of Rosenfield; however, all uppercase RH prefixes are used rather than Rh.

Two-Gene Concept of Tippett

In 1986, Tippett[130] proposed a genetic model for the Rh blood group system based on two closely linked structural *Rh* loci: D and *CcEe*. This concept complemented some biochemical data evolving at that time suggesting that two red cell membrane polypeptides carry the Rh antigens.[131] To produce the eight common *Rh* gene complexes, two alleles, D and *non-D*, are found at the first locus, and four alleles, (*ce, Ce, cE,* and *CE*) are found at the second locus. Tippett's model explains the *cis* or compound antigens we observe and also suggests that the partial D categories may represent alternate alleles at the

D locus. Mutation and unequal crossing over were offered as possible explanations for the rare and unusual *Rh* gene complexes found in the system.

Cloning of Rh DNA

In 1991, Colin et al.[127] published scientific data that finally put to rest the 50 years of theoretical debate on the genetic control of the Rh blood group system. These workers were able to show that, as previously predicted by Tippett,[130] two structural genes encode for the production of three Rh polypeptide chains. One gene is responsible for the expression of D and a second gene was responsible for the expression of Cc and Ee proteins. Phenotypes from both Rh+ and Rh− persons were subjected to southern blot analysis and using both a complete Rh cDNA clone as a probe and exon-specific probes corresponding to Rh DNA fragments, the *Rh* genome was cloned. In the Rh+ persons two genes were found present at the *Rh* locus, whereas in the Rh− persons only one gene was found. Thus, the second gene is required for the expression of the D antigenic protein. Analysis continued on genomic Rh DNA and some of these studies, as well as some earlier work, is referred to in the section on biochemical and molecular findings.

Antigens and Phenotypes

In addition to the five common Rh antigens, the products of rare variant alleles exist. Some *Rh* genes may code for various amounts of antigens or suppress, enhance or influence the expression of other gene products. Table 5-11 lists the gene products sufficiently well described to be granted an international number assignment (ISBT terminology) as a unique Rh protein epitope. The notation that represents the more common phenotypic description for some of the antigens is listed along with alternative terminology. Many of the Rh antigens are associated with each other by similar genetic and/or phenotypic features. It is expected that as more is known at the molecular level, some of these associations within the Rh system may change. Other excellent references are available for a more comprehensive discussion and understanding of the polymorphism of the Rh system.[2,131–134]

Weak D Phenotype

Weak D is the current phenotypic term[135,136] used when either a quantitative or qualitative difference in D results in a weakened expression of the antigen.

In 1946, Stratton[137] reported on variable reactivity with anti-D sera and the term D^U was used to define those red cells reacting with anti-D only when a more sensitive indirect antiglobulin test was used. Many red cells that previously tested D-negative, D^U-positive with early reagents and methods may be classified today as D-positive, using more sensitive testing techniques, including automated methods, mAbs, or potent antisera. The frequency of the weak D phenotype is relatively low, less than 1 percent.

The weak D phenotype can arise from three different genetic mechanisms: (1) a person may inherit a gene that encodes for a weakened quantitative expression of D[138,139]; (2) one gene may interact with another to modify and weaken the expression of the D antigen[140]; or (3) a gene may not encode for all the epitopes that makes up the complete D antigen.[141–145] Although in reduced amount, all epitopes of D are present in mechanisms 1 and 2 and those individuals cannot make allo-anti-D. Individuals with mechanism 3 can make allo-anti-D to their missing epitopes of D.

The weak D phenotype produced by a variant *Rh* gene that encodes a quantitatively weaker reactive D antigen[138] is more common in the black population and is usually of the genotype *cDe/cde*. Transmission of a variant gene for the weakened expression of D is rare in whites but, when present, it is more common in the genotypes *CDe/cde* and *cDE/cde*. The inherited forms of weak D generally give negative or very weak reactions with direct agglutination tests and may only be detectable by indirect antiglobulin tests.

The second genetic situation or gene interaction in which weak D[140] is observed most often is when the *D* gene is accompanied by the *Cde* haplotype represented on the red cells of the genotype *CDe/Cde* or *cDe/Cde*. The expression of D carried by one gene complex can be depressed, for unknown reasons, by the actions of the C antigen carried on the opposite paired gene complex. This weak D phenotype is an example of the *trans* position effect where the C allele is *trans* to D. The D gene can express normally in the next generation if it is not paired with a modifying C allele on the opposite chromosome. Most of the gene interaction forms of weak D are more easily agglutinated by anti-D typing sera, as compared with red cells from the gene that expresses a quantitatively weakened form of D.

In the third mechanism leading to the weak D phenotype, the gene expresses an incomplete D antigen and usually types as D-positive. Most of these D variants are not recognized until they have formed allo-anti-D. Current terminology uses weak D for all weakened expressions of D whether the differences are quantitative or qualitative. Once a weak D person makes alloimmune anti-D, the individual can then be described as D variant or partial D (see below).

It is now apparent that the weak D antigen is a poor immunogen[146]; however, accelerated destruction of weak D red cells, and severe hemolytic transfusion reactions,[147,148] can result if weak D blood is transfused to a person who is in the process of forming allo-anti-D. These observations have led to the double standard that is frequently applied when testing for weak D in blood donors and transfusion recipients. Currently, donor units that test negative on direct agglutination are further tested by the indirect antiglobulin method and if positive will be labeled Rh-positive. Conversely, weak D antiglobulin testing is not required for potential transfusion recipients. If patients are not tested for weak D, they will be classified as Rh-negative by direct testing and can be safely transfused with Rh-negative blood. Since weak D recipients rarely make anti-D when transfused with D-positive blood, and since Rh-negative blood is in shorter supply, some facilities choose to test patients for weak D and transfuse weak D recipients with Rh-positive blood. With the newer more sensitive direct agglutination methods used for D testing, most weak D patients will initially test as Rh-positive and the circumstances for finding antiglobulin weak D blood are so rare that such testing on all transfusion recipients may not prove that beneficial. Furthermore, unless the patient has anti-D, there is no easy way to determine if the weak D individual is a rare D variant (epitope deficient) who could possibly make anti-D. These differing policies for blood donors and transfusion recipients can lead to conflicting results and be confusing to people who are told that they are Rh-positive when they donate blood, but Rh-negative when they receive a transfusion. This situation can occur even more frequently among patients who are autologous blood donors.

Weak D testing plays an important role in deter-mining who should receive anti-D immunoprophy-laxis with Rh-immunoglobulin (Rhlg). Newborns of Rh-negative mothers are tested for D and weak D, and Rhlg is recommended for mothers of D-positive or weak D-positive infants in order to prevent immunization. HDN has been reported in a weak D infant of a D-negative mother previously immunized to D-positive cells.[149] However, it is generally held that pregnant women of the weak D phenotype do not require prophylaxis as the chance of immunization is so low. An argument can be made that partial D mothers may be at greater risk and should receive prophylaxis, but the decision is an individual one.

Partial D

In 1953, Argall, et al.[141] observed that a weak D-positive individual produced an alloanti-D. Other similar but rare occurrences led to the first concept that the D antigen was composed of a cluster or mosaic of genetically separate components or subdivisions. "Partial D" or "D variant" are the current phenotypic terms used to describe red cells that lack part of the D antigen mosaic. The occurrence of this phenotype is recognized when partial D individuals are immunized and make an alloanti-D to the missing piece of their antigen.

Initially, four serologic subdivisions of the D antigen were identified and named. Over time, the D antigen mosaic concept was extended and another classification system, one that divided the D antigen into "categories," emerged to define the increased complexity. Today the use of mAbs provides an additional tool to more precisely define the D antigen at the epitope level. The epitope region of the antigen consists of four to five amino acids on the linear D polypeptide that is complementary to the combining site of the antibody. These individual antigenic determinants characterize genetically different parts of the whole D antigen.

Epitope deficiency is a term that more accurately defines these partial D individuals who form alloimmune anti-D to the missing part or epitope that their RBCs lack. The alloanti-D from epitope deficient individuals can be mistaken as an autoanti-D. The antibody appears to react with most D-positive red cells except their own, since most cells from D-positive individuals contain all the epitopes of the D antigen. The significance of the alloanti-D from partial D in-

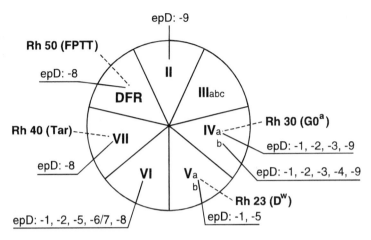

Fig. 5-2. Partial D categories with associated low-incidence antigens and missing epitopes of D.

dividuals is that it can cause a transfusion reaction or HDN. Once the patient has been determined to be D variant, Rh-negative blood should be selected for transfusion.

The classification systems for the component parts of the D antigen have evolved to the current representation in Figure 5-2. Studying antibodies to the D subdivisions, Wiener and Unger[150,151] identified four antigenic component parts, called Rh^A, Rh^B, Rh^C, and Rh^D, that were later numbered Rh12, Rh14, Rh15, and Rh16. Tippett and Sanger[142] expanded the four original subdivisions to six and notated them as categories I, II, III, IV, V, and VI. As more examples of D-positive individuals with anti-D in their sera were studied, Tippett and Sanger[143] refined some of the categories to include additional subcategories a, b, and c. It is not clearly known how the four subdivision and six category classifications correlate, since most serologic studies were performed using the category system definitions. The original Wiener alphabet terminology has become obsolete. The later revisions to the category system terminology include the deletion of category I, the addition of category VII,[152] and more recently Lomas et al.[153] proposed the addition of a new category, DFR, and the deletion of category Vc.

Some of the categories are associated with specific low-incidence marker antigens. The relationship of these low-incidence antigens to the D categories are

shown in Figure 5-2, and the antigens are further described below. The complexity of the partial D model continues to unfold as monoclonal anti-D reagents[144] are used to further characterize the categories of the D antigen. Lomas and Tippett and colleagues[154] in 1989, defined seven epitopes of D, and by 1993, the studies expanded to include nine epitopes.[155] Of the nine epitopes, the number lacking from cells of each category vary between two and five.

It is understandable that the genetic expression of the D antigen is extremely polymorphic now that it is known that D-positive individuals carry two *Rh* genes as opposed to one *Rh* gene in Rh-negative individuals. Mouro et al[156] recently determined the molecular basis of the D^{VI} category (partial D category VI) characterized by the lack of epitopes D1, D2, D5, D6/7, and D8. Using southern blot analysis, the study establishes that the D^{VI} phenotype is associated with at least two types of genomic rearrangements of the *D* gene that they call type I and II. The results of their study strongly suggest that the DNA segment of the *D* gene, encompassing exons 4, 5, and 6, is replaced in these variants by the equivalent region of the *CcEe* gene. They further propose that the D-specific amino acids encoded by these three exons (15 residues), might be critical for the reactivity with the different monoclonal antibodies characterizing epitopes D1, D2, D5, D6/7, and D8 that are carried by the normal D but not by the D^{VI} protein.

Using monoclonal reagents, it is expected that other partial D antigens may be identified that were previously undetected. The understanding of the polymorphism of the D antigen will become clearer as molecular studies continue to define the genetic relationship between the categories and their missing epitopes.

Go^a (Gonzales, D^{Cor}, Rh30)

Some partial D red cells have an associated low-incidence antigen that appears to be a substitute for the missing D component. Go^a is one such low-frequency "replacement antigen" that seems to replace the missing part of the D antigen in category IVa individuals. The Go^a antigen was first described by Alter et al.[157] in 1967 and later found to be the same antigen as D^{Cor}, described by Rosenfield et al.[158] in 1956. The Go^a antigen has only been found in the black population and it occurs with a frequency of 1.9 to 2.8 percent in American blacks. The D antigen appears slightly enhanced when Go^a is present and anti-Go^a has caused severe HDN.

D^W (Wiel, Rh23)

D^W was discovered by Chown et al.[159] in 1962 and is analogous to Go^a, as it appears to be a replacement antigen for category Va individuals. The D^W antigen has been found in 9 of 235 blacks, but in 0 of 13,000 whites.[160] The D antigen does not seem to be enhanced by the presence of D^W as it does with Go^a.

Tar (Targett, Rh40)

In 1975, Humphreys et al.[161] described a new low-incidence blood group antigen called Targett. In 1979, Lewis et al.[162] designated the antigen as Tar and provided evidence for assigning Tar to the Rh system. The Tar antigen is usually associated with a slightly weakened expression of the D antigen termed D^T and Tar is proposed as a D antigen marker for category VII individuals.[152]

FPTT (Rh50)

Lomas et al.[153] recently published studies on a new genetic determinant of D that was given the partial D category phenotypic term DFR. The DFR phenotype is associated with both the Cde and cDE gene complexes and both $CD^{DFR}e$ and $cD^{DFR}E$ are responsible for the production of the low-incidence antigen FPTT. At the date of this writing FPTT has become the newest member recognized of the Rh blood group system and has been numbered Rh50.

Cis Antigens

Cis gene products are expressed when one each of the C,c and E,e allelic pairs is inherited as a genetic unit on the same chromosome (Table 5-16) and not expressed if the genes are carried on opposite chromosomes in the trans position. These occurrences are useful in selecting a most probable genotype from the many possibilities represented by a given phenotype. Because of the existence of these "compound" antigens (as they are also known), it is believed that C,c and E,e gene products are in close spatial association on the red cell. Indeed, as we now know, the C or c and E or e are epitopes of the same gene, whereas the D epitope is a product of a second gene. Some investigators prefer to write the gene products in D, C, E order rather than C, D, E to reflect the closeness of the CE activity.

ce (f, Rh6)

The ce antibody, originally named "f" by Rosenfield and colleagues[163] in 1953, does not behave as a mixture of anti-c plus anti-e. It only reacts with red cells of individuals who have c plus e antigens in a cis position on the same haplotype. Anti-ce (f) reacts with cde and cDe cells, but not with cells of genotype CDe/cDe. Anti-ce is often found as a separable antibody along with anti-c.

Ce (rh_i, Rh7)

The cis gene product Ce^{164} is similar to ce, except both alleles, C and e, must be present on the same haplotype, either CDe or Cde for expression of the

Table 5-16. Compound or Cis Antigens Produced by Common Haplotypes

Antigens			Haplotypes		
Rh6	ce(f)	R^0	cDe	r	cde
Rh7	Ce (rh_i)	R^1	CDe	r'	Cde
Rh27	cE (rh_{ii})	R^2	cDE	r''	cdE
Rh22		R^Z	CDE	r^y	CdE

antigen. Anti-Ce is frequently found in association with anti-C. Most Rh-positive persons who make anti-C have anti-Ce as the predominant antibody, making antibody identification testing and interpretation difficult.

CE (Jarvis, Rh22); cE (rh$_{ii}$, Rh27)

Other antigens of *cis* genes, *cis* CE[165] and *cis* cE[166] are known, although the antibodies to these specificities are considerably more rare.

The G Antigen and C^G

The G (Rh12) antigen was described in 1958 by Allen and Tippett[167] from serologic observations of an antibody that appeared to recognize both the C and D antigens. The antibody reacting as anti−C+D was first thought to represent crossreactivity between the D and C antigens, but anti-CD was subsequently determined to specify a new antigen named G. The G antigen, with few exceptions, is expressed by any gene making D or C, although rare individuals D+(G−) and D−C−(G+) have been described. Whenever anti-D or anti-C are made without known exposure to the specific D or C antigen, an anti-G should be considered.

An antigen in a weakened form that almost always accompanies C, termed C^G (Rh21) has been defined by varying situations. Sera containing anti-C usually contains anti-Ce, and it has been suggested that the anti-C portion of the antisera mixture may actually represent anti-C^G. Others propose that the C^G antigen may be a product of the same gene producing the D−C−(G+) phenotype above.[168,169]

Cc and Ee Variant Antigens and Phenotypes

Usually one of the two common alleles, *C* or *c* and *E* or *e*, are present, however rare variant antigens may reside at the same genetic site encoded for by genes distinct from those determining the common alleles. Variants of the C antigen are found more frequently in whites and most notably, variants to the e antigen are found to be both frequent and complex in blacks.[170] Examples of phenotypes with weakened expression of C, c, and E antigens have been described similar to the genetic weak D phenotype.

C^W (Rh8); C^X (Rh9); E^W (Rh11)

The antigen C^W, discovered in 1946 by Callender and Race,[171] was thought for many years to simply be an allele of C, however it was determined that most genes that produce C^W also make C. Studies have also found some rare cases where the gene that produces C^W also make c. A puzzling feature of most anti-C sera is that they cannot distinguish C^W from C but can react with red cells if either the C or C^W antigen is present. The sera appear to contain an inseparable specificity, "anti-CC^W; thus, C^W red blood cells will react with most anti-C sera whether the C antigen is present or not. The C^W antigen is relatively rare, occurring in less than 2 percent of whites, and is even rarer in blacks. Since C^W is a low-incidence antigen, it appears as though C may stimulate the production of anti-C^W. Indeed, individuals immunized with C-positive, C^W-negative cells have produced anti-C^W specificity. Most antibody examples are naturally occurring since they have not developed as a result of a known stimulus. Anti-C^W has been implicated in hemolytic transfusion reactions and HDN.

The C^X antigen, discovered by Stratton and Renton[172] in 1954, is comparable in many ways to C^W. It seems likely that the genes that produce C^X also produce C. As with C^W, it is now known that C^X can also be made by genes that make c but no C. Anti-C sera will react with red cells whether the C or C^X antigen is present. The frequency of the C^X antigen of 1/1,000 is considerably lower than C^W. Studying a random population of East African blacks, Sistonen and coworkers[173] found the prevalency of C^X to be 4 out of more than 500 people tested. Anti-C^X has been implicated in a case of HDN.

The quite rare E^W antigen was first found in 1955[174] when it was implicated as a possible cause of HDN. In addition to reacting with specific anti-E^W, the E^W antigen is agglutinated by some but not all anti-E.

E^T (Rh24); c-like (Deal, Rh26)

In 1962, Vos and Kirk[175] found a naturally occurring antibody in the serum of an Australian Aborigine that appeared to have anti-E specificity. The E^T antibody, as it became known, reacts invariably with E-positive samples of white and black Americans, but with only one-half of E-positive Aborigines. Studies show that it is probably more appropriate to consider E^T a part of the e antigen rather than as a product of an *Ee* allele. Individuals of E+, E^T- phenotype can develop allo-anti-E^T.

The Deal antigen, first described by Huestis et al.[176] in 1964, appears to be a rare variant of c rather than of C. In fact, anti-Rh26 can easily be mistaken for anti-c because most examples of a c-positive red cells are Rh:26 and most c-negative cells are Rh:-26.

hr^S (Rh19) and hr^B (Rh31)

Shapiro et al., in 1960[177] and 1972,[178] reported the results of studies on anti-hr^S and anti-hr^B specificities respectively found in the sera of two South African black women, Mrs. Shabalala and Mrs. Bastiaan. Both women were e-positive and possessed an anti-e-like reactivity in their serum. The antibodies were thought to detect a component of the e antigen similar to the concept of the categories of D (see Partial D). Both hr^S and hr^B antigens are present in most e-positive red cells. Variant states of the e antigen exist predominantly in blacks, where the hr^S or hr^B component is absent. Such individuals type e-positive but, if immunized, they make an anti-e to the missing piece of their e antigen. The antibody that is produced will react with most e-positive red cells, but not their own. The hr^S cells were found to lack an e component in almost 1 percent of e-positive blacks and in 0.17 of e-positive whites in the South African population tested; however, overall, the e "mosaic" picture has proven far more complex than that of D. It has not been practical for investigators to define e subdivisions or categories for people with e-positive red cells who make e-like antibodies. Some investigators[179,180] argue that hr^S and hr^B are distinct epitopes of e found respectively within the Hr$_O$ (Rh17) and Hr^B (Rh34) high-incidence Rh antigens.

V (ce^S, Rh10); VS(e^S, Rh20); Cde Phenotype

Among blacks there are numerous qualitative and quantitative Rh variant antigens and phenotypes (Table 5-17), and some of these are quite likely to be encountered. Variants of e are fairly common among blacks, but extremely rare in whites. The nature of these antigens as defined by their antibody specificities is still somewhat controversial.

In 1955, DeNatale et al.[181] reported the first example of anti-V that defined an antigen present in about 30% of the red cells tested from a randomly selected black population. Very few whites carry the V antigen. Some consider V an example of the *cis* antigen product ce^S, as it is similar to ce(f) in that it involves the *cis* product c plus the black antigen e^S. Others disagree with this interpretation and consider V a variant antigen residing at the same genetic site as E.

In 1960, Sanger et al.[182] reported on a new antibody, anti-VS, that reacted with all V-positive red cells. It was not named for its relationship to V, but rather for the initials of the patient in whose serum it was originally found. The VS antigen is present in up to 40 percent of the black population. It was later determined that anti-VS specified the e^S component of the ce^S *cis* antigen product.

Another difference in blacks and whites at the phenotypic level is represented by the *Cde* haplotype of the *Cde/cde* genotype. The *Cde* cells of blacks react more weakly with human anti-C sera. This is probably due to the high anti-Ce component found in most anti-C sera that reacts with the e structure of the Ce cells in whites, but not with the Ce^S cells more frequently found in blacks.

Deletion Phenotypes

The rare deletion phenotypes are characterized by red cells that appear to lack the C,c and/or E,e antigens and conversely, the red cells of these phenotypes usually express strong D activity. Indeed, studies show that most deletion red cells that have been phenotyped have an increased number of D sites available per cell.[183] The deletion of the Rh activity is noted using a dash or dot in the haplotype.

Recent analysis of Rh genomic DNA[184] points out the fallacy of concluding a genotype from individuals expressing the -D-, -c^{W}D-, and Cd- phenotypes. These rare deletion individuals are found to possess normal *D* gene structure and are not found to possess gross deletion of *CcEe* genetic material. Apparently, small alterations at the *Rh* locus, not gene deletions, account for the partial or complete lack of *CcEe* gene expressions.

Other features of the D-deletion phenotypes include the absence of some very high-incidence Rh system antigens, and the presence of some very low-incidence Rh antigens. The characteristics common to the various deletion phenotypes are reviewed in

Table 5-17. High- and Low-Incidence Antigens

>99%				<1%			
More often Absent in Blacks Than in Whites				Rare in Whites, More Common in Blacks			
Rh17	Hr^0	Rh19	hr^S	Rh9	C^X	Rh10	ce^S, V
Rh18	Hr	Rh31	hr^B	Rh11	E^W	Rh20	e^S VS
Rh29	total Rh			Rh22	CE	Rh28	Hr^H
Rh34	Hr^B			Rh23	D^W	Rh42	Ce^S
Rh39	C-like			Rh30	Go^a		
Rh44	Nou			Rh32	$\overline{\overline{R}}^N$		
Rh46	Sec			Rh33	R$_0$^{Har}		
Rh47	Dav			Rh35	1114		
				Rh36	Be^a		
				Rh37	Evans		
				Rh40	Tar		
				Rh43	Craw		
				Rh45	Riv		
				Rh48	JAL		
				Rh49	STEM		
				Rh50	FPTT		

Table 5-18. As one might expect, individuals of deletion phenotypes can easily form antibodies once exposed to normal red cells through pregnancy or transfusion. Difficulties can also occur in interpretation of parentage testing results, since the common C,c and/or E,e antigens are absent.

-D-

The -D- phenotype was first described by Race et al.[185] in 1951. The gene responsible for this phenotype encodes for both the D and G antigens, although all traces of C,c and E,e antigens are lacking. The strongly enhanced D activity helps detect this rare phenotype when only routine D testing is performed.

Molecular genetic analysis of individuals homozygous for the -D- complex found no rearrangement, mutation, or deletion of the *CcEe* gene.[184] Further studies are required to determine the cause for the lack of expression of the C,c and E,e antigens in -D- individuals. Some hypotheses suggest that the altered content of the Rh polypeptides on the red cell surface may result from a regulation mechanism involving other membrane structures or may result from reduced transcriptional activity of the *CcEe* gene.

Homozygous -D- individuals lack several high-incidence antigens including Rh17 (Hr$_O$), Rh18 (Hr), and Rh34 (Hr^B), but the high-incidence Rh29 ("total-Rh") is present. The -D- individuals are easily immunized and can present significant transfusion problems. The single antibody, anti-Rh17 (Hr$_O$), is often formed and this occurrence can create transfusion problems since anti-Rh17 is compatible only with cells from -D- and Rh$_{null}$ individuals. Some im-

Table 5-18. High- and Low-Incidence Antigens Associated With D-Deletion Phenotypes

	-D-	·D·	cD–, C^{W}D –	(C)D^{IV} –
High-Incidence				
Rh29	+	+	+	+
Rh17 (Hr$_0$)	–	–	–	–
Rh18 (Hr)	–	–	–	–
Rh34 (Hr^B)	–	–	–	–
Rh44 (Nou)	–	–	–	+
Rh47 (Dav)	–	+	–	+
Low-incidence	Rh37 (Evans)			Rh30 (Go^a) Rh33 (R$_0$^{Har}) Rh45 (Riv)

mune sera of -D- individuals contain anti-e or other separable specificities.

·D·

The ·D· phenotype, discovered by Contreras and colleagues[186] in 1978, is similar to -D-, except that its D activity is not as enhanced as in -D-, and its gene encodes for a low-incidence antigen called Rh37 (Evans).[187] In fact, these phenotypes are best differentiated using anti-Rh37. The high-incidence antigen Rh47 (Dav),[188] found on all common Rh phenotypes but absent on other deletion phenotypes, is also present on ·D· cells.

C^WD-, cD-, and (C)D^{IV}-

Other rare, partially deleted phenotypes have been identified and they include C^WD-,[189] cD-,[190] and (C)D^{IV}-.[191] All three phenotypes demonstrate D, G, and Rh29 activity, weakened C,c activity, and the e antigen is absent. C^WD- and cD- red cells show strong D expression; however, (C)D^{IV}- shows depressed D activity that is typical of category IV (partial D) phenotype.

Molecular genetic analysis of individuals homozygous for the C^WD-, and cD- gene complexes reveals that that both variants carry a hybrid rearrangement of their *CcEe* gene[184] that explains the abnormal antigen profiles associated with the complexes. Segmental replacement of DNA in the *CcEe* gene may produce the CcEe hybrid protein. The altered Rh protein carries C,c epitopes with lower reactivity than normal, as well as D epitopes that are in addition to the normal D protein expressed by the *D* gene. The hybrid gene lacks the exon associated with the polymorphism of *Ee*[192] and therefore cannot produce the protein with E,e antigenicity.

(C)D^{IV}- red cells carry three low-incidence antigens—Rh30 (Go^a), Rh33 (R$_o$^{Har}), and Rh45 (Riv)—as well as the three high-incidence antigens, Rh29, Rh48 (Nou), and Rh47 (Dav). The Nou[192] antigen is found on all common Rh phenotypes and on (C)D^{IV}- cells, but is absent on -D-, cD-, and C^WD- cells.

Other High-Incidence Antigens

Individuals of the deletion phenotypes, as well as individuals of Rh$_{null}$ phenotype, can easily form antibodies to red cells of normal Rh phenotypes when stimulated through pregnancy and transfusion. These specificities often define antigens of high-incidence, determinants commonly derived from all normal *Rh* gene complexes (Tables 5-17 and 5-18). Issitt has pointed out some interesting antithetical relationships between some high and low-incidence antigens of the Rh system.[131,193]

Rh39

Rh39 is an antigen that is present on all except Rh$_{null}$ RBCs. Interestingly, the antibody, anti-Rh39, initially appears to determine a C-like specificity, but the activity can be absorbed by D deletion red cells that are phenotypically C-negative. Thus far, Rh 39 has only been found as an autoantibody.[194]

Rh46 (Sec)

Sec is the newest antigen of high-incidence to be discovered in the Rh system.[195] It has been found to be made by all common *Rh* genes but Sec is not made by *Rh-deletion* genes or those that make the low-incidence antigen, Rh32.

Duclos and LW

Both Duclos (previously Rh38)[190] and LW (previously Rh25 and now LW^a) are high-incidence antigens that earlier were assigned to the Rh system because of their phenotypic relationship with Rh. They continue to be related biochemically by their association with the Rh polypeptides in the RBC membrane.[196,197] It is now clear that they do not belong to the Rh system as their genes segregate independently and do not reside at the *Rh* locus (see LW System below).

Other Low-Incidence Antigens

Some low-incidence Rh antigens have been mentioned previously as rare alleles at the *C/E* genetic sites, as rare variants of *e*, and as genetic markers for specific categories of D (partial D). Low-incidence antigens are generally defined as occurring on less than 1 percent of red cells from most random populations. Table 5-17 lists the low-incidence antigens currently recognized in the Rh system. The low-incidence Rh antigens discussed below represent marker antigens associated with rare gene com-

Table 5-19. Low-Incidence Antigens and Depressed Phenotypes Associated With Some Rare Genes

Genes	Antigens		
	Low-Incidence	D Expression	Depressed
$\overline{\overline{R}}^N$	Rh32	Normal to slightly elevated	C,e
(C)D(e)		Increased	C,e
(C)D(e)	Rh35	Normal	C,e
R^{oHar}	Rh33	Markedly decreased	D,e

plexes (Table 5-19), as well as the newest antigens to be discovered and accepted into the Rh system. The rare genes responsible for low-incidence antigens are generally believed to be a result of a single point mutation, the product of one amino acid substitution within the Rh polypeptide.

Rh33 (R_o^{Har})

The low-incidence antigen Rh33 is found as a product of either the rare variant gene, R^{oHar} or the rare variant $D^{IV}(C)$-.[198] In 1971, Giles et al.[199] reported that the R^{oHar} gene encodes for normal amounts of c and diminished amounts of D, e, f, and Hr° and no G antigen. The D antigenic expression made by R^{oHar} is reduced and may be difficult to detect although some monoclonal anti-D reagents are able to detect the D antigen with ease. The D expression from individuals of the gene complex $D^{IV}(C)$- is easy to detect, since the D antigen appears exhaulted.

Rh32

In 1960, Rosenfield et al.[200] described a new low-incidence marker antigen, Rh32. Rh32 is encoded by a rare variant gene termed $\overline{\overline{R}}^N$, that also produces a depressed C, markedly depressed e and normal to slightly elevated levels of D antigen. The $\overline{\overline{R}}^N$ gene occurs rarely in whites but is found in 1 percent of blacks. Anti-Rh32 has been found without known stimulus, in the sera of patients with autoantibodies. Some investigators[131] consider anti-Rh32 and anti-Rh46, the antibody to the high-incidence antigen Sec, to be antithetical.

Rh35 and Rh36 (Be^a, Berrens)

In 1963, Broman et al.[201] and in 1965, Heiken and Giles[202] described two additional rare (C)D(e) gene complexes in Scandinavian whites that, along with

the rare $\overline{\overline{R}}^N$ gene, produced depressed phenotypes with common features. The genes are not identical and, in 1971, Giles and Skov[203] described an antibody that identified the low-incidence marker antigen, Rh35, that distinguishes two gene complexes. Interestingly, when Rh35 is present there are normal amounts of D antigen, and when Rh35 is absent the D antigen is enhanced.

Similar to Rh35, Rh36[204] is a low-incidence marker antigen that distinguishes between two rare variant gene complexes, (c)d(e), that otherwise encode for similar depressed phenotypes. Anti-Be^a was first reported in a case of HDN.

Rh48(JAL); Rh49(STEM); RH50 (FPTT); LOCR

The JAL[205,206] and STEM[207] antigens are among the newest members assigned to the Rh system. Investigations of their respective antibodies were initiated when they were found to be implicated in individual cases of HDN. As described above, some low-incidence antigens appear to be associated as markers for rare gene complexes (Table 5-19) and the JAL antigen similarly appears to be related as a marker for two unusual gene complexes. In whites, JAL appears to be encoded by the Ce complex and red cells of the JAL+ phenotype express a weakened C antigen. In blacks, JAL appears to be a product of the ce complex and the JAL+ phenotype exhibits a weakened c and e antigen.

Anti-STEM was initially found in the sera of a postpartum black African woman, and the STEM antigen appears to be associated with the unusual e-variant phenotypes more frequently found in blacks. Individuals of hr^S- and hr^B-phenotype are now being further characterized by the presence or absence of the STEM antigen.

FPTT (Rh50),[153] as previously discussed, appears as a low-incidence marker antigen for the new partial D phenotype, DFR. It was initially described in association with Rh33 and appears to be associated with weakened C or e phenotypes, or both.

Another newly discovered red cell antigen, LOCR,[208] appears to be phenotypically related to Rh and, with the addition of more evidence, LOCR may be assigned to the Rh system. The LOCR antigen, similar to JAL and STEM, was initially specified through an investigation of a case of HDN. Similar to some other low-incidence antigens, including JAL and FPTT, the LOCR antigen is associated with weakened phenotypic expression of some common Rh antigens, specifically c and e.

Other antisera are under investigation that contain specificities to other low-incidence antigens that appear phenotypically related to Rh. As more information accumulates, these determinants will either be ruled in or out as members of the extensive and complex Rh blood group system.

Rh_{null} and Rh_{mod} Phenotypes and Rh Deficiency Syndrome

The term Rh_{null} describes red cells that lack expression of all known Rh antigens.[209] This phenotype was first reported in an Australian Aboriginal woman by Vos et al.[210] in 1961. Although exceedingly rare, the Rh_{null} phenotype can result from two different genetic mechanisms. The *regulator* type[211] of Rh_{null} results from the homozygous inheritance of the recessive suppressor gene $X^o r$. $X^o r$ is an allele to the very common regulator gene $X^1 r$, and when present, prevents the expression of normal *Rh* genes. These regulator genes segregate independently of other Rh system genes.

A second form of Rh_{null}, an even more rare *amorphic type*, occurs in persons homozygous for a rare silent allele (r)[212] at the *Rh* locus. When $X^o r$ is heterozygous, or when one amorphic gene is passed on to the next generation, an overall depression of Rh antigens may be demonstrated in the offspring, since only Rh antigens inherited from the normal parent are expressed.

Rh_{mod} individuals have much reduced and sometimes varied Rh activity. When the Rh antigens are severely depressed, the individuals can look like Rh_{null}. The Rh_{mod} phenotype has a genetic derivation similar to the *regulator* type of Rh_{null}. A homozygous recessive suppressor gene X^Q, inherited independently of the Rh locus, is responsible for the depression of Rh activity. No suppression of Rh is noted when the X^Q gene is present in a single dose. The Rh expression of the X^Q gene appears between that of the normal $X^1 r$ and that of the Rh_{null} $X^o r$ regulator gene and, in both of these Rh_{mod} and Rh_{null} situations, the genes can pass on normal expression of Rh activity to the next generation. Although Rh_{null} and Rh_{mod} individuals appear to be similar, varying only in degree of expression, it is still

to be determined whether these situations represent inheritance of the same recessive modifying genes with different degrees of penetrance, or whether $X^o r$ and X^Q represent inheritance of different genetic alleles. Molecular DNA studies[213] using exon-specific probes deduced from the recent cloning of *Rh* genes (*CcEe* and *D*), confirmed that the Rh-deficient individuals carry normal genes at the Rh site on the chromosome and can pass on normal Rh antigenic expression in their offspring. They were further able to determine that Rh_{null} regulator variants could be either of the *DD, Dd,* or *dd* genotypes and deduced that the inhibitor genes can suppress Rh expression from chromosomes carrying either one or two of the *Rh* genes.

Studies on Rh_{null} cells have revealed some interesting relationships on the phenotypic level between Rh and other genetically independent blood group systems. Rh_{null} cells appear to have suppressed S, s, and U antigens. Glycophorin B, the carrier of Ss antigens, appears to be present in greatly reduced amount[214] and appears to be responsible for a shape change on Rh_{null} cells. This shape change makes it more difficult to detect S,s, and especially U, since the U antigen is located very close to the RBC membrane. Indeed, Rh_{null} cells appear U-negative, even when they are U-positive. Other antigens that include LW, Fy5, and the high-incidence Duclos (formerly Rh38) have shown close phenotypic association with Rh as their presence is notably missing or severely diminished in Rh_{null} cells.[215] The relationship of glycophorin B, LW, and Fy5 to the Rh proteins is proposed in a model in which these structures form a cluster on the red cell membrane surface. This Rh cluster or complex model will be discussed further in the section on biochemical and molecular findings.

The clinical importance of the Rh-deficiency phenotypes is evident from an individual's ability to produce significant RBC antibodies easily, as well as the ability to demonstrate an accompanying hemolytic anemia of varying severity. Rh_{null} individuals immunized through pregnancy or transfusion form complex alloantibodies including Rh29, Rh39, hr, Hr_O, and Rh34, as well as simple C, D, and e. Anti-Rh29, also called anti-total Rh, is directed towards all Rh antigens and the "total Rh" antibody has been implicated in HDN.

In 1967, Schmidt et al.[216] observed that Rh_{null} red cells had a surface defect and decreased red cell survival and were associated with a hemolytic anemia. With this original study and the many since performed, additional features were associated with what would become known as Rh_{null} syndrome. The features of this syndrome include the presence of cup-shaped stomatocytes, some spherocytes and the following indications of reduced red cell survival: increased reticulocyte count, reduced hemoglobin and haptoglobin, and increased bilirubin and fetal hemoglobin levels. More sophisticated studies have revealed that Rh_{null} cells have hyperactive membrane ATPase, reduced cation and water content, and relative deficiency of membrane cholesterol.[217,218]

The Rh_{mod} phenotype was described in an original case by Chown et al.[219,220] Reduced red cell survival and a hemolytic anemia are features of the Rh_{mod} phenotype, although the amount of clinical disease can vary. Usually the hemolytic anemia is less in Rh_{mod} than in Rh_{null} individuals; however, more severe forms of the clinical disease have been observed from Rh_{mod} phenotypes. The morphologic and red cell membrane abnormalities seen in Rh_{mod} red cells are similar to those of Rh_{null} cells. The more encompassing term Rh-deficiency syndrome is used to accommodate the similar clinical phenomenon observed in both the Rh_{null} and Rh_{mod} phenotypes.

A vast number of studies have been performed over the years on Rh_{null} cells. It was assumed that comparisons between the red cells that lack all known Rh antigens and the red cells of normal Rh expression could be the key to unlocking the mysteries of Rh structure and function. Since 1982[221,222] biochemical information about the red cell membrane components that carry the Rh antigens and their genetic derivation[127] began accumulating rapidly. Although much is known about the structure of the Rh polypeptide, little is known about its function. Rh cDNA cloning[223–227] suggests that the polypeptide closely resembles transporter proteins with multiple membrane bilayer-spanning domains. Kuypers et al.[228,] in 1984, reported that Rh_{null} cells show abnormal structure of phospholipids in the RBC membrane. In 1988 de Vetten and Agre[229] demonstrated that Rh polypeptides provide a site for fatty acid acylation of the red blood cell membrane and that observation further supports the theory that Rh proteins are involved in the organization of lipids within the membrane bilayer. Agre and Cartron[230] point to the membrane–structure role of Rh polypeptides as a more minor supporting role, since clinical sequelae of the Rh_{null} syndrome often are not severe. Indeed, the severity of the hemolysis and anemia varies among individuals. Rh_{null} individuals with a sufficiently compensated anemia may lead normal lives and may not even be detected in preliminary blood donor screening tests.

With all the noted abnormalities of the red cell membrane of Rh_{null} individuals, it was felt that the hemolytic anemia was a product of shortened in vivo survival of the aberrant RBCs. Observations support that the shortened survival is due to accelerated RBC clearance by the spleen, as the Rh_{null} red cells function and survive normally after splenectomy[231] and the syndrome is completely corrected.

Rh Antibodies

Most Rh antibodies result from immunization through transfusion or pregnancy. Furthermore, most of these immune IgG Rh specificities have been implicated in hemolytic transfusion reactions and HDN.

The D antigen is the most effective immunogen, followed by c and E. In fact, D is probably the most potent immunogen of all red blood cell antigens. Various studies have shown that when Rh-negative individuals are transfused with 1 or more units of Rh-positive red cells, more than 80 percent will form anti-D within 2 to 5 months. Other studies indicate that when Rh-negative recipients are transfused with 1 to 40 ml of Rh-positive red cells, 15 to 30 percent will make anti-D,[232] respectively. Although the D antigen is highly immunogenic, 20 to 30 percent of Rh-negative individuals repeatedly exposed to D will never form anti-D. These individuals are called nonresponders. Deliberate immunization studies against the C, c, E, and e antigens have shown them to be much less immunogenic than D, with less than 1 percent of individuals forming the corresponding antibody after exposure.

It is a standard practice to Rh type all donors and recipients and to give Rh-negative red cells to Rh-negative recipients. The use of Rh-positive blood for Rh-negative recipients should be restricted to acute emergencies when Rh-negative blood is not available. Once anti-D is formed, it can cause severe and even fatal HDN. If a person immunized to D carries subdetectable levels of antibody, subsequent transfusions can be dangerous and lead to delayed transfusion reactions. Donors and patients are routinely matched only for the D antigen since immunization from transfusion to the other Rh antigens is uncommon.

Because of the long-standing practice of transfusing Rh-negative individuals with Rh-negative blood, most antibodies formed as a result of transfusion are not anti-D, and most transfusion reactions are not due to D incompatibility. Since the introduction of RhIG in 1968, hemolytic disease of the newborn from anti-D has become a rare occurrence. Prior to the use of RhIG, studies indicated that 15 to 22 percent of untreated Rh-negative women eventually produced anti-D. Today, most cases of HDN are due to ABO incompatibility and are usually mild.

Other than anti-D, the Rh antibodies most commonly found in the sera of immunized patients in decreasing order of occurrence are anti-E, anti-c, anti-e, and anti-C. Anti-E is by far the most common Rh antibody. Anti-c, however, is usually IgG and causes more clinically significant problems. Anti-e is more commonly found as an autoantibody than as an alloantibody. Only 2 percent of the population is negative for the e antigen and therefore capable of producing the alloantibody.

Some Rh specificities are more likely to be found in combination with others. Anti-ce is present in most sera containing anti-c and/or anti-e. Anti-C rarely occurs alone without anti-D. Since D-positive and C-positive people usually share the G antigen, C may not be recognized as foreign in D-positive, C-negative individuals. Most anti-C sera are mixtures of anti-C and anti-Ce. Anti-c commonly occurs with anti-E in immunized people. If anti-E is present and a hemolytic reaction follows the transfusion of E-negative blood, the presence of a subdetectable level of anti-c should be suspected. Although it is not standard practice to select donor blood negative for antigens which might stimulate antibody production, some consider it advisable to select R^1R^1 (*CDe/CDe*) cells for transfusion to R^1R^1 recipients with anti-E to avoid anti-c stimulation. Since patients are more frequently exposed to c than to E, it does not follow that once anti-c is found that anti-E will more likely develop.

Most examples of Rh antibodies are IgG; however, some saline-reactive Rh specificities can be found and these more commonly include anti-E and anti-C^W. Examples of naturally occurring anti-C, anti-C^X, anti-Rh30, and anti-Rh32 have also been found. Naturally occurring anti-D may be detected in Rh-negative donors when sensitive enzyme detection methods are used.

Most of the Rh antibodies are of the subclass IgG1, followed by IgG3. Although both IgG subclasses efficiently initiate complement activation, Rh antibodies do not bind complement. The reason for this is probably that the Rh antigens are too far apart on the red cell to allow antibodies to bind close enough for complement activation. IgG3-coated red cells are cleared more efficiently in vivo than are IgG1-coated cells. IgG1 crosses the placenta more efficiently than IgG3; however, high-titer IgG3 anti-D in the serum of a pregnant woman may predict a more severe HDN due to the more rapid clearance of the coated red cells. Rh antibodies, particularly anti-C, have been known to cause delayed transfusion reactions occasionally associated with hemoglobinemia. Since Rh antibodies do not activate complement, hemoglobinemia may be the result of hemoglobin released from the cells damaged in the spleen and reticuloendothelial system.

Rh antibodies are often directed against the Rh protein responsible for warm autoimmune hemolytic anemia (WAIHA). Some have easily recognized Rh specificity, with autoanti-e being the most frequently observed.[233] Autoantibodies to c, f, E, rh_i, and G have also been found. More commonly, WAIHA autoantibodies are directed toward broader Rh specificities. These warm autoantibodies characteristically react with all normal Rh phenotypes and sometimes with D-deleted cells.

Some of the more common observations of Rh system antibodies have been addressed. The earlier cited texts[1,7] provide a more extended look into the characteristics of antibody production related to the Rh blood group antigens, and expand on the significance of these antibodies in clinical medicine.

Biochemical and Molecular Findings

Because of the notable serologic and genetic complexities of the Rh system, great efforts were undertaken to chemically isolate and identify the Rh antigenic protein(s). For many years relatively little was learned; however, during the early 1980s, an eruption of biochemical information began to emerge. The following is an attempt to briefly highlight the transition of knowledge over the past decade that includes the first isolation of the Rh protein in 1982, the peptide mapping and amino acid sequence studies of the early 1990s, and the cloning of the Rh genome. Information about the molecular biology of the Rh system continues to expand so rapidly that much of what is contained in text books becomes outdated as soon as it is in print. For a more comprehensive analysis of the Rh system at the biochemical and molecular level, the reader should refer to the citations listed at the end of the blood group section as well as the current literature.

The Rh antigens are carried on protein chains that were first partially characterized by studies of red cell membranes.[234,235] These studies show that the red cell surface is primarily composed of a lipid membrane bilayer embedded with large protein molecules. The internal cytoplasmic membrane is composed of a network of linked proteins that maintain the cell's shape and flexibility. These cytoskeletal proteins are anchored to the membrane bilayer via other transmembrane connecting proteins. The most numerous integral membrane proteins that penetrate the lipid bylayer include band 3, the anion exchanger, the glycophorins, other membrane transporters, and structural components of blood group antigens such as the clinically important Rh proteins.

Several problems interfered with the early attempts to isolate the specific membrane protein component carrying Rh. Rh antigens are not found in abundant quantity and, unlike the ABO and Lewis systems, Rh antigens appear to be red-cell bound and are not found in plasma or other body fluids. In addition, the number of Rh sites found on red cells is approximately one-tenth the number of ABO and MN sites.[236–238] Not only are there difficulties in harvesting sufficient material for study but, once the Rh proteins are removed from the membrane, they are denatured and no longer able to complex with Rh antibodies in efforts to further characterize the antigenic structures.[230,239]

During the early 1980s, several groups of investigators were able to isolate a common Rh-membrane-associated protein. These early reported findings are summarized in part in an excellent review by Issitt.[148] In 1982, two simultaneous but independent studies[221,222] were published by Moore and associates in Edinburgh, and Gahmberg and associates in Helsinki. These studies documented the first successful efforts to isolate the Rh polypeptides. A third report followed in 1983, by Ridgwell and associates[240] in Bristol, also claiming to have isolated the Rh proteins.

These investigators used techniques that involved radiolabelling RBCs and yielded proteins that were immunoprecipitated with anti-D, anti-c, and anti-E. Gahmberg[241] precipitated one protein using D-positive red cells only with anti-D. The isolates demonstrated electrophoretic mobilities from 28 to 33 kd. Moore et al.[221] suspected that the D antigen was carried on a different protein than c and E, and Ridgwell et al.[240] concluded that the Rh antigens were carried on two different membrane proteins.

Among these early studies on the isolation of Rh, it is generally agreed that the proteins that immunoprecipitated with anti-D at a molecular weight of 32 kd were likely the same. The two protein concept was supported by earlier observations[242] on the need for a thiol group for certain Rh antigen activity, and that two thiol group-containing proteins are present on RBCs of all normal Rh phenotypes and are absent on Rh$_{null}$ cells.[241]

Some of the features of the basic biochemistry of Rh began to be described as a result of these initial studies[243] and that information added more pieces to the puzzle on the structure and function of the Rh proteins within the red cell. The D peptide is an integral membrane protein that spans the red cell membrane lipid bilayer. The membrane lipids[244] probably contribute in a minor way to the antigenicity of the Rh structure by orienting the protein to allow for antibody binding. Although Rh and band 3 proteins are similar membrane-spanning proteins, Rh was determined to be non band-3 protein. A distinguishing feature of the Rh antigen bearing proteins is that the peptides are not glycosylated. In stark contrast to Rh, all other blood group systems have attached carbohydrate regardless of whether their antigenic structures are lipid or protein in nature. The Rh peptides also are not phosphorylated.

Indirect evidence soon emerged that the Rh polypeptides might serve a structural stabilizing function by attaching to the cytoskeleton.[245] By definition the cytoskeleton is not solubilized in non ionic detergents and the Rh protein was also found to be very poorly soluble.[245,246] Since the Rh polypeptide is extremely hydrophobic, it was suggested that there may be some weak linkage to the cytoskeleton. More current observations[230] on the interaction between the Rh polypeptides and the membrane skeleton support that the linkage either does not exist or is relatively weak.

Once the breakthrough to isolate the Rh proteins was accomplished, other investigations rapidly followed and information on the Rh proteins continued to escalate.[237,238,247–249] For a more comprehensive look into the work on the isolation of the Rh proteins and their defined biochemistry, the reader is referred to the literature.[133,148,230] From the mid-1980s into the early 1990s, several groups of investigators continued studies on isolated Rh proteins and two groups published findings on the cDNA sequence for an Rh polypeptide.[223,224] In 1987, workers in Baltimore[239,250–252] developed a nonimmunoprecipitation method to isolate the Rh polypeptides that proved to be highly beneficial in the advancement of investigations. The great advantage of the nonimmune method is that the yield of product for study was nearly 10 times greater than previous yields using immune precipitation methods. In 1987 information began to emerge from the Paris workers[237,238,247,249,253,254] using monoclonal Rh antibodies,[255] competitive immunoassays and flow cytometry. These studies conclude that the Rh antigens are carried on three distinct proteins. One peptide appears to carry D and G, and two additional and separate peptides carried c, and E. Further two-dimensional iodopeptide mapping studies were performed indicating that three proteins carrying D, c, and E are distinct but closely related, as they all shared some peptide fragments.[253]

Peptide mapping and sequencing studies performed by Cartron[247] in Paris and by Agre et al.[252] in Baltimore confirm the identity of the same amino acid residues at positions 2 to 16 of the N-terminal end of the polypeptides and thus corroborate that the proteins they each isolated are the same. As mapping studies on the three Rh polypeptides continued, the homology of the Rh proteins was extended to the first 21 amino acid residues and later to 41. Saboori et al.[239] suggested that amino acid substitutions beyond the identical residues probably resulted in the polymorphism of the Rh antigens.

During the late 1980s, the number of genes encoding the three Rh polypeptides was still unknown; however, at that time, additional interesting biochemical information about these polypeptides continued to be revealed.[256–258] As demonstrated by de Vetten and Agre[229] Rh polypeptides were shown to carry palmitic acid, an abundant fatty acid, at a site on the inner portion of the membrane bilayer, thus making the Rh protein one of the major red cell fatty acid-acylated proteins. This fatty acylation is implicated but not yet confirmed to play a role in Rh antigenic reactivity.

Another interesting biochemical feature of the Rh polypeptides, one that relates to antigenicity, establishes that the reactivity of D and C depends on a thiol group at or near the outer surface of the RBC membrane. The observation that the loss of a thiol group means the loss of antigen sites, amplifies the important role in antigen activity of an exofacial free sulfhydryl subsequently found on Rh polypeptides.[242] Additionally, two thiol groups are found on membrane proteins on normal red cells, but not on membranes of Rh$_{null}$ red cells.[259]

Another interesting biochemical association with Rh proteins is that of the enzyme phosphatidylserine or (PS) flippase. PS flippase is responsible for regulating the phospholipid asymmetry between the RBC membrane leaflets[260] and is found to immunoprecipitate with Rh antibodies.[261] Because of the coprecipitation it was suggested that PS flippase may be part of a cluster of proteins associated with Rh[230]; however, it is of interest to note that Rh$_{null}$ red cells show normal PS flippase activity.[262]

Similar new theories began to emerge from several sources pointing to the Rh protein involvement with other membrane biochemical structures to form a cluster at the red cell membrane surface.[247] Some of the primary members postulated to be part of this Rh cluster or complex model include the nonglycosylated Rh polypeptides,[223–225,227] Rh related glycoproteins,[226] LW glycoprotein, glycophorin B, and Duffy proteins. Cartron[247] suggested that without the presence of the Rh proteins the other structural proteins within the complex would not be appropriately incorporated within the cell membrane. This theory was generated by noting that the U, LW, and Fy5 antigens are absent from the glycoproteins of Rh$_{null}$ cells, as compared to their presence on red cells with normal Rh polypeptides.

As discussed previously, Rh proteins are unique from other blood group antigens in that they are not glycosylated. Now, as part of a cluster concept, Rh-related glycoproteins are found in association with the usual nonglycosylated Rh polypeptides. Moore and Green[263] showed a relationship between Rh polypeptides and glycoproteins that were found to carry ABH antigens but no Rh determinants. The Rh related glycoproteins coprecipitated with the Rh polypeptides using Rh mAbs in membrane studies. The glycoprotein is of the molecular weight of 45,000 to 60,000 kd, as compared to the second Rh polypeptide of molecular weight around 30,000 kd. The Rh related glycoproteins are not expressed on Rh$_{null}$ cells. The relationship of the genes expressing the associated proteins is not known, as the production of the Rh glycoprotein is controlled from a locus on chromosome 6[226] and the nonglycosylated Rh polypeptides are known to be controlled at a locus on chromosome 1.[264,265] More specifically, the localization of the *Rh* locus encoding for the nonglycosylated Rh polypeptide is confirmed by DNA studies to be on chromosome region 1p34.3–p36.1.[266]

In 1990, two basically identical studies[223,224] cloned an Rh complementary DNA (cDNA) that was indirectly determined to represent the genetic material that encodes production of Cc and/or Ee polypeptide(s). With continued cDNA analysis of Rh polypeptides, a clearer molecular structural picture developed. In 1990, Cherif-Zahar et al.[223] depicted the Rh polypeptides as mostly contained deep within the RBC membrane leaflets. At that time, the Rh protein was represented as traversing the membrane layers 13 times with small portions outside the membrane, and the N-terminus of the polypeptide was placed within the cytoplasm and the C-terminus outside the cell membrane.[259] More recently, the picture has been revised to reflect evidence that the polypeptide spans the lipid bilayer approximately 12 times with both the amino and carboxyl groups being intracellular.[267] The internal membrane spanning part of the polypeptide is a hydrophobic cylindrical alpha helix with external and some internal hydrophobic short loops connecting the domains. The molecular analysis of the Rh polypeptides has deduced a calculated molecular weight of 45.5 kd for the Rh protein rather than the electrophoretic mobility of 32 kd deduced from sodium dodecyl sulfate–polyacrylamide gel electrophoresis (SDS–PAGE) methods of evaluation.[230] Abnormal binding of SDS has been cited as the likely explanation for the difference, since increased binding of SDS is known to occur to very hydrophobic proteins.

Finally, the long-standing question as to the number of genes encoding the production of the Rh polypeptides has been answered. Using Southern blot analysis of genomic DNA from different Rh phenotypes, Colin et al.[127] in 1991 confirmed that Rh-positive individuals have two *Rh* genes, whereas Rh-negative individuals have only one. It was the *CcEe* gene that they were able to clone; and they determined this based on their recognition that it was not the *D* gene. The *D* gene was then able to be cloned by two different groups in 1992 and 1993,[227,268] confirming that one gene codes for D and the other encodes for the CcEe polypeptide(s).

There is a 92 percent sequence identity between the two *Rh* genes with a variation of 36 amino acid substitutions among 417 positions. It is proposed that the substantial sequence homology between the two *Rh* genes results from their evolutionary derivation.[269] Based on studies of Rh blood groups in anthropoid apes and monkeys, it is believed that the *Rh* locus evolved as a unique *Cc* gene that duplicated to give rise to the *D* gene. The E, e antigens arrived later as they do not reside in nonhuman primates. Since there are only two *Rh* genes, the Ee antigens can not result from duplication of the *Cc* gene but might result from some alternative splicing events[132] within the gene.

Detailed studies continue in an effort to further define the molecular genetic basis of the C,c and E,e polymorphisms.[270] We now know that the CcEe gene spans approximately 75 kb of DNA and is composed of 10 exons.[271] Mouro et al.[272] described cloning and sequencing of cDNAs and genomic DNA and found that the E and e alleles differ by a single nucleotide resulting in one amino acid substitution, whereas the C and c alleles differ by six nucleotides producing four amino acid substitutions. The reader should refer to the current literature, as knowledge of the molecular genetic structure of the Rh proteins is increasing rapidly.

With the volumes of biochemical information that is known about Rh, we still do not clearly know the functional importance of the Rh polypeptides.[269] To determine the functional role of the Rh polypeptides, Rh_{null} cells have been used in many studies as a means of demonstrating the differences between normal cells and cells that lack Rh protein. Some of these studies were described in the section on the Rh_{null} phenotype.

The Rh structures appear to most closely resemble that of transporter proteins. However, our current knowledge indicates that the Rh polypeptides appear to maintain cell stability through orientation of the phospholipids in the lipid bilayer and that they also appear to somewhat regulate the cell volume. The specific Rh antigens carried on the polypeptides do not appear to have an independent functional role. As long as a certain amount of Rh protein is present, the RBC membrane maintains normal function regardless of which of the antigens are present.

In summary, we have traversed five decades to finally synthesize and solidify the genetic theories of Rh. Simply put, two genes (*D* and *CcEe*) encode for three Rh polypeptides (D, Cc, and Ee) and the enormous polymorphism that we see arises from a small number of amino acid substitutions as shown in sequence studies. As the knowledge of the molecular biochemistry of the Rh system increases, the remaining mysteries of one of the most clinically significant blood groups will continue to unfold.

THE LW SYSTEM

Since the LW and Rh antigens are strongly related phenotypically, a discussion of the LW blood group system is often integrated with that of the Rh system. Although the two antigens were simultaneously discovered, we now know that they belong to independent blood groups and that they are controlled by genes on separate chromosomes that segregate independently.[273,274] The *LW* genes are assigned to chromosome 19 and the Rh genes are assigned to the short arm of chromosome 1.[264,265]

Indeed, the relationship between Rh and LW

started from the same point of time. The original human anti-D of Levine and Stetson[115] and the Rhesus monkey anti-D of Landsteiner and Wiener[116] were initially thought to identify the same Rh_o (D) antigen. In 1963, Levine et al.[275] described the first example of anti-LW found in a human. As it turned out, the original Rhesus monkey anti-D reacted to Levine's "new" specificity. The antigen was named LW in honor of its true early discoverers, Landsteiner and Wiener.

The close phenotypic relationship between the Rh D antigen and LW led to the original confusion between the two. The LW antigen is present in greater quantities on D-positive red cells than on D-negative cells; thus, weak anti-LW will react with D-positive but not D-negative cells. Conversely, LW antibodies react equally strong with D-negative and D-positive cord red cells. The strong LW activity on cord cells is lost when the cell population matures to its adult form. Rh_{null} cells are truly LW-negative since LW antigens are altogether lacking on Rh_{null} cells.

Early terminology of the LW system included LW_1, LW_2, LW_3, and LW_4 phenotypes, with LW_4 representing the smallest expression of the LW antigen (Table 5-20). The corresponding antibodies react in ascending order of strength. The anti-LW made in an LW_4 person reacts with LW_3, LW_2, and LW_1 cells, and the anti-LW made by an LW_3 person reacts with LW_2 and LW_1 cells.

Newer terminology evolved as further discoveries were made. In 1981, Sistonen et al.[276] reported on a new blood group antigen called Ne[a]. Ne[a] was found in approximately 5 percent of the Finnish population and in 1 percent of other Europeans tested. In 1982, Sistonen and Tippett[277] described an antithet-

Table 5-20. Genotypes That Produce Four Possible LW Phenotypes

New Terminology		Old Terminology	
Phenotype	Genotype	Phenotype	Genotype
LW (a+b−)	*LW^a LW^a*	LW₁ (LW+, D+)	*LW LW*
	LW^a LW	or	
LW (a+b+)	*LW^a LW^b*	LW₂ (LW+, D−)	*LW lw*
LW (a−b+)	*LW^b LW^b*	LW₃	*lw lw*
	LW^b LW		
LW (a−b−)	*LW LW*	LW₄	*lw lw*

ical relationship between anti-Ne^a and the anti-LW from LW$_3$ individuals. It was then proposed that anti-Ne^a would define the antigen LW^b (formerly Ne^a), and that anti-LW from LW$_3$ individuals would define the antigen LW^a (formerly LW). In this newer LW system terminology, two alleles give rise to four phenotypes: LW(a+b+), LW(a+b−), LW(a−b+), and LW (a−b−) (Table 5-20).

Only rarely is LW implicated in clinical transfusion problems. A transient form of anti-LW has been described in people whose LW antigens have been temporarily depressed.[278,279] It seems that the antibody disappears as the LW antigens resume normal levels. An autoanti-LW specificity is often found associated with one or more Rh autoantibodies.

There is now biochemical and molecular information about the LW and Rh proteins[280] that is contrary to their close phenotypic association and confirms their distinction. The LW antigens are carried on a glycoprotein(s) with molecular weight(s) of 37 to 47 kd.[281] Two dimensional iodopeptide maps[282] of the LW and D proteins clearly show that the LW glycoprotein is not simply a version of the Rh polypeptide with carbohydrate attached. Additionally, in contrast to what was previously speculated,[283] there is no biochemical precursor relationship between Rh and LW.

Recent molecular information continues to show the differences between the LW and Rh blood groups.[272,284] No structural homology is seen between the Rh and LW proteins in sequence studies and from the structural information derived from the cloning of LW cDNA. Conclusive evidence shows that these two proteins are unrelated as the *Rh* structural gene resides on chromosome 1p36 and the LW structural gene resides on chromosome 19p13. Although molecular studies have excluded a structural relationship between LW and Rh, LW protein has shown a strong resemblance to another hematologic protein. Sequence similarities have related LW and the intercellular adhesion molecules (ICAMs), which are counterreceptors for the lymphocyte function-associated antigens.[285]

Biochemical and molecular knowledge is continuing to increase at a rapid pace for the LW system as it is for Rh. Since many studies are in progress, the reader should refer to the current literature for the latest information.

OTHER BLOOD GROUPS

The ISBT has made great strides in organizing the blood group systems into a numerical nomenclature. Table 5-21 lists the blood groups systems covered in this section with their common names and ISBT nomenclature. For clarity, common names have been used as much as possible in the text discussion, to describe antibodies and antigens.

The Kell and XK (Kx) Systems

Antigens

The Kell and the XK Blood Group Systems are described together because although Kx is not a precursor to the Kell antigens as once was thought, it is related to Kell. The Kell System has 21 known antigens, making it a fairly complex system. The antigens, their ISBT numerical notation, and their frequencies are shown in Table 5-22. The Kell system thus far has four sub loci of the KEL gene producing low-prevalence and high-prevalence antithetical antigens: (1) K (KEL1) and k (KEL2); (2)Kp^a (KEL3), Kp^b (KEL4), and Kp^c (KEL21); (3)Js^a (KEL6) and Js^b (KEL7); and (4) Wk^a (KEL17) and KEL11. The antithetical partner of the fifth antigen, Ul^a (KEL10), has not yet been reported. K14 and K24 may represent a sixth sublocus of Kell.[286]

Another series of high-prevalence antigens, KEL12, KEL13, KEL14, KEL18, KEL19, and KEL22, are called paraKell antigens because they are related phenotypically but not genetically to the Kell system. Each of these antigens is absent from K$_o$ (Kell$_{null}$) red cells, undetectable on 2-aminoethyli-sothiouroniumbromide (AET)-treated red cells, and poorly expressed on Kp(a+b−) cells (which have other weakened Kell antigens). In addition, all these paraKell antigens, except KEL18, have been shown to be inherited and are located on the Kell glycoprotein. This does not prove that the paraKell antigens are produced by the Kell gene, even though it is likely they are in the Kell system. Kel23 and Kel24 can also be included in the paraKell category. Kel23 has been biochemically proved by Marsh et al.[287] to be related to the Kell system. The low-prevalence antigen KEL24 is thought to be the allele to the KEL14 antigen.[286]

Very little is known about the nature of the remaining Kell antigens, Ku (KEL5), KEL16, and Km

Table 5-21. International Society of Blood Transfusion (ISBT)

Name	Symbol	No.	001	002	003	004	005	006	007	008
						No. Within the System (to Name, Concatenate				
Lutheran	LU	005	Lu^a	Lu^b	Lu^{ab}	Lu4	Lu5	Lu6	Lu7	Lu8
Kell	KEL1	006	K	k	Kp^a	Kp^b	Ku	Js^a	Js^b	
Lewis	LE	007	Le^a	Le^b	Le^{ab}					
Duffy	FY	008	Fy^a	Fy^b	Fy^3	Fy^4	Fy^5	Fy6		
Kidd	JK	009	Jk^a	Jk^b	Jk^{ab}					
Diego	DI	010	Di^a	Di^b						
Yt	YT	011	Yt^a	Yt^b						
Xg	XG	012	Xg^a							
Scianna	SC	013	Sm	Bu^a	Sc^3					
Dombrock	DO	014	Do^a	Do^b	Gy^a	Hy	Jo^a			
Colton	CO	015	Co^a	Co^b	Co^{ab}					
Landsteiner-Wiener	LW	016					LW^a	LW^{ab}	LW^b	
Chido/Rodgers	CH/RG	017	Ch1	Ch2	Ch3	Ch4	Ch5	Ch6	WH	
Hh	H	018	H							
Kx	XK	019	Kx							
Gerbich	GE	020		Ge2	Ge3	Ge4	Wb	Ls^a	An^a	Dh^a
Cromer	CROMER	021	Cr^a	Tc^a	Tc^b	Tc^c	Dr^a	Es^a	IFC	WES^a
Knops	KN	022	Kn^a	Kn^b	McC^a	Sl^a	Yk^a			

(Data and abbreviations compiled from ISBT working parties [3][6][417].)

(KEL20). The K_o phenotype lacks expression of all Kell and paraKell antigens, possibly due to a partial deletion of the Kell gene. The antibody produced by K_o individuals defines the Ku antigen, present on all red blood cells except the K_o phenotypes.[288] The Km antigen is present on all normal Kell red cells, but absent on McLeod and K_o red cells. The KEL16 antigen may be a qualitative variant of the k antigen.[289]

The Kx (XK1) antigen is expressed most strongly on K_o red cells lacking all expression of Kell antigens and weakly on cells with normal Kell antigens. The discovery that the Kx antigen was not part of the Kell System occurred because the gene for expression of Kx was located on the X-chromosome, while the Kell gene was not.[290] The ISBT gave the system the number XK1. McLeod cells lack the Kx antigen completely and are therefore XK0.

The common Kell antigens K, k, Kp^a, Kp^b, Js^a, and Js^b are well developed at birth and, as would be expected, can stimulate antibodies that cause HDN.

Kell antigens show variability when treated with combinations of enzymes and/or chemicals. ZZAP (0.1 mol/L DTT and 0.17 percent papain) eliminates all Kell antigens, whereas AET destroys all Kell antigens except Kx, rendering the cells K_o. DTT alone in high concentration denatures all Kell antigens except Km and Kx, but in low concentration only removes Js^a and Js^b. Trypsin and chymotrypsin together destroy all Kell antigens. All these chemicals are used in research studies to segregate and identify new Kell specificities. Kell antigens are found only on red cells.[291]

Some antigens in the Kell system show occasional weak antigen-antibody reactions. One example of this weakened antigen expression occurs when the Kp^a allele is located in the *cis* position to the k and the *trans* position to the K allele, causing depression of the resulting antigens.[2] When K^o is present with the k, Kp^a, haplotype, once again the Kell antigens are weakened. Another category of weak Kell phenotypes is called K(mod),[292] named because it is analo-

Designations for Blood Group Systems and Antigen Specificities

Symbol With Number Within System, Minus Leading Zeros) For example: LU1											
009	010	011	012	013	014	015	016	017	018	019	020
Mull		Lu11	Much	Hughes	Lu14		Lu16	Lu17	Au[a]	Au[b]	Lu20
	Ul[a]	Cote	Bøc	K13	San		k-like	Wk[a]			
		Rg1	Rg2								
WES[b]	UMC										

gous to the Rh(mod) type, in which Rh antigens are extremely depressed. The genetic formation of Rh(mod) is well described, however, whereas the genetic formation of K(mod) is not. Sensitive serologic techniques show all Kell antigens to be extremely depressed. The first patient to be discovered with these weakened antigens, Day, is included in this category as are several other patients with slightly different reactivities. A final illustration of reduced Kell antigen strength was described by Daniels[293] in Gerbich and Leach types of Gerbich-negative individuals.

Antibodies

Antibodies in the Kell system are usually formed in response to transfusion or pregnancy. They are commonly IgG1 proteins reacting best using the indirect antiglobulin test, although naturally occurring Kell antibodies have been reported. Many Kell antibodies activate complement. Kell antibodies tend to react poorly in low-ionic-strength solutions.[294] Kell system antibodies may appear to show dosage but, because of the presence of depressed antigens, true dosage cannot always be determined. Autoantibodies are present in this system and are discussed further in the section on clinical considerations.

Anti-K

The first example of anti-K was discovered by Coombs et al.[295] in 1946 during the first trials of antiglobulin serum. Because K is quite immunogenic, second only to D in the Rh system, 5 to 10 percent of those individuals transfused with one unit of K-positive blood will make anti-K.[296] Since K is of low prevalence, it is not difficult to find K-negative blood for transfusion. Several examples of IgM saline-reactive anti-K have been found in individuals with no history of transfusion or pregnancy and no explanation has been found to account for them.[297,298] Other reports of IgM anti-K have been attributed to bacterial infections with *Escherichia coli, Tubercule bacillis,* and *Streptococcus faecium,* among

Table 5-22. Kell System Antigens and Antibodies

Name	ISBT Numerical Notation	% Positive White	% Positive Black	Implicated in	
				HTR	HDN
K	KEL1	9	3.5	X	X
k	KEL2	99.8	99.9	X	X
Kp^a	KEL3	2	0.1	X	X
Kp^b	KEL4	>99.9	99.9	X	X
K^u	KEL5	>99.9	>99.9	X	X
Js^a	KEL6	<1.0	19.5	X	X
Js^b	KEL7	>99.9	99.9	X	X
Ul^a	KEL10	2.6a	>0.1c		
Cote'	KEL11	>99.9			
Boc	KEL12	>99.9			
K13	KEL13	>99.9			
San	KEL14	>99.9			
"k-like"	KEL16	99.8			
Wk^a	KEL17	0.3b			
K18	KEL18	>99.9			
Sub	KEL19	>99.9			
Km	KEL20	>99.9			
Kp^c	KEL21	<0.1			
K22	KEL22	>99.9			
K23	KEL23	<0.1			X
Cls	KEL24	<2.0			

^{a} In Finns only, probably lower in other whites.

^{b} In English donors, not known in other whites.

^{c} In Others, not known in blacks.

others. The antibodies usually disappear when the infection is resolved.[299]

Antibodies to Kp^a, Js^a, Ul^a, Wk^a, Kp^c, KEL23, KEL24

Antibodies to the above antigens rarely form, due to their low prevalence in the population. When they are produced, they are usually IgG immune antibodies, reacting best at the indirect antiglobulin phase. Finding crossmatch-compatible blood for these patients is not a problem. Recently the first case of HDN attributable to anti-Ul^a was described.[300]

Antibodies to k, Kp^b, Js^b, KEL11

Individuals capable of making these antibodies are rare because the antigens are of high prevalence. There are several examples of naturally occurring

anti-Kp^b, but the rest are IgG immune. Thus far all patients forming anti-Js^b have been from the black population because of the extremely low prevalence (less than 0.1 percent) of Js^b negative individuals in the white population. Compatible blood for patients with these antibodies must be obtained from relatives or a rare donor file.

Antibodies to KEL12, KEL13, KEL14, KEL16, KEL18, KEL19, KEL20, KEL22

There is very little information available regarding the activity of these antibodies in vivo. They have generally been classified as IgG immune.[301]

Anti-Ku

This antibody is directed against cells carrying any Kell system antigen. It is produced by K$_o$ individuals who have been stimulated through transfusion or pregnancy. Very few examples have been found, and there is still some possibility that the antibody may be a mixture of anti-K11, -K12, -K14, -K18, -K19, and/or -K22. Anti Ku has been implicated as the cause of HDN.[301]

Anti-Kx

This antibody was separated from the now obsolete anti-KL along with anti-KEL20 (Km).[302] It does not react with McLeod red cells. Anti-Km reacts with all Kell cells except K$_o$ and McLeod cells. Anti-Kx reacts strongly with K$_o$ cells but shows intermediate strength with K$_o$ heterozygotes.

Genetics

During the past few years, great strides have been made in genetic research of the KELL Blood System. As previously mentioned, the *XK* gene is sex-linked and is located on the short arm of the X chromosome at Xp21.[291] The *K* gene is an autosome located on the long arm of chromosome 7 at 7q33.[291] The *K* gene, which codes for five sets of alleles, may be a series of closely linked loci or may represent a single genetic locus with five subloci. Although theoretically there are many Kell haplotypes possible, only four common ones have been seen. The most common is *k Kp^b Js^b K11*. No gene complex has been found that has more than one of the low-prevalence antigens *K, Kp^a, Kp^c, Js^a, Ul^a,* or *Wk^a*.[2]

The Kell system has a "null" phenotype similar to

that of the Rh system. When two recessive K^o genes (K^o is the silent allele at the Kell complex locus) are inherited at the Kell locus, the Ko phenotype is produced. This phenotype is devoid of all Kell antigens but it does have the Kx antigen (XK1). The Kx antigen is described more fully in the section on McLeod genetics.

As mentioned in the section on Kell antigens, the Kell system has positional effects. If the Kp^a allele is present in cis position to k and *trans* position to the K allele, the resulting antigen strength is sometimes depressed.[2,303] Another researcher found that cells from an individual with KEL11 in the heterozygous state always have a depression of most or all of the antigens produced by any gene complex that includes Kp^a.[304] Although the paraKell antigens, KEL12, KEL13, KEL14, KEL18, KEL19, KEL22, KEL23, and KEL24 are defined by antibodies not reacting with K_o cells, they do react with cells showing other Kell antigens. They are phenotypically assigned to part of the Kell system, but a genetic association has not been established.

McLeod Phenotype Genetics

Marsh et al.[302] described the genetic background of the McLeod phenotype in 1975. These workers showed that the responsible gene was linked to the X-chromosome and named it Xk. At that time four alleles were postulated at this locus, controlling the amount of Kx on red cells and granulocytes, as well as controlling chronic granulomatous disease (CGD). It is now believed that there are only two alleles at the *XK* locus: *XK1*, which produces the Kx antigen, and *XK O*, which does not produce Kx and results in the McLeod phenotype (Table 5-23). It has been shown that the XK locus (the ISBT changed the name from Xk)[6] and the locus for X-linked CGD are not the same, although they are both on the X chromosome.

Because the *XK* gene is sex linked, lyonization (the process whereby one X chromosome in females is inactivated by chance in embryonic life) occurs. If a woman inherits one abnormal variant of the *XK* gene and one normal XK gene, the woman will produce a dual population of red cells and granulocytes, some normal and some McLeod.

Biochemistry

The Kell system antigen-bearing protein has been described by Redman et al.[291] as a single glycosylated protein band weighing 93 kd. The protein has intra chain disulfide bonds that retain it in a folded configuration.[291] The Kell glycoprotein is thought to be a transmembrane glycoprotein with the cytoplasmic portion of the molecule complexed with the red blood cell cytoskeleton.[305]

K_o (Kell$_{null}$) red blood cells lack both Kell group antigens and the carrier protein that bears them. McLeod red blood cells do have Kell antigens on them but they are extremely weak. At one time it was thought that McLeod cell abnormality was caused by a Kell protein deficiency, but the membrane abnormality is now attributed to the absence of the Kx antigen.[291]

Clinical Significance

The most common antibody in the Kell system, anti-K, can cause severe HDN and both immediate and delayed hemolytic transfusion reactions (HTR). Anti-k, anti-Kp^a, anti-Kp^b, anti-Js^a, and anti-Js^b are all rare antibodies, but when present, can cause HDN and HTR. Anti-Kx has been the cause of a delayed HTR, but Kx positive granulocytes were transfused to the same patient without incident.[306]

The other Kell system antibodies have the potential to cause HDN and HTR, but because of their high or low-prevalence antigens, are seldom or never seen. Several examples of HTR have been caused by interdonor incompatibilities.[307] Table 5-22 summarizes the antibodies implicated in HDN and HTR.

Autoantibodies with Kell specificity have been estimated to occur with a frequency of 1 in 170 by Marsh et al.,[308] who found four cases in patients with

Table 5-23. XK System Alleles

Allele	Kx on Red Cell	Kell Antigens on RBCS	Chronic Granulomatous Disease
XK1	Trace or abundant (Ko)	Normal	No
XK0	No	Severely depressed (McLeod)	Yes or no

WAIHA. These autoantibodies can be either benign or pathological, and most of the autoimmune states have been reversible. In one-half of these cases, the Kell antigens were depressed, and this depression offered some protection from the hemolytic effects of the autoantibody. The mechanism of this reduction of K antigen strength is unknown. Approximately 15 percent of these individuals with WAIHA do show evidence of in vivo hemolysis—sometimes severe. When these patients with WAIHA are transfused with blood with normal expression of Kell antigens, a severe hemolytic reaction will usually occur.

McLeod Syndrome

McLeod syndrome describes the serologic, hematologic, and clinical conditions seen in individuals possessing the McLeod phenotype (Table 5-24). The abnormal red cell morphology was described 14 years after the discovery of the McLeod phenotype.[309] The acanthocytic cells are very striking, and it is suggested that all patients displaying acanthocytes be evaluated for McLeod syndrome or carrier status.

Table 5-24. McLeod Syndrome Characteristics

Hematologic
   Acanthocytes
   Increased reticulocytes
   Compensated hemolytic state
   30% reduction in membrane water permeability
   Increased phosphorylation of spectrin protein band 3 without increased intake of phosphorus (attachment of phosphate groups may affect cell shape)
Serologic
   Reduced serum haptoglobin
   Normal serum B-lipoprotein
   High levels of CK (MM isoenzyme)
   Increased LDH
   Increased carbonic anhydrase (enzyme derived specifically from muscle)
   Weakened Kell antigens
Clinical
   Enlarged spleen
   Progressive neurologic changes
   Areflexia (lack of deep-tendon reflexes)
   Choriform movements (jerky, but well-coordinated movement)
   Mild dysarthria (uncoordinated speaking muscles)
   Cardiomyopathy
   Wasting of skeletal muscles
   Neurogenic myopathy

Even female carriers will have a mixed population of these cells, due to the lyonization effect. Marsh et al.[310] discovered muscle changes in these same McLeod patients. Skeletal muscle wasting and weakness, neurological defects, and elevated CPK are found in males after the age of 40.

McLeod-type red cells have also been found to have increased phosphorylation,[311] but the reason for this phenomenon is not known. More studies are needed in order to show the relationship between biochemical changes on McLeod red cells and neurologic and muscular defects.

At one time, CGD was thought to be related to the McLeod syndrome. As previously mentioned, the gene controlling this disease is near the *XK1* gene in the p21 region of the X chromosome, as is the gene for Duchenne muscular dystrophy (DMD).[291] These diseases may be a result of deletions of portions of the X chromosome.

The Duffy System

Antigens

The Duffy system is composed of six red cell antigens: Fy^a, Fy^b, Fy3, Fy4, Fy5, and Fy6 (ISBT:FY1, FY2, FY4, FY5, and FY6). The two most significant antigens in this system are Fy^a and Fy^b because they are moderately immunogenic and their antibodies are clinically significant. These antigens are well developed at birth and are denatured by enzymes. They do not store well in saline, in solutions with low pH or ionic strength, or in the frozen state. Another antigen, Fy^x, was first thought to be distinct from other Fy antigens, but it now seems to be a rare quantitative variant of the Fy^b antigen that is found in whites and reacts weakly with anti-Fy^b.[312,313]

The Fy3 antigen is found on all red cells that have the Fy^a or Fy^b antigen but does not appear in individuals with the Fy(a−b−) phenotype. It is interesting to note that while enzymes denature Fy^a and Fy^b, the Fy3 antigen is actually enhanced. This information supports the theory that Fy3 is a separate antigen from Fy^a and Fy^b.[314]

The Fy4 antigen, which at one time was thought to be the silent antigen, Fy, is present in a double dose in the common black phenotype Fy(a−b−). It is also frequently present in a single dose in black individuals with the phenotype Fy(a+b−) or

Fy(a−b+). In the white population these phenotypes usually represent the genotypes Fy^{a}Fy^a and Fy^{b}Fy^b but in the black population the most probable genotypes are Fy^{a}Fy and Fy^{b}Fy. Theoretically, it should not be present in Fy(a+b+) individuals, although there is some evidence that it may be.[315]

The Fy5 antigen initially seems similar to the Fy3 antigen because it is present on all Fy(a+) and/or Fy(b+) red cells but is absent from all Fy(a−b−) red cells in black individuals. Upon closer scrutiny, Colledge et al.[316] demonstrated that the Fy5 antigen is not present on Rh$_{null}$ cells, although they have normal expressions of Fy^a, Fy^b, and Fy3. These unusual findings suggest a relationship between the Fy and Rh antigens, but exact mechanisms are not known.

The newest Duffy antigen specificity, Fy6, was defined by a murine mAb in 1987.[317] This antigen appears to be closely associated with the receptor site for *Plasmodium vivax*.

Antibodies

Anti-Fy^a was discovered in 1950 by Cutbush et al.[318] in the serum of a hemophiliac who had been multiply transfused. The following year, Ikin et al.[319] found the antibody to the antithetical antigen, anti-Fy^b. In 1971, Albrey et al. found anti-Fy3[314] in the serum of an Fy(a−b−) individual; anti-Fy4 was discovered by Behzad et al.[315] in 1973. So far, the few documented examples of anti-Fy5 suggest that it is only produced by black Fy(a−b−) individuals.[316] Anti-Fy^a and anti-Fy^b are usually IgG immune antibodies that react best in the indirect antiglobulin test. Several examples of the antibody have been found that are saline agglutinins, while approximately one-half of all examples bind complement. Anti-Fy^a is a relatively common antibody; anti-Fy^b is much less common. The other Duffy antibodies are extremely rare.

Genetics

Donahue et al.[320] in 1968, proved that the Duffy locus was on chromosome 1. This was the first time that a human cell blood group was assigned to an autosome. The *Rh* locus has also been assigned to chromosome 1 and Duffy and Rh are said to be syntenic, that is, on the same chromosome but with no demonstrable linkage.[321] The antigens Fy^a and Fy^b

Table 5-25. Racial Variation in Duffy Phenotypes

Phenotype	Frequency	
	% White	% Black
Fy(a+b−)	17	9
Fy(a+b+)	49	1
Fy(a−b+)	34	22
Fy(a−b−)	<0.1	68

(Adapted from Issitt,[2] with permission.)

are produced by co-dominant alleles, and since the Fy^x antigen is a weakened form of the Fy^b antigen, it is also thought to be the product of an allele. Because all Fy(a+b+) individuals are positive for the Fy3 antigen, it seems unlikely that Fy3 is an allele of Fy^a and Fy^b.

The Duffy antigens presented in Table 5-25 show how gene frequencies vary among different racial groups. At one time Fy4 was also postulated to be an allele of Fy^a and Fy^b but, because there have been cases of Fy(a+b+) cells testing weakly positive for the Fy4 antigen,[2] perhaps Fy4 is not an allele of Fy^a and Fy^b, but rather an allele of Fy3. As mentioned previously, anti-Fy5 reacts negatively with Rh null cells and weakly with −D− cells, leading to the conclusion that the Fy5 determination is formed by the interaction of the Duffy groups and Rh genes.[316] The phenotype Fy(a−b−) in blacks is formed by the presence of a double dose of the Fy4 antigen. The Fy(a−b−) phenotype has also been found in several nonblack individuals, and theoretically, this phenotype results from a genetic background different from that of blacks.

Biochemistry

Current knowledge of the Fy^a and Fy^b antigen structure suggests that antigen activity is located on a glycoprotein on the erythrocyte membrane. Hadley et al.[322] identified the protein as a broad band with a molecular weight of 40,000 daltons and a diffuse edge, which may extend the protein to 66,000 daltons. The Fy3, Fy4, and Fy5 antigens have not been identified biochemically, but since they are not denatured by enzymes, it seems likely that they are different from the enzyme-labile Fy^a and Fy^b antigens.

Clinical Significance

It is well documented that anti-Fy[a] and anti-Fy[b] can cause both immediate and delayed HTRs. Anti-Fy[a] and anti-Fy3 have been implicated in HDN, while anti-Fy[b], -Fy4, and -Fy5 have the potential to be. An important clinical finding in the Duffy system was the discovery that Fy(a−b−) human red cells were resistant to infection by *Plasmodium knowlesi*,[323] a simian malarial parasite. *P. knowlesi* is similar to the parasite *P. vivax*, which infects man but cannot be cultured in vitro. Several in vivo studies have shown that Fy(a−b−) individuals are resistant to *P. vivax*, and it is now thought that Fy6 is the probable receptor for *P. vivax* malaria.[317] Current studies of the invasion process of *P. knowlesi* show that merozoites attach to Fy(a−b−) as well as Fy(a+) and Fy(b+) erythrocytes but are unable to form a junction site to enter the cells of Fy(a−b−) individuals.[324] In west Africa, most blacks are Fy(a−b−) and are resistant to *P. vivax* malaria; this favors a natural selection theory for individuals living in areas where malaria is endemic. It is now thought that FY3 is a possible receptor for *P. knowlesi*.[325]

The Kidd System

Antigens

The Kidd system consists of the antigens Jk[a], Jk[b] and Jk3 (ISBT: JK1, JK2, JK3). The antigens Jk[a] and Jk[b] are antithetical, present only on red cells, and are well developed at birth. Occasionally, very weakened forms of these two antigens exist and can only be identified using trypsin- or papain-treated cells, although no qualitative difference has been found. The Jk3 antigen is found on all red cells that have the Jk[a] or Jk[b] antigen, but it is not present on Jk(a−b−) red cells, which lack all Kidd antigens. Marsh et al.[326] described Jk3 on neutrophilic granulocytes but Branch et al.[327] have not been able to confirm this. Table 5-26 shows the frequencies of the Kidd phenotypes by racial group.

Antibodies

Anti-Jk[a] was first discovered in 1951 by Allen et al.[328] in the serum of a woman who had given birth to an infant with HDN. Two years later, Plaut et al.[329] described anti-Jk[b] in the serum of a patient who had had a transfusion reaction. Anti-Jk3, an inseparable

Table 5-26. Frequencies of Kidd Phenotypes

Phenotype	White (%)	Black (%)
Jk(a+b−)	28	57
Jk(a+b+)	49	34
Jk(a−b+)	23	9
Jk(a−b−)	------Very rare------	

mixture of anti-Jk[a] and anti-Jk[b], was then found in the first case of the Jk(a−b−) phenotype in 1959.[330] Anti-Jk[a], the more common antibody, and anti-Jk[b] are usually IgG-immune, but IgM forms have been reported.[331] These two antibodies are probably the most difficult to identify in the blood bank. Causes for these difficulties in detection include the following: (1) these antibodies frequently show dosage to such a degree that they do not react with heterozygous cells, (2) anti-Jk[a] and anti-Jk[b] can quickly fall to undetectable levels in vivo, (3) anti-Jk[a] and anti-Jk[b] bind complement and may need complement to react in vitro, and (4) these antibodies are often present in mixtures with other antibodies, thus making identification of separate entities rather difficult. Anti-Jk[a] and anti-Jk[b] react best at the antiglobulin phase and show enhancement with enzymes, polybrene, or LISS. Kidd antibodies may also show in vitro hemolysis. Anti-Jk3 is a very rare antibody that is usually IgG immune, but an IgM example has been reported.[332]

Genetics

There are three alleles at the Kidd locus: *Jk[a]*, *Jk[b]*, and *Jk*. The genes *Jk[a]* and *Jk[b]* show autosomal codominant inheritance, while a double dose of the recessive *Jk* allele, called a silent allele, produces the Jk(a−b−) null phenotype. This phenotype lacks the Jk[a], Jk[b], and Jk3 antigens and produces anti-Jk3 more frequently. In 1986, Okubo et al.[333] reported a case in which the Jk(a−b−) phenotype showed dominant inheritance and proposed the existence of a suppressor gene, In(Jk), similar to the In(Lu) gene to explain this phenomenon. This phenotype occurs more frequently in some Polynesian ethnic groups.[334] Initially, the Kidd locus was tentatively assigned to chromosome 7,[335] with possible linkage to the Colton locus, then it was shown that Kidd was probably carried on chromosome 2,[336] but finally, Kidd has been linked to chromosome 18.[337]

Biochemistry

The Kidd antigens are thought to be membrane proteins. Sinor et al.[338] performed experiments identifying the Jk[a] protein as a single band having a MW of 50,000 daltons. Although Jk(a−b−) cells do not exhibit any anomalies like Rh or Kell$_{null}$ cells, these cells are known to be more resistant to lysis in 2M urea than are other Kidd phenotypes.[339] Since hemolysis is usually caused by water entering a cell, Edwards–Moulds and Kasschau demonstrated slow water uptake in Jk(a−b−) cells.[340] Reid[341] has theorized that Jk blood group antigens are carried on a protein that allows urea to move through the lipid bilayer of the RBC membrane. Additional investigation is required in order to explore all aspects of these phenomena with respect to the membrane structure of Jk(a−b−) cells.

Clinical Significance

Kidd antibodies can cause both immediate and delayed HTRs. As mentioned earlier, Kidd antibodies may quickly fall to undetectable levels in vivo, but with restimulation, can rapidly increase in titer and destroy all circulating antigen-positive cells. Issitt[2] reports that up to one-half of all delayed transfusion reactions are caused by anti-Jk[a] or anti-Jk[b]. Kidd antibodies can cause HDN because the antigens are well developed at birth, however most documented cases are relatively mild.

Anti-Jk[a] and -Jk[b] have been seen as autoantibodies. Examples of both benign and destructive autoanti-Jk[a] have been identified.[342,343] Autoanti-Jk[a], in the presence of aldomet and chlorpropamide, has also been responsible for cell destruction in two WAIHAs.[344,345] Ellisor et al. have described an example of autoanti-Jk[b] plus autoanti-Jk3.[346] These antibodies actually only mimicked anti-Jk[b], since absorptions with Jk(a−b−) or Jk(a+b−) cells removed all activity.

It is interesting to note that several bacterial organisms may have Jk[b]-like specificity. For example, *Streptococcus faecium* and *Micrococcus* converted Jk(b−) cells to Jk(b+),[347] while *Proteus mirabilis* stimulated autoanti-Jk[b].[348]

The Lutheran System

The Lutheran blood group system is composed of four pairs of antithetical antigens: Lu[a]/Lu[b], Lu6/Lu9; Lu8/Lu14, and Au[a]/Au[b] (ISBT: LU1/LU2, LU6/LU9, LU8/LU14, AND LU18/LU19). There are three types of "null" phenotypes: dominant, recessive, and sex-linked. The Lutheran system also has eight paraLutheran antigens and two antigens no longer thought to be related to Lutheran. Table 5-27 summarizes the antigens and also shows the ISBT numerical nomenclature used in the system.

Antigens

The more commonly encountered Lu[a] and Lu[b] antigens are not completely developed at birth and are destroyed by trypsin, chymotrypsin, and pronase. Antigen strength varies on red cells. The Lu[a] and Lu[b] antigens also occasionally show significant depression in Lu(a−b+[w]) and Lu(a+[w]b+[w]) individuals. This phenotype is denoted as Lu(w) and has been postulated to be caused by an allele of the independent suppressor gene *In(Lu)* or *SYN-1B*. Marsh called this allele *SYN-1C*.[349]

The other three sets of antithetical antigens, Lu6/Lu9, Lu8/Lu14, and Au[a]/Au[b], basically show the same antigen characteristics as Lu[a] and Lu[b]. Nine other high-prevalence Lutheran antigens, Lu4, Lu5, Lu7, Lu11, Lu12, Lu13, Lu16, Lu17, and Lu20[350] are called paraLutheran antigens because antibodies to these antigens do not react with Lu(a−b−) red cells. They are said to be phenotypically (not genetically) related to the Lutheran system.

LU(a−b−) Phenotypes

The first null Lutheran phenotype was discovered by Crawford et al.[351] and was postulated to be caused by a suppressor gene located somewhere other than the Lutheran locus. This gene, named In(Lu), showed dominance, because inheriting one gene prevented normal expression of all Lutheran antigens as well as P_1, i, In[b341] and Anton/Wj.[352,353] Successive generations showed 50 percent inheritance of the gene. The Lutheran antigens were not completely absent, because the cells could absorb and elute Lutheran antibodies; therefore, the antigens

Table 5-27. Lutheran Antigens[a]

Antithetical Pairs of Antigens Produced by Genes at the Lutheran Locus

Low Incidence	ISBT Numerical	% Frequency	High Incidence	ISBT Numerical	% Frequency
Lu^a	LU1	8	Lu^b	LU2	92
			LU^{ab}	LU3	High
Lu9 (Mull)	LU9	2	Lu6 (Jan)	LU6	High
Lu14 (Hof)	LU14	2.4	Lu8 (M.T.)	LU8	High
Lu19 (Au^b)	LU19	50	Lu18 (Au^a)	LU18	80

Antigens Phenotypically Related to the Lutheran Locus

Name	ISBT Numerical	Frequency
Lu4	LU4	high
Lu5	LU5	high
Lu7	LU7	high
Lu11 (Lull)	LU11	high
Lu12 (Much)	LU12	high
Lu13 (Hughes)	LU13	high
Lu16	LU16	high
Lu17	LU17	high
Lu20	LU20	high

must be severely depressed. This small amount of antigen prevents these individuals from producing Lutheran antibodies. According to Daniels et al.,[354] In(Lu) also weakens the expression of Kn^a, Sl^a, McC^a, Cs^a, and Yk^a. Since the *In(Lu)* gene causes depression of many antigens not within the Lutheran system, Marsh et al.[349] suggested that the gene controlling normal expression of the involved antigens be called *SYN-1A*, while the allele causing depression (formerly *In(Lu)* be called *SYN-1B*. The *Lu^w* gene could be called *SYN-1C*.

The second type of null phenotype arises when an individual inherits two recessive silent *LU* genes.[355] These individuals do not pass a normal *LU* gene to offspring, as shown by dosage studies identifying heterozygotes. Also, Lu(a−b−) individuals are absent in successive generations. These Lu(a−b−) individuals can and do make Lutheran system antibodies.

The third type of Lu(a−b−) phenotype, described recently by Normal et al.,[356] did not fit either of the above Lutheran patterns. Because all affected family members were male, the pattern was suggestive of an X-borne recessive inhibitor to Lutheran.

The proposed name was the XS locus, with XS1 as the common allele and XS2 as the rare allele causing suppression.

Antibodies

The first example of anti-Lu^a was described by Callender et al.[357] in 1945. The antibody may be naturally occurring or immune with an optimal temperature of reaction of 12° to 18°C. Anti-Lu^a may be IgM, IgG, or a mixture of IgM, IgG, and IgA.[7] Some examples bind complement and/or react at 37°C in the antiglobulin phase. The agglutination of anti-Lu^a has a characteristically mixed-field appearance with large clumps of cells floating amid unagglutinated cells. Dosage effect has also been reported.

Anti-Lu^b was discovered in 1956 by Cutbush and Chanarin.[358] Most examples of the antibody are immune and react best at the antiglobulin phase, although saline agglutinins have been found. This antibody is usually partly IgG, with IgM and IgA sometimes present.

In 1963, Darnborough et al.[355] described an antibody made by Lu(a−b−) individuals that appeared to be an inseparable anti-Lu^{ab.} It is now called anti-Lu3.

Antibodies to other Lutheran antigens have been identified. Anti-Lu6, -Lu9, -Lu8, and -Lu14 were discovered and helped to define the two pairs of antithetical antigens. Anti-Lu4, -Lu5, -Lu7, -Lu11, -Lu12, -Lu13, -Lu16, and -Lu17 define antigens still not proven to be genetically related to the Lutheran system. Anti-Au^a, originally described in 1961 by Salmon et al., and anti-Au^b found in 1989[359] are now believed to be part of the Lutheran system. All these antibodies are very rare and react best at the antiglobulin phase.

Genetics

As mentioned previously, the Lutheran system is made up of 4 sets of alleles: *Lu^a/Lu^b*, *Lu6/Lu9*, *Lu8/Lu14* and *Au^a/Au^b*. It is likely that these alleles are located at four closely linked subloci. The Lutheran system, the first system to display linkage on an autosome, is linked to the Secretor (Se) locus.[360] These genes have been found to reside on chromosome 19.[361]

Biochemistry

The biochemistry of the Lutheran system is not well defined. Originally, Marcus et al.[85] demonstrated Lu^b activity in red cell gangliosides. Subsequently, Marsh suggested that Lutheran antigen activity was associated with glycoproteins.[362] This was also supported by Parsons et al.,[363] who showed that a murine monoclonal antibody, Bric 108, recognized the Lu^b antigen on 2 glycoproteins with molecular weights of 85 and 78 kd. Finally, Daniels and Khalid[364] postulated that Lu^a, Lu^b, Lu3, Lu4, Lu6, Lu8, and Lu12 were also located on the same membrane components as those identified by Bric 108. Other discrepant results with enzymes, AET, and DTT suggest heterogeneity of Lutheran antigens.

Clinical Significance

Since the Lutheran antigens are not well developed at birth, it seems logical that HDN should be mild in nature. In fact, mild HDN has been caused by both anti-Lu^a and anti-Lu^b.[365,366] Most examples of anti-Lu^a go undetected because this antigen is not routinely present on antibody screening cells. Fortunately, anti-Lu^a has not been found to remove Lu(a+) red cells from circulation.[367] The Lu^b antigen is always present on screening cells, but because of its high prevalence, the antibody is seldom produced. Anti-Lu^b has been implicated in transfusion reactions[368] and accelerated clearance of Lu(b+) cells.[369] Blood that is Lu(b−) is difficult to locate and blood from the rare donor files may have to be obtained. Other Lutheran antibodies are of questionable clinical significance because their infrequent appearance makes investigation difficult. One case of in vivo destruction due to anti-Lu6 has been described.[370]

The Xg^a System

Antigens and Antibodies

The Xg^a (XG1) antigen was named as such because the gene that codes for its production is carried on the X chromosome. Thus far an antithetical antigen has not been found and the silent allele Xg has only been postulated. The antigen is present at birth, though it is less fully developed than adult Xg^a. Common enzymes (such as ficin, papain, and trypsin) denature Xg^a, but neuraminidase does not.

The antibody to Xg^a, first detected by Mann et al.[371] in 1962, reacts best by the indirect antiglobulin test. Most examples are IgG immune, activate complement, and do not show dosage. Since more males are Xg(a−) than are females, a larger proportion of antibody producers are male. In addition, although approximately 20 percent of all transfusions are from Xg(a+) donors, there are very few examples of anti-Xg^a, which supports the theory that the antigen is not a good immunogen.

Genetics

Because of its X-linked mode of inheritance, the phenotypic frequencies of Xg^a are much lower in males than in females (67 percent and 89 percent, respectively). The *Xg^a* gene is located on the X chromosome, which helps define its independence from other blood groups. The gene was also found through family studies to behave as a dominant character. The pedigree in Figure 5-3 illustrates this sex-linked dominant inheritance. Males who are Xg(a+) pass this on to all their daughters, but to none of their sons. Whether females pass on the Xg^a antigen depends on their zygosity and on the sex of their

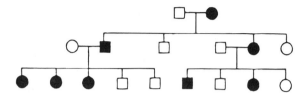

Fig. 5-3. Pedigree showing sex linkage of Xg^a □, male; ○, female; □○ lacks Xg^a; ■● has Xg^a.

offspring. One unexplained phenomenon of this blood group is that it does not support the Lyon hypothesis. If one Xg^a gene is present, all the cells from the woman carry the Xg^a antigen. One explanation for this phenomenon might be that the Lyon effect inactivates some but not all genes on the X chromosome. The Xg^a antigen has been used to type the red cells of individuals with sex-chromosome aneuploidy such as Turner's syndrome (XO), Klinefelter's syndrome (XXY), and other abnormal XY karyotypes.

Clinical Significance

Although anti-Xg^a is usually immune and can cross the placenta, it has not been implicated in HDN or HTRs. There have been reported cases of Xg(a+) red cells transfused to an individual with a potent anti-Xg^a with no increased red cell destruction in vivo.[372,373] Thus far, only one example of autoanti-Xg^a has been reported; it activated complement and caused severe hemolytic anemia in the patient,[374] who was pregnant at the time. At birth, her Xg(a+) infant had a positive direct antiglobulin test, but there was no evidence of anemia and only a mild rise in bilirubin.

The Diego System

Thus far, the Diego blood group system consists of the codominant alleles Di^a and Di^b (ISBT: DI1 and DI2) located on chromosome 17.[375] The Di^a antigen, discovered in 1955,[376] occurs rarely in whites and has the highest prevalence in people of Mongolian extraction, including South American Indians, sometimes as high as 36 percent. In 1967, Thompson et al.[377] reported finding Di^b, a high-prevalence antigen (more than 99 percent) in the white and the black population. The Di(a−b−) phenotype has not yet been reported. The antigens are well developed

at birth, with both anti-Di^a and anti-Di^b capable of causing severe HDN; there have been cases of HDN reported that are mild or subclinical.[378] Both anti-Di^a and anti-Di^b are IgG antibodies reacting best in the indirect antiglobulin test, but naturally occurring anti-Di^a has been found.[379] Anti-Di^b has occasionally shown dosage. There has been a delayed transfusion reaction due to anti-Di^b reported.[377]

The Diego blood group system is used frequently in anthropological studies, as the Di^a antigen is commonly found in individuals of Mongolian ancestry.

The Cartwright System

The Cartwright blood group system is composed of the codominant alleles Yt^a and Yt^b (ISBT: YT1 and YT2), assigned to chromosome 7.[380] The Yt^a and Yt^b antigens are located on a phosphatidylinositol-linked erythrocyte acetylcholinesterase (AChE) protein.[381] Yt^a, reported in 1956 by Eaton,[382] is a very common antigen that is found in more than 99 percent of whites. In 1964, Giles and Metaxas[383] discovered Yt^b, which is present in approximately 8 percent of whites. The Yt(a−b−) phenotype has not yet been found. The Yt^a antigen is postulated to be a strong immunogen that stimulates the antibody frequently in Yt(a−) individuals. While Yt^a is not fully developed at birth, the Yt^b antigen is.

Although both anti-Yt^a and anti-Yt^b are immune antibodies reacting best in the antiglobulin phase, only anti-Yt^a appears to show dosage. Neither antibody is associated with significant HDN. Anti-Yt^a has been reported to cause HTRs in some cases.[384] Recently anti-Yt^a has been discovered post transfusion in the serum of a Yt(a+) patient.[385] When Yt(a−) blood cannot be located for an individual with anti-Yt^a, 51-Cr-survival studies may be helpful. Such studies indicate that approximately 50 percent of Yt(a+) units will survive normally in vivo.[386] Levy et al.[387] reported twice the normal rate of RBC destruction in a patient with anti-Yt^b, using ^{51}Cr labeling. Monocyte assays also corroborate these findings. Additional studies are needed to determine reliable in vivo significance.

The Scianna System

The Scianna blood group system was described after the common antigen Sm and the rare antigen Bu^a were found to be antithetical.[388] These antigens, now called SC1 and SC2, have frequencies of greater than 99 percent and 1 percent, respectively, and are controlled by codominant alleles. The antigens are well developed at birth. The SC3 antigen is present on all red cells positive for SC1 and/or SC2. When individuals type SC: − 3, they are also SC: − 1 and SC: − 2. This "null" phenotype is thought to represent expression of a double dose of the recessive allele *SC*.[389] One interesting property of SC1 is that it can be transiently lost from red cells so that they appear SC: − 1.[2] These individuals can then produce antibodies. Only family studies can differentiate between genetic and acquired forms of SC.

In 1962, the original antibody anti-Sm, now called anti-SC1 was described by Schmidt et al.[390] Anderson et al. found anti-Bu^a, or anti-SC2, one year later.[391] These immune antibodies react best in the antiglobulin test and are capable of causing both HDN and HTRs.[392] One case of autoanti-SC1 has been reported,[393] but no signs of hemolytic anemia were detected.

The Gerbich System

Antigens

The seven Gerbich blood group system antigens, located on glycophorins C and D, consist of GE2, GE3, GE4, Wb (GE5), Ls^a (GE6), An^a (GE7), and Dh^a (GE8). GE2, GE3, and GE4 are high prevalence, while the others are all low prevalence. The glycophorin proteins are produced by a single gene on chromosome 2.[395] Although more Gerbich-negative individuals have been found among Melanesians than among any other population, the gene prevalence of the positive antigen, varying from 0.2 percent to 1.0 percent is still low.[396] Nonmelanesians are so commonly antigen-positive that gene prevalence calculations cannot be made.[396] Table 5-28 summarizes the different nomenclatures currently used to describe the phenotypes.

Properties of the Gerbich antigens include complete development at birth, variable weakening of antigen expression with enzymes (destroyed by neuraminidase), and decreased expression with DTT treatment.[397] There is speculation that the antigens are in some way associated with the Kell system, because Gerbich and Leach phenotypes of Gerbich-negative individuals show weakened Kell blood group antigens.[398]

Antibodies

Since Rosenfield et al.[399] described the first three examples of anti-Ge in 1960, many Gerbich antibodies have been reported. A numerical nomenclature was introduced after it was found that some Gerbich antibodies agglutinated cells of other Gerbich-negative individuals. Although most Gerbich antibodies are IgG, and detected by the indirect antiglobulin test, IgM saline examples have been identified.[400] Gerbich antibodies have been found in individuals with no known immunogenic stimulus,[396] but the greatest number are formed in response to pregnancy or transfusion. It is important to note that anti-GE1 is extremely rare and has only been found in early studies of Melanesian people.

Genetics and Biochemistry

The biochemistry of the Gerbich system has helped describe the genetics of this system. Red cell membranes of Gerbich-positive individuals have normal

Table 5-28. Gerbich Phenotypes/Nomenclature

Historical Name	Anstee et al.	Revised Numerical	Freq. % Random Population
Gerbich neg			
Gerbich type	Ge − Yus −	GE: − 2, − 3,4	<0.1
Yus type	Ge − Yus +	Ge: − 2,3,4	<0.1
Leach type	Ge − Yus −	Ge: − 2, − 3, − 4	^a
Melanesian type		Ge: − 1,2,3	^b
Gerbich pos			
	Ge +	Ge: 2,3,4	>99.9

^a Only five cases of Leach phenotype.
^b Melanesians only.

β- and γ-SGPs, structures that all Gerbich-negative individuals lack. Membranes from the Gerbich- and Yus-type Gerbich-negative cells show unique SGPs with polyacrylamide gel electropheresis (PAGE), while the Leach type of Gerbich-negative cells demonstrate no SGPs of any kind (a true null phenotype).[394] It is believed that an internal deletion of a part of the gene responsible for the glycophorin C and D production is responsible for the Ge and Yus type of Ge negative.[401] The gene responsible for the Gerbich SGP molecules is inherited in an autosomal, codominant manner and, as previously mentioned, is located on chromosome 2.[397]

Clinical Significance

An interesting clinical finding in the Gerbich system was the discovery by Pasvol et al.[402] that Gerbich negative red cells of the Leach type were invaded by *P. falciparum* approximately one-half as often as normal red cells. This reduction might be due to reduced oligosaccharides carried on the SGP of Gerbich-positive cells that are absent on Leach type Gerbich-negative cells. Another observation in individuals with the Leach phenotype is that a portion of their red cells show elliptocytosis and increased osmotic fragility, although this has no serious clinical sequelae. This phenomenon has been attributed to the absence of SGPs.[403]

Although there are cases of anti-Ge causing a positive direct antiglobulin test in infants, there has been no clinical evidence of HDN. Gerbich antibodies have the potential to cause HTRs, as shown by the MMA and ^{51}Cr survival studies.[404,405] In addition, two cases of severe autoimmune hemolytic anemia have been reported to be due to anti-Ge.[406,407] A third Gerbich antibody behaved like an alloantibody when the Gerbich antigen was depressed in a patient receiving gold therapy.[408]

THE DOMBROCK SYSTEM

The antigen Do[a] (DO1) of the Dombrock blood group system, with a prevalence of 67 percent, was first reported in 1965 by Swanson et al.[409] Do[b] (DO2) with a prevalence of 83 percent was described by Molthan et al.[410] in 1973. Although the Gy[a] (Gregory) and Hy (Holley) antigens and their association were discovered in 1966 and 1967, in 1992 the ISBT

elevated them and the Jo[a] antigen to the Dombrock system, giving them the abbreviations DO3, DO4, and DO5, respectively.[3] Moulds et al.[411] identified anti-Gy[a] in 1966, while Schmidt et al.[412] described anti-Hy in 1967. The Jo[a] antigen, a little known high-prevalence antigen, was found to be located on the same glycoprotein as the Do[a]/Do[b] and Gy[a]/Hy antigens.[413] This glycoprotein is one of the phosphatidylinositol-linked (PI-linked) proteins in which other blood group antigens have been found.[414] A null phenotype occurs when red cells lack DO3 and are DO: -1,-2,-3,-4,-5.[398] Both Hy and Gy[a] antigens are found with high prevalence in black and white populations. In fact, these antigens were found to be related when Moulds et al.[411] noted that all white Gy(a−) individuals were also Hy− and that the occurrence of this phenotype was greater than its statistical probability. The Hy−, Gy(a−) phenotype is only found in whites; black individuals who are Hy(a−) all type Gy(a+).

Both the Do[a] and Do[b] antigens are well developed at birth, but no clinical HDN has been reported. Both the Do[a] and Do[b] antigen reactions are enhanced with enzymes.[18] Anti-Do[a] is IgG and reacts best by the indirect antiglobulin test. It does not activate complement and may show dosage. Anti-Do[b], although only rarely described, also reacts best in the indirect antiglobulin test. Anti-Do[a] has been reported to have caused an immediate HTR.[6] Anti-Do[b] has been identified as the probable cause of both an immediate and a delayed HTR.[6]

Gy[a] and Hy antibodies are usually IgG non-complement binding and react best in the indirect antiglobulin test. The antigens are poorly expressed on cord cells, which might be the reason they have not been implicated in HDN. Although the antibodies react weakly when undiluted, they frequently have high titers, placing them in the now-outdated HTLA (high-titer, low-avidity) category. Both anti-Gy[a] and -Hy have caused transfusion reactions.[411,415,416] All anti-Jo[a] antibodies described thus far are IgG and have occurred only rarely in the black population.[18]

THE CROMER SYSTEM

The Cromer antigens have recently been recognized as a blood group system.[417] The 10 antigens of this system are carried on a PI-linked complement regulatory protein called decay accelerating factor (DAF).[418] The antigens, Cr[a] (CR1), Tc[a] (CR2), TC[b] (CR3), TC[c] (CR4), Dr[a] (CR5), ES[a] (CR6), IFC[b] (CR7), WES[a] (CR8), WES[b] (CR9), and UMC (CR10),[419] are all destroyed by chymoptrypsin but not by other proteolytic enzymes. The cells of the inherited null phenotype, Inab, carry no Cromer-related antigens and are deficient in DAF, which makes them more susceptible to lysis by complement. Seven of the antigens are high prevalence, while three are low prevalence. The *DAF* gene has been found on the long arm of chromosome 1.[417]

The antibodies of the Cromer system are mostly IgG and rather uncommon. The first example of anti-Cr[a] was found by Stroup and McCreary[420] in a black antenatal patient. Other examples of antibodies to Cromer system antigens have been discovered at different times in various ethnic populations.[418] These antibodies are mostly IgG and have not been reported as a cause of HDN or HTR. Clinical significance of the antibodies is variable, with some antibodies causing decreased red cell survival, and other showing no adverse effect when transfused.[18]

THE KNOPS SYSTEM

The Knops system consists of five antigens, Kn[a], Kn[b], McC[a], Sl[a], Yk[a] (ISBT: KN1, KN2, KN3, KN4, KN5), which were only recently defined as a single blood group system.[3] Previously these antigens were associated with so called high-titer, low-avidity antibodies and were assigned a "collection" status with Cs[a] and Cs[b]. Now they are known to be located on the C3b/C4b portion of the red cell and encoded by a gene on chromosome 1.[421] The Kn[a] antigen was described in 1978 by Molthan and Moulds.[422] The Kn[b] antigen, antithetical to Kn[a], has been described by Mallen et al.[423] Molthan[424] has also described the antigens McC[b] and McC[c]. Lacey et al.[425] studied the antibody that defined the Sl[a] antigen that Molthan first called anti-McC[c]. The Yk[a] antigen was first described by Molthan and Giles[426] and a relationship to Cs[a] was postulated. But in 1993, the ISBT removed Cs[a] and Cs[b] from the Knops blood group system and kept them in their own collection.[3]

These high-prevalence red cell antigens are well developed on cord cells and are not destroyed by enzymes. The Kn[a] and McC[a] antigens were postu-

lated to be phenotypically related when it was found that 53 percent of McC(a−) samples were also Kn(a−),[427] which is far greater than the expected 0.02 percent prevalence. Molthan[428] also established a phenotypic relationship between Kn[a], McC[a], Cs[a], and Yk[a] by finding antigen-negative individuals in much higher prevalence than expected, although Cs[a] has recently been excluded.

Anti-Kn[a] and anti-McC[a] are IgG, do not activate complement, are not inhibited by serum, and react best in the indirect antiglobulin test. Although Molthan[428] described examples of Kn[a] and McC[a] antibodies causing hemolytic reactions and extravascular red cell removal and Gandhi et al.[429] found decreased survival of Cr-labeled red cells, Marsh[18] summarized that anti-Kn[a], McC[a], and Sl[a] are benign, do not cause HTRs or HDN and can usually be ignored for clinical purposes.

THE COLTON SYSTEM

The Colton blood group system is composed of three antigens: Co[a], Co[b], and Co[ab] (often called Co3) (ISBT: CO1, CO2, and CO3). Co[a] and Co[b] are antithetical, while Co3 is present on all cells that are either Co(a+) or Co(b+). The antigens are well developed at birth and may be enhanced by enzymes. Co[a], which has a prevalence of greater than 99 percent, was discovered by Heisto et al. in 1967,[430] while Co[b], with a prevalence of 10 percent, was found by Giles et al. in 1970.[431]

The antibodies anti-Co[a], anti-Co[b], and anti-Co3 are IgG. They usually don't bind complement, and they react best using the indirect antiglobulin test. Anti-Co3 was described by Rogers et al.[432] in 1974 and is inseparable from anti-Co[a] and anti-Co[b].

Genes *Co[a]* and *Co[b]* are codominant alleles. The Co(a−b−) phenotype is present when one silent *Co* allele is inherited from each parent. Recently, Lacey et al.[433] described a Co(a+b+) phenotype that suggests that an inhibitory gene may be present. The *Co* locus is known to be on chromosome 7.[434]

Anti-Co[a] has quickly destroyed a test dose of Co(a+) cells[434] and has also caused at least one delayed HTR.[435] Anti-Co[b] has been associated with both an immediate and a delayed HTR,[436,437] as well as with accelerated destruction of a test dose of Co(b+) red cells.[438] Anti-Co[a] has caused one case of severe HDN,[439] but there are no reports of HDN related to anti-Co[b].

THE CHIDO/RODGERS SYSTEM

In 1978, O'Neill et al.[440] showed that Chido and Rodgers are plasma antigens carried on the C4d portion of the complement molecule in plasma and bind to the red cell when complement is activated. The phenotype of C4 in plasma therefore controls the Chido and Rodgers phenotype of the red cells. Giles[441,442] proposed and described the Ch and Rg blood group system nomenclature. The Chido and Rodgers antigens are frequently spoken of as two antigens, although antibodies to nine different specificities have been found. Of the nine determinants, now called Rg[a] (RG1), Rg[b] (RG2), Ch[a] (CH1), Ch[b] (CH2), CH3, CH4, CH5, CH6, and WH[6], five are high prevalence and the rest are low prevalence. The Ch[a] and Rg[a] antigens are partially destroyed by enzymes and poorly developed at birth on red cells, although the antigens are strongly present in the newborn's plasma.[443]

Individuals lacking any of the Ch/Rg determinants are capable of making antibodies against the antigens they lack. Anti-Ch[a] was first described by Harris et al.[444] in 1967; anti-Rg[a] was discovered in 1976 by Longster and Giles.[445] These antibodies are stimulated by transfusion, pregnancy, and exposure to plasma antigens through cryoprecipitate and factor VIII and sometimes have no known stimulation. The antibodies are usually IgG4, react best in the indirect antiglobulin test, do not usually bind complement, and produce loose, fragile agglutinates. They are neutralizable by serum of most antigen-positive individuals.

Both Chido and Rodgers are inherited as codominant characters and are linked to the HLA locus on chromosome 6.[446,447] The *Ch[a]* and *Rg[a]* genes control the production of C4 in the plasma. Individuals genetically deficient in C4 are usually Ch(a−), Rg(a−)[448] and have SLE (systemic lupus erythematosus) or an SLE-like syndrome.[449]

Clinically, these antibodies are benign and usually do not cause HTRs and red cell destruction. However, there have been two cases of severe anaphylactic reactions in patients with antibodies to Ch or Rg when large amounts of plasma were transfused.[450]

They pose a laboratory problem in pretransfusion testing because they may obscure clinically significant antibodies in an individual's serum. The strength of the antibodies varies greatly, and they are not always neutralized by plasma containing the antigens. Although not a clinical problem, patients with cold agglutinin disease have increased C4d on their red cells, which causes them to react strongly with anti-Ch and anti-Rg.[451]

COST COLLECTION

The Cs[a] antigen is a high-prevalence antigen found only on red cells, including cord cells. It is not destroyed by proteolytic enzymes. These antigens show a variation in strength among individuals that is not attributable to zygosity. The antithetical antigen to Cs[a], Cs[b] was discovered by Molthan and Paradis[452] in 1984.

Giles et al.[453] discovered anti-Cs[a] in 1965. The antibodies are IgG reacting best by the indirect antiglobulin test. They do not bind complement and are not neutralized by serum. Frequently this antibody is found in combination with other antibodies. This heterozygosity, as well as variation in antigen strength, make identification of this antibody difficult.

Although the Yk[a] and Cs[a] antigens are inherited as dominant mendelian characters and share a phenotypic relationship, because the prevalence of Cs(a−) and Yk(a−) together is greater than expected, the Yk[a] antigen is not included in this collection.[3]

Clinically, most investigators,[454,455] believe that anti-Cs[a] causes HTRs, although there is only one report of decreased red cell survival.[456] Anti-Cs[a] has not been reported to cause HDN, although the antigen maybe well developed at birth.

WRIGHT COLLECTION

Antigens and Antibodies

The Wr[a] (WR1) antigen is a low-prevalence antigen showing dominant inheritance and present in approximately 1 in 1,000 blood samples. Dosage studies have confirmed the high-prevalence antithetical antigen Wr[b] (WR2).[457] Because of this relationship, in 1991 the ISBT changed the status of the Wright antigens from independent antigens to a collection of antigens. Wr^b is situated in the α-helical region of glycophorin A.[458] There is a possibility that Wr^a also is located there, because individuals who are En(a−) (lack SGPs) or have hybrid SGPs are Wr(a−b−).[6] Wren et al.[458] reported no amino acid differences in glycophorin A residues from En(a+), Wr(a+b−) and Wr(b+) red cells. A true WR null condition has not been found.

The first antibody to Wr^a, reported in 1953 by Holman,[459] reacted in the indirect antiglobulin test. Since then, anti-Wr^a has been found to react as solely IgM 16 times, partly IgM nine times, and solely IgG 19 times.[460] The Wr^a antibody seems to be more common in patients with a hyperactive immune system, who are exposed to breakdown products of Wr(a−) red cells, such as recently delivered women with anti-D and patients with autoimmune hemolytic anemia.[461] Anti-Wr^b was described by Adams et al.[462] and reacts best using the indirect antiglobulin test.

Clinical Significance

Anti-Wr^a is present in approximately 1 in 100 sera and has caused both mild and severe cases of HDN.[463] Two hemolytic transfusion reactions have also been reported as due to anti-Wr^a,[464,465] although both antibodies were naturally occurring. The antibody is often found in the serum of patients who have formed other blood group antibodies, as well as in the serum of patients with autoimmune antibodies (this is not to be confused with autoanti-Wr^a, which has never been reported). In fact, Issitt states that 1 in every two or three sera of patients with autoimmune hemolytic anemia contains anti-Wr^a. Anti-Wr^b is sometimes found as an autoantibody in patients with autoimmune hemolytic anemia and has caused one fatality.[466] At one time, Wr(a−b−) cells were thought to be resistant to *P. falciparum*, but that has since been disproved.[467]

INDIAN COLLECTION

The In^a antigen was described in 1973 by Badakere et al.[468] Two years later, the In^b antigen, still frequently called Salis, was reported by Giles.[469] These antigens reside on an 80-kd membrane glycoprotein lymphocyte homing receptor called CD44.[470] Not

much is known about the antigens, but their antibodies react at 18° and 37°C and are detected best by the indirect antiglobulin test. These antibodies are destroyed by papain, ficin, and reducing agents such as 0.2 M DTT.[18] No cases of HDN or HTR have been attributed to these antibodies, although anti-In^a has been produced in response to transfusion of In(a+) blood to an In(a−b+) patient.[471]

THE Bg ANTIGENS

Antigens

The Bg antigen actually represents the HLA system of antigens on red cells. Most individuals who have the Bg^a antigen on their red cells have HLA-B7 on their leukocytes.[472] In the same way, Bg^b correlates with HLA-B17, and Bg^c with HLA-A28.[473] It has been difficult to characterize these antigens, because the strength of the antigens varies from person to person, as well as over time in one individual. HLA antigens are present in plasma, but there is no evidence that these are adsorbed onto red cells in vivo. Bg antigens are hard to detect using conventional techniques, but AutoAnalyzer methods[474] have helped develop more consistency in detection and monoclonal antibodies and flow cytometry have been used successfully in studying these antigens.[475] It is thought that all HLA antigens are represented on red cells, but some are in such small amounts that they remain undetected using current techniques. Papain treatment may enhance antigens, but the effect of other enzymes on Bg is unknown. The Bg antigens are only partially developed at birth,[473] and their inheritance is unclear.

Antibodies

The Bg antibodies were first described as detecting several low-prevalence red cell antigens, called OT, HO, DBG, and Stobo. In 1967, Seaman et al.[474] defined three specificities from these antibodies: anti-Bg^a, anti-Bg^b, and anti-Bg^c. Sera containing any of these antibodies frequently have mixtures of two or more. Pavone and Issitt[476] report that 34 percent of individuals who make other red cell antibodies also have anti-Bg antibodies, and it is thought that more sera contain Bg/HLA antibodies at an undetectable level. In the past, Bg antibodies "contaminated" reagents, because red cells with strong Bg antigens negative for the reagent antigen were not always available to test pools of antisera. Since the discovery that chloroquine diphosphate solution inactivates these antigens, contamination of reagents with anti-Bg antibodies is no longer a problem.[18] Bg antibodies usually react weakly by the indirect antiglobulin test and are IgG. They are not thought to bind complement.

Clinical Significance

In general, Bg antibodies do not cause HTRs or HDN. Strong Bg antibodies may clear a small percentage of Bg-positive red cells extravascularly at an increased rate,[477] but there is no further evidence supporting Molthan's[478] report that anti-Bg^a was responsible for a HTR involving intravascular hemolysis. Bg antibodies are more of a serologic than a clinical problem.

In certain diseases, Bg antibodies on red cells are increased. The antigen Bg^a was found to gain strength in patients with infectious mononucleosis,[479] with the rise persisting for months or even years. Increases have also been reported in patients with leukemia, lymphoma, polycythemia, and megaloblastic or hemolytic anemia, and in those with reticulocytosis.[480]

Although the presence of Bg antibodies does not always correlate with cytotoxic HLA antibodies, a case has been described where anti-Bg^a was found in an eluate from tissue of a rejected transplanted kidney.[481] Morton et al.[474] suggested that organ recipients with cytotoxic antibodies be screened for Bg antibodies using the AutoAnalyzer and that organ donors be selected accordingly.

Sd^a AND CAD ANTIGENS

The Sd^a antigen is present on red cells, in tissues, and in body fluids, with the greatest amount in urine. Although the antigen is not well developed on red cells at birth (indeed, it is not even detected on the cells until about 10 weeks of life) it is present in high concentration in infant saliva. Studies show that the antigen cannot be destroyed by enzymes, varies in strength among individuals, and is depressed on red cells during pregnancy.[482] Ninety-one percent of individuals have detectable levels of Sd^a antigen on their red cells but approximately 50 percent of those who type Sd(a−) have Sd^a in their urine; thus, the actual prevalence of Sd(a+) individuals is closer to 96 percent. The presence of the Sd^a antigen in urine is the most reliable indicator of the Sd(a+) phenotype. The Sd^x antigen, once thought to be related to Sd^a, is probably an independent antigen, renamed Rx.[483]

The Cad antigen was first found on polyagglutinable red cells. This low-prevalence antigen was previously thought to be Sd^a because Cad-positive cells reacted very strongly with anti-Sd^a. Although recent studies have identified a terminal N-acetylgalactosamine (GALNAc) common to both the Sd^a and Cad antigen, it has not been proven that they have the same structure when they are on the rbc membrane. Some categories of Cad cells were postulated to be polyagglutinable, because it was thought that all serums contained low levels of anti-Sd^a.[484] Instead, Cad cells might be polyagglutinable because all sera contain anti-Cad.[485]

Antibodies

Anti-Sd^a was reported simultaneously in 1967 by two independent investigators.[486,487] The antibody is made by approximately one-half of all Sd(a−) individuals or about 2 percent of the population.[488] It is usually found as an IgM antibody reacting at room temperature, 37°C, and in the indirect antiglobulin phase. The agglutination has a characteristic mixed-field appearance with clumps having a refractile quality. The antibody may cause complement activation. The ability to neutralize anti-Sd^a in vitro with urine containing the Sd^a antigen provides a useful tool in antibody identification.

Biochemistry and Genetics

Studies performed on the Tamm-Horsfall protein in urine revealed the biochemical structure of the Sd^a antigen[489]; that is, when an individual is Sd(a+), the Tamm-Horsfall protein carries a GALNAc-terminal sugar, which is absent in Sd(a−) individuals.

The Cad antigenic determinant is located on glycophorin A and B of red blood cells and is associated with a pentasaccharide containing a terminal GALNAc sugar.[490] This sugar is the same terminal sugar found in the Sd^a antigen, which explains why Cad-positive red cells are agglutinated by anti-Sd^a. Both

Cad and Sd^a are inherited as dominant autosomal characters. Because the Sd^a antigen is not well developed on cord cells, anti-Sd^a does not cause HDN. There are many cases cited in the literature to support the theory that anti-Sd^a does not cause HTRs. Petermans and Cole Dergent[491] reported one case of an anti-Sd^a that did result in a HTR, although the cells involved were of the strongly Sd^a antigen-positive type. Issitt[2] reports that both Sd(a+) and Sd(a−) 51Cr tagged cells were destroyed equally at an increased rate by a patient with anti-Sd^a.

Cad-positive red blood cells have been found to be resistant to in vitro invasion by the malarial parasite *P. falciparum*.[492] This resistance may occur as a result of the Cad antigen either blocking the site for parasite attachment on glycophorin A or B, or interaction with sialic acid, so the antigen is unavailable for attachment by the parasite.

JOHN MILTON HAGEN ANTIGEN

The John Milton Hagen (JMH) antigen is a high-prevalence antigen that is well developed at birth and is destroyed by enzymes. The antigen resides on a fourth PI-linked protein with a molecular weight of 76 kd.[493] The antibody, described by Sabo et al.[494] in 1978 is IgG, not inhibited by serum, and usually high-titered, although it reacts weakly undiluted. The data suggest three mechanisms by which an individual can be JMH−: (1) inheritance of a JMH-negative gene; (2) loss of the antigen in JMH+ indi-

Table 5-29. High Prevalence Antigens

Antigen	Usual Immunoglobulin of Antibody	Binds Complement	Implicated in	
			HDN	HTR
Lan	IgG		Mild	X
At^a	IgG	No		?
Jr^a	IgG	Yes	?	X
Ok^a	IgG			X
Gill	IgG		No	
AnWj				
Rx		Yes		X
Emm				
MER2				
Duclos				

Table 5-30. Low-Prevalence Antigens Not Associated With a Collection

Antigen	Implicated in HDN	Comments/References
Bi^a	Mild	
Bp^a		
By	Mild	5 examples in patients with antibody-induced hemolytic anemia
BOW		
Bx^a		
Chr^a		
ELO		
FPTT		
Fr^a	Mild	
HJK		
HOFM		
Hey		
Hg^a		
JFV	Mild	
JONES	Mild	
Je^a		
Jn^a		
Kg	Mild	
Li^a	Mild	
Milne		
Mo^a		
NFLD		
Ol^a	Mild	
Os^a		
Pt^a		Present with antibodies to other low incidence antigens
RASM	Mild	
Rd	Mild	
Rb^a		
Re^a	Mild	
Sw^a		Present with other antibodies to low incidence antigens
SWI	Mild	
To^a		Many examples (12%)
Tr^a		Often present with anti Wr^a
Vg^a		
Wd^a		
Wu		

viduals over age 50; and (3) transient depression of the antigen from disease.[398] Individuals with depressed or "lost" antigens may have a positive direct antiglobulin test as well as anti-JMH in their serum, possibly because they have a small amount of JMH antigen left on their cells. Clinically, anti-JMH does not cause HTRs or HDN and patients can usually be transfused with JMH(+) red cells.[494]

THE VEL ANTIGEN

The Vel antigen has a very high prevalence. Vel-negative individuals are slightly more common in Sweden[495] and Norway.[496] The amount of Vel antigen on red cells may vary, making typing difficult in some cases.

Anti-Vel was first described in 1952 by Sussman and Miller.[497] Anti-Vel may be partly IgM and partly IgG. Serologically, some examples do not adsorb or elute well from Vel-positive red cells. The genetic and biochemical nature of the Vel antigen is not known. Several investigators postulated that the Vel-negative phenotype is formed through two different genetic pathways.[496,498] Clinically, anti-Vel has been implicated in at least one transfusion reaction[499] and one mild case of HDN.[500] Several examples of autoanti-Vel have also been reported.[501]

OTHER ANTIGENS

Numerous other antigens exist that do not belong to known systems or collections and do not have antithetical antigens, but have nonetheless clinical significance in routine blood banking because they may cause HDN, HTRs, or incompatible crossmatches. Table 5-29 summarizes antibodies to high-prevalence antigens, while Table 5-30 shows those to low-prevalence antigens. These tables are by no means exhaustive, as new antigens are discovered every day.

REFERENCES

1. Landsteiner K: Uber agglutinationserscheinungen normalen menschlichen blutes. Klin Wochenschr 14:1132, 1901
2. Issitt PD: Applied Blood Group Serology. 3rd Ed. Montgomery Scientific, Miami, FL, 1985
3. Daniels GL, Moulds JJ, Anstee DJ et al: ISBT working party on terminology for red cell surface antigens: Sao Paulo report. Vox Sang 65:77, 1993
4. Salmon C, Cartron JP, Rouger PH: The Human Blood Groups. Masson Publishing USA, New York, 1984
5. Walker RH: Technical Manual. 11th Ed. American Association of Blood Banking, Bethesda, MD, 1993
6. Lewis M, Anstee DJ, Bird GWG et al: Blood group terminology 1990. Vox Sang 58:152, 1990
7. Mollison PL, Engelfriet CP, Contreras M: Blood Transfusion In Clinical Medicine. 9th Ed. Blackwell Scientific, Oxford, 1993
8. Economidou J, Hughes-Jones NC, Gardner B: Quantitative measurements concerning A and B antigen sites. Vox Sang 12:231, 1967
9. Doinel C, Ropars C, Salmon C: Quantitative and thermodynamic measurements on I and i antigens of human red cells. Immunology 30:289, 1976
10. Masouredis SP, Sudora E, Mahan L, Victoria EJ: Antigen site densities and ultrastructural distribution patterns of red cell Rh antigens. Transfusion 16:94, 1976
11. Masouredis SP, Sudora E, Mahan L, Victoria EJ: Immunoelectron microscopy of Kell and Cellano antigens on red cell ghosts. Haematologia 13:59, 1980
12. Masouredis SP, Sudora E, Mahan L, Victoria EJ: Quantitative immunoferritin microassay of Fy^a, Fy^b, Jk^a, U and Di^b antigen site numbers on human red cells. Blood 56:969, 1980
13. Giblett ER: A critique of the theoretical hazard of inter- vs intra-racial transfusion. Transfusion 1:233, 1961
14. Guilbert B, Dighiero G, Avremas S: Naturally occurring antibodies against nine common antigens in human sera. I. Detection, isolation, and characterization. J Immunol 128:2779, 1982
15. Cleghorn TE: The frequency of Wr^a. By and M^g blood group antigens in blood donors in the south of England. Vox Sang 5:556, 1960
16. Ramsey G: Red cell antibodies and the new immunology. Lab Med 25:90, 1994
17. Benacerraf B: Role of MHC gene products in immune regulation. Science 212:1229, 1981
18. Moulds JM, Masouredis SP (eds): Monoclonal Antibodies. American Association of Blood Banks, Arlington, VA, 1989
19. Reid ME: Associations of red blood cell membrane abnormalities with blood group phenotype. p. 257. In Garratty G (ed): Immunobiology of Transfusion Medicine. Marcel Dekkar, New York, 1994
20. Thompson JS, Tompson MW: Genetics in Medicine. 3rd Ed. WB Saunders, Philadelphia, 1980

21. Allen FH: Null types of the human erythrocyte blood groups. Am J Clin Pathol 66:467, 1967

22. Brown PJ: Basic red cell membrane structures. p. 43. In Pierce SR, Steane S (eds): Biochemistry for Blood Bankers. American Association of Blood Banks, Arlington, VA, 1983

23. Watkins WM: Biochemistry and genetics of the ABO, Lewis and P blood group systems. Adv Hum Genet 10:1, 1980

24. Goldstein IJ, Hayes CE: Lectins: carbohydrate-binding-proteins. p. 127. In Tipson RS, Horton D (eds): Advances in Carbohydrate Chemistry and Biochemistry. Plenum, New York, 1978

25. Hakomori S: Blood Group ABH and Ii antigens of human erythrocytes: chemistry, polymorphisms, and developmental changes. Semin Hematol 18:39, 1981

26. Harmening DM, Firestone D: The ABO blood group system. p. 86. In Harmening DM (ed): Modern Blood Banking and Transfusion Practices. FA Davis, Philadelphia, 1994

27. Grundbacher FJ: Changes in the human A antigen of erythrocytes with the individual's age. Nature 204: 192, 1964

28. Tilley CA, Crookston MC, Brown BL, Wherrett JR: A and B and A_1Le^b substances in glycosphingolipid fractions of human serum. Vox Sang 28:25, 1975

29. Furukawa K, Mattes MJ, Lloyd KO: A_1 and A_2 erythrocytes can be distinguished by reagents that do not detect structural differences between the two cell types. J Immunol 135:4090, 1985

30. Beattie KM: Discrepancies in ABO blood grouping. p. 129. In A Seminar on Problems Encountered in Pretransfusion Tests. American Association of Blood Banks, Washington, DC, 1972

31. Pittiglio DH: Genetics and biochemistry of A, B, H, and Lewis antigens. p. 1. In Wallace ME, Gibbs FL (eds): Blood Group Systems: ABH and Lewis. American Association of Blood Banks, Arlington, VA, 1986

32. Stamps R, Sorol RJ, Leach M et al: A new variant of blood group A: A_{pae}. Transfusion 27:315, 1987

33. Salmon CH, Lopez M, Cartron JP, Bouguerra A: Quantitative and thermodynamic studies of erythrocytic ABO antigens. Transfusion 16:580, 1976

34. Grundbacher FJ: Genetics of anti-A and anti-B levels Transfusion 16:48, 1976

35. Martensson L, Fudenberg HH: Gm genes and gamma globulin synthesis in the human fetus. J Immunol 95:514, 1965

36. Auf der Maur C, Holdel M, Nydegger UE, Rieben R: Age dependency of ABO histo-blood group antibodies: reexamination of an old dogma. Transfusion 33: 915, 1993

37. Medical Research Council: Hypogammaglobulinaemia in the United Kingdom. Report of a Medical Research Council Working Party. Lancet 1:163, 1969

38. Holburn AM: Radioimmunoassay studies of the cross-reacting antibody of human blood group O sera. Br J Haematol 32:589, 1976

39. Lundberg WB, McGinnis MH: Hemolytic transfusion reaction due to anti-A_1. Transfusion 15:1, 1975

40. Wright J, Lim FC, Freeman J: An example of auto-anti-A_1 agglutinins. Vox Sang 39:222, 1980

41. Marsh WL, Nichols ME, Oyen R et al: Inherited mosaicism affecting the ABO blood groups. Transfusion 15:589, 1975

42. Yoshida A, Yamaguchi H, Okubo Y: Genetic mechanisms of cis AB inheritance. I. A case associated with unequal chromosome crossing-over. Am J Hum Genet 32:332, 1980

43. Yoshida A, Yamaguchi H, Okubo Y: Genetic mechanisms of cis AB inheritance. II. Cases associated with structural mutation of blood group transferases. Am J Hum Genet 32:645, 1980

44. Drozda EA Jr, Dean JJ: Another example of the rare A_y phenotype. Transfusion 25:280, 1985

45. Rubinstein P, Allen FH Jr, Rosenfield RE: A dominant suppressor of A and B. Vox Sang 25:377, 1973

46. Ducos J, Marty Y, Ruffie J: A new case of A_x phenotype transmitted by A_2B subjects. Vox Sang 29:390, 1975

47. Oriol R, Pendu J, Mollicone R: Genetics of ABO, H, Lewis, X, and other related antigens. Vox Sang 51: 161, 1986

48. Salmon C, Cartron JP, Rouger P et al: H deficient phenotypes: A proposed practical classification Bombay A_h, H_z, H_m. Blood Transfus Immunohaematol 23:233, 1980

49. Watkins WM: Biochemistry and genetics of the ABO, Lewis, and P blood group systems. p. 1. In Harris H, Hirschhorn K (eds): Advances in Human Genetics. Plenum, New York, 1980

50. Tilley CA, Crookston MC, Crookston JH et al: Human blood group A- and H-specified glycosyltransferase levels in the sera of newborn infants and their mothers. Vox Sang 34:8, 1978

51. Wrobel DM, McDonald I, Race C, Watkins WM: "True" genotype of chimeric twins revealed by blood group gene products in plasma. Vox Sang 27:395, 1974

52. Frederick J, Hunter J, Greenwell P et al: The A^1B genotype expressed as A_2B on red cells of individuals with strong B gene-specified transferase. Transfusion 25:30, 1985

53. Beck ML: Blood group antigens acquired de novo.

p. 45. In Garratty G (ed): Blood Group Antigens and Disease. American Association of Blood Banks, Arlington, VA, 1983

54. Gerbal A, Maslet C, Salmon C: Immunological aspects of the acquired B antigen. Vox Sang 28:398, 1975

55. Yates AD, Greenwal P, Watkins WM: Overlapping specification of the glycosyltransferases specified by the blood-group A and B genes: a possible explanation for aberrant blood-group expression in malignant tissues. Biochem Soc Transfus 11:300, 1983

56. Reid ME, Bird GWG: Associations between human red cell blood group antigens and disease. Transfus Med Rev IV:47, 1990

57. Hardman JT: Clinical relevance of ABH and Lewis blood group systems. p. 83. In Wallace ME, Gibbs FL (eds): Blood Group Antigens and Disease. American Association of Blood Banks, Arlington, VA, 1983

58. Bird GWG: Determinants of recognition and of susceptibility to disease. p. 1. In Garratty G (ed): Blood Group Antigens and Disease. American Association of Blood Banks, Arlington, VA, 1983

59. Anstall HB: ABH antigens in disease. p. 135. In Wallace ME, Gibbs FL (eds): Blood Group Systems: ABH and Lewis. American Association of Blood Banks, Arlington, VA, 1986

60. Garratty G: Do blood groups have a biological role? p. 201. In Garratty G (ed): Immunobiology of Transfusion Medicine. Marcel Dekker, New York, 1994

61. Davidson I: Early immunologic diagnosis and prognosis of carcinoma. Am J Clin Pathol 57:715, 1976

62. Crookston MC: Anomalous ABO, H and I phenotypes in disease. P. 67. In Garratty G (ed): Blood Group Antigens and Disease. American Association of Blood Banks, Arlington, VA, 1983

63. Beck ML: The I blood group collection. p. 23. In Moulds JM, Woods LL (eds): Blood Groups: P, I, Sd^a, and Pr. American Association of Blood Banks, Arlington, VA, 1991

64. Hillman RS, Giblett ER: Red cell membrane alterations associated with "marrow stress." J Clin Invest 44:1730, 1965

65. Testa U, Rochant H, Henri A et al: Changes in i-antigen expression of erythrocytes during in vivo aging. Rev Fr Transfus Immunohematol 24:299, 1981

66. Chaplin H, Hunter VL, Malech AC, Kilzer P, Rosche ME: Clinically significant allo-anti-I in an I-negative patient with massive hemorrhage. Transfusion 25:57, 1986

67. Rubin H, Solomon A: Cold agglutinins of anti-i specificity in alcoholic cirrhosis. Vox Sang 12:227, 1967

68. Layrisse Z, Layrisse M: High incidence cold agglutinins of anti-I^T specificity in Yanomama Indians in Venezuela. Vox Sang 14:369, 1968

69. Watanabe K, Hakomori S, Childs RA, Feizi T: Characterization of a blood group I-active gangioside structural requirements for I and I specificities. J Biol Chem 254:3221, 1979

70. Joshi SR, Bahtia HM: A new red cell phenotype I-i-: red cell lacking in both I and I antigens. Vox Sang 36:34, 1979

71. Giblett ER, Crookston MC: Agglutinability of red cells by anti-i in patients with thalessaemia major and other haematological disorders. Nature 201:1138, 1964

72. McGinniss MH: The ubiquitous nature of human blood group antigens as evidenced by bacterial, viral, and parasitic infections. p. 25. In Garratty G (ed): Blood Group Antigens and Disease. American Association of Blood Banks, Arlington, VA, 1983

73. Issitt PD: Cold-reactive autoantibodies outside the I and P blood groups. p. 73. In Moulds JM, Woods LL (eds): Blood Groups: P, I, Sd^a, and Pr. American Association of Blood Banks, VA, 1991

74. Syzmanski IO, Tilley CA, Crookston MC et al: A further example of human blood group chimaerism. J Med Genet 14:270, 1977

75. Rohr TE, Smith DF, Zopf DA, Ginsberg V: Le^b-active glycolipid in human plasma: measurements by radioimmunoassay. Arch Biochem Biophys 199:265, 1980

76. Cutbush M, Giblett ER, Mollison PL: Demonstration of the phenotype Le(a+b+) in infants and in adults. Br J Haematol 2:210, 1956

77. Crookston MC, Tilley CA, Crookston JH: Human blood chimaera with seeming breakdown of immune tolerance. Lancet 2:1110, 1970

78. Schenkel-Brunner H, Hanfland P: Immunochemistry of the Lewis blood-group system. III. Studies on the molecular basis of the Le^x property. Vox Sang 40:358, 1981

79. Hammar L, Mansson S, Rohr T et al: Lewis phenotype of erythrocytes and Le^b-active glycolipid in serum of pregnant women. Vox Sang 40:27, 1981

80. Spitalnik S, Crowles J, Cox MT, Blumberg N: Detection of IgG anti-Lewis(a) antibodies in cord sera by kinetic Elisa. Vox Sang 48:235, 1985

81. Graham HA, Hirsch HF, Davies DM: Genetic and immunochemical relationships between soluble and cell-bound antigen of the Lewis system. p. 257. In Mohn JF, Plunkett RW, Cunningham RK, Lambert RM (eds): Human Blood Groups. S Karger, Basel, 1977

82. Potapov MI: Detection of the antigen of the Lewis

system, characteristic of the erythrocytes of the secretory group Le(a−b−). Probl Hematol Blood Transf 15:45, 1970

83. Posner MP, McGeorge MB, Mendez-Picon G et al: The importance of the Lewis system in cadaver renal transplantation. Transplant 41:474, 1986

84. Anstall HB, Blaylock RC: The P blood group system: biochemistry, genetics and clinical significance. p. 1. In Moulds JM, Woods LL (eds): Blood Groups: P, I, Sd^a, and Pr. American Association of Blood Banks, Arlington, VA, 1991

85. Marcus DM, Kundu SK, Suzuki A: The P blood group system: recent progress in immunochemistry and genetics. Semin Haematol 18:63, 1981

86. Tippett P: Contribution of monoclonal antibodies to understanding one new and some old blood group systems. p. 83. In Garratty G (ed): Red Cell Antigens and Antibodies. American Association of Blood Banks, Arlington, VA, 1986

87. Soderstrom T, Enskog A, Samuelsson BE, Cedergren B: Immunoglobulin subclass (IgG3 restriction of anti-P and P^k) antibodies in patients of the rare p blood group. J Immunol 134:1, 1985

88. Lopez M, Cartron J, Cartron JP et al: Cytotoxicity of anti-PP$_1$P^k antibodies and possible relationship with early abortions of p mothers. Clin Immunol Immunopathol 28:296, 1983

89. Vos GH: A comparative observation of the presence of anti-Tj^a-like hemolysins in relation to obstetric history, distribution of various blood groups and the occurrence of immune anti-A or anti-B hemolysin among aborters and nonaborters. Transfusion 5:327, 1965

90. Ben-Ismail R, Rouger P, Carme B et al: Comparative automated assay of anti-P$_1$ antibodies in acute hepatic distomiasis (fasciliasis) and in hydatidosis. Vox Sang 38:165, 1980

91. Petit A, Duong TH, Bremond JL et al: Allo-anti-corps irreguliers anti-P$_1$; et clonorchiase a Chonorchis sinensis. Rev Fr Transfus Immunohematol 24:197, 1981

92. Brown KE, Hibbs JE, Gallinella G et al: Resistance to parvovirus B19 infection due to lack of virus receptor (erythrocyte P antigen). N Engl J Med 330:1192, 1994

93. Holliman SM: The MN blood group system: distribution, serology, and genetics. p. 1. In Unger PJ, Laird-Fryer (eds): Blood group systems: MN and Gerbich. American Association of Blood Banks, Arlington, VA, 1989

94. Tippett P, Reid ME, Poole J et al: The Miltenberger subsystem: is it obsolescent? Transfus Med Rev VI: 170, 1992

95. Tokunaga E, Sasakawa S, Tamaka K et al: Two apparently healthy Japanese individuals of type M^{k}M^k have erythrocytes which lack both the blood group MN and Ss-active sialoglycoproteins. J Immunogenet 6: 383, 1979

96. Issitt PD: The MN Blood Group System. Montgomery Scientific Publications, Cincinnati, OH, 1981

97. Smith ML, Beck ML: The immunoglobulin class of antibodies with M specificity. Commun Amer Assoc Blood Banks. Atlanta, GA, 1977

98. Howard PL, Picoff RC: Another example of anti-M in an M-positive patient. Transfusion 12:59, 1972

99. Chapman J, Murphy WF, Waters AH: Chronic cold haemagglutinin disease due to anti-N-like autoantibody. Vox Sang 42:272, 1982

100. Giles CM, Howell P: An antibody in the serum of an MN patient which reacts with the M$_1$ antigen. Vox Sang 27:43, 1974

101. Ballas SK, Dignam C, Harris M, Marcolina MJ: A clinically significant anti-N in a patient whose red cells were negative for N and U antigens. Transfusion 25:377, 1985

102. Telischi M, Behzad O, Issitt PD, Pavone BG: Hemolytic disease of the newborn due to anti-N. Vox Sang 31:109, 1976

103. Cohen DW, Garratty G, Morel P, Petz LD: Autoimmune hemolytic anemia associated with IgG autoanti-N. Transfusion 19:329, 1979

104. Morel PA, Bergren MO, Hill V et al: M and N specific hemagglutinins of human erythrocytes stored in glucose solutions. Transfusion 21:652, 1981

105. Fassbinder W, Siedl S, Koch KM: The role of formaldehyde in the formation of haemodialysis-associated anti-N-like antibodies. Vox Sang 35:141, 1978

106. Lalezari P, Malamut DC, Dreisiger ME, Sanders C: Anti-s and anti-U cold reacting antibodies. Vox Sang 25:390, 1973

107. Johnson MH, Plett MJ, Conant CN, Worthington M: Autoimmune hemolytic anemia with anti-S specificity. Transfusion 18:389, 1978

108. Taliano V, Guevin RM, Hebert D et al: The rare En(a−) phenotype in a French-Canadian family. Vox Sang 38:87, 1980

109. Cartron JP, Rahuel C: Human erythrocyte glycophorins: protein and gene structure analyses. Transfus Med Rev VI:63, 1992

110. Rolih S: Biochemistry of MN antigens. p. 31. In Unger PJ, Laird-Fryer B (eds): Blood Group Systems: MN and Gerbich. American Association of Blood Banks, Arlington, VA, 1989

111. Giles CM: The identity of Kamhuber and Far antigens. Vox Sang 32:269, 1977

112. Dahr W, Kordowicz M, Moulds J et al: Characterization of the Ss sialoglycoprotein and its antigens in Rh$_{null}$ erythrocytes. Blut 54:13, 1987

113. Giblett ER: Blood group antibodies causing hemolytic disease of the newborn. Clin Obstet Gynecol 7: 1044, 1964

114. Walker W, Murray S, Russell JK: Stillbirth due to haemolytic disease of the newborn. J Obstet Gynaecol Br Emp 64:573, 1957

115. Levine P, Stetson R: Unusual case of intragroup agglutination. JAMA 113:126, 1939

116. Landsteiner K, Wiener AS: An agglutinable factor in human blood recognized by immune sera for rhesus blood. Proc Soc Exp Biol Med 43:223, 1940

117. Wiener AS, Peters HR: Hemolytic reactions following transfusions of blood of homologous group, with 3 cases in which same agglutinogen was responsible. Ann Intern Med 13:2306, 1940

118. Levine P, Katzin EM: Isoimmunization in pregnancy and the variety of isoagglutinins observed. Proc Soc Exp Biol 43:343, 1940

119. Levine P, Newark NJ, Burnham L et al. The role of isoimmunization in the pathogenesis of erythroblastosis fetalis. Am J Obstet Gynecol 42:925, 1941

120. Race RR, Sanger R: Blood Groups in Man. Blackwell Scientific, New York, 1975

121. Wiener AS: Genetic theory of the Rh blood types. Proc Soc Exp Biol Med 54:316, 1943

122. Race RR: An "incomplete" antibody in human serum. Nature 153:771, 1944

123. Fisher RA: Fitting of gene frequencies to data on the rhesus reactions. Ann Eugen 13:150, 1946

124. Fisher RA, Race RR: Rh gene frequencies in Britain. Nature 157:48, 1946

125. Race RR: The Rh genotypes and Fisher's theory. Blood 3 (suppl):27, 1948

126. Mourant AE: A new rhesus antibody. Nature 155:542, 1945

127. Colin Y, Cherif-Zahar B, Le Van Kim C et al: Genetic basis of the Rh D-positive and RhD-negative blood group polymorphism as determined by Southern analysis. Blood 78:2747, 1991

128. Lawler SD, Race RR: Quantitative aspects of Rh antigens. Proceedings International Society of Hematology. Grune & Stratton, New York, 1951

129. Rosenfield RE, Allen FH Jr, Swisher SN, Kochwa S: A review of Rh serology and presentation of a new terminology. Transfusion 2:287, 1962

130. Tippett P: A speculative model for the Rh blood groups. Ann Hum Genet 50:241, 1986

131. Issitt PD: Some Messages received from Blood Group Antibodies. p. 99. In Garratty G (ed): Red Cell Antigens and Antibodies. American Association of Blood Banks, Arlington, VA, 1986

132. Vengelen-Tyler V, Pierce SR (eds): Blood Group Systems: Rh. American Association of Blood Banks, Arlington, VA, 1987

133. Issitt PD: The Rh blood group system, 1988: eight new antigens in nine years and some observations on the biochemistry and genetics of the system, review. Transfus Med Rev 3:1, 1989

134. Issitt PD: The Rh Blood Groups. p. 111. In Garratty G (ed): Immunobiology of Transfusion Medicine. Marcel Dekker, New York, 1994

135. Moore BPL: Does knowledge of Du status serve a useful purpose? Vox Sang, suppl 1. 46:95, 1984

136. Agre PC, Davies DM, Issitt PD et al: A proposal to standardize terminology for weak D antigen. Transfusion 32:86, 1992

137. Stratton F: A new Rh allelemorph. Nature 158:25, 1946

138. Race RR, Sanger R, Lawler SD: The Rh antigen Du. Ann Eugen 14:171, 1948

139. Stratton F, Renton PH: Rh genes allelomorphic to D. Nature 162:293, 1948

140. Cappellini R, Dunn LC, Turri M: An interaction between alleles at the Rh locus in man which weakens the reactivity of the Rh$_o$ factor (Du). Proc Natl Acad Sci USA 41:283, 1955

141. Argall CI, Ball M, Trentelman E: Presence of anti-D antibody in the serum of a Du patient. J Lab Clin Med 4:895, 1953

142. Tippett P, Sanger R: Observations on subdivisions of the Rh antigen D. Vox Sang 7:9, 1962

143. Tippett P, Sanger R: Further observations on the subdivisions of the Rh Antigen D. Arztl Jugendkd 23: 476, 1977

144. Tippett P: The D antigen and high-and low frequency Rh antigens. p. 25. In Vengelen-Tyler V, Pierce SR (eds): Blood Group Systems: Rh. American Association of Blood Banks, Arlington, VA, 1987

145. Tippett P: Sub-divisions of the Rh antigen D, review. Med Lab Sci 45:88, 1988 [corrected; published erratum appears in Med Lab Sci 45:294, 1988]

146. Schmidt PJ, Morrison EG, Shohl J: The antigenicity of the Rh$_o$ (Du) blood factor. Blood 20:196, 1962

147. Vengelen-Tyler V: The Rh Blood Group Systems and Associated Disease. In Vengelen-Tyler V, Pierce SR (eds): Blood Group Systems: Rh. American Association of Blood Banks, Arlington, VA, 1987

148. Issitt PD: Biochemistry of the Rh Blood Group System. p. 105. In Vengelen-Tyler V, Judd WJ (eds): Recent Advances in Blood Group Biochemistry. American Association of Blood Banks, Arlington, VA, 1986

149. Mollison PL, Cutbush M: La maladie hemolytique chez un enfant Du. Rev Hematol 4:608, 1949

150. Wiener AS, Unger LJ: Rh factors related to the Rho factor as a source of clinical problems. JAMA 169: 696, 1959

151. Wiener AS, Unger LJ: Further observations on the blood factors RhA, RhB, RhC, RhD. Transfusion 2: 230, 1962

152. Lomas C, Bruce M, Watt A et al: Tar + individuals with anti-D, a new category D VII. Transfusion 26: 560, 1986

153. Lomas C, Grassmanm W, Ford D et al: FPTT is a low-incidence Rh antigen associated with a "new" partial Rh D phenotype, DFR. Transfusion 34:612, 1994

154. Lomas C, Tippett P, Thompson KM et al: Demonstration of seven epitopes on the Rh antigen D using human monoclonal anti-D antibodies and red cells from D categories. Vox Sang 57:261, 1989

155. Lomas C, McColl K, Tippett P: Further complexities of the Rh antigen D disclosed by testing category DII cells with monoclonal anti-D. Transfus Med 3:67, 1993

156. Mouro I, Le Van Kim C, Rouillac C et al: Rearrangements of the blood group RhD gene associated with the DVI category phenotype. Blood 83:1129, 1994

157. Alter AA, Gelb AG, Chown B et al: Gonzales (Goa), a new blood group character. Transfusion 7:88, 1967

158. Rosenfield RE, Haber G, Gibbel N: A new Rh variant. Bibl Haematol 7:90, 1956

159. Chown B, Lewis M, Kaita H: A new Rh antigen and antibody. Transfusion 2:150, 1962

160. Chown B, Lewis M, Kaita H, Phillips S: The Rh antigen Dw (Wiel). Transfusion 4:169, 1964

161. Humphreys J, Stout TD, Kaita H, Chown B: A new blood group antigen, Targett. Proceedings International Congress of Blood Transfusion, Helsinki, 1975

162. Lewis M, Kaita H, Allderdice PW et al: Assignment of the red cell antigen, Targett (Rh40), to the Rh blood group system. Am J Hum Genet 31:630, 1979

163. Rosenfield RE, Vogel P, Gibbel N et al: A "new" Rh antibody, anti-f. BMJ 1:1975, 1953

164. Rosenfield RE, Haber GV: An Rh blood factgor, rhi(Ce), and its relationship to hr(ce). Am J Hum Genet 10:474, 1958

165. Dunsford I: A new Rh antibody-anti-CE. Proceedings 8th Congress of European Society Haematology. Paper No. 491, Vienna, 1961

166. Keith P, Corcoran PA, Caspersen K, Allen FH: A new antibody; anti-Rh [27] (cE) in the Rh blood group system. Vox Sang 10:528, 1965

167. Allen FH Jr, Tippett PA: A new Rh blood type which reveals the Rh antigen G. Vox Sang 3:321, 1958

168. Levine P, Rosenfield RE, White J: The first example of the Rh phenotype rGrG. Am J Hum Genet 13:299, 1961

169. Rosenfield RE, Levine P, Heller C: Quantitative Rh typing or r-Gr-G with observations on the nature of G (Rh 12) and anti-G. Vox Sang 28:293, 1975

170. Issitt PD: An invited review: the Rh antigen e, its variants, and some closely related serological observations. Immunohematology 7:29, 1991

171. Callender ST, Race RR: A serological and genetical study of multiple antibodies formed in response to blood transfusion by a patient with lupus erythematosus diffusus. Ann Eugen 13:102, 1946

172. Stratton F, Renton PH: Haemolytic disease of the newborn caused by a new rhesus antibody, anti-Cx. BMJ 1:962, 1954

173. Sistonen P, Abdulle OA, Sahid M: Evidence for a "new" Rh gene complex producing the rare Cx (Rh9) antigen in the Somali population of East Africa. Transfusion 27:66, 1987

174. Greenwalt TJ, Sanger R: The Rh antigen Ew. Br J Haematol 1:52, 1955

175. Vos GH, Kirk RL: A "naturally-occurring" anti-E which distinguishes a variant of the E antigen in Australian aborigines. Vox Sang 7:22, 1962

176. Huestis DW, Catino ML, Busch S: A "new" Rh antibody (anti-Rh26) which detects a factor usually accompanying hr'. Transfusion 4:414, 1964

177. Shapiro M: Serology and genetics of a new blood group factor: hrB. J Forensic Med 7:96, 1960

178. Shapiro M, Le Roux M, Brink S: Serology and genetics of a new blood factor: hr B. Haematologia 6: 121, 1972

179. Moores PP: The Blood Groups of the Natal Negro People. University of Natal, Durban, Republic of South Africa (thesis) 1976

180. Moores P, Smart E: Serology and genetics of the red blood cell factor Rh34. Vox Sang 61:122, 1991

181. DeNatale A, Cahan A, Jack JA et al: A new Rh antigen common in Negroes, rare in white people. JAMA 159:247, 1955

182. Sanger R, Noades J, Tippett P, Race RR: An Rh antibody specific for V and Ris. Nature 186:171, 1960

183. Rochna E, Hughes-Jones NC: The use of purified ^{125}I-labeled anti-globulin in the determination of the number of D antigen sites on red cells of different phenotypes. Vox Sang 10:675, 1965

184. Cherif-Zahar B, Raynal V, D'Ambrosio AM et al: Molecular analysis of the structure and expression of the RH locus in individuals with D--, Dc-, and DCw- gene complexes. Blood 84:4354, 1994

185. Race RR, Sanger R, Selwyn JG: A probable deletion in a human Rh chromosome. Nature 166:520, 1950

186. Contreras M, Armitage S, Daniels GL, Tippett P: Homozygous. D. Vox Sang 36:81, 1979

187. Contreras M, Stebbing B, Blessing M, Gavin J: The Rh antigen Evans. Vox Sang 34:208, 1978

188. Daniels GL: An investigation of the immune response of homozygotes for the Rh haplotype --D-- and related haplotypes. Using cells of rare Rh phenotypes. Rev Fr Transfus Immunohematol 25:185, 1982

189. Gunson HH, Donohue WL: Multiple examples of the blood CwD-/CwD- in a Canadian family. Vox Sang 2:320, 1957

190. Tate H, Cunningham C, McDade MG et al: An Rh gene complex Dc-. Vox Sang 5:398, 1960

191. Salmon C, Gerbal A, Liberge G et al: The gene complex DIV (C)-. [In French.] Rev Fr Transfus 12:239, 1969

192. Habibi B, Perrier P, Salmon C: Antigen Nou. A new high frequency Rh antigen. Rev Fr Transfus Immunohematol 24:117, 1981

193. Issitt PD, Gutgsell NS: Some new Rh antigens: Rh43 to Rh47. Immunohematology 3:1, 1987

194. Issitt PD, Pavone BG, Shapiro M: Anti-Rh39—a "new" specificity Rh system antibody. Transfusion 19:389, 1979

195. Issitt PD, Gutgsell NS, McDowell MA et al: Studies on anti-Rh46. Blood, suppl 1. 70:110a, 1987

196. Habibi B, Fouillade MT, Duedari N et al: The antigen Duclos. A new high frequency red cell antigen related to Rh and U. Vox Sang 34:302, 1978

197. Dahr W, Kruger J: Solubilization of various blood group antigens by Triton X-100, abstracted. p. 141. In Proceedings of the Tenth International Congress of the Society of Forensic Haematogenetics, 1983

198. Issitt PD, Wren MR, McDowell MA et al: Anti-Rh33, the second separable example, also made by a person who made anti-D and has C+ red cells. Transfusion 26:506, 1986

199. Giles CM, Crossland JD, Haggas WK, Longster G: An Rh gene complex which results in a "new" antigen detectable by a specific antibody, Anti-Rh 33. Vox Sang 21:289, 1971

200. Rosenfield RE, Haber GV, Schroeder R, Ballard R: Problems in Rh typing as revealed by a single negro family. Am J Hum Genet 12:147, 1960

201. Broman B, Heiken A, Tippett PA, Giles CM: The D(C) (e) gene complex revealed in the Swedish population. Vox Sang 8:588, 1963

202. Heiken A, Giles CM: On the Rh gene complexes D--,D(C) (e), and d(c) (e). Hereditas 53:171, 1965

203. Giles CM, Skov F: The CDe rhesus gene complex; some considerations revealed by a study of a Danish family with an antigen of the Rhesus gene complex (C) D (e) defined by a "new" antibody. Vox Sang 20:328, 1971

204. Davidson J, Stern K, Strauser ER, Spurrier W: Be, a new "private" blood factor. Blood 8:747, 1953

205. Lomas C, Poole J, Salaru N et al: A low-incidence red cell antigen JAL associated with two unusual Rh gene complexes. Vox Sang 59:39, 1990

206. Poole J, Hustinx H, Gerber H et al: The red cell antigen JAL in the Swiss population: family studies showing that JAL is an Rh antigen (RH48). Vox Sang 59:44, 1990

207. Marais I, Moores P, Smart E, Martell R: STEM, a new low-frequency Rh antigen associated with the e-variant phenotyes hrs-(Rh: -18, -19) and hrB-(Rh: -31, -34). Transfus Med 3:35, 1993

208. Coghlan G, McCreary J, Underwood V, Zelinski T: A "new" low-incidence red cell antigen, LOCR, associated with altered expression of Rh antigens. Transfusion 34:492, 1994

209. Moulds JJ: Rh$_{null}$ s: amorphs and regulators. p. 63. In Walker RH (ed): A Seminar on Recent Advances in Immunohematology. American Association of Blood Banks, Washington, DC, 1973

210. Vos GH, Vos D, Kirk RL, Sanger R: A sample of blood with no detectable Rh antigen. Lancet 1:34, 1961

211. Levine P, Celano MJ, Falkowski F et al: A second example of ---/--- or Rh$_{null}$ blood. Transfusion 5:492, 1965

212. Ishimori T, Hasekura H: A Japanese with no detectable Rh blood group antigens due to silent Rh alleles or deleted chromosomes. Transf 7:84, 1967

213. Cherif-Zahar B, Raynal V, Le Van Kim C et al: Structure and expression of the Rh locus in the Rh-deficiency syndrome. Blood 82:656, 1993

214. Hermand P, Mouro I, Huet M et al: Immunochemical characterization of rhesus proteins with antibodies raised against synthetic peptides. Blood 82:669, 1993

215. Tippett P: Regulator genes affecting red cell antigens. Transfus Med Rev 4:56, 1990

216. Schmidt PJ, Lostumbo MM, English CT, Hunter OB Jr. Aberrant U blood group accompanying Rh-null. Transfusion 7:33, 1967

217. Lauf PK, Joiner CH: Increased potassium transport and ouabain binding in human Rh$_{null}$ red blood cells. Blood 48:457, 1976

218. Ballas SK, Clark MR, Mohandas N et al: Red cell membrane and cation deficiency in Rh null syndrome. Blood 63:1046, 1984

219. Chown B, Lewis M, Kaita H, Lowen B: A new cause of haemolytic anaemia? Lancet 1:396, 1971

220. Chown B, Lewis M, Kaita H, Lowen B: An unlinked modifier of Rh blood groups: effects when heterozygous and when homozygous. Am J Hum Genet 24: 623, 1972

221. Moore S, Woodrow CF, McClelland DB: Isolation of membrane components associated with human red cell antigens Rh(D), (c), (E) and Fy. Nature 295:529, 1982

222. Gahmberg CG: Molecular identification of the human Rho (D) antigen. FEBS Lett 140:93, 1982

223. Cherif-Zahar B, Bloy C, Le Van Kim C et al: Molecular cloning and protein structure of a human blood group Rh polypeptide. Proc Natl Acad Sci USA 87: 6243, 1990

224. Avent ND, Ridgwell K, Tanner MJ, Anstee DJ: cDNA cloning of a 30 kDa erythrocyte membrane protein associated with Rh (Rhesus)-blood-group-antigen expression. Biochem J 271:821, 1990

225. Le Van Kim C, Cherif-Zahar B, Raynal V et al: Multiple Rh messenger RNA isoforms are produced by alternative splicing. Blood 80:1074, 1992

226. Ridgwell K, Spurr NK, Laguda B et al: Isolation of cDNA clones for a 50 kDa glycoprotein of the human erythrocyte membrane associated with Rh (rhesus) blood-group antigen expression. Biochem J 287:223, 1992

227. Le Van Kim C, Mouro I, Cherif-Zahar B et al: Molecular cloning and primary structure of the human blood group RhD polypeptide. Proc Natl Acad Sci USA 89: 10925, 1992

228. Kuypers F, van Linde-Sibenius-Trip M, Roelofsen B et al: Rh$_{null}$ human erythrocytes have an abnormal membrane phospholipid organization. Biochem J 221:931, 1984

229. de Vetten MP, Agre P: The Rh polypeptide is a major fatty acid-acylated erythrocyte membrane protein. J Biol Chem 263:18193, 1988

230. Agre P, Cartron JP: Molecular biology of the Rh antigens, review. Blood 78:551, 1991

231. Seidl S, Spielmann W, Martin H: Two siblings with Rh$_{null}$ disease. Vox Sang 23:182, 1972

232. Mollison PL, Frame M, Ross ME: Differences between Rh(D) negative subjects in response to Rh(D) antigen. Br J Haematol 19:257, 1970

233. Weiner W, Battery DA, Cleghorn T et al: Serological findings in a case of haemolytic anemia with some general observations of the pathogenesis of this syndrome. BMJ 2:125, 1953

234. Lux SE: Spectrin-actin membrane skeleton of normal and abnormal red blood cells, review. Semin Hematol 16:21, 1979

235. Cohen CM: The molecular organization of the red cell membrane skeleton, review. Semin Hematol 20: 141, 1983

236. Merry AH, Thomson EE, Anstee DJ, Stratton F: The quantification of erythrocyte antigen sites with monoclonal antibodies. Immunology 51:793, 1984

237. Bloy C, Blanchard D, Lambin P et al: Human monoclonal antibody against Rh(D) antigen: partial characterization of the Rh(D) polypeptide from human erythrocytes. Blood 69:1491, 1987

238. Bloy C, Blanchard D, Lambin P et al: Characterization of the D, c, E, and G antigens of the Rh blood group system with human monoclonal antibodies. Mol Immunol 25:925, 1988

239. Saboori AM, Smith BL, Agre P: Polymorphism in the Mr 32,000 Rh protein purified from Rh(D)-positive and -negative erythrocytes. Proc Natl Acad Sci USA 85:4042, 1988

240. Ridgwell K, Roberts SJ, Tanner MJ, Anstee DJ: Absence of two membrane proteins containing extracellular thiol groups in Rh$_{null}$ human erythrocytes. Biochem J 213:267, 1983

241. Gahmberg CG: Molecular characterization of the human red cell Rh$_o$(D) antigen. EMBO J 2:223, 1983

242. Green FA: Erythrocyte membrane sulfhydryl groups and Rh antigen activity. Immunochemistry 4:247, 1967

243. Ridgwell K, Eyers SA, Mawby WJ, Anstee DJ, Tanner MJ: Studies on the glycoprotein associated with Rh (rhesus) blood group antigen expression in the human red blood cell membrane. J Biol Chem 269: 6410, 1994

244. Green FA: Phospholipid requirement for Rh antigenic activity. J Biol Chem 243:5519, 1968

245. Ridgwell K, Tanner MJ, Anstee DJ: The Rhesus (D) polypeptide is linked to the human erythrocyte cytoskeleton. FEBS Lett 174:7, 1984

246. Gahmberg CG, Karhi KK: Association of Rho(D) polypeptides with the membrane skeleton in Rho(D)-positive human red cells. J Immunol 133:334, 1984

247. Cartron JP: Recent advances in the biochemistry of blood group Rh Antigens. p. 69. In Rouger P, Salmon C (eds): Monoclonal Antibodies Against Human Red Blood Cell and Related Antigens. Librairie Arnette, Paris, 1987

248. Krahmer M, Prohaska R: Characterization of human red cell Rh (rhesus-) specific polypeptides by limited proteolysis. FEBS Lett 226:105, 1987

249. Bloy C, Blanchard D, Dahr W et al: Determination of the N-terminal sequence of human red cell Rh(D) polypeptide and demonstration that the Rh(D), (c), and (E) antigens are carried by distinct polypeptide chains. Blood 72:661, 1988

250. Agre P: Clinical relevance of basic research on red cell membranes, review. Clin Res 40:176, 1992

251. Saboori AM, Denker BM, Agre P: Isolation of proteins related to the Rh polypeptides from nonhuman erythrocytes. J Clin Invest 83:187, 1989

252. Agre P, Saboori AM, Asimos A, Smith BL: Purification and partial characterization of the Mr 30,000 integral membrane protein associated with the erythrocyte Rh(D) antigen. J Biol Chem 262:17497, 1987

253. Blanchard D, Bloy C, Hermand P et al: Two-dimensional iodopeptide mapping demonstrates that erythrocyte Rh D, c, and E polypeptides are structurally homologous but nonidentical. Blood 72:1424, 1988

254. Hughes-Jones NC, Bloy C, Gorick B et al: Evidence that the c, D and E epitopes of the human Rh blood group system are on separate polypeptide molecules. Mol Immunol 25:931, 1988

255. Goossens D, Champomier F, Rouger P, Salmon C: Human monoclonal antibodies against blood group antigens. Preparation of a series of stable EBV immortalized B clones producing high levels of antibody of different isotypes and specificities. J Immunol Methods 101:193, 1987

256. Avent ND, Ridgwell K, Mawby WJ et al: Protein-sequence studies on Rh-related polypeptides suggest the presence of at least two groups of proteins which associate in the human red-cell membrane. Biochem J 256:1043, 1988

257. Agre P, Smith BL, Hartel-Schenk S: Biochemistry of the erythrocyte Rh polypeptides: a review. Yale J Biol Med 63:461, 1990

258. Gahmberg CG: Biochemistry of rhesus (Rh) blood group antigens, review. J Immunogenet 17:227, 1990

259. Bloy C, Hermand P, Blanchard D et al: Surface orientation and antigen properties of Rh and LW polypeptides of the human erythrocyte membrane. J Biol Chem 265:21482, 1990

260. Zachowski A, Favre E, Cribier S et al: Outside-inside translocation of aminophospholipids in the human erythrocyte membrane is mediated by a specific enzyme. Biochemistry 25:2585, 1986 [erratum: 25:7788, 1986]

261. Schroit AJ, Bloy C, Connor J, Cartron JP: Involvement of Rh blood group polypeptides in the maintenance of aminophospholipid asymmetry. Biochemistry 29:10303, 1990

262. Smith RE, Daleke DL: Phosphatidylserine transport in Rh$_{null}$ erythrocytes. Blood 76:1021, 1990

263. Moore S, Green C: The identification of specific Rhesus - polypeptide - blood - group - ABH - active -glyco-

protein complexes in the human red-cell membrane. Biochem J 244:735, 1987

264. Ruddle F, Ricciuti F, McMorris FA et al: Somatic cell genetic assignment of peptidase C and the Rh linkage group to chromosome A-1 in man. Science 176:1429, 1972

265. Marsh WL, Chaganti RS, Gardner FH et al: Mapping human autosomes: evidence supporting assignment of rhesus to the short arm of chromosome No. 1. Science 183:966, 1974

266. Cherif-Zahar B, Mattei MG, Le Van Kim C et al: Localization of the human Rh blood group gene structure to chromosome region 1p34.3-1p36.1 by in situ hybridization. Human Genet 86:398, 1991

267. Avent ND, Butcher SK, Liu W et al: Localization of the C termini of the Rh (rhesus) polypeptides to the cytoplasmic face of the human erythrocyte membrane. J Biol Chem 267:15134, 1992

268. Cartron JP, Agre P: Rh blood group antigens: protein and gene structure. Semin Hematol 30:193, 1993

269. Colin Y, Cherif-Zahar B, Le Van Kim C et al: Recent advances in molecular and genetic analysis of Rh blood group structures, review. J Med Primatol 22:36, 1993

270. Colin Y, Bailly P, Cartron JP: Molecular genetic basis of Rh and LW blood groups. Vox Sang 67(Suppl 3):67, 1994

271. Cherif-Zahar B, Le Van Kim C, Rouillac C et al: Organization of the gene (RHCE) encoding the human blood group RhCcEe antigens and characterization of the promoter region. Genomics 19:68, 1994

272. Mouro I, Colin Y, Cherif-Zahar B et al: Molecular genetic basis of the human rhesus blood group system. Nature Genet 5:62, 1993

273. Sistonen P: Linkage of the LW blood group locus with the complement C3 and Lutheran blood group loci. Ann Hum Genet 48:239, 1984

274. Povey S, Morton NE, Sherman SL: Report of the Committee on the Genetic Constitution of Chromosomes 1 and 2. Cytogenet Cell Genet 40:67, 1985

275. Levine P, Celano MJ, Wallace J, Sanger R: A human "D-like" antibody. Nature 198:596, 1963

276. Sistonen P, Nevanlinna HR, Virtaranta-Knowles K et al: Nea, new blood group antigen in Finland. Vox Sang 40:352, 1981

277. Sistonen P, Tippett P: A "new" allele giving further insight into the LW blood group system. Vox Sang 42:252, 1982

278. Giles CM, Lundsgaard A: A complex serological investigation involving LW. Vox Sang 13:406, 1967

279. Chown B, Kaita H, Lowen B, Lewis M: Transient pro-

duction of anti-LW by LW-positive people. Transfusion 11:220, 1971

280. Bloy C, Blanchard D, Hermand P et al: Properties of the blood group LW glycoprotein and preliminary comparison with Rh proteins. Mol Immunol 26:1013, 1989

281. Mallinson G, Martin PG, Anstee DJ et al: Identification and partial characterization of the human erythrocyte membrane component(s) that express the antigens of the LW blood-group system. Biochem J 234: 649, 1986

282. Bloy C, Hermand P, Cherif-Zahar B et al: Comparative analysis by two-dimensional iodopeptide mapping of the RhD protein and LW glycoprotein rearrangements of the blood group RhD gene associated with the DVI category phenotype. Blood 83:1129, 1994

283. Race, RR: Modern concepts of the blood group systems. Ann NY Acad Sci 127:844, 1965

284. Anstee DJ, Mallinson G: The biochemistry of blood group antigens—some recent advances, review. Vox Sang, suppl 3.67:1, 1994

285. Bailly P, Hermand P, Callebaut I et al: The LW blood group glycoprotein is homologous to intercellular adhesion molecules. Proc Natl Acad Sci USA 91:5306, 1994

286. Eicher C, Kirkley K, Porter M et al: A new low frequency antigen in the Kell system: K24 (Cls), abstracted. Transfusion 25:448, 1985

287. Marsh WL, Redman CM, Kessler LA et al: A low incidence antigen in the Kell blood group system identified by biochemical characterization. Transfusion 27: 36, 1987

288. Corcoran PA, Allen FH, Lewis M et al: A new antibody, anti-Ku (anti-Peltz) in the Kell blood-group system. Transfusion 1:181, 1961

289. Marsh WL: The Kell blood group. Adv Immunohematol 4 (2) 1976

290. Lee S, Zambas E, Marsh WL et al: Molecular cloning and primary structure of Kell blood group protein. Proc Natl Acad Sci USA 88:6353, 1991

291. Redman CM, Marsh WL: The Kell blood system and the McLeod phenotype. Semin Hematol 30:209, 1993

292. Marsh WL, Redman CM: The Kell blood group system. Transfusion 30(2):158, 1990

293. Daniels GL: Studies on Gerbich negative phenotypes and Gerbich antibodies, abstracted. Transfusion 22: 405, 1982

294. Merry AH, Thomson EE, Lagar J et al: Quantitation of antibody binding to erythrocytes in LISS. Vox Sang 47:125, 1984

295. Coombs RRA, Mourant AE, Race RR: In-vivo isosensitization of red cells in babies with haemolytic disease. Lancet 1:264, 1946

296. Kornstad L, Heisto J: The frequency of formation of Kell antibodies in recipients of Kell-positive blood, p. 754. In Proceedings of the Sixth Congress of the European Society of Haematology, Copenhagen, 1957

297. Hopkins DF: Saline agglutinating anti-K and anti-k in the apparent absence of IgM antibody. Br J Haematol 19:749, 1970

298. Mukumoto Y, Konishi H, Ito K et al: An example of naturally occurring anti-Kell (K1) in a Japanese male. Vox Sang 35:275, 1978

299. Marsh WL, Nichols ME, Oyen R et al: Naturally occurring anti-Kell stimulated by *E. coli* enterocolitis in a 20-day-old child. Transfusion 18:149, 1978

300. Sakuma K, Sazuki H, Ohto H et al: First case of hemolytic disease of the newborn due to anti-Ul[a] antibodies. Vox Sang 66:293, 1994

301. Marsh WL, Reid ME, Kuriyan M et al: A Handbook of Clinical and Laboratory Practices in the Transfusion of Red Blood cells. p. 106. Moneta Medical Press, VA, 1993

302. Marsh WL, Oyen R, Nichols ME, Alen FH Jr: Kx: a leukocyte and red cell antigen associated with the Kell system. Br J Haematol 29:247, 1975

303. Allen FH, Lewis SJ: Kp[a] (Penney), a new antigen in the Kell blood group system. Vox Sang 2:81, 1957

304. Ford DS, Knight AE, Smith F: A further example of Kp[a]/Ko exhibiting depression of some Kell group antigens. Vox Sang 32:220, 1977

305. Jaber A, Blanchard D, Goossens CB et al: Characterization of the blood group Kell (K1) antigen with a human monoclonal antibody. Blood 73:1597, 1989

306. Taswell HG, Pineda AA, Brzica SM: Chronic granulomatous disease: successful treatment of infection with granulocyte transfusions resulting in subsequent hemolytic transfusion reaction, abstract ed. Transfusion 16:535, 1976

307. West NC, Jenkins JA, Johnston BR et al: Interdonor incompatibility due to anti-Kell antibody undetectable by automated antibody screening. Vox Sang 50: 174, 1986

308. Marsh WL, Oyen R, Alicea E et al: Autoimmune hemolytic anemia and the Kell blood groups. Am J Hematol 7:155, 1979

309. Wimer BM, Marsh WL, Taswell HF, Galey WR: Hematological changes associated with the McLeod phenotype of the Kell blood group system. Br J Haematol 36:219, 1977

310. Marsh WL, Marsh NJ, Moore A et al: Elevated serum

creatine phosphokinase in subjects with McLeod syndrome. Vox Sang 40:403, 1981

311. Marsh WL: Deleted antigens of the Rhesus and Kell blood group systems: association with cell membrane defects. p. 165. In Garratty G (ed): Blood Group Antigens and Disease. American Association of Blood Banks, Arlington, VA, 1983

312. Chown B, Lewis M, Kaita H: The Duffy blood group in caucasians: evidence for a new allele. Am J Hum Genet 17:384, 1965

313. Lewis M, Kaita H, Chown B: The Duffy blood group system in caucasians: a further population sample. Vox Sang 23:523, 1972

314. Albrey JA, Vincent EER, Hutchinson J et al: A new antibody, anti-Fy3, in the Duffy blood group system. Vox Sang 20:29, 1971

315. Behzad O, Lee CL, Gavin J, Marsh WL: A new anti-erythrocyte antibody in the Duffy system: anti-Fy4. Vox Sang 24:337, 1973

316. Colledge KI, Pezzulich M, Marsh WL: Anti-Fy5: an antibody disclosing a probable association between the Rhesus and Duffy blood group genes. Vox Sang 24:193, 1973

317. Nichols ME, Rubinstein P, Barnwell J, et al: A new human Duffy blood group specificity defined by a murine monoclonal antibody. J Exp Med 166:776, 1987

318. Cutbush M, Mollison PL, Parkin DM: A new human blood group. Nature 165:188, 1950

319. Ikin EW, Mourant AE, Pettenkoffer JH et al: Discovery of the expected haemagglutinin anti-Fy^b. Nature 168:1077, 1951

320. Donahue RP, Bias WB, Renwick JH: Probable assignment of the Duffy blood group locus to chromosome 1 in man. Proc Natl Acad Sci USA 61:949, 1968

321. Sanger R, Tippett P, Gavin J, Race RR: Failure to demonstrate linkage between the loci for the Rh and Duffy blood groups. Ann Hum Genet 36:353, 1973

322. Hadley TJ, David PH, McGinniss MH, Miller LH: Identification of an erythrocyte component carrying the Duffy blood group Fy^a antigen. Science 223:597, 1984

323. Miller LH, Mason SJ, Dvorak JA et al: Erythrocyte receptors for *Plasmodium knowlesi* malaria: Duffy blood group determinants. Science 189:561, 1975

324. Miller LH, Aikawa M, Johnson JG et al: Interaction between cytochalasin B-treated malarial parasites and erythrocytes: attachment and junction formation. J Exp Med 149:172, 1979

325. Hadley TJ, McGinniss MH, Klotz FW et al: Blood group antigens and invasion of erythrocytes by malaria parasites. p. 17. In Garratty G (ed): Red Cell Antigens and Antibodies. American Association of Blood Banks, Arlington, VA, 1986

326. Marsh WL, Oyen R, Nichols ME: Kidd blood-group antigens of leukocytes and platelets. Transfusion 14:378, 1974

327. Gaidulis L, Branch DR, Lazar GS et al: The red cell antigens A, B, D, U, Ge, Jk3, and Yt^a are not detected on human granulocytes. Br J Haematol 60:659, 1985

328. Allen FH Jr, Diamond LK, Niedziela B: A new blood group antigen. Nature 167:482, 1951

329. Plaut G, Ikin EW, Mourant EA et al: A new blood group antibody, anti-Jk^b. Nature 171:431, 1953

330. Pinkerton FJ, Mermod LE, Liles BA et al: The phenotype Jk(a−b−) in the Kidd blood group system. Vox Sang 4:155, 1959

331. Polley MJ, Mollison PL, Soothill JF: The role of 19S gammaglobulin blood group antibodies in the antiglobulin reaction. Br J Haematol 8:149, 1962

332. Arcara PC, O'Conner MA, Dimmette RM: A family with three Jk(a−b−) members, abstracted. Transfusion 9:282, 1969

333. Okubo Y, Yamaguchi H, Nagao N et al: Heterogeneity of the phenotype Jk(a−b−) found in Japanese. Transfusion 26:237, 1986

334. Henry S, Woodfield G: Frequencies of the Jk(a−b−) phenotype in Polynesian ethnic groups. Transfusion 35:277, 1995

335. Mohr J, Eiberg H: Colton blood groups: indication of linkage with the Kidd (Jk) system as support for assignment to chromosome 7. Clin Genet 11:372, 1977

336. McBride OW, Swan D, Leder P et al: Chromosomal locations of human immunoglobulin light chain constant region genes, abstracted. Birth Defects 18:297, 1982

337. Geitvik GA, Hoyheim B, Gedde-Dahl T et al: The Kidd (Jk) blood group locus assigned to chromosome 18 by close linkage to a DNA-RFLP. Hum Genet 77:205, 1987

338. Sinor LT, Eastwood KL, Rachel JM, et al: Dot-Blot purification of the Kidd blood group antigen, abstracted. Transfusion 26:561, 1986

339. Heaton DC, McLoughlin K: Jk(a−b−) red blood cells resist urea lysis. Transfusion 22:70, 1982

340. Edwards-Moulds J, Kasschau M: A mechanism by which Jk(a−b−) red cells resist lysis in 2M urea, abstracted. Transfusion 26:561, 1986

341. Reid ME: Associations of RBC membrane abnormalities with blood group phenotype. p. 257. In Garratty G (ed): Immunobiology of Transfusion Medicine. Marcel Dekker, New York, 1994

342. Hoffman M, Berger MB, Menitove JE: Autoimmune

hemolytic anemia due to auto anti-Jkᵃ. J Lab Clin Med 13:674, 1982

343. Issitt PD, Pavone BG, Frohlich JA et al: Absence of auto anti-Jk3 as a component of anti-dl. Transfusion 20:733, 1980

344. Patten E, Beck CE, Scholl C et al: Autoimmune hemolytic anemia with anti-Jkᵃ specificity in a patient taking aldomet. Transfusion 17:517, 1977

345. Sosler SD, Behzad O, Garratty G et al: Acute hemolytic anemia due to a chlorpropamide-dependent auto anti-Jkᵃ, abstracted. Transfusion 19:641, 1979

346. Ellisor SS, Reid ME, O'Day T et al: Autoantibodies mimicking anti-Jkᵇ plus anti-Jk3 associated with autoimmune hemolytic anemia in a primipara who delivered an unaffected infant. Vox Sang 45:53, 1983

347. McGinniss MH, MacLowry JD, Holland PV: Acquisition of Kell-like antigen by Kell-negative cells, abstracted. Transfusion 18:624, 1978

348. McGinnis MH, Leiberman R, Holland PV: The Jkᵇ red cell antigen and gram-negative organisms, abstracted. Transfusion 19:663, 1979

349. Marsh WL, Johnson CL, Mueller KA: Proposed new notation for the In(Lu) modifying gene. Transfusion 24:371, 1984

350. Levene C, Gekker K, Poole J et al: Lu20, a new high incidence "para"-Lu antigen in the Lutheran blood group system, abstracted. Rev Paul Med, suppl 1 H. 110:13, 1992

351. Crawford MN, Greenwalt TJ, Sasaki T et al: The phenotype Lu(a−b−) together with unconventional Kidd groups in one family. Transfusion 1:228, 1961

352. Crawford MN, Tippett P, Sanger R: The antigens Auᵃ, i, and P, of cells of the dominant type of Lu(a−b−). Vox Sang 26:283, 1974

353. Marsh WL, Brown PJ, DiNapoli J et al: Anti-Wj: an autoantibody that defines a high-incidence antigen modified by the In(Lu) gene. Transfusion 23:128, 1983

354. Daniels GL, Shaw MA, Lomas CG et al: The effect of In(Lu) on some high-frequency antigens. Transfusion 26:171, 1986

355. Damborough J, Firth R, Giles M et al: A "new" antibody anti-Luᵃ Luᵇ and two further examples of the genotype Lu(a−b−). Nature 198:796, 1963

356. Normal PC, Tippett P, Beal RW: An Lu(a−b−) phenotype caused by an X-linked recession gene. Vox Sang 51:49, 1986

357. Race RR, Paykoc ZV: Hypersensitivity to transfused blood. BMJ 2:83, 1945

358. Cutbush M, Chanarin I: The expected blood-group antibody, anti-Luᵇ. Nature 178:855, 1956

359. Daniels GL, Le Pennee PY, Rouger P: The red cell

antigens Auᵃ and Auᵇ belong to the Lutheran system. Vox Sang 60:191, 1991

360. Mohr J: A search for linkage between the Lutheran blood group and other hereditary characters. Acta Pathol Microbiol Scand 28:207, 1951

361. Eiberg H, Mohr J, Staub-Nielsen L et al: Linkage relationship between the locus for C3 and 50 polymorphic systems: assignment of C3 to DME-SELU linkage group: confirmation of C3-LES linkage: support of LES-DM synteny, abstracted. In Batsheva, BT (ed): Sixth International Congress of Human Genetics. Alan R Liss, New York, 1987

362. Marsh WL: Recent developments relating to the Duffy and the Lutheran blood groups. p. 108. In Walker RH (ed): A Seminar on Recent Advances in Immunohematology. American Association of Blood Banks, Washington, DC, 1973

363. Parsons SF, Mallinson G, Judson PA et al: Evidence that the Luᵇ blood group antigen is located on red cell membrane glycoproteins of 85 and 78 kd. Transfusion 27:61, 1987

364. Daniels G, Khalid G: Identification by immunoblotting of the structures carrying Lutheran and Para-Lutheran blood group antigens. Vox Sang 57:137, 1989

365. Francis BJ, Hatcher DE: Hemolytic disease of the newborn apparently caused by anti-Luᵃ. Transfusion 1:248, 1961

366. Scheffer H, Tamaki HT: Anti-Luᵇ and mild hemolytic disease of the newborn. Transfusion 6:497, 1966

367. Greendyke RM, Chorpenning FW: Normal survival of incompatible red cells in the presence of anti-Luᵃ. Transfusion 2:52, 1962

368. Greenwalt TJ, Sasaki TT, Steane EA: The Lutheran blood groups: a progress report with observations on the development of the antigens and characteristics of the antibodies. Transfusion 7:189, 1967

369. Molthan L, Crawford MC: Three examples of anti-Luᵇ and related data. Transfusion 6:584, 1966

370. Issitt PD, Valinsky J, Marsh WL et al: In vivo destruction of antigen-positive red cells by anti-Lu6, abstracted. Transfusion 27:548, 1987

371. Mann JD, Cahan A, Gelb AG et al: A sex-linked blood group. Lancet 1:8, 1962

372. Cook IA, Polley MJ, Mollison PL: A second example of anti-Xgᵃ. Lancet 1:857, 1963

373. Sausais L, Krevans JR, Townes AS: Characteristics of a third example of anti-Xgᵃ, abstracted. Transfusion 4:312, 1964

374. Yokoyama M, McCoy JE Jr: Further studies on auto anti-Xgᵃ antibody. Vox Sang 13:15, 1967

375. Spring FA, Bruce LJ, Anstee DJ et al: A red cell band

3 variant with latered stibene disulphonate binding is associated with the Diego (Di^a) blood group antigen. Biochem J 288:713, 1992

376. Levine P, Robinson EA, Layrisse M et al: The Diego blood factor. Nature 77:40, 1956

377. Thompson PR, Childers DM, Hatcher DE: Anti-Di^b first and second examples. Vox Sang 13:314, 1967

378. Zafar M, Reid ME: Review: the Diego blood group system. Immunohematology 9:35, 1993

379. Steffey N: Investigation of a probable non-red cell stimulated anti-Di^a. Red Cell Free Press 8:24, 1983

380. Zelinski T, White L, Coghlan G et al: Assignment of the Yt blood group locus to chromosome 7q. Genomics 11:165, 1991

381. Telen MJ, Rosse WF, Parker CJ et al: Evidence that several high-frequency human blood group antigens reside on phosphatidylinositol-linked erythrocyte membrane proteins. Blood 75:1404, 1990

382. Eaton BR, Morton JA, Pickles MM, et al: A new antibody, anti-Yt^a characterizing a blood group of high incidence. Br J Haematol 2:333, 1956

383. Giles CM, Metaxas MN: Identification of the predicted blood group antibody anti-Yt^b. Nature 202:1122, 1964

384. Ballas SK, Sherwood WC: Rapid in vivo destruction of Yt(a+) erythrocytes in a recipient with anti-Yt^a. Transfusion 17:65, 1977

385. Mazzi G, Raineri A, Santarossa L et al: Presence of anti-Yt^a antibody in a Yt(a+) patient. Vox Sang 66:130, 1994

386. Mohandas K, Spivack M, Delehanty CL: Management of patients with anti-Cartwright (Yt^a). Transfusion 25:381, 1985

387. Levy GJ, Selset G, McQuisten D et al: Clinical significance of anti-Yt^b. Transfusion 28:265, 1988

388. Lewis M, Chown B, Kaita H: On the blood group antigens Bu(a) and Sm. Transfusion 7:92, 1967

389. Nason SG, Vengelen-Tyler V, Cohen N et al: A high incidence antibody (anti-Sc3) in the serum of a Sc:-1, -2 patient. Transfusion 20:531, 1980

390. Schmidt RP, Griffitts JJ, Northman FF: A new antibody, anti-Sm, reacting with a high incidence antigen. Transfusion 2:38, 1962

391. Anderson C, Hunter J, Zipursky A et al: An antibody defining a new blood group antigen, Bu^a. Transfusion 3:30, 1963

392. DeMarco M, Uni L, Fields D et al: HDN due to the Scianna antibody, anti-Sc2. Transfusion 35:58, 1995

393. Tregellas WM, Holub MP, Moulds JJ et al: An example of autoanti-Scl demonstrable in serum but not in plasma, abstracted. Transfusion 19:650, 1979

394. Anstee DJ, Ridgwell K, Tanner MJA et al: Individuals lacking the Gerbich blood group antigen have alterations in the human erythrocyte membrane sialoglycoproteins β and γ. Biochem J 221:97, 1984

395. Mattei MG, Colin Y, Le Van Kim C et al: Localization of the gene for human erythrocyte glycophorin C to chromosome 2.q14-21. Hum Genet 74:420, 1986

396. Reid ME: The Gerbich blood group antigens: a review. Med Lab Sci 43:177, 1986

397. Unger PJ: The Gerbich blood groups: distribution, serology, and genetics. p. 59. In Unger P, Laird-Fryer B (eds): Blood Group Systems: MN and Gerbich. American Association of Blood Banks, Arlington, VA, 1989

398. Issitt P: Null red blood cell phenotypes: Associated biological changes. Transfus Med Rev 7:139, 1993

399. Rosenfield RE, Haber GV, Kissmeyer-Nielson JA et al: Ge, a very common red-cell antigen. Br J Haematol 6:344, 1960

400. Vengelen-Tyler V, Morel PA: Serologic and IgG subclass characteristics of Cartwright (Yt) and Gerbich (Ge) antibodies. Transfusion 23:114, 1983

401. High S, Tanner MJA, Macdonald EB et al: Rearrangements of the red cell membrane glycophorin C (sialoglycoprotein (beta)) gene: a further study of alterations in the glycophorin C gene. Biochem J 262:47, 1989

402. Pasvol G, Anstee DJ, Tanner MJA: Glycophorin C and the invasion of red cells by *Plasmodium falciparum*. Lancet 1:907, 1984

403. Reid ME, Martynewycz MA, Wolford FE et al: Leach type Ge- red cells and elliptocytosis, letter. Transfusion 27:213, 1987

404. Pearson HA, Richards VL, Wylie BR et al: Assessment of clinical significance of anti-Ge in an untransfused man. Transfusion 31:257, 1991

405. Nance SJ, Arndt P, Garratty G: Predicting the significance of red cell alloantibodies using a monocyte monolayer assay. Transfusion 27:449, 1987

406. Shulman IA, Thompson JC, Nelson JM et al: Autoanti-Gerbich causing severe autoimmune hemolytic anemia, abstracted. Transfusion 25:447, 1985

407. Reynolds MV, Vengelen-Tyler V, Morel PA: Autoimmune haemolytic anaemia associated with auto anti-Ge. Vox Sang 41:61, 1981

408. Beattie KM, Sigmund KE: A Ge-like autoantibody in the serum of a patient receiving gold therapy for rheumatoid arthritis. Transfusion 27:54, 1987

409. Swanson J, Polesky HF, Tippett P et al: A "new" blood group antigen, Do^a. Nature 206:313, 1965

410. Molthan L, Crawford MN, Tippett P: Enlargement of the Dombrock blood group system: the finding of anti-Do^b. Vox Sang 24:382, 1973

411. Moulds JJ, Polesky HF, Reid M et al: Observations on the Gy^a and Hy antigens and the antibodies that define them. Transfusion 15:270, 1975

412. Schmidt RP, Frank S, Baugh M: New antibodies to high incidence antigenic determinants (anti-So, anti-El, anti-Hy and anti-Dp), abstracted. Transfusion 7: 386, 1967

413. Spring FA: Evidence that the high incidence antigen Jo^a is carried on the glycoprotein that expresses the Gy^a and Hy antigens, abstracted. Transfus Med suppl 2. 1:59, 1991

414. Telen, Marilyn J: Red cell antigens. p. 218. In Anderson KC, Ness PM (eds): Scientific Basis of Transfusion Medicine. WB Saunders, Philadelphia, 1994

415. Beattie KM, Castillo S: A case report of a hemolytic transfusion reaction caused by anti-Holley. Transfusion 15:476, 1975

416. Hsu TCS, Jagathambol K, Sabo BH et al: Anti-Holley (Hy): characterization of another example. Transfusion 15:605, 1975

417. Lewis M, Anstee DJ, Bird GWG et al: ISBT working party on terminology for red cell surface antigens: Los Angeles report. Vox Sang 61:158, 1991

418. Daniels G: Cromer-related antigens-blood group determinants on decay-accelerating factor. Vox Sang 56:205, 1989

419. Story J: Serology and genetics of the Cromer blood group system. p. 31. In Moulds JM, Laird-Fryer B (eds): Blood Groups Chido/Rodgers, Knops/McCoy/York and Cromer. American Association of Blood Banks, Bethesda, 1992

420. Stroup M, McCreary J: Cr^a, another high frequency blood group factor, abstracted. Transfusion 15:522, 1975

421. Moulds JM, Nickells MW, Moulds JJ et al: The C3b/C4b receptor is recognized by the Knops, McCoy, Swain-Langley and York blood group sera. J Exp Med 173:1159, 1991

422. Molthan L, Moulds JJ: A new antigen, McC^a (McCoy), and its relationship to Kn^a (Knops). Transfusion 18: 566, 1978

423. Mallan MT, Grimm W, Hindley L et al: The Hall serum: detecting Kn^b, the antithetical allele to Kn^a, abstracted. Transfusion 20:630, 1980

424. Molthan L: The status of the McCoy/Knops antigens. Med Lab Sci 40:59, 1983

425. Lacey P, Laird-Fryer B, Block U et al: A new high incidence blood group factor, Sl^a and its hypothetical allele. Abstract. Transfusion 20:632, 1980

426. Molthan L, Giles CM: A new antigen Yk^a (York), and its relationship to Cs^a (Cost). Vox Sang 29:145, 1975

427. Helgeson M, Swanson J, Polesky H: Knops-Helgeson (Kn^a), a high-frequency erythrocyte antigen. Transfusion 10:137, 1970

428. Molthan L: Biological significance of the York, Cost, McCoy, and Knops alloantibodies. Rev Fr Transfus Immunohematol 25:127, 1982

429. Gandhi JG, Moulds JJ, Szymanski ID: Shortened long-term survival of incompatible red cells in a patients with anti-McCoy-like antibody. Transfusion 24: 16, 1984

430. Heisto H, van der Hart M, Madsen G et al: Three examples of a new red cell antibody, anti-Co^a. Vox Sang 12:18, 1967

431. Giles CM, Damborough J, Aspinall P et al: Identification of the first example of anti-Co^b. Br J Haematol 19:267, 1970

432. Rogers MJ, Stiles PA, Wright J: A new minus-minus phenotype: Three Co(a$-$b$-$) individuals in one family, abstracted. Transfusion 14:508, 1974

433. Lacey PA, Robinson ML, Collins DG et al: Studies of the blood of a Co(a$-$b$-$) proposita and her family. Transfusion 27:268, 1987

434. Kurtz SR, Kuszaj T, Ouellet R et al: Survival of homozygous Co^a (Colton) red cells in a patient with anti-Co^a. Vox Sang 43:28, 1982

435. Kitzke HM, Julius H, Delaney M et al: Anti-Co^a implicated in delayed hemolytic transfusion reaction, abstracted. Transfusion 22:407, 1982

436. Lee EL, Bennett CC: Anti-Co^b causing acute hemolytic transfusion reaction. Transfusion 22:159, 1982

437. Squires JE, Larison PJ, Charles WT, Milner PF: A delayed hemolytic transfusion due to anti-Co^b. Transfusion 25:137, 1985

438. Dzik WH, Blank J: Accelerated destruction of radiolabeled red cells due to anti-Colton b. Transfusion 26: 246, 1986

439. Simpson WKH: Anti-Co^a and severe haemolytic disease of the newborn. S Afr Med J 47:1302, 1973

440. O'Neill GJ, Yang SY, Tegoli J et al: Chido and Rodgers blood groups are distinct antigenic components of human complement C4. Nature 273:668, 1978

441. Giles CM: Antigenic determinants of human C4, Rodgers and Chido. Exp Clin Immunogenet 5:99, 1988

442. Giles CM: "Partial inhibition of anti-Rg and anti-Ch reagents. II. Demonstration of separable antibodies for different determinants. Vox Sang 48:167, 1985

443. Swanson JL: Serology and Genetics of Chido/Rodgers and Knops/McCoy/York blood groups. p. 1. In Moulds J, Laird-Fryer B (eds): Blood Groups: Ch/Rg, Kn/McC/Yk, Cromer. American Association of Blood Banks, Bethesda, 1992

444. Harris JP, Tegoli J, Swanson J et al: A nebulous anti-

body responsible for crossmatching difficulties (Chido). Vox Sang 12:140, 1967

445. Longster G, Giles CM: A new antibody specificity, anti-Rg^a reacting with a red cell and serum antigen. Vox Sang 30:175, 1976

446. Middleton J, Crookston MC, Falk JA et al: Linkage of Chido and HL-A. Tissue Antigens 4:366, 1974

447. Giles CM, Gedde-Dahl T Jr, Robson EB et al: Rg^a (Rodgers) and the HLA region: linkage and associations. Tissue Antigens 8:143, 1976

448. Ballow M, McLean RH, Einarson M et al: Hereditary C4 deficiency. Genetic studies and linkage to HLA. Transplant Proc 11:1710, 1979

449. Moulds JM: Incidence of Rodgers-negative individuals in sle patients. Immunology 6:92, 1990

450. Westoff CM, Sipherd BD, Wylie DE et al: Severe anaphylactic reactions following transfusions of platelets to a patient with anti-Ch. Transfusion Vol 32:576, 1992

451. Tilley CA, Romans DG, Crookston MC: Localisation of Chido and Rodgers determinants to the C4d fragment of human C4. Nature 276:713, 1978

452. Molthan L, Paradis DJ: Anti-Cs^b: the finding of the antibody antithetical to anti-Cs^a. Med Lab Sci 44:94, 1987

453. Giles CM, Huth MC, Wilson TE et al: Three examples of a new antibody, anti-Cs^a which reacts with 98% of red cell samples. Vox Sang 10:405, 1965

454. Tilley CA, Crookston MC, Haddad SA et al: Red blood cell survival studies in patients with anti-Ch^a, anti-Yk^a, anti-Ge and anti-Vel. Transfusion 17:169, 1977

455. Shore CM, Steane EA: Survival of incompatible red cells in a patient with anti-Cs^a and three other patients with antibodies to high-frequency red cell antigens, abstracted. Transfusion 18:387, 1978

456. Pineda AA, Dharkar DD, Wahner HW: Clinical evaluation of a Cr-labeled red blood cell survival test for in vivo blood compatibility testing. Mayo Clin Proc 59:25, 1984

457. Wren MR, Issitt PD: Evidence that Wr^a and Wr^b are antithetical. Transfusion 28:113, 1988

458. Wren MR, Issitt PD, Dahr W: Additional data on the relationship of Wr^b to Wr^a antigen measurement using enzyme-linked antiglobulin tests and further data on the structure of Wr^b, abstracted. Transfusion 24:425, 1984

459. Holman CA: A new rare human blood group antigen (Wr^a). Lancet 2:119, 1953

460. Lubenko A, Contreras M: The incidence of HDN attributable to anti-Wr^a, letter. Transfusion 32:87, 1992

461. Cleghorn TE: The occurrence of certain rare blood group factors in Britain. Thesis. University of Sheffield, Sheffield, UK, 1961

462. Adams J, Broviac M, Brooks W et al: An antibody in the serum of a Wr(a+) individual, reacting with an antigen of very high frequency. Transfusion 11:290, 1971

463. Drozda E: Anti-Wr^a and mild hemolytic disease of the newborn, letter. Transfusion 31:783, 1991

464. Metaxas MN, Metaxas-Buhler M: Studies on the Wright blood group system. Vox Sang 8:707, 1963

465. van Loghem JJ, van der Hart M, Land ME: Polyagglutinability of red cells as a cause of severe haemolytic transfusion reaction. Vox Sang 5:125, 1955b

466. Dankbar DT, Pierce SR, Issitt PD et al: Fatal intravascular hemolysis associated with auto anti-Wr^b, abstracted. Transfusion 27:534, 1987

467. Hermanti P, Enders B, Neunzige G et al: Wr(a+ b−) red blood cells are fully susceptible to invasion by *Plasmodium falciparum*. Lancet, 2:466, 1984

468. Badakere SS, Joshi SR, Bhatia HM et al: Evidence for a new blood group antigen in the Indian population (a preliminary report). Ind J Med Res 61:563, 1973

469. Giles CM: Antithetical relationship of anti-In^a with the Salis antibody. Vox Sang 29:73, 1975

470. Spring FA: Characterization of blood-group-active erythrocyte membrane glycoproteins with human antisera. Transfus Med 3:167, 1993

471. Joshi SF, Gupta D, Choudhuy KK et al: Transfusion-induced anti-In^a following a single unit transfusion. Transfusion Vol 33:444, 1993

472. Morton JA, Pickles MM, Sutton L: The correlation of the Bg^a blood group with the HL-A7 leukocyte group: demonstration of antigenic sites on red cells and leucocytes. Vox Sang 17:536, 1969

473. Morton JA, Pickles MM, Sutton L et al: Identification of further antigens on red cell and lymphocytes. Vox Sang 21:144, 1971

474. Seaman MJ, Benson R, Jones MN et al: The reactions of the Bennett-Goodspeed group of antibodies with 380. the auto analyser. Br J Haematol 13:464, 1967

475. Giles CM: Human leukocyte antigens (HLA) class I (Bg) on red cells studied with monoclonal antibodies. Immunology 6:3, 1990

476. Pavone BG, Issitt PD: Anti-Bg antibodies in sera used for red cell typing. Br J Haematol 27:607, 1974

477. van der Hart M, Szaloky A, van der Berg-Loonen EM et al: Presence d'antigenes HL-A sur les hematis d'un donneur normal. Nouv Rev Fr Hematol 14:555, 1974

478. Molthan L: Transfusion reaction presumably due to anti-Bg^a, letter. Transfusion 19:609, 1979

479. Morton JA, Pickles MM, Darley JH: Increase in

strength of red cell Bg^a antigen following infectious mononucleosis. Vox Sang 32:26, 1977

480. Morton JA, Pickles MM, Turner JE et al: Changes in red cell Bg antigens in haematological disease. Immunol Commun 9:173, 1980

481. Frist S, Wenz B: Eluate analysis of anti-Bg^a associated renal allograft rejection. Transfusion 1976:16, 261

482. Spitalnik S, Cox MT, Spennacchio J et al: The serology of Sd^a effects of transfusion and pregnancy. Vox Sang 42:308, 1982

483. Bass LS, Rao H, Goldstein J, Marsh WL: The Sd^x antigen and antibody: biochemical studies on the inhibitory property of human urine. Vox Sang 44:191, 1983

484. Sanger R, Gavin J, Tippett P et al: Plant agglutinin for another human blood group. Lancet 1:1130, 1971

485. Gerbal A, Lopez M, Moslet C et al: Polyagglutinability associated with the CAD antigen. Haematologia 10:383, 1976b

486. Macvie SJ, Morton JA, Pickles MM: The reactions and inheritance of a new blood group antigen, Sd^a. Vox Sang 13:485, 1967

487. Renton PH, Howell P, Ikin EW et al: Anti-Sd^a, a new blood group antibody. Vox Sang 13:493, 1967

488. Morton JA, Pickles MM, Terry AM: The Sd^a blood group antigen in tissues and body fluids. Vox Sang 19:472, 1970

489. Soh CPC, Morgan WTJ, Watkins WM et al: The relationship between the N-acetylgalactosamine content and the blood group Sd^a activity of Tamm and Horsfall urinary glycoprotein. Biochem Biophys Res Commun 93:1132, 1980

490. Blanchard D, Cartron JP, Fournet B et al: Primary structure of the oligosaccharide determinant of blood group CAD specificity. J Biol Chem 258:7691, 1983

491. Petermans ME, Cole-Dergent J: Haemolytic transfusion reaction due to anti-Sd^a. Vox Sang 18:67, 1970

492. Cartron JP, Prou O, Luilier M, Soulier JP: Susceptibility to invasion by *Plasmodium falciparum* of some human erythrocytes carrying rare blood group antigens. Br J Haematol 55:639, 1983

493. Bobolis KA, Moulds JJ, Telen MJ: Isolation of the JMH antigen on a novel phosphatidylinositol-linked human membrane protein. Blood 79:1574, 1992

494. Sabo B, Moulds JJ, McCreary J: Anti-JMH: Another high-titer, low avidity against a high frequency antigen, abstracted. Transfusion 18:387, 1978

495. Cedergren B: Rare blood in northern Sweden. p. 11. In The Book of Abstracts of the Thirteenth Congress of the International Society of Blood Transfusion. American Association of Blood Banks, Washington, DC, 1972

496. Race RR, Sanger R: Some very frequent antigens. p. 415. In Race RR, Sanger R (eds): Blood Groups in Man. 6th Ed. JB Lippincott, Philadelphia, 1975

497. Sussman LN, Miller EB: Un nouveau facteur sanguin "Vel." Rev Haematol 7:368, 1952

498. Issitt P: Some high incidence antigens that may represent independent blood group systems. p. 397. In Issitt P (ed): Applied Blood Group Serology. 3rd Ed. Montgomery Scientific Publications, Miami, FL, 1985

499. Levine P, White JA, Stroup M: Seven Ve^a (Vel) negative members in three generations of a family. Transfusion 1:111, 1961

500. Williams CK, Villiams B, Pearson J et al: An example of anti-Vel causing mild hemolytic disease of the newborn, abstracted. Transfusion 25:462, 1985

501. Becton DL, Kinney TR: An infant girl with severe autoimmune hemolytic anemia: apparent anti-Vel specificity. Vox Sang 51:108, 1986

Chapter 6

The HLA System

J. Michael Cecka

HLA antigens are a central component of the immune system. These integral membrane glycoproteins play key roles in antigen processing and in coordinating interactions between lymphocytes and macrophages, dendritic cells, other lymphocytes, and cells targeted for immune destruction. The fact that T lymphocytes recognize and respond to foreign antigens in the context of HLA molecules may also explain why even slight differences in allogeneic HLA antigens are the major barriers to transplantation of tissues and organs from one individual to another.

Early observations that sparked interest in the study of what later became HLA were made by blood bankers. Jean Dausset,[1] then Director of Laboratories at the National Blood Transfusion Center in Paris, first reported an interesting antiserum from a multiply transfused patient who was leukopenic. The serum agglutinated leukocytes from some but not all randomly selected donors. He termed the first HLA antigen "MAC." Later it was renamed HLA-2, and, as the complexity of HLA began to unfold, HLA-A2. Jon van Rood, who was then in charge of the University Hospital Blood Bank in Leiden, identified similar leukocyte-agglutinating antibodies in the serum of a multiparous woman who had a nonhemolytic transfusion reaction. He and his colleagues developed a computer system to analyze reaction patterns of leukocyte-agglutinating antibodies that

developed after transfusions or pregnancies and later identified the first allelic pair, 4a and 4b.[2] These alleles are now recognized as two strong public antigens of the HLA-B locus, Bw4 and Bw6.

From these early observations, HLA has come to be recognized as the most polymorphic genetic system in humans, including more than 100 alleles that can combine in more than 5 million ways. The HLA antigens play an important role in transplantation and may also be important in the success of reproduction, some disease processes, autoimmunity, and tolerance.

HLA is now commonly identified as an acronym for human leukocyte antigen. In fact, HLA was a compromise among members of the first Nomenclature Committee in 1967 who were considering "Hu1," as Dausset and his colleagues had begun naming antigens, and "LA," where L stood for leukocyte and A for the first locus. The rich and often entertaining history of the development of HLA during the fledgling years of the 1960s and 1970s has been recounted in the words of those who pioneered the field in *History of HLA: Ten Recollections.*[3]

The HLA system plays an increasingly important role in transfusion medicine in such areas as transplantation, the requirement of HLA-matched platelets for alloimmunized patients, and the recognition of the significance of the HLA system in transfusion-associated graft-versus-host disease (GVHD) (see Ch.

42). HLA antigenic differences, the antibodies that may be produced against them, and the cellular immune responses that may develop can have a profound effect in individual patients, beyond the febrile, nonhemolytic transfusion reactions that first interested those who studied the leukocyte-agglutinating antibodies.

THE HLA ANTIGEN MOLECULES

There are two classes of HLA molecules that differ in their tissue distribution, structure, and function. The best studied class I molecules are designated HLA-A, -B, and -C. These are transmembrane glycoproteins that consist of a heavy chain of a little more than 300 amino acids (45,000 D in molecular weight), noncovalently associated with a 12,000-D light chain (β_2-microglobulin). The heavy chain has three extracellular "domains" of approximately equal size, a transmembrane portion, and a cytoplasmic piece (Fig. 6-1). The class II molecules include HLA-DR, -DQ, and -DP, which differ from class I molecules in that they consist of two noncovalently associated polypeptide chains, designated α (35,000 D) and β (29,000 D). Both chains span the cell membrane and have two extracellular domains. Both chains have carbohydrate moieties.

TISSUE DISTRIBUTION AND EXPRESSION

The class I HLA-A and -B antigens are expressed on all nucleated cells in the body, with the highest concentration on mature lymphocytes. Red blood cells may express very low levels of these antigens as remnants from the reticulocyte or adsorbed from the plasma. HLA-A and -B antigens are also expressed on platelets. There has been debate as to whether HLA is an integral membrane protein on platelets or whether platelet HLA is adsorbed from plasma.[4,5] As much as 80 percent may be adsorbed, but 90,000 to 150,000 molecules per platelet have been reported,[6] even after treatment to remove adsorbed antigens. The amount of HLA on platelets can vary from one individual to another[7,8] and within an individual, depending on the age of the platelets.[9]

The HLA-DR antigens have a more limited tissue distribution. These are found in high concentrations on B lymphocytes, dendritic cells, monocytes, and macrophages. Expression of class II antigens can be induced by cytokines on some cells and tissues that normally do not express them.[10] Thus, T cells can display HLA-DR molecules when activated by antigens, mitogenic agents, or other cells and in some disease states.

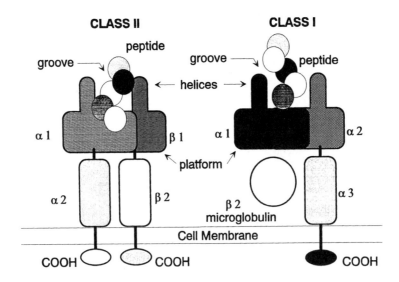

Fig. 6-1. HLA antigen structure. The HLA class I and II antigens are structurally similar transmembrane glycoproteins that acquire and display peptides derived from intra- and extracellular proteins to cells of the immune system.

STRUCTURE AND FUNCTION OF HLA MOLECULES

The HLA field has undergone an explosive period of growth and development over the past few years with the increasing application of molecular biologic techniques to the study of HLA. Nucleotide sequences are now available for nearly all known HLA specificities, many subtypes, and variants. The novel three-dimensional protein structure of HLA molecules, beginning with HLA-A2, was revealed in 1987.[11] A similar structure for class II antigens based on molecular modeling was proposed[12] and subsequently verified by the solution of the structure of HLA-DR1.[13] The structures of HLA-A68 and HLA-B27 have also been solved.[14,15] Comparisons between HLA class I structures have produced some fascinating insights into the role that HLA molecules play in the immune response.

Unlike the immunoglobulin structure, with globular domains folded about one another to form an antigen-combining site, the N-terminal domains of HLA molecules form a β-pleated sheet "platform" overlaid with two extended helices separated by a long, deep "groove." The HLA molecules carry short peptides they acquire during their assembly and transport to the cell surface. Peptides fit into the highly specialized groove formed by the α_1 and α_2 domains of the class I molecules and the α_1 and β_1 domains of the class II molecules (Fig. 6-1). In the crystallographic studies that revealed the structure of HLA, electron-dense material in the groove between the helices was not clearly resolved, suggesting that the space was not occupied by a single entity. More recent studies have shown that complex mixtures of peptides can be bound to a single HLA molecule.[16–18] Although many different peptides can occupy the groove of a particular HLA molecule, there is some selectivity conferred by "pockets" formed beneath the helices and the amino acid side chains that line the peptide site.[14] Thus, different HLA molecules exhibit some degree of specificity with regard to the peptides that can be accommodated.

The peptides that bind to the HLA class I and II molecules also differ both in their origin and in their structure. First, by virtue of the assembly of the HLA molecules and the workings of accessory proteins and polypeptides in the endoplasmic reticulum, the class I molecules are preferentially loaded with peptides derived from the breakdown of endogenous proteins from the cytoplasm of the cell (including viral proteins), whereas the class II molecules acquire their peptides in endosomes and are thus biased toward peptides derived from extracellular proteins that have been endocytosed and degraded.[19,20] Second, the class II structure accommodates longer peptides than the class I structure because the ends of the peptide-binding groove are open in the class II structure.[21] The loaded HLA molecules are exported to the cell surface where they serve as targets and restriction elements in cell interactions, leading to the various types of immune response. The HLA class I proteins can associate with the CD8 cellular marker and preferentially interact with cytotoxic T cells, and the class II proteins associate with CD4 and interact with T cells that provide "help" during the induction phase of an immune response.

ORGANIZATION OF THE HLA GENE COMPLEX

The genetic complex that encodes the HLA antigens is located on the short arm of chromosome 6. The complex has been characterized extensively through the efforts of many different laboratories. The detailed genetic map has been summarized and is regularly updated.[22] Figure 6-2 outlines the organization of those genes that encode HLA antigens and some additional associated genes. The HLA complex is slightly less than 4,000 kilobases in actual length. There are three genes that encode the classical HLA-A, -B, and -C class I antigens located at the telometric end of the complex. There are three additional class I genes that encode less well characterized HLA-E, -F, and -G molecules, and four pseudogenes designated HLA-H, -J, -K, and -L.

At least 11 genes encoding class II HLA-DR, -DQ, and -DP polypeptides and 7 pseudogenes have been identified at the centromeric end of the complex. Two additional class II genes have been identified that may encode novel class II molecules.[23] These have been designated DMA and DMB and are located between the DQ and DP regions. Each class II molecule consists of one α gene product and one β gene product, noncovalently linked. Different haplotypes may include different numbers of DR β genes and pseudogenes (the latter are indicated as

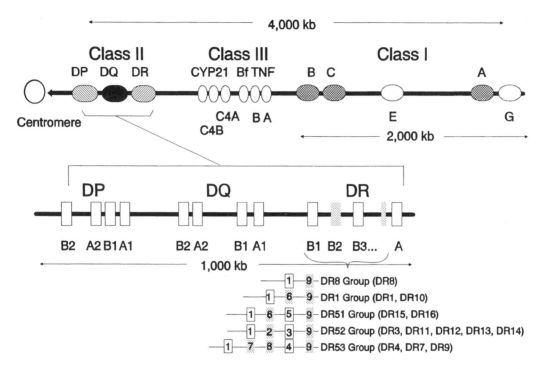

Fig. 6-2. Organization of the HLA gene complex. This abbreviated map of the human major histocompatibility complex shows the general organization of the major class I (*HLA-A, -B,* and *-C*) and class II (*HLA-DR, -DQ,* and *-DP*) genes. Structurally unrelated genes (class III) encoding tumor necrosis factor (TNF A and B); complement components Bf, C4A, and C4B; and 21-hydroxylase (CYP21), among others, separate the class I and II genes. The genetic fine structure of the class II region is illustrated in the expanded view and described in the text. Shaded boxes with no outline designate pseudogenes.

shaded boxes in Fig. 6-2). The DR8 allele is encoded by the β_1 gene. The β_9 pseudogene may also be associated with DR8-bearing haplotypes. Haplotypes with DR3, DR11, DR12, DR13, or DR14 alleles encoded by the β_1 gene are also associated with the β_2 pseudogene, the β_3 gene encoding the DR52-associated specificity, and perhaps the β_9 pseudogene. In each case, the DR specificity is determined by alleles of the β_1 gene, and the associated DR51, DR52, and DR53 specificities by the β_5, β_3, or β_4 genes, respectively.

The genes encoding the class I and II HLA antigens are separated by a series of structurally unrelated genes. Some of the more familiar of these are indicated in Figure 6-2. Tumor necrosis factor α and β molecules; complement proteins C2, C4A, and C4B; and Bf (factor B) are encoded in this intervening region. This region has been historically designated as class III because of its close association with the major histocompatibility complex in most species, but as yet, no clear structural or functional relationship between these genes and those encoding the class I and II antigens has been identified.

The HLA antigens are inherited in a simple mendelian fashion most of the time, with each child inheriting the entire linked set of genes (one haplotype) from each parent, as outlined in Figure 6-3. The antigens are codominantly expressed, so each individual should express two antigens at each locus. The direct genetic relationship is important when the degree of HLA identity is at issue. Two HLA-identical siblings are genotypically identical because they express exactly the same HLA antigens encoded by the same genes inherited from each parent. A parent and child can be phenotypically identical in their HLA types, but only one set of antigens is

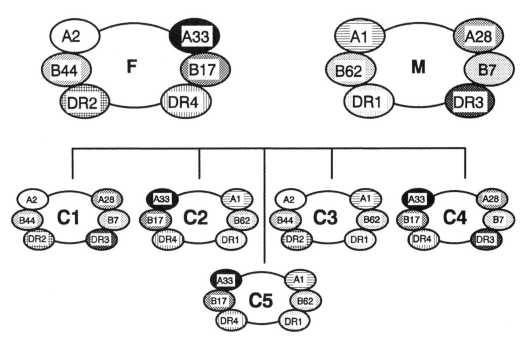

Fig. 6-3. Inheritance of HLA antigens. The HLA antigens are inherited in a straightforward mendelian fashion with each child receiving one maternal and one paternal HLA haplotype. Full siblings may share both (C2 and C5), one (C1 and C3 or C1 and C4), or no haplotypes (C1 and C2 or C1 and C5) with one another. Alleles are expressed codominantly, and crossovers occur infrequently (less than 2 percent between HLA-A and -DR).

genotypically identical. The second set of antigens may react with the same typing reagents but can differ in subtle but immunologically relevant ways. If both parents pass a gene for HLA-A2, the child is phenotypically homozygous, even though more detailed testing might identify two distinct A2 alleles. Recombination is relatively uncommon and occurs between the HLA-A and -B locus with a frequency of about 1 percent and 0.8 percent between HLA-B and -DR, respectively.

HLA TYPING

Serology

Before our current understanding of HLA had been worked out at the molecular level, a small group of serologists painstakingly began to sort out the organization and key associations of the HLA antigens through a rather unique, worldwide collaborative effort. In 1964, the pioneer serologists initiated a se-

ries of international workshops to share their knowledge, techniques, and results and to assemble a cohesive language of HLA. These workshops have been held every 2 to 4 years through the present and have expanded to include the thousands of new HLA specialists. Newer molecular technologies have also been included in the more recent gatherings.

A key early development in HLA typing was the microcytotoxicity test, introduced by Terasaki and McClelland[24] in 1964 and adopted as the standard testing method at the 1970 Workshop. The microcytotoxicity test remains the standard for serologic tissue typing today. This technique, outlined in Figure 6-4, allowed for testing using only 1 μl of serum. Sixty to 72 reactions could be tested on a tray the size of a credit card. Because the HLA typing sera were obtained primarily from placentae of multiparous women or from units of blood, volumes were very limited. The introduction of the microcytotoxicity test made it possible for sera to be shared and used for many tests at laboratories all over the world.

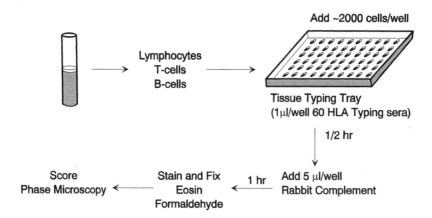

Fig. 6-4. The original microcytotoxicity test. The test outlined here used only 1 μl of each rare HLA typing serum to determine the tissue type from peripheral blood lymphocytes. By preserving these limited reagents, this test allowed HLA typing to be standardized throughout the world. Although there have been modifications and improvements, as described in the text, the microcytotoxicity test remains the standard method for tissue typing.

From 100 μl of serum, 100,000 tests could be performed. In a recent overview of the past 30 years of the microcytotoxicity test, Paul Terasaki estimated that more than 10 million tissue typings had been performed around the world using 1,000 L of sera; a remarkable feat that would have required more than 50,000 L for testing by other serologic methods. The test is versatile enough to accommodate numerous modifications. Improvements have been made in cell isolation techniques using monoclonal antibodies to lymphocyte subsets to enrich T or B lymphocytes rapidly. Enhancing antibodies can be added to the tray to increase sensitivity,[25] incubation temperatures have been modulated to detect cold-reacting antibodies,[26] and automated reading of trays developed with fluorescent vital dyes have all been incorporated into the basic test format.

The same test is used to detect anti-HLA antibodies. If one serum is added to a panel of wells, each of which contains well characterized single-donor lymphocytes, the resulting pattern of cytotoxicity can be used to describe the antibody reactivity. If the panel is large enough or is well chosen to include a representative sample of HLA alleles, antibody specificities can be identified in some cases. When discrete specificities can be identified, the results are useful in predicting crossmatch outcomes for specific kidney donors or for ordering antigen-negative

platelets. Crossmatching lymphocytes from a cadaveric kidney donor against a tray that has been loaded with sera from sensitized patients awaiting transplantation is a common application of the microcytotoxicity test for antibody.[27]

Public and Private Specificities and Cross-Reacting Groups

Anti-HLA antibodies can be grouped under two broad headings according to their pattern of reactivity as follows: (1) those that recognize a unique (private) specificity such as A28 and (2) those that react with two or more allelic products. The second category may include antibodies that cross-react with multiple antigens or antibodies that recognize specific structures shared by different alleles.

Most sera that contain anti-HLA antibodies are broadly reactive. It is rare to find an antiserum that reacts with a single, unique HLA allele. This observation might be explained if each serum contains many different antibodies, each reacting with different antigenic determinants on the HLA molecules. However, several patterns of reactivity are encountered with unusual frequency.[28] These have been referred to as cross-reacting groups or CREGS. A rather large number of CREGS have been characterized by different laboratories using a variety of techniques.[29–31] Recent efforts to correlate available HLA sequence data with reactivity patterns reveal that unique structures on the surface of the HLA molecules correlate with many patterns of antibody reactivity.[32,33] The antibodies most commonly produced against HLA antigens may be directed toward a limited number of "public" antigenic determinants shared by several HLA molecules, rather than against groups of "private" determinants, each unique to a specific HLA allele.

The HLA-B locus alleles, Bw4 and Bw6, first described by van Rood and van Leeuwen,[2] are good examples of public determinants. All B-locus antigens express either Bw4 or Bw6. An examination of the sequences of all antigens included in the Bw4 and Bw6 groups, as shown in Figure 6-5, reveals that all Bw4 sequences have the amino acid arginine at position 83 of the α_1 helix, whereas the Bw6 sequences all have a glycine at that position. All Bw6 sequences have an asparagine at position 80, one turn of the helix from position 83, and the Bw4 sequences have either threonine or isoleucine at this position. These amino acid differences are really dramatic at the molecular level. The structure of this small area of the HLA molecule is believed to be critical in determining whether anti-Bw4 or anti-Bw6 antibodies can bind.[33] Structures recognized by antibodies with private specificities may be nearby or distant on the molecule's surface. Bw4 antisera can

also react with HLA-A9 (-A23 and -A24), -A25, and -A32 antigens. These A-locus antigens also have the characteristic arginine at position 83.

The Serologically Defined Specificities

By 1984, more than 100 serologic specificities have been identified, and a few more have been recognized at more recent workshops. The serologic specificities are summarized in Figure 6-6. The list was arrived at by international agreement and reflects a process of searching for and finding new sera that would "split" existing specificities into two or more groups with ever finer resolution.[34] The earlier "parent" specificities are listed in boldface and beside their more recent splits (boxed). Discerning readers may note that the provisional "w" workshop designations have been dropped except for Bw4 and Bw6 (to distinguish them as epitopes rather than alleles), C-locus specificities (to distinguish them from complement components), and DP-locus specificities (which were originally defined by cellular tests). The Dw specificities that were determined by mixed lymphocyte reactions also retain their "w" designation. These were not included in Figure 6-6 because the Dw "alleles" are probably all explained as responses to specific combinations of DR and DQ alleles.[35] New serologic specificities will be named only if they

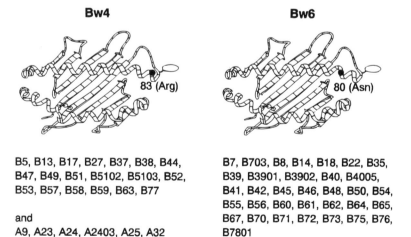

Bw4

83 (Arg)

Bw6

80 (Asn)

B5, B13, B17, B27, B37, B38, B44, B47, B49, B51, B5102, B5103, B52, B53, B57, B58, B59, B63, B77

and
A9, A23, A24, A2403, A25, A32

B7, B703, B8, B14, B18, B22, B35, B39, B3901, B3902, B40, B4005, B41, B42, B45, B46, B48, B50, B54, B55, B56, B60, B61, B62, B64, B65, B67, B70, B71, B72, B73, B75, B76, B7801

Fig. 6-5. Public HLA antigenic determinants: Bw4 and Bw6. Antisera that recognize the Bw4 and Bw6 determinants are affected by the amino acids at positions 80 and 83 in the protein sequence, shown in their approximate locations in this top view schematic of the class I molecule. The many different individual HLA antigens listed below each diagram all share the Bw4 or Bw6 determinant, respectively.

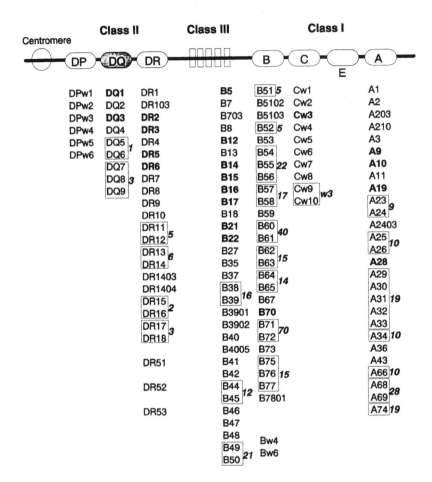

Fig. 6-6. Accepted HLA serologic specificities. HLA antigens that can be identified serologically[34] are listed according to the loci that encode the antigens (Fig. 6-2). Those specificities that have been resolved subsequently to new alleles are listed in boldface, and the "splits" of these antigens are boxed with the parent specificity indicated to the right.

identify a product with a recognized DNA allele sequence.

Frequency and Distribution of HLA Antigens

Some HLA antigens are relatively common, but others are rare. Many are found with different frequencies, depending on a person's origins.[36] The HLA-A2 antigen is fairly common and can be found in about 35 to 50 percent of any group selected at random. A1 is found in 25 percent of northern Europeans; 15 percent of blacks, Hispanics, and Chinese; but only 2 percent of Japanese. A36 and B42 are

found almost exclusively in blacks (5 and 10 percent, respectively). A43 has been found only in blacks and Japanese (less than 1 percent). B59 occurs in roughly 4 percent of Japanese but is virtually absent in whites. The differences in frequencies and distributions of the HLA antigens probably reflect the evolution of alleles under different selective pressures operating in different geographic areas. In their immunologic role in antigen processing and presentation, specific HLA antigens might have been selected by local pathogens; as a result, they are distributed differently among ethnic groups.

Obviously, the number of possible combinations of HLA antigens is very large. With the serologic HLA-A, -B, and -DR types listed in Figure 6-6 alone, it is possible to generate between 5 and 140 million distinct combinations, depending on how the broad and split antigens are counted. The task of finding two people with the same combination of antigens who are not closely related to one another is a formidable one.

Some HLA haplotypes occur more frequently than would be expected if the genes segregated independently. Because of this observation, some HLA genes are said to be in linkage disequilibrium. The most common example in the United States is the A1-B8-DR3 haplotype, which occurs in about 5 percent of whites. This is much more frequent than the 1 percent predicted on the basis of the individual antigen frequencies. Interestingly, the observation that certain combinations of HLA antigens are common may be influenced by the very large numbers of European and American tissue types that have been examined. As more and more nonwhites are typed, it appears that the occurrence of dominant haplotypes such as A1-B8-DR3 may be more the exception than the rule.

The distribution of dominant haplotypes has been recognized for some time in cases of disputed paternity when HLA was used to compute a probability of paternity.[37] The HLA system was a powerful tool for resolving questions of paternity because of the straightforward inheritance of the markers, the extensive polymorphism, and relatively low frequencies of the antigens. Given the HLA type of the child and the mother, the HLA type of the biologic father can be imputed. The exclusion probability (the likelihood of excluding a falsely accused man) is about 95 percent using the HLA-A and -B antigens. In general, it was more difficult to identify a white father with a high degree of certainty because many other whites might also satisfy the HLA criteria for paternity if the paternal haplotype were common. With the advent of DNA markers that can provide a much higher exclusion probability, fewer paternity cases are now tested by HLA typing.

Cell Exchanges and Quality of Tissue Typing

Even after 30 years, serologic HLA typing continues to evolve. Although the microcytotoxicity test mini-

mized the volumes of reagents needed, typing sera are limited, and new ones must be screened constantly. Variations in the availability and quality of typing sera could result in large differences in tissue typings from different laboratories using different sera. Several current programs monitor progress in identifying the newer HLA alleles and ensuring the quality of tissue typing by sending known samples for tissue typing to many laboratories around the world. The results of these exercises show that some HLA antigens are still difficult to type for some laboratories. Table 6-1 lists the HLA antigens that can be identified routinely by more than 95 percent of laboratories that participate in the University of California at Los Angeles (UCLA) Cell Exchange, those typed correctly by 80 to 95 percent of laboratories, and the developing specificities identified by fewer than 80 percent of laboratories reporting.[38] The more difficult antigens for many tissue typing laboratories are the class II HLA-DR antigens. Because of the limited tissue distribution, B-cell viability problems with time in shipping samples, and the potential presence of antibodies to class I antigens contaminating anti-DR sera, the quality of HLA-DR serology still lags somewhat behind that for the

Table 6-1. Identification Rate for HLA Specificities at 283 HLA Laboratories Worldwide[a]

Identification	Locus	Specificities
95–100%	A	1, 2, 3, 11, 23, 24, 28, 29, 30, 31, 32, 33
	B	7, 8, 13, 14, 18, 27, 35, 37, 39, 41[b], 42, 44, 45, 49[b], 51, 60, 62
	DR	1, 2, 3, 4, 5, 7[b], 8
80–94%	A	25, 34, 36
	B	38[b], 46, 48, 50, 52, 53, 55, 57, 59, 63, 67, 70
	DR	6, 9, 10, 11, 12
<80%	A	74[b]
	B	54, 56, 58, 61, 75, 76, 7801
	DR	14, 15, 16, 17, 18

[a] Many of the more common HLA-A, -B, and -DR antigens can be correctly and reproducibly typed by more than 95 percent of HLA laboratories around the world. HLA antigens that are less common, are frequent in nonwhites (e.g., -A34 and -A36 in blacks and -B46 and -B54 in Asians), or newer HLA specificities for which good antisera are not widely available are more difficult to identify for some laboratories.

[b] 1992 results, not tested in 1993.

(Data from Lau et al.[38])

HLA-A and -B antigens. The recent incorporation of monoclonal antibodies into some commercial tissue typing trays may reduce some of the problems caused by variability of antisera.[39] Monoclonal reagents have the advantage of essentially unlimited supply and specificities that can be very precisely established.

DNA Typing Methods

Beginning with the 1987 workshop, interest began to shift toward molecular HLA typing technologies alongside the serologic analysis. The initial emphasis was placed on typing the class II genes, HLA-DR, -DQ, and -DP because serologic reagents for the class II antigens were not as readily available or as well characterized as those for the HLA-A and -B antigens. Serologic typing was also technically more difficult because of the limited distribution of the class II antigens. Several approaches to "DNA typing" have been developed, and no single technique has yet been embraced by all laboratories working in the field.

Analyses of restriction fragment length polymorphisms (RFLP) were among the first organized forays into tissue typing at the DNA level.[40] The RFLP method uses enzymes (endonucleases) to cut DNA at specific nucleotide sequences, followed by electrophoresis to separate the fragments generated according to size. The separated fragments are blotted to a membrane and hybridized to a labeled oligonucleotide probe complementary to the gene of interest (the DR β_1 gene, for example). The size and number of bands obtained with each combination of endonucleases are characteristic for the allele.

RFLP is a cumbersome, lengthy procedure; as more nucleotide sequences have become available, techniques based on the polymerase chain reaction (PCR) have begun to play a more prominent role. The PCR reaction, as it has been used for HLA typing, uses pairs of primer oligonucleotides that correspond to sequences bracketing an informative stretch of DNA.[41] For HLA-DR typing, this might include the DR β_1 gene, which contains the most polymorphic sequences. The primers are allowed to anneal with the separated DNA strands and, in the presence of a thermostable DNA polymerase and a mixture of nucleotides, DNA synthesis is permitted for a short interval on each DNA strand, beginning from the hybridized primer. The reaction temperature is then raised to dissociate the newly formed sequences and cooled to allow the primers to anneal once again, and a new round of synthesis takes place. The newly synthesized sequences serve as templates for extension at each step. These steps are repeated through about 25 cycles, with each cycle enriching the production of the region bracketed by the primers. In effect, many copies of the particular stretch of DNA are copied. The specific sequence obtained can then be analyzed by hybridization with a panel of "sequence-specific" oligonucleotide probes designed to anneal only with the sequence of a specific allele.

Several commercial companies have developed kits that use this second approach. The kit has allele-specific oligonucleotide probes covalently attached in discrete spots to a support membrane. A specific region of the patient's DNA is amplified by PCR, labeled with biotin, and hybridized with the probes. The specifically hybridized DNA of the patient can be detected by adding enzyme coupled to streptavidin and a colorimetric substrate.

An alternative use of PCR has been developed to shorten the procedure. Rather than using primers that bracket the entire region of interest, some groups have developed primers the binding of which is dependent on allelic sequences.[42,43] In this sequence-specific primer approach, primers only anneal with DNA that express as a particular allele. At the end of the PCR cycles, only those primers specific for the individual's type generate a product. The product can be visualized directly after electrophoresis or more immediately by tests using intercalating dyes.[44] As DNA sequencing technology advances, direct sequencing of HLA genes or portions of genes amplified by PCR could assume an important role in HLA typing.

Newer HLA Nomenclature

Streamlined molecular techniques have made it possible to sequence the genes encoding HLA alleles rapidly and to deduce protein sequences from the nucleotide sequences. New guidelines were established at the 1987 workshop to incorporate the higher resolution tissue typing that can be achieved with molecular techniques. To identify class I alleles, the heavy chain locus (A, B, or C) is listed, followed by two digits corresponding to the serologic specificity and two digits with the allele designation. A fifth digit can be added to indicate further variants of an allele. If the reference is to the gene, an asterisk is inserted after the locus designation (e.g., HLA-A*210). If the reference is to the specificity associated with that gene, the asterisk is dropped (HLA-A210). For class II alleles, the nomenclature allows for specific descriptions of the multiple loci encoding the α and β chains of the class II heterodimers. These alleles are listed by the region designation, D, followed by P, Q, R, N, or O to indicate the subregion; A or B to indicate the α or β chain gene; and the number when more than one gene has been identified. *HLA-DRB1* is the β_1 gene encoding the DR β polypeptide. The alleles are assigned a four- or five-digit number, as in the class I genes.

The bulk of the early DNA typing work has been done on the class II HLA-DR, -DQ, and -DP alleles that were more difficult to type serologically. Many class I HLA-A, -B, and -C alleles have also been identified that cannot be resolved by serology, and application of DNA typing technologies to these alleles is a rapidly expanding area.

The World Health Organization Nomenclature Committee had recognized 50 HLA-A, 96 HLA-B, and 34 HLA-C alleles as of 1994.[45] The number of recognized HLA-DR (n = 127) and HLA-DQ (n = 41) α and β alleles is increasing rapidly. The level of polymorphism in the system is clearly enormous. However, little has been reported to indicate how frequently the newly defined alleles are encountered. In routine testing, the finest resolution HLA typing is not yet commonly reported because the technologies are not yet disseminated and standardized among all tissue typing laboratories.

Detailed studies of HLA sequences constitute a fascinating body of genetic literature that describes novel mechanisms for generating the enormous diversity of HLA types[33] and the evolutionary and anthropologic tracings that can be developed through studies of mixed populations,[46] primates,[47] and other mammalian species.[48] Among the major questions that still separate research from practical application of the newer typing methods is, "To what extent does the finest resolution tissue typing play an important clinical role?"

CLINICAL APPLICATIONS OF HLA

Immunologic Effects of Blood Transfusions

In 1973, Opelz et al.[49] reported an unexpected effect of blood transfusions given to patients undergoing dialysis before kidney transplantation. Rather than leading to accelerated graft loss, as was commonly expected based on the potential for immunization against HLA antigens, patients who previously had received blood transfusions had higher transplant survival rates than did those who were never transfused. Over the next several years, many transplant centers established deliberate transfusion protocols for patients awaiting a kidney transplant. The "transfusion effect" was a dominant factor in renal transplantation from the mid-1970s to the mid-1980s when the powerful immunosuppressive drug, cyclosporine, was introduced and the survival rate for nontransfused patients increased to equal that for transfused patients. The 1-year graft survival rates for transfused and nontransfused recipients of cadaveric kidney transplants are shown for each year in Figure 6-7. The shaded area shows that 90 percent of patients had been transfused before their transplant between 1981 and 1984. However, as apprehension about the potential for disease transmission through blood transfusions began to increase in the middle to late 1980s, patients became more reluctant to accept random-donor blood transfusions. As graft survival rates increased and the difference in transplant success rates between transfused and nontransfused recipients diminished, it became more difficult to justify requiring deliberate transfusions for patients who did not otherwise need them. Transplant centers began to abandon their deliberate transfusion protocols, and Figure 6-7 shows that, by 1992, only 60 percent of renal transplant recipients had ever received a blood transfusion. Recombinant erythropoetin has reduced the need for blood transfusions for many dialysis patients. Thus, the number of transplant recipients who received prior transfusions will likely decrease even more as those who have undergone dialysis for the longest periods (and were more likely to have been transfused) are transplanted.

The mechanism of the transfusion effect was never clearly established, despite intense study (see Chs. 4 and 35). Several hypotheses were put forward, in-

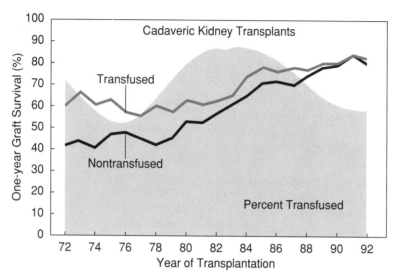

Fig. 6-7. Effect of blood transfusions on kidney transplant survival. Patients who received blood transfusions, before their cadaver donor kidney transplant had better 1-year graft survival rates (upper curve) than did those who had never been transfused (lower curve) between 1972 and 1988. The shaded area shows the percentage of patients who received pretransplant blood transfusions each year. (Data from the UCLA and UNOS Renal Transplant Registries.)

cluding induction of suppressor cells,[50] enhancing antibodies,[51] patient selection when anti-HLA antibodies produced in response to the transfusion caused a positive crossmatch against some donors,[52] and clonal deletion whereby the HLA antigens on the transplanted kidney would restimulate immune memory cells just as the highest doses of immunosuppressive drugs were administered.[53] Leukocytes were required to achieve the transfusion effect. Patients who were transfused with platelets that were filtered to remove leukocytes had significantly poorer graft survival rates than did those transfused with whole blood.[54] Because platelets express class I but not class II HLA antigens, the latter result implied that HLA-DR antigens were important to prolong graft survival. A thorough study of patients who received a single blood transfusion suggested that when one HLA-DR antigen was shared in common between the blood donor and recipient, the maximum benefit could be realized.[55] The success of donor-specific transfusions for living-related donor transplants,[56] when the donor and recipient share at least one haplotype, may also support a mechanism enhanced by having one DR antigen in common between the blood donor and recipient.

Transfusions have also been administered to women who suffer recurrent spontaneous pregnancy losses (RPL). The fetus is a transplant carrying allogeneic material from the father that must survive for a time in the mother. It was reasonable to expect that early pregnancy losses, like early kidney transplant losses, might be reduced by transfusions. The value of transfusion for the prevention of RPL is as yet incompletely evaluated because the results of only one controlled trial have been published.[57] In this study, 17 of 22 of women immunized with their husbands' leukocytes had successful pregnancies compared with only 10 of 27 who were transfused with their own washed leukocytes. However, the interpretation of such results must take into account that the probability of successful pregnancy in women with a history of three spontaneous abortions is about 60 percent without treatment (see Ch. 4). As with the effect of blood transfusions on renal transplant outcome, the mechanism of the possible beneficial effect of transfusion in women with recurrent pregnancy losses has not been explained. Antibodies that inhibit cellular immune responses[58] and noncytotoxic antibodies directed against paternal HLA antigens[59] have been reported to correlate with success.

It is unclear whether some form of inappropriate immune response against paternal HLA antigens of the fetus is responsible for the early pregnancy losses. Early reports indicated that excessive HLA compatibility between the husband and wife was associated with RPL[60] and suggested that maternal recognition of paternal HLA differences might be advantageous to fetal survival.[61] Although there has been considerable disagreement regarding the role (if any) of HLA compatibility in RPL patients, a recent study of 31 children of women undergoing leukocyte immunization showed a significant deficit of HLA-DQA1-compatible live-born children.[62]

HLA in Solid Organ Transplantation

The HLA antigens play two important roles in the success of solid organ transplants: First, they are a target for preformed antibodies in the potential recipient. Second, they are the major target of cellular rejection reactions that develop after transplantation.

One serious side effect of blood transfusions in potential transplant recipients is the risk of sensitization to HLA antigens. Preformed antidonor-HLA antibodies can produce hyperacute rejection of the transplanted kidney[63] and have also been implicated in a higher incidence of primary nonfunctioning transplanted livers.[64,65] The problem of hyperacute rejection for kidneys has been nearly eliminated by requiring a negative cytotoxic antibody crossmatch between the recipient's serum and donor's lymphocytes before transplantation, and some hospitals now also monitor anti-HLA antibodies in their heart and liver transplant candidates.

The likelihood of sensitization with relatively small numbers of blood transfusions has been a matter of some debate. Only 5 to 20 percent of male or nulliparous female patients who received fewer than 10 transfusions became broadly sensitized.[66–68] Women with prior pregnancies were at higher risk. Up to 30 percent had significant antibody production, and sensitization correlated with both the number of prior pregnancies and the number of transfusions. Exposure to allogeneic HLA antigens through a prior failed transplant also placed patients at much higher risk of sensitization when even small numbers of blood transfusions were administered. The immunizing potential of transfused blood could be nearly

eliminated by reducing HLA differences. In one study that used blood from donors who were HLA matched with the patients, anti-HLA antibodies developed in only 1 of 24 multiparous women at high risk of sensitization.[69]

The risk of hyperacute rejection makes preformed antidonor HLA antibodies a contraindication to kidney transplantation. Because most blood donors, like most organ donors, are white, blood transfusions can lead to special difficulties for blacks and Asians awaiting a kidney transplant. Nonwhites may be even more likely to respond to blood transfusions than whites because of racial differences in the distribution of HLA alleles. Blacks are more likely to produce antibodies that react with white than with black donor lymphocytes.[70,71] The problem may be more acute for black male patients than female patients because the source of immunization among male patients is more often blood transfusions from white donors, whereas female patients are sensitized by pregnancies, with the paternal HLA antigens more likely to be from a black man.[71]

Patients who receive a kidney transplant from an HLA-identical sibling donor have fewer rejection episodes, require less immunosuppression, and enjoy better graft survival rates than do patients transplanted from mismatched relatives. The effect of histocompatibility between recipients and their immediate family members as donors was established very early in the transplant experience.[72] Recipients of cadaver donor kidneys also have superior outcomes when the donor is HLA compatible.[73] The United Network for Organ Sharing (UNOS) data illustrated in Figure 6-8 show that the probability of long-term graft survival increases as the number of HLA-A, -B, and -DR antigens shared between the donor and recipient increases from zero or one through all six.

Although there is a clear benefit to graft survival for those who can receive a well matched transplant, it is rare to find two unrelated individuals with the same constellation of HLA-A, -B, and -DR antigens. The HLA types of all patients waiting for cadaveric kidney transplants in the United States are stored in the UNOS computer in Richmond, Virginia. Whenever a cadaveric organ donor is identified anywhere in the United States, the HLA type is reported and compared with those on the patient waiting list.

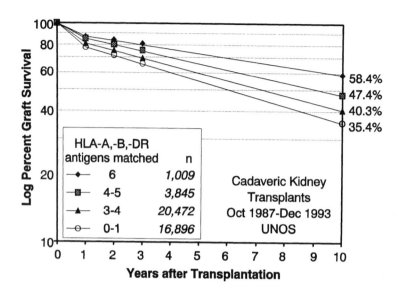

Fig. 6-8. Effect of HLA compatibility between the donor and recipient on long-term survival of cadaveric kidney transplants. These data from the UNOS Renal Transplant Registry show that cadaveric kidney transplant survival rates progressively improved as more HLA-A, -B, and -DR antigens were matched between the donor and recipient. When the graft survival rates were projected through 10 years, the survival difference for patients who received a kidney matched for all six HLA antigens and those who received a kidney matched for none or only one of six HLA antigens was 23 percent.

When a perfect HLA-A, -B, and -DR match is found, the kidney is shipped for transplantation to the HLA-matched recipient. When no match is identified, the kidney is usually allocated locally to the person waiting the longest with the next best HLA match. Even with this national effort, only 2.4 percent of patients have received kidneys with all six HLA-A, -B, and -DR antigens matched. There are many patients and donors who do not express six different HLA antigens because they are homozygous at one or more HLA loci. The kidney transplant survival rate when the patient had less than six HLA-A, -B, and -DR antigens identified but the donor expressed no antigens that were not also present in the recipient was the same as that when all six antigens were matched. The 1,009 transplants matched for six antigens in Figure 6-8 would increase to 2,400 when presumed homozygous donors and recipients were included. Still, these well matched transplants represent less than 6 percent of the kidney transplants that have been performed.

It has been possible to share kidneys for histocompatible recipients because kidneys can be stored for 30 hours or more without sustaining permanent damage.[74] Hearts and livers cannot be preserved for extended periods, and these organs have not been shared on the basis of HLA compatibility with the recipient. Nevertheless, some matched transplants do occur by chance, and a recent analysis of more than 8,000 heart transplants showed that HLA-compatible hearts also had better outcomes than did those with three or more HLA antigens mismatched.[75]

Large studies of HLA matching in liver transplant recipients have not yet been reported. One small study with very few well matched transplants reported an inverse relationship between HLA-DR incompatibilities and survival of transplanted livers.[76] The role of HLA matching in liver transplants will probably remain a matter for debate until data on a larger number of well matched liver transplants accumulate and can be studied.

Role of HLA in Allogeneic Bone Marrow Transplantation

Bone marrow transplantation has become an accepted treatment modality for a variety of hematologic malignancies, immunologic deficiencies, and genetic disorders. HLA plays a critical role in allogeneic bone marrow transplantation, affecting the transplant outcome and influencing the probability of finding a suitable donor. Because a bone marrow transplant includes a viable immune system, not only is graft rejection a possibility, but cells from the grafted marrow can also mount a rejection against the recipient. Thus, any HLA differences between the donor and recipient can lead to serious complications. GVHD occurs because T lymphocytes in the transplanted marrow respond to the HLA antigens (or to other "minor" histocompatibility antigens) of the recipient. When the patient's immune system has been severely debilitated, these cells can proliferate unchecked and cause serious damage, even death, if the GVHD is severe. GVHD occurs in roughly 40 percent of HLA-identical sibling transplants (underscoring the importance of non-HLA antigens) compared with 80 percent of transplants from phenotypically HLA-matched unrelated donors.[77–79] Graft rejection occurs in up to 15 percent of unrelated donor transplants and has been a frequent problem for patients with aplastic anemia whose pretransplant immunosuppressive regimen is less intensive than that for those with leukemia.[80,81] When the donor marrow is first depleted of T lymphocytes to prevent GVHD, the rate of graft failure also increases.[79]

Initially, allogeneic bone marrow transplants were restricted to patients with an HLA-identical sibling. This genotypic HLA match is the best possible match. In practice, an HLA-identical sibling may be available for 30 percent of potential recipients.[82] Phenotypically HLA-matched relatives, and relatives mismatched for one HLA antigen, have been used successfully for pediatric patients with immunodeficiencies[83] but have been mostly unsuccessful for leukemic patients.[84,85] Increasing HLA disparities resulted in a higher incidence of severe GVHD. HLA-mismatched relatives and unrelated donors have provided bone marrow for 12 and 15 percent of transplants reported to the International Bone Marrow Transplant Registry, respectively.[86]

The enormous diversity of HLA types makes finding a matched, unrelated donor unlikely, as was apparent from the efforts to match kidney donors and recipients. Theoretical calculations have projected that about 50 percent of patients would find an HLA-matched donor from a pool of 150,000.[87] Large volunteer bone marrow donor registries have already been established in Europe and the United States and are also developing in several Asian countries. In early 1994, a list of nearly 1,500,000 donors' HLA types were compiled by the European Bone Marrow Transplant Group from 19 registries in 16 countries. The National Marrow Donor Program (NMDP) in the United States has now recruited more than 1,200,000 potential donors and constitutes a large portion of that list.

There are logistic problems that have kept the actual success of searches through these registries below the theoretic predictions. In 1992, Bradley et al.[88] reported that only 7 percent of searches initiated through the Anthony Nolan and British Bone Marrow and Platelet Donor Panel Registries resulted in transplants. The single largest reason was failure to identify a histocompatible donor (24 percent of searches). In part, this disappointing result was due to estimations of matching that did not adequately address ethnic diversity. Most volunteer donors both in North America and Europe were white. The United States NMDP has begun an intensive recruitment program among minorities to alleviate this problem.

Hansen et al.[89] more recently reported a much better experience in searches initiated through the NMDP, with nearly 40 percent of 102 searches resulting in transplantation within 1 year. At least one HLA-A, -B, -DR-matched potential donor was identified for 57 of those patients in the initial search.

The average time to complete a search is 6 to 8 months, which further reduces the patient's chance of surviving long enough to transplant if a donor can be identified. Many delays are caused by incomplete HLA typing (only about 25 percent of volunteer donors are typed for HLA-DR), which requires that the donor be contacted after an initial search based on the HLA-A and -B type and then be tested for -DR. Storing samples of DNA may eliminate this step.

The importance of fine-resolution HLA typing that can now be achieved with DNA techniques has yet to be established for unrelated donor transplants. At least one early report hinted that differences that could not be detected by serologic typing might be important. Fleischauer et al.[90] reported that T cells that recognize an HLA-B44 subtype (that differed from the patient's -B44 at only one amino acid) were identified in a patient who rejected his unrelated donor bone marrow transplant. Preliminary analyses of the effect of HLA-DR mismatches identified by DNA typing in serologically -DR-identical transplants have been inconclusive.[91] The HLA-DP antigens do not appear to play a major role in bone marrow transplants.[92]

Post-Transfusion Graft-Versus-Host Disease

GVHD has also been recognized after blood transfusions in patients with immune deficiencies (see Ch. 42).[43] Viable lymphocytes in the transfused blood can damage tissues in the immunodeficient recipient if a response develops against the patient's HLA antigens. Post-Transfusion GVHD (PT-GVHD) can be prevented by γ irradiation, and this processing step has been recommended for blood products ordered for immunodeficient or immunosuppressed patients.[94]

PT-GVHD has also been reported in patients without overt evidence of immunodeficiency. Although these reactions have been reported infrequently, they are often fatal. Petz et al.[95] identified 39 cases in a recent survey of English language publications. In 14 of 16 instances in which HLA typing was available, PT-GVHD occurred when the blood donor was homozygous for one of the recipient's HLA haplotypes. Under these conditions, donor lymphocytes may respond to the dissimilar HLA antigens of the recipient, but because the HLA mismatch is unidirectional, the recipient's immune system does not recognize the donor lymphocytes as foreign, which allows the donor cells to escape detection.

A high proportion of PT-GVHD cases have been from Japan. Takahashi et al.[96] reported 171 cases identified through a survey of 14,000 doctors. Although tissue typing data were not included in this summary, 14 patients were younger than 1 year old and required exchange transfusions. Ten received fresh blood from their parents. The risk of a one-way HLA match in recipients of blood from first-degree relatives is estimated to be as high as 1 in 475.[97] It has been pointed out that the risk of homo-

zygosity for an HLA haplotype shared by a heterozygous recipient is also high for other blood relatives.[98] The standards of the American Association of Blood Banks now mandate that cellular blood products known to have been donated by a blood relative should be irradiated with a minimum of 25 Gy (2,500 cGy).[99]

Not all cases of PT-GVHD involved blood transfusions from immediate family members. One-way HLA matches can occur at random between unrelated individuals. Estimates of the probability that such a match would occur for the HLA-A, -B, and -DR antigens range from 1 in 500[100] to 1 in 7,174[97] for white patients and donors. Even if the lower estimate were the more reasonable, the incidence of recognized PT-GVHD in the United States is much lower than predicted if a one-way HLA match were sufficient to cause PT-GVHD. Among Japanese donors and recipients, the predicted frequency of one-way matches among unrelated individuals ranges from 1 in 312[101] to 1 in 874,[97] and the reported incidence of PT-GVHD in Japanese patients undergoing cardiovascular surgery has been estimated at one in 650.[101] Thus, the incidence in Japan seems to correlate better with predictions than in North America and Europe. Perhaps the increased frequency of PT-GVHD in Japan is caused by a key difference between transfusion practice in Japan and the United States, which is related to lymphocyte viability. In many of the cases reported from Japan, relatively fresh blood was used, often after collection on the same day.

Platelet Transfusions

Patients with a variety of hematologic malignancies undergoing chemotherapy often require platelet support during periods of thrombocytopenia, (see Ch. 16 and 32). Multiple transfusions cause many of these patients to become alloimmunized and refractory to further platelet transfusion. Varying estimates suggest that 14[102] or 38 percent[103] of patients repeatedly exposed to platelet transfusions become immunized to HLA antigens, and a fraction may have antibodies develop against platelet antigens in addition to those against HLA.[102]

Platelets from single donors matched for HLA-A and -B antigens can often be used successfully in refractory patients. A genotypically matched family member, generally a sibling, would be the best source for HLA-matched platelets. However, it may be difficult to obtain sufficient quantities from HLA-identical family members if the patient has that option, and finding unrelated donors who match exactly is frequently not possible with local pools of HLA-matched donors. A national pool of HLA-typed platelet donors could be developed, but logistically, it would be difficult to rely on such a geographically diverse donor pool for platelet-refractory patients. In practice, "HLA-matched" platelets often are not identical but rather are the best match available in a local blood bank. Many patients receive partially matched platelets, with one or more donor HLA antigens that cross-react with the patient's own. Even when the best matched platelets are used, as many as 20 percent of platelet transfusions may be ineffective in refractory patients.[104] Finer resolution HLA typing might explain these failures if there were undetected HLA differences.

Crossmatch negative platelets are also effective both for patients sensitized to HLA antigens and those with antibodies to other platelet antigens. Depending on the specificity of the patients' antibodies, many HLA antigens may not react. O'Connell et al.[105] showed that successful platelet donors selected by crossmatching for alloimmunized patients had HLA types different from those of the patients and would not have been selected as "HLA matched."

Results of a multicenter study showed that HLA-matched platelets gave somewhat better results than those selected by crossmatching alone, but only if the platelets were truly matched (i.e., contained no antigens not present in the patient, (grade A or BU).[106] Another study from the University of Virginia found the same result but concluded that ordering HLA-matched platelets provided no benefit over crossmatch-compatible platelets because more than 40 percent of products supplied as "HLA-matched" actually had at least one HLA antigen mismatched.[107] Thus, the relative merit of HLA-matched versus crossmatch-selected platelets will probably depend on the size of the donor pool and the likelihood of obtaining an HLA-matched donor for a particular patient.

Computer programs developed to predict negative crossmatches for broadly sensitized renal transplant recipients may be useful to predict which donors will be crossmatch negative for platelet-refractory patients. Crossmatch prediction programs are based on tests for antibody against panels of well characterized lymphocytes that represent most HLA types in the local donor population.[108] Ideally, using such panels, one could identify specific HLA antigens to which the patient had antibodies. Donors with those antigens could then be avoided. In practice, it is rarely that simple. Most antibodies are broadly reactive rather than having a clearly defined specificity. For this reason, most prediction programs also consider cross-reacting groups in the analysis of specificity.[109] Some go even farther, considering multiple approaches to predict probable negative HLA antigens for a particular serum.[110] It is also important to use very sensitive tests in screening for HLA antibodies to ensure the most accurate assessment of antibody specificity.[111]

In some patients, anti-HLA antibodies develop then disappear, even though the patient continues to receive transfusions. Down regulation of the anti-HLA response may result from the development of antibodies directed against the specific antigen-combining sites on the antibody molecule.[112,113] These so-called anti-idiotypic antibodies interfere with the binding of the patient's own anti-HLA antibodies. Their presence can be demonstrated by using a serum obtained after the HLA reactivity has been decreased to inhibit the HLA reactivity of an earlier serum from the same patient. When HLA antibodies disappear as a result of an active process such as anti-idiotype suppression, patients may lose their refractoriness. There is no way to predict or control which patients might develop this response.

Prevention of alloimmunization in patients likely to require platelet support is the best approach for patients who are not sensitized. Available data suggest that the rate of sensitization may be substantially reduced by using leukocyte-depleted platelets.[114] A multicenter National Institutes of Health-sponsored study is being conducted and will provide more data on this subject. Patients who are expected to require long-term support should still be HLA typed in the event that they do become sensitized during the course of their treatment.

HLA AND DISEASE ASSOCIATIONS

A number of diseases occur more frequently than would be expected in association with particular HLA types. During the 1970s and early 1980s, patients with a wide spectrum of diseases and disease states were tissue typed to determine if there were linkages with alleles of the HLA system. In 1985, Tiwari and Terasaki[115] catalogued the large body of research that had been done on HLA and disease associations, and this encyclopedic work remains a useful reference today. Although most HLA and disease associations are weak, a few were rather striking.

Nearly every patient with ankylosing spondylitis carries the HLA-B27 allele.[116] The association is so strong that HLA-B27 typing is sometimes used as a diagnostic tool for ankylosing spondylitis. Of course, ankylosing spondylitis is rare, and not everyone who has HLA-B27 has this disease. In fact, only about 2 percent do. This lack of a strong concordance is one hallmark of the HLA-associated diseases.

Juvenile (type I) diabetes is both positively and negatively associated with HLA.[117] People with HLA-DR3 and/or -DR4 are more susceptible to diabetes; those with HLA-DR2 are more resistant. More in-depth study suggests the disease association actually maps to the closely linked *HLA-DQB* gene locus and that susceptibility or resistance depends on whether the amino acid at position 57 of the DQB chain is serine, valine, or alanine (susceptible) or aspartic acid (resistant).[118] Again the genetic link between HLA and diabetes is not very strong. The concordance between monozygotic twins is less than 50 percent.[119] Environmental factors must also play an important role in the development of diabetes.

There are data suggesting a link between one environmental factor, cow's milk, and diabetes.[120] Exclusive breast feeding and delayed exposure to infant formula based on cow's milk seem to reduce the risk of diabetes. Karjalainen et al.[121] examined the antibodies to bovine albumin produced by diabetic and nondiabetic patients and found that there was a significant difference in antibody production against a 17-amino acid albumin peptide that cross-reacts with an antigen on insulin-producing β cells. Diabetic patients produced antibody to the cross-reactive determinant, but the control patients made antibodies toward other parts of the albumin molecule. Had this responsiveness been linked to the HLA-DR or -DQ type, it would have suggested a mechanism for the disease association whereby only a -DQ molecule lacking aspartate at position 57 of the β chain could present this particular peptide. However, there was no correlation between this response and HLA type.

Neonatal alloimmune thrombocytopenia is a condition that may develop as a result of immunization of the mother by paternal platelet antigens expressed in the fetus. HPA-1a (PlA^1) is the most common incompatibility associated with this condition. Among affected women with demonstrable antiplatelet antibodies, 82 to 89 percent produced antibodies against the HPA-1a antigen.[122,123] Interestingly, immunization rarely occurs as a result of platelet transfusion, but a small proportion (10 percent) of HPA-1a-negative women carrying an HPA-1a-positive fetus produce anti-HPA-1a antibody.[123] In a summary of five studies, Reznikoff-Etievant et al.[124] noted that between 75 and 95 percent of women who produced anti-HPA-1a also had HLA-DR3. That result was significantly higher than the 20 percent of controls or of the general population that has DR3. Additional studies showed that all "responders" had the supertypic HLA-DR52a allele associated with DR3.[125,126] There was no association between responsiveness to HPA-1b and HLA, which prompted the speculation that the single amino acid difference between HPA-1a and HPA-1b was critical to antigen presentation by the DR52a molecule.[127] The key allelic peptide of HPA-1a would fit in the groove of HLA-DR52a, thus explaining the HLA association with the response to HPA-1a.

FUTURE DIRECTIONS

As the molecular biologists continue to broaden our appreciation of the diversity of HLA, clinicians must struggle with the question of how important are all these differences? The challenge to those with a clinical interest in HLA will be to determine which HLA differences might be critical in particular situations. In kidney transplantation, fine-resolution matching of the HLA-DR antigens identified serologically[73] or by DNA typing[128] is not critical with modern immunosuppression. However, it would benefit long-term survival of kidney transplants to improve the level of histocompatibility even to a small degree. This would require developing new ways of looking at HLA matching so that compatible recipients could be identified even in small pools of waiting patients. Bone marrow transplantations between unrelated individuals who are HLA matched at the finest resolution for HLA-A, -B, -C, -DR, and -DQ antigens may result in fewer severe GVHD complications than those less rigorously matched, but fewer patients will be able to find a precisely matched donor. Patients with very uncommon HLA types would have a better chance if "permissible" HLA incompatibilities could be identified. The same is true for platelet-refractory patients. These problems may have similar solutions that can be investigated by expanding our focus beyond the sometimes bewildering molecular complexity of the HLA system to the immune responses patients make against HLA antigens.

REFERENCES

1. Dausset J: Leuco-agglutinins IV. Leuco-agglutinins and blood transfusion. Vox Sang 4:190, 1954
2. van Rood JJ, van Leeuwen A: Leucocyte grouping. A method and its application. J Clin Invest 42:1382, 1963
3. Terasaki PI: History of HLA: Ten Recollections. UCLA Tissue Typing Laboratory, Los Angeles, 1990
4. Kao KJ: Plasma and platelet HLA in normal individuals: quantitation by competitive enzyme-linked immunoassay. Blood 70:282, 1987
5. Liebert M, Aster RH: Expression of HLA-B12 on platelets, on lymphocytes and in serum: a quantitative study. Tissue Antigens 9:199, 1977
6. Kao KJ, Cook DJ, Scornik JC: Quantitative analysis of platelet surface HLA by W6/32 anti-HLA antibody. Blood 68:627, 1986
7. Szatkowski NS, Aster RH: HLA antigens of platelets. VI. Influence of 'private' HLA-B locus specificities on the expression of Bw4 and Bw6 on human platelets. Tissue Antigens 15:361, 1980
8. Santoso S, Mueller-Eckhardt G, Santoo S et al: HLA antigens on platelet membranes. Vox Sang 51:327, 1986
9. Periera J, Cretney C, Aster RH: Variation of class I HLA antigen expression among platelet density cohorts: a possible index of platelet age? Blood 71:516, 1988
10. Glimcher LH, Kara CJ: Sequences and factors: a guide to MHC class-II transcription. Annu Rev Immunol 10:13, 1992
11. Bjorkman PJ, Saper MA, Samraoui B et al: Structure of the human class I histocompatibility antigen, HLA-A2. Nature 329:506, 1987
12. Brown JH, Jardetzky T, Saper MA et al: A hypothetical model of the foreign antigen binding site of class II histocompatibility molecules. Nature 332:845, 1988
13. Brown JH, Jardetzky TS, Gorga JC et al: Three-dimensional structure of the human class II histocompatibility antigen HLA-DR1. Nature 364:33, 1993
14. Garret TPJ, Saper MA, Bjorkman PJ et al: Specificity pockets for the side chains of peptide antigens in HLA-Aw68. Nature 342:692, 1989
15. Madden DR, Gorga JC, Strominger JL, Wiley DC: The structure of HLA-B27 reveals nonamer self-peptides bound in an extended conformation. Nature 353:321, 1991
16. Guo H-C, Jardetzky TS, Garrett TPJ et al: Different length peptides bind to HLA-Aw68 similarly at their ends but bulge out in the middle. Nature 360:364, 1992
17. Huczko EL, Bodnar WM, Benjamin D et al: Characteristics of endogenous peptides eluted from the class I molecule HLA-B7 determined by mass spectrometry and computer modelling. J Immunol 151:2572, 1993
18. Chicz RM, Urban RG, Gorga JC et al: Specificity and promiscuity among naturally selected peptides bound to HLA-DR alleles. J Exp Med 178:27, 1993
19. Englehard VH: Structure of peptides associated with class I and class II MHC molecules. Annu Rev Immunol 12:181, 1994
20. Cresswell P: Assembly, transport, and function of MHC class II molecules. Annu Rev Immunol 12:259, 1994
21. Newcomb JR, Cresswell P: Characterization of endogenous peptides bound to purified HLA-DR molecules and their absence from invariant chain-associated alpha-beta dimers. J Immunol 150:499, 1993
22. Campbell RD, Trowsdale J: Map of the human MHC. Immunol Today 14:349, 1993
23. Kelly AP, Monaco JJ, Cho S, Trowsdale J: A new human HLA class II-related locus, DM. Nature 353:571, 1991
24. Terasaki PI, McClelland JP: Microdroplet assay of human serum cytotoxins. Nature 204:998, 1964
25. Fuller TC, Phelan D, Gebel HM et al: Antigenic specificity of antibody reactive in the anti-globulin-augmented lymphocytotoxicity test. Transplantation 34:24, 1982
26. Iwaki Y, Terasaki PI, Park MS, Billing R: Enhancement of human kidney allografts by cold B-lymphocyte cytotoxins. Lancet 1:1228, 1978
27. Delmonico FL, Fuller A, Cosimi AB et al: New approaches to donor crossmatching and successful transplantation of highly sensitized patients. Transplantation 36:629, 1983

28. Colombani J, Colombani M, Dausset J: Crossreactions in the HL-A system with special reference to Da6 crossreacting group. p. 79. In Terasaki PI (ed): Histocompatibility Testing 1970. Munksgaard, Copenhagen, 1970

29. Konoeda Y, Terasaki PI, Wakisaka A et al: Public determinants of HLA indicated by pregnancy antibodies. Transplantation 41:253, 1986

30. Rodey GE, Fuller TC: Public epitopes and the antigenic structure of the HLA molecules. Crit Rev Immunol 7:229, 1987

31. Fuller AA, Rodey GE, Parham P, Fuller TC: Epitope map of the HLA-B7 CREG using affinity-purified human alloantibody probes. Hum Immunol 28:306, 1990

32. Takemoto S, Gjertson DW, Terasaki PI: HLA matching: a comparison of conventional and molecular approaches. p. 413. In Terasaki PI, Cecka JM (eds): Clinical Transplants 1992. UCLA Tissue Typing Laboratory, Los Angeles, 1993

33. Parham P, Lawler RD, Salter CE et al: HLA-A, B, C: patterns of polymorphism in peptide-binding proteins. p. 10. In Dupont B (ed): Immunobiology of HLA. Vol. 2. Springer-Verlag, New York, 1989

34. Bodmer JG, Marsh SGE, Ekkehard DA et al: Nomenclature for factors of the HLA system 1991. Hum Immunol 34:4, 1992

35. Flomenberg N: Functional polymorphism of HLA class II gene products detected by T lymphocyte clones. p. 532. In Dupont B (ed): Histocompatibility Testing 1987. Vol. 1. Springer-Verlag, New York, 1989

36. The Central Data Analysis Committee: Allele frequencies. p. 807. In Tsuji K, Aizawa M, Sasazuki T (eds): The Data Book of the 11th International Histocompatibility Workshop. Vol. 2. Oxford University Press, Tokyo, 1991

37. Terasaki PI: Resolution for HLA testing of 1000 paternity cases not excluded by ABO testing. J Family Law 16:543, 1977

38. Lau M, Terasaki PI, Park MS: The 1993 cell typings of the international cell exchange. p. 533. In Terasaki PI, Cecka JM (eds): Clinical Transplants 1993. UCLA Tissue Typing Laboratory, Los Angeles, 1994

39. Lee JH, Lias M, Deng CT et al: Lambda monoclonal typing (LMT) procedure for HLA class I and class II typing. p. 3. In Terasaki PI (ed): Visuals of the Clinical Histocompatibility Workshop. One Lambda, Canoga Park, CA, 1993

40. Biguon JD, Semana G, Tiercy JM et al: DNA-RFLP analysis; HLA-DR beta workshop report. p. 851. In Dupont B (ed): Histocompatibility Testing 1987. Vol. 1. Springer-Verlag, New York, 1989

41. Sakai RK, Gelfand DH, Stoffel S et al: Primer-directed enzymatic amplification of DNA with a thermostable DNA polymerase. Science 239:497, 1988

42. Fernandez-Vina M, Shumway W, Stastny P: DNA typing for class II HLA antigens with allele-specific or group-specific amplification. II. Typing for alleles of the DRw52-associated group. Hum Immunol 28:51, 1990

43. Olerup O, Zetterquist H: HLA-DR typing by PCR amplification with sequence specific primers (PCR-SSP) in two hours: an alternative to serological DR typing in clinical practice including donor-recipient matching in cadaveric transplantations. Tissue Antigens 39:225, 1992

44. Chia D, Terasaki PI, Chan H et al: Direct detection of PCR products for HLA class II typing. Tissue Antigens 42:146, 1993

45. Bodmer JG, Marsh SGE, Albert ED et al: Nomenclature for factors of the HLA system 1994. Human Immunology 41:1, 1994

46. Caraballo LR, Marrugo J, Ehrlich H, Pastorizo M: HLA alleles in the population of Cartegena (Colombia). Tissue Antigens 39:128, 1992

47. Lawlor DA, Warren E, Ward FE, Parham P: Comparison of class I MHC alleles in humans and apes. p. 147. In Moeller G (ed): Immunological Reviews. Munksgaard, Copenhagen, 1990

48. Parham P, Lomen CE, Lawlor DA et al: Nature of polymorphism in HLA-A, -B, and -C molecules. Proc Natl Acad Sci USA 85:4005, 1988

49. Opelz G, Sengar DPS, Mickey MR, Terasaki PI: Effect of blood transfusions on subsequent kidney transplants. Transplant Proc 4:253, 1973

50. MacLeod AM, Mason RJ, Shewan et al: Possible mechanism of action of transfusion effect in renal transplantation. Lancet 2:468, 1982

51. Singal DP, Joseph S: Role of blood transfusions on the induction of antibodies against recognition sites on T-cells in renal transplant patients. Hum Immunol 4:93, 1982

52. Feduska NJ, Vicenti F, Amend WJ et al: Do blood transfusions enhance the possibility of a compatible transplant? Transplantation 27:35, 1979

53. Terasaki PI: The beneficial transfusion effect on kidney graft survival attributed to clonal deletion. Transplantation 37:119, 1984

54. Chapman JR, Ting A, Fisher M et al: Failure of platelet transfusion to improve human renal allograft survival. Transplantation 41:468, 1986

55. Lagaaij EL, Hennemann IPH, Ruigrok M et al: Effect

of one-HLA-DR-antigen-matched and completely HLA-DR-mismatched blood transfusions on survival of heart and kidney allografts. N Engl J Med 321: 701, 1989

56. Salvatierra O, Vicenti F, Amend WJC et al: The role of blood transfusions in renal transplantation. Urol Clin North Am 10:243, 1983

57. Mowbray JF, Liddell H, Underwood J et al: Controlled trial of treatment for recurrent spontaneous abortion by immunization with paternal cells. Lancet 1:941, 1985

58. Unander AM, Lindholm A, Olding LB: Blood transfusions generate/increase previously absent/weak blocking antibody in women with habitual abortion. Fertil Steril 44:766, 1985

59. Maruyama T, Makino T, Sugi T et al: Flow cytometric crossmatch and early pregnancy loss in women with a history of recurrent spontaneous abortions who underwent paternal leukocyte immunotherapy. Am J Obstet Gynecol 168:1528, 1993

60. Ober C: The maternal-fetal relationship in human pregnancy: an immunologic perspective. Exp Clin Immunogenet 9:1, 1992

61. McIntyre JA, Faulk WP: HLA and generation of diversity in human pregnancy. Placenta, suppl., 4:1, 1982

62. Ober C, Steck T, van der Ven K et al: MHC class II compatibility in aborted fetuses and term infants of couples with recurrent spontaneous abortion. J Reprod Immunol 25:195, 1993

63. Patel R, Terasaki PI: Significance of the positive crossmatch test in kidney transplantation. N Engl J Med 280:735, 1969

64. Karuppan S, Etriczon BG, Moeller E: Relevance of a positive crossmatch in liver transplantation. Transplant Int 4:18, 1991

65. Katz SM, Kimball PM, Ozaki C et al: Positive pretransplant crossmatches predict early graft loss in liver allograft recipients. Transplantation 57:616, 1994

66. Opelz G, Graver B, Mickey MR, Terasaki PI: Lymphocytotoxic antibody responses to transfusions in potential kidney transplant recipients. Transplantation 32:177, 1981

67. Moore SB, Sterioff S, Pierides AM et al: Transfusion-induced alloimmunization in patients awaiting renal allografts. Vox Sang 47:354, 1984

68. Martin S, Dyer PA, Manos J et al: Effect of sensitization on primary cadaveric renal allograft survival following deliberate unrelated blood transfusions. Clin Transpl 1:300, 1987

69. Scornik JC, Saloman DR, Howard RJ, Pfaff WW: Prevention of transfusion induced broad sensitization in renal transplant candidates. Transplantation 47:617, 1989

70. Kerman RH, Kimball PM, Van Buren CT et al: Influence of race on crossmatch outcome and recipient eligibility for transplantation. Transplantation 53:64, 1992

71. Lazda VA, Gaddis BM, Stormoen AJ et al: Presensitization and frequency of positive crossmatches in black and nonblack renal transplant candidates. Transplant Proc 25:2411, 1993

72. Terasaki PI, Vredevoe DL, Mickey MR: Serotyping for homotransplantation, X. Survival of 196 grafted kidneys subsequent to typing. Transplantation 5: 1057, 1967

73. Takemoto S, Terasaki PI, Cecka JM et al: Survival of nationally shared, HLA-matched kidney transplants from cadaveric donors. N Engl J Med 327:834, 1992

74. Collins GM, Bravo-Sugarman MB, Terasaki PI: Kidney preservation for transplantation. Initial perfusion and 30 hour ice storage. Lancet 2:1219, 1969

75. Opelz G, Wujciak MS: The influence of HLA compatibility on graft survival after heart transplantation. N Engl J Med 330:816, 1994

76. Markus B, Duquesnoy R, Gordon RD et al: Histocompatibility and liver transplant outcome. Transplantation 46:372, 1988

77. Gingrich RD, Ginder GD, Goeken NE et al: Allogeneic marrow grafting with partially mismatched, unrelated marrow donors. Blood 71:1375, 1988

78. Hows JM, Yin JL, Marsh J et al: Histocompatible unrelated volunteer donors compared with HLA nonidentical family donors in marrow transplantation for aplastic anemia and leukemia. Blood 68:1322, 1986

79. Beatty PG, Ash R, Hows JM, McGlave PB: The use of unrelated bone marrow donors in the treatment of patients with chronic myelogenous leukemia: experience of four marrow transplant centers. Bone Marrow Transplant 4:287, 1989

80. Beatty PG, DiBartholmeo P, Storb R et al: Treatment of aplastic anemia with marrow grafts from related donors other than HLA genotypically matched siblings. Clin Transpl 1:117, 1987

81. Champlin RE, Horowitz MM, van Bekkum DW et al: Graft failure following bone marrow transplantation for aplastic anemia: risk factors and treatment results. Blood 73:606, 1989

82. O'Reilly RJ: Allogeneic bone marrow transplantation: current status and future directions. Blood 62: 942, 1983

83. O'Reilly JR, Brochstein J, Collins N: Evaluation of HLA-haplotype disparate parental marrow grafts de-

pleted of T-lymphocytes by differential agglutination with a soybean lectin and E-rosette depletion for treatment of severe combined immundeficiency. Vox Sang 51:81, 1986

84. Beatty PG, Clift RA, Mickelson EM et al: Marrow transplantation from related donors other than HLA-identical siblings. N Engl J Med 313:765, 1985

85. Horowitz MM, Ash RC, Bach FH et al: Outcome of bone marrow transplantation using related donors other than HLA-identical siblings. Bone Marrow Transplant 4:38, 1989

86. Rowlings PA, Horowitz MM, Armitage JO et al: Report from the International Bone Marrow Transplant Registry and the North American Autologous Bone Marrow Transplant Registry. p. 101. In Terasaki PI, Cecka JM (eds): Clinical Transplants 1993. UCLA Tissue Typing Laboratory, Los Angeles, 1994

87. Beatty PG, Dahlberg S, Mickelson EM et al: Probability of finding HLA-matched unrelated morrow donors. Transplantation 45:714, 1988

88. Bradley BA, Hows JM, Gore SM et al: Current status of unrelated-donor bone marrow transplantation. p. 91. In Terasaki PI, Cecka JM (eds): Clinical Transplants 1992. UCLA Tissue Typing Laboratory, Los Angeles, 1993

89. Hansen JA, Petersdorf EW, Choo SY et al: Marrow transplants from HLA partially matched relatives and unrelated donors. Keystone Symp (in press)

90. Fleischauer K, Kernan NA, O'Reilly RJ et al: Bone marrow-allograft rejection by T lymphocytes recognizing a single amino acid difference in B44. N Engl J Med 323:1818, 1990

91. Al-Daccak R, Loisuau P, Rabian C et al: HLA-DR, DQ, and/or DP genotypic mismatches between recipient-donor pairs in unrelated bone marrow transplantation and transplant clinical outcome. Transplantation 50:960, 1990

92. Petersdorf EW, Smith AG, Mickelson EM et al: The role of HLA-DP1 disparity in the development of acute graft-versus-host disease following unrelated donor marrow transplantation. Blood 81:1923, 1993

93. Greenbaum BH: Transfusion-associated graft-versus-host disease: historical perspectives, incidence, and current use of irradiated blood products. J Clin Oncol 9:1889, 1991

94. Leitman SF, Holland PV: Irradiation of blood products. Indications and guidelines. Transfusion 25:293, 1985

95. Petz LD, Calhoun L, Yam P et al: Transfusion-associated graft-versus-host disease in immunocompetent patients: report of a fatal case associated with transfusion of blood from a second-degree relative, and a survey of predisposing factors. Transfusion 33:742, 1993

96. Takahashi K, Juji T, Miyamoto M et al: Analysis of risk factors for post-transfusion graft-versus-host disease in Japan. Lancet 343:700, 1994

97. Ohto H, Yasuda H, Noguchi M, Abe R: Risk of transfusion-associated graft-versus-host disease as a result of directed donations from relatives. Transfusion 32:691, 1992

98. Kanter MH: Transfusion-associated graft-versus-host disease: do transfusions from second-degree relatives pose a greater risk than those from first-degree relatives? Transfusion 32:323, 1992

99. McMilan KD, Johnson RL: HLA homozygosity. The risk of related-donor transfusion-associated graft-versus-host disease. Transfusion Med Rev 7:37, 1993

100. Krushall MS, Alper CA, Awdeh Z, Yunis EJ: HLA homozygous donors and transfusion-associated graft-versus-host disease (letter). N Engl J Med 322:1005, 1990

101. Takahashi K, Juji T, Miyazaki H: Post-transfusion graft-versus-host disease occurring in non-immunosuppressed patients in Japan. Transfusion Sci 12:281, 1991

102. Wernet D, Schnaidt M, Mayer G, Northoff H: Serological screening, using three different test systems of platelet-transfused patients with hematologic-oncologic disorders. Vox Sang 65:108, 1993

103. Dutcher JP, Schiffer CA, Aisner J, Wiernik PH: Long-term follow-up of patients with leukemia receiving platelet transfusion: identification of a large group of patients who do not become alloimmunized. Blood 58:1007, 1981

104. Kickler TS, Braine H, Ness PM: The predictive value of crossmatching platelet transfusions for alloimmunized patients. Transfusion 25:385, 1985

105. O'Connell BA, Lee EJ, Rothko K et al: Selection of histocompatible apheresis donors by crossmatching random donor platelet concentrates. Blood 79:527, 1992

106. Moroff G, Garratty G, Heal JM et al: Selection of platelets for refractory patients by HLA matching and prospective crossmatching. Transfusion 32:633, 1992

107. Friedberg RC, Donnelly SF, Mintz PD: Independent roles for platelet crossmatching and HLA in the selection of platelets for alloimmunized patients. Transfusion 34:215, 1994

108. Oldfather JW, Anderson CB, Phelan DL et al: Prediction of crossmatch outcome in highly sensitized dialysis patients based on the identification of serum HLA antibodies. Transplantation 42:267, 1986

109. Duquesnoy RJ, White LT, Fierst JW et al: Multiscreen analysis of highly sensitized renal dialysis patients for antibodies toward public and private class I HLA determinants. Transplantation 50:427, 1990

110. Clark BD, Leong SW: Crossmatch predictions of highly sensitized patients. p. 435. In Terasaki PI, Cecka JM (eds): Clinical Transplants 1992. UCLA Tissue Typing Laboratory, Los Angeles, 1993

111. Bryant PC, Vayntrub TA, Schrandt HA et al: HLA antibody enhancement by double addition of serum: use in platelet donor selection. Transfusion 32:839, 1992

112. Atlas E, Freedman J, Blanchette V et al: Downregulation of the anti-HLA alloimmune response by variable region-reactive (anti-idiotypic) antibodies in leukemic patients transfused with platelet concentrates. Blood 81:538, 1993

113. Reed E, Hardy M, Benvenisty A et al: Effect of antiidiotypic antibodies to HLA on graft survival in renal allograft recipients. N Engl J Med 317:1450, 1987

114. Sniecinski I, O'Donnell MR, Nowicki B, Hill LR: Prevention of refractoriness and HLA-alloimmunization using filtered blood products. Blood 71:1402, 1988

115. Tiwari J, Terasaki P: HLA and Disease Associations. Springer-Verlag, New York, 1985

116. Schlosstein L, Terasaki PI, Bluestone R, Pearson CM: High association of an HLA antigen, w27, with ankylosing spondylitis. N Engl J Med 288:704, 1973

117. Todd JA: Genetic control of autoimmunity in type 1 diabetes. Immunol Today 11:122, 1990

118. Horn GT, Bugawan TL, Long CM, Ehrlich HA: Allelic sequence variation of the HLA-DQ loci: relationship to serology and to insulin-dependent diabetes susceptibility. Proc Natl Acad Sci USA 85:6012, 1988

119. Barnet AH, Eff C, Leslie RDG, Pyke DA: Diabetes in identical twins: a study of 200 pairs. Diabetologia 20:87, 1981

120. Scott FW: Cow milk and insulin-dependent diabetes mellitus: is there a relationship? Am J Clin Nutr 51:489, 1990

121. Karjalainen J, Martin JM, Knip M et al: A bovine albumin peptide as a possible trigger of insulin-dependent diabetes mellitus. N Engl J Med 327:302, 1992

122. Mueller-Eckhardt C, Kiefel V, Grubert A et al: 348 Cases of suspected neonatal alloimmune thrombocytopenia. Lancet 1:363, 1989

123. Waters A, Murphy M, Hambley H, Nicolaides K: Management of alloimmune thrombocytopenia in the fetus and neonate. p. 155. In Nance SJ (ed): Clinical and Basic Science Aspects of Immunohematology. AABB, Arlington, 1991

124. Reznikoff-Etievant MF, Muller JY, Julien F, Patereau C: An immune response gene linked to MHC in man. Tissue Antigens 22:312, 1983

125. de Waal LP, van Dalen CM, Englefriet CP, von dem Borne AEG: Alloimmunization against the platelet-specific Zw$_a$ antigen resulting in neonatal alloimmune thrombocytopenia or posttransfusion purpura, is associated with the supertypic DRw52 antigen including DR3 and DRw6. Hum Immunol 17:45, 1986

126. Decary F, L'Abbe D, Chartrand P: The immune response to the HPA-1a antigen: association with HLA-DRw52a. Transfusion Med 1:55, 1991

127. Kuijpers RWAM, von dem Borne AEG, Mueller-Eckhardt C et al: Leucine^{33}/proline^{33} substitution in human platelet glycoprotein IIIa determines HLA-DRw52a (Dw24) association of the immune response against HPA-1a (Zw$_a$/Pl^{A1}) and HPA-1b (Zw$_b$/Pl^{A2}). Hum Immunol 34:253, 1992

128. Opelz G, Mytilineos J, Scherer S et al: Analysis of HLA-DR matching in DNA-typed cadaver kidney transplants. Transplantation 55:782, 1993

Chapter 7

Red Cell Transfusion—The Transfusion Trigger

Richard K. Spence and Scott N. Swisher

One of the central problems of transfusion medicine during the last 10 years has been how to decide when a patient requires transfusion and how much to administer in the presence of acute or chronic anemia. The problem has been particularly difficult in dealing with the anemic patient pre- and postoperatively. In the past, before the great increase in concern over transfusion-transmitted diseases, it was thought that there was little reason not to transfuse a patient to the level of 10 g/dl of hemoglobin (Hgb) preoperatively, and this was a common practice.

More recently, with increasingly stringent policies of transfusion avoidance/minimization, this problem has come into increasingly sharp focus. The problem is known generically as the *transfusion trigger*. This chapter reviews the current status of clinical investigations directed to the solution of this problem.

The National Institutes of Health Consensus Development Conference,[1] which was convened in 1988 to address the topic of perioperative red cell transfusion, focused primarily on the risks of transfusion and the need to modify our transfusion practices. It also produced recommendations for a new transfusion trigger that represented an update over the traditional 10/30 rule (i.e., Hgb level of 10 g/dl or hematocrit of 30 percent) that had existed for years. The target, or trigger, Hgb level was lowered to 8 g/dl, and guidelines for transfusion were given that directed attention toward assessment of clinical need and symptoms rather than numbers alone. Since then, much has appeared in the literature that has attempted further to define the transfusion trigger. Investigators have focused on either defining an optimal or minimally acceptable Hgb level, deriving a trigger level from oxygen transport or metabolic variables, or describing the effect of transfusion in specific clinical settings. The following section reviews and summarizes relevant information in an attempt to provide the practicing surgeon with both practical transfusion guidelines and an appreciation of the complexity of the issue (Table 7-1).

CONCEPTUAL BASIS FOR A TRANSFUSION TRIGGER

Two concepts form the basis for the use of Hgb as a transfusion trigger: the optimal Hgb/hematocrit and the minimally acceptable Hgb/hematocrit. For many years, they were considered to be one and the same. At the turn of the century, before blood transfusion was possible, surgeons tolerated low Hgb levels because there was little one could do to change them. The scientific investigation of blood-oxygen delivery mechanics was in its infancy, transfusion was a very young discipline, and little was known about optimal or minimal Hgb levels. By the 1930s, Carrel and Lindberg had demonstrated that isolated organs could survive and grow in an extremely anemic

Table 7-1. Approaches to the Transfusion Trigger

Hemoglobin/hematocrit level
Oxygen delivery/comsumption
Oxygen extraction ratio
Tissue oxygen debt
Lactate levels
Mixed venous oxygen tension/mixed venous oxygen saturation
Patient history
Cardiac status

environment, defining the minimally acceptable Hgb level for sustained life as approximately 3 g/dl.[2] During the ensuing years, as transfusion became a part of everyday practice, the optimal Hgb level was defined clinically. In 1941, less than 10 years after the first blood bank opened, Lundy recommended that all patients with preoperative Hgb levels below 10 g/dl be transfused before surgery, basing this decision on his clinical experience and understanding of oxygen transport dynamics.[3] A few years later, Clark et al.[4] provided some clinical support for the 10 g/dl level when they proposed that patients with the anemia of "chronic shock" would benefit from preoperative transfusion. The 10-g/dl Hgb level, or the 10/30 rule, for transfusion soon became a doctrine that has persisted for many years.

PHYSIOLOGIC STUDIES

Subsequent studies of the role of hematocrit, cardiac function, and oxygen transport have also supported 10-g/dl Hgb concentration as an optimal level. In vitro rheologic studies of diluted blood pumped through glass tubes at constant pressure showed that oxygen delivery (DO_2) peaks at hematocrit levels of 30 percent and then declines with progressive hemodilution.[5] Oxygen transport and survival are maximized at hematocrit levels of 30 to 40 percent in the experimental animal.[6,7] Czer and Shoemaker[8] proposed that an optimal hematocrit of 33 percent was desirable in critically ill patients but emphasized the importance of maintaining adequate blood volume status over red cell transfusion. Their patients had acute blood loss from trauma or had undergone emergency surgery. Hgb levels were confounded in

their analysis by both the nature of the critical illness and volume replacement. Even so, patients with normal compensatory mechanisms tolerated hematocrit levels as low as 18 percent. These investigators subsequently demonstrated maintenance of both cardiac output and oxygen consumption in dogs with hematocrit levels as low as 10 percent as long as volume remained normal.[9]

Several studies designed to establish an optimal Hgb concentration noted that levels lower than 10 g/dl were tolerated by most patients. Clinical studies provide further information regarding the minimally acceptable Hgb level in the form of mortality and morbidity data in anemic surgical patients. Lunn and Elwood[10] described the mortality rate in 1,584 surgical patients who received anesthesia. As the Hgb level decreased, the mortality rate increased. However, this study did not assess or control for other factors that have an effect on survival (i.e., concurrent medical problems or type of surgical procedure). Furthermore, mortality rates were not described for different Hgb levels below 10 g/dl, which make it impossible to assess the effect of severe anemia on the risk of death. In Rawstron's[11] comparison of 145 patients with preoperative Hgb levels less than 10 g/dl with a group of 412 surgical patients with Hgb levels of 10 g/dl or greater, the number of postoperative complications was similar. However, both groups received perioperative transfusions, which may have obscured a difference in operative risk. Outcomes were not stratified for Hgb levels below 10 g/dl. Alexiu et al.[12] compared the postoperative mortality and morbidity rates in patients with gastrointestinal bleeding. Sixty-nine transfused patients were compared with 72 who were resuscitated with large volumes of dextrose and normal saline. In patients not given blood, the mean preoperative hematocrit was 29 percent (range, 16 to 42 percent), dropping by the second postoperative day to a mean of 23.3 percent (range, 10 to 37 percent). There were no deaths, and the complication rate was lower than that in the transfused group. However, the number of patients with Hgb levels below 10 g/dl was not stated, and the presence of potentially confounding medical problems was not included.

Spence's group[13,14] reported two studies of anemia and the risk of postoperative morbidity and death in Jehovah's Witnesses. In the first study of

125 patients who underwent either emergency or elective surgery, the mean preoperative Hgb level in those who died was 7.6 g/dl and was significantly lower than that in the survivors (11.8 g/dl, $P<0.002$). The percentage of patients who died with preoperative Hgb levels between 0 and 6 g/dl was 61.5 percent; between 6.1 and 8 g/dl, 33.3 percent; between 8.1 and 10 g/dl, 0 percent; and greater than 10 g/dl; 7.1 percent. None of the patients with preoperative Hgb levels greater than 8 g/dl and operative blood loss less than 500 ml died (upper 95 percent confidence interval, 5 percent). However, the study was too small to describe precisely the risk of death in patients with Hgb levels between 6 and 10 g/dl. A subsequent analysis of 113 elective operations in 107 Jehovah's Witnesses showed that the mortality rate was zero with Hgb levels as low as 6 g/dl as long as blood loss was kept below 500 ml.

SIGNS AND SYMPTOMS OF ANEMIA

Because humans tolerate anemia surprisingly well, symptoms and signs caused by decreased red cell mass have limited usefulness as transfusion triggers.[15] Symptoms of exertional dyspnea do not appear in the otherwise healthy individual until the Hgb concentration reaches 7 g/dl. Even at this and lower levels, symptoms and signs are variable. Carmel and Shulman[16] reported on the correlation between symptoms and the need for transfusion in 122 medical patients with pernicious anemia. Sixty-two patients with a mean Hgb level of 5.5 g/dl were transfused, but only 34 (55 percent) had symptoms of chest pain, dyspnea at rest, syncope, or lethargy, suggesting an urgent need for additional blood. Muller et al.[17] evaluated the use of a 6-g/dl Hgb or 20 percent hematocrit transfusion trigger in 171 patients (100 children and 71 adults). Adults were more likely to demonstrate hemodynamic symptoms at this level of anemia than children, whose predominant symptoms were dyspnea and impaired consciousness. In spite of the severity of the anemia, only 54 percent of all patients were tachycardic, 32 percent were hypotensive, 27 percent had dyspnea, and 35 percent had impaired levels of consciousness.

Tolerable Versus Optimal Hemoglobin Levels

The above studies show that a Hgb value significantly lower than an optimal level of 10 g/dl is tolerated by many patients. This does not necessarily mean that a *tolerable* Hgb level should automatically be considered an *acceptable* level for use as a transfusion trigger in all patients. Conversely, it is unnecessary and potentially risky to transfuse all patients to an optimal Hgb of 10 g/dl. The main problem with a Hgb-based trigger is its lack of generalizability. Some patients can tolerate very low perioperative Hgb levels; others require supranormal values to survive, depending on diagnosis and clinical condition.

Coronary Artery Disease

The use of a minimally acceptable Hgb level as a transfusion trigger assumes that all patients are able to mobilize compensatory mechanisms equally and adequately. This may not be the case, especially in those patients with underlying coronary artery disease. The heart is more dependent on delivery for its oxygen supply than other organs, extracting approximately one-half of its delivery. When the Hgb level falls, an increase in cardiac output requires a concomitant increase in coronary artery blood flow. In the presence of critical coronary artery stenoses, the heart may be unable to respond sufficiently to meet its oxygen demands, leading to ischemia.[18] Studies in animals with normovolemic hemodilution have shown that the lower limit of cardiac tolerance for anemia lies around 3 to 5 g/dl.[18–20] Under these conditions, coronary blood flow is shifted from the endocardium to the epicardium, thereby placing subendocardial tissue at an increased risk of ischemia. The addition of an experimental coronary stenosis to this model results in depressed cardiac function at Hgb levels of 7 to 10 g/dl.

The minimally acceptable Hgb level may be that beyond which coronary artery blood flow cannot increase enough to meet myocardial oxygen demands, but this level has yet to be defined in useful clinical terms.[6] Robertie and Gravlee[6] recommend accepting a transfusion trigger of 6 g/dl in well compensated patients with no heart disease and no postoperative complications. A higher trigger, 8 g/dl, should be used in patients with stable cardiac disease and when blood loss of approximately 300 ml is expected. Older patients and those with postoperative complications who cannot increase cardiac output to compensate for hemodilution should be transfused when the Hgb level reaches 10 g/dl.

There have been few clinical studies of the effect of coexisting medical conditions on the ability of the heart to compensate for moderate or severe anemia. In a study of mortality rate and Hgb level in Jehovah's Witnesses, preoperative cardiac disease, as defined by the Multifactorial Cardiac Risk Index, appeared to worsen outcome.[14] In a smaller study of 47 patients with more severe anemia (mean Hgb level of 4.6 ± 0.2 g/dl), a history of cardiac, pulmonary, or renal disease had no association with adverse outcome.[21] Two recent reports of an increased incidence of electrocardiographic evidence of myocardial ischemia in postoperative vascular patients with hematocrits below 29 percent are worrisome, although neither accounted for the presence or severity of underlying heart disease.[22,23] All of these studies are limited by small numbers.

Oxygen Transport

Dissatisfaction with the use of either an optimal or a minimally acceptable Hgb-derived transfusion trigger have led to a search for a physiologically defined trigger based on oxygen-derived variables. In most clinical settings, oxygen consumption is relatively independent of Hgb level across a wide range of DO_2 values because of compensations made in oxygen extraction. As DO_2 decreases through a loss of Hgb, oxygen extraction should increase from a baseline of 15 to 25 percent to maintain a constant consumption. Any increase in circulating volume that improves cardiac output will also theoretically improve DO_2 regardless of Hgb level (Table 7-2). However, an improvement in DO_2 does not necessarily lead to an increase in oxygen consumption.

Wilkerson et al.[24] showed, in the exchange-transfused baboon, that oxygen consumption (VO_2) is maintained down to a hematocrit of 4 percent if left atrial pressure is held constant. These animals survived by increasing their oxygen extraction ratio (O_2ER) significantly. The investigators detected a conversion to anaerobic metabolism at a 10 percent hematocrit level, which correlated with an O_2ER of 50 percent, suggesting these two numbers might be useful as transfusion guidelines. Another study found similar results in a study of 12 nontransfused, postsurgical patients with a mean hematocrit of 7.5 percent.[25] The O_2ER was greater than 50 percent in the first 48 hours in nonsurvivors, a level that was significantly higher than that in those who lived. The hematocrit was also lower, 6.0 versus 9.6 percent, in nonsurvivors.

From the formulae for oxygen content and VO_2 (Table 7-2), it would seem that as Hgb levels increase, both DO_2 and VO_2 should increase. Although increasing Hgb level leads to higher DO_2 because of added blood volume, this does not always guarantee a rise in VO_2. Table 7-3 summarizes the major studies that have been conducted to evaluate the effect of transfusion on oxygen transport. These patients run the gamut from postoperative surgical patients[26–35] to those with recent hemorrhage,[30] burns,[31] cardiogenic shock,[33] and sepsis.[26–29,34] Pretransfusion O_2ER ranged between 24 and 48 percent, with the highest values seen in patients with cardiogenic shock. The effect of transfusion to a Hgb level of 10 g/dl on O_2ER was minimal in most patients. Moreover, although transfusion increased DO_2 in all patients, only one-half of the groups showed an increase in VO_2 with the other half showing no change. These differences may be caused by the linear relationship between DO_2 and VO_2 that exists in patients with septic and cardiogenic shock.[29] Regardless of the cause, they point out the lack of precision in the use of a predefined O_2ER or similar variable as a transfusion trigger.

Sepsis and anemia is a particularly lethal combination, as suggested by a study that included 12 septic patients with Hgb levels below 5 g/dl, all of whom died.[21] This corroborates Shoemaker et al.'s[29] finding that survival is decreased in sepsis when VO_2 is compromised, in part because of increased tissue oxygen debt and a resetting of DO_2/VO_2 interactions. Although this work suggests that transfusing to supranormal hematocrits may be beneficial, trans-

Table 7-2. Hemoglobin and Oxygen Interactions

Cardiac Output (CO) = Stroke Volume (SV) × Heart Rate (HR)

Oxygen Content (CaO_2) = (1.39 × SO_2 × Hgb + 0.003 × PO_2) × 10 ml O_2/L, where SO_2 = oxygen saturation and Hgb = hemoglobin concentration in grams per deciliter.

Oxygen Delivery (DO_2) = CO × CaO_2 ml O_2/min

Oxygen Consumption (VO_2) = CO × (CaO_2 − CvO_2) ml O_2/min

Abbreviation: CvO_2, venous oxygen content

Table 7-3. Effect of Transfusion in Critically Ill Patients

Author	Number	Diagnosis	DO$_2$ Pre	DO$_2$ Post	VO$_2$ Pre	VO$_2$ Post	O$_2$ER Pre	O$_2$ER Post	H/H Pre	H/H Post
McCormick et al.[30]	14	Blood loss	494	599	143	140	30	24	27.9	36.7
Dietrich et al.[32]	32	19 sepsis; 14 cardioshock; 3 other	410	525	119	118	30.8	23.7	8.3	10.5
Babineau et al.[26]	30	Postoperative	401	433	117	115	31	28	9.4	10.4
Marino and Krasner[27]	20	Postoperative	281	329	109	110	39	33	7.1	8.6
Robbins et al.[28]	58	ICU	331	430	115	141	36	35	8.75	
Steffes et al.[33]	21	Sepsis	532	634	145	160	27	25	9.3	10.7
Gore et al.[31]	5	Burn	882	1,060	199	206	24	20	7.5	10.5
Shoemaker et al.[29]	69	Sepsis	467	529	132	154	30	29	27.6	32.0
Shoemaker et al.[29]	132	ICU	470	562	132	156	28	28		

Abbreviations: DO$_2$, oxygen delivery; VO$_2$, oxygen consumption; O$_2$ER, oxygen extraction ratio; H/H hemoglobin/hematocrit; ICU, intensive care unit.

fusion does not always turn the tide in sepsis (Table 7-3). It may be that giving additional blood to the compromised, septic patient to improve DO$_2$ cannot compensate alone for the increased tissue oxygen debt.

METABOLIC STUDIES

Other approaches to define the transfusion trigger in metabolic terms have also had limited success. Bihari and Tinker[35] showed that patients with the adult respiratory distress syndrome may have a hidden oxygen debt unrelated to Hgb level. They used prostacyclin administration to define DO$_2$/VO$_2$ relationships in the hope of identifying those patients who would benefit from additional oxygen, but this test has not gained widespread use. Lactate levels have not been helpful in defining transfusion need. Astiz et al.[36] found no correlation between lactate level and DO$_2$ in 100 patients with either an acute myocardial infarction or sepsis. The role of mixed venous oxygen tension and mixed venous oxygen saturation as triggers have yet to be defined.

THE CHRONICALLY ANEMIC PATIENT

Many of the same observations discussed in relation to the surgical, septic, or shocked patient also apply to the decision about a transfusion regimen for the chronically anemic patient (see Ch. 19). None of the easily available laboratory measurements are of great value in dealing with this problem. The objective should be to establish a program of chronic transfusion that balances the risks of transfusion with the patient's symptoms and lifestyle needs. In addition to the risks of transmissible infection, the chronically transfused patient has the additional hazard of iron overload. This is particularly significant in the case of the congenital hemolytic anemias in which transfusion may be required at an early age in amounts sufficient to support growth and development.

The patient's age, work requirements, comorbid conditions, and ability to tolerate symptoms of anemia are factors that must be weighed in developing a program of chronic transfusion. The patient's symptoms must be evaluated carefully because it has been shown that the common symptoms of fatigue, weakness, and lassitude are poorly correlated with Hgb levels. Rather, symptoms of effort intolerance or limitation; cardiovascular and pulmonary functional symptoms; or claudication, irritability, or somnolence are more easily evaluated but may not appear until the patient has become very anemic. In most cases, a Hgb level that avoids these symptoms is desirable.

The decision about the amount of chronic transfusion should be made in discussion with a fully informed patient who understands the risks of both over- and undertransfusion. Today's patients are highly risk aversive in regard to transfusion therapy; this makes their participation in the decision mandatory. The patient's probable life expectancy based on the prognosis of an underlying disease may also be a factor in allowing a patient to make a rational decision about acceptance of chronic transfusion.

Programs of chronic transfusion should be designed around the predictable and scheduled need for transfusion rather than on the basis of Hgb monitoring and transfusion when a value thought to be too low is encountered. This results in some degree of leveling of the patient's average Hgb concentration and saves the patient repeated trips to a laboratory for Hgb determinations before transfusion.

The level of Hgb to be maintained by transfusion is usually found to be between a low of 7 g/dl pretransfusion and a high of 10 g/dl after transfusion among adults. The frequency of transfusion and the amount given at each session are the variables of the program. If two units of red cells are required about every 2 weeks in an adult to maintain a Hgb level in this range, it may be that the patient is producing few or no red cells. Transfusion requirements higher that this raise the possibility of coexisting blood loss or a hemolytic state, questions that should be investigated before a program of chronic transfusion is initiated.

CONCLUSIONS

From this analysis of the problems of defining a transfusion trigger, one can conclude that there are inadequate data to recommend a specific transfusion trigger based on either Hgb level or oxygen transport variables. The concept of a transfusion trigger or indeed any algorithmic approach to the decision to transfuse and how much to administer should probably be abandoned, at least for the present. It is possible that further study of the complex problem of the anemic state superimposed on a wide variety of pathophysiologic conditions may yield at least some more objective guidelines for dealing with this problem.

Neither optimal nor minimally acceptable Hgb levels are useful as a trigger because both frequently underestimate and overestimate transfusion need. Clinical symptoms of cardiac compromise or decreased oxygen delivery do not correlate well with Hgb levels. Oxygen transport derived transfusion triggers such as O_2ER are both organ and setting specific, with no consistent correlation with either Hgb level or red cell transfusion, and significant changes appear late in the clinical course. In the critically ill patient in whom invasive monitoring is justifiable, measurements of oxygen transport variables may be useful. The decision to transfuse should be related to a clinical assessment of the specific patient's needs and condition. The presence of cardiac, pulmonary, and atherosclerotic disease processes should be assessed and quantified when possible. Patients with coronary artery disease and pulmonary hypoxia will most likely require higher perioperative Hgb levels than do those with normal hearts and lungs to avoid ischemia and undue cardiac stress.

Furthermore, one must also recognize that the degree of anemia that justifies transfusion constantly changes because indications for transfusion should always be based on an analysis of the risks versus the benefits. As the safety of the blood supply changes, so do the indications for transfusion. The optimal transfusion trigger in 1983 to 1984 was much different than it is at present because of the extraordinary increases in the safety of the blood supply caused by the development and implementation of tests for infectious diseases and improved donor screening procedures. At present, there is increasing uneasiness that restrictive transfusion policies based on an exaggerated concern regarding the dangers of transfusion may result in significant undertransfusion of certain patients.

In general, nothing seems capable of replacing the clinical judgment of an experienced physician or surgeon who can weigh and evaluate all of the available data in arriving at the decision to transfuse.

REFERENCES

1. Perioperative red cell transfusion. NIH Consensus Development Conference Statement. 7:1, 1988
2. Diamond LK: A history of blood transfusion. p. 659. In Wintrobe MM (ed): Blood, Pure and Eloquent. McGraw-Hill, New York, 1908
3. Adams RC, Lundy JS: Anesthesia in cases of poor surgical risk. Some suggestions for decreasing the risk. Surg Gynecol Obstet 74:1011, 1942
4. Clark JH, Nelson W, Lyons C et al: Chronic shock: the

problem of reduced blood volume in the chronically ill patient. Ann Surg 125:618, 1947

5. Stehling L, Zauder HL: Acute normovolemic hemodilution. Transfusion 31:857, 1991

6. Robertie PG, Gravlee GP: Safe limits of hemodilution and recommendations for erythrocyte transfusion. Int Anesthesiol Clin 28:197, 1990

7. Chapler CK, Cain SM: The physiologic reserve in oxygen carrying capacity: studies in experimental hemodilution. Can J Physiol Pharmacol 64:7, 1986

8. Czer LSC, Shoemaker WC: Optimal hematocrit value in critically ill postoperative patients. Surg Gynecol Obstet 147:363, 1978

9. Schwarz S, Frantz RA, Shoemaker WC: Sequential hemodynamic and oxygen transport responses in hypovolemia, anemia, and hypoxia. Am J Physiol 241: HH64, 1981

10. Lunn JN, Elwood PC: Anemia and surgery. BMJ 3:71, 1970

11. Rawstron ER: Anemia and surgery. A retrospective clinical study. Aust N Z J Surg 39:425, 1970

12. Alexiu O, Mircea N, Balaban M et al: Gastrointestinal hemorrhage from peptic ulcer. An evaluation of bloodless transfusion and early surgery. Anaesthesia 30:609, 1975

13. Spence RK, Carson JA, Poses R et al: Elective surgery without transfusion: influence of preoperative hemoglobin level and blood loss on mortality. Am J Surg 59:320, 1990

14. Carson JL, Spence RK, Poses RM et al: Severity of anemia and operative mortality and morbidity. Lancet 2:727, 1988

15. Linman JW: Physiologic and pathophysiologic effects of anemia. N Engl J Med 279:812, 1968

16. Carmel R, Shulman IA: Blood transfusion in medically treatable chronic anemia. Pernicious anemia as a model for transfusion overuse. Arch Pathol Lab Med 113:995, 1989

17. Muller G, N'tita I, Nyst M et al: Application of blood transfusion guidelines in a major hospital of Kinshasa, Zaire. AIDS 6:431, 1992

18. Buckberg G, Brazier J: Coronary blood flow and cardiac function during hemodilution. Bibl Haematol 41: 173, 1974

19. Geha AS, Baue AE: Graded coronary stenosis and coronary flow during acute normovolemic anemia. World J Surg 2:645, 1978

20. Wilkerson DK, Rosen AL, Sehgal LR et al: Limits of cardiac compensation in anemic baboons. Surgery 103:665, 1988

21. Spence RK, Costabile JP, Young GS et al: Is hemoglobin level alone a reliable predictor of outcome in the severely anemic patient? Am Surg 58:92, 1992

22. Nelson AH, Fleisher LA, Rosenbaum SH: The relationship between postoperative anemia and cardiac morbidity in high risk vascular patients in the intensive care unit. Crit Care Med 21:860, 1993

23. Christopherson R, Frank S, Norris E et al: Low postoperative hematocrit is associated with cardiac ischemia in high-risk patients, abstracted. Anesthesiology 75: A99, 1991

24. Wilkerson DK, Rosen AL, Gould SA et al: Oxygen extraction ratio: a valid indicator of myocardial metabolism in anemia. J Surg Res 42:629, 1987

25. Atabek U, Alvarez R, Pello MJ et al: Erythropoietin accelerates hematocrit recovery in severe post-surgical anemia. Am Surg 61:74, 1995

26. Babineau TJ, Dzik WH, Borlase BC et al: Reevaluation of current transfusion practices in surgical intensive care units. Am J Surg 164:22, 1992

27. Marino PL, Krasner J: An interpretive computer program for analyzing hemodynamic problems in the ICU. Crit Care Med 12:601, 1981

28. Robbins J, Keating K, Orlando R, III et al: Effects of blood transfusion on oxygen consumption and oxygen delivery in critically ill surgical patients, abstracted. Crit Care Med, Suppl., 20:S113, 1992

29. Shoemaker WC, Appel PL, Kram HB: Tissue oxygen debt as determinant of lethal and non-lethal postoperative organ failure. Crit Care Med 16:1117, 1988

30. McCormick M, Feustel PJ, Newell JC et al: Effect of cardiac index and hematocrit changes in oxygen consumption in resuscitated patients. J Surg Res 44:499, 1988

31. Gore DC, DeMaria EJ, Reines HD: Elevations in red blood cell mass reduce cardiac index without altering the oxygen consumption in severely burned patients. Surg Forum XLII:721, 1991

32. Dietrich KA, Conrad SA, Cullen AH et al: Cardiovascular and metabolic response to red blood cell transfusion in critically ill volume-resuscitated nonsurgical patients. Crit Care Med 18:940, 1990

33. Steffes CP, Bender JS, Levison MA: Blood transfusion and oxygen consumption in surgical sepsis. Crit Care Med 19:512, 1991

34. Edwards JD: Oxygen transport in cardiogenic and septic shock. Crit Care Med 19:658, 1991

35. Bihari DJ, Tinker J: The therapeutic value of prostaglandins in multiple organ failure associated with sepsis. Intensive Care Med 15:2, 1988

36. Astiz ME, Rackow EC, Falk JL et al: Oxygen delivery and consumption in patients with hyperdynamic septic shock. Crit Care Med 15:26, 1987

Chapter 8

The Coagulation Cascade and Coagulation Factor Replacement in Hemophilia

Jonathan C. Goldsmith

Hemophilia is an uncommon inherited bleeding disorder that poses significant and often unpredictable health problems for those affected. Spontaneous and post-traumatic bleeding can lead to substantial morbidity and mortality rates. Time lost from school and work and the high cost of factor replacement therapy have substantial and sometimes devastating economic impact on patients and families. Care for patients with hemophilia has largely been consolidated in the United States and delivered by multidisciplinary health care teams at hemophilia treatment center (HTC) sites partially funded by the Maternal and Child Health Bureau. Cost-effective care through the use of physician extenders and prevention strategies at these HTCs has produced real gains in school attendance and employment.

COMPONENTS OF COAGULATION

Hemostasis is the result of a complex interplay of coagulation factors and inhibitors, blood platelets, the vessel wall, and its supporting structures. Each of these components is important in maintaining vascular integrity and achieving prompt cessation of bleeding after vascular injury. In what has been accepted as the traditional "cascade" hypothesis of blood coagulation, precursor forms of coagulation factors are sequentially activated to serine ester-ases.[1,2] These enzymes in turn activate other coagulation factors. A small signal is amplified by this series of enzymatic reactions. The result is the generation of milligrams of fibrin clot at a site initiated by a few micrograms of factor XIIa. Factors VIII or IX, which are deficient in hemophilia A or B, respectively, are critical intermediaries in the postulated intrinsic pathway of coagulation. Their absence or dysfunction leads to delayed or insufficient fibrin formation. This is associated with an inadequate blood clot and prolonged bleeding or delayed wound healing. Factors VIII and IX are also important in more recently proposed modifications of the cascade theory (Fig. 8-1).

In one revision of the cascade, hemostasis is initiated by factor VIIa.[3] Small amounts of factor Xa are then generated. In addition, factor VIIa crosses over to the "intrinsic pathway" and is able to produce small amounts of factor IXa. The reaction is damped off by the tissue factor pathway inhibitor unless adequate thrombin is produced. In the latter event, thrombin activates factor XI to XIa, which proceeds by way of the traditional intrinsic pathway, producing larger amounts of factor IXa. These quantities of factor IXa push the process forward. In both the traditional and revised mechanisms, thrombin also modifies factor VIII to an active form, accelerating the kinetics 100-fold.

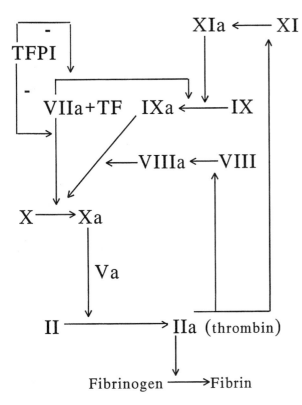

Fig. 8-1. Modified cascade of blood coagulation. Factor VIIa plays a central role in initiating coagulation in this model. Tissue factor pathway inhibitor (TFPI) plays a retarding role in reducing the influence of factor VIIa. (Modified from Broze and Gailani,[3] with permission.)

All of these reactions could theoretically take place in solution in a fluid phase. However, a more practical explanation suggests that phospholipid surfaces serve as a concentrating mechanism to bring sufficient quantities of coagulation factors together, permitting favorable reaction kinetics.[4] Surfaces are provided by blood platelets and cellular components of the vessel wall. Plasminogen, the fibrinolytic enzyme, is deposited concurrently at the time of fibrin formation. In this way, orderly clot dissolution is ensured when plasminogen is activated to plasmin. If the initial fibrin clot is too small, early dissolution occurs, and bleeding starts again.

Clinically, this last situation is manifest in hemophilia. Bleeding continues when too little clot forms initially or when the inadequate clot lyses prematurely. Early clot dissolution is seen in mild hemo-

philia and may be manifest by broad scar formation or marked by wound infections. The poor scarring in hemophilia can be distinguished from keloid formation in which there is a hypertrophic response. Historically, the diagnosis of hemophilia can be suspected in male patients with prolonged bleeding after trauma or surgery or with soft tissue or joint hemorrhages without remembered preceding injuries. There are also age-related patterns of bleeding that are helpful in establishing the diagnosis.

CLINICAL ASPECTS OF FACTORS VIII AND IX DEFICIENCIES

Uncomplicated vaginal delivery is not associated with hemorrhagic risk in the hemophilic neonate. The risk of intracranial hemorrhage is no greater than that for other term infants.[5] Infusions of factor VIII-containing materials are therefore almost never required after childbirth. In contrast, bleeding after circumcision is a common presenting symptom for infants with unsuspected hemophilia. As is typical for hemophilia, bleeding may not be profuse. However, hemorrhage continues for days and often requires red cell transfusion before the diagnosis is substantiated. These infants may also sustain prolonged bleeding from heel sticks for state-required neonatal screening tests if prolonged pressure is not applied to puncture sites. Significant soft tissue arm hemorrhages with potential neurovascular compromise can occur when well intentioned providers attempt to draw plasma samples to establish the diagnosis of hemophilia in infancy. These invasive procedures are not indicated in the child without bleeding complications. If chorionic villous sampling has been performed, verifying the existence of a hemophilic fetus, venipuncture for confirmation of the diagnosis can be delayed for several months until it is technically easier to perform. A citrated plasma sample collected from the umbilical vein at birth may also be useful in confirming the diagnosis. However, faulty technique in blood drawing and handling in the busy obstetric suite often makes these specimens less valuable.

Delayed loss of the umbilical stump may be indicative of factor XIII deficiency or dysfibrinogenemia. However, hemophiliac patients may also manifest this finding. During infancy, bleeding may be nonexistent, although bruises at sites where the boy is held may occur. These are most common on the chest and reflect caretaker thumb "imprints." Immunizations can be safely administered if a subcutaneous technique is used. Hepatitis B immunization is often initiated before hospital discharge after delivery. At the toddler stage, falls are common, and the bleeding sites reflect the affected anatomic areas. Hemorrhages into the buttocks and perineum can be large with scrotal extension. Double diapering can decrease the frequency and severity of these types of hemorrhages. Soft tissue and muscle bleeding also occurs into the legs and thighs. Intracranial hemorrhage is a risk. Use of a sponge rubber-type helmet can decrease the number of serious head bleeds. Dental eruption and frenulum tears may also bring a toddler to medical attention.

After the boy establishes his gait pattern and accomplishes running and climbing, intra-articular bleeding becomes predominant. The knees, elbows, and ankles are affected in this order of frequency. Hip and shoulder bleeds are also seen and can be more refractory to treatment because of the large size of the joint capsule. Although a few boys have symmetric bleeding, most do not. In some, a target joint develops, with the joint accounting for 80 percent of the boy's bleeding episodes. There is evidence that the first joint hemorrhage, even if promptly treated with clotting factor, initiates a process that can progress over many years to joint destruction with accompanying pain and deformity.[6] These observations have prompted many physician providers to advocate a prophylactic approach to hemophilia to prevent the initial joint hemorrhage and to convert the severe hemophiliac patient to one at decreased risk for spontaneous bleeding.[7]

Adolescents typically take on increased responsibility for recognition of bleeds and their prompt treatment. Adolescents also test limits and may expose themselves to considerable danger from bleeding through risk-taking activities such as skate boarding and motor bike riding. In addition to hemarthroses, adolescents may also encounter soft tissue bleeding and internal bleeding such as hematuria. By young adulthood, nearly all hemophiliac patients reach an age of discretion and modify their behavior patterns to avoid post-traumatic hemorrhage. Most require vocational counseling interventions to find career choices that are consistent with their present and future physical abilities. Before the advent of human immunodeficiency virus (HIV) infection, the projected life span for a hemophiliac patient was in excess of 50 years. Therefore, long-term planning is entirely appropriate in the current era of virus-safe clotting factor concentrates.

LABORATORY AND GENETIC PERSPECTIVES

Manifestations of the clinical aspects of hemophilia can be divided into three broad categories. Approximately 60 percent of hemophiliac patients are severely affected with spontaneous soft tissue and intra-articular hemorrhages. By adulthood, most of these men have one or more joints affected by an arthritic process secondary to repeated intra-articular bleeding. Fifteen percent of hemophiliac patients are moderately affected. This group has occasional spontaneous, but predictable, post-traumatic bleeding. It is normative for those moderately affected to have one arthritic joint by adulthood. The remaining 25 percent of patients are mildly affected. Unless discovered in family studies, many of these individuals escape detection until confronted by serious trauma or surgery in adulthood. They do not have spontaneous bleeding.

In the early 1950s, hemophilia A was distinguished from hemophilia B through the use of plasma mixing experiments in which blood specimens from one hemophiliac patient corrected the clotting defect in blood samples from another.[8]

Prevalence studies indicate that there are approximately four to five individuals with hemophilia A for every one affected by hemophilia B, and a total of approximately 15,500 hemophiliac patients in the United States.[9] One hemophilic birth can be anticipated for every 7,500 male births.

Traits for hemophilia A and B are inherited in an X-linked recessive manner. Approximately one-third of all hemophilia cases are the result of a spontaneous mutation. However, once established in a family, the subsequent generations are affected. All of the daughters of a hemophiliac patient are obligate carriers, and one-half of the sons of these carrier daughters express the clinical disorder. In similar fashion, the gene for hemophilia breeds true. This means that the severity of the disorder is the same

Table 8-1. Laboratory Correlation With the Clinical Severity of Hemophilia

Clinical Severity	Plasma Clotting Factor Level	Spontaneous Bleeding	Post-Traumatic Postsurgical Bleeding
Severe	<1%	Common (weekly)	Predictable
Moderate	1–5%	Occasional (monthly)	Predictable
Mild	>5–50%	Infrequent (yearly)	Predictable

in all affected male offspring. The Human Genome Project has identified the location of the genes for hemophilia A and B. The factor IX gene is carried on the distal tip of the long arm of the X chromosome.[10] The factor VIII gene is more proximal. Although missense and nonsense mutations account for many cases of hemophilia A, a more recently described inversion abnormality known as "tip-flip" may genetically explain up to 50 percent of cases.[11]

Laboratory assessment of hemophilia is based on screening tests of coagulation and confirmation by specific factor assays. Typically, a severe hemophiliac patient has a normal prothrombin time, fibrinogen determination, and platelet count. The partial thromboplastin time (PTT) is prolonged. Specific assays for factor VIII or IX with known congenitally deficient or immunologically depleted plasmas or chromogenic assays confirm the diagnosis and the severity.[12] Depending on the assay reagents, some mild hemophiliac patients may have normal PTTs. If the family and clinical history are supportive, specific factor assays are still indicated. Laboratory evaluation and clinical features tend to parallel each other. Factor VIII or IX levels less than 1 percent of normal (less than 0.01 units/ml) correlate with severe bleeding manifestations. Levels of 1 percent to less than 5 percent (0.01 to less than 0.05 units/ml) are found in those moderately affected, and factor levels of 5 to 50 percent (0.05 to 0.50 units/ml) are diagnostic of mild disease (Table 8-1).

THERAPEUTIC APPROACHES

Treatment of bleeding episodes may include conservative measures. Ice packs, rest, and splinting all play important adjuvant roles in the management of musculoskeletal and joint hemorrhages. However, factor replacement represents the standard of care. Only with temporary correction of the clotting defect can serious spontaneous bleeding be stopped or prevented, as in surgical situations.

Whole blood was the first "component" used to correct the clotting defect in hemophilia. Although whole blood supplied red cells lost in cases of external hemorrhage, it contained small amounts of missing clotting factors on a volume basis. The use of centrifugation in the early 1950s to separate plasma from cellular constituents of blood produced a transfusion material approximately twice as concentrated. The infusion of 15 to 20 ml/kg body weight was possible, especially with the concurrent use of diuretic agents. Circulating levels of factor VIII approaching 20 percent and factor IX around 10 percent could be achieved. These levels were not adequate for elective surgical interventions, but could be lifesaving in the event of central nervous system hemorrhage.

In the mid-1960s, cryoprecipitate was discovered and partly characterized.[13] If a frozen unit of plasma was thawed at 4°C, a milky precipitate remained. The precipitate could then be separated from the remainder of the plasma unit by centrifugation or siphoning. On warming to room temperature, the precipitate re-entered solution. This cryoprecipitate contained approximately 6 units/ml of factor VIII when meticulously prepared. Unfortunately, factor IX was not similarly concentrated. Cryoprecipitate concentrated factor VIII sufficiently to allow the performance of elective dental and orthopedic procedures. If stored at −18°C, cryoprecipitate would retain its factor VIII activity for up to 1 year. A few patients and families were allowed to keep cryoprecipitate in their home freezers in an early form of medically supervised home therapy.

Lyophilized clotting factor concentrates were licensed in the mid-1960s in the United States. Plasma pools collected from up to 20,000 donors represented the starting material for the purification process. Cohn fractionation procedures were used to create factor-enriched portions.[14] Ion-exchange chromatography and precipitation with neutral amino acids completed the process for factor VIII concentrates. Factor IX-rich concentrates were purified from Cohn factions with either ion-exchange chromatography or adsorption and elution from insoluble barium or calcium salts.[8] The resultant concentrates had low specific activities (less than 0.1 units/mg for factor VIII and less than 5 units/mg for factor IX), with albumin and plasma globulins as major contaminants. Low specific activities and high fibrinogen content, which many thought interfered with hemostasis, prompted the development of factor VIII concentrates of higher purity in the 1970s and early 1980s. Still, the concentrates were fairly crude.

In the early 1980s, murine monoclonal antibodies to von Willebrand factor and to antihemophilic factor (factor VIII:C) were developed.[15] In 1987, the first commercially prepared factor VIII concentrate made using these monoclonal antibody technologies was introduced for clinical use in the United States.[16,17] A second concentrate was licensed in early 1988. These high-purity factor VIII concentrates had specific activities of 2,000 to 3,000 units/mg at the end of purification. In the commercial container, the specific activity was 10 to 15 units/mg after the addition of human albumin as a stabilizer.

At the time of licensure of monoclonal antibody-purified factor VIII concentrates, phase I studies of recombinant DNA-produced factor VIII (r-AHF) were being conducted.[18] In subsequent phase II/III studies scores of previously treated and previously untreated patients gained access to r-AHF. The Food and Drug Administration granted licensure in 1992 and early 1993 to the two U.S. manufacturers.[19,20] One r-AHF is produced by coexpression of the von Willebrand factor (VWF) gene along with the factor VIII:C gene in a Chinese hamster ovary cell line system. Yield of factor VIII:C is enhanced through diminished degradation by the presence of VWF. The second r-AHF uses a baby hamster kidney cell line transfected solely with the factor VIII:C gene. There are carbohydrate differences between the two products, but efficacy in trials has been comparable. Ongoing quality control measures ensure that no animal viral agents are contained in the final product.

Factor IX-rich concentrates were also licensed in the 1960s. These prothrombin complex concentrates (PCCs) were subsequently shown to have thrombogenic properties.[21] Serious, life-threatening, deadly thromboses occurred in patients with hemophilia B. Thrombotic risk was increased by frequent dosing and by use in the setting of impaired (e.g., neonates or liver disease) or overwhelmed (e.g., perioperative) natural anticoagulant mechanisms. Activated coagulation factors in the PCCs and phospholipid contaminants probably account for the thrombotic complications.[22,23] The situation was recognized by the International Congress on Thrombosis and Hemostasis in its recommendation to add one unit of heparin to each milliliter of infused PCCs.[24] In 1991, the first coagulation factor IX concentrate was licensed. Laboratory testing in animal models revealed a two or more log reduction in thrombosis risk per administered dose.[25] Trials in surgery confirmed the clinical utility of coagulation factor IX concentrates and the absence of in vivo markers of hypercoagulability in participating patients.[26] Prothrombin and factor VII were virtually absent from the first licensed coagulation factor IX, although there was approximately 1 unit of factor X for every 10 units of factor IX. Subsequently, this product was further refined by repeating the affinity chromatography step. The resulting coagulation factor IX concentrate had a specific activity of nearly 200 units/mg. A second coagulation factor IX was purified with murine monoclonal antibody affinity chromatography. The specific activity of this factor IX exceeded 150 units/mg.[27]

INHIBITORS TO COAGULATION FACTORS

Up to 35 percent of patients with severe hemophilia A have circulating anticoagulants develop to factor VIII.[28-30] These inhibitors make replacement therapy difficult and demand individualized treatment plans. The strength of inhibitors is quantified with a 2-hour incubation with normal pooled plasma. Loss of 50 percent of the thrombin-generating activity after this incubation is defined as one Bethesda unit.[31] Approximately one-quarter of individuals with inhibitors have antibodies of a low responding variety. These are less than 10 Bethesda units and do not increase in an anamnestic fashion after factor VIII infusions. As a result, treatment for these patients usually consists of larger doses of human factor VIII, often given by continuous infusion.[32] There are two classes of licensed products designed primarily for the treatment of the other three-quarters of patients with high responding inhibitors.

The first of these is a variant of PCC in which there has been intentional, but restricted, activation of the contained clotting factors.[33,34] These activated factors can bypass pathways that require the participation of factor VIII. Sufficient quantities of thrombin are generated to produce hemostasis. When used frequently, every 6 to 8 hours, or in very large doses, greater than 100 factor IX units/kg body weight, inappropriate thrombosis can occur. A sensitive test for excessive thrombin generation such as the plasma protamine precipitation test or D-D dimer analysis should be performed 30 minutes after an infusion of these activated PCCs. If the result is abnormal, the dosing interval must be extended. A shortening of the prothrombin time is routinely encountered after infusions of these products and does not necessarily require a dosing interval adjustment. Factor IX complex concentrates are also useful but are less predictably effective than the activated PCCs.

The second class of products for the treatment of patients with factor VIII inhibitors is represented by porcine factor VIII.[35] Antihuman factor VIII antibodies tend to be species specific. Porcine factor VIII therefore circulates after infusion and can elude inactivation by the inhibitors. With the use of polyelectrolyte fractionation, a highly purified porcine factor VIII is generated from blood recovered from slaughtered animals. The resultant factor VIII has a high specific activity, 25 units/mg. In contrast to other clotting factor concentrates that are stored at 4°C, porcine factor VIII must be stored at −18°C to ensure potency. Recombinant factor VII/VIIa, an investigational agent, may be a third class of agents that could also be useful in the 2 to 3 percent of patients with hemophilia B in whom inhibitors develop to factor IX in addition to those with factor VIII inhibitors.[36]

IMPROVING CLOTTING FACTOR SAFETY

As a direct result of the acquired immunodeficiency syndrome (AIDS) epidemic, which affected more than 40 percent of those with hemophilia, viral inactivation became a top-agenda item. Improved screening of donor plasma by HIV-1 and -2 antibody, hepatitis C antibody, and alanine transaminase levels has substantially reduced the potential viral burden. Substantial gains have also been made in the purification of clotting factor concentrates, which reduced viral contamination from plasma pools. Monoclonal antibody purification techniques remove up to 10^9 viral particles/μl of plasma through partitioning. In addition, several techniques were developed to achieve sterilization of lyophilized concentrates.

Both heating and detergent solvent techniques eliminate HIV-1. In 1983, a dry heat treatment process (60°C for 60 hours) was licensed as a way to reduce hepatitis transmission. Although unsuccessful for hepatitis, the process eventually was validated for HIV elimination.[37] Other dry heat treatments were used for factor IX complex concentrates ranging from 60°C for 144 hours to 80°C for 72 hours. Some less intense dry heating processes were inadequate, and HIV infections were not prevented. Other methods for viral inactivation were developed based on the principle that viral contaminants are more sensitive to physical inactivation in hydrated forms. Heating for 20 hours at 60°C in n-heptane rendered HIV, but not hepatitis viruses, noninfectious.

A more successful process is a modification of pasteurization or heating for 10 hours at 60°C in a liquid state. This technique appears to render clotting factor concentrates noninfectious for HIV and hepatotrophic viral agents.[38] Another effective method is solvent detergent treatment with either tri-N-butyl phosphate (TNBP)-polysorbate 80 or TNBP-Triton-X100, which inactivates lipid-enveloped viral agents, including HIV, hepatitis B, and hepatitis C. Nonenveloped agents such as hepatitis A and parvovirus are not inactivated by the process.[39] One of the licensed coagulation factor IX concentrates uses a unique process for viral inactivation. Viral inactivation is attained through the used of sodium thiocyanate treatment and partitioning by murine monoclonal antibody purification and ultrafiltration (Tables 8-2 and 8-3).

MEDICAL MANAGEMENT OF HEMOPHILIA

Principles of Coagulation Factor Replacement

The central concept in replacement therapy in hemophilia is early infusion of a sufficient amount of clotting factor to stop the bleeding. Follow-up infu-

Table 8-2. Currently Available Factor VIII Products

Product Name	Manufacturer	Method of Viral Inactivation	Hepatitis Safety Studies in Humans With this Product
Intermediate- and high-purity factor VIII products derived from human plasma			
Profilate OSD	Alpha	Solvent-detergent (TNBP and polysorbate 80)	No
Koate-HP	Miles	Solvent-detergent (TNBP and polysorbate 80) 27°C, 6 hr	No
New York Blood Center FVIII-SD	New York Blood Center	Solvent-detergent (TNBP and cholate) ≥24°C, 6 hr	Yes
Humate P	Behringwerke (Distributed by Armour)	Heated in solution (pasteurized), 60°C 10 hr	Yes
Immunoaffinity purified factor VIII products (ultrapure) derived from human plasma			
Monoclate P	Armour	Pasteurized (60°C, 10 hr)	Yes
Hemofil M	Baxter-Hyland	Solvent-detergent (TNBP/Triton-X100) ≥25°C, ≥10 hr	Yes
Coagulation FVIII Method M	Manufactured by Baxter-Hyland for American Red Cross	Solvent-detergent (TNBP/Triton-X100) ≥25°C, ≥10 hr	No
Recombinant DNA-produced factor VIII products			
Recombinate	Baxter-Hyland	None	Yes
Bioclate	Armour	None	Yes
Kogenate	Miles	None	Yes
Helixate	Armour	None	Yes
Porcine factor VIII			
Hyate C	Porton Products	None	Yes

Abbreviation: TNBP, tri(n-butyl) phosphate.

Table 8-3. Currently Available Factor IX Products

Product Name	Manufacturer	Method of Viral Inactivation	Hepatitis Safety Studies in Humans With this Product
Coagulation factor IX			
AlphaNine-SD	Alpha	Solvent-detergent TNBP/Polysorbate 80 24–30°C, ≥6 hr	No
Mononine	Armour	Ultrafiltration sodium thiocyanate	Yes
Factor IX complex concentrates			
Konyne 80	Miles	Dry heat, 80°C 72 hr	No
Proplex T	Baxter-Hyland	Dry heat, 68°C 144 hr	No
Profilnine HT (wet method)	Alpha	Heated in N-heptane solution 60°C, 20 hr	No
Bebulin	Immuno	Vapor heated (10 hr, 60°C, 1,190 mbar + 1 hr, 80°C, 1,375 mbar)	Yes
Activated factor IX complex concentrates (inhibitor treatments)			
Autoplex	Baxter-Hyland	Dry heat, 68°C 144 hr	No
FEIBA	Immuno	Vapor heated (10 hr, 60°C, 1,190 mbar + 1 hr, 80°C, 1,375 mbar)	No

Abbreviations: TNBP, tri(n-butyl) phosphate

sions are then indicated to maintain clot stability and to promote wound healing. Dosing of clotting factor is determined by the seriousness of the bleeding episode, the nature and severity of the clotting defect, and the pharmacokinetic properties of the infused coagulation factor.

Antihemophilic factor is a large molecule of at least 150,000 D molecular weight. As a result, it is primarily distributed intravascularly. To achieve a level of 100 percent of normal or 1.0 unit/ml, a dose equivalent to 1 unit/ml of plasma volume must be infused. This can be approximated by the following formula:

$$50 \times \text{weight (in kilograms)}$$

In smaller children, the volume of distribution is occasionally approximately 10 percent larger. To ensure correct dosing, plasma factor VIII levels should be evaluated 10 to 15 minutes after the completion of the infusion and adjustments made as indicated. Clinically available plasma-derived and recombinant factor VIII concentrates typically have half-lives of at least 8 and usually 12 to 14 hours. Individual differences in distribution and metabolism can account for the variations.

These differences in pharmacokinetic properties are especially important when surgery is planned. In the 2 weeks before elective surgical procedures it is prudent to perform a half-life and recovery study to rule out the presence of an inhibitor and to determine precise individual pharmacokinetic character-

istics. A 50 percent correction or 25 units/kg is infused after obtaining a zero time baseline factor VIII level. A peak plasma level is determined 10 to 15 minutes after completion of the infusion, and follow-up time points are drawn at 1, 2, 4, 8, and 24 hours after the infusion. Recovery is expressed as the peak level divided by the expected level (50 percent) times 100. The half-life is derived from the plot of $\log_{10}$ factor VIII level versus time as a linear function (Table 8-4).

The principles of factor IX dosing are the same as those for factor VIII; however, the specifics are different. Factor IX with a molecular weight of 55 kD is predominantly distributed extravascularly. Therefore, most of an infused dose is not evident when plasma factor IX assays are performed. The following formula allows the calculation of a factor IX dose needed to achieve a 50 percent correction or 0.5 units/ml of plasma volume of factor IX:

$$35 \times \text{weight (in kilograms)}$$

Again, in small children, the space of distribution may be 10 to 15 percent larger. Plasma factor IX assays are needed to evaluate the response. Preoperative half-life and recovery studies are performed as outlined above for factor VIII with the following important differences. The initial dose is 20 units/kg. Plasma samples are obtained before the test infusion, 10 to 15 minutes after the infusion is completed, and then at 1, 4, 8, 24, and preferably 48

Table 8-4. A Guide to Factor Dosing in Hemophilia A

Type of Hemorrhage	Initial Dose	Follow-Up Dosing[a]
Hemarthrosis	25–40 U/kg	Occasionally for 1 day
Soft tissue/muscle	25–40 U/kg	For 2–3 days or more
Epistaxis	25–40 U/kg + Antifibrinolytic therapy for 7–10 days	Occasionally
Hematuria	25–40 U/kg + Fluids and bed rest	Occasionally
Central nervous system	50 U/kg	For 14–21 days
Major surgery		
Soft tissue	50 U/kg	For 10–14 days
Orthopaedic	50 U/kg	For 3–9 weeks
Retroperitoneal	50 U/kg	For 10–21 days

[a] 25 U/kg are infused at frequencies varying from every 8 to every 24 hours.
See text for specific recommendations.

Table 8-5. A Guide to Factor Dosing in Hemophilia B

Type of Hemorrhage	Initial Dose	Follow-Up Dosing[a]
Hemarthrosis	15–20 U/kg	Occasionally for 1 day
Soft tissue/muscle	15–20 U/kg	For 2–3 days or more
Epistaxis	15–20 U/kg followed by antifibrinolytic therapy for 7–10 days	Occasionally. Omit antifibrinolytic therapy if dose repeated
Hematuria	15–20 U/kg + fluids and bed rest	Occasionally
Central nervous system	35–40 U/kg	For 14–21 days
Major surgery		
Soft tissue	35 U/kg	For 10–14 days
Orthopaedic	35 U/kg	For 3–9 weeks
Retroperitoneal	35–40 U/kg	For 10–21 days

[a] 7.5–15 U/kg are infused at frequencies varying from every 12 to every 24 hours. See text for specific recommendations.

hours. Factor IX has a half-life of approximately 20 hours in most patients. (Table 8-5).

Hemophilia A

In hemophilia A, for treatment of a knee, elbow, or ankle hemarthrosis, a single infusion of clotting factor usually suffices. A dose of 25 units/kg of factor VIII, if given within 6 hours of the onset of patient-perceived symptoms, is sufficient in more than 90 percent of instances. During an acute hemarthrosis, splinting to rest an affected joint and ice application to limit swelling serve as useful adjuncts. Chronically involved joints with radiographic or functional abnormalities may require repeated infusions to stop bleeding and restore joint function. Soft tissue and intramuscular bleeding also require repeated infusions. For hemophilia A, in general, one-half of the initial dose is administered every 8 to 12 hours for 1 to 2 days. Hospitalization is often indicated for the management of retroperitoneal and iliopsoas bleeding to ensure plasma factor VIII levels more than 80 percent for at least several days and to provide a supervised environment for bed rest. In major surgery such as a laparotomy or joint replacement, when using intermittent factor VIII dosing, the trough level of factor VIII should be 80 percent or more for the first 3 to 5 postoperative days. Similarly, the trough level should be 50 percent or more for the next 3 to 5 days. In the case of soft tissue surgery, replacement therapy should be continued for a total of 10 to 14 days. This can be achieved after hospital discharge by once daily infusions of 25 units/kg of

factor VIII. Orthopaedic cases are different and, as in the case of total knee replacement, can require daily factor VIII dosing to 50 percent (25 units/kg) for a total of 3 weeks followed by thrice-weekly replacement for an additional 3 to 9 weeks during rigorous rehabilitation. The initial 1 to 2 weeks of replacement therapy for factor VIII in the surgical setting can also be administered by continuous infusion. After a loading dose of factor VIII of 50 units/kg, a continuous infusion of 2 to 3 units/kg/h is provided. Unfavorable troughs, which lead to postoperative hemorrhage, are avoided, and some saving in the total number of infused factor VIII units can be achieved. Intracranial hemorrhage is also effectively managed by continuous infusion therapy for 7 to 10 days followed by daily intermittent infusions of 25 to 40 units/kg/day for an additional 2 weeks.

Hemophilia B

Factor IX dosing for hemarthroses is achieved by infusing 15 to 20 units/kg for a correction equal to 30 percent of normal. If bleeding continues and repeated doses are required, 5 to 10 units/kg can be infused every 12 to 24 hours. For soft tissue or intramuscular bleeding after a loading dose of 15 to 20 units/kg, one-quarter of the initial dose is infused every 12 to 24 hours for 1 to 2 days. In surgery, the preoperative loading dose should be 35 units/kg. Doses of 7.5 to 10 units/kg are then administered every 12 hours for the first 3 to 5 postoperative days to keep the trough factor IX level over 30 percent. In the succeeding 3 to 5 days, 5 to 7.5 units/kg are infused to attain a trough factor IX level more than 20 percent. After hospital discharge, 15 to 20 units of factor IX are given daily to complete a total of 10 to 14 days. For orthopaedic cases, the daily infusions are continued to the twenty-first postoperative day. Twice-weekly infusions then may be required for an additional 3 to 9 weeks during physical therapy. Although coagulation factor IX, not factor IX complex concentrate (PCC), has been given by continuous infusion, it is not approved for use by this delivery system.[40]

The Use of Desmopressin, Aminocaproic Acid, and Tranexamic Acid Acid

Replacement therapy in mild hemophilia A can often be accomplished with desmopressin (DDAVP).[41] When administered by intravenous infusion (0.3 µg/kg), subcutaneous injection (0.4 µg/kg), or intranasal insufflation (300 µg if more than 50 kg or 150 µg if less than 50 kg), DDAVP can increase factor VIII levels three- to fivefold over baseline. Levels in excess of 30 to 50 percent can be achieved, which are sufficient to treat post-traumatic soft tissue and joint hemorrhages. Menorrhagia in carrier women with subnormal factor VIII levels can also be reduced by the administration of DDAVP. Dental procedures, including extractions, can frequently be safely performed after DDAVP. Occasionally, repeat doses of DDAVP are indicated for maintenance of a factor VIII level postoperatively. In many individuals, these can be administered daily for several days. However, in some patients, a tachyphylaxis phenomenon is seen with loss of response to DDAVP. Monitoring of peak factor VIII levels 2 hours after starting an infusion identifies these nonresponders. Recombinant factor VIII can then be substituted. Small children receiving doses of DDAVP are at risk for the development of hyponatremia and seizures.[42] Anesthetized adults unable to regulate their salt and water intake are also at risk. Thrombosis has also been a rare complication in adults.[43]

The presence of fibrinolytic activity on mucous membranes leads to early clot dissolution. When the initial clot is small or poorly formed, as occurs in hemophilia, inhibition of fibrinolytic activity can be clinically useful. In dental surgery, when frenulum tears occur, and often when there is epistaxis in the absence of an anatomic cause, use of aminocaproic acid or tranexamic acid can be effective.[44,45] Aminocaproic acid at a dose of 50 mg/kg orally every 6 hours or tranexamic acid 25 mg/kg orally every 8 hours for 7 to 10 days can stop oral and ear, nose, and throat bleeding. These agents are especially useful for oral surgery when they are used after an initial factor or DDAVP infusion.

von Willebrand's Disease

Factor VIII:C (the antihemophilic factor or factor VIII coagulant) circulates in plasma in a noncovalent association with VWF. The VWF is important for platelet adhesion to subendothelium and promotion of platelet thrombi.[46] Von Willebrand's disease (VWD) is the result of a quantitative partial deficiency (type 1), severe deficiency (type 3), or qualitative deficiency (type 2) of VWF (Table 8-6).[47] There is a concomitant reduction in factor VIII:C in most patients and a prolongation of the bleeding time. It has been estimated that from 1 in 2,000 to as many as 1 in 100 individuals is affected by VWD.[48] In general, VWD is inherited in an autosomal dominant fashion, with the gene carried on chromosome 12. Fewer than 10 percent of identified patients have type 3. Platelet-associated forms of VWD and complex deficiencies of VWF multimers have also been described.

The treatment of VWD differs from that of hemophilia A. DDAVP is the preferred therapy for most patients with VWD. Dosing is the same as in mild hemophilia A (see above). Notable exceptions to the use of DDAVP are in those with type 2B or type 3 VWD. Type 2B is associated with normal levels and multimeric composition of platelet-associated VWF. This situation can lead to a hypercoagulable state if DDAVP is administered. Patients with type 3 disease lack VWF and therefore do not respond to DDAVP. Therapy based on plasma-derived blood products is

Table 8-6. Types of von Willebrand Disease

Type	Inheritance	von Willebrand	Treatment
1	Autosomal dominant	Quantitative reduction	DDAVP
2	Autosomal dominant	Qualitative abnormality	DDAVP or Humate-P
3	Autosomal recessive	Absent	Humate-P

Abbreviation: DDAVP, desmopressin.

preferred for all treatment indications for these two groups of patients and for others with VWD undergoing major surgical procedures. VWF-rich, virus-inactivated clotting factor (Humate-P) is infused at a dose of 40 units/kg of factor VIII:C with the dual goal of increasing the factor VIII:C level to normal and shortening the bleeding time. Follow-up infusions are given as frequently as every 4 to 6 hours postoperatively at a dose of 10 units/kg, depending on the severity of the hemorrhage or surgery. Frequent dosing is required to maintain plasma levels of the VWF and achieve correction of the bleeding time. After the first 3 to 5 postoperative days, the dosing frequency is reduced to every 8 to 12 hours for 3 to 5 days and then every 12 to 24 hours for 3 to 5 additional days to complete 10 to 14 days of infusion therapy.

COMPLICATIONS OF THERAPY

Historically, clotting factors were associated with reactions in some individuals. Febrile, urticarial, anaphylactoid, and anaphylactic reactions occurred infrequently. The use of the currently available more highly purified factors is rarely accompanied by these side effects. Older less purified factors also contained significant titers of antiblood group substances A and B. Hemolysis was occasionally seen in recipients with type A, B, or AB blood, especially if repeated or continuous infusions were administered.

As mentioned above, clotting factor concentrates are manufactured from plasma donor pools from up to 20,000 individuals. As a result, before implementation of donor screening and virus-inactivation procedures, many hemophiliac patients were infected by transfusion-transmitted agents. More than 40 percent of hemophiliac patients were infected with HIV and in excess of 70 percent have been infected with hepatitis C virus.[49,50] Of the HIV-infected hemophiliac patients, more than 3,000 have AIDS based on the pre-1993 definition, which required the occurrence of an opportunistic infection or malignancy. Evidence exists that this progression can be slowed through the use of more highly purified factor VIII concentrates.[51] HIV-infected hemophiliac patients have participated in National Institute of Allergy and Infectious Diseases (NIAID)-sponsored investigational studies and have benefited from antiretroviral interventions and opportunistic infection

prevention strategies.[52] HIV infection seems to function as a cofactor, accelerating hepatitis C infection, which has resulted in an apparent increased number of deaths in hemophiliac patients of hepatic failure.[53] Although studies in hepatitis C-infected hemophiliac patients are limited, biochemical and histologic benefits of interferon-α have been demonstrated.[54] Studies of hepatitis C virus burden and serotypes may clarify the role of antiviral interventions.

FISCAL CONSTRAINTS AND SOLUTIONS

Current costs of therapeutic products make hemophilia the most expensive chronic disorder in the United States. With the average wholesale price for antihemophilic factor in excess of $1.00/unit, typical annual costs for clotting factor for an adult are $50,000 to $100,000/year. Medical care services, including preventive aspects, at HTCs, add 5 to 10 percent to the annual costs. Unfortunately, the substantial price of plasma-derived or recombinant clotting factors may be the legitimate result of research and development, viral inactivation, and donor screening expenses. Developments in gene therapy for hemophilia may change the financial outlook if market forces for clotting factor do not in the next few years. Initial experiments in hemophilic dogs have demonstrated the feasibility of gene therapy for hemophilia B.[55] Application of current and proposed gene insertion technologies could produce durable cures for hemophilia by the end of the twentieth century.

Improvements in the current plasma-derived clotting factors are a direct result of the complications and catastrophes of transfusion therapy in the early 1980s. These improved clotting factor concentrates provide a safe and effective replacement therapy for hemophilia A and B. Recombinant DNA-produced factor VIII has also favorably expanded the treatment horizon. Implementation of curative strategies could make replacement therapy by intermittent intravenous infusions obsolete by the end of this century.

REFERENCES

 1. Davie EW, Ratnoff OD: Waterfall sequence for intrinsic blood clotting. Science 145:1310, 1964
 2. MacFarlane RG: An enzyme cascade in the blood clot-

ting mechanism and its function as a biochemical amplifier. Nature 202:498, 1964

3. Broze GJ, Gailani D: The role of factor XI in coagulation. Thromb Haemost 70:72, 1993
4. Mann KG, Nesheim ME, Church WR et al: Surface dependent reactions of the vitamin K dependent enzyme complexes. Blood 76:1, 1990
5. Goldsmith JC, Kletzel M: Risk of birth related intracranial hemorrhage in hemophilic newborns: results of a North American study. Blood, suppl. 76:421A, 1990
6. Larsson A, Nilsson IM, Blombäck M: Current status of Swedish hemophiliacs: a demographic survey. Acta Med Scand 212:195, 1982
7. Carlsson M, Berntorp E, Sjorkman S, Lindvall K: Pharmacokinetic dosing in prophylactic treatment of hemophilia A. Eur J Haematol 51:247, 1993
8. Thompson AR: Factor IX concentrates for clinical use. Semin Thromb Hemost 19:25, 1993
9. Kasper C, Mannucci PM, Bulyzhenkov V et al: Hemophilia in the 1990's: principles of management and improved access to care. Semin Thromb Hemost 18:1, 1992
10. Chance PR, Dyer KA, Kurachi KA et al: Regional localization of the human factor IX gene by molecular hybridization. Hum Genet 65:207, 1983
11. Hoyer LW: Hemophilia A. N Engl J Med 330:38, 1994
12. Barrowcliffe TW: Standardization and assay. Semin Thromb Hemost 19:73, 1993
13. Poole JC, Hershgold EE, Pappenhager AR: High potency antihaemophilic factor concentrate prepared from cryoglobulin precipitate. Nature 203:312, 1964
14. Cohn EJ: The separation of blood into fractions of therapeutic value. Ann Intern Med 26:341, 1947
15. Kasper CK, Lusher JM: Recent evolution of clotting factor concentrates for hemophilia A and B. Transfusion 33:422, 1993
16. Hrinda ME, Feldman F, Schreiber AB: Preclinical characterization of a new pasteurized monoclonal antibody purified factor VIIIC. Semin Hematol 27:19, 1990
17. Brettler DB, Forsberg AD, Levine PH et al: Factor VIII concentrate purified from plasma using monoclonal antibodies: human studies. Blood 73:1859, 1989
18. White GC, McMillan CW, Kingdon HS, Shoemaker CB: Use of recombinant antihemophilic factor in the treatment of two patients with classic hemophilia. N Engl J Med 320:166, 1989
19. Schwartz RS, Abildgaard CF, Aledort LM et al: Human recombinant DNA derived antihemophilic factor (factor VIII) in the treatment of hemophilia A. N Engl J Med 323:1800, 1990
20. Bray GL: Current status of clinical studies of recombinant factor VIII (Recombinate) in patients with hemophilia A. Transfusion Med Rev 6:252, 1992
21. Aronson DL: Factor IX complex. Semin Thromb Hemost 7:28, 1979
22. White GC, Roberts HR, Kingdon HS, Lundblad RL: Prothrombin complex concentrates: potentially thrombogenic materials and clues to the mechanism of thrombosis in vivo. Blood 49:159, 1977
23. Giles AR, Nesheim ME, Hoogendoorn H et al: The coagulant active phospholipid content is a major determinant of in vivo thrombogenicity of prothrombin complex (factor IX) concentrates in rabbits. Blood 59:401, 1982
24. Menache D, Roberts HR: Summary report and recommendations of the task force members and consultants. Thromb Haemost 33:645, 1977
25. Herring SW, Abildgaard C, Shitanishi KT et al: Human coagulation factor IX: assessment of thrombogenicity in animal models and viral safety. J Lab Clin Med 121:394, 1993
26. Goldsmith JC, Kasper C, Blatt PM et al: Coagulation factor IX: successful surgical experience with a purified factor IX concentrate. Am J Hematol 40:210, 1992
27. Kim HC, Matts L, Eisele J et al: Monoclonal antibody purified factor IX—comparative thrombogenicity to prothrombin complex concentrate. Semin Hematol 28:15, 1991
28. Addiego J, Kasper C, Abilgaard C et al: Frequency of inhibitor development in haemophiliacs treated with low-purity factor VIII. Lancet 342:462, 1993
29. Rosendal FR, Nieuwenhuis HK, van den Berg HM et al: A sudden increase in factor VIII inhibitor development in multitransfused hemophilia A patients in The Netherlands. Blood 81:2180, 1993
30. White GC, McMillan CW, Blatt PM et al: Factor VIII inhibitors: a clinical overview. Am J Hematol 13:335, 1982
31. Kasper CK, Aledort LM, Counts RB et al: A more uniform measurement of factor VIII inhibitors. Thromb Haemost 34:875, 1975
32. Gordon EM, Al-Batjini F, Goldsmith JC: Continuous infusion of monoclonal antibody purified factor VIII: rational approach to serious hemorrhage in patients with allo-/autoantibodies to factor VIII. Am J Hematol 45:142, 1994
33. Sjamsoedin LJM, Heijnen L, Mauser-Bunschoten EP et al: The effect of activated prothrombin complex concentrate (FEIBA) on joint and muscle bleeding in patients with hemophilia A and antibodies to factor VIII. N Engl J Med 305:717, 1981
34. Lusher JM, Blatt PM, Penner JA et al: Autoplex versus proplex: a controlled, double-blind study of effective-

ness in acute hemarthroses in hemophilics with inhibitors to factor VIII. Blood 62:1135, 1983

35. Kernoff PBA, Thomas ND, Lilley PA et al: Clinical experience with polyelectrolyte fractioned porcine factor VIII concentrate in the treatment of hemophilics with antibodies to factor VIII. Blood 63:31, 1984

36. Macik BG, Lindley CM, Lusher JM et al: Safety and initial clinical efficacy of three dose levels of recombinant activated factor VII (rFVIIa): results of a phase I study. Blood Coagul Fibrinolysis 4:521, 1993

37. Colombo M, Mannucci PM, Carnelli V: Transmission of non-A, non-B hepatitis by heat-treated factor VIII concentrate. Lancet 2:1, 1985

38. Soumela H: Inactivation of viruses in blood and plasma products. Transfusion Med Rev 7:42, 1993

39. Morfini M, Longo G, Rossi Ferrini P et al: Hypoplastic anemia in a hemophiliac first infused with a solvent detergent treated factor VIII concentrate: the role of human B19 parvovirus. Am J Hematol 39:149, 1992

40. Goldsmith JC, Gordon EM: Treatment of hemophilia B: serendipitous use of continuous infusion coagulation factor IX. Thromb Res 70:265, 1993

41. Mannucci PM: Desmopressin: a nontransfusional form of treatment for congenital and acquired bleeding disorders. Blood 75:1448, 1988

42. Shepherd LL, Hutchinson RJ, Worden EK et al: Hyponatremia and seizures after intravenous administration of desmopressin acetate for surgical hemostasis. J Pediatr 114:470, 1989

43. Mannucci PM, Lusher JM: Desmopressin and thrombosis. Lancet 2:675, 1989

44. Walsh PN, Rizza CR, Mathews JM et al: Epsilon aminocaproic acid therapy for dental extractions in haemophilia and Christmas disease: a double blind controlled trial. Br J Haematol 20:463, 1971

45. Ramstrom G, Blomback M: Tooth extractions in haemophiliacs. Int J Oral Surg 4:1, 1975

46. Ruggeri ZM, Zimmerman TS: Von Willebrand factor and von Willebrand disease. Blood 70:895, 1987

47. Sadler JE: A revised classification of von Willebrand disease. Thromb Haemost 71:520, 1994

48. Rodeghiero R, Castaman G, Dini E: Epidemiological investigation of the prevalence of von Willebrand's disease. Blood 69:454, 1987

49. Kroner B, Rosenberg PS, Aledort LM et al: HIV-1 infection incidence among persons with hemophilia in the United States and western Europe 1978–1990. J Acquir Immune Defic Syndr 7:279, 1994

50. Brettler DB, Alter HJ, Dienstag JL et al: The prevalence of antibody to HCV in a cohort of hemophilic patients. Blood 76:254, 1990

51. Seremetis SV, Aledort LM, Bergman GE et al: Three year randomised study of high purity or intermediate purity factor VIII concentrates in symptom free HIV seropositive haemophiliacs: effects on immune status. Lancet 342:700, 1993

52. Goldsmith JC: Medical management of children and adolescents with hemophilia. p. 747. In Pizzo P, Wilfert C (eds): Pediatric AIDS. Williams & Wilkins, Baltimore, 1994

53. Eyster ME, Diamondstone LS, Lien JM et al: Natural history of hepatitis C virus infection in multitransfused hemophiliacs: effect of coinfection with human immunodeficiency virus. J Acquir Immune Defic Syndr 6: 602, 1993

54. Makris M, Preston FE, Triger DR et al: Interferon alpha for chronic hepatitis C in haemophiliacs. Gut 34:suppl. 2:S121, 1993

55. Kay MA, Rothenberg S, Landen C et al: In vivo gene therapy of hemophilia B: sustained partial correction in factor IX deficient dogs. Science 262:117, 1993

Red Cell Compatibility Testing: Clinical Significance and Laboratory Methods

Ira A. Shulman and Lawrence D. Petz

The transfusion of whole blood and blood components may be complicated by a hemolytic transfusion reaction (HTR). When an HTR is acute in onset, a patient may experience hemoglobinemia, hemoglobinuria, renal dysfunction, coagulation abnormalities, shock, and in some cases even death. Pretransfusion red blood cell compatibility testing is a process designed to minimize the chance that a patient will experience an HTR.

The first segment of this chapter briefly reviews the history of compatibility testing. Next we review the procedures involved in compatibility testing, including a discussion of the efficacy of various media used to enhance agglutination (low-ionic-strength solutions, [LISS], Polybrene, polyethylene glycol [PEG]); the advantages and disadvantages of using nonspecific versus polyspecific antiglobulin reagents; the use of solid-phase red cell adherence assays or column agglutination technologies; the safety of omitting the antiglobulin phase of the crossmatch following a negative type and screen procedure; and a discussion of compatibility test procedures that are unnecessary. This segment concludes with recommendations for routine compatibility testing that can serve as a framework for developing compatibility testing protocols in one's own laboratory.

The next segment reviews the clinical significance of various red cell alloantibodies and describes approaches to the difficult problem of transfusing patients when compatible blood cannot be made available, as in some patients with multiple alloantibodies.

This chapter concludes with a review of a number of special considerations in compatibility testing including weakly reacting forms of the D antigen, the potential for conversion of ABO blood groups, donor erythrocyte destruction in the absence of serologic evidence of alloimmunization, the use of bioassays to determine the clinical significance of red cell alloantibodies, the relationship of compatibility testing to fatal hemolytic transfusion reactions, compatibility testing for patients who will be subjected to hypothermia, and misleading results caused by the administration of antilymphocyte globulin and intravenous immunoglobulin.

Compatibility testing for patients with acquired hemolytic anemias and for emergency transfusions is discussed in Chapters 20 and 22, respectively.

ORIGINS OF THE COMPATIBILITY TEST

A review of the early 20th century origins of the compatibility test is fascinating.[1–3] Many blood bankers have the impression that modern concepts of pretransfusion testing followed quickly and logically upon Karl Landsteiner's reports of the discovery of the ABO groups in 1900 and 1901.[4,5] As emphasized by Rosenfield,[2] this was certainly not the case. Indeed, very few persons noticed Landsteiner's reports, and blood transfusion in the early part of this century was developed without blood typing.

Alexis Carrel, a Nobel Prize recipient for the development of end-to-end blood vessel anastomosis, suggested that this surgical technique might be useful for blood transfusion; the method was actually employed successfully until 1913. George Crile, later famous for his thyroid surgery, was trained by Carrel and became the best-known transfusionist of the day. He performed hundreds of direct anastomosis transfusions and published a book on the subject in 1909.[6] However, he never performed ABO typing! Crile did, however, search for hemolysis prior to transfusion, apparently using methods that had been described for blood compatibility between goats.

ABO typing prior to transfusion was first used in 1907 when Richard Weil suggested it to his fellow intern, Reuben Ottenberg. However, as Ottenberg[7] has pointed out, surgeons resented requests for pretransfusion laboratory tests and often proceeded without them—the first recorded instance of a difference of opinion between surgeons and blood transfusionists. The only benefit of this obstinacy was that it allowed Ottenberg to observe that immune hemolysis in vivo often far exceeded anything to be observed in vitro. This problem still occasionally plagues serologists in spite of the enormous efforts that have been put forth in pretransfusion testing.

In 1914 and 1915 there were several descriptions of the use of sodium citrate as an anticoagulant for human blood.[8-11] Weil's report was unique among these in that it contained two other very important observations. One was that citrated whole blood could be refrigerated safely for at least several days—the first suggestion for blood banking. The other observation was that serologic tests for compatibility did not require separate serum and erythrocyte samples, but that citrated whole blood of both patient and donor could be mixed. Weil's proportions were 1:1, 9:1, and 1:9. These mixtures were placed in narrow tubes; after 1 hour of incubation, both agglutination and hemolysis were sought as indications of incompatibility. Rous and Turner[12] improved Weil's compatibility test; the value of pretransfusion testing was further documented in 1921 by Unger,[13] who described five cases of serious reactions to ABO-compatible transfusions for which test results using the Rous-Turner method had been positive.

The discovery in 1940 of the rhesus (Rh) blood group system[14] allowed the recognition of the fact that hemolytic transfusion reactions could follow the transfusion of Rh-positive blood cells into Rh-negative recipients. It was subsequently recognized that agglutination methods for demonstration of Rh antibodies in the sera of sensitized individuals were inadequate, in that 40 to 50 percent of the subjects in whom sensitization was later confirmed by the birth of an erythroblastotic child or by a hemolytic transfusion reaction showed negative test results for anti-Rh agglutinins.

In 1944, an explanation for such failures was found independently by Wiener and by Race. Race[15] found additional evidence of Rh sensitization that he called an "incomplete antibody" that did combine with the antigen, the Rh-positive red cell, but failed to cause agglutination in the saline suspension of cells in the test tube. Wiener[16] also recognized the failure of agglutination of Rh-positive cells after incubation with the serum of some sensitized individuals. He demonstrated it as follows: to the usual mixture of a 2 percent suspension of Rh-positive cells in saline and unknown serum from the sensitized person, he added 1 drop of an anti-Rh serum known to be capable of agglutinating the test cells. The difference in degree of agglutination of this system, after incubation at 37°C and centrifugation, from the expected 4+ agglutination was the degree of inhibition of "blocking" caused by the unknown serum. Diamond and Abelson[17] showed that the combination of ordinary agglutination plus the "blocking test" was much more satisfactory than agglutination alone in that the combination demonstrated the presence of Rh antibody in 92 percent of their cases of sensitization.

Modern Antibody Detection Methods

The year 1945 was notable for the publication by Diamond and Denton,[18] pointing out that albumin was a more satisfactory medium for suspending test cells than was saline. These investigators reported that some "incomplete" antibodies that reacted with or "sensitized" red cells did not cause them to agglutinate in saline but did cause agglutination of the red cells suspended in albumin-containing media.

Also in 1945, Coombs and colleagues[19] reported the use of antiglobulin serum for the detection of weak or "incomplete" Rh antibodies. Dr. Coombs, a veterinarian, later explained that the antiglobulin test was first described by Carlo Moreschi in 1908 for bacterial agglutination.[20] Coombs and co-workers rediscovered the test while deliberately searching for ways to demonstrate "incomplete" red cell antibodies.[20]

In 1947, Morton and Pickles[21] reported that treatment of red cells with the proteolytic enzyme trypsin caused agglutination of cells sensitized with "incomplete" antibody. Subsequently, other proteolytic enzymes were found to react similarly. Low[22] worked with the enzyme papain from papayas, Haber and Rosenfield[23] used an extract from figs called ficin, and Pirofsky and Mangum[24] used bromelin extracted from pineapples. Enzyme techniques are often included among the tests used for difficult antibody identification problems and for reference laboratory procedures.

In 1964 and 1965, there were reports[25,26] of evaluations of the addition of bovine serum albumin (BSA) to the incubation medium before antiglobulin testing. This procedure was said to increase the sensitivity of the antiglobulin test.

In more recent years, other methods and reagents have been evaluated in an effort to increase the sensitivity and specificity of antibody detection including the use of LISS, the anticomplement component of antiglobulin serum, Polybrene, PEG, and solid-phase, microtiter, or column agglutination technology (CAT).

COMPATIBILITY TEST PROCEDURES

The process of pretransfusion RBC compatibility testing consists of a number of defined steps, as listed in Table 9-1.

ABO/Rh Testing of Donor Blood

The mislabeling of a donor blood container with a wrong ABO/Rh designation may result in a severe hemolytic transfusion reaction or in sensitization of a transfusion recipient to the D antigen. To prevent these adverse outcomes of transfusion, the ABO/Rh of donor blood must be determined using proper reagents and techniques.[27] Donor blood must not be

Table 9-1. Compatibility Test Procedures

1. ABO/RH testing of donor blood
2. Testing the donor's blood for antibodies
3. Patient specimen acquisition and storage
4. Review of records
5. ABO/Rh testing of potential transfusion recipients
6. Testing the patient's blood for antibodies
7. Antibody identification, if indicated
8. A major crossmatch

labeled with an ABO designation unless both ABO forward and reverse grouping results agree, and donor blood must not be labeled Rh negative unless a test to detect a weak expression of D (weak D or D^u) has been performed, with a negative result. The blood group label of a whole blood/RBC container must be verified by the performance of a second ABO determination (a forward grouping is sufficient for this purpose); if a container has been labeled Rh negative, its Rh status must be verified by a second Rh determination, although a repeat test for weak D is not required.

These verification steps are important since, in one study, nearly 15 in every million whole blood/RBC units collected were discovered to have been labeled with the wrong ABO, and nearly 1 in every 50,000 units labeled "Rh negative" were discovered to be Rh positive.[28]

Verification of Rh status is not required for a donor blood that is labeled Rh positive. Even if an Rh-negative donor blood were mislabeled Rh positive, no harm would be expected to result; the mislabeled unit would probably be given to an Rh-positive individual, but Rh-positive patients may safely receive Rh-negative blood transfusions.

The blood group label of a fresh frozen plasma (FFP), cryoprecipitate, or platelet unit does not need to be verified. However, if the blood group label of a whole blood/RBC unit is discovered to be wrong, the facility responsible for the labeling error must be notified immediately, so that other components that were made from the same blood donation can be recalled. An effort must be made to discover the cause of the labeling error and prevent a recurrence. Until a labeling problem is resolved, the blood and components in question must not be transfused.

Testing the Donor's Blood for Antibodies

The passive transfer of donor antibodies by transfusion can result in the development of a positive direct and/or indirect antiglobulin test (IAT) in the recipient,[29] the hemolysis of the recipient's red blood cells (RBCs),[30] or the hemolysis of transfused RBCs.[31,32] To avoid these problems, a blood donor with a history of a prior transfusion or pregnancy should be tested for unexpected red cell antibodies.[27] However, most laboratories find it simpler to test all blood donors for unexpected antibodies; the testing may be accomplished by any method that will detect clinically significant antibodies. Antibody screening methods used for donor blood testing do not need to be as sensitive as those used for patient pretransfusion testing. The use of an IAT is optional, the sera of several donors may be pooled before testing (each serum is tested individually if the pool tests positive), and reagent red cells used in the antibody detection test may be pooled.

A donor blood does not need to be retested to verify that unexpected red cell antibodies are absent in the donor plasma. However, since infants under 4 months of age must not be transfused with plasma-rich blood components that contain clinically significant unexpected antibodies,[27] it might be prudent to repeat donor antibody detection testing when plasma-rich components are intended for very young infants, if the method used for screening the donor blood is known to miss detecting a significant percentage of clinically significant antibodies.

Patient Specimen Acquisition and Storage

Specimen Acquisition

In one study, approximately one out of six ABO-incompatible transfusions were caused by a mislabeled specimen used for pretransfusion compatibility testing.[33] In order to minimize a clerical error in specimen acquisition and labeling, a phlebotomist must be trained to identify each patient correctly and to label each specimen and associated paperwork accurately. Some laboratories require that the ABO and Rh test results of at least two different specimens must agree before a group specific whole blood or RBC unit may be issued for transfusion.[34] Most ABO hemolytic transfusion reactions occur because the red cell unit is not properly matched to the patient at the time of transfusion.

A key element in the identification process is the patient's identification band, which is used to establish identification when a blood sample is drawn and when the patient is transfused. Identification band errors can contribute to this problem or cause significant delays in transfusion. In one study, approximately 67,000 identification band errors were detected during 2.5 million phlebotomies (median error rate = 2.2 percent).[35] Approximately one-half of the errors (49 percent) were due to a missing identification band. Other errors included more than one identification band containing different information (18 percent), incomplete information (17 percent), erroneous data (9 percent), illegible data (6 percent), and patient identification bands containing another patient's information (0.5 percent).

Ten percent of the hospitals had an error rate of 11 percent or greater. A hospital's error rate was unrelated to bed size, type of hospital, or who performed the phlebotomy. Rather, the error rate was related to hospital policies. The most important factor in maintaining a low identification band error rate was the routine monitoring for such errors by the phlebotomy staff. In approximately 5 percent of hospitals, a mandatory written order was required to remove an identification band. In 24 percent of hospitals, a written incident report was generated whenever an error was found. These two policies, although used by only a minority of hospitals, were the second and third most important factors associated with a low identification band error rate. Most (90 percent) phlebotomy staffs immediately notified a nurse or ward clerk about an identification band error, and this policy was the fourth most important factor.

Most hospitals permitted a site other than the wrist to be used for placement of an identification band; 73 percent permitted placement on an ankle and 30 percent on the patient's bed, chart, or room wall. In general, these practices were associated with lower identification band error rates. It seems that a formal designation of an alternate site for the identification band probably decreases confusion as to where to place the band when a wrist is not available. However, except for very limited circumstances (e.g., in the surgical suite), a policy that routinely permits

Table 9-2. Recommendations for Minimizing the Risk of Identification Band Errors

1. Establish and use a written protocol for patient identification.
2. Have phlebotomists check identification bands continuously.
3. Have phlebotomists immediately notify nursing or the ward clerk to correct identification band errors.
4. Delay phlebotomy until errors are corrected.
5. Generate an incident report for each identification band error.
6. Send periodic reports on errors to appropriate hospital services and overseeing committees.
7. Have identification bands placed by admission personnel.
8. Designate the ankle as an alternative placement site.
9. Strongly discourage identification band removal for any reason.

a physical separation of the identification band from the patient (i.e., placement on a room wall) should not be endorsed for fear of increasing the risk of a transfusion error. Table 9-2 lists recommendations that may minimize the risk of identification band errors.

Specimen Storage

Once a specimen has been collected, it must be handled and stored properly, to prevent deterioration. Transfusion decisions should not be based on tests performed on specimens too old to reflect the patient's true antibody status. It had previously been required or recommended when testing patients who had been transfused or pregnant within the preceding 3 months, that blood samples be obtained either on the same day, within 2 days, or within 48 hours of the scheduled transfusion. More recently, the standards of the American Association of Blood Banks (AABB)[27] allow the time limit in these circumstances to be extended to three days (also, special considerations apply for recipients under 4 months of age, see p. 231).

The use of three day old samples in pretransfusion testing is convenient for some patients. For example, a patient scheduled for a Monday surgery could be phlebotomized on a Friday instead of over a weekend. Also, using 3-day-old samples significantly de-

creases the number of phlebotomies necessary for patients who need repeated transfusions and decreases the workload for the transfusion service. However, such a policy increases the chance of not detecting an emerging alloantibody. Based on one study, it was estimated that the routine use of a 3-day-old specimen for pretransfusion testing could miss an apparently clinically significant antibody in one of about 3,000 recently transfused patients.[36] Blood bank directors must consider this small added risk in deciding whether to establish a policy of using specimens obtained within 2 or within 3 days of transfusion.

Heddle et al.[37] performed a retrospective review of post-delivery antibody records to determine the frequency of new red cell alloantibody production and transfusion during pregnancy. A total of 17,568 pregnancies were reviewed and the prevalence of clinically significant antibody production during pregnancy was 42/17,568, or 0.24 percent (95 percent confidence interval, 0.17–0.32). Only 15 women received transfusions (0.09 percent), and none of the women with new alloantibody formation during their pregnancies required transfusion; hence, new alloantibody production and the need for transfusion appear to be independent events. The probability of these events occurring together was 1 in 500,000 deliveries. These investigators concluded that screening the obstetric patient for antibodies every 3 days appears to be excessive, except perhaps in patients at high risk of bleeding, such as those with placenta previa or abruptio placenta. However, the Standards Committee of the AABB has retained the 3-day interval for antibody detection, apparently feeling that the data reported by Heddle et al.[37] made a stronger case against performing frequent compatibility tests for patients who have only a 0.09 percent chance of requiring a transfusion, than for extending the 3-day interval.[38]

Review of Records

The past records of a potential transfusion recipient must be checked and compared with current ABO/Rh results, and examined for a history of a clinically significant red cell antibody or other transfusion related problem.[27] Whenever a discrepancy is discovered between current and past ABO/Rh results, the usual cause is an error in patient identification or specimen labeling, although technical and clerical errors committed within the laboratory may also be responsible. At one institution where most specimens for blood bank testing were drawn by nonlaboratory personnel (physicians, medical students, nurses), nearly one in 1,500 patient specimens showed ABO/Rh test results that differed from the record (unpublished data).

When confronted with a patient has a history of a clinically significant antibody, it is prudent to select donor units that lack the corresponding antigen, even when current antibody detection and crossmatch tests are negative. Many clinically significant antibodies become undetectable over time, only to reappear following the transfusion of red cells bearing the corresponding antigen. In one study, 29 percent of clinically significant red cell antibodies became undetectable on at least one follow-up screening,[39] and anti-Jk[a] and anti-C became undetectable in 59 percent and 45 percent of follow-up screenings, respectively.

ABO/Rh Testing of Potential Transfusion Recipients

The ABO and Rh of an intended blood transfusion recipient must be determined using approved reagents and proper technique. Unlike the testing of a donor blood, when performing Rh testing on a potential transfusion recipient, an appropriate control should be run to prevent mistyping an Rh-negative patient as Rh-positive due to rouleaux, autoagglutination, or some other cause.[27] In addition, if a potential transfusion recipient has RBCs that do not react with anti-D, the RBCs do not need to be tested for a weak D antigen. As a result, a patient may be designated Rh negative, even if the RBCs are weak D positive. However, no adverse outcome will result, since such a patient may be transfused with Rh-negative or Rh-positive blood.[40]

With the exception of testing infants under 4 months old (see p. 231), forward and reverse ABO grouping results should match; a discrepancy, if discovered, must be resolved. If a current ABO/Rh test result is discrepant with a prior result, a clerical or technical error must be ruled out as the cause. If it is determined that a current specimen was mislabeled, a search for a second mislabeled specimen should be undertaken, since a reciprocal labeling error could involve another patient.

Testing the Patient's Blood for Antibodies

When a potential transfusion recipient is tested for unexpected RBC antibodies, the methods used should be those that will demonstrate clinically significant antibodies.[27] However, regulations and accreditation guidelines allow for considerable flexibility in antibody screening methodology. An institution should choose the antibody screening method best suited to its local needs. Test sensitivity should be balanced against specificity, as the provision of timely efficient service might be hampered by methods that detect too many irrelevant antibodies. The sensitivity and specificity of the antibody screening test depend at least in part on the factors listed in Table 9-3.

Sample Being Tested: Serum Versus Plasma

Serum is the preferred sample for antibody detection testing, although some workers prefer to use EDTA-anticoagulated plasma.[41] When plasma is used, rouleaux formation and fibrin clot formation are more likely to occur, and both can mimic agglutination and cause false-positive results.[42] Furthermore, some plasma anticoagulants (e.g., EDTA) in-

Table 9-3. Factors Determining the Sensitivity and Specificity of Antibody Screening Techniques

1. Sample being tested (serum versus plasma)
2. Ratio of sample volume to indicator reagent RBC volume
3. Use of media to enhance agglutination (e.g., low-ionic-strength saline [LISS], polybrene, polyethylene glycol)
4. Use of monospecific versus polyspecific antiglobulin reagents
5. Antigenic composition of the indicator reagent RBCs
6. Use of chemically modified indicator reagent RBCs
7. Phase(s) at which the test is checked to detect agglutination and hemolysis
8. Use of visual aids to detect agglutination
9. Use of a direct antiglobulin test (DAT) and autocontrol
10. Use of a control system to detect false-negative indirect antiglobulin test results
11. Use of slide, tube, solid-phase, microtiter, or column agglutination technology

hibit complement activation, which in turn can cause some clinically significant antibodies (e.g., some anti Jk[a]) to escape detection[43] (see p. 207).

When a patient's blood sample contains heparin, the serum may fail to clot or may clot slowly. In such a case, thrombin or protamine sulfate reagents (with or without added snake venom) may be added to the sample to accelerate clotting.[40] However, if a clot accelerating reagent is used, it must show the absence of contaminating red cell alloantibodies, to avoid unexpected positive test results.[44,45]

Ratio of Sample Volume to Indicator Reagent RBC Volume

The sensitivity of the antibody detection test may be increased when the amount of serum in the test system is increased or when the concentration of RBCs in the test system (the RBC suspension) is decreased.[28] Taswell and coworkers[46] showed that the volume of serum dispensed in 2 drops is insufficient to provide an optimum ratio of antibody to antigen in some cases. These investigators found some alloantibodies detectable only when the volume of serum was increased to 3 or more drops. However, if 4 or more drops of serum are used, it may be necessary to perform additional washes prior to performing the IAT phase of the antibody screening procedure. If inadequate washing occurs, the sensitivity of the test system in the antiglobulin test phase may be decreased. Also, if LISS is being used in the test system, the use of extra drops of serum may adversely affect the ionic strength of the test medium and cause a decrease in test sensitivity.

Use of Media to Enhance Agglutination

Low-Ionic-Strength Solutions

In 1964, two groups of investigators reported on the significance of suspending red cells used for antibody detection media with a salt solution of low ionic strength.[47–50] These investigators indicated that the rate of association of anti-D with D-positive RBCs can be increased 1,000-fold by lowering the salt concentration of the medium in which the reaction takes place from 0.17 to 0.03 M. In detecting a wide variety of blood group antibodies by the IAT, the use of a low-ionic-strength medium resulted in a reduction of the incubation time from 1 hour to 5 minutes; moreover, the titer of a wide range of antibodies was

increased. However, some false-positive results were also noted,[51,52] and low-ionic-strength media were not applied to routine compatibility testing at that time, even by the blood bankers who authored the original reports.

Interest in this methodology was suddenly awakened in 1974 by the report of Low and Messeter,[53] who reported that the LISS method had been routinely used in the blood bank at University Hospital in Lund, Sweden, since 1967. They used a 5-minute incubation time and stated that the percentage of samples in which antibodies were detected increased, the reactions were more clear cut and easier to interpret, and nonspecific reactions were negligible when the salt concentration was at least 0.03 M.

Further reports followed at a rapidly increasing rate.[54–64] In general, there is agreement that the use of low-ionic-strength media allows for detection of red cell antibodies in the antiglobulin test after only 10 minutes of incubation with a sensitivity somewhat greater than incubation in albumin media for 15 to 30 minutes. Also, somewhat stronger reactions than with albumin-suspended cells are obtained with a significant percentage of sera.

For example, when using 30 selected weak antibodies, 100 percent were detected after only a 10-minute incubation in LISS (Table 9-4). A significant percentage of antibodies were missed when using saline or albumin techniques, especially with incubation times shorter than 30 minutes. Indeed, after incubation for 10 minutes, only 50 percent of the weak antibodies were detected in saline and 63 percent in albumin. After a 15-minute incubation, 20 percent were still missed in albumin; examples of Rh, Duffy, and Kidd antibodies were not detected.[56] In testing 130 antibodies of various specificities and potency, 44 percent were found to give enhanced reactions in LISS in the antiglobulin test (Table 9-5). In tests with 57 antibodies that reacted by agglutination at room temperature, no important differences were noted among LISS, saline, or albumin-suspending media.

A prospective study[58] of 5,009 sera sent for compatibility testing compared results in LISS with the albumin and enzyme techniques. Incubation in LISS for 10 to 15 minutes at 37°C detected all antibodies that were detected by nonpapainized red cells, except for three anti-I(IH) antibodies reacting at room

Table 9-4.   Reactivity in Antiglobulin Test of 30 Selected Weak Antibodies,[a] Using Red Cells Suspended in Saline, Albumin, and LISS

Incubation (37°C)(min)	Antibodies Detected (%)			Antibodies Detected in LISS Only[b]
	SAL	ALB	LISS	
5	43	47	77	Jk^a (2), fy^a (3), Fy^b, D, e, k
10	50	63	100	Jk^a (2), Fy^a (3), Fy^b, D (2), C, E, e
15	77	80	100	Jk^a, Fy^a, Fy^b, D, C, E
30	90	90	100	Fy^a, Fy^b, D, C
60	100	100	100	None

Abbreviations: SAL, saline; ALB, albumin.

[a] Seven Rh, seven Kell, five Jk, 7 Fy, and 4 Le.

[b] No antibodies were detected in SAL and ALB, but not in LISS at any incubation period.

temperature only and one anti-IH, one anti-P$_1$, and one unidentified antibody reacting when room temperature incubation preceded 37°C incubation. Pre-papainized red cells yielded 16 additional positive reactions, but in only three could specificity be determined (weak anti-Le^a).

Molthan and Strohm[65] reported a hemolytic transfusion reaction due to anti-Kell undetectable in LISS but detectable when using saline or albumin-suspended RBCs. Two of 15 additional anti-Kell antibodies available to the authors also failed to react when using commercial LISS-additive test systems. Lalezari[66] has also pointed out that sensitization in

low-ionic-strength media accelerates antigen-anti-body reactions, with the possible exception of Kell system antibodies.

Although "false-positive" or nonspecific reactions and the detection of clinically insignificant cold antibodies occur somewhat more frequently with LISS than with saline or albumin techniques, they may not be a significant problem, especially if the room temperature incubation phase of the crossmatch is omitted.[58] Further reports have described variations of the techniques, such as the use of polycation aggregation[67] and of albumin in LISS.[68]

Polybrene

The use of a cationic polymer, hexadimethrine bromide (polybrene) for the detection of red cell antibodies was first reported in 1967.[69,70] Several automated and manual modifications were subsequently described.[71–74] The manual Polybrene test has been found to be simple, rapid, and sensitive.[71,73–77]

Mintz and Anderson[78] compared the Polybrene test, including an antiglobulin phase (P-AHG), with saline and albumin–antiglobulin tests for pretransfusion testing. A total of 10,084 pretransfusion blood samples from approximately 6,000 patients were tested. The P-AHG method detected 153 antibodies for which the authors provided antigen-negative cross-match-compatible blood for transfusion—97.5 percent of all such antibodies detected. Their routine methods detected 147 of the alloantibodies—93.6 percent of the total. Although the P-AHG method did not detect 4 of 19 anti-K antibodies, it identified 10 other alloantibodies that were

Table 9-5.   Comparison of the Strength of the Reaction of Antibodies, When Using Red Cells Suspended in Saline, Albumin, or LISS[a]

Antibodies	%
130 Antibodies reactive in antiglobulin test (37°C) (Rh, Fy, Kell, Lu, S, s, Jk, Kp, Js, Ge, Di, Xg, Yt, Vel, Bg, Le)	
Stronger reactions in LISS than in SAL	44
Stronger reactions in LISS than in ALB	31
Strongest reactions in ALB	6
Strongest reactions in SAL	0
57 Agglutinating antibodies (22–25°C) (A, B, M, N, I, H, Le, P$_1$)	
Stronger reactions in LISS than in SAL	26.5
Stronger reactions in LISS than ALB	19.4
Stronger reactions in SAL than in LISS	23
Stronger reactions in ALB than in LISS	23

Abbreviations: ALB, albumin; LISS, low-ionic-strength solutions; SAL, salines.

[a] Incubation time, 10 min in LISS, 30 min in SAL or ALB.

not detected by the routine tests. The reduced sensitivity of low-ionic-strength media to anti-K has also been noted by others.[65,71,79] Of the antibodies detected by the P-AHG method, 86 percent were detected with Polybrene before the addition of antiglobulin. Mintz and Anderson indicated that the P-AHG method is comparable to the saline-antiglobulin and albumin-antiglobulin methods for the detection of alloantibodies for which they provide antigen-negative units. They also pointed out that the Polybrene method, particularly without AHG, has significant limitations in detecting ABO incompatibility with A_2 and B donor cells; they recommended an additional method, such as the "immediate-spin" saline crossmatch, to help ensure the detection of ABO incompatibility.

Polyethylene Glycol

PEG, a high-molecular-weight polymer, has been shown to potentiate antigen–antibody reactions.[80] A number of reports have suggested that the use of PEG to enhance agglutination is superior to the use of more conventional methods for the detection of clinically significant antibodies.[80–85]

Nance and Garratty[80] tested 25 weakly reactive antibodies by PEG, Polybrene, and LISS methods. Sixty-four percent of the reactions were strongest in PEG, 28 percent reacted equally in PEG as in Polybrene or LISS, and 8 percent reacted weaker in PEG than in Polybrene or LISS. The false-positive rate with the use of PEG and anti-IgG was 1.5% with the use of random sera.

Shirey et al.[81] compared PEG with LISS techniques by testing 500 patient samples in parallel, 100 of which were known to contain antibodies in the Rh, Kell, Duffy, Kidd, and MNSs systems. In 34 percent of samples with known antibodies, PEG antiglobulin reactions were stronger than LISS antiglobulin reactions, and in 66 percent they were equal to those of LISS. Of 400 samples without detectable antibodies, 16 demonstrated inconclusive PEG reactions for a false-positive rate of 1.3 percent. It was concluded that PEG demonstrated a relatively high false-positive rate but was more sensitive than LISS in detecting clinically significant antibodies.

Wenz and Apuzzo[84] reported that the use of PEG, rather than BSA, resulted a reduced rate of positive IATs because of a reduced detection rate of clinically

insignificant antibodies, particularly Lewis system antibodies. However, the detection of antibodies related to the Rh and Kidd systems increased significantly, while the detection of other significant antibodies remained stable. The net result of using PEG was a decrease in the overall workload.

de Man and Overbeeke[82] compared PEG and albumin antiglobulin techniques by testing antibodies in the serums of 362 different patients. Agglutination in the PEG method was stronger in 70.2 percent, identical in 27.3 percent, and weaker in 2.5 percent. These investigators concluded that the PEG antiglobulin test is superior to the albumin antiglobulin test.

Use of Monospecific Versus Polyspecific Antiglobulin Reagents

There have been numerous reports of red cell alloantibodies that were not detectable with anti-IgG antiglobulin serum but that were detected with the anticomplement component of antiglobulin serum.[86–92] These antibodies may cause shortened red cell survival.[86,87,91,92] Also, reports have indicated that complement-fixing blood group antibodies are frequently detected at a higher dilution and/or higher titer score when a polyspecific antiglobulin serum is used, rather than a monospecific anti-IgG, even though the concentration of anti-IgG was the same in the monospecific antiserum as in the polyspecific antiserum as determined by titration tests.[88,93] This was reviewed by Petz and Garratty[86] in 1978 and by Garratty[92] in 1984. Unfortunately, however, polyspecific antiglobulin serum may result in some positive reactions that are not caused by clinically significant red cell alloantibodies.

In an effort to evaluate these variables, Petz et al.[43] prospectively studied 39,436 sera. Antibody detection was compared using anti-IgG or polyspecific antiglobulin serum in association with LISS or albumin reagents. Agglutination reactions were observed after an immediate spin phase, after incubation at 37°C, and in the IAT; incubation at room temperature was not performed. Negative reactions were confirmed by microscopic examination.

Four Jk^a antibodies were detected with polyspecific, but not with anti-IgG antiglobulin serum using albumin- or LISS-suspended RBCs. An additional Jk^a antibody was detected only with polyspecific antiserum when using LISS, but not with albumin. In addition, five antibodies of anti-Kell, -Jk^a, and -Fy^a specificities were detected in the indirect antiglobulin test when using LISS-suspended red cells, but not when using albumin; these positive results were obtained with anti-IgG or with polyspecific antiglobulin serum.

These investigators also determined the number of unwanted "false-positive" reactions obtained when using the polyspecific or anti-IgG antiglobulin serum with albumin- or LISS-suspended red cells. False-positive reactions were defined as those due to antibodies of no definable specificity (usually very weak and reactive with some, but not all, panel cells) or as antibodies that are optimally reactive in the cold and considered to be of no clinical significance (e.g., anti-I, -IH, -Le^b, -P$_1$, -M). The data are displayed in Table 9-6.

It is evident that some clinically significant antibodies are detected with the anticomplement component of antiglobulin serum, but not by anti-IgG. However, some test systems yield a relatively high incidence of false-positive reactions. For example, if one uses polyspecific antiglobulin serum and LISS,

a room temperature incubation, and reads all reactions microscopically, it is probable that an inordinate number of clinically insignificant reactions would be detected. Several strategies can be used to deal with this information.

When using polyspecific antiglobulin serum and LISS, 90 percent of the false-positive reactions were found to be positive only by microscopic examination.[43] However, there is no requirement for confirming negative agglutination test responses by microscopic examination, as discussed below.

Also, if the first step in evaluating a weakly positive reaction is the repeat of the test using serum and red cells that have been warmed to 37°C before mixing, about 60 percent of the weak reactions will become negative.[43] This will negate the necessity of attempting to identify the cause of the positive reaction. This step alone reduces the number of antibody identifications to manageable levels when using polyspecific antiglobulin serum with albumin, while still allowing for the detection of a large majority of the "complement-only" alloantibodies.

In summary, one must balance the advantage of detecting clinically significant "complement-only"

Table 9-6. Comparison of Polyspecific Antiglobulin Serum and Anti-IgG Antiglobulin Serum With Albumin or LISS for Red Cell Alloantibody Detection in 39,436 Serum Samples

Test System	No. of Clinically Significant Antibodies Not Detected When Using Anti-IgG AGS With Albumin	Prevalence of Clinically Significant Antibodies Not Detected When Using Anti-IgG AGS With Albumin	Percentage of False-Positive Reactions due to Cold Antibodies or "Nonspecific" Reactions	No. of False-Positive Reactions in 39,436 Sera	Ratio of False-Positive Reactions to Number of Clinically Significant Antibodies Not Detected When Using IgG AGS With Albumin
Polyspecific AGS with albumin	4	1/9,859	0.26	103	26
Polyspecific AGS with albumin prewarmed	4	1/9,859	0.17	67	17
Anti-IgG AGS with LISS	5	1/7,887	0.14	55	11
Polyspecific AGS with LISS	10^a	1/3,944	1.41	556	56
Polyspecific AGS with LISS	10^a	1/3,944	0.61	241	24
Anti-IgG AGS with albumin	—	—	0.10	39	—

Abbreviations: AGS, antiglobulin serum; albumin, 22% albumin; polyspecific, AGS containing anti-IgG and anti-C3; Anti-IgG, AGS containing anti-IgG only; prewarmed serum and red cells warmed to 37°C prior to mixing.

^{a} Five antibodies detected only with polyspecific AGS.

alloantibodies with the disadvantages resulting from using an antiglobulin serum containing anticomplement. The only significant disadvantage is the cost of investigating false-positive reactions, the frequency of which will be related to the source of the antiglobulin serum, the way the tests are read (e.g., microscopically versus macroscopically), the use of LISS versus albumin, and whether room temperature incubation is employed. For example, one may effectively use polyspecific antiglobulin serum in association with albumin-suspended RBC, but with the omission of room temperature incubation and microscopic examination of agglutination reactions.

Antigenic Composition of Indicator Reagent RBCs

Eighteen antigens (Table 9-7) must be present (but not necessarily in double-dose expression) on reagent RBCs licensed by the Food and Drug Administration (FDA) for antibody screening.[94]

In addition to the required 18, most high-incidence antigens are present on the reagent RBCs. Low-incidence antigens are often missing from reagent RBCs; therefore, antibody screening tests generally fail to detect antibodies directed at these antigens, unless by chance the screening cells used possess the low-incidence antigen.[95]

Reagent RBCs suitable by FDA regulation for antibody screening are offered commercially as a set of two or three vials, with each vial containing RBCs from a different individual. In 1992 the College of American Pathologists (CAP) surveyed more than 4,500 laboratories that performed immunohematologic testing to determine what percentage used a two-vial set versus a three-vial set, when performing

Table 9-7. Antigens Required by the FDA to Be Present on Reagent RBCs

System	Antigens
Rhesus	D, C, E, c, e
Kell	K, k
Duffy	Fy^a, Fy^b
Kidd	Jk^a, Jk^b
Lewis	Le^a, Le^b
P	P_1
MNSs	M, N, S, s

antibody screening. Of the laboratories that performed antibody screening, but not antibody identification, 67 percent used a two-vial set; however, of the laboratories that performed both antibody screening and antibody identification, a little more than 45 percent used a two-vial set, whereas more than 54 percent used a three-vial set.[96,97]

The reagent RBCs from different vials must not be pooled and then used for testing a patient for unexpected red cell antibodies, as the pooling could decrease the sensitivity of the test to detect certain antibodies.[98–100] Because some antibodies react stronger with RBCs that express a double-dose of a corresponding antigen, vendors provide antibody screening cell sets that express certain antigens at double-dose strength.[101,102]

Use of Chemically Modified Indicator Reagent RBCs

Chemical treatment of antibody screening reagent RBCs by proteolytic enzymes (ficin, papain, bromelin) will increase test sensitivity for certain antibodies (e.g., Rhesus, Kidd). However, enzyme treatment of RBCs weakens or totally destroys other RBC antigens (e.g., Duffy, MNS).[40] Consequently, antibody screening should not be performed using only enzyme-treated reagent RBCs.

The enhanced sensitivity of the enzyme method in detecting some weak alloantibodies is balanced by increased detection of benign insignificant antibodies. Issitt et al.[103] reported the results of an extensive retrospective study on samples from 10,000 recently transfused patients in which 35 samples were found to contain an antibody that reacted with ficin-treated red cells but was not demonstrable by LISS–IAT. In those 35 patients, the specificity of the antibody was such that each patient would have been transfused with antigen-negative blood, had the antibody reacted in LISS–IAT. Tests on red cells from the units that were already transfused showed that 19 patients had received 32 antigen-positive units. One patient experienced a delayed hemolytic transfusion reaction 7 days after transfusion with a drop in hemoglobin from 10.7 to 7.5 g/dl, but with an uneventful recovery. Also found in the 10,000 patients were 28 clinically insignificant antibodies, 77 sera with antibodies too weak to identify, and 216 autoantibodies that reacted only with ficin-treated red cells. Issitt et al. concluded that the use of protease-treated red cells for routine pretransfusion tests creates far more work than the accrued benefits justify.

Phase(s) at Which the Test is Checked to Detect Agglutination and Hemolysis

Current practice standards do not require that an immediate spin phase, room temperature phase, or 37°C incubation phase of an antibody screening test be read for agglutination or hemolysis. Only the IAT phase of an antibody screening test must be read. However, three of the traditional methods of antibody screening (saline-AHG, LISS-AHG, and albumin-AHG) have been shown to be more sensitive at detecting clinically important (and unimportant) antibodies when the 37°C phase of testing is read for agglutination and hemolysis. About 1 to 2 percent of antibodies with a clinically significant specificity might be detectable only if a reading of the 37°C incubation step is done when one of these three methods is used.[39,98,104,105] However, the omission of the 37°C reading might not be deleterious when using other techniques, such as PEG, which is routinely read only in the IAT phase.

Judd et al.[104] reviewed data from 87,480 tests for unexpected antibodies that used LISS, a 10-minute incubation at 37°C and anti-IgG antiglobulin serum. In 103 tests, antibodies of potential clinical significance were found (63 E, 27K, 5 Jk^a, 4 D, 3 cE, and 1 C) only at the 37°C incubation phase. The IAT became positive in subsequent samples with 27 of these antibodies. These investigators concluded that elimination of the 37°C reading for agglutination and hemolysis should not be undertaken lightly.

Use of Visual Aids to Detect Agglutination

It is standard practice to use a mirror with slight magnification or an illuminated background to aid in the detection of agglutination. The sensitivity of antibody detection testing can be further increased when a microscopic examination is performed to detect very weak RBC agglutination. However, there is no requirement that a macroscopically negative antibody screening test be checked microscopically for agglutination. In order to evaluate the importance of such a protocol, a 64-month study was done in which 209,722 antibody screening tests were performed, with each negative IAT result checked microscopically for agglutination.[28] Only seven pa-

tients were transfused with blood that had to be specially phenotyped as a result of discovering significant alloantibodies during microscopic examination of the IAT. These seven patients represented about 0.02 percent of the more than 30,000 patients transfused during the study period. One must question whether the effort and expense necessary to detect these very weak antibodies justifies the use of microscopic examination.

Use of a Direct Antiglobulin Test and Autocontrol

A DAT or autocontrol is often included as part of routine pretransfusion recipient testing, although this practice is not mandated by the AABB Standards. The rationale is that antibodies may be detected in a eluate from the DAT-positive RBC at a time that they are not detectable in the serum, thereby identifying previously undiagnosed autoimmune hemolytic anemia, immune aberrations associated with drug therapy, or occult alloantibody formation stimulated by recently transfused red cells. The effectiveness of such a policy has been questioned.

In 1986, Judd and coworkers reported a follow-up of their earlier experiences and reported results with the pretransfusion DAT in 65,049 blood samples from prospective transfusion recipients.[106,107] These investigators used an anti-IgG antiglobulin serum and found 3,570 positive test responses (5.49 percent). They performed elution studies on 778 samples, as these patients had been transfused within the preceding 14 days. In only six cases did the eluate contain an alloantibody when the corresponding serum lacked unexpected alloantibodies, as determined by routine pretransfusion studies. Three additional weakly reactive clinically significant alloantibodies were detected solely through additional serum tests performed on DAT-positive samples.

Huh and Lichtiger[108] performed a study of 14,548 pretransfusion samples and found no alloantibodies in the eluate that were not also detectable in the serum.

Stec et al.[109] include an autologous control as a routine part of serum antibody screening procedures at their institution but found that only four of 638 (0.6 percent) eluates gave results unavailable by serum testing alone. These workers recommend a red cell elution study only if there is clinical evidence of hemolysis, if the patient has received red cell transfusion within the previous 3 months, if a transfusion reaction is reported, or if there is a significant change in DAT results or the appearance of unexpected reactivity during serum testing.

Oberman et al.[110] pointed out that elimination of the DAT or autocontrol engenders less risk than does elimination of the antiglobulin crossmatch after a negative type and screen, and in both instances the risk is minimal. Nevertheless, Bator et al.[111] reported a survey of 170 hospitals and indicated that the autocontrol is frequently used as part of routine compatibility test procedures. These investigators suggested that laboratories should reassess the need for these policies.

Use of a Control System to Detect False-Negative IAT Results

A control system using RBCs sensitized with IgG must be applied to each IAT interpreted as negative to detect false-negative results that may be due to failure to add antiglobulin reagent, failure to wash away sufficient residual immunoglobulin before adding of antiglobulin reagent, or use of a faulty antiglobulin reagent (i.e., one that has been neutralized). If a licensed test system is being used that does not allow the addition of IgG sensitized cells to each negative antiglobulin test, controls must be used as recommended by the manufacturer.[27]

Use of Solid-Phase Red Cell Adherence or Column Agglutination Technologies

Solid-phase red cell adherence (SPRCA) assays and column agglutination (gel or bead media) are alternative methods to the standard slide and tube test that are currently available.[112–115]

SPRCA assays have evolved from a number of techniques as an alternative to conventional hemagglutination assays.[115] Hemagglutination assays suffer from occasional problems of rouleaux formation and the need for special potentiators and techniques for atypical antibody detection. Further problems encountered are caused by hemolysis, lack of an objective end point, and difficulty in automating hemagglutination test procedures. SPRCA methods using antibody-coated wells and cell-coated wells allow for batch red cell antigen typing and antibody detection (both ABO and unexpected antibodies).

Advancements in cell monolayer immobilization and drying enable SPRCA to compare favorably in sensitivity and specificity with traditional hemagglutination-based assays. One of the main advantages of dried SPRCA assays over hemagglutination is the labor savings. Improvements in solid-phase RBC immobilization include the use of automated cell washers that reduce labor time and exposure to potential infectious disease agents in the patient sample. Dried SPRCA reagents also improve the reliability and quality of SPRCA tests.

Column agglutination technology (CAT) is a new method for separating agglutinated from unagglutinated red cells; it may be applied to several elements of compatibility testing, including ABO/Rh and other red cell antigen typings, DAT and IAT, antibody detection testing, antibody identification, and crossmatching.

The basis of the procedure is the sieving effect of either a column of gel or glass bead microparticles to separate agglutinated from nonagglutinated RBCs in a small tube. When a centrifugal force is applied, unagglutinated red cells are forced to the bottom of the column, while movement of agglutinated red cells through the column is impeded. Strongly positive reactions form agglutinates that remain suspended near the top of the column, while weakly positive reactions form small agglutinates that remain suspended in the column at an intermediate position.

When mixed-field agglutination is present, as when testing with anti-A the red cells of a group A patient who has been transfused with group O RBC, the agglutinated A cells will be at or near the top of the column, while the unagglutinated or O RBCs will be at the bottom. A similar phenomenon will occur if blood is tested from an Rh-positive patient who has recently been transfused with Rh-negative RBCs. That is, when the patient's RBCs are tested with anti-D, the Rh-positive RBCs will form a strongly positive reaction at the top of the column, while the Rh-negative RBCs will form a negative reaction at the bottom of the column. The amount of RBCs at the bottom of the column will be in direct proportion to the amount of Rh-negative RBCs still in the patient's circulation.

There are many potential advantages for the gel test methodology as compared to tube techniques. The gel test allows procedures, reactions and their interpretations to be more standardized, since very specific quantities of serum and cells are placed in the microtubes, incubated and centrifuged for set times, and evaluated more objectively. Reactions may be stable for hours, so they can be confirmed by supervisory personnel; the results can be photocopied for documentation. Institutions, especially those that have a large infant and pediatric population and that have to work with small sample volumes may find CAT testing advantageous because of the small sample requirements. Finally, this technology eliminates the need for washing anti-globulin tests and increases the biosafety of performing the test.

The most significant limitation of a CAT method is the need to retain a test tube procedure for true STAT testing requests. This is because the 10-minute centrifuge time required to perform CAT testing is fixed, and the turnaround time for a single patient sample may be greater by CAT testing than by tube methods.

Antibody Identification

When an antibody screening test detects a red cell antibody in a patient's serum, the next step is to identify its specificity and clinical significance. The technical aspects of identification of the specificity of unexpected antibodies are reviewed elsewhere,[40] and the determination of the antibody's clinical significance is reviewed below.

Major Crossmatch

Current standards of the AABB[27] mandate that a major crossmatch using donor cells from the originally attached whole blood or component segment and the recipient serum or plasma shall be done before administration of whole blood and RBC components, except for urgent blood requirements. However, if no clinically significant unexpected antibodies were detected in an appropriately performed screening test that included the use of an antiglobulin test, and there is no record of detection of such antibodies, only the test methods that demonstrate ABO incompatibility are required. ABO incompatibility may be demonstrated by such methods as the "immediate spin" crossmatch or a "computer crossmatch."

The decision regarding whether to use a crossmatch with an antiglobulin test following a negative antibody screening test depends on analysis of the safety of antibody screening methods ("Type and Screen") for detecting clinically significant antibodies.

Safety of the Type and Screen Procedure

The safety of the type and screen procedure was evaluated by Boral and Henry,[116] who examined 12,848 blood specimens with the type and screen as well as the crossmatch and detected 283 antibodies in 247 patients. The reagent screening cells used were able to detect 96.11 percent of the antibodies. They calculated that if the antigen frequencies corresponding to those antibodies not detected by the screening cells were taken into consideration (i.e., the incompatibility frequencies) the type and screen was 99.99 percent effective in preventing the transfusion of serologically incompatible blood.

Similarly, Oberman and colleagues[117] reported a retrospective study of 82,647 crossmatches performed on serum from approximately 13,950 patients. They concluded that had blood been released without an antiglobulin crossmatch after a negative type and screen, there would have been a probability of one in 1,744 that a "clinically significant" but extremely weak recipient antibody would have gone undetected.

A review of the literature regarding clinically significant antibodies coupled with information concerning antigens not usually contained on commercially available screening cells suggests that few clinically important antibodies will be missed by an appropriately designed serum screening test.

Table 9-8 lists those antibodies that have been implicated as causes of hemolytic transfusion reactions or hemolytic disease of the newborn and that are reactive with antigens not usually contained on commercially supplied antibody detection cells.[118–154] However, there is no evidence indicating that antibodies that cause hemolytic disease of the newborn will necessarily cause hemolytic transfusion reactions; indeed, only nine of these antibodies have been reported to have caused hemolytic transfusion reactions.[120,131,136,137,139,147,148,151,153,154] Further-

Table 9-8. Antibodies Reported to Have Caused
Hemolytic Transfusion Reaction or
Hemolytic Disease of the Newborn and
That Recognize Antigens Not Usually
Present on Commercially Supplied
Antibody Detection Cells

Antibody	No. of Reported Examples Causing		Reference(s)
	HTR	HDN	
Anti-f (ce); Rh:6	0	2	118, 119
Anti-rh₁ (Ce); Rh:7	1[b]	0	120
Anti-Cʷ; Rh:8	0	4	119, 121–124
Anti-Cˣ; Rh:9	0	2	125, 126
Anti-Eʷ; Rh:11	0	2	127, 128
Anti-Goª (Gonzales); Rh:30	0	2	123, 129
Anti-Evans	0	1	123
Anti-Zd	0	1	130
Anti-Beª (Berrens)	0	4	123
Anti-Kpª (Penny)	1[a]	1	131, 132
Anti-Jsª (Sutter)	2	1	131, 133, 134
Anti-Luª (Lutheran)	1[b]	1	120, 135
Anti-Wrª (Wright)	2	4	136, 137, 123
Anti-Diª (Diego)	0	5	123, 138
Anti-Kamhuber (Far)	1	0	139
Anti-Rd (Radin)	0	5	140
Anti-Vʷ (Verweyst)	0	1	123
Anti-Miª (Miltenberger)	0	2	123
Anti-Hut (Hutchinson)	0	2	123
Anti-Mur (Murrell)	0	2	123
Anti-Hill (Hill)	0	1	123
Anti-By (Batty)	0	1	141
Anti-Good	0	1	123, 142
Anti-Heibel	0	1	143
Anti-Htª (Hunt)	0	1	123
Anti-Becker	0	1	144
Anti-Ven	0	1	145
Anti-Rm	0	1	146
Anti-Doª (Dombrock)	1	1	148, 149
Anti-Doᵇ (Dombrock)	2	0	147, 154
Anti-Reª (Reid)	0	1	150
Anti-Coᵇ	3	0	151–153

Abbreviations: HTR, hemolytic transfusion reaction; HDN, hemolytic disease of the newborn.

[a] Only one example reported to Grove-Rasmussen, but no documentation in the literature (see text).

[b] Reaction was of the delayed type (see text).

more, a critical review of these latter reports reveals inadequate documentation in many instances.

More recently, further data concerning the safety of abbreviated compatibility testing have been published.[110,155–160] Oberman et al.[110] found nine unexpected antibodies of clinical significance in 31,320 pretransfusion blood samples from 8,969 patients whose screening test for unexpected antibodies was nonreactive (anti-C, -c, -Jkᵇ, and three examples of each anti-E and anti-Jkª). Three of the antibodies were found retrospectively to manifest a positive screening test result. Another antibody was not detected by the antibody screening test due to an error in preparation of the screening RBCs.

Shulman et al.[155] issued blood to 19,818 patients without performing the antiglobulin phase of the crossmatch. In all cases, the antibody screening test response was negative. Only eight antibodies of potential clinical significance were found when the antiglobulin phase of the crossmatch was subsequently performed (anti-Jkª, -V, -Leᵇ, passively transfused anti-A, and four examples of anti-Leª). None of the patients with potentially hemolytic antibodies demonstrated a symptomatic transfusion reaction, although the patient with anti-Jkª received only 10 ml of red cells because the antibody was identified soon after release of the unit for transfusion.

A study by Pinkerton and colleagues[161] demonstrated that the routine use of an immediate spin crossmatch for a patient with no evidence of clinically significant red cell alloantibodies did not significantly increase the occurrence of a delayed hemolytic transfusion reaction (DHTR).

Heddle et al.[162] performed a prospective study in which patients requiring red cell transfusion had a type and screen performed and, if the antibody screen was negative, the antiglobulin crossmatch was omitted. Following the transfusion of the blood, the antiglobulin crossmatch was performed to look for any potential incompatibility. A total of 2,404 patients were transfused 10,899 red cell concentrates. The antiglobulin crossmatch performed after the transfusion indicated that 168 units (1.5 percent) would have been incompatible if the antiglobulin crossmatch had been performed before the transfusion. In only 27 transfusion episodes was the antiglobulin crossmatch on blood transfused positive due to an IgG antibody, and none of the patients receiving this blood had clinical or serologic evidence of hemolysis. It was concluded that the antiglobulin phase of the crossmatch can be omitted from pretransfusion testing without putting patients at risk.

Nevertheless, some investigators have reported up to a 10% increase in the risk of a DHTR when the immediate spin crossmatch was used routinely.[163] However, even if the use of an immediate spin crossmatch resulted in a modest increase in the occurrence of a DHTR, patient safety might not be compromised since a DHTR tends to be mild and is rarely a cause of serious morbidity.[164]

A small increase in risk also exists that an acute hemolytic transfusion reaction (AHTR) will occur if an immediate spin crossmatch is used as the crossmatch method. In a recent survey, the per crossmatch risk of an AHTR occurring in association with a "compatible" immediate spin crossmatch was estimated at approximately one in 250,000[165] (one out of every 30,000–40,000 patients transfused following a compatible immediate spin crossmatch developed an AHTR with hemoglobinemia and hemoglobinuria). In that survey and in other reported cases of AHTR following the use of an immediate spin crossmatch, reactions have been caused by clinically significant unexpected antibodies that escaped detection in an antibody screening test. Most of these reactions could have been avoided had an IAT been included in the crossmatch method.[165,166] Therefore, it might be argued that the routine use of an immediate spin crossmatch might increase slightly the risk of an AHTR and could increase the risk of an ABO-incompatible transfusion. By contrast, the use of an immediate spin crossmatch might allow for significant simplification and streamlining of the compatibility testing routine, which in turn might result in fewer errors and a reduction in the overall risk of an AHTR.[167]

The benefit-to-risk ratio of using an immediate spin crossmatch will depend on the method of antibody screening, the population being tested, and other factors unique to different institutions. Therefore, workers contemplating its use should weigh the economic advantages against the potential risks at their own institution. At the authors' institutions, we have chosen not to perform the antiglobulin crossmatch after a negative type and screen when there is no record of prior detection of unexpected antibodies.

Immediate Spin Crossmatch

The most commonly used procedure to demonstrate ABO compatibility is an immediate spin crossmatch. However, studies have shown that this method does not always detect ABO incompatibility, especially between group B patient sera and group A_2B donor RBCs.[168–171] Other ABO incompatibilities can also be missed, even when the patient is group O.[172] The discrepancy between ABO typing results and the results of the immediate-spin crossmatch is generally attributable to the higher potency of blood group typing reagents than that of some patients' serum antibodies. However, prozoning may also be responsible for such errors when red cells in diluents lacking EDTA are used, indicating that the immediate-spin crossmatch has the potential to miss very potent antibodies.[173]

Crossmatch error due to failure of the immediate-spin technique has only rarely been reported,[172] probably because this would occur only if a "clerical" mistake resulted in the selection of a unit of the wrong type for crossmatching and this error happened to result in a false-negative immediate-spin crossmatch. Taking into account the probability of such an event, Park[174] projected that the likelihood of missed ABO incompatibility between group B patients and group A_2B red cells due to limitation of the immediate-spin technique to be less than 1 in 2 million units.

The great majority of reports indicate that the immediate-spin crossmatch after a negative type and screen provides a high degree of safety in a cost-effective manner as has been demonstrated by extensive experience.[110,117,155–158,162,175,176]

"Computer Crossmatch"

Present AABB Standards for Blood Banks and Transfusion Services[27] indicate that a computer can be used to release red cells to a patient without a serologic crossmatch. This procedure is often called a "computer crossmatch." The conditions for using a computer crossmatch are as follows:

1. The system in use must have been validated on

site to prevent release of ABO-incompatible blood. Computer system specifications provided by a vendor are not sufficient; each institution must document the capabilities and safeguards of its own system.

2. The computer can be used to select units only for recipients for whom the only pretransfusion requirement is demonstration of ABO compatibility. It cannot be used for patients with current or previous clinically significant unexpected antibodies.

3. There must have been at least two separate determinations of the recipient's ABO group. Ideally, this should reflect tests done on two different specimens from the patient. In many settings, however, requiring and obtaining two separate specimens could delay provision of needed care and engender confusion or practices that endanger instead of protect the patient. The requirement for two ABO determinations can be met in any of three different ways: by testing two different specimens drawn on the current admission; by comparing results on the current specimen with historical records; or, if no previous records exist, and only one specimen is available, by testing the current specimen twice and comparing the results.

4. The system must include complete data about the donor unit, (i.e., unique alphanumeric identifier, the component name, the ABO group and Rh type, and the interpretation of the ABO confirmatory test). Data about the recipient is also necessary (i.e., the identification number and ABO group and Rh type).

5. The system must contain, and there must be documentation that it contains, logic to alert the user to data discrepancies for either donor unit or recipient, and to ABO incompatibilities between donor unit and recipient.

6. There must be a method to verify that data have been correctly entered into the system. This means an opportunity for the user to review and give positive verification of recorded material before it is permanently entered. Thus results cannot be accepted if captured by automatic interfacing with analytical instruments or by unverified manual entry.

When a computer crossmatch is used, careful attention must be paid to the selection of ABO grouping reagents. For instance, the use of polyclonal anti-A and anti-B may result in anomalous results, although ABO grouping discrepancies associated with the use of polyclonal grouping reagents are easily recognized and are generally not difficult to resolve. However, the use of currently available murine monoclonal reagents may be associated with grouping problems that are novel.

Monoclonal anti-A may recognize the B(A) phenomenon associated with synthesis of A blood group determinants by patients with high levels of the B-gene-specified transferase, alpha-D galactosyltransferase.[177,178] Also, several manufacturers formulate monoclonal anti-B from a murine monoclonal antibody (mAb), called ES4, that is exquisitely sensitive for acquired-B antigens.[179] Examples of potentially serious consequences that may occur through use of such reagents have been reported, particularly when serum ABO test results are also in error.[180,181] Because the safety of the computer crossmatch relies on the accuracy of the blood group of record, and because of the inherent grouping problems when some mAbs are used for ABO testing, the use of polyspecific reagents for the initial ABO/Rh determination of all blood samples submitted for pretransfusion testing has been recommended.[182]

Use of a computer crossmatch may be economically advantageous. Significant time savings can be accrued by replacing an immediate spin crossmatch with a computer crossmatch. Less time is needed to procure and prepare donor RBCs for testing, and fewer clinically insignificant antibodies are detected, thus requiring fewer antibody identification procedures. About one in 1,000 immediate spin crossmatches have been shown to give false-positive results, due mostly to rouleaux, anti-A_1, and cold agglutinins.[183] The false-positivity rate is lower when donor cells are washed before the immediate spin crossmatch is done, but testing takes longer. Additional benefits of using a computer crossmatch include job simplification, absence of unwanted negative tests due to weak anti-A and/or anti-B, the ability to reduce the specimen volume requirements for pretransfusion testing, and reduced exposure of staff to biohazardous materials. Furthermore, a computer crossmatch system matches for Rh as well as

ABO and can prevent release of platelets of the wrong ABO/Rh or plasma products that are incompatible with the intended recipient's RBCs. There is also an added measure of patient safety that arises from duplicate testing for ABO/Rh; such testing safeguards against technical and computer entry errors.

As data become available regarding the safety of using a computer crossmatch, it may be proven that computers can at least equal, if not exceed, the safety of using a serologic crossmatch test. If a computer crossmatch finds acceptance in practice, one ramification might be more widespread centralized compatibility testing. If a patient's serum does not need to come in contact with donor red cells, it would be easy to envision more out-of-hospital testing of units and patients. Also, computer links between the blood center and the hospital might someday allow direct access to the donor blood group results.

Unnecessary Compatibility Test Procedures

In recent years, there has been continued emphasis on examining the value of many compatibility test procedures. The reasons for these evaluations are essentially twofold: one is economics, and the other is an ongoing desire to provide good service in a timely fashion. The underlying philosophy that has allowed for the development of more cost-effective compatibility test procedures is that it is impractical to apply all possible serologic tests to each aspect of compatibility testing. For example, by explicitly permitting the use of plasma, the AABB Standards[27] imply that antibodies detectable only with the anti-complement component of antiglobulin serum may be ignored. By permitting omission of antiglobulin crossmatching on patients with a negative antibody screening test result, the Standards imply that the rarely encountered antibodies against antigens absent from antibody screening cells may be ignored. The FDA requires the presence of a certain number of antigens on screening cells but makes no requirements as to homozygosity. These policy statements place certain kinds of serologic events in the category of allowable risk.[184–186]

Accordingly, it is appropriate to examine procedures carefully that are performed in the blood bank, to evaluate whether they truly add a significant degree of safety at a justifiable cost. A number of suggestions may be made regarding elimination of

Table 9-9. Suggestions for Elimination of Unnecessary Procedures Commonly Performed in Blood Banks

Donor units
  Do not confirm the Rh type of Rh-positive units.
  Do not rescreen donor units for antibody.
  Use anti-A,B to confirm group O donor units, rather than using anti-A and anti-B.
  Eliminate the routine use of the DAT.
  Do not use an Rh control when testing Rh-negative donor units.

Patient testing
  Eliminate the use of anti-A,B on all recipients or use the anti-A,B only on group O recipients.
  Eliminate A_2 and O cells for reverse grouping.
  Eliminate the D^u tests on recipients excluding prenatal, postpartum, and cord blood samples.
  Eliminate the use of Rh control when using a chemically modified anti-D, except on blood group AB.
  Eliminate the room temperature antibody screen and the room temperature crossmatch.
  Eliminate the antihuman globulin crossmatch if the antibody screen is negative and there is no history of antibody formation.
  Eliminate the autocontrol and DAT during the crossmatch.
  Eliminate the evaluation of all positive DAT results by the use of elution procedures. An appropriate protocol should be established defining which positive DAT results need further evaluation.
  Eliminate screening for units negative for Le^a, Le^b, P_1, A_1, or Lu^a when these antibodies are not reactive at 37°C.

commonly performed procedures (Table 9-9). It is of value to examine the evidence relating to some of these aspects of pretransfusion testing.

Minor Crossmatch

The minor or "indirect" crossmatch is a test between the donor serum or plasma and the recipient red cells. Its performance has been the subject of considerable controversy for many years. Today, the minor crossmatch is considered obsolete and has been replaced by requirements for deliberate screening for the detection of significant blood group antibodies contained in the donor serum. Minor crossmatching is not even mentioned in the current Standards for Blood Banks and Transfusion Services of the AABB,[27] and it is not supported by any recent literature.

Donor Antibodies

In 1977, Giblett[187] reviewed the data relating to the necessity of testing the serum of all donors for the presence of unexpected antibodies. She concluded that the policy of using the antiglobulin test to screen the serum of all blood donors seems overconservative, time-consuming and unnecessarily expensive.

Nevertheless, the 16th edition (1994) of Standards for Blood Banks and Transfusion Services of the AABB[27] states, "Serum or plasma from donors with a history of transfusions or pregnancy should be tested for unexpected antibodies, preferably at the time of processing." Even this number of tests would appear wasteful except, perhaps, in Rh-negative donors, and further refinements in the indications for and techniques of donor antibody screening should be considered. However, it is unnecessary for transfusion services to repeat the testing of donor units.

Cold-Reactive Antibodies

In Giblett's 1977 report,[187] she pointed out, in an essentially parenthetical manner, that her experience indicated that there was no need to be concerned with alloantibodies that do not react at 37°C. This conclusion was thought to be justified by the fact that in vivo hemolysis was not observed in association with cold-reacting alloantibodies such as anti-A_1, -P_1, -M, -N, -Lu^a, during a 20-year period. During this time, over a million units of blood were transfused. On the rare occasions that antibodies of these specificities are found to react at 37°C (i.e., when cells and serum are warmed to 37°C and are then combined and incubated at that temperature), crossmatch-negative blood (or blood lacking the specific antigen) is still considered appropriate.

It is evident that Giblett's statements were made as the result of retrospective impressions rather than on the basis of a carefully constructed prospective study. Nonetheless, her conclusions are consistent with the experimental observations of Mollison et al.,[188] and convincing data refuting her statements have not been published. Current Standards for Blood Banks and Transfusion Services of the AABB[27] indicate that methods of testing for unexpected antibodies in serum or plasma "shall include *37°C incubation* preceding an antiglobulin test using reagent red blood cells that are not pooled." There

is no requirement for routine detection of cold-reactive antibodies.

Direct Antiglobulin Test and Autocontrol

A DAT or autocontrol frequently is included as part of routine pretransfusion recipient testing to detect previously undiagnosed autoimmune hemolytic anemia, immune aberrations associated with drug therapy, or occult alloantibody formation stimulated by recently transfused red cells. However, such a practice is not mandated by accrediting agencies, and it is our opinion that it can reasonably be omitted from routine compatibility test procedures.

RECOMMENDATIONS FOR ROUTINE COMPATIBILITY TESTING

On the basis of the aforementioned information, it seems reasonable to make the following recommendations concerning some aspects of routine testing while recognizing that numerous alternative approaches for many aspects of compatibility testing are acceptable.

1. The unnecessary procedures listed in Table 9-9 should be eliminated.
2. A minor crossmatch is superfluous.
3. An autocontrol/DAT is unnecessary as a part of routine compatibility test procedures.
4. Eluates should be performed when a patient has a positive DAT response only if the test was performed to evaluate suspected immune hemolysis, including suspected hemolytic transfusion reactions.
5. The antibody screening test may be performed by using incubation at 37°C and an antiglobulin test. Although a screening test using red cells suspended in normal saline for 30 to 60 minutes and anti-IgG antiglobulin serum will only rarely miss important antibodies, the use of a more sensitive test procedure is advisable. This can include the use of red cells suspended in albumin or LISS and/or the use of polyspecific antiglobulin serum. The routine use of enzyme-treated red cells for compatibility testing does not seem indicated.
6. If no clinically significant unexpected antibodies are detected in an appropriately performed anti-

body screening test that includes an antiglobulin test, and there is no record of previous detection of such antibodies, only serologic testing to detect ABO incompatibility should be done, such as an immediate spin crossmatch (or a "computer crossmatch").

7. Whenever the antibody screening test response is positive, antibody identification tests should be performed by using sensitive methods, and a major crossmatch using an antiglobulin test should be performed on each red cell product transfused.

8. Extraordinary measures are appropriate to prevent clerical errors at specimen collection, in the laboratory, and at the time of administration of the blood.

CLINICAL SIGNIFICANCE OF RED CELL ALLOANTIBODIES

Many factors may influence whether a red cell antibody is clinically significant, that is, will cause hemolysis in vivo. These are summarized in Table 9-10. Unfortunately, as yet there is no recognized in vitro characteristic or group of characteristics that can be used to indicate the in vivo significance of all red cell antibodies. Serologic characteristics of an antibody correlated empirically with past clinical experience has provided most of our present knowledge. In addition, red cell survival studies have contributed significantly. The two serologic characteristics that have proved most helpful in predicting in vivo significance are an antibody's specificity and its ability to react in vitro at 37°C. The following discussion reviews the clinical significance of some red cell alloantibodies; additional information is included in Table 9-8 (see also Ch. 5).

Clinically Significant Antibodies

Antibodies that react at 37°C and that cause a significant majority of hemolytic transfusion reactions are antibodies of the ABO, Rh, Kell, Kidd, and Duffy blood group systems and S and s antibodies of the MNSs system (Table 9-11, group I). The incidence

Table 9-10. Factors That May Influence the Clinical Significance of Red Cell Antibodies

Specificity
Thermal range of antibody
Number of antigen sites on red cell membrane
Mobility of antigens within membrane
Class of immunoglobulin
Subclass of IgG
Quantity of antibody-sensitizing red cells
Equilibrium constant of antibody
Presence of blood group antigenic substances in donor plasma
Ability of antibody to activate complement
Amount of blood transfused
Activity of recipient's reticuloendothelial system

Table 9-11. Clinical Significance of Some Red Cell Alloantibodies[a]

Group I. Clinically significant antibodies
    ABO
    Rh
    Kell
    Duffy
    Kidd
    Ss
Group II. Benign antibodies
    Chido/Rodgers (Ch^a/Rg^a)
    Xg^a
    Bg
    "HTLA"
    Cs^a
    Kn^a
    McC^a
    JMH
Group III. Clinically insignificant if not reactive at 37°C; possibly significant when reacting at 37°C
    Lewis (Le^a/Le^b)
    M, N
    P_1
    Lutheran (Lu^a/Lu^b)
    A_1
Group IV. Antibodies that are sometimes clinically significant
    Yt^a
    Vel
    Ge
    Gy^a
    Hy
    Sd^a
    York (Yk^a)

[a] Other antibodies that have been reported to cause shortened red cell survival on rare occasions are listed in Table 9-8 (see also Ch. 5).

Table 9-12. Antibodies Detected in Blood Transfusion Recipients in Four Studies

	Grove-Rasmussen and Huggins[305] (1973)[a]	Tovey[306]	Spielman et al.[119] (1974)	Walker[307] (1977)	Total	Order of Frequency
Anti-D	8,772	3,002	245	778	12,797	1
Anti-E	1,079	231	45	118	1,473	3
Anti-c	619	154	14	53	840	5
Anti-e	86	20	0	2	108	8
Anti-C (together with D)	2,156	28	52	163	2,399	2
Anti-Kell (K, k)	978	174	41	181	1,374	4
Anti-Duffy (Fy^a, Fy^b)	372	72	16	55	515	6
Anti-Kidd (Jk^a, Jk^b)	141	17	12	13	183	7
Anti-Ss	0	9	0	0	9	9
Others (e.g., Le^a, Le^b, Wr^a M, N, P$_1$, unidentified)	1,177	0	72	184	1,433	
Total	15,380	3,707	497	1,547	21,131	

^{a} Does not include antibodies when detected together with other antibodies (except for anti-C, when present with anti-D)

(From Garratty,[308] with permission.)

of these antibodies in blood transfusion recipients as determined in four large studies is indicated in Table 9-12.

When antibodies of group I are found, or if the patient's record indicates that these antibodies have been present in the past, it should be assumed that incompatible blood will lead to a hemolytic transfusion reaction, and red cells negative for the appropriate antigen should be transfused. Even here, it must be realized that serious hemolysis will not necessarily ensue if red cells carrying these antigens are given. The severity of hemolysis caused by antibodies that are considered clinically significant varies strikingly. Anti-A and anti-B antibodies usually, but not always, cause immediate symptomatic transfusion reactions that in some cases may even be fatal. Some antibodies in the Rh, Kell, and Kidd blood group systems may cause serious degrees of hemolysis, whereas in other instances only modest shortening of red cell survival occurs, and there are no important clinical sequelae.

Experience derived from transfusing such subjects out of absolute necessity in life-threatening situations, as in liver transplantation, when supplies of compatible blood are exhausted, has indicated that the anticipated hemolysis may not occur or may be minimal and cause tolerable morbidity[189] (see Ch.

35). Thus, every effort should be made to supply antigen-negative blood, but one must keep in mind that some extraordinary circumstances require transfusion of incompatible blood, even to patients with antibodies of specificities in group I of Table 9-11 (see case example later in chapter).

Benign Antibodies

Other alloantibodies are "benign" or cause only minimal red cell destruction even though they react at 37°C; some of these are listed in group II. Hemolytic transfusion reactions caused by antibodies of group II have not been reported.[190] Also, red cell survival studies using ^{51}Cr-labeled incompatible red cells have been performed in patients with anti-Cs^a, -Kn^a, -McC^a, -Ch^a, and -JMH; the results have indicated completely normal survival or have demonstrated destruction of only a small portion of the test dose of labeled red cells.[190] It is an appropriate policy to transfuse red cells having the pertinent antigen, regardless of in vitro incompatibility, in patients who have group II antibodies.[190]

Antibodies That Are Usually Benign

The significance of some other antibodies that had been thought capable of causing hemolytic transfusion reactions has been reassessed. Experience has indicated that antibodies that are reactive in vitro only at temperatures below 37°C are clinically benign,[187] and many examples of the antibodies in group III react only in the cold. Thus, cold-reactive antibodies, such as anti-A_1, -P_1, -M, -N, and -Lu^a, can safely be ignored.[187] Even when antibodies of these specificities react at 37°C, their in vivo significance is uncertain, but they should be considered to be of potential clinical significance, and antigen-negative blood or crossmatch-compatible blood should be transfused.[190,191]

Lewis Antibodies

Lewis antibodies are included among those in group III; they are particularly common and justify special comment. Lewis antibodies are frequently encountered, but as pointed out by Giblett[187] and Oberman et al.,[117] only a small proportion of anti-Le^a can cause significant red cell destruction, and only one hemolytic transfusion reaction attributed to anti-Le^b has been reported.[192] Waheed et al.[193] evaluated the effects of a policy of transfusing patients with Lewis antibodies on the basis of major crossmatch compatibility testing that did not necessarily result in the selection of Le(a−) and/or Le(b−) blood for patients with corresponding antibodies in the serum. They transfused 230 units of blood to 33 patients who had Lewis antibodies or a previous history of Lewis antibodies. (Waheed et al. did supply antigen-negative blood for patients who had antibodies that demonstrated hemolysis in vitro, although they presented no data to indicate that even these antibodies cause shortened red cell survival of cross-match-negative blood.) The medical record of each transfused patient was reviewed to determine the response to the transfusion and to note any evidence of transfusion reactions. No immediate or delayed hemolytic transfusion reactions were detected, and the patients did not develop antibodies of higher thermal amplitude or titer as a result of the transfusions. However, the one report of a delayed hemolytic transfusion reaction caused by anti-Le^b occurred in a patient who received a transfusion of Le^b-positive red cells that were compatible in a crossmatch procedure that utilized anti-IgG antiglobulin serum and saline-suspended RBCs.[192]

Considerable time, energy, and expense can be saved by transfusing patients with Lewis antibodies on the basis of crossmatch compatibility alone; this seems a reasonable policy based on the data of Waheed et al.[193] and the experience of others.[191,194] Indeed, the policy at the UCLA Medical Center, in transfusing patients with Lewis antibodies, regardless of their in vitro characteristics, is to transfuse crossmatch-negative blood without typing the donor units for Lewis antigens. This approach is also strongly endorsed by others,[191,193,194] except that some prefer to provide antigen-negative blood when a Lewis antibody causes hemolysis in vitro.[193,194]

Antibodies That Are Sometimes Clinically Significant

Antibodies in group IV are inconsistent in regard to their in vivo significance. When an antibody of one of these specificities is detected, one possible course of action is to perform an in vivo compatibility test. For example, red cell survival studies in patients with anti-Yt^a have indicated rapid destruction of incompatible cells in some patients,[195–198] whereas in other cases the antibody has seemed incapable of red cell destruction.[195,196,199,200] One would like to avoid the search for antigen-negative blood since only about 0.2 percent of blood donors are Yt(a−); thus, one would need to screen about 1,000 donors to find two units of Yt(a−) blood. If the red cell survival demonstrates normal survival, the probability of an acute symptomatic hemolytic transfusion reaction is very low, so if transfusion is urgently needed, antigen-positive blood may be transfused.

Similarly, several studies have indicated normal red cell survival of incompatible blood in patients with anti-Sd^a,[201–203] but there is one report of a hemolytic transfusion reaction.[204] Also, there is one report of short red cell survival caused by anti-Yk^a,[205] whereas a previous report indicated a lack of clinical significance of an example of anti-Yk^a, even though it was present in a titer of more than 1:1,000.[206] Also, some examples of Vel, Ge, Gy^a, and Hy cause in vivo red cell destruction, while others are harmless.[190]

However, even if the red cell survival test demonstrates acceptable survival when antibodies of group IV are involved, the blood bank should make every effort to obtain compatible blood. This should include searching rare donor files and typing family members, especially siblings. Autologous transfusion would be a safe approach, if feasible. These measures are indicated because an acceptable red cell survival in an in vivo crossmatch procedure only ensures a high probability of the lack of an immediate symptomatic transfusion reaction and does not ensure against shortened red cell survival, which may be heightened by an anamnestic response leading to a hemolytic transfusion reaction (see the section on In Vivo Compatibility Testing).

SUMMARY OF CLINICAL DECISION MAKING WHEN A PATIENT WHO HAS RED CELL ALLOANTIBODIES REQUIRES TRANSFUSION

When a red cell alloantibody is present that reacts at 37°C, the following approach is recommended:

1. *Group I.* If the antibody is expected to be clinically significant (e.g., has a specificity listed in group I of Table 9-11), antigen-negative blood should be transfused, except in an extreme emergency.
2. *Group II.* If the antibody reacts at 37°C but is an antibody listed in group II of Table 9-11, antigen-positive blood may be transfused, even though it is incompatible in vitro.
3. *Group III.* For antibodies of group III, crossmatch-negative blood may be issued without the necessity of ensuring that the blood is negative for the antigen in question.
4. *Group IV.* For antibodies of group IV, an effort should be made to obtain antigen-negative blood from rare donor files (through reference laboratories) and/or by typing of family members. Consideration should be given to autologous transfusion, including the freezing of the patient's red cells for long-term storage. If antigen-negative blood cannot be obtained, an in vivo survival study may be performed. If this study reveals acceptable survival of an aliquot of incompatible red cells, blood may be transfused with a low probability of an immediate symptomatic hemolytic transfusion reaction.

If the in vivo survival study involving group IV antibodies demonstrates short survival or cannot be performed and there is no time to obtain antigen-negative blood, a clinical decision is required and is based on the primary physician's assessment of the urgency of the transfusion and the transfusion medicine specialist's assessment of the

probability of a serious hemolytic transfusion reaction. If the urgency of the clinical situation truly requires emergency transfusion, it is necessary to proceed. If practical, slow administration of a small volume of red cells (15 to 20 ml of packed red cells over 30 minutes) should be begun, carefully monitoring the patient for symptoms, and obtaining a blood sample from the patient after 30 minutes to observe for hemoglobinemia. Continued clinical observation and follow-up blood samples for hemoglobinemia, perhaps after each unit, will allow for repeat assessment of the results of the transfusion. Even if the transfusion is well tolerated, the volume of red cells transfused should be kept as small as possible because of the possibility of an anamnestic reaction that may lead to a delayed hemolytic transfusion reaction. Some very urgent clinical situations may necessitate less detailed monitoring, as indicated in the following case example.

TRANSFUSION IN THE PRESENCE OF MULTIPLE ALLOANTIBODIES

The risk of transfusing incompatible blood should only be considered when the risk of not transfusing incompatible blood outweighs the risk of transfusing it. This problem most commonly arises when a patient has multiple red cell alloantibodies.[207] The following case summary illustrates appropriate management of one such instance[208] (see Ch. 35).

A pregnant 28-year-old woman with severe abdominal pain was suspected of having an abdominal pregnancy. The patient had three previous pregnancies and multiple blood transfusions following an automobile accident 8 years earlier. Compatibility tests revealed that the patient was group A, Rh positive; an anti-K antibody reactive in the IAT using anti-IgG antiglobulin serum was identified in the patient's serum.

An exploratory laparotomy was performed, at which time a viable fetus weighing 970 g was removed from the abdominal cavity. It was deemed necessary to leave the placenta in situ because it was adherent to the serosal surfaces of the uterus, right fallopian tube, transverse colon, liver, posterior portion of the pelvis, and omentum. Five units of group

A Rh-positive and K-negative compatible red cells were transfused intraoperatively.

Evidence of a delayed hemolytic transfusion reaction was present by the 10th postoperative day. Her hematocrit dropped over a period of 2 days from 35 to 24 percent without evidence of bleeding; the DAT was positive; and anti-Fy^a, anti-Jk^b, anti-hr″ (e), anti-rh′ (C), and anti-S were present in addition to the previously identified anti-K. All 5 units of blood previously found to be compatible and transfused during the exploratory laparotomy were reactive in vitro, with one or more of the newly detected red cell alloantibodies. The hematocrit continued to fall to 20 percent, and the patient developed tachycardia and hypotension. Two units of compatible blood were obtained from a supply of frozen rare donor blood. The post-transfusion hematocrit was 27 percent, but dropped shortly afterward to 14 percent, because of sudden acute massive hemorrhage from partial placental separation. An emergency laparotomy was performed with removal of the placenta, uterus, and fallopian tubes.

Five additional units of compatible blood were obtained, but the patient continued to bleed profusely. When all compatible units had been transfused, 6 incompatible units were requested by the attending surgeon. It was the surgeon's opinion that without further transfusions the patient would expire. The 6 incompatible units were chosen to be negative for the Fy^a, Jk^b, and K antigens because it was felt that these had the greatest potential for causing severe hemolysis. Two units were positive for S, e, and C; 2 units were positive for C and e; and the remaining 2 units were positive for e. The patient's serum resulted in $1+$ to $2+$ agglutination in the IAT with each of the 6 units. In addition to the 13 units of red cells, she also received 6 units of fresh frozen plasma and several liters of non-blood volume expanders.

Her immediate postoperative hematocrit was 31 percent, and she received 2 additional units of compatible red cells, after which the hematocrit was 36 percent. The total and direct serum bilirubin levels, which were 0.9 and 0.3 mg/dl, respectively, prior to the hemorrhage, rose to 8.1 and 3.2 mg/dl, respectively, 8 hours after transfusion of the 6 incompatible units. Care was taken to observe and maintain the patient's renal output. Renal function remained normal, and there was no evidence of intravascular he-

molysis or disseminated intravascular coagulation (DIC). The fate of the transfused incompatible red cells was followed by testing for the C, e, and S antigens. S-positive red cells were detectable for 6 days, C-positive for 8 days, and e-positive for 10 days. She recovered from her hemorrhage and was ultimately discharged.

SPECIAL CONSIDERATIONS

Weakly Reacting Forms of the D Antigen

Red cell samples that react weakly with anti-D have in the past been called D^u, but the term "weakly reacting" D is now preferred, because D^u suggests a definable phenotype.[209] Some weakly reacting Ds are due simply to a quantitative reduction in D antigen. For example, in subjects with the haplotype *CDe/cde*, D is expressed more weakly than in *CDe/cde* subjects; in such cases, presumably all the epitopes of D are present. In other weakly reacting Ds, "partial Ds," one or more of the eight known epitopes of D are missing. The kind of partial D with the smallest number of D epitopes, "category VI," which has only epitopes D3 and D4, is now known to have two possible genetic backgrounds: in one, exons 4, 5, and 6 of the *D* gene are deleted; in the other, presumably because of chromosomal misalignment, they are replaced by exons 4, 5, and 6 of the *Cc/Ee* gene. The findings suggest that exons 4, 5, and 6 of the *D* gene are critical for the reactivity characterizing the epitopes D1, D2 D5, D6/7, and D8.

The Rh type of donor blood is determined with anti-D; if the initial tests are negative, the blood must be tested using a method designed to detect weak D. When either test is positive, the blood must be labeled "Rh positive."

The test for weak D is unnecessary when testing a transfusion recipient[27] because if a patient who is weak D positive is mistakenly typed as Rh-negative, no harm is done by transfusion of Rh-negative blood. If a patient is known to be weak D positive, opinions vary among transfusion medicine specialists as to whether transfusion of Rh-negative blood is necessary. Weak D-positive persons who are "partial Ds" can theoretically form anti-D of limited specificity but this is a rare event.

Conversion of ABO Blood Groups

Since the most serious risk of hemolytic transfusion reactions concerns ABO incompatibility, transfusion practice could be made much safer and compatibility testing procedures shortened if red cells to be transfused were group O. Efforts to change the ABO blood groups by removal of the A and B surface antigens in vitro have been undertaken since the early 1970's when the biochemical reactions of their production was understood.[210] Schenkel-Brunner and Tuppy[211] demonstrated that these immunodeterminant sugars could be modified in vitro. These workers showed that group O red cells exposed to the genetically determined specific transferases which conferred the A determinant, N-acetylgalactosamine (GalNAc) or the B determinant galactose (Gal) acquired these sugars and the related immunological characteristics.[211] This work suggested that red cell immunoreactivity could be modified in vitro and that it was possible to remove these terminal sugars from carbohydrate chain of the glycoprotein or glycolipid, which bound the determinants to the cell surface.

Efforts were made to find glycosidases that could efficiently remove the terminal sugars under conditions that would not be injurious to the cells. To be suitable for use in transfusion, the treated cells should have essentially all the characteristics of normal group O cells in terms of survival, immunologic reactivity and metabolic and gas transport functions. A number of α-galactosidases (B-Zyme) are possible candidates for this conversion, but relatively fewer α-N-acetylgalactosaminidases (A-Zyme).

The greatest progress to date has been made with removal of the B antigen. Goldstein et al.[212] purified a B-Zyme from green coffee beans that has sialidase activity, which is capable of removal of the B determinant sugar. The conditions of exposure include pH 5.5 to 5.6 for 2.25 hours at 26°C.[212] This enzyme has been cloned and efficiently expressed. Using this approach, these investigators successfully transfused volunteer normal subjects of group A and O with transfusions or exchange transfusions of up to 3 units of B to O enzyme-converted red cells without adverse events. Survival and function of the transfused red cells have been normal, and there is little evidence of enhanced production of anti-B in the recipients.[213,214]

Less progress has been made in removing the A antigen. Not only has an efficient glycosidase been difficult to identify, but the problem is complicated by the discovery of a second type of carbohydrate chain, the type 3, which has a second GalNAc, the second or internal A determinant, behind the usual terminal galactose–fucose groups. This internal determinant may be difficult to remove without causing major changes in the entire carbohydrate chain.[215] To be of real value in improving the logistics of blood banking, this problem will have to be overcome.

Group B cells converted to O can be frozen and recovered successfully. This may be useful in stockpiling bloods for emergencies or for use in remote locations, as in military requirements. Losses in processing are about 10 percent due mainly to processing to remove white cells and platelets. A system could be envisioned in which some group A and B bloods are converted to group O shortly after drawing, with cost savings by reducing the practice of overdrawing donations to ensure the usual expected excess need for group O bloods. This should further reduce outdating, although this is already at a relatively low level in the United States at present due to improved national logistical programs.

In Vivo Compatibility Tests

Transfusion services are occasionally faced with the dilemma of providing safe blood for a patient for whom it is difficult to obtain a negative crossmatch. In some of these instances, the antibodies causing the incompatibility may be of dubious clinical significance (see p. 220). In this situation, in vivo compatibility testing has been advocated by some and is based on measuring the survival of an aliquot of red cells. The most sensitive method is the use of a small volume (e.g., 0.5 to 1 ml) of radiolabeled red cells. The usual method uses ^{51}Cr, and the details of the methodology are given elsewhere.[40,205,216] Other methods use technetium-99m (^{99m}Tc),[217,218] indium-113m (^{113m}In),[219] or double labeling with ^{99m}Tc and ^{III}In.[220,221] Methods not involving radioactive isotopes include flow cytometry[222,223] and an enzyme-linked antiglobulin test (ELAT).[224]

The results of such tests may be of distinct value but must be interpreted appropriately.[195] When survival at 60 minutes is within normal limits (i.e., 99 ± approximately 5 percent) the red cells can be regarded as compatible, and it is probable that, if 1 unit of red cells from which the aliquot had been taken is transfused, there will be no immediate symptomatic hemolytic transfusion reaction. The data of Silvergleid et al.[196] are in agreement with this statement. Twenty-nine of their 42 ^{51}Cr survival studies revealed that the 1-hour survival rate was 94 percent or greater, and none of these patients who were subsequently transfused had evidence of hemolysis.

However, if survival of the radiolabeled red cells is less than normal, interpretation of the results is less clear. The International Committee for Standardization in Haematology commented that, if survival is at least 70 percent at 1 hour, the "deduction" is that the concentration of the offending antibody is very low, so the destruction of a large volume of incompatible red cells either will be negligible or will take place only slowly.[216] Indeed, a limited body of data supports such a deduction.[225,226] However, as emphasized by Perkins[227]: "This statement by a prestigious international committee often is taken too literally by inexperienced personnel. They expect approximately normal survival of the complete unit if more than 70 percent of the labeled cells remain in the circulation at 1 hour and consider transfusion to be contraindicated if the percentage of cells surviving at that point is less than 70 percent. Neither of these assumptions is necessarily correct."

Indeed, Burton and Mollison[228] demonstrated in red cell survival studies performed in rabbits that the difference in survival of small and large doses of incompatible red cells diminished when the concentration of the antibody increased. Studies in humans indicate that survival of 70 percent or more of a small aliquot of radiolabeled red cell at 1 hour may be associated with severe hemolysis when an entire unit is transfused. For example, Silvergleid et al.[196] reported one patient with warm antibody autoimmune hemolytic anemia who had a 1-hour RBC survival of 87 percent, a pretransfusion hematocrit level of 10.5 percent, a post-transfusion hematocrit of 20.6 percent, but a hematocrit of only 10 percent just 16 hours post-transfusion. Another patient, with paroxysmal cold hemoglobinuria, had a 1-hour survival rate of Tj(a+) red cells of 87 percent and was transfused with 0.5 units of blood; the survival rate after 48 hours was only 53 percent. Other patients reported by Silvergleid et al. in whom the 1 hour sur-

vival rate of ^{51}Cr-labeled red cells was 87 to 94 percent had no evidence of post-transfusion hemolysis. Thus, it is not possible to predict the survival of red cells given in therapeutic amounts after a 1-hour survival that is less than normal.[229] Mollison[230] recommends that when the observed survival rate at 60 minutes is less than 97 percent further samples should be taken after an interval of an hour or two, or even after 24 hours, if this is practicable. Similarly, Pineda et al.[205] emphasized that normal RBC survival values at 1 hour do not exclude the possibility of severe hemolysis 24 hours later. Thus, they recommend that if a 1-hour test result is normal, the procedure should be extended routinely to 24 hours.

Another approach to predicting the survival of a unit of red cells on the basis of the survival of a small aliquot of labeled red cells is to infuse the labeled red cells with the full unit.[231,232] This may be appropriate for patients requiring chronic red cell transfusion after an initial in vivo survival study has been performed over a short period. One must also keep in mind that it is not possible to predict whether antibody production will be stimulated by transfusion and result in AHTR or DHTR when RBC are subsequently transfused.

Some proponents of the use of ^{51}Cr red cell survival studies point out that an "acceptable" in vivo compatibility test, variously defined as greater than 70 to 85 percent at 1 hour,[27,196,216] will provide sufficient confidence that an acute life-threatening symptomatic hemolytic transfusion reaction will not occur, even if the ultimate survival of the transfused cells is not normal. This appears to be the major clinical value of an in vivo compatibility test in patients who have antibodies of uncertain clinical significance.

It is also true that even poor survival of radiolabeled test cells does not necessarily preclude transfusion. For example, Mayer et al.[233] described 16 patients in whom an aliquot of red cells had a 24-hour survival rate of less than 70 percent. Life-threatening conditions necessitated transfusing 11 of these patients, and only one suffered complications directly attributable to the transfusion. Data are not available to determine the rate of destruction of a test dose of red cells that would be predictive of an acute symptomatic hemolytic reaction.

Other investigators have performed in vivo compatibility studies using a simpler method.[234] This involves the testing for grossly visible evidence of hemoglobinemia following infusion of 10 to 15 ml of donor red cells (25 to 40 ml of whole blood) over a 30-minute period and has been referred to as the "pigment method." This is an extension of good routine transfusion practice, in which close observation of the patient is made during the administration of the first portion of a unit of blood. In the event of rapid red cell destruction, the patient may exhibit mild to moderate symptoms. Since the intravascular lysis of as little as 5 ml of red cells will raise the plasma hemoglobin concentration of an adult recipient by approximately 50 mg/dl, an amount easily detectable by gross visualization, the failure to observe hemoglobinemia suggests that immediate catastrophic hemolysis will not occur with infusion of the entire unit of blood.[234] Also, after a negative test result, it is feasible to perform another in vivo test as frequently as deemed necessary if subsequent transfusions are needed. One can make an argument for using the pigment method even in instances in which one performs a survival study using radiolabeled red cells, especially if such a study indicates that the survival rate of the labeled cells is less than 97 percent at 1 hour. This is true because the survival of a larger aliquot of red cells cannot be predicted well when the 1-hour survival of a small aliquot is less than normal. The advantages of the pigment method are that it is simple and does not require experience with radiolabeling techniques. Disadvantages are that some symptoms may develop if there is very rapid hemolysis of the test dose; it is also probable that modest degrees of shortened red cell survival will not be detected.

Finally, the problem arises as to the management of patients with poor in vivo compatibility test responses. Auto-transfusion is a safe approach, if feasible. If the patient's serum antibody is against a high-frequency antigen, blood from family members or from a rare donor file may be needed. In urgent situations, transfusion can be carried out with the knowledge that an immediate symptomatic hemolytic reaction appears to be unlikely if survival of a small aliquot of cells at 1 hour is greater than 70 percent. For extreme life-threatening emergencies, utilization of blood that one expects may be hemo-

lyzed rapidly is nevertheless warranted, particularly, as such dire expectations are not always realized.[233]

The interpretation of in vivo survival studies in patients who have autoimmune hemolytic anemia is further discussed in Chapter 20.

Donor Erythrocyte Destruction in the Absence of Serologic Evidence of Alloimmunization

Since 1957, a number of reports have appeared that describe rapid destruction of transfused red cells despite apparent in vitro compatibility between the recipient serum and donor erythrocytes.[195,235–243] In spite of increasing sensitivity of serologic techniques, the problem continues to be recognized and reported in the modern literature.[218,244–247] Other cases not reported are known in many blood centers and transfusion services.

The phenomenon can be evoked quite easily in dogs by following the fate of repeated transfusions from the same donor of ^{51}Cr-labeled red cells that are not recognized as antigenically different by typing with the limited number of sera that detect canine erythrocyte antigen systems.[248] After several such transfusions, shortening of red cell life span in vivo has been observed in about 10 percent of animals so challenged. In about one-half of these responders, serologic evidence of alloimmunization has been found, but the specificities of many of these antibodies have been incompletely investigated. They are difficult to work with in the laboratory because of the weak reactions they produce; in some instances, they may be parts of already recognized systems.

In the case of humans, it was recognized shortly after the implementation of practical methods for determining the life span of donor red cells in vivo that in some instances apparently compatible donor red cells disappeared more rapidly than expected.[195] There may be an initial phase of normal survival lasting 10 or more days, followed by a phase of accelerated destruction, suggesting that the transfusion has induced an immune response; this type of curve has been called a "collapse" curve (Fig. 9-1). In other instances accelerated destruction of transfused red cells begins at transfusion (Figs. 9-2 and 9-3).

Accelerated red cell destruction in the absence of demonstrable antibodies may be a serious clinical

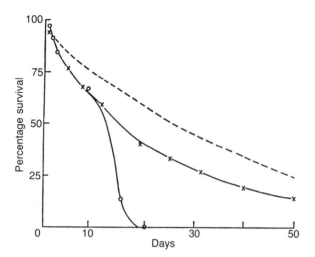

Fig. 9-1. Survival of ^{51}Cr-labeled red cells from two newborn infants following injection into a normal adult. Small samples of blood were taken from two infants, the first aged 35 hours and the second aged 50 hours. The samples were mixed with acid-citrate-dextrose (ACD) and then labeled with ^{51}Cr in the usual way. o——o, Cr survival of red cells from the first infant; 2 ml of red cells was labeled; x——x, Cr survival of red cells from the second infant; 8 ml of red cells was labeled. The interval between the two injections was 34 days. The dotted line shows the normal Cr survival curve observed when red cells from normal adults are labeled with ^{51}Cr in the same way. (From Mollison et al.,[188] with permission.)

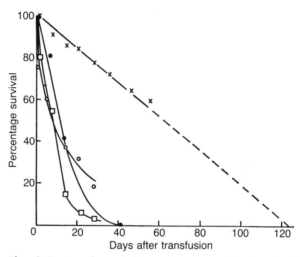

Fig. 9-2. Accelerated destruction of transfused red cells starting at the time of transfusion; no antibody demonstrable in vitro. ●——●, Survival of red cells from a particular donor as estimated by the method of differential agglutination; □——□, survival of red cells from the same donor on a subsequent occasion as estimated by labeling with ^{51}Cr; o——o, further estimate using ^{51}Cr as a label; x——x, survival of donor's own red cells in her own circulation as estimated with ^{51}Cr. All results are corrected for Cr elution. (From Mollison et al.,[188] with permission.)

problem and may be difficult or impossible to resolve. In some instances, the accelerated destruction occurs as a DHTR during the early stages of an immune response.[249] In these patients, antibody often becomes detectable in the patient's serum in subsequent days or weeks.

A much more difficult problem is presented by those patients in whom accelerated red cell destruction occurs repeatedly, but in whom antibody is never detected. Most commonly, attempts to find a compatible donor fail. For example, a patient described by Heisto et al.[239] developed hemoglobinuria 6 days after the transfusion of 2,800 ml of blood. Tests were subsequently carried out with red cells from eight different donors. The red cell survival as measured by the ^{51}Cr half-life varied from 14 days to less than 24 hours. Incidentally, the administration of large doses of prednisone did not prevent rapid cell destruction.

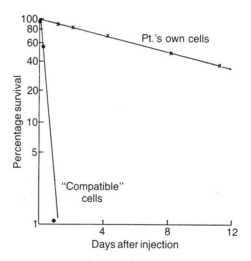

Fig. 9-3. Very rapid removal from the circulation of transfused cells compatible by all the usual serologic tests. For comparison, the survival of the patient's own red cells is shown. (From Mollison et al.,[188] with permission.)

In a patient with sickle cell disease who had undergone 58 blood transfusions, rapid destruction of transfused red cells occurred repeatedly.[243] Seventeen measurements of in vivo red cell survival were performed, and all were abnormal except for one occasion, when red cells from a sibling survived normally. However, a repeat transfusion from the same donor 6 months later survived normally for only 5 to 7 days. Subsequently, the donor's cells disappeared rapidly from the circulation. In another case described by Vullo and Tunioli,[250] red cells from the patient's father survived better than those from another donor.

Davey et al.[242] described a patient in whom anti-c was suspected because transfusion of 4 units of crossmatch-compatible red cells resulted in a severe delayed hemolytic transfusion reaction and the only common antigen lacking on the patient's cells and present on the donor's cells was c. Anti-c could not be detected in vitro, but the ^{51}Cr survival rate of c-positive red cells was 1 percent at 24 hours, while the survival rate of c-negative red cells was 80 percent at 24 hours. Eight c-negative units were transfused without evidence of a hemolytic reaction.

Similarly, Baldwin et al.[251] studied a patient who had several clinically severe hemolytic transfusion reactions. Sensitive antibody detection tests failed to reveal a red cell alloantibody other than anti-Bg^a. The tests used included a capillary technique; low-ionic strength Polybrene; low-ionic strength Polybrene antiglobulin test; low-ionic strength antiglobulin test for IgG, IgM, and IgA; a solid-phase test for both DAT and an indirect IgG antiglobulin test; an ELAT; a ^{125}I-linked anti-IgG (radioimmunoassay [RIA]); and a mononuclear cell phagocyte assay. The patient was group O, R_2R_2, and ^{51}Cr survival studies demonstrated destruction of red cells with the Rh antigen hr″(e). Survival of hr″(e)negative red cells was near normal, and the patient was successfully transfused with hr″(e)negative units of red cells.

Garratty et al.[246] described 17 patients who had a hemolytic transfusion reaction but who had no detectable antibodies. Ten of the 17 had marked hemolysis as indicated by the presence of hemoglobinuria. By using a battery of sensitive tests, antibodies were detected in four patients. Two patients had anti-C, two had anti-E, and one had anti-Jk^a. No hemolytic transfusion reactions occurred when blood lacking the respective antigens was transfused. Of the various test procedures used, only the 4 percent ficin capillary test and the Polybrene method were of any value.

Harrison et al.[218] reported a patient who had experienced repeated asymptomatic intravascular hemolytic reactions following the transfusion of red cells possessing the C antigen. Extensive serologic investigations never detected a red cell alloantibody. However, red cell survival studies with ^{99}Tc demonstrated rapid destruction of red cells with the C antigen while red cells lacking the C antigen appeared to survive normally. Transfusion of 2 units of red cells that were C negative were well tolerated. The authors also reviewed the literature. Table 9-13 summarizes the cases included in that review.

It is widely assumed that hemolysis of donor red cells in the absence of demonstrable serum antibody has an immunologic basis. This viewpoint has been strengthened by observations made in certain patients with what clinically appears to be autoimmune hemolytic anemia but who have negative DAT results. They may also lack other usual laboratory evidence of red cell-bound autoantibodies. Nevertheless, Gilliland[252] showed that increased amounts of immunoglobulin (IgG) are bound to the surface of these patients' red cells. This was accomplished by employing a sensitive quantitative method of measurement of red cell-bound IgG. Normal human red cells have fewer than 35 molecules of IgG per cell. Usually, several hundred molecules of IgG antibody per red cell are required for a positive antiglobulin test result, the precise number depending on the characteristics of the red cell, the red cell antibody, and the antiglobulin serum.[253] The "Coombs-negative" acquired hemolytic anemia patients usually have red cell burdens of IgG within the range of 50 to 400 molecules per cell.[252,253] These observations indicate that, under certain circumstances, even very small amounts of bound red cell IgG can be associated with increased red cell destruction in vivo. These methods have not been applied frequently to the problem of incompatibility between donor and recipient without serologically demonstrable antibody.

Alternatively, red cell destruction by cellular immunity may provide an explanation of this phenomenon. Antibody-mediated cellular immunity is an at-

Table 9-13. Summary of Cases of Hemolytic Transfusion Reaction Without Detectable Antibody

Case	Age	Sex	Diagnosis	Symptoms and Signs	Onset After Transfusion	Possible or Inferred Specificity	Reference
1	46	F	Reticulum cell sarcoma	Hemoglobinuria, fever	After 350 ml	e	236
2	50	F	Gastric ulcer	Hemoglobinuria	Next morning	C^w, C	237
3	54	M	Waldenström's macroglobinemia	Hemoglobinuria, fever with rigors	Shortly after	Jk^b, Le^b	238
4	58	M	Gastric tumor	Hemoglobinuria	6 days	C, e	239
5	36	F	Ruptured IUP	Hemoglobinuria, jaundice	NA	C, e	240
6	36	F	Ulcus ventriculi	NA	NA	NA	241
7	32	F	Anemia	NA	NA	NA	241
8	50	F	Curettage	NA	NA	NA	241
9	43	F	Cesarean section	NA	NA	NA	241
10	45	F	Anemia	Hemoglobinuria, malaise	10 days	c^a	242
11	48	F	Multiple myeloma	Hemoglobinuria, fever, and chills	11 days	e^a	245
12	57	F	Gastrointestinal bleeding	Hemoglobinuria, fever, and chills	NA	C^a	251
13	55	M	Lung carcinoma	Hemoglobinuria	4	C^a	218

Abbreviations: IUP, intrauterine pregnancy; NA, not applicable.
[a] Inferred by red cell survival studies.

tractive possible mechanism. In this hypothetical instance, donor red cells minimally "identified" by a small increase in surface-bound IgG interact with reticuloendothelial cells, which then hemolyze them by cellular cytotoxicity. It may also be possible that cell-mediated hemolysis, independent of antibody, may be responsible for red cell destruction. However, antibody-independent cell-mediated lysis has never been documented for red cell antigens.[251]

Bioassays to Determine the Clinical Significance of Red Cell Alloantibodies

A number of investigators have studied the in vitro interaction of antibody-sensitized red cells with mononuclear phagocytic cells.[254,255] The method involves the separation of mononuclear phagocytic cells, usually from the peripheral blood, and measuring the adherence and/or phagocytosis by these cells

of antibody-sensitized red cells. Such studies have provided significant information regarding the mechanisms of hemolysis,[256–261] and correlations have been made between in vitro results and in vivo hemolysis in autoimmune hemolytic anemias[259] and hemolytic disease of the newborn.[262] More recently, efforts have been made to develop an assay that would be useful in predicting the in vivo significance of red cell alloantibodies in patients who require transfusion and who have antibodies of dubious clinical significance.

Schanfield et al.[263] studied two antibodies (anti-Yt^a and anti-Hy^a) that had caused hemolytic disease of the newborn and obtained positive results in his test system. Twenty-five clinically insignificant antibodies and 6 antibodies of unknown significance gave negative results.

Working with 86 antibodies of 11 specificities, all

of which were expected to be clinically significant except for 5 anti-Lu[b], Hunt et al.[264] demonstrated a relationship between the antibody titer score and monocyte interaction. Forty-three antibodies interacted with monocytes in vitro, but antibodies yielding moderate- or low-titer scores often did not give positive results, including anti-D, anti-K, and anti-Jk[a]. Some antibodies of high-titer score also gave negative reactions. Their data were also consistent with previous work indicating that only antibodies of IgG1 or IgG3 subclasses were capable of producing interaction with monocytes. However, no information was provided concerning a correlation of test results with in vivo survival of red cells.

Branch et al.[265] tested 148 red cell alloantibodies of specificities generally considered of clinical significance. Only 53 percent mediated significant phagocytosis in vitro. The use of target cells homozygous for the antigen in question, the addition of fresh complement in the antibody-sensitization procedure, and use of autologous and allogeneic monocyte–macrophages appeared necessary for optimal results. Using the combined data of two reports,[265,266] in vivo clinical significance or a lack of clinical significance was documented for a total of 17 antibodies (4 anti-Ge; 2 each of anti-M, -Vel, and -Jk[a]; and 1 each of anti-Lan, Co[a], -D, -Jk[b], Yt[a], and -Yt[b]). Evidence from in vivo observations indicated that 10 of the antibodies were clinically significant and 7 were not. In each instance, the in vitro monocyte–macrophage phagocytosis assay correlated with the known in vivo clinical significance or lack of significance.

Garratty and coworkers also studied the correlation of monocyte monolayer assays and red cell survival in a variety of clinical settings,[267] including a study of red cell alloantibodies of uncertain clinical significance.[268] The significance of 12 antibodies (3 anti-Lan, 3 anti-Ge, 5 anti-Yt[a], and 1 anti-Yt[b]) was determined by red cell survival studies or by transfusion of incompatible blood. In each instance, the results of the monocyte–monolayer assay agreed with the clinical assessment of the significance of the antibody. Thus, the limited available information correlating in vitro assays with in vivo red cell survival indicates an excellent correlation. However, it is of concern that numerous examples of antibodies that one expects to be of clinical significance (e.g., Rh,

Kell, Kidd, Duffy) give negative results.[264,265] It is possible that not all such antibodies are clinically significant or that the assay systems used are not reliable.[266] It will be difficult to acquire extensive data regarding this point because in vivo testing is only justifiable when it is necessary to transfuse incompatible blood. Furthermore, if transfusion of incompatible blood is performed, the antibody may change its characteristics as a result of an anamnestic response to the transfused red cells.

Engelfriet et al.[269] pointed out that bioassays that are used to determine the significance of a "difficult" antibody may have an even more important application, that is, predicting the severity of hemolytic disease of the newborn. These investigators conclude that the antibody-dependent cellular cytotoxicity (ADCC) tests and the chemiluminescence test have the best predictive value for this purpose.

Relationship of Compatibility Testing to Fatal Hemolytic Transfusion Reactions

Ironically, perfecting the serologic aspects of compatibility testing would only prevent a very small minority of fatal hemolytic reactions, according to several surveys. In December 1975, it became mandatory to report immediately to the FDA "when a complication of blood collection or transfusion is confirmed to be fatal" in the United States. Several investigators have taken advantage of the opportunity to review such data confidentially under the Freedom of Information Act.[270–273] Schmidt[271] categorized 22 fatal hemolytic reactions that occurred during 1976–1978 as the primary cause of a patient's death and as being due to donor–patient red cell incompatibility. All 22 cases were due to problems of ABO mismatch, and in all cases the cause was a clerical identity error rather than a serologic error. In some cases the clerical error occurred in the laboratory, but in most (i.e., 17) it was a case of proper preparation of the right blood being given to the wrong patient. Most errors occurred in the intensive care unit or in the surgical suite. Honig and Bove[270] reviewed similar data.

Sazama[274] reported on transfusion associated deaths that were reported to the FDA for the period 1976–1985. Excluding deaths due to hepatitis or acquired immunodeficiency syndrome (AIDS), there were 256 deaths, 158 of which were due to acute

Table 9-14. Errors in Cases of Acute Hemolytic Reactions

Collection and ordering	
Sample drawn from wrong person	4
Misidentification of clot or requisition	9
Blood bank	
Confusion of samples or records	16
Wrong unit release	9
Serologic mistake	20
Blood given to wrong person	
In surgical suites	22
Other	55
Error unclear	10
No error	13
Total	158

(Modified from Sazama,[274] with permission.)

hemolysis. Of these, 131 were due to the transfusion of ABO-incompatible products. The errors that occurred in cases of acute hemolytic reactions are listed in Table 9-14. A comparison of this 10-year summary with the 3-year analysis of Honig and Bove found that the single most remarkable change that occurred was an increase in errors classified as "blood given to wrong person." This category accounted for 77 of the 158 errors.

Although errors in administration of blood are usually referred to as "clerical errors," Sazama concluded that many represented instead a management system error. This type of error includes the absence of proper written procedures and/or training of persons held responsible for the deaths, as well as a failure properly to assign responsibility for certain aspects of transfusion (e.g., clearing the operating room's blood-holding refrigerator between patients).

Linden et al.[33] reported that among 1,784,000 transfusions of red cell components in New York State that there were 92 cases of erroneous transfusion (1/19,000). There were 54 ABO-incompatible transfusions (1/33,000); three of these were fatal (1/600,000). Correction for underreporting of ABO-compatible errors resulted in an estimate of one per 12,000 as the true risk of transfusion error. Forty-three percent of the errors occurred as a result of failure to identify the patient and/or unit prior to transfusion, and 11 percent resulted from phlebotomist error, while the blood bank was responsible for 25 percent of errors and contributed, with another hospital service, to 17 percent.

It is evident that more impact can be made on the problem of fatal hemolytic transfusion reactions by preventing clerical and managerial errors rather than from improved serologic techniques. Extraordinary measures to prevent these errors are warranted. At some institutions, each blood transfusion recipient must be typed twice, with two independently obtained blood specimens.[34] Thus, if the blood transfusion service's records do not indicate that a patient has been previously typed, a second sample is obtained. This policy is practical even for patients admitted for same-day surgery and is effective in preventing errors in collecting and ordering. However, this policy obviously cannot prevent administration of the blood to the wrong patient which is the more common error leading to a fatal hemolytic reaction. To prevent such errors, it is wise to monitor transfusionist practices.

Monitoring Transfusionists' Practices

Recently, workers have looked to quality management approaches to improve transfusionist practice and to reduce risk to patients. Some institutions require periodic, real-time, on site transfusion reviews to assure that written procedures are up to date and practices used are acceptable. At the Los Angeles County–University of Southern California Medical Center a quality assessment/quality improvement (QA/QI) program was created to improve compliance with good transfusion practices. This program required a major commitment of resources from hospital administration to the performance of an expanded, formal, comprehensive monitoring program.[275]

The transfusion policies and procedures were extensively reviewed at various professional levels, educating the staff that a problem existed. Over a 2-year period, 200 transfusions were audited for compliance with institutional policy. The monitoring of the procedures provided educational opportunities. The staff was made aware of the rationale for the procedure and the possible consequences if errors occurred. When variances were identified, the involved staff was responsible for generating a corrective action plan. If an action plan was not forthcom-

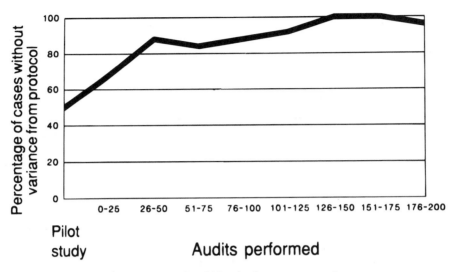

Fig. 9-4. Results of blood administration audits.

ing, reminders were initiated until resolution was reached.

At the beginning of the QA/AI process, monitoring of blood administration practices revealed that a variance from institutional blood administration policy occurred during 50 percent of blood and component transfusions. As a result of the QA/QI process, the percentage of transfusions with an associated variance from institutional policy dropped to nearly zero (Fig. 9-4). Therefore the study demonstrated that this approach could improve transfusion safety by (1) continual reinforcement of policies and procedures to ensure necessary knowledge, (2) corrective action by personnel involved in variances from acceptable performance, and (3) close monitoring of actions and documentation of inappropriate practice to motivate an appropriate behavior by the staff.

COMPATIBILITY TESTING IN SPECIFIC CLINICAL SITUATIONS

Some clinical situations require special consideration regarding compatibility testing. Several are considered elsewhere, such as compatibility testing in autoimmune hemolytic anemia (see Ch. 20) and emergency surgery and massive transfusion (see Ch. 22).

Compatibility Testing for Neonates

As pointed out in the Standards for Blood Banks and Transfusion Services of the AABB,[27] modifications of routine requirements for compatibility testing are advisable for the neonatal (under 4 months of age) recipient. These recommendations take into account both the low incidence of red cell alloantibody formation, in spite of repeated transfusions during the neonatal period[276,277] and the need to minimize the volume of blood drawn for laboratory testing in this patient group.

The Standards indicate that an initial pretransfusion specimen must be tested in order to determine the infant's ABO/Rh and for the presence of unexpected RBC antibodies (a sample from the infant's mother may be used in place of the infant's sample for antibody screening). The Rh determination and the antibody screening test must be done as for any potential transfusion recipient; however, for the ABO testing, only grouping with anti-A and anti-B reagents is required, as serum typing results might be confusing due to transplacental maternal ABO antibody. No repeat ABO/Rh testing is necessary for the remainder of an infant's hospital stay, provided the only red cells transfused during the hospital stay are ABO compatible and Rh negative or of the infant's original Rh type.

If the red cells selected for transfusion of the infant

are not group O, the infant's serum (plasma) must be tested using an IAT for anti-A or anti-B, as appropriate. The red cells used in the IAT must be either reagent cells (i.e., ABO serum typing cells) or donor cells (i.e., a major crossmatch); if testing for anti-A, the cells used must be group A_1. If no anti-A or anti-B is detected, no subsequent crossmatching is necessary during the remainder of the infant's hospital stay, unless the antibody screen demonstrates clinically significant red cell antibodies. However, if anti-A or anti-B is detected, only RBCs compatible with the anti-A or anti-B should be transfused.

If the infant is non-group O and has received blood components containing anti-A or anti-B directed against its own A or B antigens, the infant must be tested for anti-A or anti-B (either using reagent RBCs or by a crossmatch as described above) prior to receiving any non-group O RBCs. If the initial antibody screen detects potentially clinically significant unexpected RBC antibodies, units selected for transfusion do not need to be crossmatched but must not contain the corresponding antigen until the unexpected antibody is no longer demonstrable in the infant's serum (plasma). Finally, infants must not be transfused with blood or components that contain clinically significant unexpected antibodies.

Hypothermia

Concern has arisen regarding the necessity of detecting cold antibodies in patients who undergo hypothermia during bypass surgery. In 1969, Wertlake et al.[278] reported a single case in which a cold antibody resulted in hemolysis after surgery under hypothermia. In 1985, one of the authors of that report commented, "That rare event 15 years ago did not cause me then to institute crossmatching in the cold nor does it now, several thousand cases later."[279] An anonymous comment in the AABB Newsbriefs (August 1986) states, "With the passage of time and the performance of innumerable transfusions to patients undergoing hypothermia, it has become apparent that omitting the room temperature phase of antibody screening and crossmatching does not imperil the patient." The commentator concludes "if you are still performing room temperature testing on patients scheduled for hypothermia, you can discontinue the practice without conflicting with accepted standards of practice nationwide or subjecting your

patients to increased risk." Similar conclusions based on extensive experience have been reached by Schmidt.[279] Thus, although recommendations have been made to perform compatibility test procedures in the cold routinely for patients undergoing surgery with induced hypothermia,[280] no data are available to support the necessity of such a policy.

The aforementioned recommendations seem appropriate in regard to red cell alloantibodies. However, if a patient has autoimmune hemolytic anemia caused by a cold antibody (cold agglutinin syndrome [CAS]), it seems logical to avoid hypothermia because of the risk of exacerbating hemolysis. Although surprisingly few complications caused by cold autoagglutinins during cardiac surgery have been reported,[279,280] Bedrosian and Simel[281] reported a patient with well-compensated chronic CAS who had an acute hemolytic crisis during an elective herniorrhaphy in a cool operating room. The patient's hematocrit decreased from 36 percent to a low of 12.6 percent. Other instances of exacerbation of CAS with exposure to cold, although not associated with surgery, have been well documented.[282,283]

Perhaps more important concerns are the cold-mediated effects of erythrocyte agglutination within the coronary microcirculation. This might lead to inadequate distribution of cardioplegic solution, poor myocardial protection, and perioperative infarction, an event that occurs in 1 to 10 percent of patients undergoing bypass surgery and whose etiology is often unclear. Peripheral vasoconstriction and renal failure may also occur after open heart surgery without precise determination of the cause.[284]

When measures have been taken to avoid the potential hematologic and cardiac consequences of cold exposure in patients with cold agglutinins, the reported results have been excellent. Park and Weiss[285] reviewed 13 reported cases of cardiac surgery in patients with cold hemagglutinin disease that were reported between 1968 and 1985. In all patients with a known cold agglutinin, the systemic temperature was maintained above the thermal reactivity of the cold antibody. Techniques of myocardial preservation included cold crystalloid cardioplegia, normothermic ischemic arrest, warm crystalloid cardioplegia washout followed by cold cardioplegia, and warm blood–potassium cardioplegia.

Diaz et al.[280] recommend complete coronary

washout with cold crystalloid cardioplegia and maintenance of systemic perfusion with core temperature just above the critical temperature of the cold antibody.

Blumberg et al.[286] described a patient who did not have hemolytic anemia but who had a cold agglutinin with a titer of 8 at 37°C, 4 at 30°C, 64 at room temperature, and 2,024 at 4°C. During cardiac bypass surgery, systemic hypothermia was not employed and a clear potassium-containing cardioplegic solution was used. Before the introduction of 4°C cardioplegic solution into the aortic root, 37°C solution was used as a flush. Cardioplegia was then maintained by infusion of 4°C solution for the 1.6 hours of cardiopulmonary bypass. Before reintroduction of blood into the chilled heart after bypass, a 37°C cardioplegic solution flush was administered. There was no evidence of in vivo agglutination or hemolysis.

In the case reported by Park and Weiss,[285] the patient had a cold agglutinin titer of 1/10,000 at 4°C and 1/5,000 at 20°C but did not have evidence of hemolysis. Plasmapheresis was performed 1 day before surgery and produced "an eight-fold reduction in titers." Body temperature was maintained above 35°C throughout coronary artery bypass grafting, which was performed during a 72-minute normothermic cardiopulmonary bypass at 36 to 37°C. No ventricular fibrillation occurred, and no hemolysis, hemagglutination, myocardial infarction, or organ damage resulted.

Klein et al.[287] used plasma exchange before surgery for a patient with an anti-I cold agglutinin, although the patient had no evidence of immune hemolysis. The antibody reacted strongly with RBCs at 15°C, 22°C, and after papain treatment at 37°C; in addition, it agglutinated several panel cells in saline at 30°C and occasionally reacted with saline-suspended cells at 37°C. The titer at 22°C was reduced by plasma exchange from 1:4 to 1:1. During surgery, body temperature was lowered with the core temperature measured with an esophageal sensor of 29°C. There were no adverse effects during or after hypothermia. As Klein and colleagues point out, they could not be sure that difficulties would have developed had plasma exchange not been performed.

However, plasma exchange may be only minimally effective as in the case reported by Beebe et al.[288] Beginning 10 days before surgery, the patient received plasmapheresis every other day for five total treatments with each treatment exchanging 1.25 plasma volumes with an equal volume of 5 percent albumin. The cold agglutinin titer decreased from 1 in 4,096 to 1 in 512 the day before surgery, but on the morning of surgery, the cold agglutinin titer had rebounded to 1 in 1,024. The patient had chronic CAS but was managed throughout surgery for splenectomy and cholecystectomy by intraoperative forced air convection warming; esophageal and peripheral temperatures were maintained above 37°C throughout surgery and she did not have an exacerbation of her hemolysis.

Since cold agglutinins may be detected in the serums of almost all individuals, the critical problem is to decide which characteristics of a given patient's cold agglutinin would warrant special precautions during surgery. This question cannot be answered precisely, but special precautions concerning cardioplegia procedures and systemic cooling would seem important when a patient has a cold antibody-induced immune hemolytic anemia because of well-documented exacerbations of hemolysis described as a result of exposure to cold in such patients[282,283] and the potential for adverse cardiac events. Although cold-reactive antibodies are not characterized in detail in the blood transfusion service, if the antibodies have a high enough thermal amplitude to cause autoimmune hemolytic anemia, they will ordinarily be detected by routine compatibility test procedures. Furthermore, the diagnosis of CAS may be made from clinical and immunohematologic findings.

For patients without hemolytic anemia, but who have a cold agglutinin, the thermal amplitude and titer of the antibody are probably the best guides to possible complications during surgery. Although cold agglutinins reactive at room temperature might seem to be of potential significance during hypothermic surgical procedures, there is an impressive lack of reports of complications caused by such antibodies, even though they are very common.[279] Less common are antibodies that are strongly reactive at temperatures of 30°C or above. In these cases, modification of surgical techniques to use such procedures as normothermic cardioplegia and avoidance of deep systemic hypothermia may be warranted.

However, unless there is a protocol to characterize cold antibodies in patients scheduled for hypothermic surgery, such antibodies may not be noted by blood bank technologists, since detection and characterization of cold-reactive antibodies are not necessary for routine red cell transfusion. Simple screening tests would suffice, so that elaborate compatibility test procedures and antibody characterization would only rarely need be performed.

Antilymphocyte Globulin, Antithymocyte Globulin, and Intravenous Immunoglobulin

Antilymphocyte and Antithymocyte Globulin

The use of immunosuppressive agents such as antilymphocyte globulin and antithymocyte globulin may create problems in serologic tests.[289-294] These reagents are prepared by immunizing horses, goats, or rabbits; pooling the plasma; and absorbing it with human red cells and platelets. In spite of extensive absorption, antibodies reactive with human red cells may remain in the final preparation. Human red cells sensitized with these antibodies will yield a positive antiglobulin test result because antihuman globulin reagents have antibodies that cross-react with the antibodies of animal origin. Consequently, during compatibility test procedures, these antibodies may be detected on the red cells and in the serum of recipients, where they cause incompatible crossmatches, positive antibody detection test results, and positive DAT responses.

A number of potential solutions to this problem have been proposed, one of which is the absorption of antiglobulin reagents with human red cells coated with the panagglutinin of the antilymphocyte globulin.[289-291] Three absorptions may be necessary for successful removal of the unwanted antibodies. There was no loss of potency of the antihuman globulin reagents against red cells coated with weakly reactive human red cell alloantibodies. However, titrations of the antihuman globulin reagents were not performed.

An alternative approach is to neutralize the antihuman globulin with the antilymphocyte globulin reagent.[292] Although this results in a reduction in titer of the antiglobulin reagent, weakly reactive red

cell alloantibodies were still detectable when using the absorbed serum.

Judd[293] indicates that the absorption of antihuman globulin reagents with horse serum (not antilymphocyte globulin) is preferable. He recommends adding 0.2 ml of horse serum to 10 ml of antihuman globulin. The absorbed antiglobulin reagent should be tested against IgG-coated cells to ascertain that there has been no inhibition of anti-IgG. Also, if antilymphocyte globulin is to be used in a patient for whom transfusion is likely to be needed, it is preferable to obtain a specimen for compatibility testing in advance, as the antilymphocyte globulin may interfere with compatibility testing for at least 12 to 24 hours, regardless of the method used to circumvent this problem.

Intravenous Immunoglobulin

Intravenous immunoglobulin (IVIg) is widely used in a variety of clinical disorders (see Ch. 45). There are a number of reported occurrences of positive DATs,[295-301] IATs,[301,302] and immune hemolytic anemia[303,304] due to red cell alloantibodies in the IVIg preparation. One must be aware of this potential effect of IVIg, since the development of such antibodies may confuse and complicate serologic testing of transfusion candidates.[297]

REFERENCES

1. Rosenfield RE: Early twentieth century origins of modern blood transfusion therapy. Mt Sinai J Med 41:626, 1974
2. Rosenfield RE: The past and future of immunohematology. Philip Levine award lecture. Am J Clin Pathol 64:569, 1975
3. Oberman HA: The crossmatch. A brief historical perspective. Transfusion 21:645, 1981
4. Landsteiner K: Zur Kenntnis der antifermentativen, lytischen und agglutinierenden Wirkungen des Blutserums und der Lymphe. Zentralbl Mikrobiol 27:375, 1900
5. Landsteiner K: Uber agglutinationserscheinungen normalen menschlichen Blutes. Wein Klin Wochenschr 14:1132, 1901
6. Crile GW: Hemorrhage and Transfusion. Appleton & Lange, East Norwalk, CT, 1909
7. Ottenberg R: Reminiscences of the history of blood transfusion. J Mt Sinai Hosp 4:264, 1937

8. Agote L: Nuevo procedimiento para la transfusion del sangre. An Inst Mod Clin Med 1:3, 1915

9. Hustin A: Principe d'une nouvelle methode de transfusion. J M, Bruxelles 12:436, 1914

10. Lewishon R: A new and greatly simplified method of blood transfusion. Med Rec 87:141, 1915

11. Weil R: Sodium citrate in the transfusion of blood. JAMA 64:425, 1915

12. Rous P, Turner JR: A rapid and simple method of testing donors for transfusion. JAMA 64:1980, 1915

13. Unger LJ: Precautions necessary in selection of a donor for blood transfusion. JAMA 76:9, 1921

14. Landsteiner K, Wiener AS: Agglutinable factor in human blood recognized by immune sera for rhesus blood. Proc Soc Exp Biol Med 43:223, 1940

15. Race RR: An "incomplete" antibody in human serum. Nature 153:771, 1944

16. Wiener AS: A new test (blocking test) for Rh sensitization. Proc Soc Exp Biol 56:173, 1944

17. Diamond LK, Abelson NM: The demonstration of anti-Rh agglutinins, an accurate and rapid slide test. J Lab Clin Med 30:204, 1945

18. Diamond LK, Denton RL: Rh agglutination in various media with particular reference to the value of albumin. J Lab Clin Med 30:821, 1945

19. Coombs RRA, Mourant AE, Race RR: A new test for the detection of weak and "incomplete" Rh agglutinins. Br J Exp Pathol 26:255, 1945

20. Coombs RR: History and evolution of the antiglobulin reaction and its application in clinical and experimental medicine. Am J Clin Pathol 53:131, 1970

21. Morton JA, Pickles MM: Use of trypsin in the detection of incomplete anti-Rh antibodies. Nature 159:779, 1947

22. Low B: A practical method using papain and incomplete Rh-antibodies in routine Rh blood-grouping. Vox Sang 5:94, 1955

23. Haber G, Rosenfield RE: Ficin treated red cells for hemagglutination studies. p. 45. In Anonymous: PH Anderson—Papers in Dedication of his 60th Birthday. Copenhagen, Munksgaard, 1957

24. Pirofsky B, Mangum MEJ: Use of bromelin to demonstrate erythrocyte antibodies. Proc Soc Exp Biol 101:49, 1959

25. Griffitts JJ, Frank S, Schmidt RP: The influence of albumin in the antiglobulin crossmatch. Transfusion 4:461, 1964

26. Stroup M, MacIlroy M: Evaluation of the albumin antiglobulin technique in antibody detection. Transfusion 5:184, 1965

27. Klein HG: Standards for Blood Banks and Transfusion Services. American Association of Blood Banks, Bethesda, MD, 1994

28. Shulman IA: Controversies in red blood cell compatibility testing. p. 171. In Nance SJ (ed): Immune Destruction of Red Blood Cells. American Association of Blood Banks, Arlington, VA, 1989

29. Kaplan HS: The positive direct antiglobulin test resulting from passively acquired antibody. In Wilson MJ (ed): Clinical Aspects of the Positive Direct Antiglobulin Test. American Association of Blood Banks, Washington, DC, 1980

30. Zoes C, Dube VE, Miller HJ, Vye MV: Anti-A$_1$ in the plasma of platelet concentrates causing a hemolytic reaction. Transfusion 17:29, 1977

31. Franciosi RA, Awer E, Santana M: Interdonor incompatibility resulting in anuria. Transfusion 7:297, 1967

32. Reiner AP, Sayers MH: Hemolytic transfusion reaction due to interdonor kell incompatibility. Report of two cases and review of the literature. Arch Pathol Lab Med 114:862, 1990

33. Linden JV, Paul B, Dressler KP: A report of 104 transfusion errors in New York State. Transfusion 32:601, 1992

34. Rippee C, Morgan-Gannon S: Increasing detection of mislabeled specimens to reduce risk of mistransfusion. Transfusion 22:461, 1982

35. Renner SW, Howanitz PJ, Bachner P: Wristband identification error reporting in 712 hospitals. A College of American Pathologists' Q-Probes study of quality issues in transfusion practice. Arch Pathol Lab Med 117:573, 1993

36. Shulman IA, Nelson JM, Nakayama R: When should antibody screening tests be done for recently transfused patients? Transfusion 30:39, 1990

37. Heddle NM, Klama L, Frassetto R et al: A retrospective study to determine the risk of red cell alloimmunization and transfusion during pregnancy. Transfusion 33:217, 1993

38. Widmann FK: Too much pretransfusion testing? editorial. Transfusion 33:186, 1993

39. Reisner R, Taswell HF, Williamson KR: Is an albumin phase necessary for antibody detection? Transfusion, Suppl. 28:40S, 1988

40. Walker RH: Technical Manual. American Association of Blood Banks, Bethesda, MD, 1993

41. Westhoff CM, Sipherd BD, Toalson LD: Using specimens collected in EDTA for transfusion service testing. Transfusion, Suppl. 33:25S, 1993

42. Benson K: Coins and clumps: rouleaux formation vs. agglutination. ASCP Check Sample Continuing Education Program. TM 89-6, 1989

43. Petz LD, Branch DR, Garratty G et al: The significance of the anticomplement component of antiglobulin serum (AGS) in compatibility testing. Transfusion 21:633, 1981

44. Shulman IA, Meyer E, Seymour M et al: Blood Bank serologic problems caused by human thrombin. J Med Technol 8:455, 1986

45. Shirey RS, Ciappi AB, Kickler TS et al: Compatibility testing problems associated with bovine thrombin-treated plasma. Immunohematology 9:19, 1993

46. Taswell HF, Pineda AA, Moore SB: Hemolytic transfusion reactions: frequency and clinical laboratory aspects. p. 71. In Bell CA (ed): A Seminar on Immune-Mediated Cell Destruction. American Association of Blood Banks, Washington, DC, 1981

47. Hughes-Jones NC, Polley MJ, Telford R et al: Optimal conditions for detecting blood group antibodies by the antiglobulin test. Vox Sang 9:385, 1964

48. Elliot M, Bossom E, Dupuy ME, Masouredis SP: Effect of ionic strength on the serologic behavior of red cell isoantibodies. Vox Sang 9:396, 1964

49. Atchley WA, Bhagavan NV, Masouredis SP: Influence of ionic strength on the reaction between anti-D and D-positive red cells. J Immunol 93:396, 1964

50. Hughes-Jones NC, Gardner B, Telford R: The effect of pH and ionic strength on the reaction between anti-D and erythrocytes. Immunology 7:72, 1964

51. Mollison PL, Polley MJ: Uptake of gamma-globulin and complement by red cells exposed to serum at low ionic strength. Nature 203:535, 1964

52. Stratton F, Rawlinson VI: Interaction between human serum complement and normal human red cells at low ionic strength. Nature 207:305, 1965

53. Low B, Messeter L: Antiglobulin test in low-ionic strength salt solution for rapid antibody screening and cross-matching. Vox Sang 26:53, 1974

54. Moore HC, Mollison PL: Use of a low-ionic-strength medium in manual tests for antibody detection. Transfusion 16:291, 1976

55. Wicker B, Wallas CH: A comparison of a low ionic strength saline medium with routine methods for antibody detection. Transfusion 16:469, 1976

56. Garratty G, Petz LD, Webb M, Yam P: Evaluation of low ionic strength saline (LISS) as a red cell suspending medium for the detection of alloantibodies. Clin Res 26:347, 1978

57. Garratty G, Petz LD, Hafleigh E et al: Evaluation of low ionic strength solution (LISS) for compatibility testing including a prospective study comparing saline, albumin, and enzyme techniques. Transfusion 18:648, 1978

58. Hafleigh EB, Svoboda RK, Grumet FC: LISS technique without room temperature phase. Extensive transfusion experience. Transfusion 18:649, 1978

59. Rock G, Baxter A, Charron M, Jhaveri J: LISS—an effective way to increase blood utilization. Transfusion 18:228, 1978

60. Herron R, Smith DS: Use of low ionic strength salt solution in compatibility testing, letter. J Clin Pathol 31:1116, 1978

61. Fitzsimmons JM, Morel PA: The effects of red blood cell suspending media on hemagglutination and the antiglobulin test. Transfusion 19:81, 1979

62. Lown JA, Barr AL, Davis RE: Use of low ionic strength saline for crossmatching and antibody screening. J Clin Pathol 32:1019, 1979

63. Greendyke RM, Banzhaf JC, Inglis J: A comparison of six procedures for compatibility testing. Transfusion 19:782, 1979

64. Langley JW, McMahan M, Smith N: A nine-month transfusion service experience with low-ionic-strength saline solution (LISS). Am J Clin Pathol 73:99, 1980

65. Molthan L, Strohm PL: Hemolytic transfusion reaction due to anti-Kell undetectable in low-ionic-strength solutions. Am J Clin Pathol 75:629, 1981

66. Lalezari P: The manual hexadimethrine bromide (Polybrene) test. Effects of serum proteins and practical applications. Transfusion 27:295, 1987

67. Rosenfield RE: Low ionic incubation and polycation aggregation ("LIP") to augment hemagglutination in test tubes. In Thirty-first Annual Meeting, New Orleans, AABB Abstracts of Volunteer Papers, 1978

68. Leikola J, Perkins HA: Red cell antibodies and low ionic strength: a study with enzyme-linked antiglobulin test. Transfusion 20:224, 1980

69. Lalezari P: A polybrene method for the detection of red cell antibodies. Fed Proc 26:756, 1967

70. Lalezari P: A new red cell method for the simultaneous detection of hemagglutinins and leukoagglutinins. p. 419. In Curtoni ES, Mattiuz PL, Tusi RM (eds): Histocompatibility Testing. Munksgaard, Copenhagen, 1967

71. Lalezari P: The manual hexadimethrine bromide (polybrene) test. Effects of serum proteins and practical applications. Transfusion 27:295, 1987

72. Lee CL, Ho E: A three-step test for rapid detection of erythrocyte antigens and antibodies. J Lab Med 5:47, 1974

73. Lalezari P, Jiang AF: The manual polybrene test: a simple and rapid procedure for detection of red cell antibodies. Transfusion 20:206, 1980

74. Rosenfield RE, Shaikh SH, Innella F et al: Augmenta-

tion of hemagglutination by low ionic conditions. Transfusion 19:499, 1979

75. Fisher GA: Use of the manual Polybrene test in the routine hospital laboratory. Transfusion 23:152, 1983

76. Steane EA, Steane SM, Montgomery SR, Pearson JR: A proposal for compatibility testing incorporating the manual hexadimethrine bromide (Polybrene) test. Transfusion 25:540, 1985

77. Maynard BA, Smith DS, Farrar RP et al: Anti-Jk^a, -C and -E in a single patient, demonstrable only by the manual Polybrene test (MPT): incompatibility confirmed by 51-Cr studies. Transfusion 27:546, 1987

78. Mintz PD, Anderson G: Comparison of a manual hexadimethrine bromide-antiglobulin test with saline- and albumin-antiglobulin tests for pretransfusion testing. Transfusion 27:134, 1987

79. West NC, Jenkins JA, Johnston BR, Modi N: Interdonor incompatibility due to anti-Kell antibody undetectable by automated antibody screening. Vox Sang 50:174, 1986

80. Nance SJ, Garratty G: A new potentiator of red blood cell antigen-antibody reactions. Am J Clin Pathol 87:633, 1987

81. Shirey RS, Boyd JS, Ness PM: Polyethylene glycol versus low-ionic-strength solution in pretransfusion testing: a blinded comparison study. Transfusion 34:368, 1994

82. de Man AJ, Overbeeke MA: Evaluation of the polyethylene glycol antiglobulin test for detection of red blood cell antibodies. Vox Sang 58:207, 1990

83. Wenz B, Apuzzo J: Polyethylene glycol improves the indirect antiglobulin test. Transfusion 29:218, 1989

84. Wenz B, Apuzzo J: Use of polyethylene glycol in the blood bank, correspondence. Transfusion 30:767, 1990

85. Slater JL, Griswold DJ, Wojtyniak LS, Reisling MJ: Evaluation of the polyethylene glycol-indirect antiglobulin test for routine compatibility testing. Transfusion 29:686, 1989

86. Petz LD, Garratty G: Antiglobulin sera—past, present and future. Transfusion 18:257, 1978

87. Sherwood GK, Haynes BF, Rosse WF: Hemolytic transfusion reactions caused by failure of commercial antiglobulin reagents to detect complement. Transfusion 16:417, 1976

88. Wright MS, Issitt PD: Anticomplement and the indirect antiglobulin test. Transfusion 19:688, 1979

89. Neppert J: Plasma or serum, letter. Transfusion 20:116, 1980

90. Howell P, Giles CM: A detailed serological study of

five anti-Jk^a sera reacting by the antiglobulin technique. Vox Sang 45:129, 1983

91. Howard JE, Winn LC, Gottlieb CE et al: Clinical significance of the anti-complement component of antiglobulin antisera. Transfusion 22:269, 1982

92. Garratty G: The significance of complement in immunohematology, review. Crit Rev Clin Lab Sci 20:25, 1984

93. Issitt PD: The antiglobulin test and the evaluation of antiglobulin reagents. p. 4. In Advances in Immunohematology. Spectra Biologicals, Oxnard, CA, 1977

94. Title 21, Code of Federal Regulations 21:660.33, 1989

95. Mitten EA, Gregory KR, Schmidt PJ: Double failure of the type and screen. Am J Clin Pathol 87:252, 1986

96. Shulman IA: 1992 CAP Surveys. Comprehensive Transfusion Medicine Survey, 1992. Set J-C. Interlaboratory Comparison Program. College of American Pathologists, Northfield, IL, 1992

97. AuBuchon JP: 1993 CAP Surveys. Comprehensive Transfusion Medicine Survey, 1993. Set J-A. Interlaboratory Comparison Program. College of American Pathologists, Northfield, IL, 1993

98. Shulman IA, Nakayama R, Calderon C: The sensitivity of antibody detection testing using pooled vs. unpooled reagent RBCs. Immunohematology 7:16, 1991

99. Shulman IA, Kiyabu M, Nelson JM et al: The use of pooled antibody screening red cells during pretransfusion compatibility testing. Lab Med 17:407, 1986

100. De Silva M, Contreras M: Pooled cells versus individual screening cells in pre-transfusion testing. Clin Lab Haematol 7:369, 1985

101. Shulman IA, Nelson JM, Okamoto M, Malone SA: The dependence of anti-Jk^a detection on screening cell zygosity. Lab Med 16:602, 1985

102. Shulman IA, Yaowasiriwatt M, Saxena S, Nelson JM: Influence of reagent red cell zygosity on anti-Fy^a detection. Lab Med 20:37, 1989

103. Issitt PD, Combs MR, Bredehoeft SJ et al: Lack of clinical significance of "enzyme-only" red cell alloantibodies. Transfusion 33:284, 1993

104. Judd WJ, Steiner EA, Oberman HA, Nance SJ: Can the reading for serologic reactivity following 37°C incubation be omitted? Transfusion 32:304, 1992

105. Pestaner J, Shulman IA: Is it safe to omit the 37°C reading from pretransfusion compatibility testing? Am J Clin Pathol 101:361, 1994

106. Judd WJ, Butch SH, Oberman HA et al: The evaluation of a positive direct antiglobulin test in pretransfusion testing. Transfusion 20:17, 1980

107. Judd WJ, Barnes BA, Steiner EA et al: The evaluation of a positive direct antiglobulin test (autocontrol) in pretransfusion testing revisited. Transfusion 26:220, 1986

108. Huh YO, Lichtiger B: Evaluation of a positive autologous control in pretransfusion testing. Am J Clin Pathol 84:632, 1985

109. Stec N, Shirey RS, Smith B et al: The efficacy of performing red cell elution studies in the pretransfusion testing of patients with positive direct antiglobulin tests. Transfusion 26:225, 1986

110. Oberman HA, Barnes BA, Steiner EA: Role of the crossmatch in testing for serologic incompatibility. Transfusion 22:12, 1982

111. Bator S, Litty C, Dignam C et al: Current utilization of the direct antiglobulin test investigation: results of a hospital survey, letter. Transfusion 34:457, 1994

112. Plapp FV: New techniques for compatibility testing. Arch Pathol Lab Med 113:262, 1989

113. Beck ML, Plapp FV, Sinor LT, Rachel JM: Solid-phase techniques in blood transfusion serology. Crit Rev Clin Lab Sci 22:317, 1986

114. Lapierre Y, Rigal D, Adam J et al: The gel test: a new way to detect red cell antigen-antibody reactions. Transfusion 30:109, 1990

115. Sinor LT: Advances in solid-phase red cell adherence methods and transfusion serology. Transfus Med Rev 6:26, 1992

116. Boral LI, Henry JB: The type and screen: a safe alternative and supplement in selected surgical procedures. Transfusion 17:163, 1977

117. Oberman HA, Barnes BA, Friedman BA: The risk of abbreviating the major crossmatch in urgent or massive transfusion. Transfusion 18:137, 1978

118. Levine P, White J, Stroup M et al: Haemolytic disease of the newborn probably due to anti-f. Nature 185:188, 1960

119. Spielmann W, Seidl S, von Pawel J: Anti-ce (anti-f) in a CDe-cD-mother, as a cause of haemolytic disease of the newborn. Vox Sang 27:473, 1974

120. Croucher BEE, Crookston MC, Crookston JH: Delayed haemolytic transfusion reactions simulating auto-immune haemolytic anaemia. Vox Sang 12:32, 1967

121. Lawler SD, Van Loghem JJ: Rhesus antigen C^w sensitization causing in hemolytic disease of the newborn. Lancet 2:473, 1947

122. Anderson GH, Fenton E: A case of anti-Cw sensitization resulting in hemolytic disease of the newborn. Can Med Assoc J 89:28, 1963

123. Race RR, Sanger R: Blood Groups in Man. Blackwell Scientific, Oxford, 1975

124. Monaghan PW: Hemolytic disease of the newborn due to anti-C^w (rh^w). Lab Med 8:33, 1977

125. Stratton F, Renton PH: Haemolytic disease of the newborn caused by a new rhesus antibody, anti-c^x. BMJ 1:962, 1954

126. Finney RD, Blue AM, Willoughby ML: Haemolytic disease of the newborn caused by the rare Rhesus antibody anti-c^x. Vox Sang 25:39, 1973

127. Greenwalt TJ, Sanger R: The Rh antigen Ew. Br J Haematol 1:52, 1955

128. Grobel RK, Cardy JD: Hemolytic disease of the newborn due to anti-E^w. A fourth example of the Rh antigen, E^w. Transfusion 11:77, 1971

129. Alter AA, Gelb AG, Chown B et al: Gonzales (Go^a), a new blood group character. Transfusion 7:88, 1967

130. Svanda M, Prochazka R, Kout M, Giles CM: A case of haemolytic disease of the newborn due to a new red cell antigen, Zd. Vox Sang 18:366, 1970

131. Grove-Rasmussen M: Routine compatibility testing: standards of the AABB as applied to compatibility tests. Transfusion 4:200, 1964

132. Jensen KG: Haemolytic disease of the newborn caused by anti-Kpa. Vox Sang 7:476, 1972

133. Donovan LM, Tripp KL, Zuckerman JE, Konugres AA: Hemolytic disease of the newborn due to anti-Js^a. Transfusion 13:153, 1994

134. Taddie SJ, Barrasso C, Ness PM: A delayed transfusion reaction caused by anti-K6. Transfusion 22:68, 1982

135. Francis BJ, Hatcher DE: Hemolytic disease of the newborn apparently caused by anti-Lu^a. Transfusion 1:248, 1961

136. van Loghen JJ, van der Hart M, Bok J, Brinkerink PC: Two further examples of the antibody anti-Wr^a. Vox Sang 5:130, 1955

137. Metaxas MN, Metaxas-Buhler M: Studies on the Wright blood group system. Vox Sang 8:707, 1963

138. Graninger W: Anti-Di^a and the Di^a blood group. Antigen found in an Austrian family. Vox Sang 31:131, 1976

139. Speiser P, Kuhbock J, Mickerts D et al: "Kamhuber" a new human blood group antigen of familial occurrence, revealed by a severe transfusion reaction. Vox Sang 11:113, 1966

140. Rausen AR, Rosenfield RE, Alter AA et al: A "new" infrequent red cell antigen, Rd (radin). Transfusion 7:336, 1967

141. Simmons RT, Were SOM: A "new" family blood group antigen and antibody (By) of rare occurrence. Med J Aust 2:55, 1955

142. Frumin AM, Porter M, Eichman MF: The good factor

as a possible cause of hemolytic disease of the new-born. Blood 15:681, 1960

143. Ballowitz L, Fiedler H, Hoffmann C, Pettenkofer H: "Heibel" a new rare human blood group antigen, revealed by a haemolytic disease of a newborn. Vox Sang 14:307, 1968

144. Elbel H, Prokop O: Ein neues erbliches antigens als ursache gehaufter Fehlgeburten. Z Hyg 132:120, 1951

145. Van Loghem JJ, van der Hart M: Een zeldzaam voor-komende Bloedgroep (Ven). Bull Cen Lab Bloed Transfus Dienst Ned Rode Kruis 2:225, 1952

146. van der Hart M, Bosman H, Van Loghem JJ: Two rare human blood group antigens. Vox Sang 4:108, 1954

147. Moheng MC, McCarthy P, Pierce SR: Anti-Do[b] impli-cated as the cause of a delayed hemolytic transfusion reaction. Transfusion 25:44, 1985

148. Kruskall MS, Greene MJ, Strycharz DM et al: Acute hemolytic transfusion reaction due to anti-dom-brock(a). Transfusion 26:545, 1986

149. Polesky HF, Swanson J, Smith R: Anti-Do[a] stimulated by pregnancy. Vox Sang 14:465, 1968

150. Guevin RM, Taliano V, Fiset D et al: [The Reid anti-gen, a new private antigen.] [in French.] Rev Fr Transfus 14:455, 1971

151. Lee EL, Bennett C: Anti-Co[b] causing acute hemolytic transfusion reaction. Transfusion 22:159, 1982

152. Squires JE, Larison PJ, Charles WT, Milner PF: A delayed hemolytic transfusion reaction due to anti-Co[b]. Transfusion 25:137, 1985

153. Dzik WH, Blank J: Accelerated destruction of radiola-beled red cells due to anti-Colton[b]. Transfusion 26:246, 1986

154. Halverson G, Shanahan E, Santiago I et al: The first reported case of anti-Do[b] causing an acute hemolytic transfusion reaction. Vox Sang 66:206, 1994

155. Shulman IA, Nelson JM, Saxena S et al: Experience with the routine use of an abbreviated crossmatch. Am J Clin Pathol 82:178, 1984

156. Shulman IA, Nelson JM, Kent DR et al: Experience with a cost-effective crossmatch protocol. JAMA 254:93, 1985

157. Dodsworth H: Safety of the abbreviated cross-match in association with sensitive serum screening. Clin Lab Haematol 11:249, 1989

158. Mintz PD, Haines AL, Sullivan MF: Incompatible crossmatch following nonreactive antibody detection test. Frequency and cause. Transfusion 22:107, 1982

159. Dodsworth H, Dudley HA: Increased efficiency of transfusion practice in routine surgery using pre-op-erative antibody screening and selective ordering

with an abbreviated cross-match. Br J Surg 72:102, 1985

160. Havemann H, Lichtiger B: Identification of previous erythrocyte alloimmunization and the type and screen at a large cancer center. A 4-year retrospective review. Cancer 69:252, 1992

161. Pinkerton PH, Coovadia AS, Seigel C: Audit of the use of packed red blood cells in association with seven common surgical procedures. Transfus Med 2:231, 1992

162. Heddle NM, OHoski P, Singer J et al: A prospective study to determine the safety of omitting the anti-globulin crossmatch from pretransfusion testing. Br J Haematol 81:579, 1992

163. Shulman IA: Safety in transfusion practices. Red cell compatibility testing issues. Clin Lab Med 12:685, 1992

164. Ness PM, Shirey RS, Thoman SK, Buck SA: The dif-ferentiation of delayed serologic and delayed hemo-lytic transfusion reactions: incidence, long-term sero-logic findings, and clinical significance. Transfusion 30:688, 1990

165. Shulman IA: The risk of an overt hemolytic transfu-sion reaction following the use of an immediate spin crossmatch. Arch Pathol Lab Med 114:412, 1990

166. Judd WJ, Steiner EA, Abruzzo LV et al: Anti-i causing acute hemolysis following a negative immediate-spin crossmatch. Transfusion 32:572, 1992

167. Shulman IA, Odono V: The risk of overt acute hemo-lytic transfusion reaction following the use of an im-mediate-spin crossmatch, correspondence. Transfu-sion 34:87, 1994

168. Berry Dortch S, Woodside CH, Boral LI: Limitations of the immediate spin crossmatch when used for de-tecting ABO incompatibility. Transfusion 25:176, 1985

169. Lamberson RD, Boral LI, Berry-Dortch S: Limita-tions of the crossmatch for detection of incompatibil-ity between A$_2$B red blood cells and B patient sera. Am J Clin Pathol 86:511, 1986

170. Shulman IA, Nelson JM, Lam HT, Meyer E: Unrelia-bility of the immediate-spin crossmatch to detect ABO incompatibility, correspondence. Transfusion 25:589, 1985

171. Shulman IA, Meyer EA, Lam HT, Nelson JM: Addi-tional limitations of the immediate spin crossmatch to detect ABO incompatibility, letter. Am J Clin Pa-thol 87:677, 1987

172. Shulman IA: ABO incompatibility missed by saline immediate spin compatibility testing, letter. Transfu-sion 21:469, 1981

173. Judd WJ, Steiner EA, Oberman HA: Reverse ABO

typing errors due to prozone: how safe is the immediate spin-crossmatch? Transfusion 27:527, 1987

174. Park H: Limitation of the immediate-spin crossmatch, correspondence. Transfusion 25:588, 1985

175. Schmidt PJ, Samia CT, Gregory KR, Leparc GF: Rational reduction in pretransfusion testing. Lab Med 17:467, 1986

176. Heisto H: Pretransfusion blood group serology. Limited value of the antiglobulin phase of the crossmatch when a careful screening test for unexpected antibodies is performed. Transfusion 19:761, 1979

177. Yates AD, Feeney J, Donald AS, Watkins WM: Characterisation of a blood-group A-active tetrasaccharide synthesised by a blood-group B gene-specified glycosyltransferase. Carbohydr Res 130:251, 1984

178. Beck ML, Yates AD, Hardman J, Kowalski MA: Identification of a subset of group B donors reactive with monoclonal anti-A reagent. Am J Clin Pathol 92:625, 1989

179. Beck ML, Kowalski MA, Kirkegaard JR, Korth JL: Unexpected reactivity with monoclonal anti-B reagents, correspondence. Immunohematology 8:22, 1992

180. Beck ML, Kirkegaard J, Korth J, Judd WJ: Monoclonal anti-B reagents and the acquired B phenotype, letter. Transfusion 33:623, 1993

181. Beck ML, Kirkegaard JR, Pierce SR: Monoclonal blood grouping reagents: boon or burden? Transfusion 33:624, 1993

182. Butch SH, Judd WJ, Steiner EA et al: Electronic verification of donor-recipient compatibility: the computer crossmatch. Transfusion 34:105, 1994

183. Meyer EA, Shulman IA: The sensitivity and specificity of the immediate-spin crossmatch. Transfusion 29:99, 1989

184. Garratty G: Abbreviated pretransfusion testing editorial. Transfusion 26:217, 1986

185. Zuck TF: Greetings—a final look back with comments about a policy of a zero-risk blood supply, editorial. Transfusion 27:447, 1987

186. Dinman BD: The reality and acceptance of risk. JAMA 244:1226, 1980

187. Giblett ER: Blood group alloantibodies: an assessment of some laboratory practices. Transfusion 17:299, 1977

188. Mollison PL, Engelfriet CP, Contreras M: Blood Transfusion in Clinical Medicine. Blackwell Scientific, Oxford, 1993

189. Ramsey G, Cornell FW, Hahn L et al: Red cell antibody problems in 1000 liver transplants. Transfusion 27:552, 1987

190. Issitt PD: The clinical significance of some anti-red cell antibodies. Adv Pathol 1:395, 1982

191. Garratty G: Mechanisms of immune red cell destruction, and red cell compatibility testing. Hum Pathol 14:204, 1983

192. Weirr AB, Woods LE, Chesney C, Neitzer G: Delayed hemolytic transfusion reaction caused by anti-Le^{bH} antibody. Vox Sang 53:105, 1978

193. Waheed A, Kennedy MS, Gerhan S, Senhauser D: Transfusion significance of Lewis system antibodies: success in transfusion with crossmatch-compatible blood. Am J Clin Pathol 76:294, 1981

194. Perkins HA, Mallory D, Bergren M, Frank B: Lewis incompatibility, correspondence. Transfusion 22:346, 1982

195. Mollison PL, Engelfriet CP, Contreras M: Blood Transfusion in Clinical Medicine. Blackwell Scientific, Oxford, 1993

196. Silvergleid AJ, Wells RF, Hafleigh EB et al: Compatibility test using chromium-labeled red blood cells in crossmatch positive patients. Transfusion 18:8, 1978

197. Bettigole R, Harris JP, Tegoli J, Issitt PD: Rapid in vivo destruction of Yt(a+) red cells in a patient with anti-Yt^a. Vox Sang 14:143, 1968

198. Gobel U, Drescher KH, Pottgen W, Lehr JH: A second example of anti-Yt^a with rapid in vivo destruction of Yt(a+) red cells. Vox Sang 27:171, 1974

199. Eaton RR, Morton JA, Pickles MM, White KA: A new antibody, anti-Yta, characterizing a blood group of high incidence. Br J Haematol 2:333, 1956

200. Dobbs JV, Prutting DL, Adebahr ME et al: Clinical experience with three examples of anti-Yt^a. Vox Sang 15:216, 1968

201. Macvie SI, Morton JA, Pickles MM: The reactions and inheritance of a new blood group antigen, Sd^a. Vox Sang 13:485, 1967

202. Renton PH, Howell P, Ikin EW et al: Anti-Sd^a, a new blood group antibody. Vox Sang 13:493, 1967

203. Colledge KI, Kaplan HS, Marsh WL: Massive transfusion of Sd(a+) blood to a recipient with anti-Sd^a, without clinical complication. Transfusion 13:340, 1973

204. Peetermans ME, Cole-Dergent J: Haemolytic transfusion reaction due to anti-Sd^a. Vox Sang 18:67, 1970

205. Pineda AA, Dharkar DD, Wahner HW: Clinical evaluation of a ^{51}Cr-labeled red blood cell survival test for in vivo blood compatibility testing. Mayo Clin Proc 59:25, 1984

206. Tilley CA, Crookston MC, Haddad SA, Shumak KH: Red blood cell survival studies in patients with anti-Ch^a, anti-Yk^a, anti-Ge, and anti-Vel. Transfusion 17:169, 1977

207. Brzica SM Jr, Pineda AA, Taswell HF: Blood transfusion for the patient who is difficult to transfuse. Mayo Clin Proc 52:160, 1977

208. Thompson JC, Shulman IA, Nelson JM et al: Life-saving incompatible blood transfusion. Lab Med 18: 385, 1987

209. Mollison PL: The genetic basis of the Rh blood group system. Transfusion 34:539, 1994

210. Watkins WM: Biochemistry and Genetics of the ABO, Lewis, and P blood group systems, review. Adv Hum Genet 10:1, 1980

211. Schenkel-Brunner H, Tuppy H: Enzymatic conversion of human O into A erythrocytes and of B into AB erythrocytes. Nature 223:1272, 1969

212. Goldstein J: Conversion of ABO blood groups, review. Transfus Med Rev 3:206, 1989

213. Lenny LL, Hurst R, Goldstein J, Galbraith RA: Transfusions to group O subjects of 2 units of red cells enzymatically converted from group B to group O. Transfusion 34:209, 1994

214. Lenny LL, Hurst R, Goldstein J, Galbraith RA: Multi-unit transfusions to group O and A subjects of red cells enzymatically converted from group B to group O. Blood, suppl 1. 84:469a, 1994

215. Clausen H, Levery SB, Nudelman E et al: Repetitive A epitope (type 3 chain A) defined by blood group A_1 specific monoclonal antibody TH-1: chemical basis of qualitative A_1 and A_2 distinction. Proc Natl Acad Sci USA 82:1199, 1985

216. International Committee for Standardization in Haematology: Recommended methods for radioisotope red cell survival studies. Br J Haematol 45:659, 1980

217. Holt JT, Spitalnik SL, McMican AE et al: A technetium-99m red cell survival technique for in vivo compatibility testing. Transfusion 23:148, 1983

218. Harrison CR, Hayes TC, Trow LL, Benedetto AR: Intravascular hemolytic transfusion reaction without detectable antibodies: a case report and review of literature. Vox Sang 51:96, 1986

219. Morrissey GJ, Gravelle D, Dietz G, et al: In vivo red blood cell compatibility testing using indium-113m tropolone-labeled red blood cells. J Nucl Med 29: 684, 1988

220. Marcus CS, Myhre BA, Angulo MC et al: Radiolabeled red cell viability. I. Comparison of ^{51}Cr, ^{99m}Tc, and ^{111}In for measuring the viability of autologous stored red cells. Transfusion 27:415, 1987

221. Marcus CS, Myhre BA, Angulo MC et al: Radiolabeled red cell viability. II. ^{99m}Tc and ^{111}In for measuring the viability of heterologous red cells in vivo. Transfusion 27:420, 1987

222. Valinsky JE, Marsh WL, Bianco C: Flow cytometric procedure for estimation of transfused erythrocyte survival "in vivo." Transfusion 25:478, 1985

223. Postoway N, Nance S, O'Neill P, Garratty G: Comparison of a practical differential agglutination procedure to flow cytometry in following the survival of transfusion red cells. Transfusion 25:453, 1985

224. Kickler TS, Smith B, Bell W et al: Estimation of transfused red cell survival using an enzyme-linked antiglobulin test. Transfusion 25:401, 1985

225. Mollison PL, Johnson CA, Prior DM: Dose-dependent destruction of A_1 cells by anti-A_1. Vox Sang 35: 149, 1978

226. Chaplin H: Studies on the survival of incompatible cells in patients with hypogammaglobulinaemia. Blood 14:24, 1959

227. Perkins HA: The ^{51}Cr in vivo crossmatch test. p. 51. In Butch S (ed): Clinically Significant and Insignificant Antibodies. American Association of Blood Banks, Washington, DC, 1979

228. Burton MS, Mollison PL: Effect of IgM and IgG isoantibody on red cell clearance. Immunology 14:861, 1986

229. Mollison PL: Determination of red cell survival using 51-Cr. p. 45. In Bell CA (ed): A Seminar on Immune Mediated Cell Destruction. American Association of Blood Banks, Washington, DC, 1981

230. Mollison PL: Survival curves of incompatible red cells. An analytical review, review. Transfusion 26:43, 1986

231. Baldwin ML, Ness PM, Barrasso C et al: In vivo studies of the long-term ^{51}Cr red cell survival of serologically incompatible red cell units. Transfusion 25:34, 1985

232. Davey RJ: Long-term ^{51}Cr survival of serologically incompatible red cell units, correspondence. Transfusion 25:589, 1986

233. Mayer K, Chin B, Magnes J et al: Further experiences with the in vivo crossmatch and transfusion of Coombs incompatible red cells. p. 49. In Seventeenth Congress of the International Society of Hematology and 15th Congress of the International Society of Blood Transfusion Book of Abstracts, Paris, July 23–29, 1978

234. Chaplin H: Special problems in transfusion management of patients with autoimmune hemolytic anemia. In Bell CA (ed): A Seminar on Laboratory Management of Hemolysis. American Association of Blood Banks, Washington, DC, 1979

235. Jandl JH, Greenberg MS: The selective destruction of transfused "compatible" normal red cells in patients with splenomegaly. J Lab Clin Med 49:233, 1957

236. Stewart JW, Mollison PL: Rapid destruction of apparently compatible red cells. BMJ 1:1274, 1959

237. Heisto H, Myhre K, Vogt E, Heier AM: Hemolytic transfusion reaction due to incompatibility without demonstrable antibodies. Vox Sang 5:538, 1960

238. Kissmeyer-Nielsen F, Bjorn Jensen K, Ersbak J: Severe hemolytic transfusion reactions caused by apparently compatible red cells. Br J Haematol 7:36, 1961

239. Heisto H, Myhre K, Borresen W et al: Another case of hemolytic transfusion reaction due to incompatibility without demonstrable antibodies. Vox Sang 7:470, 1962

240. van der Hart M, Englefriet CP, Prins HK, Van Loghem JJ: A haemolytic transfusion reaction without demonstrable antibodies in vitro. Vox Sang 8:363, 1963

241. Van Loghem JJ, van der Hart M, Moes M, von dem Borne AEG: Increased red cell destruction in the absence of demonstrable antibodies in vitro. Transfusion 5:525, 1965

242. Davey RJ, Gustafson M, Holland PV: Accelerated immune red cell destruction in the absence of serologically detectable alloantibodies. Transfusion 20:348, 1980

243. Chaplin H, Cassell M: The occasional fallibility of in vivo compatibility tests. Transfusion 2:375, 1962

244. Benedetto AP, Harrison CR, Blumhardt R et al: ^{Tc}99m red blood cells for the study of rapid hemolytic processes associated with heterologous blood transfusions. Clin Nucl Med 9:561, 1984

245. Halima D, Postoway N, Brunt D, Garratty G: Hemolytic transfusion reactions (HTR) due to a probable anti-C, not detectable by multiple techniques. Transfusion 22:405, 1982

246. Garratty G, Vengelen-Tyler V, Postoway N et al: Hemolytic transfusion reactions (HTR) associated with antibodies not detectable by routine procedures. Transfusion 22:629, 1982

247. Maynard BA, Smith DS, Farrar RP et al: Anti-Jk^a, -C, and -E in a single patient, demonstrable only by the manual Polybrene test (MPT): incompatibility confirmed by ^{51}Cr studies. Transfusion 27:546, 1987

248. Swisher SN, Young LE, Trabold H: In vitro and in vivo studies of the behavior of canine erythrocyte-isoantibody systems. Ann NY Acad Sci 97:15, 1962

249. Pineda AA, Brzica SM Jr, Taswell HF: Hemolytic transfusion reaction. Recent experience in a large blood bank. Mayo Clin Proc 53:378, 1978

250. Vullo C, Tunioli AM: The selective destruction of "compatible" red cells transfused in a patient suffering from thalassaemai major. Vox Sang 6:583, 1961

251. Baldwin ML, Barrasso C, Ness PM, Garratty G: A clinically significant erythrocyte antibody detectable only by ^{51}Cr survival studies. Transfusion 23:40, 1983

252. Gilliland BC: Coombs-negative immune hemolytic anemia. Semin Hematol 13:267, 1976

253. Petz LD, Garratty G: Acquired Immune Hemolytic Anemias. Churchill Livingstone, New York, 1980

254. LoBuglio AF, Cotran RS, Jandl JH: Red cells coated with immunoglobulin G: binding and sphering by mononuclear cells in man. Science 158:1582, 1967

255. Huber H, Fudenberg HH: Receptor sites of human monocytes for IgG. Int Arch Allergy Appl Immunol 34:18, 1968

256. Huber H, Douglas SD, Fudenberg HH: The IgG receptor: an immunological marker for the characterization of mononuclear cells. Immunology 17:7, 1969

257. Huber H, Douglas SD, Nusbacher J et al: IgG subclass specificity of human monocyte receptor sites. Nature 229:419, 1971

258. Von dem Borne AE, Beckers D, Engelfriet CP: Mechanisms of red cell destruction mediated by non-complement binding IgG antibodies: the essential role in vivo of the Fc part of IgG. Br J Haematol 36:485, 1977

259. van der Meulen FW, van der Hart M, Fleer A et al: The role of adherence to human mononuclear phagocytes in the destruction of red cells sensitized with non-complement binding IgG antibodies. Br J Haematol 38:541, 1978

260. Fleer A, Van Schaik MLJ, von dem Borne AEGK, Engelfriet CP: Destruction of sensitized erythrocytes by human monocytes in vitro. Effects of cytochalasin B, hydrocortisone and colchicine. Scand J Immunol 8:515, 1978

261. Fleer A, van der Meulen FW, Linthout E, von dem Borne AEGK: Destruction of IgG-sensitized erythrocytes by human blood monocytes: modulation of inhibition by IgG. Br J Haematol 39:425, 1978

262. Nance S, Nelson J, O'Neill P, Garratty G: Correlation of monocyte monolayer assays, maternal antibody titers, and clinical course in hemolytic disease of the newborn (HDN). Transfusion 24:415, 1984

263. Schanfield MS, Stevens JO, Bauman D: The detection of clinically significant erythrocyte alloantibodies using a human mononuclear phagocyte assay. Transfusion 21:571, 1981

264. Hunt JS, Beck ML, Tegtmeier GE, Bayer WL: Factors influencing monocyte recognition of human erythrocyte autoantibodies in vitro. Transfusion 22:355, 1982

265. Branch DR, Gallagher MT, Mison AP et al: In vitro determination of red cell alloantibody significance using an assay of monocyte–macrophage interaction

with sensitized erythrocytes. Br J Haematol 56:19, 1984

266. Branch DR, Gallagher MT: Correlation of in vivo alloantibody significance or insignificance with an in vitro monocyte–macrophage phagocytosis assay, correspondence. Br J Haematol 61:783, 1985

267. Garratty G: Predicting the clinical significance of alloantibodies and determining the in vivo survival of transfused red cells. p. 91. In Judd WJ, Barnes A (eds): Clinical and Serological Aspects of Transfusion Reactions. American Association of Blood Banks, Arlington, VA, 1982

268. Nance SJ, Arndt P, Garratty G: Predicting the clinical significance of red cell alloantibodies using a monocyte monolayer assay. Transfusion 27:449, 1987

269. Engelfriet CP, Overbeeke MA, Dooren MC et al: Bioassays to determine the clinical significance of red cell alloantibodies based on Fc receptor-induced destruction of red cells sensitized by IgG, review. Transfusion 34:617, 1994

270. Honig CL, Bove JR: Transfusion-associated fatalities: review of Bureau of Biologics reports 1976–1978. Transfusion 20:653, 1980

271. Schmidt PJ: Transfusion mortality; with special reference to surgical and intensive care facilities. J Fla Med Assoc 67:151, 1980

272. Myhre BA: Fatalities from blood transfusion. JAMA 244:1333, 1980

273. Camp FR Jr, Monaghan WP: Fatal blood transfusion reactions. An analysis. Am J Forensic Med Pathol 2:143, 1981

274. Sazama K: Reports of 355 transfusion-associated deaths: 1976 through 1985. Transfusion 30:583, 1990

275. Shulman IA, Lohr K, Derdiarian AK, Picukaric JM: Monitoring transfusionist practices: a strategy for improving transfusion safety. Transfusion 34:11, 1994

276. Floss AM, Strauss RG, Goeken N, Knox L: Multiple transfusion fail to provoke antibodies against blood cell antigens in human infants. Transfusion 26:419, 1986

277. Ludvigsen CW Jr, Swanson JL, Thompson TR, McCullough J: The failure of neonates to form red blood cell alloantibodies in response to multiple transfusions. Am J Clin Pathol 87:250, 1987

278. Wertlake PT, McGinniss MH, Schmidt PJ: Cold antibody and persistent intravascular hemolysis after surgery under hypothermia. Transfusion 9:70, 1969

279. Schmidt PJ: Cold agglutinins and hypothermia, letter. Arch Intern Med 145:578, 1985

280. Diaz JH, Cooper ES, Ochsner JL: Cold hemagglutination pathophysiology: evaluation and management of patients undergoing cardiac surgery with induced hypothermia. Arch Intern Med 144:1639, 1983

281. Bedrosian CL, Simel DL: Cold hemagglutinin disease in the operating room. South Med J 80:466, 1987

282. Colmers RA, Snavely JG: Acute hemolytic anemia in primary atypical pneumonia produced by exposure and chilling. N Engl J Med 237:505, 1947

283. Niejadlik DC, Lozner EL: Cooling mattress induced acute hemolytic anemia. Transfusion 14:145, 1974

284. Shahian DM, Wallach SR, Bern MM: Open heart surgery in patients with cold-reactive proteins. Surg Clin North Am 65:315, 1985

285. Park JV, Weiss CI: Cardiopulmonary bypass and myocardial protection: management problems in cardiac surgical patients with cold autoimmune disease, review. Anesth Analg 67:75, 1988

286. Blumberg N, Hicks G, Woll J et al: Successful cardiac bypass surgery in the presence of a potent cold agglutinin without plasma exchange, letter. Transfusion 23:363, 1983

287. Klein HG, Faltz LL, McIntosh CL et al: Surgical hypothermia in a patient with a cold agglutinin. Management by plasma exchange. Transfusion 20:354, 1980

288. Beebe DS, Bergen L, Palahniuk RJ: Anesthetic management of a patient with severe cold agglutinin hemolytic anemia utilizing forced air warming. Anesth Analg 76:1144, 1993

289. Lapinid IM, Steib MD, Noto TA: Positive direct antiglobulin tests with antilymphocyte globulin. Am J Clin Pathol 81:514, 1984

290. Jarrell B, Besarab A, Burke JF et al: Effect of antilymphoblast globulin on Coombs' reactions. Transplantation 37:621, 1984

291. Swanson JL, Issitt CH, Mann EW et al: Resolution of red cell compatibility testing problems in patients receiving anti-lymphoblast or anti-thymocyte globulin. Transfusion 24:141, 1984

292. Ballas SK, Draper EK, Dignam CM: Pre-transfusion testing problems caused by anti-lymphocyte globulin and their solution. Transfusion 25:254, 1985

293. Judd J: Methods in immunohematology. Montgomery Scientific, Miami, 1988

294. Wick MR, DeLong EN, Moore SB: Passively acquired antibody directed at human erythrocytes seen during therapy with Minnesota antilymphoblast globulin. Vox Sang 48:229, 1985

295. Oberman HA, Beck ML: Red blood cell sensitization due to unexpected Rh antibodies in immune serum globulin. Transfusion 11:382, 1971

296. Niosi P, Lundberg J, McCullough J et al: Blood group

antibodies in human immune serum globulin. N Engl J Med 285:1435, 1971

297. Steiner EA, Butch SH, Carey JL, Oberman HA: Passive anti-D from intravenous immune serum globulin, letter. Transfusion 23:363, 1983

298. Robertson VM, Dickson LG, Romond EH, Ash RC: Positive antiglobulin tests due to intravenous immunoglobulin in patients who received bone marrow transplant. Transfusion 27:28, 1987

299. Warrier I, Lusher JM: Intravenous gamma globulin treatment for chronic idiopathic thrombocytopenic purpura in children. Am J Med 76:193, 1984

300. Huh YO, Liu FJ, Rogge K et al: Positive direct antiglobulin test and high serum immunoglobulin G values. Am J Clin Pathol 90:197, 1988

301. Lichtiger B, Rogge K: Spurious serologic test results in patients receiving infusions of intravenous immune gammaglobulin. Arch Pathol Lab Med 115:467, 1991

302. Garcia L, Huh YO, Fischer HE, Lichtiger B: Positive immunohematologic and serologic test results due to

high-dose intravenous immune globulin administration, letter. Transfusion 27:503, 1987

303. Copeland EA, Strohm PL, Kennedy et al: Hemolysis following intravenous immune globulin therapy. Transfusion 26:410, 1986

304. Kim HC, Park CL, Cowan JH et al: Massive intravascular hemolysis associated with intravenous immunoglobulin in bone marrow recipients. Am J Pediatr Hematol Oncol 10:69, 1988

305. Grove-Rasmussen M, Huggins CE: Selected types of frozen blood for patients with multiple blood group antibodies. Transfusion 13:124, 1973

306. Tovey GH: Preventing the incompatible blood transfusion. Haemetologia 8:389, 1974

307. Walker RH: Is a crossmatch utilizing the indirect antiglobulin test necessary for patients with a negative antibody screen? In Current Topics in Blood Banking. University of Michigan, Ann Arbor, 1977

308. Garratty G: Clinically significant antibodies reacting optimally at 37°C. p. 29. In Butch S (ed): Clinically Significant and Insignificant Antibodies. American Association of Blood Banks, Washington, DC, 1979

Chapter 10

Blood Donor Screening: Principles and Policies

Steven Kleinman

The obligation for blood centers to evaluate each prospective blood donor to decide on eligibility is twofold: (1) to ensure that the donated unit will not cause any adverse consequences for transfusion recipients, and (2) to ensure that the donor will not suffer any adverse reactions as a result of the donation.[1,2] Over the past decade, procedures used to evaluate donors have changed dramatically. The increased awareness of potential spread of infectious disease by blood transfusion has resulted in much more elaborate donors screening for the purpose of protecting the blood transfusion recipient.[3,4] At the same time, experience from autologous donation programs has lessened concern about adverse donor reactions.[5]

Assessment of the prospective donor's eligibility to donate is determined by a suitably qualified person, usually a nurse, medical technologist, physician's assistant, or phlebotomist. A physician is not routinely involved in eligibility decisions on individual donors. Rather, the responsibilities of the blood center physician are to ensure that appropriate standard operating procedures exist and are being followed and to evaluate donors with unusual histories. The blood center's donor eligibility procedures must be in accord with recommendations of the Food and Drug Administration (FDA) (as stated in the Code of Federal Regulations (CFR) or in memos to blood establishments[6]) and should also adhere to the Standards

of the American Association of Blood Banks (AABB).[1,2] In addition, individual states may have legal requirements pertaining to donor eligibility.

This chapter focuses primarily on donor selection and screening procedures for protection of the transfusion recipient. The rationale for policies is discussed and, when available, data to evaluate the efficacy of these policies are presented. In addition, procedures for protection of the donor are reviewed.

PROTECTION OF THE RECIPIENT

When it is suspected that an infectious agent may be transmitted by transfusion, the initial line of defense, is to formulate non-laboratory-based donor deferral policies using epidemiologic data derived from high-risk populations.[3] After this initial step, donor screening procedures are often implemented nationwide following recommendations of the Food and Drug Administration (FDA) or the AABB.[1,6] Given the current regulatory, political, and legal climate, once a procedure is implemented it is difficult to rescind it, even if there is no good evidence for its effectiveness. Because screening procedures tend to become permanent, it is important to evaluate their value carefully by pilot studies in blood donor populations before widespread implementation. If this is not done adequately, the result will be the addition of procedures that do little or nothing to increase transfusion safety but will result in deferral of safe donors. Recently, there has been a trend to perform such evaluations before instituting new donor interview questions.[7,8]

For diseases for which there are no routine laboratory tests (Creutzfeld-Jacob disease, Chagas disease, babesiosis), donor screening procedures are the only method available for increasing transfusion safety. For those infectious diseases for which routine blood donor testing is performed, donor screening procedures are important, in that they provide protection during the window period of infection when donors may be infectious but seronegative.

While there are distinct advantages to eliminating donors with possible risks of disease transmission, this approach has its share of negative consequences. Because donor deferral criteria often have poor specificity, a large number of safe donors will be deferred.[9] While this dilemma has been well recognized, there is no available algorithm to decide if a given procedure or screening question should be implemented. Such decisions attempt to balance the following factors: the extent of disease transmission, the severity of the consequences of such disease to the recipient, the expected sensitivity (effectiveness) of the procedure, and the number of donors lost by implementation of the procedure.

Methodologic Considerations for Evaluating Donor Screening Procedures

To assess the expected effectiveness of a new donor screening method or to compare the relative efficacy of two alternative screening methods, it is necessary to be aware of some basic methodolgic concerns that influence study design, analysis, and interpretation.[4]

If we apply a donor screening procedure to a population of potential blood donors, that population will be divided into deferred donors and acceptable donors. The deferred donor population will contain donors who are infectious and who are appropriately deferred (true-positive deferrals), as well as donors who are not infectious (false-positive deferrals). Classification of these two subpopulations of deferred donors is crucial to evaluating the procedure's effectiveness. Although it is possible to obtain information regarding true-positive and false-positive deferral status by performing laboratory testing on deferred donors, this is rarely done because obtaining a blood sample from a population of deferred donors is logistically complex and too time-consuming. (One donor screening procedure, confidential unit exclusion, is an exception in that donations from these individuals are collected and tested.) Furthermore, given the rare occurrence of some markers in the donor population (i.e., human immunodeficiency virus [HIV] seroprevalence of 0.0067 percent in the second half of 1992),[10] it would be necessary to perform a huge study with tens of thousands of observations in order to obtain statistically valid results. In the absence of laboratory test information on deferred donors, we must base our evaluation of the usefulness of a donor screening procedure on the total number of deferred donors. An illustrative example is provided by a recent study that attempted to compare alternate methods of donor information presentation and donor questioning with regard to HIV risk.[11] Although the investigators were able to demonstrate that a particular intervention led to the deferral of more donors, they did not perform HIV antibody testing on the deferred donors; hence, they did not demonstrate that the additional deferrals enhanced transfusion safety.

Among the population of acceptable donors, there will also be two subpopulations: those donors who are not infectious for the particular agent (i.e., the true-negative donors on the donor screening procedure), and a much smaller subpopulation of donors who will have passed the donor screening procedure but who will be infectious for the agent (false-negative donors on the screening procedure). For an infectious agent for which no routine laboratory tests are performed, it will not be possible to distinguish false negative from true negative donors. By contrast, for infectious agents such as HIV, for which we perform routine laboratory testing, we will be able to classify some donors as false-negative in the donor screening process; that is, these donors will be HIV seropositive and their units will not be transfused. However, there is also a second subpopulation of false negative donors, those who are infectious but negative on laboratory testing. Although this population is difficult to identify, it is a vitally important population to study, since it is their units that will be transfused and that may cause recipient infection.[12]

An illustrative example will clarify the above discussion. Donors with risk factors for HIV infection who are either HIV seropositive or who are HIV sero-negative, but in the window period, would both be examples of donors that were not appropriately deferred by donor screening. The HIV window period donors would be the most important group to study, as it is this group of donors who may actually transmit infections to recipients. However, most studies of HIV screening procedures have focused on interviews with HIV-seropositive donors, since they are approximately 10 times more prevalent than window period donors and are easily identified.[13]

Using this theoretical framework, we can formulate a strategy that will allow us to compare the effect of two different donor screening interventions; for example, the use of two different formats for presenting HIV risk factor questions. Ideally, we would measure the number of false-negative donors with products released for transfusion (i.e., the HIV-seronegative but infectious donor) that result from each procedure. Unfortunately, this is usually not possible because of the small numbers of such donors and the sophisticated laboratory testing that would be needed to establish the presence of infection during the window period. Alternatively, if our study were large enough, we could measure changes in the HIV-seropositive donor rate and infer that such changes would be predictive of similar changes in the rate of HIV-infectious but -seronegative donors. However, it is difficult to make this measurement due to the low prevalence of HIV-seropositive donors. Furthermore, the HIV-seropositive donor rate may also be influenced by variables other than our donor screening procedures (e.g., a media report that heightens the public's desire to obtain HIV test results). As a third alternative, we could measure the increase in deferred donors. Using this approach, we would then infer that an increased number of deferred donors means an increased number of potentially infectious donors. However, because we are dealing with a very low prevalence condition, our measured changes in the donor deferral rate may be misleading; even questions with high specificity will result in the identification of many more false-positive than true-positive donors.[9] Therefore, in comparing the number of donors deferred by several alternate interventions, we may actually be measuring the relative cost of the interventions to the blood donor col-

lection system (i.e., deferral of otherwise acceptable donors), rather than measuring a relative improvement in blood donation safety.

In summary, since the rate of deferred donors is the only measurement that can be easily obtained, this measure has been frequently used in studies of donor screening procedures. The reasoning is that better compliance with our deferral criteria will make the blood supply safer based on the implicit assumption that these deferral criteria actually enhance transfusion safety. However, if such criteria are inappropriate or outdated, better application of the criteria will not have such an effect.

Mechanisms for Selecting Safe Donors and Safe Units for Transfusion

Table 10-1 outlines procedures implemented to enhance transfusion safety; these procedures are discussed below with regard to theoretical rationale, as well as past, present, and future applications. When available, data to support the use of the procedures are given.

Exclusion of Donor Groups or Donor Sites

Because of the known spread of hepatitis between individuals inhabiting particular types of institutions, blood collection agencies do not collect blood at prisons or at homes for the mentally retarded.[14,15] In an effort to decrease the risk of acquired immunodeficiency syndrome (AIDS) transmission, blood col-

Table 10-1. Donor Selection and Screening Procedures

Timing	Procedure
Predonation	1. Exclusion of donor groups or donor sites
	2. Elimination of donation incentives
	3. Donor education
At donation site prior to donation	4. Self-exclusion in response to written material
	5. Health history interview
	6. Donor deferral registry[a]
	7. Confidential unit exclusion (CUE)
Postdonation	8. Telephone callback
	9. Donor deferral registry[a]

[a] This mechanism can be used either to disqualify the donor at the collection site or to discard the collected unit before release from the blood center.

lection agencies do not collect from groups or institutions that are known to comprise male homosexuals.[16] These policies were initially instituted as primary protective safety measures prior to the development of laboratory testing for the infectious agents of hepatitis and AIDS. Despite routine laboratory testing, these policies still remain prudent in order to eliminate donors with acute infection who are in the seronegative window period. On epidemiologic grounds, such persons would be expected to be more prevalent in these settings than in the general population.

Elimination of Donor Incentives

The primary example of a donor incentive associated with disease transmission is the payment of cash in exchange for blood donation. Because of this, in 1978, the Food and Drug Administration (FDA) instituted regulations that required the labeling of a blood unit as either volunteer or paid.[17] The regulation reads, in part, as follows:

> A paid donor is a person who receives monetary payment for a blood donation. A volunteer donor is a person who does not receive monetary payment for a blood donation. Benefits, such as time off from work, membership in blood assurance programs and cancellation of non replacement fees, that are not readily convertible to cash, do not constitute monetary payment within the meaning of this paragraph.[17]

These regulations sparked extensive discussions about the most appropriate definition of volunteer; this is a debate which has still not been resolved.[18,19] At about the same time that the FDA established its regulation, several states passed legislation virtually prohibiting the use of commercial donor blood.[17]

These regulatory and statutory requirements were instituted in response to data indicating that commercial blood donors were more likely than volunteer blood donors to transmit hepatitis to recipients. This conclusion was supported by several lines of evidence: higher rates of hepatitis B surface antigen (HBsAg) positivity in commercial donors, higher rates of hepatitis B and non-A, non-B (NANB) hepatitis in recipients of paid versus volunteer donor blood and, most definitively, documentation in a well-studied cohort of transfusion recipients that the elimination of commercial blood resulted in substantially fewer cases of post-transfusion hepatitis.[20–23] An analysis of the transition from commercial donor blood to volunteer blood in the state of New Mexico indicated that almost 100 percent of the commercial donor population ceased to donate with the removal of the cash incentive.[24] These data substantiated that the cash incentive was apparently the sole motivator for donation in this large group of commercial donors.

While paid blood donors are now very uncommon, the U.S. plasma industry still depends on commercial donors. It is of interest that seropositivity rates among this donor population for newly implemented blood screening tests (human T-cell lymphotropic virus, type I [HTLV-I] and hepatitis C virus [HCV]) are markedly higher than among volunteer blood donors,[25,26] mimicking the situation identified in the 1970s with regard to commercial blood donors and HBsAg testing. It thus appears that a significant percentage of commercial donors (of blood in the 1970s and currently of plasma) are likely to have relatively high rates of infection with multiple infectious disease agents. Some of these agents may escape detection because of limitations of existing laboratory tests or because the agents have not yet been well recognized or characterized.

Although the increased risk of blood from commercial donors has been documented, it has also been recognized that it is not the actual act of payment that makes commercial donors unsafe; rather, it is a consequence of the financial incentive attracting donors from a population (i.e., donors of a lower socioeconomic class) that has a higher rate of infectious disease.[27,28] Two recent reports have indicated that populations of paid donors, which were drawn from different segments of society than were the commercial donors of the 1960s and 1970s, were no less safe than volunteer donors.[29,30] In one recent study of carefully screened repeat paid pletepheresis donors in the midwest, the infectious disease marker rate was equivalent to that of the same blood centers' volunteer blood donor population, suggesting that both groups may have equivalent safety.[30] However, extrapolating these results to other populations of paid donors does not appear appropriate, given the use of special donor selection criteria at the study blood center. These criteria required a previous whole blood donation, an orientation session, and an eight week waiting period before donors were accepted into the paid plateletpheresis program.[31]

An incentive would be expected to be detrimental to the safety of the blood supply if it results in the recruitment of a population group that has a higher risk of transmitting infectious disease than that of the general blood donor population. If such an "unsafe" population of donors is recruited, the combined application of donor screening procedures and laboratory testing will be unable to lower the risk to that of the general donor population for two reasons. First, since a significant percentage of donors who are infected with HIV, HTLV, or HCV have no recognized risk factor, even after careful postdonation interviews, donor screening procedures will not be able to identify and defer such individuals.[13,32-35] The second factor relates to the deferral of those donors who, on postdonation interview, admit to risk factors for infection that would have resulted in their deferral. Some of these donors may knowingly give untruthful answers to interview questions, motivated by the desire to obtain the offered donor incentive.[36-38]

Currently there are no data to assess whether the use of other donor incentives (e.g., time off from work, gifts, a monetary credit for blood nonreplacement fees, participation in a group assurance plan, or working toward recognition as a multigallon donor) have an influence on blood safety.[39] However, one recent study has demonstrated that donors who received a special tee shirt from a rock radio sponsored blood drive had higher rates of several infectious disease markers, higher rates of hits on the donor deferral registry, and higher rates of medical deferral for a history of self-injected drug use.[40] It is unclear whether these rates were due to the tee-shirt incentive or to the publicity given the blood drive by the rock radio station. There are conflicting data about whether donor incentives are effective recruitment techniques.[41] Several studies have suggested that incentives are more effective in attracting blood donation by persons who have never previously donated than in influencing repeat donations in previous donors.[39] If this proves to be the case, this finding may have implications for how we think about the use of incentives. If an incentive attracts a large percentage of first-time donors from a different population group than the usual first-time donor, one might hypothesize that transfusion safety could be compromised. By contrast, if incentives are used to solicit more frequent donations from repeat donors, they may be less likely to be detrimental to transfusion safety.

One type of incentive that has been used by blood centers to increase collections is the provision of a public health screening program, such as cholesterol testing, to blood donors.[42,43] The issue of whether such a program affects transfusion safety has not been studied. However, this issue could be completely eliminated from consideration if blood centers were to perform cholesterol testing for deferred, as well as for acceptable, blood donors.[44]

The issue of appropriate donor recruitment techniques and the definition of acceptable donor incentives continue to be debated. The American Association of Blood Banks and organizations such as the U.S. National Bone Marrow Donor Registry, and internationally, the Council of Europe, have recently issued updated policies on this subject.[45,46]

An additional mechanism of safeguarding the blood supply by removing a rather unique donor incentive for a particular high-risk population to donate blood was the establishment of alternative testing sites for HIV antibody in 1985. In order to prevent donation from occurring for the purpose of obtaining HIV test results, federal and state governments established alternative test sites at which free and anonymous anti-HIV testing could be obtained.[47] Data from such programs indicate that HIV-seropositive rates were significantly higher than those found at blood centers.[48] Although it is uncertain how many alternative test site clients would have donated blood if there were no other way to obtain HIV test results, at least two studies have indicated that some percentage would have done so.[48,49] More recently, 15 to 29 percent of HIV-seropositive donors, when interviewed postdonation, indicated that their motivation for donation was to obtain their HIV antibody test result.[36-38] On the basis of these results, blood centers must continue to educate their prospective donors that blood should not be donated if the motivation is to obtain HIV antibody test results.

Selection of Donors Through Education and Donor Self-Exclusion

This approach became widely used in 1983 with the recognition that AIDS could be transmitted by blood transfusion.[3,4,50] Specific groups of individuals were identified as being at high risk of AIDS (i.e., male homosexuals with multiple partners and intravenous drug users who shared needles). Blood centers made extensive efforts through the use of the media and through discussion with gay community leaders to inform the public that individuals with such risk factors should not donate blood. Community education was augmented by distribution of written information concerning donor eligibility at donor recruitment. Also in 1983, written material provided to blood donors at the collection site was modified to include a description of risk factors for AIDS.[51] Donors were instructed that if one of the risk factors applied to them, they should not proceed with the donation process. There are data to indicate that these donor screening mechanisms were effective in decreasing the risk of AIDS transmission. A survey of gay men indicated that many who had donated before the recognition of the AIDS epidemic subsequently ceased their donation behavior.[52] Data from New York City, Los Angeles and San Francisco indicated that there were decreased donations from the populations at highest risk of transmitting AIDS infection.[9,53–55]

Health History Interview: General Considerations

Health history interview questions designed to defer donors who present increased risk of infectious disease transmission can be broadly grouped into several categories.[3] Table 10-2 presents the diseases for which the various categories of questions have been applied based on known epidemiologic risk factors.

Several methods have been used to conduct health history interviews: these include the oral approach, the self-administered written approach, and the combined approach. In the oral approach, the donor interviewer asks the donor all health history questions and records the responses on the donor card. In the self-administered approach, the donor checks off yes or no answers after reading each question. In the combined approach, the donor may self-administer some questions and respond orally to others, or the donor may self-administer all questions and then respond a second time to selected questions orally presented by the donor interviewer. Regardless of the approach, if the donor gives answers that could potentially affect his eligibility, the donor interviewer needs to document a more detailed explanation of the donor's response.

Until recently, there has been little standardization of donor questioning throughout different blood centers in the United States. In 1991, a consortium of California blood centers reported on their 3-year effort to design and implement a uniform medical donor history card.[56] The process of generating the card resulted from consensus building among the medical directors of the various blood centers, with the final questions being approved by the Center for Biologic Evaluation and Research (CBER) of the FDA. Limitations of this approach were an inability to pretest the questions in donor populations before their implementation and the reliance on medical directors rather than social scientists or communication experts to design questions. More recently, the AABB has developed a uniform donor history card, also approved by FDA, which is available to be used by any blood collection center in the United States.[2] It should be noted that there are no data to evaluate whether the use of a uniform

Table 10-2. Health History Interview Questions

Category	Disease Prevented
Medical history of a specific disease	AIDS, hepatitis, malaria, Chagas disease, babesiosis
Medical symptoms compatible with a specific disease	AIDS, bacteremia, viremia
Blood exposure by needlestick injury or blood transfusion	AIDS, hepatitis
Medical treatment	Creutzfeldt-Jakob disease
Sexual or drug use activities of donor or sexual partner(s)	AIDS, HTLV-I/II, hepatitis
Previous residence in or visit to endemic area	Malaria

card has resulted in enhanced transfusion safety. Nevertheless, the implementation of the uniform history card may produce two other benefits: a greater understanding of donation requirements by each blood center, and possible legal protection if a given blood center's procedures are legally challenged.

Although interview questions have become more standardized, it has become apparent that there is not uniformity in the standard operating procedures used when a donor gives an affirmative answer that requires further evaluation. Since the ultimate decision as to whether to accept a particular donor rests on medical judgement, such standardization is inherently difficult. Subtle psychological factors may subconsciously influence decision making. In problematic situations, it is sometimes easier for staff to accept rather than reject a blood donor; rejection may make the donor feel bad, may make the donor anxious about his or her infectious disease status, and in the case of directed donors, may be perceived by the donor as a denial of a right to donate.[57,58] Obviously, it is incumbent upon nursing and medical staff to make the proper safety decisions and not to be unduly influenced by these other psychological factors.

Health History Interview: Specific Aspects

In addition to asking the right questions during the donor interview, it is necessary to obtain the right answers. Post-donation interviews with HIV- and HCV-seropositive donors indicate the difficulty in getting donors to admit a history of risky sexual behavior or past intravenous drug use prior to donating.[32,59] Some of this difficulty may be unavoidable, given the strong psychological denial donors may have about HIV risk.[36] By contrast, it is possible that improvements in the donor screening process may result in eliciting risk behavior from an additional percentage of donors.[11] Table 10-3 lists some of the

Table 10-3. Issues in Optimizing Donor Health History Screening

1. Privacy of Interview
2. Donor comprehension of written material
3. Need for interpreters
4. Interviewer training and competency
5. Time constraints

important parameters that can be examined to potentially increase the quality of the answers given in the donor health history interview.

Because the health history interview involves questions of a delicate nature, it is important to ensure that the interview is conducted in a private and confidential fashion.[2] This can often times be difficult in the blood mobile setting. Two studies have documented that most donors felt that privacy during the history interview was adequate.[36,60] In one study of HIV-seropositive donors, 31 percent felt a lack of privacy during the donor interview, with 20 percent stating that they would have changed their answers to interview questions if they had been in a more private situation.[36] A second study, conducted with routine blood donors, found that 14 percent of donors on blood mobiles perceived their privacy was inadequate.[60] This study evaluated interventions designed to increase privacy, establishing that the use of acoustic paneling mounted on health history tables or the use of background white noise reduced the transmission of donor speech from the health history interview table to other sites in the blood mobile. However, despite these objective improvements in reducing sound transmission, donors' perception of privacy was unaffected. It is somewhat disturbing that a significant minority (14 to 31 percent) of donors in these studies believed that privacy was inadequate. It is possible, but unproven, that such perceptions might affect donor responses to sensitive sexual or drug-use behavior questions on the donor interview. Therefore, it remains important to devise methods to provide greater privacy or to alter the perception of those donors who feel their privacy is inadequate.

One approach to the health history interview that may address donors' privacy concerns and may result in eliciting more truthful risk behavior information is the use of a computer interactive interview. In one study of 272 donors, the subjects stated that they had a feeling of increased privacy compared to the usual interview format.[61] In addition, the rate of HIV-related deferrals for HIV-related symptoms or risk behaviors was significantly increased when compared to the usual interview format. Similar deferral data were obtained from a larger study of 2,600 donors, which has been presented to the FDA Blood Products Advisory Committee but has not yet been published in the peer-reviewed literature.[62] Unfortunately, data from both studies need to be interpreted cautiously due to inherent limitations in study design. Because of FDA requirements, both studies required that the group given the computer interview also be screened by standard health history screening techniques. In addition, in the published study, the computer interview was given anonymously, that is, without the donor providing any identifying information, making this situation very different from the standard health history interview. Despite these flaws, these preliminary results should encourage further investigations of this potentially new approach.

It has been recognized that donor comprehension of predonation written materials can often pose a problem. In the past, this material has often been written at an educational level that required a high degree of reading comprehension. More recently, attempts have been made to rewrite such material at a lower grade level. Another solution to this problem is to place less reliance on the use of written material. Toward this end, the AABB and FDA have recommended that, in the case of HIV risk factors, a verbal discussion take place between the interviewer and the donor.[63,64] In addition to presenting HIV risk factor information to the donor, this verbal discussion serves the purpose of emphasizing the significance and importance of this information.

Another potential problem encountered at the donation site occurs when the donor does not speak English well or at all. In this setting, it is important to administer the questionnaire in the donor's native language and to use an interpreter to assist in the interview. However, the use of an interpreter poses problems if the interpreter is either a relative or a fellow employee. Since many HIV risk questions are of an extremely personal nature, this creates a situation in which the donor may not give a truthful history to the interpreter. Currently there is no consensus as to how to solve this problem; one possible solution is not to accept such donors unless an independent interpreter is used.[4]

Several additional factors are currently receiving increasing attention due to blood centers' need to comply with the FDA's Good Manufacturing Practice regulations. These factors are the adequacy of training for donor room personnel, the level of accredita-tion of such staff, and the level of staff competency. In the interview setting, competency would apply to building rapport with the donor so as to be able to effectively solicit information during the interview. While it is plausible that the attitudes of interviewers with regard to sexual behavior may have an impact on their ability to elicit truthful sexual behavior histories, there are no data to address this issue.

The goal of maximizing donor throughput at the collection site, which is important both for productivity and for donor convenience, may also affect the quality of the donor interview. Despite pressures to process donors quickly, it is important that the donor be given sufficient time to think carefully about answers to interview question, particularly since it may be necessary to recall behaviors from many years ago.[65]

In summary, each blood collection organization must carefully examine its own operations and devise procedures that maximize the ability to obtain correct answers from donors.

Donor Deferral Registries

Donor deferral registries were originated in an effort to decrease the risk of transfusion-associated hepatitis at a time when other more specific methods were unavailable. More recently, their use has been extended to include donors who might transmit HIV and other infections.[6,66,67]

These registries are computer, microfiche, or manual files of names and identifying information from donors who have been deferred for specified reasons. Individual blood centers have established in-house (local) donor deferral registries to comply with a section of the Code of Federal Regulations that states that persons who have ever tested positive for HBsAg or anti-HIV should no longer be accepted as blood donors.[6,67] The rationale of donor deferral registries is that individuals with a previous positive test result may revert to a negative test result at a later date, despite the fact that they could still transmit disease. This situation could occur because of either a biologic phenomenon or a testing error. Donor deferral registries have expanded to include the names of donors who have previously volunteered information (i.e., history of intravenous drug use, hepatitis, or high-risk AIDS activity) that should have permanently excluded them as blood donors.

Donors who volunteer such information at one visit may be tempted to withhold the information at a subsequent visit, especially if their self-assessment is that the history ought not to have precluded them as blood donors.

Since donors may not always donate to the same blood collection agency, some states have created statewide donor deferral registries that include the names of donors deferred at any blood collection agency within the state.[66] The American Red Cross (ARC) uses a national system in which donors who are entered into specific categories of the deferral registry of an individual ARC region also have their names included in a national registry.[66,67] Because of donor confidentiality concerns, donor deferral registries that extend beyond an individual blood center do not list the reason for donor entry into the registry.

Over the past 10 years, the size and complexity of donor deferral registries have increased enormously. For example, the national component of the ARC donor deferral registry contains more than 20 separate deferral categories and over 300,000 donor names.[66,67] It has been estimated that there may be up to 3 million entries in donor deferral registries throughout the United States.[66] The problems associated with managing such expanded deferral registries have also increased dramatically, creating a major source of difficulty in complying with FDA regulations. These regulations and blood center standard operating procedures require that if a donor is listed in certain permanent deferral categories, namely anti-HIV positive or history of intravenous drug use, on a donor deferral registry, additional donations from that individual should not be distributed for transfusion. Difficulties in complying with this requirement have resulted in much publicity about blood centers erroneously releasing blood products, despite the fact that such released products have been shown to be uninfected with any transmissible agents.

Problems encountered in managing donor deferral registries include (1) the difficulty in obtaining accurate information that uniquely identifies a donor; (2) the existence of multiple records for the same donor because of conflicting information obtained on separate donations; (3) the need to move donors from one category of the registry to another;

and (4) the fact that some information leads to permanent deferral, while other data only result in deferral if the phenomena (e.g., a positive anti-HBc test) occurs on two occasions.[66]

The donor deferral registry can be used in one of two ways. At some blood centers, the donor's name is checked against the deferral registry prior to donation; no blood is collected if the donor is listed on the registry. At other blood centers, blood is collected, but the donor deferral registry is checked before the unit is placed into inventory; the unit is quarantined and destroyed if the donor's name is found on the registry.

Maintenance and continuous use of statewide or national donor deferral registries are time-consuming, logistically complex, and expensive. Unfortunately it has remained difficult to assess whether such massive efforts afford significant increases in safety to the blood transfusion recipient.

Telephone Callback

A further safeguard intended to increase transfusion safety is the mechanism of telephone callback.[3] At blood donation, donors receive instructions that they may call the blood center sometime after the donation to report additional pertinent medical history information. Telephone callbacks fall into two general categories. Most often, donors call back to report the development of an acute illness, such as fever, upper respiratory tract infection, or a gastrointestinal disorder, occurring from several hours to several days postdonation. In some cases, donors call back to indicate risk factors for HIV infection that might not have been disclosed at the time of donation.

Blood centers must have established policies for deciding how to evaluate postdonation telephone information. In general, if such information would have caused the donor to be deferred, and if the blood center receives such a phone call before transfusion of the donor's blood components, those components will be retrieved and destroyed. More problematic is what to do if blood components from such a unit have already been transfused. In such cases, the hospital transfusion service medical director must decide whether to inform the recipient's physician that a recent blood transfusion has a higher-than-usual risk of transmitting infection. In the case of a unit transfused from a donor who reports HIV risk factors, such information should be expected to produce anxiety in the recipient. Furthermore, since HIV antibody testing will be unable to resolve the situation definitively for several weeks to several months, this anxiety may not be easily alleviated. In my opinion, the best way to handle such a situation is for a blood center physician or designee to recontact the donor who volunteered the information and attempt to obtain a specific and accurate history. This may allow the hospital transfusion service medical director to better estimate the likelihood of risk to the recipient. Using this information, the decision as to when and whether to notify the recipient's physician and/or the recipient and the details of the specific notification message can be determined on a case-by-case basis. Unfortunately, there are no clear-cut guidelines as to how to handle these situations.

There are no controlled studies and little available data to assess the impact of the telephone callback mechanism on preventing HIV transmission. One recently analyzed set of data reviews an 8-year experience with telephone callback in San Francisco; the community blood center averaged 24 donor initiated callbacks per year in which donors revealed HIV-related risk factors that they had not disclosed at the time of donation.[68] Despite these risk factors, all such donated units tested HIV seronegative. On follow-up investigation, it was found that donors in two cases subsequently seroconverted for HIV. Although these data suggest that telephone callback may have some effect on eliminating infectious HIV window period units, it is not possible to evaluate the extent of this impact.

Confidential Unit Exclusion

The procedure known as confidential unit exclusion (CUE) was introduced at many blood centers following a 1986 FDA recommendation stating that at donation, donors should be offered a procedure by which they could designate confidentially whether or not their blood should be transfused to others.[69] The rationale for CUE was to provide an opportunity for those donors who felt pressured to donate by such groups as peers, fellow employees, and employers at a workplace or community blood drive to indicate that their blood should not be transfused. The CUE procedure works as follows. After the health history interview but before donation of the unit, each blood donor indicates whether his or her unit should or should not be used; if a donor neglects to make any indication, the unit will not be used.

Numerous small studies have attempted to evaluate the sensitivity, specificity, or predictive value of the CUE procedure.[70–77] Assessments of the efficacy of CUE have focused primarily on the frequency of its use by HIV-seropositive donors. These data have been somewhat conflicting and have led to differing conclusions about the value of the CUE procedure. Furthermore, those studies in which follow-up interviews were performed with donors who chose the CUE option have consistently established that most donors selecting this option did so as a result of either misunderstanding or error.[74–78] These latter findings have prompted suggestions that the CUE procedure be modified to make it more understandable to blood donors, in an effort to improve its specificity.[71,74] Several modifications to the CUE procedure have occurred since 1986. Many centers have switched from the use of a manual ballot separated from the donor card to the use of a peel-off barcoded sticker that the donor affixes to the history card. There have also been simplifications in the wording of the CUE form, clearer written and oral instructions as to the purpose of CUE, and clearer instructions as to how to complete the process correctly.

The rate of use of the CUE procedure has decreased from 7 per 1,000 donations in the early years[70,79,80] to 2 to 4 per 1,000 in more contemporary reports.[77,79,80] It is probable that some of this decrease has resulted from improvements in the CUE procedure. Other factors that may have also contributed are fewer persons with HIV risk presenting at the donation site or a greater number of deferrals of such individuals during the health history interview.

Recently, two large studies have attempted to reevaluate whether CUE is a useful procedure.[79,80] In addition to looking at whether HIV seropositive donors excluded their blood from transfusion, these two studies were able to analyze whether donors who were demonstrated to seroconvert for HIV (i.e., HIV-seronegative donation followed by HIV-seropositive donation) used the CUE option on their preseroconversion sample. This is the most relevant group for evaluation of CUE's effect on transfusion safety because, unlike HIV-seropositive units, these units would otherwise be transfused to recipients if the CUE procedure were not in place.[73,79]

Investigators from the Centers for Disease Control (CDC) have compiled data on the use of CUE at preseroconversion donation of 322 HIV-seroconverting donors at 40 blood centers from January 1987 through December 1990.[79] These workers found that 3.4 percent of such donations were excluded; however, 9 of the 11 exclusions came from one center (New York Blood Center) that has consistently shown results for the CUE procedure that differ from the rest of the United States.[53,71] If these data from New York Blood Center are eliminated, the data from the remaining 39 centers indicate that two of 246, or 0.8 percent, of HIV-seroconverting donors used this option.

The Retrovirus Epidemiology Donor Study analyzed the CUE process in 1.5 million donations made at five blood centers in 1991 and 1992.[80] These investigations found that 8 percent of 169 HIV-seropositive donations were excluded and that one of eleven HIV-seroconverting donors used this option on their preseroconversion unit.

If the aggregate data from HIV-seroconverting donors are analyzed, it appears evident that the CUE procedure does very little to enhance blood transfusion safety. Nevertheless, despite its ineffectiveness in the target group of HIV window period donors, several studies have demonstrated that donors who use CUE have higher rates of seropositivity for many infectious disease markers[76,79–81] and that some individuals who use CUE admit to HIV risk factors.[75,78] For these reasons, many still advocate retaining CUE as part of the donation process.

In 1992, the FDA analyzed the then available data on CUE sensitivity and specificity and concluded that the CUE procedure was no longer mandatory, and its use was left to the discretion of each individual blood center.[64] Currently some blood centers that previously used the CUE procedure have discontinued it.

Donor Selection for Prevention of Transmissible Agents or Conditions

Human Immunodeficiency Virus

The latest revision of FDA recommendations for screening prospective donors for prevention of HIV transmission was issued in April 1992.[64] These recommendations state that prospective donors:

1. Must receive both oral and written information concerning HIV (AIDS) risk factors and the potential for HIV transmission through donated blood. This information should include informing the donor that in early HIV infection a donor may be infectious and capable of transmitting HIV despite a negative test for HIV antibody.
2. Should be given specific information as to how they can obtain an HIV antibody test at a site other than the donor center.
3. Should be told that all units of donated blood will be tested for HIV antibody and, if positive, the donor will be notified of the test result and his name will be placed on a donor deferral registry.
4. Should be advised not to donate if symptoms which may be compatible with HIV infection are present. These symptoms include persistent fevers, night sweats, unexplained weight loss, persistent cough or shortness of breath, persistent diarrhea, swollen lymph nodes that persist for greater than 1 month, the presence of whitish oral lesions, or the presence of bluish purple spots on the skin or in the mouth.
5. Should be asked direct health history questions about behaviors that put them at risk of HIV. It is preferable that these questions be asked orally.

The specific information to be obtained from donors during the donor interview includes the following:

1. Have you ever had clinical or laboratory evidence of AIDS or HIV infection?
2. For men: Have you had sex with another man, even once since 1977?
3. Have you ever injected intravenous drugs?
4. Have you engaged in sex in exchange for money or drugs since 1977?
5. Have you received clotting factor concentrates for hemophilia or other clotting disorders?

If a donor answers yes to any of the above questions, he or she needs to be permanently deferred as a blood donor.

The donor should also be asked questions regarding behaviors during the previous 12-month interval. A yes answer to any of these questions will lead to a temporary deferral, which is removed 12 months after the last potential exposure. The following questions are asked:

> In the past 12 months, have you had sex with a person who has HIV infection or AIDS?
>
> In the past 12 months, have you had sex with a person who currently or previously used intravenous drugs?
>
> For women only: In the past 12 months, have you had sex with a man who has had sex with another man (i.e., a man who is bisexual)?
>
> In the past 12 months, have you had sex with a prostitute?
>
> In the past 12 months, have you had sex with a person receiving clotting factor concentrates?
>
> In the past 12 months, have you had syphilis or gonorrhea?
>
> In the past 12 months, have you had a blood transfusion?
>
> In the past 12 months, have you had an accidental needle stick injury or a blood splash to a mucous membrane or to nonintact skin?

At the conclusion of the medical history, donors must sign a consent that specifically states that they understand that they should not donate blood if they are at risk of HIV infection.

Rationale for the Current Criteria

Use of Orally Presented Donor Informational Material and Interview Questions

When donor screening procedures for preventing AIDS were first implemented in the early to mid-1980s, most blood centers in the United States did not ask donors direct questions about sexual orientation or behavior (i.e., a question from the nurse to the donor, such as "Have you ever had sex with another male?").[4] At the time, there were no available data to indicate that more explicit questioning might result in deferral of an increased number of high-risk persons; indeed, one hypothesis was that direct questioning about a person's sexual orientation might lead to untruthful answers because of concerns about maintaining the confidentiality of information.[4,16] A more direct approach also posed the

possibility of embarrassing or offending potential blood donors.

During the late 1980s, the donor interview process was re-evaluated on the basis of information obtained from interviews with HIV-seropositive donors and a much more open societal attitude toward discussing issues of sexual orientation and sexual behavior. A retrospective study demonstrated that asking donors direct oral questions about sexual behavior resulted in a fivefold increase in HIV-related deferrals from 1.46 to 7.31 donors per month at one blood center.[82] A second blood center conducted a survey concerning donors' attitudes toward being asked such explicit sexual behavior questions. Of 1,204 regular blood donors who responded, more than 90 percent endorsed the use of these questions, while only 1 percent felt that the questions might cause them to stop donating.[82] Subsequently, a prospectively designed study was performed at two U.S. blood centers to address the effectiveness of donor screening procedures, including revised donor information brochures, the use of an AIDS information video, and the use of a set of behavior oriented direct questions asked orally by the health historian. This study strongly suggested that the use of direct behavior-oriented oral questions led to a statistically significant increase in donors deferred for HIV risk behavior.[11] A second study, performed by the ARC, compared deferral rates in three groups, each of approximately 4,000 donors, using direct behaviorally oriented questions, indirect comprehension questions, and more generalized written interview questions; this study reached a similar conclusion with regard to the benefit of direct oral questioning.[83] The current FDA and AABB recommendations suggest, but do not require, that direct questions be asked orally.[64,84]

Use of Specific Questions on the Health History Interview

With the implementation of anti-HIV testing in 1985, anti-HIV-positive blood donors were identified, notified of their test results, and interviewed. These interviews revealed that although many HIV-seropositive donors were men who had sex with other men, they did not consider themselves to be at risk of HIV infection.[85] It became apparent that a person might respond very differently if asked whether he were a member of a specific group (i.e., a homosexual man), as opposed to being asked if he had ever engaged in a specific behavior (i.e., having sex with another male). The FDA therefore recommended in September 1985 that "any male who has had sex with another male since 1977" should not donate blood.[86] The recommendation emphasized that individuals who had had only a single homosexual experience should refrain from donating.

Three additional studies, summarized in Table 10-4, have examined the reasons why HIV-seropositive donors with known risk factors donated blood.[36–38] The CDC Multicenter Study included 512 donors (304 of whom had HIV risk factors) from 20 blood centers; the ARC Multicenter Study included 80 donors with HIV risk factors from three geographic areas; and the National Institutes of Health (NIH) study included 98 donors with HIV risk factors from Washington, DC. These studies show a similar profile of motivations for donation by HIV-seropositive donors. One major reason for donating was the donors' self-assessment that they were not at risk of HIV infection; CDC data indicated that many of donors were in psychological denial about their HIV risk. A second motivation for dona-

tion was social or peer pressure to donate; in the CDC study this pressure came from an employer or fellow employees, rather than from the blood center, in 75 percent of cases. Another group of donors was at least partially motivated to donate in order to obtain their HIV antibody test results. Some persons who donated indicated that they misunderstood the accuracy of the HIV antibody tests; some donors concluded that their donations were safe because they had previously tested HIV antibody negative, while other donors felt they would not be jeopardizing recipients since, if they were infectious, the HIV antibody test would inevitably be positive and their blood would not be used. Data from these studies contributed to a revision of donor questioning to include more specific HIV risk questions. These changes are reflected in current FDA recommendations and in the AABB's uniform donor history card.[2,64]

A preponderance of data has demonstrated that the theoretical possibility of long-term persistent HIV infection in the absence of detectable HIV antibody does not exist.[87–89] These data have demonstrated that seroconversion for HIV is highly likely to occur within 6 months of HIV exposure and that HIV nucleic acid cannot be detected in HIV antibody-negative individuals from high-risk groups at risk of latent HIV infection. Thus, HIV risk behaviors that can be defined as ending at a specific point in time (i.e., sex with a particular person who demonstrated HIV risk behaviors, an accidental exposure to blood, a blood transfusion) should only defer a prospective donor until serologic testing can definitively prove that the individual is free of HIV infection. In order to be absolutely certain that the required time for seroconversion has elapsed, a 12-month deferral interval for these behaviors has been selected. Other behaviors, such as male-to-male sex or past intravenous drug use, still require a lifetime deferral. The rationale (unproven) for these permanent deferrals is that such behaviors represent lifestyle choices that are not likely to be limited to defined time intervals.

As heterosexual transmission of HIV infection becomes more common in the United States,[90] it is to be anticipated that such a shift will be reflected in the demographics of HIV-seropositive blood donors. Thus far, no dramatic changes have occurred. In a CDC study of HIV-seropositive donors from 20

Table 10-4. Motivations for Donation by HIV-1 Antibody-Positive Blood Donors

Reasons	CDC Multicenter[a] (%)	ARC Multicenter (%)	NIH Wash, DC (%)
Denial of risk	NA	61	26
Social pressure	27	29	15
Wanted to get test results	15	29	26
Previous HIV-seronegative test	9	NA	NA
Positive test would stop blood from being transfused	10	NA	14
Misunderstood the pamphlet	7	NA	6
Other	32	NA	13

Abbreviations: ARC, American Red Cross; CDC, Centers of Disease Control; NIH, National Institutes of Health; HIV-1, human immunodeficiency virus type 1; NA, data not available.

[a] Some donors gave more than one reason.

blood centers, the number of seropositive donors who acquired their HIV infection by heterosexual exposure did not increase significantly when 1990–1991 data were compared to data from 1988–1989.[32] ARC data indicate that the rate of HIV-seropositive female donors has remained constant from 1988–1992; however, a slightly decreasing rate of HIV seropositive male donors has resulted in an increased percentage of females among all HIV-seropositive donors.[10]

The risk of heterosexual spread of HIV has been addressed by several items in the most recent FDA recommendations.[64] Several potential heterosexual risk exposures are a cause for 12-month deferrals; these include sex with an intravenous drug user, sex with a prostitute, sex with a bisexual man, or sex with a person using clotting factor concentrates. In the early years of the AIDS epidemic, donors who had immigrated to the United States from a country (e.g., Haiti and sub-Saharan Africa countries) in which heterosexual activity played a major role in the transmission of HIV infection were permanently deferred.[3,4] With the advent of HIV-2 antibody testing as a safeguard against transmitting HIV-2, an HIV strain more prevalent in parts of Africa, deferral policies based on geographic factors were no longer necessary and were discontinued.[91] This change in policy occurred concurrent with the recognition that heterosexual spread of HIV might be expected to increase in the U.S. population. As a protection against this occurrence, the FDA, in its most recent recommendations, added a history of syphilis or gonorrhea to the list of 12-month deferrals. The rationale for this policy is the assumption that having acquired either of these sexually transmitted diseases would indicate that a prospective donor had an increased risk of acquisition of HIV through heterosexual activity.

A recent study evaluated the impact of a proposed change in deferral criteria for heterosexual exposure to HIV.[32] This study analyzed the responses of HIV-seropositive donors with regard to their number of sexual partners in the last year and during their lifetime; furthermore, similar response data were cited from surveys of noninfected donors. It was concluded that the implementation of the proposed deferral criteria would be very nonspecific, leading to deferral of high percentages of noninfected do-

nors while providing only a marginal increase in blood safety.

It is well established that HIV is not transmitted by casual contact; therefore, persons who have had close contact with individuals who are anti-HIV positive or who have AIDS should not be deferred as blood donors.[92] If a person admits to living in the same household as an HIV-infected person, the potential for sexual or body fluid contact with that individual should be determined; if such contact has not occurred, the donor should not be deferred.

Hearsay Evidence of HIV Risk: A Dilemma

On occasion, donor interviewers may acquire information that is difficult to evaluate because it has been obtained from a third party, such as a spouse, a sex partner, or a fellow worker (hearsay evidence).[4] For example, a third party may assert that a particular donor is at risk of HIV infection (i.e., is homosexual), even though the donor has responded that he is not at risk. In this situation, the blood center will need to decide whether to use the collected unit and whether to defer the donor from future donations. The AABB has recommended that blood centers have written procedures indicating how such information will be assessed for validity.[93] In such a case, the blood center is faced with fulfilling two obligations: protecting the safety of a potential transfusion recipient, and avoiding false placement of a donor on a computerized deferral list based on a third-party accusation. One possible approach to this dilemma is for a blood center physician or a senior nursing staff member to reinterview the donor. It can be explained to the donor that additional information has prompted the need to reassess the donor's eligibility. The physician can emphasize the importance of truthful history in protecting recipient safety and can review HIV risk factor information with the donor. The physician can obtain answers to explicit HIV risk questions from the donor. If the donor admits to risk, he can be deferred. On the other hand, if the donor denies all HIV risk, the physician will need to make a decision as to whether to believe the donor or the third party. Unfortunately, there are no precise guidelines as to how such a decision should be made. My belief is that when the third-party evidence is not convincing, and when the donor insists that he has been truthful, the correct procedure is to advise the donor that he is eligible to make future donations. The donor will be reinterviewed and retested for HIV antibody on subsequent donations, thereby providing some degree of confirmation of their safety.

Revisions of Health History Questions: The Future

At least three areas of continued monitoring are necessary to ensure that HIV-related donor deferral criteria are optimally effective for preventing potentially HIV-infected persons from donating; these are continued observation of HIV-seropositive donor demographics, continued assessment of the risk factors and motivation for donation of HIV-infected donors, and evaluation of whether donor history questions are successful in eliminating persons with known HIV risk factors. The first two of these items are undergoing continued assessment by the multicenter CDC HIV Seropositive Donor Study. The third item, the effectiveness of donor history questions, is being addressed by the National Heart, Lung, and Blood Institute (NHLBI)-sponsored Retrovirus Donor Epidemiology Study, which is conducting anonymous detailed questionnaire surveys of sexual and drug-use behavior among recent blood donors who successfully completed the donation process.

Hepatitis

Federal guidelines for preventing transfusion-transmitted hepatitis were established decades ago in the Code of Federal Regulations (CFF).[6] The current regulations require the following deferral policies: (1) donors with a history of viral hepatitis are permanently deferred, (2) donors with a history of close contact with someone who has viral hepatitis are deferred for 12 months after their last potential exposure, and (3) donors who have received a blood transfusion are deferred for 12 months.[94] (Although the CFR indicates a 6-month deferral for these categories, subsequent FDA memos to blood establishments have changed this deferral to 12 months.[94] This change was based upon establishing consistency with HIV deferral time intervals, as well as the observed lag period to HCV seroconversion following HCV exposure using first-generation HCV tests.[95]) In addition, a person testing positive for HBsAg or known to have previously tested positive for HBsAg is also permanently deferred as a blood donor.

Recently, the FDA has clarified that a history of viral hepatitis applies only to clinical disease and that deferral is not required when the donor's history is based solely on a positive serologic test result (i.e., anti-HBc or anti-HBs) that indicates past exposure to HBV.[96] Furthermore, the permanent deferral requirement for a history of viral hepatitis no longer applies to an episode of viral hepatitis occurring before the age of 10.[97] This recent change in FDA policy is based on epidemiologic evidence that viral hepatitis in childhood, occurring before the onset of sexual activity, is almost exclusively due to infection with the hepatitis A virus (HAV).[98] Since HAV infection does not induce a chronic carrier state, it is evident that persons who acquired HAV in the remote past do not pose a hazard to transfusion recipients.[99] This type of reasoning raises the issue of whether donors with a history of HAV at any age should be acceptable as blood donors.[100,101] Although medical knowledge supports the safety of donations from these individuals, such a policy would be of limited value, as it would be difficult to prove definitively that a particular past episode of viral hepatitis was due to HAV. Because of this problem in establishing accurate diagnosis, it is still required that donors who present with a stated history of HAV above age 10 be deferred.

In the past, blood collection agencies deferred all donors with a history of jaundice.[102] Currently, the policy at most blood centers is to question the donor concerning the etiology of the jaundice and to accept those donors whose history of jaundice is related to the neonatal period or to obstructive biliary tract disease. Other related donor deferral criteria for potential hepatitis risk are based on the known parenteral routes of spread of HBV and HCV. Persons who have ever injected intravenous drugs by needle have long been deferred as blood donors due to hepatitis risk; the importance of this criterion has been reemphasized with the advent of the HIV epidemic.

Donors with a history of tatoos are deferred for 12 months due to the possibility of hepatitis spread by contaminated needles.[1,2] By contrast, donors who have had needle exposure through ear piercing, skin piercing, acupuncture, or electrolysis should not automatically be deferred. Rather, it should be evaluated whether these procedures were performed using disposable sterile needles, as is often the case if the procedure is done in a professional setting. If it cannot be verified that sterile technique was followed, consideration should be given to deferring such donors for 12 months.

Donors receiving hepatitis B immunoglobulin (HBIG) should be deferred for 12 months after such administration due to the underlying hepatitis B exposure risk. By contrast, donors receiving hepatitis B vaccine do not need to be deferred unless the vaccine was given for a recent exposure to HBV.

According to FDA regulations, donors who have had close contact with a patient with acute viral hepatitis should be deferred for 12 months.[94] Clearly, sexual contact is included in this definition; it is less clear how to define nonsexual close contact. One commonly used definition is the sharing of household, kitchen, or toilet facilities, as would occur with living in the same household.[4] In the case of HBV, this definition appears reasonable in that it has been demonstrated that HBV can rarely be transmitted from an acutely infected patient to a nonintimate household contact, probably through nonsexual contact with body fluids.[103] Data for nonsexual household transmission of HCV are more equivocal, and it is unclear whether nonsexual contacts of such patients pose a risk to recipients.[104] Nevertheless, the FDA requires deferral of such prospective donors. Persons who occasionally eat a meal or visit a patient who has viral hepatitis may have little hepatitis risk; medical judgement should be used to determine whether a particular donor with this type of history should be deferred.

FDA requirements do not apply to sexual or close contacts of asymptomatic or symptomatic chronic carriers of HBV and HCV. Given the high rates of sexual and body fluid transmission of HBV, the same 12-month deferral criteria should be applied to donors who have close contacts with chronic HBV carriers. With regard to HCV, newer data suggest that sexual transmission occurs with a high enough frequency to make it prudent to defer sexual partners of HCV carriers for 12 months following their last exposure.[105] Deferral policies for close, nonsexual contacts of HCV carriers are more problematic, given the scarcity of reproducible clinical data.[104]

Other Infectious Diseases

Specific donor history questions regarding a donor's travel to, or emigration from, a malarial endemic area are used to defer donors who may be at risk of transmitting malaria.[1,2,106] Donors are also questioned as to a past history of Chagas disease or babesiosis.[1,2]

Creutzfeld-Jacob disease (CJD) is a rare, fatal, degenerative neurologic disease with a long asymptomatic latent period.[107] The etiologic agent is either a virus or a prion.[108] Although transmission has not been documented secondary to blood transfusion, human-to-human transmission has occurred by tissue transplantation.[109] The concern for blood transfusion safety arises from the fact that persons who have received therapeutic injections of cadaver-derived pituitary human growth hormone have developed CJD, raising the possibility that other recipients of this hormonal product may have become asymptomatic chronic carriers of the CJD agent.[110,111] To eliminate possible risk to transfusion recipients, all prospective donors are asked whether they have ever received human growth hormone.[107,112,113] If it can be established that the growth hormone was pituitary derived (i.e., the injection was given before the availability of recombinant growth hormone in 1985), the donor is permanently deferred.

Another potential fatal complication of transfusion is bacterial infection.[114] Bacteria can be introduced into the donor unit at collection if the donor is bacteremic, if the skin site is not properly decontaminated, if there is an undetected abscess adjacent to the phlebotomy site, or through introduction of a small skin plug in the phlebotomy needle.[114–116] Examination of the skin at the venipuncture site is conducted before phlebotomy and strict requirements for ensuring the sterility of the site are adhered to by the phlebotomist. Blood is not collected from persons who are febrile at donation, who state that they do not feel well, or who are taking systemic antibiotics. In the past, blood centers have temporarily deferred donors with a history of dental procedures for up to 72 hours because of the high frequency of postprocedure bacteremia. These criteria have been liberalized with the recognition that many other types of trauma to mucous membranes that are not evaluated at donation may also cause bacteremia.[117] Most recently, it has been recommended that donors need only be deferred for 24 to 72 hours after particular traumatic types of dental procedures, such as root canals and tooth extractions.[2,114]

Unlike other infectious diseases, the risk of bacterial infection also applies to candidates for autologous donation, due to the ability of gram-negative rods to multiply at refrigerator temperatures and to secrete endotoxin into the blood bag.[118] For this reason, autologous donors who are taking antibiotics or who give a history of recent or concurrent medical procedures are evaluated for the possibility of bacteremia and are deferred accordingly.

Donors are asked if they have had a previous history of syphilis or gonorrhea during the past 12 months. This question has the purpose of decreasing the risk of HIV transmission, rather than preventing the transmission of the disease in question. There is no requirement to ask donors about other types of venereal disease, such as herpes simplex virus (HSV), genital warts, or *Chlamydia.*

Donors who have received certain types of live, attenuated viral vaccines are deferred for 2 weeks (except rubeola, which is a 4-week deferral). Donors receiving toxoid or killed viral vaccines are not deferred.[2]

Over the past decade, experience with transfusion-transmitted viruses such as HIV and HCV has clearly demonstrated that, in the absence of laboratory testing, asymptomatic donors with chronic latent viral infection may endanger recipients.[3,4] Concern for this type of circumstance may lead to deferral of donors with unusual histories (i.e., chronic fatigue syndrome in quiescence, treated Dengue fever), despite the fact that there is no definitive evidence of their potential infectivity.

Other Risks to the Recipient

Most medications taken by donors pose no known risks to recipients. In most cases, only small quantities of drugs will be present in a unit of blood, and the drug will undergo significant dilution in the recipient's plasma volume. However, some drugs may pose a risk due to their demonstrated teratogenic potential at low plasma concentrates. Three such medications (all in FDA pregnancy category X) have been identified by the FDA as potentially dangerous to recipients: these are etretinate (Tegison) used for severe psoriasis, isotretinoin (Accutane) used for severe cystic acne, and finasteride (Proscar) used for symptomatic benign prostatic hypertrophy.[113] Deferral periods for Accutane and Proscar are one

month whereas deferral for etretinate is permanent because of its demonstrated presence in plasma several years following cessation of use.

As stated by the FDA, it is the responsibility of each blood center to determine policies for deferral of donors taking other medications, giving consideration to the possible effects of the medication on the recipient or to a fetus who might be exposed to the drug during a maternal transfusion.

One common class of medications that almost always results in donor deferral is systemic antibiotics, provided that the donor is on the medication for prophylaxis or treatment of local or systemic bacterial infection. Donors on other medications are evaluated to determine if their underlying medical condition poses a threat to their ability to tolerate the donation successfully.

Donors with a history of malignancy pose a theoretical risk to recipients. Since many recipients are immunosuppressed, it may be possible that malignant cells circulating in a donor's blood could engraft and multiply in a recipient. In order to decrease the possibility of this occurrence, donors are questioned about a history of cancer. Until recently, a positive answer would result in permanent deferral unless the cancer was known to be low grade, fully excised, incapable of hematogenous spread (i.e., basal cell cancer of skin, cervical carcinoma in situ). This conservative approach has now been modified in some blood centers so that a donor who has a history of a solid organ tumor and has been symptom and treatment free for 5 years is considered clinically cured and is eligible to be a blood donor. Donors with a history of hematologic malignancy are still permanently deferred.

PROTECTION OF THE DONOR

Phlebotomy Procedure and Informed Consent

A donor must give informed consent prior to undergoing a blood donation.[1,2,44] The consent process begins with the donor reading a pamphlet concerning the process of blood donation. This written material should indicate that (1) approximately 450 ml of blood will be collected through a vein in the antecubital fossa (elbow); (2) additional blood will be collected for laboratory testing; (3) complications of donation, such as fainting, light-headedness, hematoma, or even nerve damage may occur; (4) infectious disease testing of donated blood will be performed; and (5) the donor will be notified of any abnormal results of medical significance. In addition, the written material must include a description of HIV risk factors. The donor's informed consent is obtained at completion of the health history interview, after the donor has had an opportunity to ask questions about the donation process. The donor's signature on the health history card confirms that the donor understands the donation process, certifies that all questions have been answered truthfully, and gives the blood center permission to use the donated unit as it deems fit.[44]

General Considerations

Several steps of the donation process help to assure that the donor's health is protected. The donor answers health history questions, undergoes a monitoring of vital signs, sometimes called a physical examination, and has a hemoglobin and/or hematocrit evaluation.

The major considerations influencing deferral criteria that protect the donor are (1) establishing that the donor does not fall into a group that is likely to have an increased risk of immediate post-donation reactions, (2) establishing that the donor is unlikely to have a post-donation reaction that is especially severe or prolonged or for which his cardiovascular status does not permit him to adequately compensate, and (3) ensuring that the donor does not acquire iron deficiency through phlebotomy.

While deferral criteria designed to protect the blood donor are sometimes decided on theoretical grounds, some specific criteria are amenable to controlled scientific studies. The general methodology of these studies is to monitor the rate and severity of the two major post donation reactions (i.e., vasovagal reactions and acute hypovolemic reactions) in donors with a specific characteristic and to compare these data with reaction rates in control donors. Since it has been demonstrated that subpopulations of acceptable donors may vary as much as 20-fold in reaction rates (from 6.4 percent in first-time female donors ages 18 to 30 to 0.3 percent in repeat male donors above age 50), there may be a wide tolerance limit before concluding that reaction rates in a group

of potentially deferable donors are unacceptably high.[119] Studies quantitating rates of donor reactions have established that donors older than 65 years of age, and donors taking various types of antihypertensive medication can safely donate[120-123]; these studies led to revision of previous more restrictive criteria.

Specific Donor Requirements

Age

Each state has established laws concerning the minimum acceptable age limit for donation. This age generally is 17 or 18; donors who are legally minors need written consent of a parent or guardian. The upper age for blood donation has changed over the past decade. Previously, this upper age limit had been set at 65 by many states and by national blood banking organizations such as the ARC. However, with the continued aging of the population, improvements in the health status of older individuals, and the general societal change in attitude toward older people, studies have been performed to reexamine the scientific basis for this policy.[119,120] These studies documented that persons over the age of 65 who met all other donation criteria actually had lower rates of post-transfusion reactions than those of donors in some other age groups. In addition, older donors did not develop any greater frequency of severe or life-threatening reactions. Similar findings have been documented in autologous donors older than 65 of age.[124] One large blood center in a retirement community has reported their experience with more than 50,000 donations in allogeneic donors from age 65 to 85; although they described two cardiac events in donors, these appeared to be temporally unassociated with donation.[125] On the basis of these data, most blood centers no longer impose an upper age limit for donor eligibility.

Health History Questions About Conditions Affecting the Donor

Donors are asked questions concerning a history of cardiovascular, pulmonary, liver, or other severe disease. Each blood center has a policy regarding the acceptability of donors with affirmative answers to any of these questions. In general, donors with coronary artery disease, cardiac valvular disease, arrhythmia, significant cerebrovascular disease, or congestive heart failure are deferred, as are donors with any active pulmonary disease impairing gas exchange. Some centers have tended to become somewhat less stringent in these deferral policies based on their experience with autologous donors who have successfully completed the donation process despite medical conditions that would have previously deferred them as allogeneic donors.[5,125]

A guideline for determining the suitability of donors who have undergone recent surgery in the absence of blood transfusion is to accept such persons when healing is complete and when they have resumed full activity. Donors who are pregnant are deferred during pregnancy and for 6 weeks after delivery. Donors with seizure disorders are acceptable provided that they have had no seizures within the past 12 months with or without medication. This policy appears reasonable as there are no data linking the convulsive activity associated with seizure disorders to the convulsive activity that may occur secondary to ischemia from a post-donation vasovagal reaction.[126]

Vital Signs

In order to reduce the risk of acute hypovolemic reactions, most blood centers defer donors who weigh less than 110 pounds; at this weight, phlebotomy of 450 ml of blood results in a decrease of 13 percent of the donor's blood volume.[119] Not surprisingly, the rate of donor reactions has been demonstrated to be inversely proportional to body weight, with the highest reaction rates in donors weighing 110 to 119 pounds.[119] Some blood centers will collect slightly smaller units from donors weighing 100 to 110 pounds.

Donors with temperature above 37.5°C (99.5°F) are deferred from donation. Donors with blood pressure above 180 systolic or 100 diastolic, donors with pulse rates outside the established limits of 50 to 100 beats per minute, and donors with an arrhythmia detected on pulse examination are usually deferred based upon uncertainties about their cardiovascular status. Exceptions may be made upon the discretion of the medical director. One common exception is for athletes in whom lower pulse rates are an indication of enhanced cardiovascular conditioning.

Hemoglobin Screening

The major purposes for determining the donor's hemoglobin concentration prior to donation is to ensure either that the donor does not have preexisting anemia or that the donor will not be made anemic by the blood donation.[2] A related purpose for hemoglobin screening is to protect donors from becoming iron deficient as a result of phlebotomy.[127]

Normal values for hemoglobin in the adult population are expressed either as a mean ±2 SD or as 5 percent and 95 percent, respectively, of reference ranges for age and sex. Using these definitions, standard limits for normal hemoglobin in U.S. adults are 14 to 18 g/dl in males and 12 to 16 g/dl in females.[128] Despite these definitions of normal, symptoms of anemia do not occur unless the hemoglobin is significantly lower than the normal range (i.e., less than 8 g/dl). Iron deficiency, defined as the depletion of body iron stores, may exist in the absence of overt anemia. Iron deficiency is uncommon in males with low or low-normal hemoglobin concentrations but is relatively common in females with such findings.[129–131] Total body iron stores are estimated to be 1000 mg in males but only 399 to 500 mg in females, and iron loss is substantial in menstruating females.[128] Hence, females may be thrown into negative iron balance by blood donation, which depletes the body of approximately 200 to 250 mg iron per donated unit.[127]

Since the largest percentage of donor deferrals occur in donors who fail the hemoglobin screening requirement, interest has developed in assessing the appropriateness of the hemoglobin cutoff level.[127] However, it has been difficult to establish the appropriate lower limits for acceptable hemoglobin levels with any scientific validity. The acceptable minimal hemoglobin level in the United States is 12.5 g/dl for both males and females, as mandated by FDA requirements.[6] The AABB now has identical requirements; previously, the AABB required a minimum hemoglobin level of 13.5 g/dl for males and 12.5 g/dl for females.[129] During the last decade, several studies have attempted to assess the appropriate minimum hemoglobin level by determining the ability of proposed cutoffs to detect donors with iron deficiency in the absence of overt iron deficiency anemia.[132,133] These studies used receiver operating curves to maximize both sensitivity and specificity of prospective hemoglobin cutoff values. The studies concluded that optimal minimum hemoglobin levels were 12.5 g/dl for males and either 12.0 g/dl or 11.5 g/dl for females. The 11.5 g/dl cutoff for females has been used in Australia and more recently in Canada.[134,135] However, a recent re-evaluation of the Canadian experience with the 11.5 g/dl standard has concluded that this value allows too many women with iron deficiency anemia to donate; these investigators suggested the lower limit for females be set at 12.5 g/dl.[134]

In order to arrive at the appropriate minimal hemoglobin standard, it is essential to decide whether such a limit is designed to prevent iron depletion without accompanying microcytic iron deficiency anemia. There are conflicting data regarding the consequences of depletion of storage iron without anemia; some investigators claim that work performance and subjective well-being are affected, while others dispute these findings.[129,136,137] Unfortunately, all proposed minimum hemoglobin levels are poorly predictive of body iron stores.[129,130] If the intent were to ensure that donors not become iron depleted, it would be necessary to perform a more direct test for measurement of iron metabolism, such as serum ferritin or zinc protoporyphin.[131,138] However, serum ferritin levels are not readily usable in the blood donor setting due to the complexities and expense of the assay whereas zinc protoporyphin has poor sensitivity for detecting iron deficiency in the absence of overt anemia.

The assessment of donor hemoglobin levels is further complicated by differences that result from the method of obtaining the sample.[129] Blood donor hemoglobin concentrations are routinely determined by capillary samples obtained from a finger pad or earlobe, usually by means of an automated lancet. Alternatively, venipuncture samples may be used. Most studies have shown that sampling by capillary methods give values that are higher than those obtained by venous sampling.[138,139] In addition, direct comparison studies show that samples obtained from earlobe punctures give higher hemoglobin values than fingerstick samples[139,140]; these findings are reflected by a higher hemoglobin deferral rate at blood centers using fingerstick rather than earstick sampling.[127,140]

The hemoglobin screening method employed by most blood centers is an indirect method using a copper sulfate solution at a particular specific gravity. A drop of the donor's blood is allowed to drop through the copper sulfate solution; if the drop of blood sinks to the bottom of the copper sulfate within the allowable time limit, it is concluded that the donor has met the minimum hemoglobin standard. Since it is well known that many donors with normal hemoglobin levels will have abnormal copper sulfate results, a failure to qualify on the copper sulfate test does not automatically lead to donor deferral.[2,130] For these donors, another drop of capillary donor blood is retested by a more quantitative method, either a spun microhematocrit or a cynamomethemoglobin methodology; if the sample is above a hematocrit of 38 percent or a hemoglobin of 12.5 g/dl, the donor is accepted for donation.[2]

Frequency of Donation

According to FDA regulations, an individual may not donate whole blood more frequently than every 56 days (8 weeks). However, it is possible for the medical director (or other designated physician) to accept a donor more frequently, provided that the physician makes the decision on a case by case basis, follows procedures in the CFR and provides adequate documentation on the donor record.

The rationale for the limit on frequency of donation is to prevent donors from being made iron deficient due to excessive phlebotomy. While this requirement appears to protect males from becoming iron deficient, data show that many premenopausal women will become iron deficient if they donate at this frequency[129,138]; hence, many authorities have recommended either a reduced donation frequency for women (i.e., two to three times per year) or the ingestion of oral iron supplements.[127,129,138]

CONCLUSION

Optimal donor screening procedures represent a balance between maximizing safety for both recipient and donor and minimizing the unnecessary deferral of safe blood donors. Given the importance of recipient safety, decisions about donor screening policies tend to favor the use of less specific procedures, in an effort to enhance transfusion safety. In some cases, such enhancement can be demonstrated; in other cases, it is inferred from indirect evidence; and in still other cases, data may be completely lacking. Donor screening policies can be evaluated scientifically providing that the inherent limitations of the methodology used in this type of operational research are recognized. Additional attention to quality assurance of donor screening procedures is warranted due to the difficult logistical situations that exist in some blood collection settings.

REFERENCES

1. Widmann FK (ed): Standards for Blood Banks and Transfusion Services. 15th Ed. American Association of Blood Banks, Bethesda, MD, 1993

2. Walker RH (ed): AABB Technical Manual. 11th Ed. American Association of Blood Banks, Bethesda, MD, 1993

3. Kleinman S: Donor screening procedures and their role in enhancing transfusion safety. p. 207. In Smith D, Dodd RY (eds): Transfusion-Transmitted Infections. American Society of Clinical Pathologists, Chicago, 1991

4. Kleinman S: Donor selection and screening procedures. p. 169. In Nance SJ (ed): Blood Safety, Current Challenges. American Association of Blood Banks, Bethesda, MD, 1992

5. Goldfinger D, Capon S, Czer L: Safety and efficacy of preoperative donation of blood for autologous use by patients with end-stage heart or lung disease who are awaiting organ transplantation. Transfusion 33: 336, 1993

6. US Department of Health and Human Services, Food and Drug Administration. The Code of Federal Regulations US Government Printing Office, Washington, DC, 1994

7. Grossman BJ, Kollins P, Lau PM et al: Screening blood donors for gastrointestinal illness: a strategy to eliminate carriers of Yersinia enterocolitica. Transfusion 31:500, 1991

8. Appleman MP, Shulman IA, Saxena S, Kirchhoff LV: Use of a questionnaire to identify potential blood donors at risk for infection with *Trypanosoma cruzi*. Transfusion 33:61, 1993

9. Kaplan HS, Kleinman SH: AIDS: Blood donor studies and screening methods. p. 297. In Barker LF, Dodd RY (eds): Infection, Immunity and Blood Transfusion. Alan R Liss, New York, 1985

10. US Department of Health and Human Services; Centers for Disease Control and Prevention: National HIV Serosurveillance Summary. Results through 1992. Vol. 3. US Public Health Service, Washington, DC, 1993

11. Mayo DJ, Rose AM, Matchett SE et al: Screening potential blood donors at risk for human immunodeficiency virus. Transfusion 31:466, 1991

12. Kleinman S, Secord K: Risk of human immunodeficiency virus (HIV) transmission by anti-HIV negative blood: estimates using the lookback methodology. Transfusion 28:499, 1988

13. Petersen LR, Doll LS: Human immunodeficiency virus type 1-infected blood donors: epidemiologic, laboratory and donation characteristics. Transfusion 31:698, 1991

14. Schafer IA, Mosley JW: A study of viral hepatitis in a penal institution. Ann Intern Med 149:1162, 1958

15. Krugman S, Friedman H, Latimer C: Hepatitis A and B: serologic survey of various population groups. Am J Med Sci 275:249, 1978

16. American Association of Blood Banks, American Red Cross, Council of Community Blood Centers: Joint statement on acquired immune deficiency syndrome related to transfusion. January 13, 1983

17. Barker LF: International forum: which criteria must be fulfilled for a donation or a donor to be considered voluntary? Vox Sang 34:363, 1978

18. Morris JP: International forum: which criteria must be fulfilled for a donation or a donor to be considered voluntary? Vox Sang 34:369, 1978

19. Beal RW, van Aken VG: Gift or good? Vox Sang 63: 1, 1992

20. Cherubin CE, Prince AM: Serum hepatitis specific antigen (SH) in commercial and volunteer sources of blood. Transfusion 11:25, 1971

21. Szmuness W, Prince AM, Brotman B, Hirsch RL: Hepatitis B antigen and antibody in blood donors: an epidemiolgic study. J Infect Dis 127:17, 1973

22. Allen JG, Dawson D. Saymor WA et al: Blood transfusion and serum hepatitis: use of monochloroacetate as an antibacterial agent in plasma. Ann Surg 150: 455, 1959

23. Alter HJ, Holland PV, Purcell RH et al: Post transfusion hepatitis after exclusion of commercial and hepatitis B antigen positive donors. Ann Intern Med 77: 691, 1972

24. Surgenor DM, Cerveny JF: A study of the conversion from paid to altruistic blood donors in New Mexico. Transfusion 18:54, 1978

25. Canavaggio M, Leckie G, Allain JP et al: The prevalence of antibody to HTLV-I/II in United States

plasma donors and in United States and French hemophiliacs. Transfusion 30:780, 1990

26. Dawson GJ, Lesniewski RR, Stewart JL et al: Detection of antibodies to hepatitis C virus in U.S. blood donors. J Clin Microbiol 29:551, 1991

27. Mosley JW, Galambos JT: Viral hepatitis. p. 500. In Schiff L (ed): Diseases of the liver. JB Lippincott, Philadelphia, 1975

28. Kahn RA: Donor screening to prevent posttransfusion hepatitis. p. 99. In Keating LJ, Silvergleid AJ (eds): Hepatitis. American Association of Blood Banks, Washington, DC, 1981

29. Taswell HA: Directed, paid and self donors. p. 137. In Clark GM (ed): Competition in Blood Services. American Association of Blood Banks, Arlington, VA, 1987

30. Strauss RG, Ludwig GA, Smith MV et al: Concurrent comparison of the safety of paid cytapheresis and volunteer whole-blood donors. Transfusion 34:116, 1994

31. Huestis DW, Taswell HF: Donors and dollars, editorial. Transfusion 34:96, 1994

32. Petersen LR, Doll LS, White CR et al: Heterosexually acquired human immunodeficiency virus infection and the United States blood supply: considerations for screening of potential blood donors. Transfusion 33:552, 1993

33. Operskalski EA, Schiff ER, Kleinman SH et al: Epidemiologic background of blood donors with antibody to human T-cell lymphotropic virus. Transfusion 29:746, 1989

34. Lee HH, Swanson P, Rosenblatt JD et al: Relative prevalence and risk factors of HTLV-I and HTLV-II infection in US blood donors. Lancet 337:1435, 1991

35. Kolho EK, Krusius T: Risk factors for hepatitis C virus antibody positivity in blood donors in a low-risk country. Vox Sang 63:192, 1992

36. Doll LS, Petersen LR, White CR et al: Human immunodeficiency virus type 1-infected blood donors: behavioral characteristics and reasons for donation. Transfusion 31:704, 1991

37. Leitman SF, Klein HG, Melpolder JJ et al: Clinical implications of positive tests for antibodies to human immunodeficiency virus type 1 in asymptomatic blood donors. N Engl J Med 321:917, 1989

38. Williams A, Kleinman S, Lamberson H et al: Assessment of the demographic and motivational characteristics of HIV seropositive blood donors. Paper presented at the Third International Conference on AIDS, Washington, DC, June 1987

39. Mayo DJ: Evaluating donor recruitment strategies. Transfusion 32:797, 1992

40. Read EJ, Herron RM, Hughes DM: Effect of nonmonetary incentives on safety of blood donations. Transfusion, suppl. 33:45S, 1993

41. Piliavin JA: Why do they give the gift of life?: a review of research on blood donors since 1977. Transfusion 30:444, 1990

42. Murray C: Evaluation of on-site cholesterol testing as a donor recruitment tool. Transfusion, suppl. 28:56S, 1988

43. Rzasa M, Gilcher R: Cholesterol testing: incentive or health benefit? Transfusion, suppl. 28:56S, 1988

44. Kleinman SH, Shapiro A: The agreement to donate blood: Presenting information to blood donors and obtaining consent. p. 29. In Smith DM, Carlson KB (eds): Current Scientific/Ethical Dilemmas in Blood Banking. American Association of Blood Banks, Arlington, VA, 1987

45. Director of Recruitment Development, National Marrow Donor Program: Policy regarding donor incentives at time of recruitment. Memorandum to donor center and recruitment group coordinators and donor center medical directors. November 22, 1993

46. Council of Europe: Guide to the preparation use and quality assurance of blood components. p. 12. Strasbourg, Council of Europe Press, 1992

47. Mason JO: Alternative sites for screening blood for antibodies to AIDS virus. N Engl J Med 313:1157, 1985

48. Forstein M, Page PL Coburn TJ: Alternative sites for screening blood for antibodies to AIDS virus. N Engl J Med 313:1158, 1985

49. Snyder AJ, Vergeront JM: Safeguarding the blood supply by providing opportunities for anonymous HIV testing. N Engl J Med 319:374, 1988

50. Dodd RY: Donor screening for HIV in the United States. p. 143. In Madhok R, Forbes CD, Evatt BL (eds): Blood, Blood Products and AIDS. Chapman & Hall, London, 1987

51. Director, Office of Biologics Research and Review, Food and Drug Administration: Recommendations to decrease the risk of transmitting acquired immune deficiency syndrome (AIDS) from blood donors. Memorandum to all establishments collecting human blood for transfusion. March 24, 1983

52. Seage GR III, Barry MA, Landers S et al: Patterns of blood donations among individuals at risk for AIDS, 1984. Am J Public Health 78:576, 1988

53. Pindyk J, Waldman A, Zang E et al: Measures to decrease the risk of acquired immunodeficiency syndrome transmission by blood transfusion. Transfusion 25:3, 1985

54. Perkins HA, Samson S, Busch MP: How well has self-exclusion worked? Transfusion 28:601, 1988

55. Busch MP, Young MJ, Samson SM et al: Risk of human immunodeficiency virus transmission by blood transfusions prior to the implementation of HIV antibody screening in the San Francisco Bay Area. Transfusion 31:4, 1991

56. Kolins J, Silvergleid AJ: Creating a uniform donor medical history questionnaire. Transfusion 31:349, 1991

57. Piliavan JA: Temporary deferral and donor return. Transfusion 27:199, 1987

58. Sayers MH: Duties to donors. Transfusion 32:465, 1992

59. Maclennan S, Barbara JA, Hewitt et al: Screening blood donations for HCV. Lancet 339:131, 1992

60. Popovsky MA, McCarthy S, Schwab A, Dempessey-Hart D: Privacy of donor screening: perception vs. reality. Transfusion, suppl. 31:67S, 1991

61. Locke SE, Kowaloff HB, Hoff RG et al: Computer-based interview for screening blood donors for risk of HIV transmission. JAMA 268:1301, 1992

62. CCBC Newsletter: Interactive Computerized Donor Screening Study Results Insufficient to Recommend Adoption by Blood Centers, FDA Panel Concludes. p. 2. October 1, 1993

63. American Association of Blood Banks: Statement and recommendations of the American Association of Blood Banks regarding donor history questions. Memorandum to institutional members. July 29, 1989

64. Recommendations for the prevention of human immunodeficiency virus (HIV) transmission by blood and blood products. Center for Biologics Evaluation and Research, Washington, DC, rev April 1992

65. Mosley JW: Who should be our blood donors? Transfusion 31:684, 1991

66. Sherwood WC: Donor deferral registries. Transfus Med Rev 121, 1993

67. Grossman BJ, Springer KM: Blood donor deferral registries: highlights of a conference. Transfusion 32:868, 1992

68. Samson SA, Edmiston RK, Busch MP, Perkins HA: How well has donor call-back worked? Transfusion, suppl. 33:35S, 1993

69. Department of Health and Human Services, Food and Drug Administration: Additional recommendations for reducing further the number of units of blood and plasma donated for transfusion or for further manufacture by persons at increased risk of HTLV-III/LAV infection. October 30, 1986

70. Ciavetta J, Nusbacher J, Wall A: Donor self-exclusion patterns and human immunodeficiency virus antibody test results over a twelve month period. Transfusion 29:81, 1989

71. Loiacono BR, Carter GR, Carter CS et al: Efficacy of various methods of confidential unit exclusion in identifying potentially infectious blood donations. Transfusion 29:823, 1989

72. Busch MP, Perkins HA, Holland PV et al: Questionable efficacy of confidential unit exclusion, letter. Transfusion 30:668, 1990

73. Petersen LR, Busch MP: Confidential unit exclusion: how should it be evaluated? Transfusion 31:870, 1991

74. Kean CA, Hsueh Y, Querin JJ et al: A study of confidential unit exclusion. Transfusion 30:707, 1990

75. Wolles S, Galel S: Value of confidential unit exclusion. Transfusion, suppl. 33:80S, 1993

76. Kessler D, Valinsky JE, Bianco C: Sensitivity and Specificity of confidential unit exclusion (CUE)—Does it work? Transfusion, suppl. 33:35S, 1993

77. Menitove JE, Lewandowski C, Ashworth LW et al: Confidential unit exclusion process continues to identify donors with an increased frequency of HIV seropositivity. Transfusion, suppl. 31:69S, 1991

78. Kleinman S, Crawley P: An assessment of HIV related donor screening procedures. Transfusion, suppl 28:42S, 1988

79. Petersen LR, Lackritz E, Lewis WF et al: The effectiveness of the confidential unit exclusion system. Transfusion 34:865, 1994

80. Korelitz JJ, Williams Ae, Busch MP et al: Demographic characteristics and prevalence of serologic markers among donors who use the confidential unit exclusion process: The Retrovirus Epidemiology Donor Study. Transfusion 34:870, 1994

81. Nusbacher J, Chiavetta J, Naiman R, et al: Evaluation of a confidential method of excluding blood donors exposed to human immunodeficiency virus: studies on hepatitis and cytomegalovirus markers. Transfusion 27:207, 1987

82. Silvergleid AJ, Leparc GF, Schmidt PJ: Impact of explicit questions about high-risk activities on donor attitudes and donor referral patterns-results in two community blood centers. Transfusion 29:362, 1989

83. Gimble JG, Friedman LI: Effects of oral donor questioning about high-risk behaviors for human immunodeficiency virus infection. Transfusion 32:446, 1992

84. American Association of Blood Banks: Statement and recommendations of the American Association of Blood Banks regarding donor history questions.

Memorandum to institutional members. July 29, 1989

85. Schorr JB, Berkowitz a, Cumming PD, et al: Prevalence of HTLV-III antibody in American blood donors. N Engl J Med, 313:384, 1985

86. Director, Office of Biologics Research and Review, Food and Drug Administration. Revised definition of high risk groups with respect to acquired immunodeficiency syndrome (AIDS) transmission from blood and plasma donors. Memorandum to all registered blood establishments. September 3, 1985

87. Sheppard HW, Dondero D, Arnon J, Winkelstein W Jr: An evaluation of the polymerase chain reaction in HIV-1 seronegative men. J AIDS, 4:819, 1991

88. Eble BE, Busch MP, Khayam-Bashi H et al: Resolution of infection status of HIV-seroindeterminate and high-risk seronegative individuals using PCR and virus-culture: Absence of persistent silent HIV-1 infection in a high-prevalence area. Transfusion 32: 503, 1992

89. Jackson JB: Human immunodeficiency virus (HIV) indeterminate western blots and latent HIV infection. Transfusion 32:497, 1992

90. Brookmeyer R: Reconstruction and future trends of the AIDS epidemic in the United States. Science 253: 37, 1991

91. O'Brien RT, George JR, Holberg SD: Human immunodeficiency virus type 2 infection in the United States: epidemiology, diagnosis, and public health implications. JAMA 267:2775, 1992

92. Friedland GH, Saltzman BR, Rogers MF et al: Lack of transmission of HTLV-III/LAV infection to household contacts of patients with AIDS or AIDS related complex with oral candidiasis. N Engl J Med 314: 344, 1986

93. American Association of Blood Banks: Association Bulletin #93-4: Statement and recommendations of the American Association of Blood banks \regarding management of hearsay information about blood donors. Memorandum to institutional members. December 2, 1993

94. Director, Center for Biologics Evaluation and Research, Food and Drug Administration: Revised recommendations for testing whole blood, blood components, source plasma and source leukocytes for antibody to hepatitis C virus encoded Antigen (anti-HCV). Memorandum to all registered blood establishments. April 23, 1992

95. Alter HJ, Purcell RH, Shih JW, et al: Detection of antibody to hepatitis C virus in prospective followed transfusion recipients with acute and chronic non-A, non-B hepatitis. N Engl J Med 321:1494, 1989

96. Director, Center for Biologics Evaluation and Research, Food and Drug Administration: donor suitability related to laboratoty testing for viral hepatitis and a history of viral hepatitis. Memorandum to all registered blood establishments. December 22, 1993

97. Director, Center for Biologics Evaluation and Research, Food and Drug Administration: Exemptions to permit persons with a history of viral hepatitis before the age of eleven years to serve as donors of whole blood and plasma: alternative procedures, 21 CFR 640. 120 Memorandum to all registered establishments. April 23, 1992

98. Trepo c: International forum: should donors with a history of jaundice still be rejected? Vox Sang 41:110, 1981

99. Sheretz RJ, Russell BA, Reuman PD: Transmission of hepatitis A by transfusion of blood products. Arch Intern Med 144:1579, 1984

100. Alter HJ: Discussion: transfusion associated hepatitis. In Polesky HF, Walker RH (eds). Safety in Transfusion Practices. p. 32. College of American Pathologists, Skokie, IL, 1980

101. Polesky HF, Hanson M: Tests for viral hepatitis markers in blood donors. p. 17. In Polesky HF, Walker RH (eds): Safety in Transfusion practices. College of American Pathologists, Skokie, IL, 1980

102. Aach RD: International forum: should donors with a history of jaundice still be rejected? Vox Sang 41:110, 1981

103. Perillo RP, Gelb L, Campbell C et al: Hepatitis B antigen, DNA polymerase activity, and infection of household contacts with hepatitis B virus. Gastroenterology 76:1319, 1979

104. Alter MJ: The detection, transmission, and outcome of hepatitis C virus infection. Infect Agents Dis 2:155, 1993

105. Seeff, LB, Alter HJ: Spousal transmission of the hepatitis C virus? Ann Intern Med 120:807, 1994

106. Director, Center for Biologics Evaluation and Research, Food and Drug Administration: Recommendations for deferral of donors for malaria risk. Memorandum to all registered blood establishments. July 26, 1994

107. Holland PV: Why a new standard to prevent Creutzfeldt-Jakob disease? Transfusion 28:293, 1988

108. Prusiner SB: Prions and neurodegenerative diseases. N Engl J Med 317:1571, 1987

109. Rapaport EB: Iatrogenic Creutzfeldt-Jakob disease. Neurology, 37:1520, 1987

110. Gibbs CJ Jr, Joy A, Heffner R et al: Clinical and pathologic features and laboratory confirmation of Creutzfeldt-Jakob disease in a recipient of pituitary

derived human growth hormone. N Engl J Med 313: 734, 1985

111. NIDDK Fact Sheet: Human growth hormone and Creutzfeldt-Jakob disease. NIH Publication No. 86-2793. National Institutes of Health, Washington DC, December 1987

112. Director, Office of Biologics Research and Review, Food and Drug Administration: Deferral of donors who have received human pituitary derived growth hormone. Memorandum to all registered blood establishments. November 25, 1987

113. Acting Director, Office of Blood Research and Review, Center for Biologics Evaluation and Research, Food and Drug Administration: Deferral of blood and plasma donors based on medications. Memorandum to all registered blood establishments. July 28, 1993

114. Goldman M, Blajchman MA: Blood product-associated bacterial sepsis. Transfus Med Rev 5:73, 1991

115. Blajchman MA, Ali AM: Bacteria in the blood supply: an overlooked issue in transfusion medicine. p. 213. In Nance SJ (ed); Blood Safety: Current Challenges. American Association of Blood Banks, Bethesda, MD, 1992

116. Anderson KC, Lew MA, Gorgone BC et al: Transfusion-related sepsis after prolonged platelet storage. Am J Med 81:405, 1986

117. Ness PM, Perkins HA. Transient bacteremia after dental procedures and other minor manipulations. Transfusion 20:82, 1980

118. Richards C, Kolins J, Trindade CD: Autologous transfusion-transmitted Yersinia enterocolitica. JAMA 268:1541, 1992

119. Tomasulo PA, Anderson AJ, Paluso MB et al: A study of criteria for blood donor deferral. Transfusion, 20: 511, 1980

120. Pindyck J, Avorn J, Kuriyan M et al: Blood donation by the elderly. JAMA 257:1186, 1987

121. Simon TL, Rhyne RL, Wayne SJ, Garry PJ: Characteristics of elderly blood donors. Transfusion 31:693, 1991

122. Pisciotto P, Sataro P, Blumberg N: Incidence of adverse reactions in blood donors taking antihypertensive medications. Transfusion 22:530, 1982

123. Kleinman S, Neth CR, Thompson PR: Safety of blood donation by donors taking beta blocking agent for hypertension. Transfusion 23:433, 1983

124. McVay PA, Andrews A, Kaplan EB et al: Donation reactions among autologous donors. Transfusion 30: 249, 1990

125. Schmidt PJ: Blood donation by the healthy elderly. Transfusion 31:681, 1991

126. van der Linder GJ, Siegenbeek van Heukelmon LH, Meinardi H: Blood donation, a risk for epileptic patients? Vox Sang 51:148, 1986

127. Keating LJ: Should donor hemoglobin standards be lowered? Con. Transfusion 29:259, 1989

128. Baker WF Jr, Bick RL: Iron deficiency anemia. In Bick RL (ed): Hematology Clinical and Laboratory Practice. CV Mosby, St. Louis, 1993

129. Garratty G: Should donor hemoglobin standards be lowered?: Pro. Transfusion 29:261, 1989

130. Lloyd H, Collins A, Walker W et al: Volunteer blood donors who fail the copper sulfate screening test. What does failure mean, and what should be done? Transfusion 28:46, 1988

131. Morse, EE, Cable R, Pisciotto P et al: Evaluation of iron status in women identified by copper sulfate screening as ineligible to donate blood. Transfusion 27:238, 1987

132. Ali AM, McAvoy AT, Ali MAM et al: An approach to determine objectively minimum hemoglobin standards for blood donors. Transfusion 25:286, 1985

133. Ali AM, Goldsmith CH, McAvoy AT et al: A prospective study evaluating the lowering of hemoglobin standards for blood donors. Transfusion 29:268, 1989

134. Pi DW, Krikler SH, Sparling TG, et al: Reappraisal of optimal hemoglobin standards for female blood donors in Canada. Transfusion 34:7, 1994

135. Raftos J, Schuller M, Lovric VA: Iron stores assessed in blood donors by hematofluorometry. Transfusion 23:226, 1983

136. Dallman PR: Manifestations of iron deficiency. Semin Hematol 19:19, 1982

137. Rector WG, Fortunin NJ, Conley CL: Non-hematologic effects of chronic iron deficiency. A study of patients with polycythemia vera treated solely with venesection. Medicine (Baltimore) 62:382, 1982

138. Gordeuk VR, Brittenham GM, Bravo J et al: Prevention of iron deficiency with carbonyl iron in female blood donors. Transfusion 30:239, 1990

139. Avoy DR, Canuel ML, Otton BM, Mileski EB: Hemoglobin screening in prospective blood donors. Transfusion 17:261, 1977

140. Coburn TJ, Miller WV, Parrill WD: Unacceptable variability of hemoglobin estimation on samples obtained from ear punctures. Transfusion 17:265, 1977

Autologous and Designated Donor Programs

Arthur J. Silvergleid

In response to increasing public and professional awareness of and concern about the potential infectious disease complications of allogeneic blood transfusion, interest in alternative transfusion programs of all forms mushroomed in the early 1980s. By 1986, predeposit autologous transfusion programs were available at most hospital-based or community blood banks, and intraoperative and trauma blood salvage programs, thanks to emerging technology, were equally widely adopted. Autologous transfusion programs, always in the shadow of the more traditional allogeneic blood banking, had clearly moved to center stage. It is the purpose of this chapter to review the predominant form of autologous transfusion, preoperative autologous donation (PAD) and to provide details of the essential components of a successful and safe program. In addition, another consequence of public fear of acquired immunodeficiency syndrome (AIDS), directed (or designated) donation programs, is reviewed.

AUTOLOGOUS TRANSFUSION

Autologous transfusion may be used as a general term to describe any procedure whereby previously donated or shed blood is transfused—or reinfused—into the donor/patient. Most commonly, this involves donation, in vitro storage, and subsequent transfusion of the previously donated units. Other forms of autologous transfusion include preoperative hemodilution (the withdrawal of 1 or 2 units of blood immediately preoperatively, with volume replacement by crystalloid solutions and subsequent reinfusion of the units initially removed) and blood salvage (the recovery of blood that is shed perioperatively with return of the blood to the same patient). (For a discussion of hemodilution and blood salvage, see Ch. 24.)

Preoperative Donation

The most widely available form of the autologous option is the preoperative collection, storage, and retransfusion of donated blood. First described by Grant[1] in 1921, PAD (also called predeposit) was basically ignored until the publication of the extensive experience of Milles et al.[2] Newman et al.,[3] and others in the 1960s revived interest in such programs. During the 1970s, PAD programs gradually increased in popularity and availability; a survey taken in 1981 by the American Association of Blood Banks (AABB) indicated that, between 1974 and 1981, the number of AABB member institutions offering PAD programs increased fourfold.[4] Since the recognition of the AIDS epidemic in 1981, the rise in interest in autologous transfusion programs of all forms, particularly PAD programs, has been extraordinary. Programs already in existence before 1981 have experienced anywhere from a 2- to 10-fold increase in participation; the number of blood centers and hospitals that make such programs available has vastly increased.

According to the 1990 AABB survey, approximately 6 percent of all blood collected by AABB member institutions in 1989 was intended for autologous use.[5] Similar data were reported in 1993 by Northfield Laboratories, Inc. Their survey of blood collection activity by 184 community blood centers showed that autologous collections increased 23 percent per year from 1988 through 1992, at which time they represented 5.7 percent of total collections.[6] Wallace et al.[7] also reported a marked increase in autologous donations (a 65 percent increase between 1987 and 1989) but commented that only 54 percent of units were transfused into the patients who preoperatively deposited them.

Benefits of Predeposit Programs

Benefits accrue both to the donor/patient who participates in a PAD program and to the institution or community that provides the service. For the donor/patient, the most obvious benefit is freedom from concern about the infectivity of the blood and thus its safety; autologous blood represents the safest possible blood for transfusion. Complications of transfusion, such as disease transmission; hemolytic, febrile, or allergic transfusion reactions; alloimmunization to erythrocyte, leukocyte, platelet, or protein antigens; and graft-versus-host disease are eliminated by transfusing autologous blood, provided the donor is not bacteremic at the time of donation and/or there are no clerical errors resulting in the inadvertent transfusion of the wrong unit of blood.[8–10] Also, erythropoiesis may be stimulated by repeated phlebotomies, thus enabling the patient to regenerate hemoglobin at an accelerated rate postoperatively.

The hospital or community blood bank that provides a PAD program also derives benefits from the provision of this service. The most tangible benefit is the generation of additional blood from a group of individuals who would not normally be a part of the donor pool. An intangible benefit to the center or hospital is the goodwill that attends the provision of this medically indicated and much desired program.

Drawbacks/Limitations

PAD programs are not without some drawbacks. Among the most important is the fact that donor/patients require substantially more time and attention than do regular donors. Not only are autologous donors often less healthy than volunteer donors, but they are also highly likely to be first-time donors. Thus, in addition to the increased clerical time required to process an autologous donor through donor registration, there is an increased requirement for professional time to explain the procedure, draw the unit, and treat a greater number of donor reactions. Units that require special handling (additional labels, separate storage, or early delivery) are more expensive to collect, and, in addition, they must be maintained in a patient-specific inventory at the transfusing institution. Furthermore, units that are not needed by the donor/patient are generally not transfused to other patients but, instead, are wasted. All of these factors contribute to the higher cost of autologous units of blood compared with that of allogeneic units. The impact of this higher cost is compounded by the fact that current reimbursement programs (including Medicare) either deny the medical necessity of PAD programs or ignore the well-documented increase in costs.[11]

In the event that surgery is postponed or canceled, some units will be lost through outdating or have to be frozen at increased expense, with some loss of red cells. Finally, there is the potential, as with any transfusion, for clerical error, resulting in the donor/patient receiving allogeneic blood rather than the predeposited autologous units.[10]

Indications

Before 1981, PAD programs were targeted at specific patient groups, including those undergoing orthopaedic or plastic surgery or those with past or potential transfusion-related problems. Examples of the latter are patients with multiple antibodies, an antibody to a high-frequency antigen, or a history of severe transfusion reactions. In the late 1980s, when concern about the safety of the blood supply was at its peak, and in response to statutes in several states (e.g., the Gann Act[12] in California). Many patients contemplating an elective surgical procedure during which the necessity for a blood transfusion was even a remote possibility opted to participate in a PAD program. As a result, the actual utilization of predonated units by autologous donor/patients declined from 85 to 90 percent in 1980 (author's experience) to between 40 and 58 percent, according to a number of studies published 10 years later.[5,13] This decline in utilization is attributable in part to what many experts consider to be overutilization of the autologous option in situations in which the likelihood of sufficient blood loss to justify a transfusion was minimal.

As a general guideline, patients who are in relatively good health, who can tolerate iron replenishment, and who are contemplating a surgical procedure during which the likelihood of blood loss in excess of 500 to 1,000 ml is equal to or greater than 5 to 10 percent are good candidates for PAD programs. Others have suggested that autologous donation is indicated for any patient scheduled for elective surgery for whom crossmatched blood is recommended by the local hospital maximal surgical blood order schedule.[14,15]

The number of units to predeposit depends on the anticipated blood loss, an amount which varies, even for the same procedure, among surgical teams in different hospitals. Therefore, the number of units to be drawn for a given procedure cannot be generalized but instead must be determined by the hospital and, even more specifically, by the surgical team. Recently, Axelrod et al.[16] suggested a method for making this calculation, which was labeled "SOP-CAB," the acronym for "schedule of optimal preoperative collection of autologous blood." With their method—individualizing it for each surgical team and/or hospital—one could approximate the number of autologous units to draw to prevent the need for allogeneic blood in any given percentage (e.g., 90 to 95 percent) of patients. This is a sensible way to approach this complex, highly emotionally charged situation. Unfortunately, satisfying the transfusion needs of a large percentage of patients results in a high percentage of wasted units (see section on Cost-Effectiveness of Preoperative Autologous Donation). On the other hand, given the still incompletely allayed concerns about blood safety, it will not be an easy task to convince either patients or surgeons to eschew the autologous option in those situations in which the likelihood of requiring a transfusion is remote at best. That is one of the challenges of the 1990s.

Community Blood Bank versus Hospital-Based Programs

PAD programs are offered by both community blood centers[17] and hospital-based blood banks.[18] Initial concerns about the ability of a blood center geared toward batched processing to provide individualized treatment to autologous donor units were allayed during the 1980s. Given the increased participation by patients and donors in autologous and directed donor programs, community blood banks quickly became experienced with blood products that require special handling.

Hospital-based predeposit programs have one slight advantage over community blood center programs, that is, hospital-based programs can provide predeposit services to some higher-risk donor/patients who might not be encouraged to donate at the community blood center.[19] Patients in this category include pregnant women, elderly or debilitated patients, or those with moderate to severe coronary artery disease. Although such patients have been shown in several studies to be at low risk from the autologous donation, it is nevertheless reassuring both for the patient and for hospital donor room personnel to know that any emergency medical problem can be managed by utilizing the full resources of the hospital.

Hospital-based programs also differ from community blood bank-based programs in that predeposited blood that does not leave the collecting facility need not undergo complete infectious disease screening (see below), which helps control costs to some degree. Obviously, this option is not available to a community blood center because the Food and Drug Administration (FDA) requires that all units of blood be tested for a variety of infectious disease markers except those that are drawn and transfused at the same site. Even this policy is under review, and the option of not testing locally drawn autologous units may be rescinded.

PROGRAM SPECIFICS
Physician Request

All participants in PAD programs enter into the program at the request of their physician, usually the surgeon or anesthesiologist who will perform the surgery. Physicians certify that they are familiar with or have examined the patient and believe that the phlebotomy will pose no undue risks. Occasionally, surgeons refer the patient to a family practitioner, internist, or cardiologist for such certification. The final decision as to the acceptability of the donor/patient ultimately rests with the blood bank medical director; however, release by the attending physician is an important component of the decision process.

Iron Supplementation

An important aspect of patient management for patients participating in PAD programs is iron replacement. Several early studies indicated that enhanced erythropoiesis could effectively be achieved after two to three weekly phlebotomies, provided that the patient was receiving an iron supplement.[20] The recommended dose of iron is 300 mg of ferrous sulfate, orally three times daily, if tolerated. Patients should begin oral iron supplements as soon as surgery is scheduled, preferably days to weeks before the first phlebotomy, and should continue them until hospitalization. This recommendation is valid even though more recent studies do not demonstrate increased levels of erythropoietin or erythropoiesis, unless the phlebotomy schedule is significantly more intense than that in current common practice.[21,22]

Scheduling

The most practical schedule for obtaining more than 1 unit of autologous blood is to draw units at weekly intervals, with the last unit withdrawn preferably 1 week, although no fewer than 72 hours, before surgery. This 72-hour interval is based on a conservative estimate of the time required for a healthy individual to compensate for the acute volume and protein deficit caused by 1 unit phlebotomy. Given allowable shelf lives of 35 days (CPDA-1) or 42 days (AS-1 or AS-3), weekly phlebotomies enable the patient to donate up to 5 or 6 units of blood on such a schedule. If more units are expected to be needed for surgery, as many units as are needed may be obtained on a weekly schedule; those units that will need to be stored beyond the storage limit for liquid-stored blood will need to be stored frozen.

In unusual circumstances, individuals can tolerate a more intense donation schedule (e.g., every 3 or 4 days), although this is rarely necessary. On the other hand, for individuals unable to tolerate frequent phlebotomies and for whom surgery may safely be delayed for up to 6 months, a schedule of monthly phlebotomies may be practical. For these individuals, the predonated blood would have to be stored frozen and thawed and deglycerolized before transfusion. More details about frozen autologous blood can be found later in this chapter.

Informed Consent

Autologous donors, just as volunteer donors, must sign an informed consent form as a prerequisite to donating blood. If the donor/patient is a minor, a parent or guardian must give consent. The consent form should outline as completely as possible the advantages, nature, and purposes of autologous transfusion; the risks involved; and the possibility of complications. In the event that autologous blood is processed completely and is therefore potentially available for transfusion to others, specific permission for release of unused autologous blood should be obtained from the donor/patient. In addition, it is advisable to have patients sign an authorization for the release of laboratory test results to their physician if it is indicated.

Donor Criteria

Autologous donors need not meet all the criteria established to protect allogeneic recipients or donors. However, if blood from an autologous donor would not be acceptable for transfusion to an allogeneic recipient, either by virtue of the medical history or an abnormal laboratory test result, that unit must be labeled "for autologous use only." On the other hand, if the autologous donor would not normally be allowed to donate because of concern for the donor's well-being (e.g., a donor with coronary artery disease) but the blood, once collected, would be acceptable for transfusion to an allogeneic recipient, such a unit need not necessarily be restricted to autologous use.

Certain factors that are strictly defined for allogeneic donors, including age, weight, and hemoglobin level, are evaluated with greater flexibility for the autologous donor. Donor/patients ranging in age from childhood through their eighties and nineties have participated in PAD programs. For example, in 1987, we reported our experience with 180 pre-teenage and teenage donor/patients who participated in a community blood bank-based autologous transfusion program. We documented the safety and effectiveness of such a program in these youthful donors.[23] Others have also reported favorable experiences with autologous blood transfusion in a pediatric population.[24] Similarly, strict weight requirements, instituted primarily to protect the donor while allowing for the withdrawal of enough blood to provide for a therapeutic dose of red blood cells to a recipient, may be waived for the autologous donor. Underweight donors should have proportionately smaller units withdrawn, generally limiting the amount donated to less than 12 percent of the estimated blood volume. To determine the correct amount to draw from an underweight donor/patient, a relatively simple calculation (e.g., amount to draw/ 450 ml = donor weight/110 lb) may be made. Once the volume of blood to be drawn is determined, a second calculation (volume to draw/450 ml = amount of anticoagulant/63 ml) can be used to determine the appropriate amount of anticoagulant to leave in the primary container. A multiple satellite bag configuration allows one to remove excess anticoagulant without sacrificing the integrity of the closed collecting system and preserves the sterile storage interval.

Minimal criteria for hemoglobin level (110 g/L and/or hematocrit 33 percent) for the autologous donor have been defined.[25] These values are fairly liberal, and as a result it is unusual for a presumably healthy donor to be unable to complete a donation program consisting of three or fewer donations. Occasionally, the second or third donation may have

to be delayed, although even this is relatively rare. Table 11-1 enumerates mean hematocrit levels at the first, second, third, and subsequent donations for patients in each of three age categories: teenage, middle-age adults (45 to 65 years old), and elderly adults (older than age 65).

One situation in which lower than normal hemoglobin levels in an autologous donor may have an impact is in the circumstance in which autologous blood is completely processed and, if appropriate, made available for allogeneic use if not required by the donor/patient. Although red blood cell units prepared from blood with low hemoglobin/hematocrit values are acceptable when returned to an autologous donor/patient, such units do not constitute an adequate dose for an allogeneic recipient. An acceptable guideline in this circumstance is to consider the lowest acceptable levels for an allogeneic donor, a hematocrit of 38 percent or a hemoglobin level of 125 g/L, to be the cutoff below which units should be labeled "for autologous use only."

Thus, many patients who do not meet all of the standards of a normal blood donor may participate in an autologous blood donation program.[19,23] However, logic dictates that there are patients for whom the risk of donation is greater than the risk of allogeneic blood transfusion. The criteria for determining appropriate candidates for autologous donations vary greatly from one blood bank to another. It is difficult to define precise standards, especially because the incidence rates of post-transfusion hepatitis and AIDS are only estimates and the data concerning the risk of donation in high-risk patients are not extensive.

If we acknowledge the relative paucity of data,

Table 11-1. Mean Hematocrit at Each Donation

Age Category	Sex	Number of Donations				
		1	2	3	4	5
Teenage	Male	44 (53)[a]	41 (45)	38 (22)	37 (7)	36 (1)
	Female	41 (141)	37 (114)	36 (43)	38 (6)	37 (1)
Middle-age	Male	44 (34)	42 (28)	39 (13)		
	Female	41 (66)	38 (44)	37 (7)		
Elderly	Male	43 (47)	41 (36)	42 (5)		
	Female	42 (50)	38 (40)	37 (11)		

[a] The number in parenthesis indicates the number of donors in that sample. Hematocrits have been rounded to the nearest whole number.

there have been several studies that provide some reassurance regarding the ability of even higher risk autologous donors to tolerate the donation process. These studies involve both normal and higher risk autologous donors in either the hospital or nonhospital setting. Both Mann et al.[19] and Owings et al.[26] evaluated high-risk autologous donations made in a hospital setting and concluded that the process was safe. Similarly, AuBuchon and Popovsky[27] reviewed the records of 5,660 out-of-hospital autologous donations, in 886 (16 percent) of which the donor did not meet the usual medical criteria for an allogeneic donation.[27] Donation by persons not meeting routine criteria was followed by a higher reaction rate than that by donors without any variance (4.3 percent versus 2.7 percent), although most reactions were minor and tended to occur most often in individuals who were younger than age 17, were female, weighed less than 110 pounds, or had experienced a reaction at the time of a prior donation. More than 99 percent of donors with a history of cardiovascular disease did not experience a reaction.

Data somewhat in conflict with the above was obtained by Spiess et al.[28] who performed hemodynamic monitoring (blood pressure, heart rate, cardiac output, lead II electrocardiogram, and pulse oximetry) during preoperative blood donations by 123 high-risk patients. This study's special monitoring detected a significant number of adverse hemodynamic changes that might not have been recognized by conventional observations of donors' symptoms or other subjective responses. Among the observed findings were systolic and diastolic hypotension, orthostatic hypotension, tachycardia, arrhythmias, and ST-T wave changes. This report suggests that, although clinically apparent reactions may not appear to be of a magnitude to be problematic, there is evidence that hemodynamically compromised patients may be at enhanced risk from the donation process. These findings are particularly pertinent in light of the data by Birkmeyer et al.[29], which indicate that even a small fatality risk (1 per 101,000 donations) negates all health benefits associated with blood donation by patients awaiting coronary artery bypass graft surgery.

Based on the above, special consideration should be given before medical clearance for donation to patients with atherosclerotic cardiovascular disease,

those with congestive heart failure of any cause, or those who are receiving medications that would inhibit compensatory cardiovascular responses such as β-blocking agents, nitrates, and so forth. Examples of patients who should be excluded from donating on the basis of these considerations are as follows: patients with unstable angina or angina at rest, those who have had a myocardial infarction within the last 3 months, those in congestive heart failure, those with aortic stenosis, those with significant ventricular arrhythmias, those with transient ischemic attacks, and those with marked hypertension.

Other patients who should be excluded from donating are those with infections, if there is any potential for a bacteremia. Intermittent seeding of a donor's blood with a few organisms is possible, as has been documented in patients with indwelling vascular lines and Foley catheters, and can occur after dental extractions, sigmoidoscopy, and barium enema. Although most bacteria do not proliferate in the cold, some psychrophilic organisms, *Yersinia enterocolitica*, for example, may reach peak concentrations in blood within 1 or 2 weeks of storage at 4°C and have been associated with fatal reactions when infused after prolonged (≥ 3 weeks) storage at 4°C.[30] Gross contamination of blood may not be visible to the naked eye, and the organisms may not show up by direct Gram staining or wet hanging drop methods.[31]

Abbreviated Medical History

Collection facilities that practice crossover of autologous units acceptable for allogeneic transfusion must perforce subject autologous donor/patients to the same medical history questions asked of allogeneic donors. On the other hand, if crossover is not practiced, it makes sense to streamline the medical history, tailoring it to prevent complications from the donation process with additional consideration for possible bacterial contamination. The logic for streamlining is compelling, that is, it should help make the process more cost-effective and it makes little sense to ask embarrassing questions about a donor/patient's sexual activities when the answers will have no impact on the disposition of the collected unit.

Several alternative streamlined questionnaires have been published;[32] however, as yet, there is no agreed on uniform streamlined questionnaire. In our center, autologous donor/patients are simply asked the following four questions:

Do you have an infection, cold, or flu today?

List all medications you are taking.

Have you ever had hepatitis, lung or kidney disease, or other chronic illness?

Have you ever had a heart condition, heart attack, heart surgery, or stroke?

Information gleaned from the donor/patient's responses is used to ask follow-up questions or to make a decision about eligibility. Given the value of streamlining the medical history for PAD programs that do not practice crossover, it is anticipated that some attention will shortly be directed towards developing uniformity in this important aspect of the PAD process.

CONTROVERSIAL AREAS

In this next section, several aspects of the provision of PAD services for which no consensus has been reached are addressed. These include extent of testing (of autologous units), release of potentially infectious units to the donor/patient, participation by patients known to be infectious for hepatitis or AIDS, crossover, the role of erythropoietin, and cost-effectiveness.

Extent of Testing

An important question of policy that must be addressed by anyone establishing a PAD program is the extent of testing to which autologous units will be subjected. In this regard, there are two opposing viewpoints, each of which is briefly considered here.

Minimal Testing

One approach for handling predeposited autologous blood (available only if the blood will not leave the facility in which it is collected) is subjecting the blood to minimal or no testing. Such blood is simply ABO and Rh grouped, labeled with the name of the donor/patient, and provided for transfusion as whole blood (generally) or red blood cells (occasionally). There are several advantages to this approach. The

first and most obvious is a reduction in processing costs. Considering that donor units intended for allogeneic transfusion must, in addition to ABO and Rh grouping, be tested for syphilis, antibody to human immunodeficiency virus (HIV) types 1 and 2 (anti-HIV-1 and anti-HIV-2), antibody to hepatitis C virus (anti-HCV), antibody to human T-cell lymphotropic virus type I (anti-HTLV-I), hepatitis B surface antigen (HB_sAg), antibody to hepatitis B core antigen (anti-HB_c), and alanine aminotransferase (ALT) and also screened for unexpected red cell antibodies, there are substantial savings to be realized by avoiding such testing. In addition, hospital transfusion services wishing to develop an autologous transfusion program can avoid the necessity for obtaining a separate donor center licensure provided that they do not process allogeneic donor units, make autologous units available for allogeneic transfusion, or transfer units to another facility.

In contrast, when autologous blood will be transfused outside the collecting facility, the first unit from a given donor during a 30-day period must, according to the FDA[33] and the AABB,[25] be subjected to infectious disease testing, including a syphilis screen, anti-HIV-1 and 2, HB_sAg, anti-HCV, and anti-HB_c. As in the above situation, such incompletely tested blood cannot be made available for allogeneic use if it is not required by the donor/patient.

An administrative benefit of minimal processing is the fact that bookkeeping and recordkeeping are simplified. Because the blood is unavailable for transfusion to anyone other than the autologous donor/patient, there is little concern about tracking the unit to determine its ultimate disposition; units not transfused to a donor/patient are simply discarded by the hospital transfusion service.

A very important but perhaps somewhat controversial benefit of minimal processing is the fact that, by not processing the unit fully, one can avoid the awkward and sometimes confusing problems created by testing and the subsequent finding of abnormal laboratory test results. Considering the number of tests routinely performed on donated blood and the increasing number of participants in PAD programs, one can confidently predict that between 1 in 10 and 1 in 20 autologous donor/patients will have at least one abnormal laboratory test result. Abnormal laboratory test results create problems in several ways. How do you confirm the abnormal result? If the result is a positive by enzyme-linked immunosorbent assay for anti-HIV, is there time to confirm this by a more specific test, such as the Western blot or indirect fluorescent antibody technique? How do you protect the donor/patient's confidentiality while discharging your ethical responsibility to inform the patient's physician and health care workers that the blood might be infectious? Are the patient's physicians and health care workers capable of interpreting the test results properly? Should potentially infectious blood (e.g., HB_sAg positive, anti-HIV positive, or anti-HCV positive) be allowed into the system in view of the even remote possibility that an error might result in that unit being transfused to someone other than the autologous donor/patient (see below)? And then, lastly, how and what do you tell the donor/patient who is already concerned about the upcoming surgery?

Complete Testing

As cogent as the arguments may be in favor of minimal testing, equally compelling arguments are advanced by those convinced that autologous units should be processed to the same degree as units intended for allogeneic transfusion. One straightforward argument is that it is cleaner administratively to process all donated units in the same manner. Particularly in a large institution, it is wise, if possible, to avoid exceptions to standard operating procedure; if only certain units are handled in other than the routine manner, the possibility for error increases.

Furthermore, if donated blood is not tested for all infectious disease markers and it is to be shipped from one institution to another, it should be transported as if it were infectious. The transportation of infectious units of blood, or partially untested units, should be done in consideration of the fact that such units constitute a potential biohazard. The shipping of all partially untested units of blood under biohazard conditions constitutes a significant administrative burden.

A third argument in favor of complete testing of autologous blood is that it allows for the possibility of crossover, including crossover of components not set aside for the donor/patient. Given the fact that

approximately 50 percent of autologous blood is not utilized by the donor/patient, one could imagine that hundreds of thousands of units of such blood would annually be made available by way of crossover. However, in the early 1990s, crossover as a practice in the United States was virtually eliminated (see below) for all practical purposes, eliminating crossover as a justification for performing complete infectious disease testing on autologous blood.

The major point in favor of complete processing is that it enables the collecting facility to make appropriate decisions about the disposition of potentially infectious units. As alluded to earlier, some collecting facilities choose to discard units testing positive for anti-HIV, HB_sAg, and anti-HCV rather than allow them into the system because the potential always exists for a clerical error, resulting in transfusion of the unit to a person other than the donor/patient.[8–10] Other facilities, although they may allow such units to be released for transfusion to the autologous donor/patient only, prefer to be able to alert their processing staff and the transfusion team about the abnormal test result. Whereas it can be argued that all blood units should be handled as though they were infectious, it is also true, human nature being what it is, that extra diligence can be achieved when information is available that indicates that a particular unit of blood has a greater potential for infectivity.

Release of Infectious Units

A second controversial issue in the management of a PAD program is the disposition of units that test positive for an infectious disease marker. Because there are no firm guidelines from the AABB or FDA regarding this issue, practice varies considerably from institution to institution. Although some institutions release all units back to the donor/patient regardless of the infectious disease test results, others do not release units that test positive for anti-HIV-1 or 2, HB_sAg, or anti-HCV. Even among those centers reluctant to release infectious units, anti-HB_c, anti-HTLV-I or II, an elevated ALT level, or a positive serologic test for syphilis are generally considered less significant and do not by themselves affect the decision to release. It should be noted that both FDA and AABB require a written statement from the receiving transfusion service and the attending physician that anti-HIV-1-positive, anti-

HIV-2 repeatedly reactive, or HB_sAg confirmed reactive units are acceptable in order for such units to be shipped from the collecting to the transfusing facility.

The rationale for a liberal release policy is to protect donor/patients from the adverse consequences of allogeneic blood exposure, regardless of their own infectious disease status. In partial support of this approach, it has been reported that allogeneic mononuclear cells may have a deleterious effect on HIV-infected patients.[34]

On the other hand, the rationale for not releasing potentially infectious units is to protect health care workers and prevent transmission of an infectious disease to another patient should the known infectious unit be inadvertently transfused to the wrong patient. Regardless of how tight the control, errors in release and in transfusion are not completely preventable. In response to a 1992 College of American Pathologists' survey (J-C), 34 of 3,886 (0.9 percent) of laboratories admitted issuing an autologous unit of whole blood or red blood cells for the wrong patient; on 20 occasions, the unit was actually transfused into the wrong patient![35] Also, Linden[10] reported further instances of autologous blood errors and incidents, including two instances in which patients received the blood of another patient. Such data, few as there are, support the position (endorsed by the author) of not releasing potentially infectious units.

Adopting the nonrelease position creates its own set of logistic dilemmas. The most troublesome of which is how to handle units (donor/patients) with a repeat reactive infectious disease test. Can the decision to release or discard be made on the basis of the screening test alone? Should confirmatory testing always be done? Is there time before surgery to obtain confirmatory testing? Should additional units be drawn before obtaining confirmatory testing? There are no simple answers to these questions. Although some indication of the likelihood that a screening test result is a true positive may be gleaned from the sample to cutoff ratio, this is far from absolute.

Participation by Known Infectious Donors

This controversial area is a corollary of and flows naturally from the preceding one. Just as there is disagreement on how to handle infectious units, there is an identical lack of consensus as to whether or not to allow the known infectious donor (anti-HIV-1 or 2, HB_sAg, or anti-HCV positive) to participate in PAD programs.

Mintz[36] presented thoughtful arguments regarding civil rights issues, the Americans With Disabilities Act, and safety issues (the special hazards of allogeneic blood in HIV-positive patients[34] and concluded that patients infected with HIV must be permitted to provide and receive autologous blood.

On the other hand, Petz and Kleinman[37] disagreed based on a review of the relative risks of a policy of allowing HIV-infected persons to participate in autologous blood programs compared with the risks engendered by excluding such persons as autologous donors. If an HIV-positive patient is not allowed to donate autologous blood, the major risk to that patient is HCV transmission by allogeneic transfusion.[38] Such transmission occurs about once in 5,000 units (see Ch. 38), although only about 10 percent of patients have microscopic evidence of cirrhosis develop, thus resulting in a possibility of symptomatic liver disease after transfusion of 1 in 50,000 units.

In contrast, if known HIV-positive units are accepted into the inventory for autologous transfusion but one is inadvertently transfused to the wrong person, there is a 90 percent probability that the recipient will become infected with HIV and thus have a fatal disease. Because the probability of transfusing the wrong unit has been estimated to be about 1 in 12,000,[9] the risk of severe morbidity and death as a result of receiving an HIV-positive unit into the inventory is greater than the risk of symptomatic disease caused by transfusion of allogeneic blood. They therefore concluded that a greater good was served by excluding known HIV-infected patients from participation in autologous blood programs. This issue is distinctly different from the question of allowing untested units to be used in an autologous program. If untested autologous units are transfused, the risk of HIV transmission from a transfusion error is about 1/120,000,000 since it is the product of the independent risk of transfusion to the wrong person (about 1/12,000) and the rate of HIV seroprevalence in autologous units (about 1/10,000).[39] However, when patients known to be seropositive for HIV are allowed to donate, the HIV seroprevalence of these units is 100 percent and the risk of HIV transmission in this case is 12,000 × 1, or 1/12,000.

Such a conclusion does not necessarily apply to patients who have positive tests for other infectious diseases, and a decision analysis approach should be used to develop a policy regarding each infectious disease marker.[40] We believe that it is preferable to exclude patients from autologous blood programs if their test results for anti-HIV or HB$_s$Ag are confirmed positive.

Crossover

Autologous blood that is drawn from a donor/patient who meets all criteria for the collection of allogeneic blood (including medical history screening and laboratory testing) may be crossed over into the allogeneic blood supply. Although there are many arguments to support crossover, including increasing the total available blood supply, possibly reducing the overall cost of autologous blood programs, and avoiding the waste of a valuable resource, crossover had—for all practical purposes—become virtually obsolete by the early 1990s. Whereas 65 percent of autologous programs practiced crossover in 1987, only 2 percent of autologous blood collected in 1989 to 1990 was made so available.[5,41] The primary reasons for the lack of enthusiasm for crossover are concerns about the safety of autologous blood and concerns about logistic barriers to accurate administration of a program flexible enough to encompass crossover.

In terms of safety, legitimate concerns have been raised regarding the donors/patients' understanding of the nature of their illnesses, such that an accurate medical history could be obtained and appropriate decisions regarding crossover made. In addition, unresolved questions persist about donor motivation and therefore whether autologous blood is comparably safe as true volunteer blood. Finally, much has been written regarding the relative safety of autologous blood, as determined by the frequency of viral markers in autologous blood donors. Unfortunately, little agreement exists regarding approaches to statistical analysis, such as whether to compare donors or donations, what constitutes comparable populations, or even whether the frequency of viral markers is an adequate measure of safety in a viral marker-negative cohort of donors.[42–44]

Safety issues aside, there are substantial logistic barriers to crossover. Among them are the reluc-

tance of many surgeons to release autologous blood until so late in its dating period that it is difficult to guarantee its use for another patient; the necessity to make a separate determination for each unit donated as to its eligibility for crossover; and, finally, the geometric increase in the complexity of record-keeping and billing for a relatively small return in terms of the number of units added to the system.

For these reasons, crossover is not a viable solution to the problem of decreasing the expense of autologous or PAD programs. Indeed, Kruskall et al.[32] suggested that resources could actually be saved if what little crossover is done were eliminated. The author agrees with this statement and believes that the more appropriate response to the increase in wastage that has accompanied the increase in participation is to educate physicians and patients better concerning appropriate donation policies to minimize overcollection as much as possible.

Role of Erythropoietin

One of the more exciting scientific advances in the past decade was the isolation, purification, and, ultimately, genetic engineering of clinically useful quantities of recombinant human erythropoietin (r-huEPO). Much important work has been done to evaluate and define the parameters for use of r-huEPO and a great number of studies have focused on its value in the perioperative setting, both as an adjunct and as an alternative to preoperative autologous donation. Although a complete analysis of the emerging data is not within the scope of this chapter, several conclusions can be drawn and suggestions for further analysis offered. Published studies have indicated the following. First, r-huEPO given preoperatively to iron-replete donors does result in increased red blood cell production and collection potential. Unfortunately, no clinical benefit accrued to the erythropoietin-treated donors, as their exposure to allogeneic blood was no different from that of nontreated donors.[45] Second, aggressive blood collection by itself could substitute for exogenous erythropoietin therapy in nonanemic blood donors.[46] Third, iron availability was rate limiting in the response to exogenous r-huEPO (even when total body iron stores were adequate).[47] Fourth, the effective dose range for r-huEPO was 12,000 to 18,000 units/week given subcutaneously.[48] Fifth, donor/patients most likely to be unable to complete a prescribed preoperative donation schedule—and therefore most likely to benefit from exogenous r-huEPO—were anemic individuals, those with small blood volumes, and those with low body iron stores.[49] Sixth, r-huEPO was able to decrease allogeneic blood exposure in patients who were anemic at the time of their first donation.[50] Seventh, r-huEPO was able to reduce allogeneic blood transfusion needs in some patients to whom it was given as an alternative to transfusion.[51–53] Eighth, much as in routine autologous programs, substantial wastage of autologous blood was documented.[49,54,55] In analyzing the data, one conclusion seems clear, that is, that r-huEPO will play a more restricted role in perioperative blood conservation than initially predicted. Its routine use in autologous donors would appear to be unjustified. Rather, its use should be restricted (1) to serving as an adjunct to PAD in anemic patients and in those with small blood volumes who are unable to donate enough blood to meet their anticipated needs and (2) to correct anemia preoperatively in selected patients (i.e., those who, for religious reasons, refuse transfusions). Further studies, including careful analysis of cost-effectiveness, should be done to establish the usefulness of r-huEPO as an alternative to transfusion (autologous or allogeneic) in selected patients. Finally, given the excessive wastage of autologous blood, considerable thought should be given to a patient's likelihood to require blood before subjecting them either to r-huEPO or routine PAD.

Cost-Effectiveness of Preoperative Autologous Donation

In the early 1990s, a variety of factors, among them the increasing safety of allogeneic blood, the tremendous waste of unused autologous blood, and public concern over the rising costs of health care, stimulated some workers to analyze the cost-effectiveness of autologous blood protocols relative to other prophylactic and therapeutic interventions. With the use of models based on decision trees representing all the possible transfusion-related outcomes in cohorts of autologous blood donors and nondonors undergoing a variety of surgical procedures and calculation of the ratio of cost per quality-adjusted life expectancy increase in years (QALY), they were able

to demonstrate that phenomenal costs were associated with modest returns for most patients participating in PAD programs. In one study of the cost-effectiveness of PAD in orthopaedic procedures, the cost for a QALY gained varied (depending on the procedure, the institution, and the amount of blood routinely transfused for that procedure) between $40,000 and $1,467,000.[56] In that same study, the estimated average benefit of PAD was less than 0.2 days of quality-adjusted life expectancy increase per patient.

In another study by the same authors, this time in patients undergoing coronary artery bypass graft surgery, the average cost of PAD was $508,000 to $909,000 per QALY saved, depending on the number of units donated.[29] Moreover, although the authors conceded that the actual risk of PAD is uncertain, even a small fatality risk (greater than 1 in 101,000 units) associated with blood donation by patients awaiting coronary artery bypass grafts would negate all life expectancy benefits of PAD.

Etchason et al.[57] calculated the incremental cost-effectiveness of substituting autologous for allogeneic blood in two procedures with high probabilities of requiring transfusion (total hip replacement and coronary artery bypass graft surgery) and two with low transfusion probabilities (abdominal hysterectomy and transurethral resection of the prostate). Even with rather conservative estimates of the transmission rates of infectious diseases by transfusion of allogeneic blood, the substitution of autologous for allogeneic blood resulted in little expected health benefit, that is, 0.0002 to 0.00044 QALY (1.8 to 3.8 hours) saved per unit. The variation in effectiveness is a function of the differences in the life expectancies of the average patient (related to average age) undergoing each procedure. Cost-effectiveness ratios (cost per QALY saved) ranged from $235,000 to more than $23 million (Table 11-2). These cost estimates do not compare favorably with most other accepted medical interventions.

These investigators also analyzed the impact of strategies suggested to reduce costs such as reduction in testing,[32] crossing over of unused units, and using collection schedules to provide for an optimal number of donated units.[16] No strategy was able to lower the ratio to less than $87,000/QALY saved, with most estimates being above $135,000/QALY

Table 11-2. Results of Baseline Analysis of Cost-Effectiveness of Autologous Blood Donation in Four Surgical Procedures

Procedure	Total Hip Replacement	Coronary Artery Bypass Grafting	Abdominal Hysterectomy	Transurethral Prostatectomy
Mean age of patient (yr)	62	67	49	68
% of donated units wasted	16	28	74	96
Incremental costs ($ per unit transfused)	68	107	594	4,783
Incremental effectiveness (QALY per unit transfused)	0.00029	0.00022	0.0044	0.00020
Cost-effectiveness ($ per QALY)	235,000	494,000	1,358,000	23,643,000

Abbreviation: QALY, quality-adjusted life-year.
(From Etchason et al.,[57] with permission.)

saved, even for procedures with a high probability of a need for transfusion.

The greater expense of autologous blood is primarily related to the fact that a significant number of units are wasted. Reducing wastage would seem a logical means to eliminate this expense, but efforts to do this are surprisingly limited in effectiveness even for procedures with a high probability of requiring transfusion because of the significant variation in transfusion requirements for a given surgical procedure. This is demonstrated in Figure 11-1, which illustrates the actual transfusion requirements in 115 patients who underwent hip replacement surgery. Although the median number of units trans-

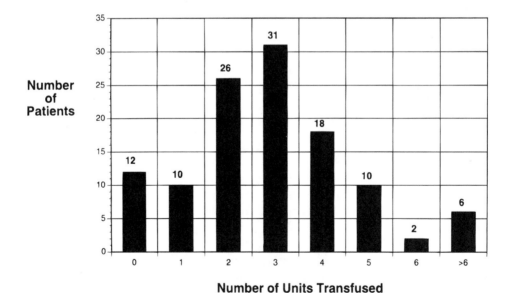

Fig. 11-1. The actual number of units of red blood cells transfused to 115 patients who underwent hip surgery. Note that, if all 115 patients had donated 3 units of autologous blood (345 units donated), 26 patients would each have wasted 1 unit (26 units), 10 patients would have wasted 2 units (20 units), and 12 patients would have wasted all 3 units (36 units), for a total of 82 wasted units. Thus, the wastage rate would be 82 of 345 or 24 percent. Accordingly, a high wastage rate of donated blood is inherent in preoperative autologous donation programs.

fused was 3, if each patient had donated 3 autologous units (a total of 345 units), 26 patients would have wasted 1 unit, 10 patients would have wasted 2 units each, and 12 patients would have wasted all 3, for a wastage rate of 24 percent (82 of 345). Goodnough and Marcus[58] also reported on the marked variability of transfusion needs for patients undergoing elective orthopaedic surgery. Accordingly, it seems unreasonable to expect that wastage rates can be reduced significantly below 20 percent unless there is undercollection or overtransfusion of autologous units.

For surgical procedures with a low probability of transfusion requirement, a high wastage rate is obviously unavoidable if such patients donate autologous blood. For example, if 50 percent of patients require blood for a given surgical procedure, the wastage rate will be 50 percent if all patients donate one unit.

Even with wastage rates as low as 15 percent, the cost-effectiveness of autologous blood donation is more than $100,000 per QALY saved for patients at age 15, and the cost-effectiveness ratios increase rapidly for older patients or when wastage rates are higher (Table 11-3). Using Table 11-3, one can calculate the cost-effectiveness of autologous blood donation in any circumstance if the patient's age and the expected wastage rate for a given procedure are known. For example, if a 20-year-old woman with an uncomplicated pregnancy donates 1 unit of autologous blood and the probability of requiring transfusion is 2 percent, the cost-effectiveness of autologous donation in that setting is $16,300,000 per QALY saved.

It appears that however one chooses to define the upper limit of cost-effective medical care ($30,000, $50,000, or $100,000), the cost of PAD almost always exceeds that number with room to spare. The primary reasons for this were described above, that is, the increasing safety of the allogeneic blood pool and the increased collection costs and wastage associated with autologous blood. Nevertheless, despite the high societal cost and minimal benefits of PAD, it is highly unlikely, given its intangible value to patients and its acceptance as a standard of care by physicians, that PAD will be abandoned on economic grounds. Individual patients, motivated by anxiety over what they perceive as the risks of allogeneic transfusions, may be willing to pay the added costs of autologous donation themselves. Alternatively, if patients are informed accurately about the risks of allogeneic transfusion and therefore the minimal benefit of autologous donation, especially when the expectation of transfusion need is not high, many may choose not to donate. Whether society will be willing to continue to expend scarce resources on autologous donation while more cost-effective practices are not universally available is yet to be answered. Although there is currently no consensus or absolute standard by which the effectiveness of a medical intervention can be judged to be worth its cost, carefully performed analyses of cost-effectiveness should be used as one important method to

Table 11-3. Cost-Effectiveness of Autologous Blood Donation Assuming Various Wastage Rates and Patient Ages

Age (yr)	Percent of Units Wasted				
	98	75	50	25	15
15	15,800,000[a]	1,020,000	371,000	156,000	105,000
20	16,300,000	1,050,000	382,000	161,000	109,000
30	17,700,000	1,130,000	414,000	174,000	118,000
40	20,000,000	1,280,000	468,000	197,000	133,000
50	24,100,000	1,540,000	564,000	237,000	160,000
60	31,600,000	2,030,000	741,000	312,000	211,000
70	46,600,000	2,990,000	1,090,000	459,000	310,000

[a] In dollars per quality-adjusted life-year.
(From Etchason et al.,[57] with permission.)

rank various health care practices for the expenditure of limited health care resources.

Much as in the other controversial issues surrounding PAD, there remains honest disagreement over the most appropriate ways to enhance the cost-effectiveness of PAD. Because the higher processing cost of autologous blood contributes heavily to its overall cost-ineffectiveness, some have argued that testing of autologous units should be eliminated;[32] others maintain that testing is important both from the standpoint of assuring uniformity in the handling of all donated units (and thereby reducing the risk of error) and to enable decisions to be made regarding the disposition of infectious units.[59] In addition, some have argued that crossover should be reinstituted on a wider scale to decrease wastage;[60] others contend that complete elimination of crossover would lead to cost savings by allowing for the streamlining of the medical history and the elimination of the need to perform infectious disease testing.[32]

About one issue, however, there is virtual uniformity, that is, the absolute necessity to decrease inappropriate utilization of PAD in circumstances in which the likelihood of a transfusion being required is remote at best. Transfusion medicine specialists need to educate their surgical colleagues, anesthesiologists, lawmakers, the media, health care insurers, and the general public regarding the diminishing risks of allogeneic blood and the great expense of autologous blood. The others, in turn, need to reassure anxious patients that the autologous option is not always the most appropriate one. Finally, unnecessary transfusion—either autologous or allogeneic—must be avoided at all times.

Frozen Autologous Blood

Freezing of red blood cell units, with an allowance for extended storage, has an important, albeit limited, role in traditional predeposit programs. One important application is for the donor who will need more units than can be collected during the period for liquid storage of blood. Another less common application is for donors who cannot tolerate frequent phlebotomies (see the previous section on Scheduling).

Another increasingly important application of red cell freezing technology is for the patient whose surgery is postponed beyond the normal expiration date of the predonated units. In these situations, where delay is unavoidable, it is becoming common practice to rejuvenate and freeze the short-dated units to prevent their outdating.

There are two reasons for individuals to predonate red blood cell units for frozen long-term storage in the absence of any immediate or defined need. One of these is eminently practical; the other is a subject of debate. For the individual who has a rare blood type, with compatible donors on the order of 1 in 100 or less, providing a repository of frozen autologous units may be lifesaving. For the individual predonating units to be frozen primarily out of concern for the safety of the community blood supply, the acknowledged benefits are less obvious. Arguments raised against widespread development of repositories of frozen autologous blood include tremendous cost; the possibility that, in an emergency, particularly if it occurs in a different geographic locale, the blood will not get to the donor/patient in a timely fashion; and concerns that, if enough individuals withdraw from the community blood donor pool to provide only for themselves, the community's blood supply will be severely curtailed. It is clear that the considerable cost involved in providing frozen autologous blood has limited interest in such programs.

Predeposit of Components

Although red blood cells represent the component prepared for most patients participating in PAD programs, other components, including fresh frozen plasma, cryoprecipitate (as a source of fibrinogen and/or fibrin sealant), platelets, fresh platelet-rich plasma, and bone marrow or peripheral blood stem cells, may also be harvested, stored, and transfused in the appropriate circumstance. Fresh frozen plasma is only rarely indicated, but it is simple to prepare either at the time of whole blood donation or by plasmapheresis if there is concern that large-volume transfusion will lead to coagulopathy. Similarly, cryoprecipitate may be prepared easily enough and is more and more often specifically requested as the key ingredient in fibrin sealant.[61] Platelets may be predeposited in two different clinical settings. In the first, which utilizes apheresis technology, a large number of autologous platelets with or without fresh plasma may be collected before or at the time of surgery, stored, and reinfused as needed. In the second setting, patients with acute leukemia or other malignancy in remission could also donate platelets by apheresis and have the platelets stored frozen for subsequent transfusion when the remission ends and the patient is made thrombocytopenic by additional chemotherapy.[62] Because many transfused patients will eventually have refractoriness to donor (including HLA-matched) platelets, their own platelets, harvested during remission, can be life sustaining.

With a combination of techniques, it has become possible to harvest large numbers of bone marrow or peripheral blood stem cells, and, if necessary, treat them to remove residual cancer or leukemia cells, store them frozen, and reinfuse them after treating the patient with extremely high tumor-ablative doses of chemotherapy or radiotherapy.[63,64] By harvesting bone marrow primarily from patients with malignancies that have not invaded the marrow or by treating the harvested marrow or peripheral blood to remove residual malignant cells, one could provide the patient with a life-preserving stem cell inoculum after delivering what would ordinarily be a fatally high dose of chemotherapy or radiotherapy.

Labeling and Serologic Testing of Predeposited Blood

Predeposited autologous blood must be labeled to reflect all testing that has been done. Blood that has not been processed completely should have that information indicated on the special autologous tag. In addition, such blood should bear the statement "for autologous use only—may not be issued to another patient" or some similar statement, either on the autologous tag or directly on the bag itself. Information required on the autologous transfusion tag includes the patient's name, a unique identifying number (e.g., the hospital registration or social security number), the ABO and Rh group, and the date of expiration of the unit. Units that have been completely processed and are acceptable for allogeneic transfusion if not required by the donor/patient can have the special tag removed (although the fact that the unit was donated for autologous use must remain clearly in evidence even though the donor/patient's identity is removed) and be placed in the general inventory after they have been released by the patient's physician; most hospitals attempt to obtain this release approximately 48 hours after uncomplicated surgery.

Pretransfusion compatibility testing can obviously be abbreviated for the autologous donor/patient. It is recommended, however, that an ABO, Rh, and antibody screen be performed on a patient specimen just as if the patient were to be provided with allogeneic blood. This practice is encouraged for the following two reasons: (1) it permits consistent application of standard procedures and (2) it alerts the transfusion service to any potential crossmatching problems should the patient subsequently need allogeneic blood. Also, the ABO group of the labeled autologous unit must be confirmed by the transfusion facility. Finally, although a crossmatch is optional, it is recommended that an immediate-spin crossmatch be performed before issuing the blood as a precaution against a clerical or labeling error.

Indications for Transfusion of Autologous Blood

Because autologous blood is safer than allogeneic blood, there is a tendency to use more liberal indications for transfusion in patients who have predeposited autologous units.[65–67] Indeed, some physicians transfuse autologous blood "regardless of the patient's postoperative hematocrit and clinical status."[65] Although there is general agreement on the relative safety of autologous blood, the potential for an adverse outcome to transfusion is not eliminated merely because patients will receive their own blood. Hemolysis secondary to inadequate handling,[68] sepsis resulting from bacterial contamination,[69] and transfusion of the wrong unit as a result of misidentification[10,35] are (fortunately rare) potential complications not avoided by the autologous transfusion. A less rare and important complication is pulmonary edema resulting from hypervolemia. These potential complications make it imperative that autologous blood be transfused wisely and only when specifically indicated. In certain situations, it may be reasonable to relax the transfusion "trigger" (e.g., by transfusing a postpartum patient with a hemoglobin ≤ 10 g/L rather than ≤ 8 g/L), but it is never reasonable to transfuse an autologous unit simply because it is available or would otherwise be discarded. Transfusing to replace iron lost in the donation process, to promote wound healing or general well-being, or to normalize the hemoglobin level is of arguable benefit and should generally be avoided. Preoperatively deposited blood provides good insurance for the patient from whom significant blood loss at surgery is a real possibility. Should the anticipated blood loss not occur, the preoperatively deposited blood becomes a risk, albeit slight, rather than a benefit and should be treated accordingly.

DESIGNATED DONOR PROGRAMS

Widespread interest in directed, designated, or recipient-specific donations is, with rare exceptions, a direct response to the concerns about blood safety raised by the acquired AIDS epidemic. Before 1983, recipient-specific donations occurred and were considered medically indicated in the following three clinical settings: (1) red cell transfusions from a prospective kidney donor to the prospective recipient, usually three transfusions of 200 ml each, at 2-week intervals;[70] (2) apheresis-harvested platelet concentrates from HLA-matched family members or nonrelated donors for the refractory, thrombocytopenic patient;[71] and (3) washed maternal platelets for thrombocytopenic infants with isoimmune neonatal thrombocytopenia.[72] For each of these clinical situations, there were solid data indicating the clinical benefits to be derived from using a designated donor.

Since the onset of the AIDS epidemic and particularly since it became clear that the disease could be transmitted by blood transfusion, concern on the part of prospective transfusion recipients led to a strong movement for more widespread adoption of designated donor programs. For whatever reasons, perhaps largely because of failure of blood banks to establish sufficient credibility to reassure them (perhaps an impossible task), more patients became convinced that they could select safer donors than could a blood center. In a survey taken for the AABB in January 1986, 81 percent of respondents believed that, if they needed blood, they would prefer to receive it from directed donors.[73] Even when cautioned that such an approach might lead to serious blood shortages, 36 percent still indicated that they would not accept random donor blood. The blood banking industry has been widely split on this issue.

Although the three major blood bank organizations, the AABB, American Red Cross, and the Council of Community Blood Centers, have officially discouraged the use of directed donations, virtually every blood collection agency in the United States now offers them. In addition, in several states, provision of directed donor services is mandated by legislation enacted primarily to protect the patient's right to be offered this transfusion option. In the next two sections, the arguments for and against directed donor programs are briefly discussed.

Arguments Against Directed Donations

The objections to directed donations can be summarized as follows. First, directed donations are, on average, no safer than random volunteer donations. Second, directed donors may be under excessive pressure to donate and may therefore be unwilling to disclose details of their medical history that would disqualify them from donating (i.e., directed donations may actually be less safe). Third, directed donors are most often first-time donors and, as a result, have a higher frequency of positive infectious disease screening tests results. Fourth, directed donor programs may foster the mistaken notion that there are two levels of blood safety, with directed blood acknowledged by the blood banking community to be safer. Fifth, handling of directed donor units places an administrative and logistic burden on the blood bank and hospital that increases expenses and may lead to handling errors. Sixth, legal hazards might be created, such as the loss of donor anonymity or the implied warranty to process and deliver a specified unit of blood for transfusion. Seventh, surgical schedules may be subject more to the vagaries of supply of directed units rather than to strict medical necessity. Eighth, concern arises that severe blood shortages might result if members of the volunteer donor pool withheld their donations to conserve them until they could be directed to a relative or friend.

Arguments for Directed Donations

The arguments raised against directed donations in 1983 have not changed; however, it is now possible to evaluate accumulated data to test the validity of some of those arguments.

Table 11-4. Seroprevalence of Infectious Disease Markers at Blood Centers, 1991–1992 (Rates per 100,000 Donations)

	First Time Donors		
	Directed (n = 30,778)	Community (n = 384,276)	P
Anti-HIV-1 or 2	13.0	31.0	NS
Anti-HTLV-I	78.0	33.6	<0.0001
STS	61.7	54.1	NS
HB$_s$Ag	363.9	182.9	<0.0001
Anti-HCV	661.1	588.6	NS

Abbreviations: HIV, human immunodeficiency virus; STS, serologic test for syphilis; HB$_s$Ag, hepatitis B surface antigen; HTLV, human T-cell lymphotropic virus; HCV, hepatitis C virus; NS, not significant.

1. A very large body of data has been collected concerning the safety of directed donations as part of the Retrovirus Epidemiology Donor Studies (REDS) (Kleinman SH: personal communication, May 23, 1995). The data were collected at five geographically and demographically diverse blood centers under the sponsorship of the National Heart, Lung, and Blood Institute of the National Institutes of Health. Seropositivity for various infectious disease markers was measured in 30,778 first-time directed donors and compared with 384,276 first-time (allogeneic) community donors (Table 11-4). Results of tests that are specific markers for infectious diseases indicated that there were no significant differences in the prevalence of positive test findings in directed donors compared with community donors for anti-HIV-1 or 2, the serologic test for syphilis, or anti-HCV, but there was a significantly higher prevalence of positive test results in directed donors for anti-HTLV-I (relative risk 2.32) and HB$_s$Ag (relative risk 1.99).
2. Directed donors, although they may be under pressure to donate, are also presumably concerned enough about the recipient as someone they know that they would avoid donating once apprised of the potential harm of their donation. Indeed, analysis of the REDS data indicated that essentially all differences between directed and community donors were explained by differences in the demographics of the two groups (age, sex, ethnic group, and so forth). Because none of the variation was explained on the basis of being a directed rather than a community donor, the authors concluded that their data did not provide evidence that directed donors give less reliable histories. (Kleinman SH: personal communication, May 23, 1995)
3. A comparison of the prevalence of positive test results for infectious disease markers in directed donors compared with those in the total community donor population has led to erroneous conclusions because directed donors are largely first-time donors, whereas community donors are frequently repeat donors. It is scientifically invalid to compare such dissimilar populations of donors and to conclude that a difference in prevalence of infectious disease markers can be interpreted to indicate a difference in safety between the two groups.
4. The blood banking community, through education and communication, is responsible for countering the idea that there are two levels of blood safety.
5. The logistics of providing a directed donor program, particularly for a community blood center, may seem overwhelming if unreasonable time-frame demands are coupled with the necessity to perform an ever-increasing number of blood processing tests. However, the logistics of providing directed donor units are comparable to those of providing predeposited autologous units, and the two programs can successfully be organized in a parallel fashion.
6. With regard to the legal concerns raised earlier, there are equally compelling reasons to believe that offering a directed donor program might relieve the blood bank of some legal issues, particularly in states where legislation mandating blood banks to accept and process directed donations has been passed. If a blood bank does not offer such a program, individuals who have acquired a transfusion-related infectious disease may be induced to institute litigation.
7. Although there have been numerous last-minute conferences held to discuss the availability or lack of availability of directed donor units, this author has yet to see a medically indicated procedure canceled for lack of such blood.

8. As has been stated above, directed donors are often (60 to 70 percent) first-time donors, a fact confirmed in numerous studies.[74] Thus, concerns that the donor pool would shrink have not been confirmed. In fact, advocates of directed donor programs are convinced that many new donors are coming to the blood bank to make a directed donation and hope that effective marketing of this service, combined with recruitment efforts to enlist these donors into the regular donating pool, will expand rather than contract the community's donor base.

9. Finally, offering a directed donor program provides a service actively sought and much appreciated by patients. Even while expressing concerns about the medical justification, the blood bank can reap rich dividends in patient and community goodwill by providing such a service.

TECHNICAL CONSIDERATIONS

Because directed donor programs are being offered throughout the United States, certain technical and logistic questions need to be addressed so that programs can be designed to provide optimal patient care with minimal inconvenience for the blood bank. These include physician involvement, informed consent/confidentiality, pretyping, donor eligibility criteria, special considerations for related donors, crossover, scheduling, and time constraints.

Physician Involvement

A very important aspect of a successful designated donor program is physician involvement. A physician's request should be required before the blood bank draws any designated donors for a patient, and the physician should be kept informed of the status of collected units, especially if some donated units are not acceptable for transfusion. Communication between the blood bank and the hospital physician staff, particularly regarding details of the directed donor program, may prevent such problems as unreasonable timeframe demands or requests to use unprocessed directed donor blood (an unacceptable practice) from developing.

Informed Consent/Confidentiality

Directed donors, like autologous donors, should sign a special consent and release form. The important elements to incorporate on this form include the donor's acknowledgment of the risks of blood donation; the donor's consent to release the blood into the general community supply if it is either not needed by or is incompatible with the intended recipient; and the donor's acknowledgment that it is not possible to guarantee with absolute certainty that the blood will in fact be given to the intended recipient, with, perhaps, as a list of the possible reasons why this might be so. In addition, the donor should be reminded that all results of processing tests are strictly confidential. This latter is occasionally a source of concern or contention when the blood bank does not release a directed unit for transfusion and information as to the reason is sought by the patient. In this situation, the blood bank is unfortunately placed in the awkward position of having to placate an irate patient or physician while protecting the donor's confidentiality. Nevertheless, because it is absolutely essential to protect the donor's confidentiality in this regard, it may be necessary to inform the intended recipient that not all units drawn may be released for transfusion, nor may it be possible in all cases for the blood bank to offer a complete explanation. As a further safeguard of donor confidentiality, it is recommended that the donor's name not appear on the designated donor tag; instead, a code can be used that is interpretable only by blood bank staff.

In addition to requiring designated donors to sign a consent and release form, it is also prudent to request similar consent from the intended recipient. In addition to including all of the elements of the form discussed above, many centers require that the recipient or a designated representative provide a list of acceptable donors before releasing any units (or even collecting them).

Pretyping

Should prospective designated donors be pretyped, ABO and Rh, for compatibility with the intended recipient? For the hospital-based donor facility, pretyping may be viewed as a generally compensated service to hospital patients. For the community blood center or a larger hospital-based donor facility, on the other hand, pretyping can create logistic problems. Among the problems created by pretyping are a lack of trained and/or credentialed staff to perform nonroutine blood testing; lack of information about the ABO and Rh groups of the intended recipient; and perhaps most important, a potential loss of donors and available units if incompatible designated donors decide not to donate.

Donor Eligibility Criteria

There are a number of issues related to designated donor participants and their selection, qualifications, and relationship to the intended recipient. Most fully developed directed donor programs accept all designated donors regardless of their relationship to the intended recipient. An exception to this is the virtual universal refusal to provide blood from a husband to his wife if she is in the childbearing stage of her life. In addition, although parent-to-child directed donations are generally accepted and even occasionally mandated, some concern has been expressed that such donations might allosensitize the recipient and prejudice a subsequent response to family blood products. Directed donors must meet all criteria established for protection of the recipient; this includes an acceptable medical history and normal infectious disease screening test results.

Rare exceptions to this policy may be medically justifiable. For example, if a patient is severely thrombocytopenic and is refractory to platelet transfusions as a result of alloimmunization, a sibling may be the optimal and, at times, the only feasible source of compatible platelets for this life-threatening situation.

Special Considerations for Related Donors

In 1989, attention was drawn to the fact that one of the potential adverse consequences of receiving blood from related donors was the development of often fatal graft-versus-host disease.[75–77] This was particularly likely if the donor was homozygous for an HLA haplotype shared with the recipient. Based on the initial reports of this syndrome, the AABB recommended that directed donor blood from first-degree relatives should be irradiated to abrogate the capacity of the transfused lymphocytes to initiate and produce clinically significant graft-versus-host disease. Subsequent reports provided additional data,[77–79] and irradiation is now required for all donor units known to be from a blood relative[25] rather than simply those donated by first-degree relatives.

The currently recommended dose is 25 Gy (2,500 rads) delivered to the center of the radiation field, with a minimum of 15 Gy (1,500 rads) to peripheral portions of the field. According to the FDA, red blood cell-containing units so irradiated must be transfused within the lesser of the original allowable dating period or 28 days from the time of irradiation (see Ch. 42).[80]

Crossover

Most collection facilities that provide directed donor services crossover unused directed donor blood into the general inventory. This can be accomplished because directed donors must meet all criteria for allogeneic transfusion. The REDS data provide good information on which to make an informed decision as to whether or not crossover is justified. This is an important question because Wallace et al.[7] reported that 55 percent of directed donor units are never transfused, indicating that a significant number of transfusion services do not crossover directed donor units.

As indicated in Table 11-4, the prevalence of positive test results for anti-HTLV-I and HB_sAg was higher in first-time directed donors compared with first-time community donors. The relative risk of a positive test result for HB_sAg was about 2, and the implication of this is that directed donors are twice as likely to transmit hepatitis B as are community donors. Because the probability of transmitting hepatitis B by blood donated by community donors has been estimated to be about 1 in 200,000 units,[81] the probability regarding directed donations would be 1 in 100,000 units. In other words, for each 200,000 units of community blood transfused, there would be one instance of hepatitis B transmission, whereas for each 200,000 units of directed donor blood transfused, there would be two instances of hepatitis B transmission. Thus, if one were to discard directed donor units because of concern regarding an increased risk of infectious disease transmission, one would need to discard 200,000 units to prevent one instance of hepatitis B transmission. If the cost of a unit of blood is $100.00, then the cost of preventing an instance of transmission of hepatitis B by discarding designated donor units rather than crossing them over would be $20,000,000. Therefore, discarding directed donor units does not seem justifiable.

Although the REDS data indicate that the prevalence of a positive test result for anti-HTLV-I was also higher in directed donors, this is not clinically important regarding the question of crossover because of the low prevalence of positive test findings and the low rate of development of disease in patients positive for anti-HTLV-I.

Scheduling

Compressed collection schedules, which are appropriate for the autologous donor, should not, with rare exceptions, be applicable to the designated donor. One exception might occur when a parent donates for an infant who requires chronic transfusion support. In this situation, in which small quantities of relatively fresh blood are required at stable intervals, it may be prudent to draw less than full units of blood at more frequent intervals than the current 8-week standard. Such an approach protects the donor from iron depletion and the recipient from exposure to multiple donors, and is therefore recommended. In fact, so compelling is the argument regarding decreasing patient exposure to blood from multiple donors, that eloquent pleas have been made to create a classification of donor that is a variation of a directed donor, a so-called "dedicated donor."[82] Dedicated donors are committed to providing repeated donations of specific components for a single recipient—thereby reducing or obviating the need for that patient to receive components from multiple donors. Goldfinger[83] and Brecher et al.[84] also pointed out the evident advantages in reducing the number of donors to whom a patient is exposed by allowing certain directed donors to donate whole blood more than once every 8 weeks. Although no allowances have been made in the Standards for Blood Banks and Transfusion Services[25] to enable dedicated donors to donate more frequently, persuasive arguments have been made that such allowances are in the best interests of the patients in need of, and fortunate to have, a dedicated donor.

Another exception to rigid adherence to donor scheduling might be for the designated donor who is providing apheresis-harvested platelets or granulocytes. Here again, because limiting the recipient's exposure to blood products is of significant benefit,

donors may be allowed to donate at more frequent intervals. A note of caution is worth mentioning with regard to directed apheresis donors, that is, considering the expense of the procedure, the importance of the component, and the time involved in harvesting it, it would be most unfortunate to have to discard an apheresis-harvested component because of an abnormal infectious disease screening test result, such as a positive HB_sAg, anti-HIV, or anti-HCV. It would also be unfortunate to have to cancel a planned procedure at the last minute when it was discovered that the donor had either an unacceptable medical history or inadequate veins. One way to avoid the aforementioned complications is to insist that all prospective directed apheresis donors who have not previously been blood donors come to the blood bank at least 24 hours before the planned procedure to allow blood center personnel to explain the procedure, evaluate the potential donor's medical history and veins, and draw a tube of blood for complete preprocessing. Although preprocessing is an additional expense because processing will have to be repeated on the day of actual donation, according to AABB Standards for Blood Banks and Transfusion Services,[25] it is far less costly in the long run than discarding an apheresis component critically needed by the patient.

Time Constraints

A final consideration for directed donor programs is the fact that time constraints must be established to provide a service without creating logistic problems for the blood bank or unrealistic expectations for the patient. Given the time required to process, label, and deliver 1 unit of blood to the hospital transfusion service, it is unrealistic to consider a directed donor program for urgent blood needs. Each blood bank must establish guidelines concerning how soon blood will be available after donation (e.g., 24 to 48 hours). Obviously, directed donor blood cannot be available for emergency transfusion. Although generally used for elective surgery, it is occasionally useful for medical patients when transfusion needs are predictable (e.g., in some patients with hematologic or oncologic conditions). It is important to limit the time during which directed units will be held for the intended recipient after surgery. Here, a limit of 1 week but no more than 2 weeks seems appropriate. By restricting this period, the blood bank can protect the community from experiencing a blood shortage resulting from a high percentage of reserved units. In the opinion of this author, those directed units not used by the intended recipient within 1 to 2 weeks after donation should be released into the general inventory unless there is a compelling reason not to do so.

REFERENCES

1. Grant FC: Autotransfusion. Ann Surg 74:253, 1921
2. Milles G, Langston HT, Dalessandro W: Autologous transfusion. p. 76. In The John Alexander Monograph Series. Charles C Thomas, Springfield, 1971
3. Newman MM, Hamstra R, Block M: Use of banked autologous blood in elective surgery. JAMA 218:861, 1971
4. Sandler SG: Overview. p. 1. In Sandler SG, Silvergleid AJ (eds): Autologous Transfusion. A Technical Workshop. American Association of Blood Banks, Bethesda, 1983
5. Devine P, Postoway L, Hoffstadter DM et al: Blood donation and transfusion practices: the 1990 American Association of Blood Banks institutional membership questionnaire. Transfusion 32:683, 1992
6. Forbes JM, Laurie ML: The Northfield Blood Collection Report: Community Blood Center Collections, 1988–1992. Northfield Laboratories, Inc, Evanston, 1993
7. Wallace EL, Surgenor DM, Hao HS et al: Collection and transfusion of blood and blood components in the United States, 1989. Transfusion 33:139, 1993
8. Sazama K: Reports of 355 transfusion-associated deaths: 1976 through 19185. Transfusion 30:583, 1990
9. Linden JV, Paul B, Dressler KP: A report of 104 transfusion errors in New York State. Transfusion 32:601, 1992
10. Linden JV: Autologous blood errors and incidents. Transfusion, suppl. 34:28S, 1994
11. Yomtovian R, Kruskall MS, Barber JP: Autologous-blood transfusion: the reimbursement dilemma. J Bone Joint Surg 74A:1265, 1992
12. California State Bill 37(SB-37): The Paul Gann Memorial Blood Act. Effective date 1/1/90
13. Goodnough LT, Saha P, Hirschler NV, Yomtovian R: Autologous blood donation in nonorthopaedic surgical procedures as a blood conservation strategy. Vox Sang 63:96, 1992
14. Kruskall MS, Glazer EE, Leonard SS et al: Utilization and effectiveness of a hospital autologous preoperative blood donor program. Transfusion 26:335, 1986
15. Toy PTCY, McVay PA, Strauss RG et al: Transfusion 32:562, 1992
16. Axelrod FB, Pepkowitz SH, Goldfinger D: Establishment of a schedule of optimal preoperative collection of autologous blood. Transfusion 29:677, 1989
17. Silvergleid AJ: Autologous transfusions: experience in a community blood center. JAMA 241:2724, 1979
18. Kruskall MS: Establishment of an autologous transfusion program in a transfusion service. p. 57. In Sandler SG, Silvergleid AJ (eds): Autologous Transfusion. A Technical Workshop. American Association of Blood Banks, Bethesda, 1983
19. Mann M, Sacks HJ, Goldfinger D: Safety of autologous blood donation prior to elective surgery for a variety of potentially "high-risk" patients. Transfusion 23:229, 1983
20. Zuck TF: Donor response to predeposit autologous transfusion phlebotomy. p. 51. In Dawson RB (ed): Autologous Transfusion. A Technical Workshop. American Association of Blood Banks, Bethesda, 1976
21. Kickler TS, Spivak JL: Effect of repeated whole blood donations on serum immunoreactive erythropoietin levels in autologous donors. JAMA 260:65, 1988
22. Biesma DH, Draaijenhagen RJ, Poortman J et al: The effect of oral iron supplementation on erythropoiesis in autologous blood donors. Transfusion 32:162, 1992
23. Silvergleid AJ: Safety and effectiveness of predeposit autologous transfusions in preteen and adolescent children. JAMA 257:3403, 1987
24. Novak RW: Autologous blood transfusion in a pediatric population. Clin Pediatr 27:184, 1988
25. Klein HG (ed): Standards for Blood Banks and Transfusion Services. 16 Ed. American Association of Blood Banks, Bethesda, 1994
26. Owings DV, Kruskall MS, Thurer RL, Donovan LM: Autologous blood donations prior to elective cardiac surgery: safety and effect on subsequent blood use. JAMA 262:1963, 1989
27. AuBuchon JP, Popovsky MA: The safety of preoperative autologous blood donation in the nonhospital setting. Transfusion 31:513, 1991
28. Spiess BD, Sassetti R, McCarthy RF et al: Autologous blood donation: hemodynamics in a high-risk patient population. Transfusion 32:17, 1992
29. Birkmeyer JD, AuBuchon JP, Littenberg B et al: Cost-effectiveness of preoperative autologous donation in coronary artery bypass grafting. Ann Thorac Surg 57:161, 1994
30. Stenhouse MAE, Milner LV: *Yersinia enterocolitica*: a hazard in blood transfusion. Transfusion 22:396, 1982
31. Tabor E, Gerety RJ: Five cases of Pseudomonas sepsis

transmitted by blood transfusion (letter). Lancet 1: 1403, 1984

32. Kruskall MS, Yomtovian R, Dzik WH et al: On improving the cost-effectiveness of autologous blood transfusion practices. Transfusion 34:259, 1994

33. Parkman PD: Guidance for Autologous Blood and Blood Components. Food and Drug Administration, Bethesda, 1989

34. Busch MP, Tzong-Hae L, Heitman J: Allogeneic leukocytes but not therapeutic blood elements induce reactivation and dissemination of latent human immunodeficiency virus type 1 infection: implications for transfusion support of infected patients. Blood 80: 2128, 1992

35. College of American Pathologists: Comprehensive Transfusion Medicine Survey. Set J-C, 1992

36. Mintz PD: Participation of HIV-infected patients in autologous blood programs. JAMA 269:2892, 1993

37. Petz LD, Kleinman S: HIV-infected patients participating in autologous blood programs (letter). JAMA 270: 2181, 1993

38. Carson JL, Russell LB, Taragin MI: The risks of blood transfusion: the relative influence of acquired immunodeficiency syndrome and non-A, non-B hepatitis. Am J Med 92:45, 1992

39. Yomtovian R, Kelly C, Bracey SK et al: Procurement and transfusion of human immunodeficiency virus-positive or untested autologous blood units: issues and concerns: a report prepared by the Autologous Transfusion Committee of the American Association of Blood Banks. Transfusion 35:353, 1995

40. Dzik WH, Devarajan S: Should autologous blood that tests positive for infectious diseases be used or discarded? Transfusion 29:743, 1989

41. Anderson BV, Tomasulo PA: Current autologous transfusion practices: implications for the future. Transfusion 28:394, 1988

42. Starkey JM, MacPherson JL, Bolgiano DC et al: Markers for transfusion-transmitted disease in different groups of blood donors. JAMA 262:3452, 1989

43. AuBuchon JP, Dodd RY: Analysis of the relative safety of autologous blood units available for transfusion to homologous recipients. Transfusion 28:403, 1988

44. Kruskall MS, Popovsky MA, Pacini DG et al: Autologous versus homologous donors: evaluation of markers for infectious disease. Transfusion 28:286, 1988

45. Goodnough LT, Price TH, Friedman KD et al: A phase III trial of recombinant human erythropoietin therapy in nonanemic orthopedic patients subjected to aggressive removal of blood for autologous use: dose, response, toxicity, and efficacy. Transfusion 34:66, 1994

46. Goodnough LT, Price TH, Rudnick S, Soegiarso RW:

Preoperative red cell production in patients undergoing aggressive autologous blood phlebotomy with and without erythropoietin therapy. Transfusion 32:441, 1992

47. Rutherford CJ, Schneider TJ, Dempsey H et al: Efficacy of different dosing regimens for recombinant human erythropoietin in a simulated perisurgical setting: the importance of iron availability in optimizing response. Am J Med 96:139, 1994

48. Hayaski JI, Kumon K, Takanashi S et al: Subcutaneous administration of recombinant human erythropoietin before cardiac surgery: a double-blind, multi-center trial in Japan. Transfusion 34:142, 1994

49. Goodnough LT, Rudnick S, Price TH et al: Increased preoperative collection of autologous blood with recombinant human erythropoietin therapy. N Engl J Med 321:1163, 1989

50. Mercuriali F, Zanella A, Barosi G et al: Use of erythropoietin to increase the volume of autologous blood donated by orthopedic patients. Transfusion 33:55, 1993

51. Levine EA, Gould SA, Rosen AL et al: Perioperative recombinant human erythropoietin. Surgery 106:432, 1989

52. Canadian Orthopedic Perioperative Erythropoietin Study Group: Effectiveness of perioperative recombinant human erythropoietin in elective hip replacement. Lancet 341:1227, 1993

53. Levine EA, Rosen AL, Sehgal LR et al: Treatment of acute postoperative anemia with recombinant human erythropoietin. J Trauma 29:1134, 1989

54. Graf H, Watzinger U, Ludvik B et al: Recombinant human erythropoietin as adjuvant treatment for autologous blood donation. BMJ 300:1627, 1990

55. Biesma DH, Kraaijenhagen RJ, Marx JJM, van de Wiel A: The efficacy of subcutaneous recombinant human erythropoietin in the correction of phlebotomy-induced anemia in autologous blood donors. Transfusion 33:825, 1993

56. Birkmeyer JD, Goodnough LT, Aubuchon JP et al: The cost-effectiveness of preoperative autologous blood donation for total hip and knee replacement. Transfusion 33:544, 1993

57. Etchason J, Petz L, Keeler E et al: The cost effectiveness of preoperative autologous blood donations. Transfusion 332:719, 1995

58. Goodnough LT, Marcus RE: Erythropoietin and preoperative blood donation. N Engl J Med 322:1157, 1990

59. Silvergleid AJ: All blood collected should be tested for infectious disease markers. p. 177. In Maffei LM, Thurer RL (eds): Autologous Blood Transfusion: Cur-

rent Issues. American Association of Blood Banks, Bethesda, 1988

60. Myhre BA: Crossing over of autologous and directed donor blood. Ann Clin Lab Sci 22:343, 1992

61. Gibble JW, Ness PM: Fibrin glue: the perfect operative sealant? Transfusion 30:741, 1990

62. Schiffer CA, Aisner J, Wiernik PH: Frozen autologous platelet transfusion for patients with leukemia. N Engl J Med 229:7, 1978

63. Dicke KA, Spitzer G, Peters L: Autologous bone-marrow transplantation in relapsed adult leukemia. Lancet 1:51, 1979

64. Reiffers J, Marit G, Vezon G et al: Autologous blood stem cell grafting in hematological malignancies. Present status and future directions. Transfusion Sci 13: 399, 1992

65. Love TR, Hendren WG, O'Keefe DD, Daggett WM: Transfusion of predonated autologous blood in elective cardiac surgery. Ann Thorac Surg 43:508, 1987

66. Woolson ST, Marsh JS, Tanner JB: Transfusion of previously deposited autologous blood for patients undergoing hip-replacement surgery. J Bone Joint Surg [Am] 69:325, 1987

67. Wasman J, Goodnough LT: Autologous blood donation for elective surgery: effect on physician transfusion behavior. JAMA 258:3135, 1987

68. Cregan P, Donegan E, Gotelli G: Hemolytic transfusion reaction following autologous frozen and washed red cells. Transfusion 31:172, 1991

69. Richards C, Kolins J, Trindade CD: Autologous transfusion-transmitted *Yersinia enterocolitica*. JAMA 268: 1541, 1992

70. Salvatierra O, Jr, Iwaki Y, Vincenti F et al: Incidence, characteristics, and outcome of recipients sensitized after donor-specific blood transfusion. Transplantation 32:528, 1981

71. Lohrmann H, Bull MI, Decter JA et al: Platelet transfusions from HL-A compatible unrelated donors to alloimmunized patients. Ann Intern Med 80:9, 1974

72. Pearson HA, McIntosh S: Neonatal thrombocytopenia. Clin Haematol 7:111, 1978

73. Hamilton, Frederick, and Schneiders, Inc: AABB Public Opinion Poll, December 1985. American Association of Blood Banks, Bethesda, 1985

74. A survey summary of directed donations in California. CBBS Today 4(1):7, 1986

75. Jugli T, Takashi K, Shibata Y et al: Post-transfusion graft versus host disease in immunocompetent patients after cardiac surgery in Japan. N Engl J Med 321:56, 1989

76. Thaler M, Shamiss A, Orgad S et al: The role of blood from HLA-homozygous donors in fatal transfusion-associated graft versus host disease after open heart surgery. N Engl J Med 321:25, 1989

77. Petz LD, Calhoun L, Yam P et al: Transfusion-associated graft-versus-host disease in immunocompetent patients: report of a fatal case associated with transfusion of blood from a second-degree relative, and a survey of predisposing factors. Transfusion 33:742, 1993

78. Kanter MH: Transfusion-associated graft versus host disease: do transfusions from second degree relatives pose a greater risk than those from first degree relatives? Transfusion 32:323, 1992

79. Perkins HA: Should all blood from related donors be irradiated? Transfusion 32:302, 1992

80. Quinnan GV, Jr: Recommendations Regarding License Amendments and Procedures for Gamma Irradiation of Blood Products. Food and Drug Administration, Bethesda, 1993

81. Dodd RY: The risk of transfusion-transmitted infection (editorial). N Engl J Med 327:419, 1992

82. Strauss RG, Wieland MR, Randels MJ, Koerner TAW: Feasibility and success of a single-donor red cell program for pediatric elective surgery patients. Transfusion 32:747, 1992

83. Goldfinger D: Directed blood donations: Pro. Transfusion 29:70, 1989

84. Brecher ME, Moore SB, Taswell HF: Minimal-exposure transfusion: a new approach to homologous blood transfusion. Mayo Clin Proc 63:903, 1988

Home and Outpatient Transfusion Programs

Cherie S. Evans

HEALTH CARE DELIVERY: CHANGING PARADIGMS

The Hospital Model

Throughout most of recorded history, medical care has been provided in the home. It was not until the middle of the twentieth century that the focus shifted to the hospital, largely as a result of the increasingly complex and costly technology of modern medical care, which mandated centralization. Eventually, hospital-based care came to represent the "gold standard" for health care delivery. As malpractice litigation grew both in the volume of cases and the magnitude of awards, physicians became unwilling to accept the potentially higher liability of prescribing any but the simplest therapy in the outpatient setting, much less the home. As early as 1947, however, it was recognized that the pendulum had swung too far, and efforts began to move medical care out of the hospital. The first hospital-based home care program was started at Montefiore Hospital in New York City and was referred to as the "hospital without walls".[1] Going a step beyond the visiting nurse programs set up in the 1800s by philanthropic women's societies, this program provided a full array of services and included physicians, nurses, and therapists. This pioneering program is now mirrored in outpatient care programs provided by an increasingly varied array of infusion nursing agencies, surgery centers, dialysis centers, urgent care centers, and so forth, as the trend continues today.

Economic Forces

In the last 15 years, recognition at a national level of the critical need to control health care expenditure has accelerated rapidly. By 1995, some economists predict health care expenditure will be 15 percent of the gross national product, roughly 1 trillion dollars.[2] Concern over our nation's ability to continue to allocate such a disproportionate amount to health care has led to significant changes in reimbursement for health care providers. To provide more health care options in less expensive outpatient settings, reimbursement for in-home medical care became available through the Medicare and Medicaid programs in the mid-1960s. Unfortunately, reimbursement for physicians was so low that there was little, if any, incentive for them to supervise care in the home. This was a significant obstacle to the trend away from hospital-based care because physicians traditionally made most of the decisions about health care delivery options. In 1982, the Tax Equity and Fiscal Responsibility Act expanded reimbursement for outpatient services by expanding coverage for chronic outpatient care and incorporating hospice care as a covered service.[3] Implementation

295

of the diagnosis-related group system made it imperative for hospitals to develop mechanisms to limit the length of inpatient admissions and re-evaluate the necessity of expensive technologies and services. As a result, hospitals and health care plans became much more aggressive in directing their staff and participating in physicians' choices regarding the use of the home and outpatient care option.[4] Finally, in the 1990s, it became a presidential mandate to contain health care costs, even if that would require a complete reorganization of our country's mechanisms of health care delivery.

Societal Forces

There are more than financial reasons for us to move medical care out of the hospital whenever possible. There has been a significant change in the patient population. Those older than age 65 represent an ever-increasing proportion of our patients. In addition to this simple increase in numbers, many of these patients have debilitating conditions, requiring either chronic care or more prolonged care after an acute illness or surgery. This is a population for whom mobility is often a problem. Therefore, transfer to a hospital may require special transportation facilities, discomfort, or even the risk of injury. These patients are likely to be less affluent and to be living on fixed incomes, making cost-effectiveness critical. For such patients, obtaining medical care in the home may be their only viable option.

The arrival of the acquired immunodeficiency syndrome (AIDS) epidemic has almost overwhelmed many city's health care budgets. Cities such as San Francisco and New York expect a substantial proportion of their hospital beds will be required for the care of these patients alone.[5,6] This is a patient population who requires a wide variety of infusion therapies, from parenteral nutrition to antibiotics to transfusions. Yet much of the care these patients require is adaptable to the outpatient or home setting if there are mechanisms developed to facilitate delivery of the care. Many of the agencies caring for these patients, recognizing both the market opportunity and the advantages for their patients, have established successful outpatient and home care programs that provide all of these therapy modalities.[7]

Another trend in health care delivery is the rapidly increasing use of free-standing "surgicenters" for

surgical procedures that do not require the full facilities of a hospital.[8] In most cases, these centers handle only elective surgery, making the use of autologous blood a potential option. These surgical facilities often approach a hospital and/or a regional blood bank to have the patient's blood collected, stored, and transported. Because there is always a chance of unanticipated bleeding during a procedure, an increasing number of surgicenters also desire a source of allogeneic units. In fact, one national voluntary accreditation agency, the Accreditation Association for Ambulatory Health Care, in their standards for outpatient surgery services, state that the service must demonstrate that "procedures have been developed for obtaining blood and blood products on a timely basis."[9] In view of the fact that an increasing number of health care payers are using such accreditation to qualify ambulatory care facilities for reimbursement, there is an added impetus for the center to incorporate transfusion into their program.

Ever since the 1970s, consumer activists have focused attention on the need for more patient involvement in health care decisions.[10] If health care providers are to survive in an increasingly competitive market, they need to be cognizant of this trend. An increasing number of patient "consumers" are asking for less institutionalized approaches to health care that are convenient, personalized, and affordable. In response to this demand for convenience, many dialysis centers began performing transfusions for patients at the time they come in for their dialysis therapy; however, the current widespread use of erythropoietin therapy for patients with end-stage renal disease has greatly decreased the transfusion requirements of this patient population.

The New Paradigm

Responding to these needs requires a change in our underlying assumptions about complex or high technology medical care (i.e., that it is only safe and of the highest quality when provided in a hospital). This belief persists despite considerable precedent for the successful provision of high technology therapy with its attendant risks in outpatient and home settings. Hemophiliac patients have been transfused at home for decades.[10] Outpatient hemodialysis and chemotherapy are routine. Nursing agencies are providing a growing array of infusion therapies in the home, including antibiotics, pentamidine, and γ globulin. Both surgery and emergency care are now frequently performed in free-standing centers. In this environment, the old belief that it is too risky to transfuse blood outside of a hospital seems untenable.

ADMINISTRATIVE ISSUES

Legal Concerns

Unlike hospital-based transfusion, there are no established standards or regulations from any regulatory body or accrediting agency for outpatient or home transfusion. There are guidelines for home transfusion therapy from the Scientific Section Coordinating Committee of the American Association of Blood Banks (AABB); however, these cover only the most basic aspects of such a service.[11] It was the belief of the committee that this was an area in which the AABB was unlikely to be able to exert any control, making "standards" unrealistic. Many states have written regulations for inpatient transfusion that may be applicable to the outpatient setting; examples are the requirement that transfusions be given on the order of a physician or that only licensed personnel may administer them.[12] Therefore, it is advisable that anyone setting up a home transfusion service should carefully review their own state's regulations to find any that may apply.

As with any form of medical care, the higher the degree of risk from the therapy is, the higher is the level of accountability. It is well known that transfusion, in the best of circumstances, carries a degree of risk; furthermore, it has been argued that this risk is increased by some ill-defined amount when transfusions are provided outside of a hospital. Currently, there is no case law, and therefore no precedent, to determine who will be liable for any real or perceived negligence if an adverse transfusion reaction occurs in an outpatient or home setting. This has been of particular concern for regional blood centers and hospitals that provide home and outpatient transfusion services in conjunction with separate entities such as nursing agencies, doctors' offices, dialysis centers, and so forth. Because of this legal uncertainty, many centers have consulted liability experts and have been advised that a contract between the blood center and the transfusing facility is essential. This contract should clearly delineate the responsibilities of each of the involved parties.

In addition, some blood centers have been advised to attempt to divorce themselves from any activity that might be construed as official approval of those elements of the program for which the blood center is not directly responsible. This advice, if accepted, would result in a change in the relationship between most blood centers and the home transfusion agencies in which blood center personnel review in detail the agencies' policies and procedures, often extensively revising them. Some blood centers are also actively involved in providing continuing education and even perform inspections of the agencies.[13] A few centers have been advised that these practices might be construed to imply some form of official certification by the blood center, in effect, that the agency's procedures and staff were "approved," thereby increasing the blood center's vicarious liability.

This "hands-off" approach has not been widely accepted by blood centers or hospitals because of a concern that, at a minimum, it will result in a failure to fulfill the transfusion service's responsibility for quality assurance (QA), as required of transfusion services by both the AABB and the Joint Commission on Accreditation of Healthcare Organizations (JCAHO).[14] At this time, the most common approach for any organization that provides blood to another facility for outpatient or home transfusion is to have their medical and technical staff review the policies and procedures of that facility to ensure they meet at least minimal standards for transfusion practice. This also includes a review of the certification and continuing education required for the transfusionist and a review of the program for disposal of biohazardous materials. It is important that agencies that perform transfusions have medical directors and that they be involved in reviewing transfusion policies, transfusion appropriateness, and adverse outcomes. Whether or not the medical director needs to be licensed by the state in which the transfusion is performed may vary from state to state.

Another important issue to consider is the original qualifications and subsequent continuing education of the staff that administers the transfusions. Reliance on "paramedical" staff has increased greatly in hospitals as a part of their cost-containment efforts. In some outpatient settings, such as surgicenters where there is a physician present at the time of the transfusion, staffing similar to that seen in hospitals seems reasonable. However, in most dialysis centers and in the home, the "transfusionist" is operating essentially independently and is therefore likely to be held to a higher level of professional accountability. This may be offset somewhat by having specific orders from the attending physician for all potential significant complications that may arise and by ensuring that the physician is available by telephone for immediate consultation. In addition, agencies generally prefer to employ nurses with recent acute care training and experience and to provide continuing education programs that explicitly address transfusion issues.

Informed Consent

The AABB recommends that informed consent should be obtained before any elective transfusion.[15] In some states, such as California, state law requires that patients be informed of risks of transfusion and its alternatives before nonemergency transfusions.[16] Adequate documentation of informed consent requires written documentation that the patient has been informed of significant adverse reactions to transfusions, has been told about alternatives to allogeneic transfusion, and has been given the information that the outpatient setting makes the risk greater.[17] Documentation should also include a statement that the patient consents to the transfusion. Obtaining informed consent in the home transfusion setting is the responsibility of the patient's attending physician. When the transfusions are performed by a nursing agency and a copy of the informed consent is not available on site, the transfusionist should ascertain that the risks and benefits of the transfusion were previously explained to the patient. Some nursing care agencies may require that an additional informed consent be part of their records.

Organizational Approaches

Two major approaches to home and outpatient transfusion have emerged in the last decade. Both reflect the changes that have been taking place in the traditional relationships among health care providers. On the one hand, hospitals that have previously focused their attention on centralized inpatient services are looking outward into the community to determine how they may best position themselves to provide therapy in the community setting, as dictated by current market forces and the demand for cost containment.[18] Hospitals have the option of providing compatibility testing and blood components and then contracting with the outpatient facilities and/or nursing agencies that will perform the actual transfusion or of providing the complete service, employing their own hospital nurses.

The second approach is for a regional blood center to extend its traditional role as a collection, storage, and distribution facility and establish a transfusion service, often through the reference laboratory.[19] Blood centers can also choose to provide full-service transfusion programs by performing transfusions at the blood center itself or by employing donor collection personnel to administer the transfusions elsewhere. It is more common, however, for a blood center to choose to provide only compatibility testing and blood components and contract with other agencies to administer the transfusions.

Both of these approaches have advantages and disadvantages, which are summarized in Table 12-1. Hospital-based programs should have the advantage of having an established mechanism for QA of inpatient transfusions, which they may directly apply to their outpatient or home program. This involves expanding the scope of their transfusion committee and establishing audit criteria appropriate to the setting in which the transfusions will be performed. If they choose to employ their own nurses, they have a high degree of control of the certification and training of the transfusionists. Most hospital programs, however, only provide transfusions for the patients of physicians on the hospital's medical staff, which can present a problem. In many areas with predominantly hospital-based outpatient transfusion programs, nursing agencies that provide transfusions in the home may end up dealing with several different hospitals, each of which has different forms and procedures. Confusion may result, which increases the chance of error. In addition, surgicenters often have difficulty obtaining any blood services from their local hospital. Typically, these are centers

Table 12-1. Organizational Approaches to Out-of-Hospital Transfusion Services

I. Hospital-based out-of-hospital transfusion services
A. Advantages
1. Mechanism in place for transfusion service quality assurance assessment
a. Transfusion committee in existence
b. Audit criteria already developed
2. Laboratory and nursing personnel may be from same facility
3. Additional income for laboratory
B. Disadvantages
1. Provides transfusion only for patients of physicians on own medical staff
2. Not routinely set up to ship components
3. May not be able internally to fill special orders (cytomegalovirus negative, irradiated, washed, leukocyte reduced)
II. Regional blood center-based transfusion service
A. Advantages
1. Centralization: a single set of forms and procedures, despite multiple nursing agencies, ordering physicians, and hospitals
2. Special orders: equipped to provide special requests on a routine basis
3. Shipping of all components is routine
4. Additional income for laboratory
B. Disadvantages
1. No standing transfusion committee
2. Large time commitment to review procedures of each agency or facility for which blood is provided
3. Quality assurance needs for auditing practice and inspections more difficult to meet

(From Evans,[19] with permission.)

established by one or more physicians in a community who previously treated their patients in the hospital with which they are now competing. It is not unusual for the hospital administration to take a jaundiced view of facilitating the surgicenter's success by providing transfusion services.

When a regional blood center establishes a transfusion service, it has the advantage of centralization and, therefore, uniformity, regardless of how many different physicians, agencies, or outpatient facilities use the service. Any special processing orders (cytomegalovirus negative, filtered, irradiated, and so forth) that may need to be filled are routine for a blood center. In addition, blood centers already have a validated and quality-controlled mechanism for packaging and shipping blood that may be used. Of more difficulty for a blood center is the issue of QA because there is no pre-existing transfusion committee. Despite concerns about vicarious liability, the blood center cannot avoid the need to have a sufficient QA program to ensure that at least minimal requirements are met.

Because of difficulties with obtaining blood from the local hospital, surgicenters often turn to the regional blood center for blood services. It is becoming common for blood centers to supply autologous blood to the surgicenters in their area. The blood center draws the units, stores them, and then ships them to the surgicenter on the day of surgery. Most blood centers do not, however, provide emergency access to allogeneic units for surgicenters. Unlike hospitals, the crossmatching and transfusion service capability in a blood center is generally not staffed to handle emergencies or supply blood after hours or on weekends. In addition, most blood centers believe that patients so unstable that they have an urgent need for blood should be transferred to a hospital for treatment.

QUALITY ASSURANCE

A formal program of QA is mandated by accrediting agencies such as the JCAHO and the AABB, which define the requirements for transfusion services.[14] From a legal viewpoint, QA programs seem even more necessary in the home transfusion setting where the risks of transfusion are increased. In the absence of established standards for outpatient and home transfusions, each transfusion service must set its own criteria for acceptable practice. In hospitals, this can be done through the transfusion committee; in blood centers, it usually becomes the responsibility of the medical director. At a minimum, there should be criteria set for patient selection, appropriateness of component and amount transfused, administration technique, reaction evaluation, and biohazardous waste disposal. Once the service is established, transfusion practice needs to be monitored over time to ensure that the agreed-on criteria are being met. If a large volume of outpatient transfusions is anticipated, a facility may choose to audit only a subset of transfusions. For many transfusion services, however, the volume is sufficiently low and the perceived liability sufficiently high that all outpatient transfusions are audited for compliance with the QA criteria.

For facilities the personnel of which perform all aspects of the transfusion service (i.e., laboratory functions and blood administration), these criteria can be applied to their outpatient transfusions in a manner analogous to that for their inpatient transfusions. This mechanism of auditing for compliance with preset criteria and reviewing the records of any transfusions with adverse outcomes was proved over the last two decades in hospitals to be a successful QA mechanism. However, for hospitals and blood banks that choose to perform only compatibility testing and provide blood components, setting up an effective QA program is one of the most difficult challenges they face because two independent organizations each represent a portion of the "transfusion service." Auditing transfusions is not a major problem. However, as a result of auditing, if problems are found, it may be difficult to implement successful corrective action. A system of concurrent review of appropriateness of transfusion is one approach that was proved to be effective in hospitals and may also be applied to an outpatient system.[20] In this system, the blood center or hospital transfusion service requires that the transfusion request include the indication for transfusion and current supporting clinical and laboratory data. The technologist receiving such a request has predetermined guidelines for acceptance of the request. Any request not falling within these guidelines is referred to the transfusion service physician before compatibility testing is done or units are identified. This physician evaluates the request, if necessary consulting with the involved agency or attending physician, and determines whether the request is appropriate. If the answer is yes, the reasons can be documented on the written request and the components supplied. If the request is not considered acceptable by the transfusion service, a mechanism to resolve such differences in opinion must be in place. If such differences cannot be resolved (i.e., an inadequate method of sample identification was used), the transfusion service should be prepared to deny the request. Given the increased risk involved in transfusion in an outpatient setting, a firm commitment to the pre-established criteria seems prudent. The blood bank also

needs to decide how to handle incomplete or inaccurate requests, sample labels, or patient identification. Even when the units in question are autologous, the need to prevent injury caused by clerical errors remains.

The blood center should also be involved in the evaluation of any transfusion reactions that occur. Depending on circumstances, this may be a retrospective review of records for a patient who was transferred directly to the hospital but may also include involvement in the serologic workup of the patient. Consideration needs to be given to how this evaluation would be coordinated in the event that the pre-transfusion sample would provide useful information and the serologic evaluation is being done by another laboratory.

MEDICAL ISSUES
Patient Selection

Patients who are appropriate candidates for outpatient dialysis or surgery would likely be appropriate patients for transfusion were such needed. Home transfusions are another matter because a physician is unlikely to be present and sophisticated medical facilities are not immediately available in the event of a severe transfusion reaction. The ideal patient who is undergoing home transfusion has a chronic medical condition, is in good fluid balance, and has a stable cardiorespiratory system. Typical conditions are listed in Table 12-2.[21] Only patients for whom

Table 12-2. Patient Selection for Out-of-Hospital Transfusion

Typical Conditions
1. AIDS/AIDS-related complex
2. Anemia of chronic renal disease
3. Hemoglobinopathies
4. Anemia associated with malignancy
5. Chronic gastrointestinal bleeding
6. Refractory anemia
7. Myelosclerosis, myelodysplasia, myelophthisic states
8. Bone marrow failure
9. Thrombocytopenia
10. Coagulation factor deficiency
11. Output surgery

Abbreviation: AIDS, acquired immunodeficiency syndrome.
(From Evans,[19] with permission.)

the expected benefits of transfusing in the home are sufficient to warrant the increased risk should be chosen. Most home transfusion programs consider mere convenience to be an insufficient reason. In addition, Medicare requires "homebound" status for reimbursement. Typically, elderly individuals for whom transportation is difficult or expensive are candidates if they are in otherwise stable condition. Home therapy is also frequently sought for pediatric patients because hospitalization is particularly disruptive for children. Providing medical care in the home also helps reinforce a sense of independence and self-worth in chronically ill individuals of any age.

In addition to evaluating the appropriateness of the patient for home transfusion, the home should also be evaluated. Despite the fact that a well-run program takes every step possible to prevent adverse transfusion reactions, such may still occur. The patient, therefore, needs to be in a home with a telephone and adequate, rapidly available emergency assistance. In many urban areas, there is a rapid emergency response mechanism already in place. In more rural areas, the adequacy and availability of emergency services needs to be carefully evaluated. Another competent adult should be available for the entire period of the transfusion and for at least 30 to 60 minutes thereafter. If the patient should have a reaction, this is the individual who will contact the patient's physician, relay information, and arrange for emergency transportation, if necessary.

One frequently quoted criterion for patient selection for home transfusion, which is questioned by some, is that the patient should have no clinically significant alloantibodies. However, as experience with home transfusion has grown, services are becoming more comfortable with selecting antigen-negative units for such patients as long as the antibody specificities are clearly identified and the patient has a well-documented transfusion history. This does not mean that it would be appropriate to transfuse patients with unresolved serologic findings or in the presence of an autoantibody when the absence of underlying alloantibodies cannot be convincingly proved.

Another questionable criterion for patient selection for home transfusion is that the patient have previously received a transfusion of a similar component in the hospital with no adverse reaction. A growing number of reputable home transfusion programs no longer adhere to this requirement. The two most serious reactions that are likely to occur as a result of transfusion are anaphylaxis and acute hemolysis. The infusion agencies that would be performing the transfusion already provide any number of treatment modalities more likely to cause anaphylaxis than transfusion. Their staff is well versed in the management of this complication. In regard to a fatal acute hemolytic reaction, the most likely cause is transfusion of an ABO-incompatible unit as a result of a clerical error.[22] It is reasonable to assume that such errors are more likely to occur on the first transfusion because there is no historical type recorded to cross-reference. There are a number of approaches used to prevent such errors. Some institutions choose to administer only type O packed cells for the first transfusion of a patient at home. Others use a check sample system for the first unit. Such a check sample system is outlined in Figure 12-1. Even in the event of a sample mix-up involving the sample used for compatibility testing for a patient new to the laboratory, this system should ensure that the

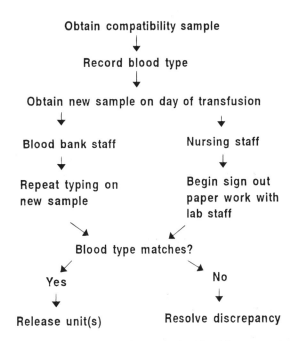

Fig. 12-1. Check sample system for blood being used in home transfusion.

unit transfused is at least the correct ABO type. After the first transfusion, the patient's record is used to cross-check the ABO type.

Patients being transfused in surgicenters have often had autologous units drawn. Although this is the safest form of blood transfusion, a clerical error could still be lethal. To prevent such errors, some programs use a commercially available packaging system to prevent use of the blood other than that for the patient from which it was drawn. After blood collection, the unit is placed in a sealed bag with a lock that can only be opened by a specific code number.[23] That number is imprinted on an armband that is affixed to the patient's wrist at the time of the phlebotomy. The major problem reported with this approach has been convincing patients to keep the armband on until they come back for their surgery. Another approach for patients with autologous units is to take a photograph of the patient at the time of collection, which is affixed to the unit and compared with the patient at the time of transfusion.

Component Selection

Because minor febrile or urticarial transfusion reactions are more troublesome in the outpatient setting than in the hospital, most physicians choose to premedicate their patients with an antihistamine and/or antipyretic. In addition, leukocyte-reduced cellular components are often chosen for allogeneic units. This is usually done by filtration, either in the blood bank or at the bedside. It has been suggested that no more than 2 units of packed red blood cells should be given in any 24-hour period in the home as a mechanism to avoid volume overload.[24] For services that wish to standardize their therapy in an effort to minimize involvement by the transfusion service director, this approach, although conservative, may be a reasonable choice. However, services that deal with young, volume-depleted patients with AIDS frequently transfuse 3 or even 4 units at a time in an effort to keep the cost in both time and money to a minimum. These patients tolerate such transfusions extremely well. On the other hand, even 2 units may be excessive if a frail, elderly, chronically anemic patient were being transfused who might be better served by 1 unit/day over several days. Ideally, transfusion services make such decisions on a case-by-case basis.

Certain components are never given in an outpatient setting. Whole blood is not indicated when a stable patient is transfused. If the patient is sufficiently unstable to make a whole blood transfusion appropriate, the patient needs to be transported to a hospital. Granulocytes are also contraindicated. Any patient septic enough to require such treatment needs inpatient care. The components most commonly given are packed red blood cells and platelets. In some areas, there is also a growing use of autologous bioadhesive preparations ("fibrin glue") in surgicenters. Although less frequent, there are also appropriate uses for cryoprecipitate and fresh frozen plasma for outpatients.

TRANSFUSION SERVICE PROCEDURES

Obtaining Patient Samples

The sample for compatibility testing may be drawn in the home, outpatient office, or clinic for patients receiving allogeneic transfusion. For patients receiving autologous units, the sample is the pilot tube attached to the unit of blood. In labeling this sample, the critical process of patient identification begins. Generally, the patient sample is labeled with the patient's name, a unique identifying number, the date of the phlebotomy, and the initials of the phlebotomist. Studies continue to demonstrate that the most common source of fatal transfusion reactions is a clerical error leading to an ABO-mismatched transfusion.[22] Positive identification of the patient and the unit(s) of blood is no less important in the outpatient setting than in the hospital. The information on this label must be an exact match to the information on the request for the transfusion. Any inaccurate or missing information on the sample label or request should invalidate the sample.

It is equally important to ensure absolute identification of the patient. The AABB recommends the use of a wristband identification system, such as that used in hospitals.[11] This wristband is placed on the patient at the time the compatibility sample is drawn and remains there until the transfusion is administered. Wherever the transfusion is performed, there should be two competent individuals to cross-check the patient's identification, blood type, and unit expiration date. In the home, this is often done by the friend or member of the family who will be staying throughout the transfusion to assist the nurse should the need arise. This two-person verification should not be omitted in any other outpatient setting.

Transportation of Components

Transportation for blood components intended for outpatient transfusion is not significantly different that that for components going to hospitals. The mechanism needs to be validated and quality controlled on some periodic basis to ensure temperatures are maintained, as expected. Both hospitals and blood centers typically ship units packed in such a way that the temperature is known to be maintained for a specific period. The transfusing agency or facility knows that the components are not to be unpacked until immediately before transfusion to maintain the temperature in the correct range. As an added assurance, temperature-sensitive devices that change color if the temperature is too low or too high may be attached to the unit(s).

Administration

Blood components are generally administered in outpatient settings with the use of standard hospital equipment and protocols. The most significant difference is the intensity with which these transfusion are monitored, particularly in the home setting where the nurse usually remains with the patient through the entire transfusion and for as long as 1 hour afterward. Nursing services typically require that vital signs be checked as often as every 5 minutes during the first 15 minutes and every 15 minutes thereafter. Many nurses use this time to educate the patient and/or caregiver on the post-transfusion protocol and about other aspects of their medical care.

The simplicity of the process generally facilitates error-free performance of any medical procedure, including transfusion. Transfusion service directors in hospitals have years of experience with the difficulties inherent in monitoring staff adherence to approved protocols and quality control when blood warmers are used in departments not under the control of the clinical laboratory. In view of this experience and the fact that outpatient transfusions should not need to be given so quickly that the temperature of the blood is critical, the use of these devices outside of the hospital should be discouraged, if not interdicted. In addition, infusion pumps are rarely indicated in outpatient settings, particularly in the home. The one exception would be the transfusion of a small child for whom the rate of transfusion is more critical.

Post-Transfusion Protocol

Because outpatients will not be directly monitored by medical personnel after the transfusion, education of the patient and/or a caregiver about possible signs and symptoms of a delayed transfusion reaction is essential. At a minimum, instructions should cover circulatory overload, delayed hemolysis, and transfusion-transmitted infections, including hepatitis and AIDS. The patient should receive specific instructions about whom to contact in the case any unexpected symptoms occur. Someone with medical expertise should be available on an around-the-clock basis to respond to such a patient inquiry. A written copy of these instructions should be left with the patient or caregiver.

Any equipment that has been in contact with blood is considered potentially biohazardous and must be disposed of in accordance with all federal and state regulations. Blood banks are required to be able to track any biohazardous materials that originate with them all the way to their ultimate use or disposal. At a minimum, the blood bank should require a copy of the contract the nursing agency or outpatient facility has with an approved biohazardous waste company or a hospital for the disposal of all such contaminated materials. In the case of home transfusion, it is also essential to be certain that anything in the home that inadvertently was contaminated with blood has been disinfected. Even equipment that has not actually been in contact with blood may best be handled as if biohazardous. It would be best if anything that might potentially be identified as being related to the transfusion is not discovered in residential refuse.

REFERENCES

1. Koren MJ: Home care—who cares. N Engl J Med 314: 917, 1986
2. Burner ST, Waldo DR, McKusick DR: National health expenditures projections through 2030. Health Care Financing Rev 14:1, 1992

3. Bulkin W, Lukashok H: Rx for dying: the case for hospice. N Engl J Med 318:376, 1988
4. Feldstein PJ, Wickizer TM, Wheeler JR: Private cost containment. N Engl J Med 318:1310, 1988
5. Weinberg DS, Murray HW: Coping with AIDS: the special problems of New York City. N Engl J Med 317:1469, 1987
6. Chen RT, George MA, Rutherford GW et al: Use of hospital by patients with AIDS in San Francisco. N Engl J Med 319:1671, 1988
7. Rogatz P, Ungvarski P, Hinkelman M: Coping with AIDS. N Engl J Med 381:1621, 1988
8. Moxley JH, Roeder PC: New opportunities for out-of-hospital health services. 310:193, 1984
9. Accreditation Handbook for Ambulatory Health Care. 1994–95 ed. Accreditation Association for Ambulatory Health Care, Skokie, IL, 1993
10. Rabiner SF, Telfer MC, Fajardo R: Home transfusions of hemophiliacs. JAMA 221:885, 1972
11. Beck ML, Grindon AJ: Home transfusion therapy. Transfusion 26:296, 1986
12. Guilday TJ: Legal considerations of home blood transfusions. p. 41. In Snyder EL, Menitove JE (eds): Home Transfusion Therapy. American Association of Blood Banks, Arlington, Virginia, 1986
13. Evans CS, Moore H, Perkins H: A home transfusion service established by a regional blood bank and a home care agency. Transfusion, suppl. 28:57S, 1988
14. Standards Committee American Association of Blood Banks: Standards for Blood Banks and Transfusion Services. 16th Ed. American Association of Blood Banks, Bethesda, Maryland, 1994
15. Widmann FK: Informed consent for blood transfusion: brief historical survey and summary of a conference. Transfusion 30:460, 1990
16. Paul Gann Blood Safety Act, California State Health & Safety Code, Section 1645, 1991
17. Silberstein LE: Quality assurance for out-of-hospital transfusion programs. p. 53. In Kurtz SR, Summers S, Kruskall MS (eds): Improving Transfusion Practice: The Role of Quality Assurance. American Association of Blood Banks, Arlington, Virginia, 1989
18. Bachert LB: Making home transfusions work. Med Lab Observer 19:42, 1987
19. Evans CS: Out-of-hospital transfusion: a regional blood center approach. In Fridey JL, Kasprisin CA, Issitt LA (eds): Out-of-Hospital Transfusion Therapy. American Association of Blood Banks, Bethesda, Maryland, 1994
20. Toy PT: Prospective vs retrospective transfusion audits at hospitals. p. 1. In Kurtz SR, Summers S, Kruskall MS (eds): Improving Transfusion Practice: The Role of Quality Assurance. American Association of Blood Banks, Arlington, Virginia, 1989
21. Marek K, McVan B: Home transfusion therapy: a new home care service. p. 13. In Fisher K, Gardner K (eds): Quality and Home Health Care: Redefining the Tradition. Joint Commission on Accreditation of Healthcare Organizations, Chicago, IL, 1987
22. Sazama K: Reports of 355 transfusion-associated deaths: 1976 through 1985. Transfusion 30:583, 1990
23. Wenz B, Burns ER: Improvement in transfusion safety using a new blood unit and patient identification system as part of safe transfusion practice. Transfusion 31:401, 1991
24. DePalma L, Synder EL: Medical aspects of home transfusion. p. 23. In Snyder EL, Menitove JE (eds): Home Transfusion Therapy. American Association of Blood Banks, Arlington, Virginia, 1986

Chapter 13

Blood Product Preparation and Administration

Loni Calhoun

Blood components and derivatives are prepared from blood collected by whole blood (WB) or apheresis donation. The components of whole blood (red cells [RBC], white cells, platelets [PLT], and plasma) are separated by differential centrifugation and can be further modified or packaged to meet special patient needs. ABO compatibility is considered when components are selected for transfusion and, except for cytomegalovirus (CMV) and human T-cell lymphotrophic virus type I, they usually carry the same disease risks as the whole blood from which they were separated.

In contrast, blood derivatives (albumin solutions, immune serum globulins, and concentrated coagulation factors) are prepared by more extensive processing of large pools of donor plasma. They are given without regard to ABO compatibility and, depending on the manufacturing process, have a significantly decreased risk of disease transmission.

Those responsible for the transfusion of blood components and derivatives should have a basic understanding of the products they request and handle: content and indications of use; preparation, storage, and compatibility requirements; administration and patient care requirements; and adverse effects that may result. This chapter reviews the more general and practical aspects of blood preparation and administration. The reader should refer to Sections IV through VI of this book for thorough discussions on the indications, dose, and adverse effects of transfusion.

COMPONENT MANUFACTURING PROCESS

WB for component or derivative production is collected from healthy blood donors who have been screened with a medical history and physical examination and who meet current acceptability standards. Essential to good component production are a clean venipuncture site to minimize bacterial contamination and a good flow rate to ensure maximum levels of coagulation factors in the starting product.

Anticoagulants and Preservatives

WB is collected into sterile Food and Drug Administration (FDA)-approved blood bags that contain a premeasured amount of anticoagulant-preservative (AP) solution. Standard blood bags contain enough AP solution to collect and store 450 ml of whole blood, plus or minus 10 percent, or 45 ml.

A correct balance of AP solution to blood prevents clotting and ensures maximal function and viability of blood cells and plasma proteins during storage. If a donation does not proceed in routine fashion and only 300 to 405 ml are collected, only the red cells can be used, and they must be labeled as a low-volume unit.[1] If less than 300 ml is to be collected, the amount of anticoagulant needed should be calcu-

Table 13-1. Contents of Food and Drug Administration-Approved Anticoagulant-Preservative and Additive Solutions

| Content (g/volume) | Primary Bag | | Adsol System | | Nutricell System | | Optisol System | |
	ACD-A (67.5 ml)	CPDA-1 (63 ml)	Primary Bag CPD (63 ml)	Additive AS-1 (100 ml)	Primary Bag CP2D (63 ml)	Additive AS-3 (100 ml)	Primary Bag CPD (63 ml)	Additive AS-5 (100 ml)
Trisodium citrate	1.48	1.66	1.66	—	1.66	0.588	1.66	—
Dextrose	1.65	2.01	1.61	2.20	3.22	1.10	1.61	0.900
Citric acid	0.54	0.206	0.206	—	0.206	0.042	0.206	—
Monobasic sodium phosphate	—	0.140	0.140	—	0.140	0.276	0.140	—
Adenine	—	0.017	—	0.27	—	0.030	—	0.030
Mannitol	—	—	—	0.75	—	—	—	0.525
Sodium chloride	—	—	—	0.90	—	0.410	—	0.877
Shelf life (days)	21	35	21	42	21	42	21	42

Abbreviations: ACD-A, acid-citrate-dextrose anticoagulant; CPDA-1, citrate-phosphate-dextrose-adenine anticoagulant; CPD, citrate-phosphate-dextrose anticoagulant; AS, additive solution.

lated (see below), and the excess should be transferred into an attached satellite bag before collection begins.

Amount of anticoagulant needed (in milliliters)

$$= \frac{\text{milliliters of blood to be collected}}{450 \text{ ml}}$$

$\times$ milliliters of anticoagulant in bag

The FDA approves AP solutions and collection systems using 75 percent recovery of transfused RBC after 24 hours in circulation as the criterion of acceptance.[2] AP solutions used for WB collection and extended storage of RBC are summarized in Table 13-1.

Component Fractionation

Because RBC, PLT, and plasma have different specific gravities (1.08 to 1.09, 1.03 to 1.04, and 1.023 respectively),[2,3] they can be separated from one another by differential centrifugation. The optimal centrifugation time and rotor speed for the large high-speed centrifuges used in component fractionation are determined by preparing components under different conditions to find the best time and speed combinations that produce the highest yields.

To simplify fractionation, blood is collected into a primary bag that has one, two, or three satellite

bags attached with integral tubing. Such sets provide a "closed" system of separation, that is, any portion of the original unit can be transferred from one bag to another without breaking the sterile integrity of the system. Alternatively, a sterile connecting device can be used to attach additional satellite bags as needed. These devices connect tubing (and hence their bags) without compromising sterility or expiration.

Set selection is based on intended use and inventory needs. A quad set with three attached satellites is the most expensive but most versatile; it can be used to make RBC, PLT, or fresh frozen plasma (FFP) and then cyroprecipitated antihemophilic factor (CRYO) from 1 unit of WB or FFP and three pediatric aliquots of RBC or any other four-bag combination of components.

The separation of WB into its component parts is summarized in Figure 13-1. Typically, WB intended for platelet harvest is maintained at room temperature (20 to 24°C) and platelet-rich plasma is separated within 8 hours of collection. Platelets then are concentrated into a smaller volume of plasma (40 to 60 ml), which will still maintain a pH above 6.0 throughout storage. Concentrates of platelets may also be harvested from the WB "buffy coat" (white cell/platelet layer)[4] or collected by apheresis (the product known as Platelet Pheresis [PLT-P]). The

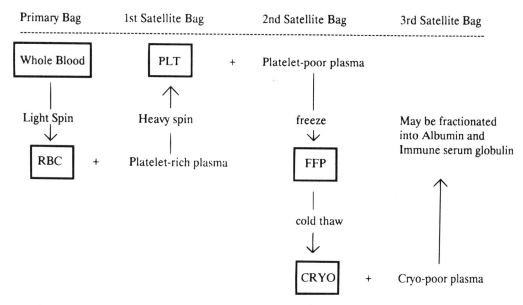

Fig. 13-1. Fractionation of whole blood into primary blood components using a Quad-set.

remaining platelet-poor plasma can be labeled and used as FFP if it is placed at $-18°C$ or colder within 8 hours of collection.

FFP can be thawed in the cold anytime within its 1-year shelf life and separated into CRYO (a cold precipitate of factor VIII, fibrinogen, and other plasma proteins) and CRYO-poor plasma, which may be kept as plasma or may be added back to the primary RBC bag to make a modified WB component. The CRYO must be refrozen within 1 hour of separation if it is not needed for immediate transfusion.

Both FFP and plasma that does not meet FFP criteria (i.e., not frozen within 8 hours or CRYO-poor plasma) can be fractionated into plasma derivatives by a modification of the cold ethanol precipitation process developed by Cohn et al.[2,5] This process uses combinations of ethanol concentrations, ionic strength, pH, and temperature to precipitate sequentially and purify different plasma proteins. Plasma can also be converted into viral-inactivated clotting factor concentrates.

A solvent-detergent process to prepare viral-inactivated plasma is under review for licensure by the FDA at the time of this writing. If approved and put into production, it may become the plasma product of choice over FFP (see Ch. 43).

White cells can be separated from units of freshly collected WB, but final yields are low compared with granulocyte collections by leukapheresis.[6–8] This kind of special WB processing is generally performed only when a young infant has urgent needs and leukapheresis products are not available.

Shelf Life and Storage

As long as sterility is maintained and blood bag seals are not broken, storage is limited only by the viability and stability of the individual component. These characteristics vary not only with the AP solution used but also with the conditions of storage. Not all blood components store equally well under the same conditions. Storage requirements and dating limits are set by the FDA[9] to ensure product quality and are summarized in Table 13-2. Blood components require strictly controlled and monitored environments. They can be used up to midnight on their date of expiration unless otherwise indicated.

RBC separated in a closed system are given the same expiration as their original WB counterpart, even though up to 275 ml of the plasma and AP solution are removed. If an approved additive solution (AS) is added within 72 hours of collection, RBC shelf life can be extended to 42 days. RBCs can also be transfused or frozen up to 3 days after their expi-

Table 13-2. Component Storage Temperatures and Shelf Life

Temperature (°C)	Component	Shelf Life
20–24	Platelets	3–5 days[a]
	Platelets, pooled	4 hr[b]
	Platelets, Pheresis	24 hr or 5 days[a]
	Granulocytes	24 hr
	CRYO, thawed	6 hr
	CRYO, thawed/pooled	4 hr[b]
1–6	Whole blood	21–35 days[c]
	RBC	21–42 days[c]
	RBC, washed	24 hr[b]
	F-RBC, deglycerolized	24 hr[b]
	FFP, thawed	24 hr[b]
	Liquid plasma	24 hr
		5 days more than the RBC unit
≤ − 18	FFP	1 yr
	CRYO	1 yr
	Plasma	5 yr
≤ − 65	F-RBC (40% glycerol)	10 yr
≤ − 120	F-RBC (20% glycerol)	10 yr

Abbreviations: CRYO, Cryoprecipitate; RBC, red blood cells; F-RBC, frozen RBC; FFP, fresh frozen plasma.

[a] Depending on the plastic bag or procedure used.

[b] If sterility is compromised during preparation.

[c] Depending on the anticoagulant-preservative used.

ration date if they are treated with an approved "rejuvenation" solution known to restore 2,3-diphosphoglyceric acid (2,3-DPG) and adenosine triphosphate levels.[2] Blood labels will indicate such rejuvenation.

If the seal is broken during preparation and sterility is compromised (i.e., an "opened" system), products stored between 1 and 6°C must be transfused within 24 hours; those stored between 20 and 24°C must be transfused as soon as possible and not after 4 hours. The new expiration date and time will be placed on the bag label. Opened-system products that are to be frozen must be placed in the freezer within 6 hours of breaking the seal. When thawed, they too are assigned a 4- or 24-hour shelf life, depending on storage temperature.

Refrigerated Storage

Blood refrigerators are specially designed to maintain the required 1 to 6°C temperature range throughout their interior space. They must have a system to monitor the temperature continuously and

record it at least once every 4 hours.[1] The monitoring sensor is placed in a container that has heat transference characteristics similar to the smallest unit of blood being stored. To confirm that the monitoring device is accurate, most blood banks compare daily the recorded temperatures against one or two manually read thermometers also stored in the refrigerator.

Blood refrigerators need an alarm system with an audible signal to alert the staff when temperatures reach the storage limits of 1 and 6°C. Such alarms should be battery operated or have separate electrical circuits and power failure alarms in case power to both the alarm and refrigerator is lost. The alarm system must be checked periodically to ensure that it is in good working order. Written instructions should be posted so that all staff know the action to take when it sounds.

A blood refrigerator must be clean, well lit, and organized so that allogeneic stock units are not confused with unprocessed, quarantined, or autologous units, and crossmatched units can be easily found. Allogeneic stock units should be grouped by ABO-Rh to avoid selection errors in emergency situations;[10] autologous stock and crossmatched units are grouped alphabetically by patient name.

Frozen Storage

Like blood refrigerators, blood freezers must have a design to maintain proper temperature throughout the entire interior and a system to monitor temperature continuously and record it every 4 hours. Thermometers placed in containers with small volumes of antifreeze should be stored in the freezer and manually checked daily to confirm recorder accuracy. Freezers must also have an alarm with an audible signal to alert the staff before temperatures become too warm, and it too must be periodically checked.

Frozen Plasma

Plasma freezers must maintain temperatures colder than − 18°C, but temperatures colder than − 30°C provide even better factor VIII preservation. Studies have shown that 40 percent of factor VIII activity is lost in large pools of plasma stored at − 20°C for periods up to 2 years, whereas plasma stored at − 30°C and − 40°C retains 90 percent activity.[11]

Frozen Red Cells

Frozen RBC stored at temperatures colder than − 65°C with a cryoprotective agent are licensed with a 10-year shelf life, even though no controlled studies exist to establish a maximal time for storage.[2] Indeed, units stored up to 21 years have been transfused with success.[12,13]

Several different freezing methods are in use. Frozen RBC prepared with high concentrations of glycerol (about 40 percent weight/volume) are stored at − 65°C or colder in supercold mechanical freezers that maintain temperatures closer to − 80°C near the wall so that the − 65°C limit is not compromised near the top where it may be warmer. Frozen RBC with a low concentration of glycerol (about 20 percent weight/volume) for cryoprotection require liquid nitrogen storage (− 120°C or colder). Because these units do not tolerate temperature changes, alarm sensors are placed in the liquid nitrogen tank somewhere above the minimal height so that the alarm sounds before the temperature of the gas phase goes above − 120°C.

Room Temperature Storage

Components that need 20 and 24°C storage can be laid on a countertop or table in any room that meets this temperature requirement; however, ambient temperature must be recorded every 4 hours during storage time. Because room temperature can fluctuate significantly, "environmental chambers" have been developed to provide controlled and monitored room temperatures. These chambers are equipped with continuous recording devices and alarms much like blood refrigerators and freezers.

Platelets

Although PLT are licensed by the FDA for 72-hour storage at 1 to 6°C with optional agitation or for up to 5 days at 20 and 24°C with continuous agitation, data show that PLT stored within the latter temperature range have superior function and viability and are the component of choice.[14,15]

Function, viability, and shelf life depend on a complex combination of temperature, method of production, PLT count, RBC and white cell contamination, the volume of plasma or resuspending fluid, the gas transport properties of the storage bag, the method of agitation, and pH.[14–17] A decline in pH, related to normal cell glycolysis and the production of lactic acid and carbon dioxide, triggers disc-to-sphere shape change in PLT, pseudopod formation, and platelet granule release. When the pH drops below 6.0, the shape change becomes irreversible, and in vivo recovery and survival is markedly reduced. The decrease in pH varies with the number of PLT and contaminating white cells and the buffering capacity of the suspending fluid or plasma.

Maintenance of pH also depends on the permeability of the storage bag to oxygen and carbon dioxide. PLT stored in standard blood bags made of polyvinyl chloride (PVC) and a 2-diethylhexyl phthalate (DEHP) plasticizer have a shelf life of only 3 days. Plastics with better gas permeability are now in common use: polyolefin with no plasticizer (Fenwal PL732 bag, Baxter Healthcare Corp, Fenwal Division, Deerfield, IL), PVC with a trimellitate non-DEHP plasticizer (Fenwal PL1240 and Bayer CLX bags, Bayer-Biological Products, Covina, CA), PVC with a 2-DEHP plasticizer (Terumo XT612, Terumo Medical, Somerset, NJ), and PVC with a butyrl-trihexylcitrate plasticizer (Fenwal PL2209). Platelets prepared in these bags are licensed for 5-day storage.

Gentle agitation during storage is needed to facilitate gas exchange within the bag and reduce the formation of platelet aggregates, even though the shear stress associated with agitation contributes to platelet activation and lysis. Three kinds of agitators have been developed and evaluated: flatbeds,[18–21] circular (end-over-end) rotators,[22] and elliptical (side-over-side) rotators.[22] Most combinations of bag/rotator storage are suitable for 5-day preservation, but some perform better than others. For example, polyolefin bags without plasticizer (Fenwal PL732) work best with circular rotators or flatbed agitators, and PVC bags with plasticizer (Fenwal PL1240 and Bayer CLX) work best with circular or elliptical rotators. Platelet storage in Fenwal PL732 bags with 6-rpm elliptical rotation is not recommended.[22] Agitation is not critical for platelets stored 1 to 6°C because the cold temperature decreases metabolism and carbon dioxide production.

Granulocytes

Granulocytes are best transfused as soon as possible after collection but may be stored between 20 and 24°C for up to 24 hours.[1] Their storage capability is both fragile and complex. Locomotion is the most labile function that limits storage. Chemotaxis is well enough preserved up to 8 hours but is impaired by 24 hours. Microbial killing and phagocytotic activity is well preserved.[23]

Currently, granulocytes are stored without agitation.[24] McCullough et al.[25] reported that agitation during storage can decrease chemotaxis and the microbial killing function of granulocytes and increase the hemolysis of any RBC present. However, Miyamato and Sasakawa[26] evaluated the effect of 80-rpm horizontal rotation on granulocytes prepared from WB buffy coats and found no hemolysis or significant changes in cell count, morphology, phagocytosis, or microbial killing; they recommend gentle agitation to preserve a pH of 7.2.

Derivative Storage

Expiration dates and storage requirements vary with the specific derivative and are detailed in the package instructions. Manufacturers do not recommend frozen storage, especially for products stored in glass bottles. Freezing may cause IgG molecules to aggregate and small cracks to develop in glass that then permit bacterial entry. Most recommend that any unused portion of a derivative be discarded after 3 or 4 hours to reduce the risks of contamination.

Donor Testing

A sample of donor blood, not exceeding 30 ml, is collected at the time of donation and tested in accordance with state and federal regulations. These tests are identified in the FDA required *Circular of Information for the Use of Human Blood and Blood Components,* a pamphlet provided by blood suppliers that should be made available to all transfusionists.

The ABO group is determined with anti-A, anti-B, A_1 cells, and B cells. Rh type is determined with anti-D and an appropriate control system to detect false-positive results. RBC that type D− are tested for weak D (D^u) antigen expression. Units testing positive for D or weak D are labeled "Rh positive." Those negative for both tests are labeled "Rh negative." Routine testing for other antigens is neither required nor encouraged. Any and all discrepancies must be resolved before the unit is released to stock.

Donors who have been pregnant or transfused are screened for unexpected clinically significant antibodies. When such antibodies are found, the plasma portion of the unit is not used for transfusion. Techniques for detecting donor antibodies need not be as sensitive as those used for testing recipients; a pooled screening cell reagent can be used to test pools of several (two to five) donor sera. If the pool is nonreactive, all donors in the pool are considered negative. If the pool is positive, all sera in the pool are retested individually.

Tests currently required to prevent disease transmission are listed in Table 13-3. Units that test repeatedly reactive or positive for these tests cannot be used for allogenic transfusion. Instead, they are appropriately discarded, and the donors are notified of their abnormal results as national, state, and local practice dictate. See Section V for a complete review

Table 13-3. Current Donor Disease Testing

Test	Implemented	Purpose
Serologic test for syphilis	(1920s)	Determines previous exposure to syphilis; surrogate test for high-risk behavior.
HBsAg	(early 1970s)	Detects hepatitis B surface antigen.
Anti-HIV	March 1985	Detects antibody to the human immunodeficiency virus, types 1 and 2.
ALT	November 1986	Detects alanine aminotransferase; surrogate test for hepatitis C.[a]
Anti-HBc	Initiated: 1987 Licensed: March 1991	Detects antibody to hepatitis B core antigen; surrogate test for hepatitis C; high prevalence in HIV+ individuals.
Anti-HTLV	November 1988	Detects antibody to human T-cell lymphotropic virus, type I.
Anti-HCV	May 1990	Detects antibody to hepatitis C virus.

[a] 1995, ALT no longer required.

of transfusion-transmitted infectious diseases. Currently, testing donors for antibody to CMV is optional.

Disease test methods are constantly improving. When new tests are required, blood banks make every effort to "back-test" all units in their existing inventories as quickly as possible. Because such testing is usually not possible on older frozen RBC units, some facilities freeze a corresponding aliquot of donor serum on all frozen RBC units to make them easier to test fully should this situation occur.

Labeling

Blood bag labels should conform to FDA requirements and follow uniform labeling guidelines.[9] Essential label items include the product's name and identity, ABO/Rh type, and the manufacturer's identity. Although label information must be eye readable, machine-readable bar codes can be added for computerized processing and inventory control. Blood labels also reference the *Circular of Information for the Use of Human Blood and Blood Components.*

Every effort is made to reduce errors during the labeling process. The work area should be quiet, with minimal distractions. Many blood banks incorporate manual or computerized "doublecheck" systems into their procedure to verify label accuracy. Although previous records and results are never used to label a unit, they are checked to confirm the unit's ABO/Rh type and acceptability before the label is applied.

Laboratories must establish safeguards to make sure untested products are not issued for transfusion. If a product must be released before testing is complete, its label must clearly indicate the tests not done and carry the statement "for emergency use only." Records should document the urgent circumstances.

Transport and Shipping

Two factors must be considered when preparing blood for transport and shipping: (1) optimal storage temperature should be maintained to ensure product quality and (2) packaging methods should ensure the safety of transport personnel.[2] In addition, all units must be inspected before transport and, if abnormal in appearance, should be quarantined for further evaluation.

Units transported short distances within a facility (i.e., from the hospital blood bank to the patient's room) need no special packaging as long as the temperature of the blood does not exceed storage or transport limits. For example, RBC temperature must be maintained between 1 and 10°C during transport. An RBC removed from 5°C storage will reach the upper limit of 10°C in 30 minutes if transported at an ambient temperature of 25°C.[27] If temperature maintenance is a concern, blood can be packaged in an insulated container with ice or other appropriate coolant. Such systems, if used, must be periodically monitored for function, and transport staff must be appropriately trained.

For long-distance shipping and when shipments are handled by personnel not under the direct authority of the shipper, blood units (including untested units from healthy donors) are shipped as "biologic products" for which the government has established minimal packaging requirements.[28,29] Individual carrier services may have additional requirements. Containers should be able to maintain temperatures and withstand leakage, pressure, and other conditions incidental to ordinary handling. Packing methods must be monitored periodically to ensure proper temperature maintenance.

Autologous Requirements

Units intended for autologous transfusion should be tested and labeled according to the American Association of Blood Banks (AABB) *Standards for Blood Banks and Transfusion Services* unless these are superseded by FDA requirements.[1] The ABO and Rh type must be determined, but antibody screening and disease testing are optional for units collected and transfused within the same facility. If blood is to be shipped outside the collecting facility, disease testing must be done on at least the first unit from a given donor during a 30-day period.

Units must carry the patient's name, an identification number (in the absence of a hospital number, a birthdate or social security number is acceptable), the ABO and Rh type, transfusing hospital, and, if the blood does not meet all allogenic donor criteria, a label prominently stating "For autologous use only."

When the results of testing for hepatitis B surface antigen (HBsAg), hepatitis C virus, and human immunodeficiency virus (HIV) are confirmed to be pos-

Table 13-4. Summary of Blood Components and Derivatives

Component	Contents	Volume	QC Requirements	Indications	Contraindications	Dose	Transfusion Considerations
Whole Blood (WB)	450 ml of donor blood plus AP solution. Few viable PLT or WBC. ↓ Factor V and VIII. Hct: 30–40%, WBC: 10^9	~500 ml	450 ± 45 ml of donor blood	Acute hypovolemia; massive transfusion, exchange transfusion	Condition responsive to a specific component.	As needed for replacement: Adults: 1 unit ↑ Hct 3% ↑ Hgb 1 g/dl Infants: 3 ml/kg ↑ Hgb 1 g/dl	Must be ABO identical, crossmatch compatible. Infuse as fast as patient tolerates
Red Blood Cells (RBC)	CPD, CPDA-1: WB with 200–250 ml of plasma removed. Hct: 70–80% AS: WB with most plasma removed and 100 ml of AS added. Hct: 50–60%.	CPD, CPDA-1: ~250 ml AS: ~350 ml	Hct must be ≤80%	Symptomatic anemia	Pharmacologically treatable anemia	Same as WB	Must be ABO compatible, crossmatch compatible. Allow 10 min of preparation time if packed just before issue. Infuse within 4 hr or as patient tolerates.
Red Blood Cells, Washed (W-RBC)	RBC washed with 1–2 L of normal saline to remove non-RBC elements. Depending on method: RBC ↓ 20%, WBC ↓ 85%, plasma ↓ 99%	~300 ml	Plasma removal. WBC count if used as leukocyte reduced.	Symptomatic anemia plus history of repeated allergic/febrile reactions; paroxysmal nocturnal hemoglobinuria	Pharmacologically treatable anemia	Same as WB	Must be ABO compatible, crossmatch compatible. Allow 20–30 min preparation time. Infuse as RBC.
Red Blood Cells, Frozen-Deglycerolized (F/D-RBC)	RBC frozen with glycerol, which is washed away before transfusion. Contains >80% original RBC, 10^7 WBC, minimal plasma, resuspended in normal saline.	200–300 ml	80% recovery of original RBC mass after deglycerolization; <1% residual glycerol (420 mOsm); <300 mg of residual free Hgb. WBC count if used as leukocyte reduced.	Prolonged storage for rare or autologous units. Symptomatic anemia, see W-RBC.	Pharmacologically treatable anemia	Same as WB	Must be ABO compatible, crossmatch compatible. Allow ~1 hr preparation time. Infuse as RBC.
Platelets (PLT)	>5.5 × 10^{10} PLT plus plasma, hemostatic levels of clotting factors, 10^8 WBC, trace to 0.5 ml of RBC.	~50 ml	>5.5 × 10^{10} PLT, pH 6.0 at end of storage. Prepared within 8 hr of WB collection.	Bleeding related to thrombocytopenia or PLT dysfunction. Low PLT count.	Hemostatic problem not related to PLT.	To ↑PLT count by 50,000/μl: Adults: 1 U/10 kg of body weight. Infants: 5 ml/kg of body weight.	Should be ABO compatible with patient RBC if possible. Allow 10–20 min to pool before transfusion. Infuse 5–10 ml/min or as patient tolerates.

Component	Composition/Content	Volume	Tests	Indications	Contraindications	Dosage	Special Instructions
Platelets, Pheresis (PLT-P)	>3×10^{11} PLT plus plasma, hematostatic levels of clotting factors, 10^6–10^8 WBC, trace to 5 ml of RBC.	300–500 ml	3×10^{11} PLT, pH 6.0 at end of storage.	See PLT. Refractory patients needing HLA-matched, crossmatch compatible, or HLA antigen negative PLT. Helps ↓ donor exposures.	Hemostatic problem not related to PLT.	1 U = 6–8 PLT or 1 hemostatic dose for adults.	Should be ABO compatible with patient's RBC if possible. Allow 1 hr if volume reduction is needed. Infuse 5–10 ml/min or as patient tolerates.
Red Blood Cells or Platelets, Leukocyte Reduced	RBC or PLT/PLT-P with ↓ WBC: <5×10^8 to ↓ febrile transfusion reactions; <5×10^6 to ↓ alloimmunization and CMV transmission.	~ to original component.	WBC counts; 80% recovery of RBC.	RBC or PLT indications plus history of repeated febrile transfusion reactions; patient at risk from becoming refractory to PLTs; patient at risk for CMV infection.	See RBC or PLT contraindications	See RBC or PLT	See RBC or PLT. Allow 30–60 min if prepared before transfusion.
Granulocytes	Apheresis: 1×10^{10} WBC in fresh plasma; PLT and RBC varies with collection method. *Buffy coat:* 10^9 WBC in fresh plasma, heavy RBC contamination	Apheresis: 200–400 ml Buffy coat: 30–50 ml	WBC counts	Severe neutropenia or WBC dysfunction with infection unresponsive to antibiotic therapy.	Effective antibiotic therapy available.	Adults: 1 or more U daily until WBC >500/µL. Infants: 10^9 WBC daily.	Should be ABO compatible with patient serum; crossmatch compatible if >5 ml of RBC present. Do not transfuse with depth microaggregate or leukocyte-removal filters. Transfuse slowly over 2–4 hr.
Fresh Frozen Plasma (FFP)	Plasma plus AP solution from 1 U of WB. Contains ~400 mg fibrinogen and 200 U of other clotting factors.	200–250 ml	Separate and place in freezer within 8 hr of WB collection.	Bleeding related to clotting factor deficiencies where factor concentrates are not available or are contraindicated: multiple deficiencies, severe liver diseases, warfarin reversal, TTP, DIC	Deficiency corrected with pharmacologic agent or factor concentrate; volume expansion; nutrition source.	10 ml/kg of body weight. 15 ml/kg may be needed for initial dose.	Should be ABO compatible. Allow 15–30 min to thaw. Infuse 5–10 ml/min or as patient tolerates.

(Continued)

Table 13-4. *(Continued)*

Component	Contents	Volume	QC Requirements	Indications	Contraindications	Dose	Transfusion Considerations
Plasma; Liquid Plasma	Plasma plus AP solution. Contains ~200 U of stable clotting factors. May have ↓ factors V, VIII and fibrinogen.	180–300 ml	Must be separated from WB before 5 days postexpiration.	See FFP	Know factor V or VIII deficiency.	Same as FFP	Same as FFP
Cryoprecipitated Antihemophilic Factor (CRYO)	80–120 U of factor VIII. 150–250 mg of fibrinogen, 30–50 mg of fibronectin, and 40–70% of the original plasma vWF and 30% factor XIII. Resuspended in donor plasma.	5–15 ml	Factor VIII: C (80 U) Fibrinogen assay optional.	Bleeding related to hemophilia A, von Willebrand's disease, factor XIII or fibrinogen deficiency or dysfunction; fibrin sealant for topical hemostasis in surgery; bleeding related to uremia, uncertain.	Safer or more concentrated therapy is available. Clotting defect not known.	Based on plasma volume and desired factor level. 8–10 bags = 2 g of fibrinogen.	Consider alternative therapies. Should be ABO compatible if possible. Allow 5–10 min to thaw and 15 min to pool. Transfuse 5–10 ml/min or as patient tolerates.
Factor VIII Concentrates	Lyophilized concentrate of factor VIII; activity units are on label. Consult manufacturer: only some may contain vWF.	10–30 ml	—	Treatment for moderate to severe factor VIII deficiency (hemophilia A)	Bleeding not associated with factor VIII deficiency. Monoclonal product: hypersensitivity to mouse protein.	Based on plasma volume and desired factor level: 1 U/kg ↑ activity level 2%.	Reconstitute per manufacturer's directions. Give IV by syringe push.
Factor IX Concentrates (Prothrombin Complex)	Lyophilized concentrates of factor IX plus some factors II, VII, and X; protein C; and ABO antibody, depending on method of preparation.	10–30 ml	—	Treatment for severe factor IX deficiency (hemophilia B) or specific factor deficiencies.	Bleeding not associated with specific factor deficiencies. Patients with liver disease or those at risk from thrombosis.	Based on plasma volume and desired factor level: 1 activity U/kg ↑ activity level 1%.	Reconstitute per manufacturer's directions. Give IV by syringe push.
Albumin; Plasma Protein Fraction (PPF)	Albumin: 5% or 25% protein solution; ~96% albumin, 4% globulin. PPF: 5% protein solution; ~83% albumin, 17% αβ globulin. All products have Na content ~145 mEq/L.	50 or 250 ml	—	Large, acute colloid losses occurring with hypovolemic shock or severe burns; blood pressure support during hypotensive episodes.	Nutritional hypoproteinemia; chronic hypoalbuminemia; or when crystalloids can be as effective. 25% albumin is not for dehydrated patients or those at risk of circulatory overload.	Shock: determined by patient's condition and response. Burns: as needed to maintain protein level of 5.2 g/dl.	No filter required. Do not infuse PPF intra-arterially or >10 ml/min. PPF has been reported to cause hemolysis when mixed with older RBC.

Product	Composition	Volume		Indications	Contraindications	Dose	Special Notes
Immune Serum Globulin (ISG)	IM preparations: 16-g/dl protein solution. IV preparations: 5-g/dl protein solution. Primarily IgG, some IgM and IgA.	Varies	—	Prophylactic passive immunity for immuno-incompetent patients or those at risk of disease. Thrombocytopenia associated ITP, AIDS, Kawasaki syndrome. IVIG is indicated for high-dose therapy or patients who cannot tolerate IM injection.	Known severe anaphylactic reaction to plasma.	Depends on therapeutic indication, patient size, and type of product given.	No filter required. Must be given via designated IM or IV route.
Rh Immune Globulin (RhIG)	ISG containing purified anti-D. Full dose vial: ~300 μg of anti-D Mini dose vial: ~50 μg of anti-D	~1 ml, depending on concentration of IgG	—	To prevent Rh-negative individuals from becoming sensitized to D antigen after exposure to Rh-positive RBC by pregnancy or transfusion. Rh-positive patients with thrombocytopenia related to ITP or AIDS.	Recipient is already sensitized to D. Fetus or newborn is known to be Rh negative.	20 μg of RhIG/1 ml of RBC exposure: full dose protects against 15 ml of RBC, minidose protects against 2.5 ml of RBC. Termination of pregnancy within first 12 weeks: 1 minidose. All other situations: 1 full dose or more as indicated.	No filter required. Give IM per manufacturer's directions. At delivery, assess for fetal-maternal hemorrhage.

Abbreviations: AP, anticoagulant-preservative; PLT, platelets, pheresis; WBC, white blood cells; Hct, hematocrit; CPD, citrate-phosphate-dextrose anticoagulant; CPDA-1, citrate-phosphate-dextrose-adenine anticoagulant; RBC, red blood cells; WB, whole blood; Hgb, hemoglobin; CMV, cytomegalovirus; CRYO, cryoprecipitate; vWF, von Willebrand factor; TTP, thrombotic thrombocytopenic purpura; DIC, disseminated intravascular coagulation; PPF, plasma protein fraction; IV, intravenous, IM, intramuscular; ISG, immune serum globulin; RhIG, Rh immune globulin; ITP, idiopathic thrombocytopenic purpura; AIDS, acquired immunodeficiency syndrome; IVG, intravenous immune globulin.

itive, a biohazard label is affixed to the unit. If autologous units that test positive for any disease marker are shipped, the transfusing facility will be notified in advance. In some cases (i.e., when HB_sAg or HIV is confirmed), the transfusing facility and the patient's physician will be asked to provide written approval for shipment.

If patients do not use their autologous units and it is acceptable for homologous transfusion, standard testing, acceptability, and labeling requirements must be met, and all patient identity marks must be removed.

Quality Assessment

Facilities that prepare blood components must comply with the FDA's good manufacturing practices and monitor the variables involved in production: reagents, equipment, personnel, and the blood products themselves.[2] Reagents are tested each day of use, and equipment is checked periodically for proper function. Personnel performance is documented by observation, annual review, and competency evaluation programs. These variables, plus general laboratory procedures, are also evaluated with the use of national proficiency samples.

Component quality is demonstrated by testing representative samples to make sure that they meet the product definition and/or by documenting the method of production. Standard quality control requirements are summarized in Table 13-4. Routine sterility testing is not required but may be desirable when special components are made or when a unit is found to have an abnormal appearance on inspection. Such testing should be performed under conditions that can detect the cryophilic organisms associated with contaminated blood.

BLOOD PRODUCT DESCRIPTIONS

The separation of WB into blood components and derivatives allows the blood bank to maintain a stock inventory of different products to meet specific transfusion needs. Frequently used components and derivatives are described in Table 13-4 with a brief summary of indications/contraindications of use and general transfusion considerations.

To understand the appropriate use and total effect of a blood component or derivative better, the clinician must keep in mind "real product" content. For example, a unit of WB contains more than RBC for oxygen delivery and plasma for volume expansion. Although blood stored more than 24 hours between 1 and 6°C has few viable PLT and granulocytes, some functioning lymphocytes persist throughout storage. Stable coagulation factors II, VII, IX, and X and fibrinogen are also well maintained. Heat-labile coagulation factors V and VIII decrease with time and are not considered adequate to correct specific deficiencies in bleeding patients, but levels of 30 percent for factor V and 15 to 20 percent for factor VIII have been reported in WB stored 21 days.[30,31] The AP solution plus the natural metabolic changes that take place during storage also result in biochemical alterations unique to in vitro storage (see Ch. 25 and 41). These changes are not significant in most transfusion situations.

Most units of PLT contain more platelets, often 6 to 8×10^{10}, than standards require. PLT plasma has hemostatic levels of coagulation factors; activity levels of 47 and 68 percent have been reported for factors V and VII, respectively, in PLT stored 72 hours at 22°C.[32] Each bag also contains a small volume (trace to 0.5 ml) of RBC and a significant number (about 10^8) of white cells, but this number in both PLT and PLT-P can vary tremendously, depending on preparation and handling methods.[33–36]

Meeting Special Patient Needs

Common components may need to be modified to meet special patient needs. These are summarized below and presented in detail in other chapters of this book. Physicians should be aware of the time required to prepare these components for transfusion. Some procedures significantly alter expiration date. If they are not used by the patient for whom they were intended, the blood bank will attempt, if appropriate, to use them for other patient orders rather than let them expire.

Irradiated Blood

Blood components that contain viable lymphocytes are irradiated to reduce the risk of graft-versus-host disease in susceptible patients, which include those who have undergone bone marrow or peripheral blood progenitor cell transplantation, those with congenital immunodeficiencies, and those who are temporarily immunocompromised: patients undergoing chemotherapy; fetuses receiving intrauterine transfusion; newborns receiving exchange transfusion; and recipients of blood donated by blood relatives (see Ch. 42).

The recommended dose of γ radiation is a minimum of 25 Gy targeted to the central portion of the blood container, with no less than 15 Gy targeted to the outer portions.[1] This dose abrogates lymphocyte growth without causing significant damage to the in vitro and in vivo functions of PLT and granulocytes within their approved storage periods. RBC, however, show a doubling of supernatant potassium levels within 1 to 2 days of irradiation, a ratio that persists throughout storage.[37] Because of this damage, the shelf life of irradiated RBC is limited to the originally assigned expiration date or 28 days from the date of irradiation, whichever comes first.[1] Bag labels will reflect this modification.

Blood is irradiated using self-contained cesium-137 or cobalt-60 irradiators or cobalt-60 teletherapy units. This process may take as little as a few minutes or up to several hours, depending on the size of the γ-ray source and the location and availability of the equipment.[37] Physicians should keep preparation time in mind when writing blood orders.

Leukocyte-Reduced Red Blood Cells and Platelets

Patients at risk from HLA alloimmunization, who may require prolonged PLT therapy and become refractory, or those who are already immunized and experience febrile nonhemolytic reactions should receive leukocyte-reduced RBC and PLT components. Leukocyte reduction may also benefit patients by reducing the risks of CMV transmission[38,39] and bacterial contamination.[40] Current standards require leukocyte reduction methods to reduce the total white cell count in a blood bag to below 5×10^8, if the intent is to prevent febrile nonhemolytic transfusion reactions, but below 5×10^6 to prevent HLA alloimmunization or CMV infection.[1]

Many methods have been used to reduce the number of leukocytes in RBC and PLT components with varying degrees of efficiency: centrifugation, buffy coat removal, saline washing, freezing and deglycerolization, and filtration.[41–43] Only modern third-generation leukocyte-removal filters reliably provide 99.9 percent (log 3) or greater white cell removal so that the final product meets the 5×10^6 require-

ment. These filters contain multiple layers of synthetic nonwoven fibers that selectively retain white cells while allowing RBC and/or PLT to pass through. Selective retention is based on cell size, surface tension characteristics, surface charge density differences between blood cells, and possibly, cell-to-cell interactions and cell activation and adhesion properties.[44] Leukocyte-removal filters for RBC and PLT filtration are not identical and not interchangeable.

Special filter and set configurations are commercially available for prestorage filtration, laboratory filtration before issue, or bedside use. Manufacturer's directions must be followed carefully, and filters must be used only for their intended product. White cell counts should be performed periodically to ensure the performance of the sets or systems in use. Because routine automated methods for counting white cells are not sensitive enough to monitor product quality, more effective high-volume manual counting chambers or flow cytometric procedures are recommended.[45,46]

Washed Red Blood Cells and Platelets

Washing a unit of RBC with 1 to 2 L of sterile normal saline removes about 99 percent of plasma proteins, electrolytes, and antibodies. Overriding the photo cell on automated wash machines or taking care to remove the buffy coat during manual washes can reduce the white cell count 10-fold, but this level of removal is insufficient to prevent HLA sensitization. Washed RBC units reduce the incidence of febrile and urticarial reactions and, if washed with large enough volumes of saline, anaphylactic reaction.[2]

Procedures for washing PLT with normal saline[47,48] or saline buffered with ACD-A or citrate[49,50] recover about 90 percent of the original PLT and reduce the plasma content about 95 percent. The white cell count in these units is not significantly altered, so washed PLT may be beneficial for patients experiencing severe allergic reactions but may not reduce febrile reactions. Studies show that saline washing does not significantly alter clot retraction ability; PLT size distribution; PLT morphology; hypotonic shock recovery; or aggregation response to arachidonic acid, collagen, adenosine diphosphate, and epinephrine. These data parallel in vivo observations that show similar post-transfusion increments with washed and unwashed platelets. Pineda et al.[49] observed that washed labeled PLT, regardless of the wash solution, have decreased in vivo recovery, but those that are recovered have normal survival. Platelets washed with ACD-A buffered saline are reported to have better recovery than those washed in unbuffered saline. Those washed in unbuffered saline (pH 4.5 to 5.5) contained substantially more IgA protein than did PLT washed in citrate-buffered saline (pH 6.5 to 6.8).[50]

Resuspending and storing PLT in balanced salt solutions, including the commercially available intravenous solution Plasmalyte-A (Baxter Healthcare Corp, Deerfield, IL), has also been shown to maintain and, in some cases, improve PLT quality.[51–53]

Volume-Reduced Platelets

Rarely, a patient who needs PLT transfusion is not able to tolerate the volume of plasma, plasma protein, or chemical contents of PLT or PLT-P products. To remedy this, the PLT or PLT-P can be centrifuged shortly before transfusion and excess plasma removed (70 to 80 percent, if needed). Centrifuged PLT must be allowed to rest at room temperature, without agitation, for 20 to 60 minutes before being resuspended in the remaining plasma and transfused. These manipulations produce a 15 to 55 percent loss of PLT, depending on the centrifugation force and time.[2]

Volume-reduced PLT should be transfused as soon as possible after preparation. Pisciotto et al.[54] report acceptable in vitro storage characteristics in PLT volume reduced to 20 to 25 ml and stored in syringes up to 6 hours at 20 to 24°C. However, volume-reduced syringe preparations should not be left in infant incubators for extended times because rapid pH drops were noted at temperatures of 37°C.

Aliquot Preparations

When a less than full unit of blood or blood component is needed for transfusion, it is preferable to split the contents into smaller aliquots and issue just the volume needed (storing the rest for later transfusion) than it is to send the entire bag and have the unused portion discarded. Such maneuvers help conserve the blood supply and reduce the number of donors a patient is exposed to when multiple small-volume transfusions are needed, as in neonatal practice.

Ideally, aliquots are transferred from the "mother unit" into integrally attached satellite bags or bags connected by a sterile connecting device (see component fractionation above) so that component dating is not shortened. Small aliquots can also be drawn into syringes using resealable medical injection site couplers or into bags connected by opened port, but this changes the dating of the mother unit and all aliquots prepared from it to 24 hours or less. Aliquot containers should contain the volume of component the patient needs plus the estimated volume that will be lost to the infusion set and tubing. Container labels should parallel those on their larger counterparts, but this may be difficult because of size. Photocopying and reducing the label on the mother unit can help blood banks meet this requirement.

Alternative methods of maintaining inventories of small-volume RBC include collecting half-units every 4 weeks from cooperative donors or routinely collecting the maximum 495 ml of WB from donors and transferring 30 to 60 ml to an attached empty satellite bag for use as a separate pediatric unit.[2]

Fibrin Sealant

The fibrinogen in CRYO has been used in cardiovascular surgery as a topical hemostatic fibrin sealant or fibrin glue.[55] The contents of one to two bags of thawed CRYO are drawn into a syringe and applied to the bleeding surface simultaneously with topical thrombin (usually of bovine origin) that has been drawn into a second syringe. The fibrinogen reacts with the thrombin to form a fibrin clot.

Some patients exposed to fibrin sealant have developed inhibitors to bovine thrombin and human factor V. These inhibitors result in abnormal thrombin time assays that use bovine thrombin reagents and have been considered responsible for postoperative bleeding.[56]

PRETRANSFUSION PROCEDURES

The Physician's Order

The administration of blood components or derivatives begins with the physician's assessment of patient need and a written order specifying the product to be given, the amount or volume, and special administration requirements, if needed. This order, when forwarded to the laboratory by form or computer, must indicate the patient's first and last name, hospital identification number, the product requested, and the date of transfusion. The laboratory should refuse to accept requests with inadequate or illegible information. Telephone orders are accepted in urgent situations but should be followed up with a standard request.

Providing the patient's age or birthdate, diagnosis, and the requesting physician's name is very helpful if questions arise during testing. Nursing and laboratory staff are trained to verify the order and check it against the patient's current clinical status and laboratory data whenever possible. All questions are clarified with the physician before transfusion is started.

Coupled with the physician's decision to transfuse is the responsibility to obtain informed consent and to explain the treatment along with its benefits, risks, and alternative therapies. This communication between patient and physician must be documented in an acceptable manner (see Ch. 14). Some states have passed legislation that requires physicians to inform their patients of the risks and alternatives to allogeneic transfusion (e.g., autologous and directed donation) unless there is an emergency or medical contraindication.

Specimen Requirements

Proper identification of the sample is the first step in transfusion safety. The information on the transfusion request is compared with the patients' identification bands and tube labels, and patients are asked to identify themselves. Any discrepancy in the information must be resolved before the specimen is drawn. Hospitals must establish a procedure for emergency situations when an identification band is not immediately available. Special blood bank identification systems have been developed to meet this need and are commercially available.

Tube labels must carry the patient's first and last name, hospital identification number, and collection date, and there must be a mechanism for identifying the phlebotomist.[1] The labels and/or request form must be signed or initialed. The label is placed on the tube before the phlebotomist leaves the bedside.

Serum or plasma can be used for compatibility testing, but serum is preferred for most test systems

(see Ch. 9). Care must be taken to avoid hemolysis during collection because free hemoglobin can mask antibody-induced hemolysis in compatibility tests. The volume of serum needed depends on the number of tests performed, the methods used, and the patient's hematocrit level; a routine 3-unit crossmatch order can be completed with a 5-ml clotted specimen. However, most blood banks request 10-ml specimens to standardize collection procedures and avoid having to draw more if a compatibility problem is encountered. Infant sample requirements are discussed later in this chapter.

If a patient has been transfused or pregnant within the past 3 months, the specimen used for pretransfusion testing must be drawn within 3 days of the intended transfusion so that it reflects the patient's current alloantibody status.[1] For convenience, because this information often is not known, most blood banks set a 3-day limit for all specimens. If it is known with certainty and documented that the patient has not been recently transfused or pregnant, the specimen may be used for an extended time. This can be helpful in managing preadmission specimen collections, especially for patients admitted for same-day surgery.

All patient specimens are stoppered and stored between 1 to 6°C for at least 7 days after transfusion so that they are available for additional testing if a patient has a delayed reaction. Samples of blood from units transfused, usually a segment from the donor bag, must also be saved 7 days post-transfusion. If a segment is not set aside when the unit was placed in inventory or crossmatched, the blood bank will remove one at the time of issue.

Laboratory Testing

Compatibility testing must be performed before all RBC transfusions. The reader should refer to Chapter 9 for a complete discussion of this topic. Pretransfusion testing is not required for non-RBC products such as plasma and PLT, but the patient's ABO/Rh type should be known if compatible products are needed.

Physicians should become familiar with the compatibility policies and time requirements of their facility's blood bank. If blood is urgently needed before testing is complete, the physician can authorize its immediate release by signing an emergency release request.

Blood Selection

ABO compatibility is the single most important factor in selecting blood for transfusion because the accidental transfusion of group A or B RBC into someone with pre-existing anti-A or anti-B can cause an immediate and severe hemolytic transfusion reaction. Rh compatibility is the second most important factor because the D antigen is very immunogenic and anti-D can cause severe hemolytic disease of the newborn. ABO and Rh compatibility guidelines are given in Table 13-5. After ABO and Rh selection criteria are met, the hospital's inventory control policies are considered.[2] It is prudent to select the oldest units first to avoid having them expire unused.

ABO Compatibility

WB, which contains both RBC and plasma, must be ABO identical with the patient. When donor RBC and plasma are separated, more selection options are available. RBC products need only be compatible with the patient's serum, and plasma products should be compatible with the patient's RBC whenever possible.

Although it is ideal to give ABO-identical PLT, few blood banks have the inventory to do this exclusively. When ABO-identical PLT are not available, any ABO group can be provided (see Ch. 16). Incompatible PLT plasma generally causes no ill effects, although the patient may develop a positive direct antiglobulin test result and, rarely, immune hemolysis. These same considerations apply to CRYO.

ABO-identical granulocyte components are preferred because they are contaminated with RBC and contain a significant volume of plasma. Any bag that contains more than 5 ml of RBC should be ABO compatible with the patient's serum and crossmatched like standard RBCs.

Rh Compatibility

Rh-positive individuals can receive Rh-positive or Rh-negative RBC components. Rh-negative individuals should receive only Rh-negative red cells to avoid becoming sensitized to the D antigen. Rarely, Rh-negative patients who do not have anti-D are given Rh-positive blood when Rh-negative blood is not available and transfusion is urgent. Preferably, this practice is limited to male patients and women beyond their childbearing years. Rh sensitization of premenopausal female patients should be avoided, if at all possible.

FFP and CRYO do not contain RBC. The Rh type may appear on their unit labels, but it need not be considered in their selection. Although PLT do not carry Rh antigen, Rh-negative recipients can become sensitized from contaminating red cells.[57] Although the risk of this occurring is small, blood banks give Rh-negative platelets to Rh-negative recipients whenever possible, especially to Rh-negative female patients who might bear children. If Rh-positive platelets must be transfused, physicians can consider giving Rh immune globulin to prevent immunization. One standard vial of Rh immune globulin provides protection for 30 or more bags of PLT prepared from WB donations or 3 to 6 bags of PLT-P, depending on the volume and final hematocrit of the PLT-P.

Component Preparation

Some blood components require additional preparation before they can be transfused (Table 13-4). Because these steps take time to complete and can

Table 13-5. ABO and Rh Compatibility Guidelines

Patient's Blood Group	Antigens on Red Cells	Antibodies in Serum	Compatible Red Cell Products	Compatible Plasma Products
A	A	Anti-B	A, O	A,AB
B	B	Anti-A	B,O	B,AB
AB	A and B	—	AB,A,B,O	AB only
O	—	Anti-A and anti-B	O only	O,A,B,AB
Rh-positive	D	—	Rh-positive, Rh-negative	—
Rh-negative	—	Anti-D if sensitized	Rh-negative	—

significantly shorten a product's shelf life, they must be carefully coordinated with the expected time of transfusion. Every effort is made to begin component preparation early enough so that it is ready when needed but not so early that it expires before use.

To prepare frozen FFP and CRYO for transfusion, the bags are thawed at temperatures of 30 to 37°C with gentle agitation. Circulating water baths are most commonly used, but microwave ovens have been successfully adapted to thaw FFP.[58,59] The thawing process may take up to 0.5 hour, depending on component volume and the number of units being thawed at one time. After thawing, FFP is stored between 1 and 6°C to preserve clotting factors V and VIII; CRYO is stored between 20 to 24°C to prevent reprecipitation and subsequent loss of the concentrated factors during transfusion.[60] These temperatures are not ideal for factor VIII storage; so the shelf life is shortened to 24 and 6 hours, respectively. Data suggest that CRYO storage can be extended to 24 hours if it is used as a source of fibrinogen.[60]

Before frozen RBCs can be transfused, they must be thawed, and the cryoprotectant must be removed, a process called deglycerolization. Deglycerolized RBC expire in 24 hours because they are prepared in an opened system. This time might be extended if sterile "closed" systems were available.[61]

Blood banks often pool ABO-identical units of PLT or CRYO into one bag for easier administration when an order for multiple units is received. Pools can take 10 to 20 minutes to prepare and routinely expire in 4 hours because of the potential for bacterial contamination. However, pools of 1-day-old PLT prepared with a sterile connecting device have been shown to be stored satisfactorily up to 5 days, provided that the final container is appropriate for the increased volume and PLT number.[62]

Patient Preparation

Patients should be told of the events that will occur during transfusion to reduce their anxiety. They should also be instructed to report any changes or symptoms during and after a transfusion, but this does not substitute for careful patient observation.

Before sending for the unit of blood, venous access should be established, according to accepted practice. If a pre-existing intravenous line is used, it must be checked for patency and signs of extravasation or infection. A saline drip can be used to maintain the line, but if the patient is volume restricted, the line can be capped off with a heparin lock until it is needed. Because a transfusion may take several hours, the patient should be made as comfortable as possible before starting.

The medical record must be checked for special instructions and premedication requirements. Most patients do not require premedication, but those with a history of allergic reactions may be given antihistamines in advance. The practice of routinely giving antipyretics to patients who have had a febrile reaction is controversial. Fever-reducing drugs can mask this symptom of hemolytic reactions, although they should not affect concurrent changes in blood pressure, pulse, or respiration.

Blood Issue

Patient caretakers should not send for the unit of blood until the patient is ready and the necessary equipment has been assembled. Transfusion services should have blood delivery policies in place and appropriate training programs for the staff assigned to this function.

Many laboratories require that two individuals, a laboratory staff member and the individual transporting the unit, confirm donor and patient identity and compatibility before it leaves the blood bank. The unit is inspected at this time for any unusual physical appearance that might indicate bacterial contamination: purple cells; purple, brown, or red plasma; a zone of hemolysis above the cell mass; visual clots or murkiness.[2] Any problem discovered must be resolved before the unit is issued.

Blood bank records must document the unit's identity, the person issuing the unit, the transporter or person receiving the unit, the visual inspection, and the date and time of issue. If the transfusion is delayed, the unit should be returned to the blood bank for proper storage and later reissue. Returned units are accepted for storage and reissue only if the container's closure has not been disturbed and transport temperature ranges have been maintained. The allowable "return time" is usually within 30 minutes of blood issue (see the previous section on Transport and Shipping).[27]

TRANSFUSION EQUIPMENT

Intravenous therapy has become a highly sophisticated technology.[63,64] Standards of practice for intravenous care are set by the Centers for Disease Control and Prevention, the Intravenous Nurses Society, equipment manufacturers' recommendations where applicable, and, to some extent for blood transfusion, the AABB. Many patients have pre-existing intravenous lines for chemotherapy, antibiotics, and total parenteral nutrition (TPN). Nurses have learned to adapt these lines to accommodate blood transfusion. Physicians likewise must be aware of what is in use so they can give appropriate guidelines.

Needles and Catheters

Many venous access devices are marketed for intravenous therapy and blood administration. Selection depends on venous integrity, the frequency and duration of treatment, and the administration requirements and toxicity cautions of the therapy being given.[63] All therapy needs are considered when venous access is established.

Peripheral Vein Access

Stainless steel needles are used for short-term or single-dose therapy because they are easy and less painful to insert, even though needle points can traumatize a vein and cause intravenous infiltration. Needles come in a variety of sizes and designs. They may be siliconized for smoother insertion or heparinized to reduce clot formation or have flexible wings for better insertion control and anchoring. Winged or butterfly sets have integrated extension tubing to help reduce the risks of contamination and infiltration.

Over-the-needle catheters have a plastic cannula that fits snugly over an introducing needle. Once positioned in the vein, the needle is removed, leaving only the flexible catheter. Although slightly more painful to insert, an over-the-needle catheter causes less trauma to the vein for short-term peripheral therapy. Peripheral vein catheters are changed every 48 to 72 hours.

Central Vein Access

Central vein (CV) catheters are used for medium- to long-term therapy (1 to 6 weeks) or when solutions are toxic or irritating to the vein lining and require immediate dilution. They are made of PVC, Teflon, polyurethane, or silicone and come in a variety of styles.

In-the-needle catheters are positioned in CVs by way of peripheral vein-introducing needles that are removable after placement. Percutaneous catheters are placed through special introducing needles and guidewires using an infraclavicular approach to the subclavian vein. Indwelling tunneled catheters and totally implanted ports are surgically implanted silicone catheters designed for long-term therapy. With proper care, they may last up to several years. Indwelling tunneled catheters are tunneled under the skin so that the external infusion port is distanced from the point of CV entry. With totally implanted ports, both the infusion port and the CV catheter are subcutaneously implanted, and a special noncoring needle is used to access the port.

Many of the above catheters are available in a multilumen design, with each lumen having its own infusion port. This allows the simultaneous infusion of incompatible fluids, including blood, without mixing. Blood samples may be drawn from CV catheters if they are properly flushed before and after collection.

Catheter Size

A needle or catheter should be large enough to achieve good flow rates but not so large that it causes mechanical damage to the vein. Eighteen gauge is commonly used for routine transfusion, with 23 gauge being used if veins are small.

Strict guidelines limiting needle or catheter size are not warranted.[65] Blood can be infused safely through very small devices, but one should expect slower flow rates. If the rate achievable with gravity is too slow, the product may be diluted with saline, may be split, or may be used with an infusion pump. Data gathered during infusion pump analyses indicate no significant change in hemolysis as needle size varies from 18 to 27 gauge when this single variable is evaluated.[66-68] The potential for hemolysis depends on a complex combination of factors, including blood viscosity and age, the resistance within the total set, flow rate, and applied pressure.[65]

Connecting Devices

The use of an extension tube and a stopcock or connecting device between the infusion set and the needle or catheter gives the infusionist additional working room and reduces the risk of infection, phlebitis, and infiltration from movement. Connectors (Y-shaped, T-shaped, and three- or four-way stopcocks) also make the infusion line more versatile. However, their selection and use should be carefully monitored because some allow several solutions to flow at one time and not all fluids are compatible with blood. Hospital guidelines are needed for indications of use and maintenance. All connections should be securely fastened with Luer locks or taped to prevent loosening or contamination.

Intermittent injection caps can be used to cap off a catheter not in use. These "heparin locks" may be used for blood transfusion, provided that the line is flushed first with saline. This removes the heparin and confirms the patency of the line. Short connecting needles are recommended to avoid damage to the injection cap and catheter.

Infusion Sets

Blood derivatives are administered according to their package insert and may not require a filter or special infusion set. Blood components, on the other hand, must be transfused through a sterile, pyrogen-free transfusion set and must be filtered to remove potentially harmful clots and debris that may form during collection or storage.

The manufacturers of blood administration sets recommend they be changed every 24 hours or after a specified number of units (4 to 10). In practice, hospitals may change them after every transfusion or limit their use to a several units and/or several hours (4 to 6) for patient safety. Trapped protein and debris provide a medium for potential bacterial growth; as filtered particles accumulate, the flow rate decreases. Multiple blood components given back-to-back through the same set should be ABO compatible with one another. Blood sets should not be used for the subsequent infusion of other intravenous fluids. Blood in the line may be incompatible with the solution and may adversely alter its pH and/or therapeutic value.

Standard Blood Sets

Standard blood administration sets have in-line filters (170 to 260-μm pore size), drip chambers, and tubing; set configurations vary with manufacturer. Priming instructions are printed on the package. For optimal performance and flow rate, filters should be completely wetted, and drip chambers should be filled no more than one-third to one-half full. After the chamber and filter are primed, blood is allowed to flow through the tubing to expel unwanted air. Priming volumes vary with design, from 30 to 80 ml.

Single-lead or straight sets are most commonly used and can be primed directly with blood. Double-lead or Y sets are preferred when saline is needed for component dilution or for flushing the line. Set design may also include in-line hand pumps and large-bore tubing for rapid transfusions, volumetric chambers or bags for accurate volume measurement, and multiple medical injection sites if other lines must be connected. The practice of "piggybacking" other lines into the blood line should be discouraged.

Component Sets

Component sets and syringe-push sets are designed for FFP, PLT, and CRYO transfusions, but they may also be used for very small RBC transfusions. Gravity-drip component sets, with both straight and Y configurations, have small drip chambers and 170-μm filters, plus shorter tubing with no in-line rubber surfaces. Their small priming volume (10 to 30 ml) minimizes component loss if the set is not flushed with saline after transfusion.

Syringe-push sets have a priming volume of 4 to 6 ml and a Y configuration for syringe and blood bag attachment. The 170-μm in-line filter, located within the tubing, is not always apparent. Once attached, the syringe must not be removed from the set; the contents must be pushed through the intravenous end for the product to be filtered.

Special Filters

Refer to the leukocyte-reduction section for a discussion of third-generation leukocyte-removing filters (see p. 317). These filters have special priming and use requirements; some also have flow rate restrictions and are not recommended for use with infusion pumps or pressure devices. Manufacturers' directions must be carefully followed for optimal filter performance.

Second-generation microaggregate filters (MAF) were developed earlier to remove the very small aggregates of degenerating PLT, leukocytes, and fibrin that form progressively during storage and pass through standard filters. Screen-type MAFs contain woven polyester that physically blocks particles larger than the 40-μm pore size. Depth-type MAFs are packed with Dacron, polyester wool, or polyurethane foam, which adsorbs particles larger than 10 to 40 μm.

MAFs are intended for RBC filtration. Their use with FFP, PLT, and CRYO components may not be contraindicated, but their large priming volume can retain considerable amounts of these components if they are not thoroughly flushed with saline after use. Depth-type MAFs must not be used for granulocyte transfusions.

The clinical significance of microaggregate filtration has been reviewed.[69,70] The routine use of MAFs for transfusion is not justified, even in massive transfusion situations. Their use in cardiopulmonary bypass surgery may be prudent to reduce postoperative morbidity from arteriolar emboli, and specialized intra-arterial line MAFs are available for these procedures. MAFs are also used to filter salvaged autologous blood in surgery before reinfusion. Their role in preparing leukocyte-reduced RBC to prevent febrile nonhemolytic transfusion reactions has been replaced by the more efficient leukocyte-removal filters. MAFs are less expensive than leukocyte-removal filters, and they can be used to prepare RBC with less than 5×10^8 residual white cells using a spin-cool-filter procedure.[71] However, the logistics of preparation and the range of residual white cells (1.1 to 11×10^8) in spin-cool-filter units make this use of MAFs less desirable.

Pediatric MAFs are still used to filter small aliquots for neonatal/pediatric transfusion because of their convenience, availability, and small priming volume, not for the need to remove microaggregates. Caution is needed for MAFs with very small stainless steel screen filters. They can occlude quickly and have been reported to cause excessive hemolysis.[72]

Blood Warmers

Routine warming of blood is not needed. Infusing 1 to 3 units of refrigerated blood drop by drop over several hours causes no harm. Patients who may benefit from warmed blood include (1) adults receiving multiple transfusions at rates greater than 50 ml/kg/hr, (2) young children infused at rates greater than 15 ml/kg/hr, (3) infants receiving exchange or large-volume transfusions, (4) patients receiving rapid infusions through CV catheters, and (5) patients with high-titer cold agglutinins active in vitro at 37°C.[73]

Massive, rapid transfusions of cold blood (1 to 6°C) can induce adverse physiologic changes associated with hypothermia, including cold-induced coagulopathies and cardiac arrhythmias, leading to cardiac arrest.[74,75] Hypothermia is defined as a core body temperature less than 35°C in adults or below 36.5°C in small infants,[75] temperatures not uncommonly seen in surgical and trauma patients.

In an early comparison review of blood warmers, Russell[74] suggested a worst-case scenario, that is, a patient cooled to 35°C who needs a transfusion at rates of 150 ml/min. Blood warmed to 32°C and given this fast was calculated not to lower the cardiac temperature below 34°C. Thus, warming refrigerated blood to 32°C at 150-ml/min flow rates became the desirable standard for warming equipment. Modern techniques and surgical procedures, however, may require flow rates of almost 1 L/min, and this has forced improvements in warming methods and requirements.

Presently, the AABB recommends that blood be warmed as it passes through the transfusion set using a system with a visible thermometer and, ideally, an audible alarm. Blood must not be warmed above 42°C.[1] Thermostatically controlled water baths and dry heat warmers with electric warming plates meet these standards, but adequate warming is difficult to achieve with flow rates above 150 ml/min. New countercurrent or high-volume heat exchangers circulate heated water through outer and/or inner water jackets while blood flows through a separate chamber. These units have good warming efficiency and very low resistance to flow and are well suited for warming blood at rates approaching 1 L/min.

Rapid warming can also be achieved by adding an "equal volume" of 70°C saline to 4°C RBC in the blood bag without adversely affecting osmotic fragility, plasma hemoglobin or plasma potassium levels, or red cell survival in vivo.[76,77] Average-sized RBC units (305 ml) equilibrate at 36 to 38°C less than 30 seconds after beginning the admixture with 250 ml of saline, warmed in a monitored warming oven.[78] This method is appropriate only for rapid, immediate transfusion. Once warmed, the red cells can cool quickly (3°C in 5 minutes) and deteriorate rapidly.[79]

Regardless of the system used, quality control procedures must ensure that blood is not warmed above 42°C. Excessive warming can cause hemolysis and endanger the patient. Using uncontrolled equipment (i.e., tubs filled with hot water from the tap, warming blankets, or saline bags heated by microwave) should be discouraged. Although microwave ovens have been used successfully to thaw FFP, their use in warming RBC has resulted in cell damage and hemolysis.[80,81]

Pressure Devices

Rapid transfusion often requires faster flow rates than gravity alone can provide. The simplest and most common device to increase the rate is to use a blood administration set with in-line pump that is squeezed by hand. To achieve maximal rates, large-bore needles are recommended with their use.

Alternatively, a pressure bag with sphygmomanometer can be used. The bags are like pressure cuffs except that they completely enclose the blood bag between a mesh panel and an air bladder so that pressure is evenly applied. These devices must be carefully monitored during use. Pressures greater than 300 mmHg can cause the seams of the blood bag to rupture or leak. Also, as the blood bag empties, the pressure against it will decrease, and the flow rate will slow unless the air bladder is reinflated.

Newer designs encase the blood bag and air bladder in a hard-sided box and feature high-efficiency foot pumps or regulators to keep the system pressurized as the blood bag deflates. They also feature automatic release valves to prevent overinflation and provide quick deflation when blood bags must be changed.

Infusion Control Devices

Infusion control devices are categorized as controllers or pumps.[63,64] Controllers rely on gravity alone to deliver the fluid, and sound an alarm when the actual rate differs from the selected rate. They offer little advantage in blood transfusion and may add unnecessary expense.

Pumps generate a positive pressure on the infusion fluid to maintain the selected infusion rate (0.1 to 999 ml/hr), and an alarm sounds when they can-

not maintain it. Syringe pumps have a screw drive mechanism to advance the plunger on a syringe. Rates are controlled by the drive speed and syringe size. Peristaltic pumps have linear or rotary roller bars that occlude the tubing and push fluid along the line. Volume is controlled by roller speed and tubing diameter. In piston cassette/diaphragm pumps, fluid is pulled into a refillable chamber and then pushed to the patient in short, intermittent bursts. Peristaltic and cassette pumps may require special infusion sets supplied by the manufacturer.

Most transfusions proceed well with gravity alone. However, when an accurate slow infusion rate is needed and/or a viscous blood component must be transfused through a small needle or catheter, pumps may indeed be required to overcome infusion line resistance and maintain flow.

Many models have been evaluated for blood transfusion use under a variety of transfusion conditions.[66–68,70,82–85] Their use is not contraindicated, although some RBC damage may occur. This damage is not related to the pump mechanism or specific model as much as it is related to total system variables, including age and viscosity of the blood, rate and degree of pressure used, needle size, and even temperature of the blood. Observed increases in hemolysis are usually insignificant and should not cause problems to the patient. Available data show that pump use for PLT and granulocyte transfusion is also acceptable.[86,87]

Ideally, facilities should evaluate the pumps they intend to use with their own in-house practices.[85] Before an infusion control device is selected for blood transfusion, the manufacturer's specifications and recommendations should be reviewed. Does the manufacturer approve their use with blood? Are there obvious contraindications? Devices with rate alarms that sound when opaque fluids are used are not suitable. When rapid rates and high pressure are needed, the pump's PSI rating (the maximal pressure that a pump will exert before its occlusion alarm sounds) should be checked against the pressure needed to infuse the blood and the pressure tolerance of the blood filter being used.

Intravenous Solutions

Drugs or medications, including those intended for intravenous use, must never be added to blood components.[1] Drugs that have an excessively high pH or are hypotonic can hemolyze RBC, or the blood component may buffer the drug and alter its therapeutic effect. If the entire unit is not transfused, the patient will not receive the prescribed dose, or if the patient experiences a reaction, it may be difficult to assess whether the blood or the drug was responsible.[73]

The only solution that may be added to blood without question is normal saline, 0.9 percent sodium chloride injection USP. However, other solutions intended for intravenous use may mix with blood in the tubing or be added to blood if they have been approved for this use by the FDA or if there is adequate documentation that this practice is safe and efficacious.[1] Some isotonic, calcium-free electrolyte solutions (pH 7.4) meet these requirements.[88–90]

Some solutions are not compatible with blood. Five percent dextrose in water causes RBC to clump and hemolyze.[90–92] Lactated Ringer's and other solutions that contain calcium can cause small clots to form in the tubing. TPN solutions are extremely hypertonic and also readily hemolyze RBC. When blood is transfused through a line already primed with a solution, 25 percent of that solution remains in the tubing 10 minutes after the blood is started; 10 percent remains after 30 minutes.[91] Thus, prolonged contact can occur between blood and other solutions, even when not intended. To reduce this contact when blood is piggybacked into an existing intravenous line, other fluid therapies are stopped, and the tubing is flushed with normal saline.

BLOOD ADMINISTRATION PROCEDURES

Recipient Identification

Procedures to identify the transfusion unit with the intended recipient must define the information to be checked and by whom and how the check is documented. This can be considered a three-step procedure, and the same two responsible individuals (physicians and/or nurses) should participate in all three steps. A transfusion must never begin until the identification is complete and found to be accurate. Any discrepant information or question must be resolved before proceeding further.

Step 1

Two individual should verify the following items on the transfusion request, the blood bag label and attached compatibility tags, and the patient's chart as appropriate by reading aloud to one another and checking:

1. The patient's name and hospital identification number. Check the spelling and numbers carefully.
2. The donor number and component name. Was the correct component received? If irradiated, leukocyte-reduced, or CMV-negative blood was requested, do labels indicate this fact?
3. The patient's and donor's ABO and Rh types. Are they compatible? This requires that the personnel responsible for blood product infusion understand without question the rules of compatibility.
4. The product's expiration date and time. These must still be current. If the product has undergone special preparation, its expiration will change. The new time should be clearly indicated on the label.
5. The appearance of the blood. Does the product appear normal? The laboratory should have checked for signs of contamination, but this should be re-examined before the infusion is started.
6. Special instructions. Are special instructions attached, such as the need for a special filter or a blood warmer?

Step 2

These same individuals must verify in the recipient's presence that the name and hospital or blood bank number on the identification band is identical to that on the transfusion request and compatibility record. If possible, patients are asked to identify themselves.

Problems sometimes arise in surgery when identification bands are inaccessible or removed. Procedures must be developed to ensure that this identification step is not compromised. Hospital identification bands may be taped to the patient's forehead or foot. The patient's name and number can be written or taped on the body, using indelible ink if necessary.

Step 3

Both individuals must sign the transfusion form and add the date and time of the verification to show that the checks were properly completed. The transfusion should be started immediately thereafter. If this cannot be done, the identity check should be repeated when the infusion is started.

Monitoring the Patient

Any change in the patient's clinical condition during transfusion may signal a transfusion reaction. Existing symptoms and initial vital signs (temperature, pulse, blood pressure, and respiration rate) should be documented at the start of transfusion, just before connecting the blood bag. Although fever is not a contraindication for transfusion, thought should be given to postponing the transfusion until the fever subsides. If the start of the transfusion is delayed, the unit should be returned to the blood bank promptly. The use of other refrigerators for temporary storage is poor practice because of undocumented temperature control.

The patient should be observed for 5 to 15 minutes during the initial "test dose" phase of the transfusion. Serious, life-threatening transfusion reactions can appear quickly, and immediate action must be taken if this occurs. After the first 25 to 50 ml has been infused, the patient's clinical status and vital signs are rechecked and documented again. If everything still appears to be satisfactory, the chance of a serious reaction is greatly reduced, and continual monitoring is no longer necessary. The patient's status should still be observed every 0.5 to 1 hour, or as the patient's condition warrants, up to several hours post-transfusion. All these observation data must be appropriately documented in the medical record.

Infusion Rates

Blood products can be given as fast as the patient tolerates or requires them, but care must be taken to avoid circulatory overload. Rates will vary with the patient's blood volume, cardiac status, and hemodynamic condition.[24] Otherwise healthy adults may tolerate rates up to 100 ml/min, whereas patients with chronic anemia and cardiovascular compromise may only tolerate rates of 2 ml/min. PLT, FFP, and CRYO are given at rates of about 5 to 10 ml/min. Granulocytes are infused slowly, between 2 and 4 hr/unit, to reduce the adverse symptoms often associated with granulocyte transfusion. Blood derivative package directions should be consulted for their infusion rate guidelines.

Slow infusion rates, 25 to 50 ml during the first 15 minutes, are used at the start so that, if an acute reaction does occur, the dose administered is minimal. Thereafter, if the "test dose" is tolerated, the infusion rate is increased so that the product is infused within a reasonable time. Most transfusions are completed within 2 hours. The maximal time a transfusion may take is not supported by scientific data, but a 4-hour limit is commonly used to reduce the risk of bacterial proliferation.[2]

Infusion rates are calculated using the infusion system's "drop per milliliter" rating (10 to 20 for most blood sets). The infusion rate should be checked periodically when the patient is monitored for reaction symptoms. If blood flows more slowly than needed, the following steps may be taken.[2]

1. Elevate the blood bag. It should be at least 3 to 4 feet above the patient's heart to overcome routine venous pressures.
2. Check the patency of the needle.
3. Check the blood bag and administration set filter for clots.
4. Dilute CPD/CPDA-1 RBCs with 50 to 100 ml of normal saline if the patient is able to accept the added fluid and NaCl.

When it is known in advance that very slow infusion rates are required, the laboratory can be asked to split the product into two or more aliquots. Each aliquot can be infused over the usual 4-hour maximum time.

Transfusion Completion

The transfusion is completed when all relevant data are documented in the medical record and on the transfusion form. The empty blood bag, with infusion set and fluids if attached, must be disposed of as a contaminated item in accordance with hospital policy. Many facilities now provide specific written instructions on post-transfusion care to inpatients and outpatients. These instructions outline relevant symptoms and the action to take if they are noted.

Transfusion Reactions

Any adverse effect caused by transfusion may be considered a transfusion reaction. Some are mild; others are life-threatening. All recognized ones should be documented and reported. Personnel attending the patient during transfusion need to understand the importance of reactions, their causes, and their associated symptoms. A full discussion can be found in Chapter 41.

Hospital procedures should specify the course of action to take when a reaction is suspected. Ideally, this information is on the transfusion form accompanying the blood bag so that it is available at the bedside. An appropriate immediate response is summarized below.

1. Stop the transfusion immediately. Disconnect the infusion set with attached blood and fluids from the needle and catheter.
2. Establish a "keep-open" drip of normal saline using new infusion equipment.
3. Document vital signs if they have not already been taken, and check the blood labels and record against the patient's identification band to confirm clerical accuracy.
4. Notify the responsible physician so that treatment, if necessary, can begin.
5. Notify the blood bank and describe the signs and symptoms.

The blood bank may request additional samples for investigation: a post-transfusion clotted specimen, drawn atraumatically, with proper labels and forms; the remainder of the suspect unit with attached intravenous set, needles removed and tubing tied; and a copy of the completed transfusion form. The transfusion need not be stopped in all cases. When circulatory overload is suspected, slowing the rate of infusion may resolve the problem. If only hives are noted, the patient may be medicated and the unit restarted with the agreement of the responsible physician.

PEDIATRIC TRANSFUSION ISSUES

Children, with their small blood volumes, small veins, and special needs, present a transfusion challenge to physicians, nurses, and laboratory staff.

Blood banks must be prepared to provide frequent, small-volume transfusion products with minimal demand for test sample and minimal waste of blood inventory but also with minimal donor exposures.

Compatibility Testing

Blood banks categorize children into two age groups: (1) neonates and infants younger than 4 months old and (2) those who are 4 months and older. This classification relates to immune maturity and compatibility test requirements. Children aged 4 months and older are considered immunologically competent and are tested as adults, whereas infants younger than 4 months rarely make antibodies and require less testing (see Ch. 9).[1]

For each hospitalization during the first 4 months, an initial pretransfusion specimen is tested for ABO/Rh RBC antigens and screened for unexpected antibodies. If the antibody screen result is negative, no crossmatching or repeat testing is necessary throughout the hospital stay. If the antibody screen finding is positive for clinically significant antibodies, units selected for crossmatch must either be antigen negative for the antibody in question or crossmatch compatible by antiglobulin methods.

Before group A, B, or AB infants are given RBC other than group O; their serum should also be tested for anti-A and anti-B using antiglobulin methods. If antibody is detected, the units selected must be ABO compatible, but crossmatching is not required. This test for anti-A/-B must be repeated if the infant receives any ABO-incompatible plasma and subsequent nongroup O RBC are needed.

Pretransfusion testing is not required for plasma or platelet requests, but the child's ABO/Rh type must be known before compatible products can be selected. Type-identical products are given to young infants whenever possible to avoid transfusing incompatible plasma antibody.

Specimen Requirements

Cord blood, if available, can be used for initial pretransfusion testing within the early neonatal period. It represents a larger volume of blood than can be collected peripherally and saves the baby additional blood loss. Even so, venous samples collected by heel stick are preferred because of concerns over cord specimen identification and contamination with

Wharton's jelly, which causes false-positive reactions. Volume requirements vary with institutional procedures and the infant's hematocrit; 1 ml is usually sufficient for routine initial testing.

Mother's serum, whether collected in-house or transported from another facility along with the infant, also can be used for initial antibody screening and is very useful if identification studies are needed. Such specimens must be properly labeled and link the mother's identity to the baby. Sufficient volume should be drawn; a 10- to 15-ml clotted specimen may be needed for antibody identification.

Component Selection Issues

Blood selection guidelines for children after infancy parallel those for adults, but very young infants have special blood needs. Although there are no universal standards, most facilities arbitrarily select a "fresh RBC" less than 7 days old for an infant's initial small-volume transfusion and then continue to use it for subsequent transfusions to that same infant until the unit expires or is fully transfused. Fresh blood is usually not necessary for small-volume transfusions[93,94] but can be important in large, massive transfusion situations because of 2,3-DPG, potassium, and pH changes during storage.

RBC for intrauterine fetal transfusion and exchange transfusion are traditionally the freshest units available (7 days old or less) that are crossmatch compatible with mother's serum. Group O Rh-negative units are selected for transfusion when infant fetal type is not known. If a specified hematocrit (50 percent for the neonate) is needed, units of WB can be volume reduced, or RBC can be resuspended with albumin or FFP by established formulas.[2] Units known to lack hemoglobin S are recommended for massive or exchange transfusion when infants are severely hypoxic or acidotic.[1]

RBC units that contain AS are used for pediatric transfusion. However, AS-RBC are not used routinely for newborns because of concerns about reactive hyperinsulinemia, renal toxicity, and diuresis-associated fluctuations in cerebral blood flow, which could be triggered by the higher concentrations of dextrose, adenine, and mannitol in AS units. A clinical comparison of CPDA-1 and AS-1 (Adsol, Baxter Healthcare Corp, Deerfield, IL) RBC show them to be equally effective in the small-volume transfusion setting with no apparent untoward effects.[95]

In an effort to evaluate additive risks, Luban et al.[96] calculated the amounts of additives that would be transfused along with AS-1 RBC in theoretical neonatal clinical settings and related these findings to the toxicology of the additives. They suggest that AS-RBC present no problems when used for a small-volume transfusion (10 ml/kg/hr) of premature infants, even if given once daily over an extended period, but recommend entire units not be used in massive transfusion settings (i.e., exchange transfusion, cardiac bypass surgery, and extracorporeal membrane oxygenation). The risk potential for extremely premature neonates, those with severe renal or hepatic insufficiency, or those requiring multiple transfusions daily is unknown, and it may be prudent to remove the AS medium by centrifugation or washing before transfusion.[96]

Infants with very low birth weights (less than 1,200 g at birth and usually less than 29 weeks of gestational age) may benefit from receiving CMV-seronegative cellular components when they or their mothers are CMV antibody negative or this information is not known.[97] Leukocyte-reduced RBC or PLT may safely be substituted if CMV-seronegative units are not available, but routine use of leukocyte-removal filters for neonatal transfusions is not justified.[98]

Blood Administration

Before any transfusion is started, children who have an ability to understand should be given an appropriate explanation of what is happening so they can participate without fear. Parent education is also essential so that they do not contribute to the child's anxiety. Nurses must be especially observant of children unable to communicate and must be prepared to evaluate minor changes in vital signs, respiratory distress, or cardiac status as a potential consequence of transfusion.

Intravenous access can be difficult to achieve and maintain in very small infants and children who are not able to cooperate. Umbilical vessels may be cannulated in the newborn. Feet or scalp veins are used for peripheral access for infants who are not yet walking, with the saphenous or subclavian vein for CV access. Small veins require small needles: 23- to 25-

gauge needles or 22- to 24-gauge catheters are traditionally chosen.

Although standard straight blood administration sets are commonplace in the pediatric setting, sets with in-line calibrated chambers that more accurately measure volume or component/syringe-push sets with smaller priming volumes may be preferred. Sets are primed directly with blood and not flushed after transfusion because children often have saline or volume restrictions.

Physicians should not routinely request more blood than can be given within several hours. The infusion rate varies with the child's condition, rate of blood loss, venous access device, and component viscosity. Acceptable replacement rates in infants are 5 to 10 ml/hr/kg. With rapid blood loss or in massive transfusion situations, rates as fast as 1.5 ml/min/kg may be used, but patients should be carefully monitored for drops in ionized calcium levels and blood pressure.[99] Slow infusion requirements, coupled with small intravenous lines and the viscosity of some RBC components, makes the use of infusion pumps commonplace in pediatric critical care units. Although any device approved for blood transfusion can be used, those designed for pediatric use, with 0.1-ml infusion increments, are ideal.

Even though very young infants cannot regulate their temperature as well as older children, it is usually not necessary to warm small-volume transfusions given slowly. If warming is critical, aliquots may be placed in the infant's incubator for 30 minutes.[100] Blood in small containers quickly warms to ambient temperature, especially during passage through the infusion tubing.

The mechanics of transfusing warm aliquots in cold surgical suites are not so simple. Conventional warming equipment can be adapted to small-volume transfusions by using smaller pediatric warming coils, shortened tubing, and/or attaching a stopcock to the warmer's exit port and filling syringes of warmed blood as needed. Caution must be taken to avoid contaminating the stopcock and to ensure that the blood resting in the warmer does not warm above 42°C with prolonged exposure. These approaches are unsatisfactory to some because of the blood lost to the priming volume of the warming system.

It is tempting but dangerous to place small aliquots of blood or blood tubing in a warm uncontrolled environment (i.e., between heated saline bags or warming blankets). Such practices can result in excessive heating and hemolysis.[101] Even phototherapy units and infrared radiant warmers operating at full power have been associated with RBC damage.[74,102]

REFERENCES

1. Klein HG (ed): Standards for Blood Banks and Transfusion Services. 16th Ed. American Association of Blood Banks, Bethesda, 1994
2. Walker RH (ed): Technical Manual. 11th Ed. American Association of Blood Banks, Bethesda, 1993
3. Walker R: Preparation of blood components. p. 49. In Myhre B (ed): ASCP Workshop on Quality Control in Blood Banking. American Society of Clinical Pathologists, Chicago, 1971
4. Hogman CF: New trends in the preparation and storage of platelets. Transfusion 32:3, 1992
5. Cohn EJ, Strong LE, Hughes WL et al: Preparation and properties of serum and plasma proteins. IV. A system for the separation into fractions of the protein and lipoprotein components of biological tissues and fluids. J Am Chem Soc 68:459, 1946
6. Wheeler JG, Abramson JS, Ekstrand K: Function of irradiated polymorphonuclear leukocytes obtained by buffy coat centrifugation. Transfusion 24:238, 1984
7. Rock G, Zurakowski S, Baxter A, Adams G: Simple and rapid preparation of granulocytes for the treatment of neonatal septicemia. Transfusion 24:510, 1984
8. Goldfinger D, Medici MA, Hsi R et al: Preparation and in vitro function of granulocyte concentrate for transfusion to neonates using the IBM 2991 blood processor. Transfusion 23:358, 1983
9. Code of Federal Regulations, Food and Drugs, Title 21, Parts 600 to 799. U.S. Government Printing Office, Washington, DC, 1994
10. Shulman IA, Kent D: Unit placement errors: a potential risk factor for ABO and Rh incompatible transfusions. Lab Med 22:194, 1991
11. Rock G: Factor VIII concentrates. p. 127. In Cash JD (ed): Progress in Transfusion Medicine. Vol. 2. Churchill Livingstone, New York, 1987
12. Umlas J, Jacobson M, Kevy SV: Suitable survival and half-life of red cells after frozen storage in excess of 10 years. Transfusion 31:648, 1991
13. Valeri CR, Pivacek LE, Gray AD et al: The safety and therapeutic effectiveness of human red cells stored at −80 C for as long as 21 years. Transfusion 29:429, 1989

14. Slichter SJ: Optimum platelet concentrate preparation and storage. p. 1. In Garratty G (ed): Current Concepts in Transfusion Therapy. American Association of Blood Banks, Arlington, 1985

15. Rowley K, Snyder EL: Platelet storage. p. 46. In Cash JD (ed): Progress in Transfusion Medicine. Vol. 2. Churchill Livingstone, New York, 1987

16. Dzik WH, Cusack WF, Sherburne B, Kickler T: The effect of prestorage white cell reduction on the function and viability of stored platelet concentrates. Transfusion 32:334, 1992

17. Rao GHR, Escolar G, White JG: Biochemistry, physiology, and function of platelets stored as concentrates. Transfusion 33:766, 1993

18. Snyder EL, Koerner TAW, Jr, Kakaiya R et al: Effect of mode of agitation on storage of platelet concentrates in PL-732 containers for 5 days. Vox Sang 44: 300, 1983

19. Snyder EL, Bookbinder M, Kakaiya R et al: 5-Day storage of platelet concentrates in CLX containers: effect of type of agitation. Vox Sang 45:432, 1983

20. Champion AB, Chong C, Carmen RA: Storage of platelets on flatbed agitators in polyvinylchloride blood bags plasticized with tri (2-ethylhexyl) trimellitate. Transfusion 27:399, 1987

21. Snyder EL, Ferri P, Brown R et al: Evaluation of flatbed reciprocal motion agitators for resuspension of stored platelet concentrates. Vox Sang 48:269, 1985

22. Snyder EL, Pope C, Ferri PM et al: The effect of mode of agitation and type of plastic bag on storage characteristics and in vivo kinetics of platelet concentrates. Transfusion 26:125, 1986

23. Huestis DW, Glasser L: The neutrophil in transfusion medicine. Transfusion 34:630, 1994

24. American Association of Blood Banks: Circular of Information for the Use of Human Blood and Blood Components. American Association of Blood Banks, Bethesda, 1994

25. McCullough J, Weiblen BJ, Peterson PK, Quie PG: Effects of temperature on granulocyte preservation. Blood 52:301, 1978

26. Miyamoto M, Sasakawa S: Studies on granulocyte preservation. III. Effect of agitation on granulocyte concentrates. Transfusion 27:165, 1987

27. Myhre BA: Quality Control in Blood Banking. John Wiley & Sons, New York, 1974

28. United States Postal Service: Mailability of etiologic agents. Federal Register 54(156):33823, 1989

29. Code of Federal Regulations, Title 42, Part 72. Interstate shipment of biological material that contains or may contain etiologic agents. U.S. Government Printing Office, Washington, DC, 1993

30. Bowie EJW, Thompson JH, Owen CA: The stability of antihemophilic globulin and labile factor in human blood. Mayo Clin Proc 39:144, 1964

31. Counts RB, Haisch C, Simon TL et al: Hemostasis in massively transfused trauma patients. Ann Surg 190: 91, 1979

32. Simon TL, Henderson R: Coagulation factor activity in platelet concentrates. Transfusion 19:186, 1979

33. Champion AB, Carmen RA: Factors affecting white cell content in platelet concentrates. Transfusion 25: 334, 1985

34. Schoendorfer DW, Hansen LE, Kenney DM: The surge technique: a method to increase purity of platelet concentrates obtained by centrifugal apheresis. Transfusion 23:182, 1983

35. Strauss RG, Halpern LN, Eckermann I: Comparison of autosurge versus surge protocols for discontinuous-flow centrifugation plateletpheresis. Transfusion 27:499, 1987

36. Mintz PD, Cullis HM, Pearson TH: A technique to reduce lymphocyte contamination of plateletpheresis products collected with a centrifugal blood cell separator. Transfusion 27:159, 1987

37. Baldwin ML, Jefferies LC (eds): Irradiation of Blood Components. American Association of Blood Banks, Bethesda, 1992

38. Gilbert GL, Hayes K, Hudson IF, James J: Prevention of transfusion acquired cytomegalovirus infection in infants by blood filtration to remove leukocytes. Lancet 1:1228, 1989

39. Bowden RA, Slichter SJ, Sayers MH et al: Use of leukocyte-depleted platelets and cytomegalovirus-seronegative red blood cells for prevention of primary cytomegalovirus infection after marrow transplant. Blood 78:246, 1991

40. Nusbacher J: *Yersinia enterocolitica* and white cell filtration. Transfusion 32:597, 1992

41. Lane TA, Anderson KC, Goodnough LT et al: Leukocyte reduction in blood component therapy. Ann Intern Med 117:151, 1992

42. Pietersz RNI, Steneker I, Reesink HW: Prestorage leukocyte depletion of blood products in a closed system. Transfusion Med Rev 7:17, 1993

43. Rebulla P, Porretti L, Bertolini F et al: White cell-reduced red cells prepared by filtration: a critical evaluation of current filters and methods for counting residual white cells. Transfusion 33:128, 1993

44. Dzik S: Leukodepletion blood filters: filter design and mechanisms of leukocyte removal. Transfusion Med Rev, 7:65, 1993

45. Lutz P, Dzik WH: Large-volume hemocytometer chamber for accurate counting of white cells (WBCs) in WBC-reduced platelets: validation and application for quality control of WBC-reduced platelets prepared by apheresis and filtration. Transfusion 33: 409, 1993

46. Vachula M, Simpson SJ, Martinson JA et al: A flow cytometric method for counting very low levels of white cells in blood and blood components. Transfusion 33:262, 1993

47. Buck SA, Kickler TS, McGuire M et al: The utility of platelet washing using an automated procedure for severe platelet allergic reactions. Transfusion 27:391, 1987

48. Vesiling GW, Simpson MB, Shifman RE et al: Evaluation of a centrifugal blood cell processor for washing platelet concentrates. Transfusion 28:46, 1988

49. Pineda AA, Zylstra VW, Clare DE et al: Viability and functional integrity of washed platelets. Transfusion 29:524, 1989

50. Sloand EM, Fox SM, Banks SM, Klein HG: Preparation of IgA deficient platelets. Transfusion 30:322, 1990

51. Rock G, White J, Labow R: Storage of platelets in balanced salt solutions: a simple platelet storage medium. Transfusion 31:21, 1991

52. Bertolini F, Rebulla P, Porretti L, Murphy S: Platelet quality after 15-day storage of platelet concentrates prepared from buffy coats and stored in a glucose-free crystalloid medium. Transfusion 32:9, 1992

53. Shimizu T, Shibata K, Kora S: Plasma-depleted platelet concentrates prepared with a new washing solution. Vox Sang 64:19, 1993

54. Pisciotto PT, Snyder EL, Napychank PA, Hopfer SM: In vitro characteristics of volume-reduced platelet concentrate stored in syringes. Transfusion 31:404, 1991

55. Gibble SW, Ness PM: Fibrin glue: the perfect operative sealant? Transfusion 30:741, 1990

56. Banninger H, Hardegger T, Tobler A et al: Fibrin glue in surgery: frequent development of inhibitors of bovine thrombin and human factor V. Br J Haematol 85:528, 1993

57. Goldfinger D, McGinnis MH: Rh incompatible platelet transfusion—risks and consequence of sensitizing immunosuppressed patients. N Engl J Med 284:942, 1971

58. Rock G, Tackaberry ES, Dunn JC, Kashyap S: Rapid controlled thawing of fresh-frozen plasma in a modified microwave oven. Transfusion 24:60, 1984

59. Mead JH, Boucock BP, Russell RE et al: Water environment microwave thawing. Am J Clin Pathol 85:510, 1986

60. Spivey MA, Jeter EK, Lazarchich JK, Spivey LB: Postfiltration factor VIII and fibrinogen levels in cryoprecipitate stored at room temperature and at 1 to 6°C. Transfusion 32:340, 1992

61. Myhre BA, Marcus CS: The extension of 4°C storage time of frozen-thawed red cells. Transfusion 32:344, 1992

62. Moroff G, Holme S, Dabay MH et al: Storage of pools of six and eight platelet concentrates. Transfusion 33:374, 1993

63. Weinstein SM: Plumer's Principles & Practice of Intravenous Therapy. 5th Ed. JB Lippincott, Philadelphia, 1993

64. Phillips LD: Manual of I.V. Therapeutics. FA Davis, Philadelphia, 1993

65. Luban NLC: Mechanical devices in pediatric transfusion. p. 69. In Luban NLC, Kolins J (eds): Hemotherapy in Childhood and Adolescence. American Association of Blood Banks, Arlington, 1985

66. Herrera AJ, Corless J: Blood transfusions: effect of speed of infusion and of needle gauge on hemolysis. J Pediatr 99:757, 1981

67. Gibson JS, Leff RD, Roberts RJ: Effects of intravenous delivery systems on infused red blood cells. Am J Hosp Pharm 41:468, 1984

68. Lau P, Miller FP: Comparisons of mechanical infusion pumps and needle size on blood flow and hemolysis. Lab Med 18:98, 1987

69. Snyder EL, Bookbinder M: Role of microaggregate filtration in clinical medicine. Transfusion 23:460, 1983

70. Ciavarella D, Snyder E: Clinical use of blood transfusion devices. Transfusion Med Rev 2:95, 1988

71. Parravicini A, Rebulla P, Apuzzo J et al: The preparation of leukocyte-poor red cells for transfusion by a simple cost-effective technique. Transfusion 24:508, 1984

72. Longhurst DM, Gooch WM III, Castillo RA: In vitro evaluation of a pediatric microaggregate blood filter. Transfusion 23:170, 1973

73. Pisciotto PT (ed): Blood Transfusion Therapy, A Physician's Handbook. 3rd Ed. American Association of Blood Banks, Arlington, 1989

74. Russell WJ: A review of blood warmers for massive transfusion. Anaesth Intensive Care 2:109, 1974

75. Iserson KV, Huestis DW: Blood warming: current application and techniques. Transfusion 3:558, 1991

76. Wilson EB, Knauf MA, Iserson KV: Red cell tolerance of admixture with heated saline. Transfusion 28:170, 1988

77. Iserson KV, Knauf MA: Confirmation of high blood flow rates through 150 μ filter/high-flow tubing. J Emerg Med 8:689, 1990

78. Iserson KV, Knauf MA, Anhalt D: Rapid admixture blood warming: technical advances. Crit Care Med 18:1138, 1990

79. Linko K, Palosaari S: Warming of blood units in water bath and cooling of blood at room temperature. Acta Anaesthesiol Scand 23:97, 1979

80. Staples PJ, Griner PF: Extracorporeal hemolysis of blood in a microwave blood warmer. N Engl J Med 285:317, 1971

81. Linko K, Hynynen K: Erythrocyte damage caused by the Haemotherm Microwave Blood Warmer. Acta Anaesthesiol Scand 23:320, 1979

82. Thompson HW, Lasky LC, Polesky HF: Evaluation of a volumetric intravenous fluid infusion pump for transfusion of blood components containing red cells. Transfusion 26:290, 1986

83. Gurdak RG, Anderson G, Mintz PD: Evaluation of IVAC infusion pump model 560 for delivery of red blood cells, abstracted. Transfusion 26:556, 1986

84. Burch KJ, Phelps SJ, Constance TD: Effect of an infusion device on the integrity of whole blood and packed red blood cells. Am J Hosp Pharm 48:92, 1991

85. Criss VR, DePalma L, Luban NLC: Analysis of a linear peristaltic infusion device for the infusion of red cells to pediatric patients. Transfusion 33:842, 1993

86. Snyder EL, Ferri PM, Smith EO, Ezekowitz MD: Use of electromechanical infusion pump for transfusion of platelet concentrates. Transfusion 24:524, 1984

87. Snyder EL, Malech HL, Ferri PM et al: In vitro function of granulocyte concentrates following passage through an electromechanical infusion pump. Transfusion 26:141, 1986

88. Ryden SE: Compatibility of blood with intravenous solutions. p. 33. In Marnett BL, Brzica SM (eds): From Vein to Vein, A Seminar for Phlebotomists and Transfusionists. American Association of Blood Banks, Washington, DC, 1976

89. Miripol J, Symbol R: A comparison of the hemolytic effects of solutions used to dilute red cells, abstracted. Transfusion 22:414, 1982

90. Dickson DN, Gregory MA: Compatibility of blood with solutions containing calcium. S Afr Med J 57:785, 1980

91. Ryden SE, Oberman HA: Compatibility of common intravenous solutions with CPD blood. Transfusion 15:250, 1975

92. Stautz RL, Nelson JM, Meyer EA, Shulman IA: Compatibility of ADSOL-stored red cells with intravenous solutions. Am J Emerg Med 7:162, 1989

93. Strauss RG: Transfusion therapy in neonates. Am J Dis Child 145:904, 1991

94. Strauss RG, Sacher RA, Blasina JF et al: Commentary on small-volume red cell transfusion for neonatal patients. Transfusion 30:565, 1990

95. Goodstein MH, Locke RG, Wlodarczyk D et al: Comparison of two preservation solutions for erythrocyte transfusions in newborn infants. J Pediatr 123:783, 1993

96. Luban NLC, Strauss RG, Hume HA: Commentary on the safety of red cells preserved in extended-storage media for neonatal transfusions. Transfusion 31:229, 1991

97. Preiksaitis JK: Indications for the use of cytomegalovirus-seronegative blood products. Transfusion Med Rev 5:1, 1991

98. Strauss RG: Selection of white cell-reduced blood components for transfusion during early infancy. Transfusion 33:352, 1993

99. Kevy SV: Guidelines for blood ordering. p. 1. In Luban NLC, Kolins J (eds): Hemotherapy in Childhood and Adolescence. American Association of Blood Banks, Arlington, 1985

100. Luban NLC, Midesell G, Sacher RA: Techniques for warming red blood cells packaged in different containers for neonatal use. Clin Pediatr 24:642, 1985

101. Wu NW, Foung SKH, Hoopes P et al: Microwave heat-induced hemolysis (letter). Clin Pediatr 24:645, 1985

102. Strauss RG, Bell EF, Snyder EL et al: Neonates transfused under radiant warmers may receive damaged erythrocytes, abstracted. Transfusion 25:468, 1985

Transfusion Medicine in a Hospital Setting

Lawrence D. Petz and Scott N. Swisher

One should be aware that "blood banking" is an archaic term.[1] During the last quarter of a century, a complex clinical and research discipline has quietly emerged from blood banking. This new discipline projects a different image and deservedly has acquired a new name: "transfusion medicine."

The ever-increasing scope and complexity of transfusion medicine necessitates greater direct clinical involvement by the director of transfusion medicine in the hospital and outpatient setting. The morbidity and occasional deaths associated with blood transfusion require that blood products be used only for appropriate indications. The director of transfusion medicine must have the expertise to evaluate the use of blood products and must devote time and energy to consulting with primary physicians to ensure that transfusion practices are appropriate. The transfusion committee must also play a prominent role in establishing policies and in monitoring their implementation.

The regional blood center has also changed. Most centers are now run by professional managers whose goals are to maintain adequate supplies of blood and to distribute blood to hospitals in a cost-effective manner. However, one unfortunate consequence of the emphasis on management and on good manufacturing practices has been to isolate some blood centers from the medical aspects of transfusion. The best safeguard is to retain the managerial compo-

nent while expanding the medical expertise within the regional center.

With more than 20 blood components and products now available, a physician with special expertise in transfusion medicine should assist with the selection of the appropriate blood component and advise on the evaluation and management of suspected transfusion complications. Directors of hospital transfusion services must have relevant knowledge and experience in a wide range of topics related to transfusion medicine. These topics have been reviewed by the Curriculum Committee of the Transfusion Medicine Academic Award Group[2] and include the scientific basis of transfusion, the management of blood donation, preparation of blood components, pretransfusion testing, appropriate transfusion of blood components, adverse effects of transfusion, autoimmunity, transplantation, and therapeutic apheresis.

The transfusion medicine specialist must be available to make clinical observations, to contact the responsible physician about findings, and to make suggestions for further testing or therapy. In short, transfusion medicine is a subspecialty, and the director has become a clinical consultant.[1]

AUTOMATIC SPECIAL CASE CONSULTATIONS

A systematic approach to clinical consultations is one mechanism that can assist primary physicians in providing optimal care for the patient who requires a

Table 14-1. Situations Requiring Automatic Consultation

1. A patient suffers a transfusion reaction
2. There is a request for the emergency release of uncrossmatched blood
3. An adult patient's red cell transfusions exceed 8 U in 8 hr
4. Inventory dictates that Rh-negative patients receive Rh-positive blood or platelets
5. A patient receives more than 6 U of fresh frozen plasma in 24 hr
6. Blood fewer than 7 days old is requested for an adult patient
7. Washed red cell preparations are requested
8. Blood products screened for antibodies to the cytomegalovirus are requested
9. Irradiated blood products are requested
10. Fewer than 3 or more than 12 U of platelets are requested for an adult patient
11. A patient receives platelet transfusions on 3 consecutive days
12. HLA-matched platelets are requested
13. A patient has severe reactions to platelet concentrates
14. Fresh platelet concentrates are requested
15. Cryoprecipitate is requested for a patient who does not have hemophilia A or von Willebrand's disease
16. Granulocyte concentrates are requested
17. Varicella-zoster immune globulin is requested
18. There is an unusual or extraordinary request for blood, components, or services

(From Tomasulo et al.,[3] with permission.)

transfusion. Several prototypic consultation services have already been described at both hospitals and regional blood centers.[3,4] Tomasulo et al.[3] developed a list of situations that require automatic consultation (Table 14-1). Each director of transfusion medicine should develop a similar list, which is modified according to local needs. Most of the situations listed involve complex transfusion medicine settings.

The consultation list may be used in several ways. It describes circumstances that require notification of the director of transfusion medicine by the blood bank staff. The clinician can be contacted either by telephone or at the patient's bedside. When used by the hospital transfusion audit committee, the list can help identify general problems in transfusion practice that require further evaluation. It also is an ideal source of guidance for trainees in transfusion medicine.

Although the list was designed for hospital consultations, the regional blood service can use a similar mechanism to identify situations that require communication with the hospital's director of transfusion medicine.

Use of a consultation list should be part of the transfusion service's standard operating procedure. This would formalize the educational process and help develop the teamwork necessary to provide the most appropriate transfusion support. Medical directors and technical staffs must support the use of the list and should educate the hospital staff about the information gained from it. The goal of these efforts is that all concerned recognize that transfusion medicine specialists are valuable consultants available to physicians who care for patients undergoing transfusion.

Transfusion medicine specialists should emphasize their consulting roles to ensure appropriate use of blood and blood products. Regularly scheduled transfusion medicine ward rounds, preferably daily, provide needed contact with primary physicians and make the availability of the consultation service more evident. Tact and forewarning are necessary when performing automatic, unsolicited consultations. Each situation should be evaluated in a positive and supportive fashion before an opinion is delivered.

The proposed system of automatic consultation has been accepted and used successfully in a number of medical centers. Popovsky et al.[4] described a formally organized consultation service with daily visits to patients of mutual interest to blood bank physicians and primary clinicians. Automatic consults were performed as were consultations conducted at the direct request of clinicians. The most frequent reasons for consultations were clarification or amplification of the clinical history (34 percent), evaluation of transfusion reactions (27.2 percent), and assessment of serologic problems (18.2 percent). The consultations resulted in diagnostic, management, and therapeutic recommendations for a wide variety of medical problems. The authors indicated that a blood bank consultation service is feasible, is enlightening for the blood bank and clinicians, and contributes to patient care.

The format is only one part of a systematic transfusion medicine consulting and educational service. Other activities should include educational programs, case conferences, and visiting lectures, all of which complement the automatic consultation program.

HOSPITAL TRANSFUSION COMMITTEE

A hospital transfusion committee should be appointed according to institutional procedures as a permanent professional committee of the medical board or other appropriate body. Representation should reflect local conditions but should include the director of transfusion medicine (medical director of the blood bank). It could also include the director of laboratories, a generalist, a surgeon, representatives of transplant teams, an internist, a hematologist-oncologist, an anesthesiologist, a pediatrician (perhaps with an interest in neonatal care), an obstetrician, representatives of the hospital administration, the nursing department, and other groups especially concerned with transfusion, such as dialysis or hepatitis surveillance staff.

The transfusion committee should review all transfusion practices and services within the institution and should regularly issue recommendations and reports of surveillance to its parent organization. Its activities should include frequent reviews of all adverse reactions to transfusions; transfusion and blood waste statistics; blood bank laboratory proficiency and accreditation surveys; and the adequacy of transfusion service personnel, facilities, and equipment. The committee can establish guidelines to reserve (crossmatch) blood for elective surgical procedures (e.g., a maximal surgical blood order schedule, as discussed in detail in Ch. 22) and decide how safely to minimize the time during which blood will be held in a reserved status. The committee, working with the transfusion service medical director, can serve a vital function in the education of clinical staff, identification of problem areas, promotion of optimal transfusion practices, and maintenance of an appropriate relationship with the regional blood center.

The greatest single responsibility of the hospital transfusion committee should be to play a central role in promoting and monitoring the safe and effective use of blood and blood products.[5,6] The transfusion committee must demonstrate assertive yet sensitive leadership while conducting blood use audits. When utilized appropriately, audit reviews are among the most powerful tools available for physician education, and they can lead to measurable changes in the standards and quality of practice within a hospital.

TRANSFUSION AUDITS

Goals of Medical Practice Audits

Medical practice audits can achieve a variety of goals. It is important that a transfusion committee establish defined objectives before beginning the process of medical practice audits. Appropriate goals include (1) modification of physician behavior in the area of transfusion therapy; (2) improvement of the standards of practice within a hospital; (3) identification and implementation of more cost-effective procedures; (4) compliance with regulatory agencies, such as the Joint Commission on Accreditation of Healthcare Organizations (JCAHO), which require audits and quality assurance activities; (5) provision of data for the hospital credentials committee or risk management department on the performance of individual physicians; (6) provision of data to the risk management or legal office regarding departments or areas of the hospital in which therapeutic misadventures are exposing the institution to the risk of malpractice litigation; (7) establishment and enforcement of a uniform standard of transfusion practice throughout the hospital; and (8) monitoring of the therapeutic and adverse effects of transfusion.

The report of Salem-Schatz et al.[7] suggests that there is, indeed, a need for systematic auditing of practices in transfusion medicine. They conducted a face-to-face survey of 122 general surgeons, orthopaedic surgeons, and anesthesiologists in three hospitals and determined that there were widespread deficiencies in physicians' knowledge of transfusion risks and indications. Attending physicians routinely had lower knowledge scores than did residents, yet they exhibited more confidence in their knowledge. Residents indicated that they frequently ordered transfusions that they judged unnecessary because a more senior physician suggested that they do so.

The JCAHO indicates that blood and blood components usage evaluation can prompt effective analysis, evaluation, and continuous improvement in each of four key sets of processes: (1) ordering of appropriate blood or blood components; (2) distribution, handling, and dispensing of blood and blood components; (3) administration of blood and blood components; and (4) monitoring of the effects of blood and blood components on patients so that appropriate modifications may be undertaken in a timely manner. The Standards of the American Association of Blood Banks[8] also state that all transfusing facilities shall use a peer-review program that documents the monitoring of transfusion practices for all categories of components.

It is not intended that all individual units transfused be evaluated. Blood usage review is carried out by using predetermined clinically valid criteria to screen all cases and by using peer review to evaluate all variations from the criteria to determine whether the variations are justified.

Development of Criteria

Although universally accepted indications for transfusion of various blood components are not available, a plethora of guidelines have been published in recent years.[9-20] Furthermore, Coffin et al.,[19] Silberstein et al.,[11] and Stehling et al.[16] described in detail how such guidelines may be used as a basis for the peer review process.

Transfusion guidelines should address the criteria for administering each of the major blood components, specially processed components (e.g., white cell reduced or irradiated), and autologous blood. There may be separate criteria for adult and pediatric patients.[16] Procedures such as therapeutic hemapheresis and perioperative blood recovery may be included in the review process. In addition, the transfusion committee may choose to audit individual services or procedures (e.g., coronary artery bypass surgery,[21] wristband identification errors,[22] errors in the administration of blood,[23] and the appropriate use of informed consent for transfusion.[24,25])

The transfusion committee should either develop criteria themselves or create an ad hoc subcommittee

to make recommendations. To achieve credibility with the clinical staff, the audit criteria must be developed by a representative group of physicians in the institution. If audit criteria are to be used initially by nonphysician reviewers in selecting charts for more detailed review, it is especially important that medical records personnel or quality assurance auditors are involved in the committee from its inception. If they are not, criteria may be developed in a form that is not usable by nonphysicians, who must rely on the written audit standards in screening charts for later review.

There must be a clear understanding that audit criteria are not to be used in a rigid or strict manner to distinguish between "good" or "bad" transfusion practices. Instead, audit criteria should ordinarily be used as a screening mechanism to identify those transfusion events most likely to have been inappropriate. The "cutoff" values used in the criteria are relatively arbitrary points selected mainly to exclude from review those cases in which the transfusion was probably appropriate. The criteria should be written in as brief and clear a manner as possible and should define a level of performance that is so acceptable to the committee that no further review of the medical record is necessary.

It is important that the chairman of every clinical department be notified in writing of the precise goals and plans for the audit process. The departmental chairmen should then be invited to provide input, perhaps by attending meetings or by sending a representative from the department. The audit criteria should be approved by the departmental chairmen before initiating the audits.

Examples of Criteria

Criteria may be developed with varying degrees of complexity. Examples of simple but effective screening criteria for appropriate use of red cells, platelets, granulocytes, fresh frozen plasma, and cryoprecipitate are given in Table 14-2.

Some medical centers also include an assessment of the outcome of each transfusion in their medical practice audit criteria. For example, a patient who receives a transfusion with red blood cells must have a hemoglobin value or hematocrit level drawn within 24 hours of the end of the transfusion episode, and patients receiving fresh frozen plasma must have a

Table 14-2. Examples of Transfusion Medicine Audit Criteria

Red cell transfusion
Symptomatic anemia in a normovolemic patient, regardless of hemoglobin level
Acute loss of ≥15% of estimated blood volume
Preoperative hemoglobin ≤9 g/dl and operative procedure associated with expected blood loss requiring transfusion
Hemoglobin ≤9 g/dl in a patient being treated by a chronic transfusion regimen

Platelets
Platelet count <20,000/μl in a patient with a hypoproliferative thrombocytopenia
Platelet count <50,000/μl in a patient who is actively bleeding or who is scheduled for surgery or an invasive procedure
Platelet count <50,000/μl in a patient with disseminated intravascular coagulation
Platelet count <100,000/μl in a patient who has excessive bleeding within 48 hr of cardiopulmonary bypass

Granulocytes
Bacterial infection unresponsive to 48 hr of appropriate antibiotic therapy in patients with marrow hypoplasia and neutrophil counts of <500/μl
Bacterial infection or progressive fungal infection in patients with severe neutrophil dysfunction

Fresh Frozen Plasma
Prothrombin and partial thromboplastin times >1.5 times the mean normal value in a patient who is actively bleeding or who is scheduled for surgery or an invasive procedure
Warfarin overdose in a patient with major bleeding or impending surgery

Cryoprecipitate
Fibrinogen <100 mg/dl in a patient who is actively bleeding or who is scheduled for surgery or an invasive procedure, von Willebrand's disease or, in selected patients, hemophilia unresponsive to desmopressin

determination of prothrombin time (PT) and activated partial thromboplastin time (PTT) or a specific coagulation factor assay within 4 hours after completion of the transfusion.[6] Criteria may be established to indicate the appropriate level of the measured blood component after transfusion (e.g., the hemoglobin should be less than 11 g/dl after a transfusion of red blood cells or whole blood, and the platelet count should be 30,000/μl greater than the pretransfusion level after a platelet transfusion). Some trans-

fusion committees use the discharge hematocrit level as a clinical indicator for the blood transfusion audit.[18]

Still other examples of transfusion medicine audit criteria include a list of exceptions to the stated criteria, explanatory instructions, and definitions.[5] However, a detailed list of exceptions usually indicates that the transfusion committee has forgotten the purpose of the criteria and has attempted to draft all-inclusive, detailed standards rather than to provide screening criteria. Exceptions may also appear in audit criteria because a physician specialist group refuses to permit inclusion of their "unique" patients in the criteria that apply to others.

Depending on how the review of transfusion is implemented, the transfusion committee may need to develop an algorithm that can be used by medical records personnel to identify records in need of review by the committee. An example of a blood transfusion review algorithm for red blood cells is given in Figure 14-1, and an example for platelet transfusion review is given in Figure 14-2.

Also, it is useful to review a sample of accepted records in a given category from time to time to fine tune the criteria and to ensure that nothing of importance is being missed.

Methods of Implementation

A number of descriptions of the means of implementing transfusion medicine audits have been published.[5,6,10,16] Methods have been developed for prospective audit (reviewing blood requests before the release of blood products),[11] concurrent review (performed within 1 to 2 days of the transfusion),[3,16] and retrospective review (days to weeks after transfusion).[10,11,16]

Toy[26] described the combined use of prospective and concurrent reviews. When platelets or fresh frozen plasma are ordered, the blood bank technologist obtains the patient's laboratory data from the computer. Requests that do not meet screening criteria require the approval of the blood bank physician. In addition, a retrospective review of each transfusion is performed by a technologist the day after the transfusion. For every patient transfused in the previous 24 hours, the technologist generates from the hospital computer the results of laboratory tests performed the day before, the day of, and the day after

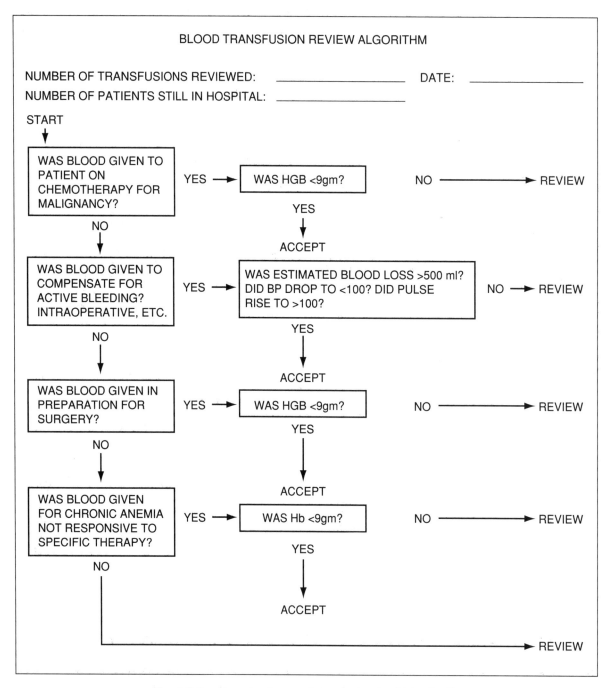

Fig. 14-1. Algorithm for transfusion audit of red blood cells.

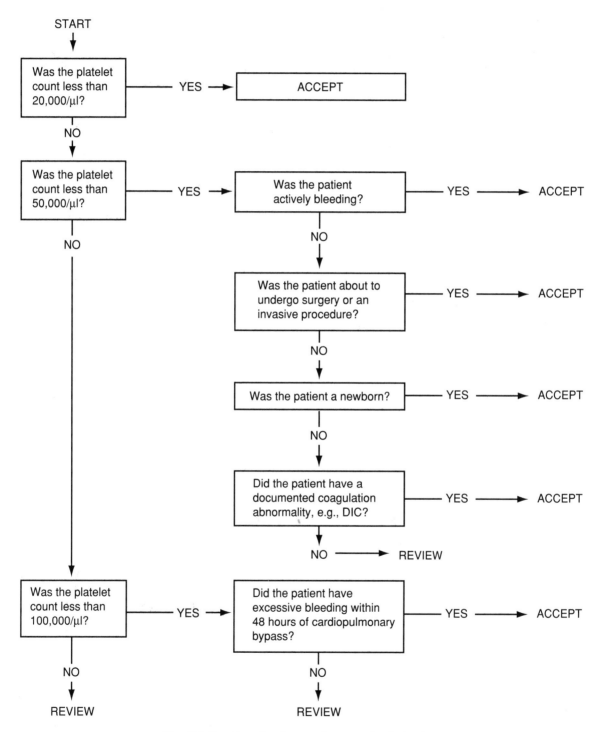

Fig. 14-2. Algorithm for transfusion audit of platelets.

blood was issued to that patient. Test results requested include the hemoglobin concentration, hematocrit, mean corpuscular red blood cell volume, PT, PTT, platelet count, and fibrinogen concentration. The printout includes the patient's age and room. The technologist then records on the test printout the patient's diagnosis, if it was written on the blood request slip, and the time and type of blood components issued. Cases that do not meet screening criteria are referred to the blood bank resident. This review takes approximately 1 hour/day of technologist time.

When a case is referred to the blood bank resident, the medical record of the patient is reviewed. The patient is usually still in the hospital. If the case meets criteria for appropriate transfusion, no further action is taken. If the transfusion was inappropriate, the case is discussed with the blood bank director and the physician who ordered the transfusion. Inappropriate cases are recorded and reviewed again by the chief resident or by a transfusion committee member. This review takes the blood bank resident or transfusion committee member approximately 1 hour/day and the blood bank director approximately 2 hours/week.

Once a month, the results are reported to the transfusion committee. In cases of inappropriate transfusion, the committee sends a letter to the attending physician with copies to the house staff. Clinicians who repeatedly use blood inappropriately are reported by the committee to their chief of service. If a clinician disagrees with the committee decision, a one-on-one discussion with the transfusion committee chairman usually resolves the disagreement.

In institutions without the computer capability described above, it is not possible to perform the initial review of the appropriateness of transfusions in the blood bank. In this case, records of patients who have been transfused can be reviewed by medical record room personnel using algorithms such as those in Figures 14-1 and 14-2. The algorithms should describe a set of indications for transfusion commonly encountered in the hospital and a set of criteria that probably justify a particular transfusion and exempt it from specific review and evaluation by the transfusion committee. If the particular criteria are not met when the record is examined by the medical record room personnel, the case is referred for review by the professional committee for its judgment and appropriate action.

Ideally, records of all patients who receive a transfusion of any blood product should be examined by the medical record room personnel. If this is impossible, a carefully selected stratified sample should be selected by a predetermined program for analysis. This should cover records from all services that have used transfusions during the review interval and all staff members who have ordered blood. Outpatient transfusion clinics should be included. It is usually preferable to conduct the review monthly to keep its findings in step with current practice in the institution. This also permits questionable cases to be fresh in the memories of those involved when discussions of the appropriateness of a transfusion are required.

It should be emphasized that medical record room personnel do not exercise the professional judgment of a physician; they are only responsible for examining the record to see whether the audit criteria have or have not been met in an individual case in which a transfusion has been administered.

Medical records that indicate compliance with the criteria are not reviewed further by the transfusion committee. Charts that do not pass this review are assigned to a physician member of the group. The medical records auditors should be told when to stop referring charts, depending on how many charts the committee wishes to review. Physician members of the transfusion committee then review each referred chart. If a transfusion has been found to be probably inappropriate, the responsible physician should be so notified and requested to respond formally to the finding. The option to appear at a committee meeting for discussion of the matter should usually be offered. In most instances, the matter can be settled at this point.

If the inappropriate transfusion has resulted in an unfavorable outcome for the patient or if the same physician is repeatedly cited for inappropriate practices, an appearance before the committee should be required. If an agreement cannot be reached or if the same issue arises again in the future, the responsible head of the service and/or chief of staff should be informed so that the staff as a whole may assume its responsibility in the matter. The staff may then exercise its discipline, if required. This is rarely needed if proceedings are handled in a nonadversarial, educational way.

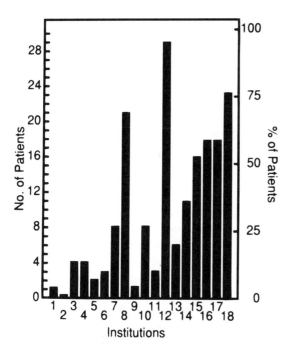

Fig. 14-3. Number (percentage) of patients transfused with plasma among 30 consecutive first-time coronary artery bypass graft patients at 18 institutions. (From Goodnough et al.,[21] with permission.)

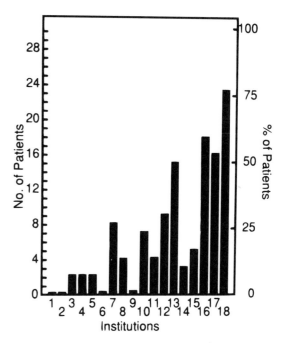

Fig. 14-4. Number (percentage) of patients transfused with platelets among 30 consecutive first-time coronary artery bypass graft patients at 18 institutions. (From Goodnough et al.,[21] with permission.)

Another method of implementing a transfusion medicine audit is to audit patients undergoing a particular surgical procedure. For example, Goodnough et al.[21] in collaboration with the Transfusion Medicine Academic Award Group, audited 540 patients undergoing elective first-time coronary artery bypass grafts at 18 institutions. They determined that blood component usage for such surgery differs widely among institutions and that the variability is accounted for in part by unnecessary transfusions in otherwise routine, uncomplicated coronary artery bypass graft procedures. Examples of this variability are given in Figures 14-3 and 14-4. Note that, in some institutions, fewer than 10 percent of patients were transfused with plasma or platelets, whereas in other institutions, greater than 75 percent of such patients were so transfused.

Effectiveness of Reviews

Measurable benefit should result from appropriately conducted blood usage reviews. Such benefit has been documented in a number of published reports.

Shanberge[9] surveyed the use of fresh frozen plasma on a daily basis and supplemented this with an educational program for the attending and house staffs. He reported that, in the first 2 years, these steps resulted in a 77 percent decrease in the number of units of fresh frozen plasma transfused (Fig. 14-5). At the beginning of the project, 2 to 3 hours were spent each day reviewing and discussing plasma. Subsequently, the process required only 1 to 2 hours/week. Similarly, Solomon et al.[27] reported that efforts to modify the use of fresh frozen plasma resulted in a 52 percent decrease in usage.

Simpson[28] reported that the use of concurrent audits and consultation for platelet transfusion resulted in a 56 percent reduction in use during a time when the patient load increased 38 percent in the two principal platelet concentrate user groups. Three years after implementation of the audit system, only 8 percent of the platelet transfusion requests were considered inappropriate, in contrast to a 54 percent incidence at the outset.

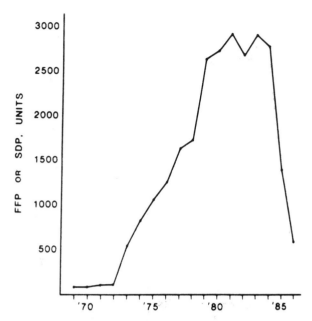

Fig. 14-5. Fresh frozen plasma usage at William Beaumont Hospital from 1969 through 1986 (abscissa). (From Shanberge,[9] with permission.)

Lichtiger et al.[29] reported that transfusion audits performed over a 4-year period reduced transfusion of red blood cells by 18.6 percent, platelet concentrates by 44.1 percent, and fresh frozen plasma and cryoprecipitate by 56.6 percent.

Soumerai et al.[30] performed audits of transfusion practices before and after brief, focused educational outreach visits by transfusion medicine specialists and reported a substantial improvement in the appropriateness of blood product use in surgery. They further concluded that savings in blood use for surgical services probably exceeded program costs.

Giovanetti et al.[31] reported that a survey regarding transfusion practice in elective surgery indicated that overrequest, overtransfusion, excessive reconstitution of whole blood (i.e., concurrent transfusion of red cells and fresh frozen plasma), and underuse of predeposit were found in all 10 surgical departments of the hospital. After implementation of a quality assurance program, there was a reduction of about two-thirds in overtransfusion, whereas overrequest, reconstitution of whole blood, and predeposit rates remained unchanged. These results indicate that significant effort and education are

sometimes required to make transfusion practices optimal.

Toy[26] listed several outcome measurements that can be compiled monthly while performing medical practice audits. These are (1) the number of inappropriate transfusion events and (2) the number of units transfused. Another outcome measurement is the percentage of orders altered as a result of screening at the time the order was requested.

System Audits

Another category of audits consists of system audits that deal primarily with the operational effectiveness of a transfusion service, emphasizing such monitoring parameters as the outdate rate, the crossmatch to transfusion (C/T) ratio, or workload and productivity figures.[5] Thus, a systems audit reviews managerial and operational data to determine whether broad aspects of transfusion therapy are appropriate. As part of their audit function, the transfusion committee should decide specifically which parameters are to be monitored on a regular basis and then direct the hospital administration and blood bank staff to modify their records systems to facilitate the gathering of the required data. Considerable judgment must be exercised to select the most useful parameters while minimizing the administrative burden placed on the blood bank by the additional record keeping.

It is easier to devise a list of key indicators that are to be monitored (Table 14-3) than it is to provide reasonable standards for these indicators.[5] Indeed, standards applicable to all hospitals are not currently available for most of these indicators. Therefore, transfusion services wishing to assess their performance must begin with an analysis of their own local experience as the basis for acceptable values. Furthermore, although much has been written about appropriate values for outdate, C/T ratio, workload, and productivity, there remain significant philosophic and practical objections to the imposition of such uniform standards on all transfusion services, ignoring their differences in size, mission, and patient mix.

Unless sophisticated data processing capabilities are present in the transfusion service, many of these indicators are best monitored only when a problem seems apparent in a particular area. However, it is

Table 14-3. A Suggested List of Key Indicators for Systems Audits

1. Units transfused—total number of whole blood, RBCs, platelet concentrates, apheresis platelets, granulocyte apheresis units, fresh frozen plasma, cryoprecipitate, coagulation factor concentrates, Rh immune globulin, cryopreserved red cells, washed RBCs, leukocyte-poor RBCs, etc.

2. Patients transfused—total number of patients receiving each product and component listed in item 1.

3. Units transfused per patient transfused

4. Relative percentage of whole blood versus RBCs

5. Crossmatch-to-transfusion ratio

6. Outdate rate

7. Transfusion reactions

8. Workload and productivity

9. Hours worked per unit transfused or patient transfused—in many transfusion services, this parameter may be a more valid indicator of the efficiency of operations than the value obtained from traditional workload-productivity figures.

10. Uncrossmatched units—the number and percentage of units issued uncrossmatched

11. Fresh unit requests

12. Turnaround time—the total time required between receipt of transfusion request and availability of the unit for transfusion to the patient. This may be examined for stats, routines, and operative requests.

13. Stat requests. The number and percentage may be analyzed by ward, service, requesting physician, and diagnosis; distribution of requests by day of week, shift, and hour may be revealing in some situations.

14. Units returned unused. The number and percent of units that are signed out from the transfusion service and later returned unused; analysis by ward, clinical service, and requesting physician may be informative.

15. Age distribution of units

16. Surgical cancellations because of unavailability of blood

17. Late requests for preoperative crossmatches. The number and percent of preoperative requests that are received by the transfusion service after the deadline for submission of requests; analysis by ward, service, and physician may be important.

18. Distribution of requests. The number of units requested by day of week, shift, or hour.

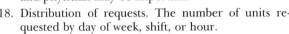
Abbreviations: RBC, red blood cells.

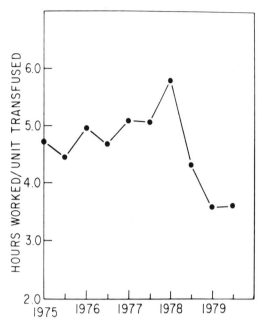

Fig. 14-6. Hours worked per red blood cell (RBC) unit transfused at Walter Reed Army Medical Center. Even when compiled properly, College of American Pathologists (CAP) workload and productivity methods do not permit detection of excessive or unnecessary testing in a laboratory. By the simple method of dividing the total hours worked or paid by the total number of units transfused, a rough index of efficiency may be obtained. A series of comprehensive management changes in 1978 were designed to eliminate duplication and unnecessary testing at Walter Reed Army Medical Center. Using RBC units as the denominator, the policy changes were associated with a 30 percent reduction in the number of hours of technologist time required to provide a given level of cell support. (From Simpson,[5] with permission.)

valuable to monitor a number of the indicators regularly, probably on a monthly basis with quarterly, semiannual, and annual summaries.

One example of the effectiveness of a systems audit is illustrated in Figure 14-6.[5]

SAME-DAY ADMISSIONS FOR SURGERY

Efforts to control the cost of medical care have led to encouragement of physicians to reduce the duration of hospitalization. One method to accomplish this is to admit patients on the morning of the day of scheduled surgery. Such a policy has the potential to increase the risk of transfusion unless special precautions are put in place. Moore et al.[32] determined that, during a 4-month period, serologic problems arose in 70 of 2,859 patients who were admitted on the day of surgery. In 36 of the 70 cases, the sample arrived at the blood bank about the time of the beginning of the operation; in 19 of these 36 cases, the operation had begun before serologic resolution, and in 7 of these 19, the antibody was found to be of hemolytic potential. Although none of the patients in their series required urgent transfusion before completion of the blood bank workup, the potential risk is obvious and unacceptable in elective surgical situations.

To respond to the expanding use of same-day admissions, we have developed a policy at the University of California Los Angeles Medical Center that takes advantage of the fact that, if a patient has not been transfused or pregnant within the preceding 3 months, there is no requirement that a sample be obtained from the patient within 3 days of the scheduled transfusion. For each patient scheduled for same-day admission, we require that a sample of blood for type and screen be obtained (unless there is no expected need for transfusion) and that a simple blood bank history form be completed by the patient in advance of surgery as part of the preoperative workup. The form asks only the following questions: (1) have you had a blood transfusion within the last 3 months and, if yes, when was the transfusion and (2) have you been pregnant within the last 3 months?

If the patient has not been transfused or pregnant within the previous 3 months, we use the specimen that was obtained during the preoperative workup for compatibility testing, providing that it was submitted within 30 days of surgery. A type and screen is performed on the day the specimen is received. If there is any potential problem for obtaining compatible blood for the patient, the ambulatory surgical center is notified both with a phone call and in writing. In some cases with complex serologic problems, it is necessary to obtain an additional specimen from the patient.

If a patient has been recently transfused or pregnant, the requirement for obtaining a specimen within 3 days is followed. Even here, an antibody screening test performed days to weeks in advance is advisable to identify existing serologic problems.

Most transfusion services (including ours) have thought that the difficulties in obtaining a reliable history make it easier to implement a policy of obtaining a specimen for compatibility testing within 3 days of transfusion for all patients. However, our policy regarding same-day admissions has worked well and has minimized last minute workups, thereby contributing to patient safety.

REFERENCES

1. Klein HG: Transfusion medicine. The evolution of a new discipline. JAMA 258:2108, 1987
2. Cable R, Thal S, Fink A, Calhoun L, Petz LD, the Transfusion Medicine Academic Award Group: A comprehensive transfusion medicine curriculum for medical students. Transfusion (in press)
3. Tomasulo PA, Lenes BA, Noto TA et al: Automatic special case consultations in transfusion medicine. Transfusion 26:186, 1986
4. Popovsky MA, Moore SB, Wick MR et al: A blood bank consultation service: principles and practice. Mayo Clin Proc 60:312, 1985
5. Simpson MBJ: Criteria for transfusion practices. p. 60. In Wallas CH, Muller VH (eds): The Hospital Transfusion Committee. American Association of Blood Banks, Arlington, 1982
6. Grindon AJ, Tomasulo PA, Bergin JJ et al: The hospital transfusion committee. Guidelines for improving practice. JAMA 253:540, 1985
7. Salem-Schatz SR, Avorn J, Soumerai SB: Influence of clinical knowledge, organizational context, and practice style on transfusion decision making. Implications for practice change strategies. JAMA 264:476, 1990
8. Klein HG: Standards for Blood Banks and Transfusion Services. American Association of Blood Banks, Bethesda, 1994
9. Shanberge JN: Reduction of fresh-frozen plasma use through a daily survey and education program. Transfusion 27:226, 1987
10. Murphy S: Guidelines for platelet transfusion (editorial). JAMA 259:2453, 1988
11. Silberstein LE, Kruskall MS, Stehling L et al: Strategies for the review of transfusion practices. JAMA 262:1993, 1989
12. Erstad BL, Gales BJ, Rappaport WD: The use of albumin in clinical practice (review). Arch Intern Med 151:901, 1991
13. Welch HG, Meehan KR, Goodnough JT: Prudent

strategies for elective red blood cell transfusion. Ann Intern Med 116:393, 1992

14. American College of Physicians: Practice strategies for elective red blood cell transfusion. Ann Intern Med 116:403, 1992

15. Contreras M, Ala FA, Greaves M et al: Guidelines for the use of fresh frozen plasma. British Committee for Standards in Haematology, Working Party of the Blood Transfusion Task Force. Transfusion Med 2:57, 1992

16. Stehling L, Luban NLC, Anderson KC et al: Guidelines for blood utilization review. Transfusion 34:438, 1994

17. Lundberg GD: Practice parameter for the use of fresh-frozen plasma, cryoprecipitate, and platelets. Fresh-Frozen Plasma, Cryoprecipitate, and Platelets Administration Practice Guidelines Development Task Force of the College of American Pathologists. JAMA 271:777, 1994

18. Goodnough LT, Vizmeg K, Riddell J, 4th, Soegiarso RW: Discharge haematocrit as clinical indicator for blood transfusion audit in surgery patients. Transfusion Med 4:35, 1994

19. Coffin C, Matz K, Rich E: Algorithms for evaluating the appropriateness of blood transfusion. Transfusion 29:298, 1989

20. Murphy MF, Brozovic B, Murphy W et al: Guidelines for platelet transfusions. British Committee for Standards in Haematology, Working Party of the Blood Transfusion Task Force. Transfusion Med 2:311, 1992

21. Goodnough LT, Johnston MF, Toy PT: The variability of transfusion practice in coronary artery bypass surgery. Transfusion Medicine Academic Award Group. JAMA 265:86, 1991

22. Renner SW, Howanitz PJ, Bachner P: Wristband identification error reporting in 712 hospitals. A College of American Pathologists' Q-Probes study of quality issues in transfusion practice. Arch Pathol Lab Med 117:573, 1993

23. Shulman IA, Lohr K, Derdiarian AK, Picukaric JM: Monitoring transfusionist practices: a strategy for improving transfusion safety. Transfusion 34:11, 1994

24. Widmann FK: Informed consent for blood transfusion: brief historical survey and summary of a conference. Transfusion 30:460, 1990

25. Willett DE: The duty to warn about transfusion risks. Arch Pathol Lab Med 113:307, 1989

26. Toy PTCY: Monitoring transfusion practice. p. 85. In Kolins J, McCarthy LJ (eds): Contemporary Transfusion Practice. American Association of Blood Banks, Arlington, 1987

27. Solomon RR, Clifford JS, Gutman SI: The use of laboratory intervention to stem the flow of fresh-frozen plasma. Am J Clin Pathol 89:518, 1988

28. Simpson MB: Concurrent audits and consultation for platelet transfusion. Transfusion 26:593, 1986

29. Lichtiger B, Fischer HE, Huh YO: Screening of transfusion service requests by the blood bank pathologist: impact on cost containment. Lab Med 19:228, 1988

30. Soumerai SB, Salem-Schatz S, Avorn J et al: A controlled trial of educational outreach to improve blood transfusion practice. JAMA 270:961, 1993

31. Giovanetti AM, Parravicini A, Baroni L et al: Quality assessment of transfusion practice in elective surgery. Transfusion 28:166, 1988

32. Moore SB, Reisner RK, Losasso TJ, Brockman SK: Morning admission to the hospital for surgery the same day. A practical problem for the blood bank. Transfusion 27:359, 1987

Chapter 15

Medicolegal Considerations

Karen Shoos Lipton and Edward L. Wolf

This chapter reviews the legal issues associated with the practice of transfusion medicine, specifically those involving legal liabilities arising from injury to recipients of blood transfusions. A broad overview such as this is complicated by four factors, which, taken together, preclude an exhaustive survey of the field.

First, both the legal principles implicated in the practice of transfusion medicine and the specific operation of those principles depend on the specific person or entity whose conduct is being challenged. Certain broad rules equally applicable to the blood collector, the hospital, and the treating physician can be identified. Other rules reflect the specific role occupied by each of these entities in the rendition of health care.

Second, as an attribute of our federal system, the laws governing legal liability in this field vary from one jurisdiction to another throughout the United States. On some issues, there is substantial unanimity among jurisdictions, such that, given a particular set of facts, the same result would obtain everywhere. On others, there is sharp conflict between the rules applied by the various states, or there are subtle, but legally significant, differences. In the latter situations, facts that establish legal liability in one jurisdiction may not give rise to such liability in another, even where both jurisdictions purport to apply the same rule. In light of this variety, the cases cited throughout this chapter as support for various propositions are generally offered for purposes of illustration, rather than as definitive statements of prevailing law throughout the United States.

Third, because so much of the law associated with transfusion medicine has evolved only since the late 1980s, the law is in flux. In many states, key issues have not been resolved; in others, the law with regard to a particular issue may appear settled, only to shift in a dramatic and unexpected manner.

Finally, the enormous range of legal liabilities associated with the provision of blood services makes broad pronouncements difficult. Claims can be asserted by donors, recipients, or third parties. Allegations can involve nerve damage, bacterial contamination, viral transmission, inadequately performed investigations of potential post-transfusion infections, provision of incorrect test results, and any number of other issues. The parties against whom liability is asserted can be not only blood collectors, physicians, and hospitals, but also employers, sex partners, and manufacturers of allegedly defective consumer products or industrial machinery.

Given these limitations, and the overriding limitation of space, it is still possible to state the generally applicable law, to summarize the critical aspects in which the law may differ among jurisdictions, to describe how the law applies to the different parties engaged in transfusion medicine, and to identify remaining areas of legal uncertainty. While the discussion focuses primarily on liabilities involving claims of recipients arising from the transmission of disease—particularly human immunodeficiency virus (HIV) infection—through transfusion, the legal issues considered would be relevant to virtually any claim asserted in connection with the provision of blood services.

APPLICATION OF FAULT-BASED PRINCIPLES

Under traditional concepts of tort law, a claim that a person sustained injury due to the acts of another could only succeed where the injured party was able to show that the other party was at fault. The injured party, the plaintiff, was required to establish either that the defendant intended to cause an injury or that the defendant acted in an unreasonable manner, with the foreseeable result being injury to another.

These theories of tort liability are "fault-based" and, under them, plaintiffs can recover only if they can show that their injury is the result of the defendant's harmful conduct, whether intentional or negligent. Imposition of this requirement, however, often results in denial of recovery to plaintiffs who are indisputably and seriously injured. To provide compensation in such circumstances, theories of "liability-without-fault" were developed and expanded. Liability-without-fault enables individuals injured by a product to receive compensation, with the cost of that compensation reflected in the price of the product, most often one that is mass produced and marketed, or otherwise treated as a cost of doing business.[1]

As the theory of strict product liability gained acceptance, plaintiffs argued that it, and related theories of liability-without-fault (e.g., the one that deems all sales transaction to include certain "implied warranties," the injury-causing breach of which can be the basis for legal recovery),[2] should be applied to the provision of blood services. Under this theory, if a "defective" blood component transmitted hepatitis, an injured recipient could recover damages even where the blood collector, hospital, or physician had taken all reasonable measures to provide a safe unit for transfusion. In other words, the receipt of a blood component in the course of medical treat-

ment would, under tort law, be considered indistinguishable from the purchase of furniture, an automobile or a prescription pharmaceutical.

In an early and influential case, the highest state court in New York confronted an attempt to impose liability-without-fault against blood collectors and ruled that the conduct at issue involved the rendition of a medical service to a patient, rather than the placement of a product into the stream of commerce for sale to a consumer.[3] The court in that case, and most others that subsequently considered the issue, rejected application of theories asserting liability-without-fault in connection with injuries arising from the provision of blood services. These cases recognize that the collection of blood or blood components from a donor, as well as its subsequent testing, processing, labeling, and distribution, all require complex judgments about substances that, as biologic agents, are inherently variable, incapable of being rendered uniform, and essential to a recipient's medical treatment.[4]

While a few cases reached a contrary result,[5,6] these holdings found general acceptance in most jurisdictions, albeit often through very different legal analyses.[7,8] They have since been codified by "blood shield" statutes that, beginning in the 1970s, have been enacted in virtually every state. Although formulations of statutory blood shields vary, all provide, in essence, that liability against blood collectors cannot be imposed in the absence of fault.[9,10] In other words, lawsuits arising from the transmission of disease as a result of a blood transfusion "sound in negligence," regardless of the defendant—blood collector, hospital, or a provider of medical care.

ELEMENTS OF NEGLIGENCE

Successful prosecution of a negligence claim requires a plaintiff to establish the elements of the tort: that the defendant owed a *duty* to the plaintiff, that there was a *breach* of that duty, that the breach was the *proximate cause* of the injury, and that there is in fact a legally compensable *injury*.[11] Issues involving the elements of proximate cause and injury, which are not dependent on the identity of a specific defendant, tend to be the same for the blood collector, the treating physician, and the hospital and are considered first.

Causation and Injury

Proximate Cause

Unreasonable conduct, no matter how egregious, cannot give rise to legal liability unless the conduct caused injury; absent this causal relationship between the conduct and the injury, there can be no finding of negligence. Issues surrounding causation in transfusion-transmitted infection generally arise in one of two contexts.

In the first context, causation issues arise over the requirement that the plaintiff be infected as a result of the transfusion at issue, and not as a result of some prior or subsequent exposure. For patients transfused with multiple units or over a long period of time, this can be a significant obstacle to recovery. This obstacle frequently surfaces in litigation by HIV-infected plaintiffs who allege that they received factor VIII that was fractionated through a process that failed to inactivate transmissible disease, or that came from donors who were inadequately screened or from donations that were not properly tested. In many of these cases, where the defendant is alleged to have acted unreasonably in responding to the risk that acquired immunodeficiency syndrome (AIDS) could be transmitted by blood products, a review of medical records or test results from preserved samples will establish that the plaintiff was actually infected with HIV before the point at which AIDS or its causative agent was identified as potentially bloodborne. Under this scenario, the plaintiff will be unable to establish proximate cause since, even if a defendant had taken the precautions in question, the plaintiff would have been infected by an earlier exposure. Even in the absence of evidence about a particular plaintiff, published data may suggest a probability that such prior exposure occurred.[11a]

This same absence of causation also exists in cases involving transfusions of blood collected subsequent to implementation of a screening test for the HIV antibody. Reliance on a volunteer donor pool, which in general has a lower incidence of disease markers than that of the overall population, combined with donor screening criteria and implementation of testing for HIV antibody, has dramatically reduced the number of HIV-infected donors, with no similarly dramatic mitigation of the incidence of HIV infection among the population at large.[12] As a result, patients admitted to some hospitals in certain high-risk areas are many times more likely to be already infected with the HIV virus—whether they know it or not—than are the donors of blood they might receive. Particularly for plaintiffs whose histories may include high-risk behaviors, the issue of causation may be formidable, even if the possibility of an infected donor cannot be excluded or if such a donor is identified. The same issue may also arise in a case alleging transmission of hepatitis C or some other agent with a relatively high incidence throughout the nontransfused population.[13]

In the second context, the issue centers around the requirement that the plaintiff demonstrate that the injury would not have occurred in the absence of the unreasonable conduct. This is a common issue in litigation involving infections transmitted before the existence of a feasible serologic test for the causative agent. For example, a plaintiff contending that certain additional questions should have been asked of potential blood donors cannot establish proximate cause if the infected unit came from a donor who, although infected, would have provided an acceptable response.[14] Similarly, a claim that a surrogate test for AIDS should have been implemented will fail if the surrogate test would not have identified and excluded the allegedly infected unit.[15]

Another issue surrounding proximate cause is as significant as, but less precise than, the issues previously discussed. As the word "proximate" suggests, the relationship between the injury and the unreasonable act that allegedly caused it cannot be unduly attenuated. Some level of attenuation, however, will not prevent plaintiff from establishing proximate cause. If a blood collector fails to defer a donor who volunteers that he has engaged in high-risk behavior for HIV and that donor's blood, which is in the serologic window period, is released and infects a recipient, the relationship between the unreasonable act—the failure to defer as an HIV risk—and the injury—transmission of HIV—is clear and proximate. If the hypothetical donor in the HIV window period had instead volunteered that a member of his household was recently diagnosed with viral hepatitis and the blood collector, in violation of its own procedures, failed to defer him, the relationship becomes less clear. Had the blood collector acted reasonably with regard to a donor who was known to be at risk of one infectious disease—hepatitis—that donor would not have been allowed to donate, and the plaintiff would not have been infected with a different infectious agent—HIV. Although the relationship is more attenuated, legal authority does exist for the proposition that proximate cause would be established by such facts.[16]

Extending the hypothetical, if the unit that transmits an infection is drawn from a donor who should have been considered unsuitable because of a low hematocrit, the relationship becomes even more attenuated. It may seem intuitively unfair to impose liability if HIV is transmitted by transfusion of a unit of blood from a donor who should have been deferred because of transient anemia or some other reason relating to the donor's protection. At some point, a court would also likely find the relationship between injury and breach too remote to satisfy the proximate cause inquiry. Articulating a rationale for determining when that point is reached is extremely difficult, both because the rules applied vary among jurisdictions and because the exercise is so dependent upon the facts of each specific case.[11] In light of that difficulty, potential defendants must assume that any wrong in connection with a transfusion can be the basis for legal liability, should that transfusion result in injury.

Injury

Not every harm visited upon a person is a legally cognizable injury. Most of the harms potentially associated with the receipt of a blood transfusion are the type for which compensation has traditionally been provided. Nonetheless, and despite the judicial, legislative, and societal trend over the last century to expand the range of harms that give rise to a legal cause of action, some courts have declined to recognize as compensable certain harms arising out of transfusions.

As a general proposition, blood recipients who are infected with agents known to cause disease have sustained legally cognizable injuries, even if they have not yet developed symptoms associated with the disease.[17] This is true, even with respect to agents that may result, in most cases, in only subclinical exposure with no adverse health effect. Of course, with regard to certain such agents, the lack of association between an infection and a subsequent disease state may substantially reduce the damages arising from an injury, or the relatively benign nature of the in-

jury and the lack of data suggesting a probability that it will progress to a more serious injury may lead courts to permit potential plaintiffs to defer suit until manifestation of the more severe condition.[18] But, while the reduction in damages may diminish an asymptomatic plaintiff's incentive to bring and prosecute a lawsuit, it probably does not constitute a defense to one.

Harm, however, that is related solely to a recipient's lack of knowledge that he or she is infected is not legally compensable unless that lack of knowledge is the cause of additional harm. This situation most commonly arises in cases involving delayed or failed notifications of individuals who received transfusions that transmitted infections. The injury in such a situation is not the recipient's infection: that was a *fait accompli* before the notification was or should have been undertaken.

In such cases, the injury, if any, must lie in something that a recipient could and would have done, had he or she received timely and appropriate notification. For instance, a recipient may already have known of her infection before what would have been a timely notification—either from test results or manifestation of illness. Similarly, after notification, a recipient still may not have receive treatment for her infection—either because such treatment was unavailable (as might be the case with hepatitis C) or because the recipient's asymptomatic condition did not warrant it (as might be the case with HIV). In these cases, there has been no legally compensable injury.[19] In sum, simply being deprived of knowledge of one's infection, does not constitute an independent compensable injury; a finding of such injury requires plaintiff to show that, had the fact of infection been communicated, some additional harm could have been avoided.

Similarly, liability arising from a recipient's fear that he or she may have exposed others to the infectious agent and liability to third parties who fear that such exposure occurred between the time notification should have occurred and the time it actually did occur are not generally treated as legally cognizable injuries. While the law with regard to such claims varies across jurisdictions, the general view is that the emotional distress occasioned by the uncertainty of not knowing whether an infection has been transmitted to a third party is not a compensable injury, unless the infection has in fact been transmitted. In other words, most courts to consider the issue have determined that neither the distress caused by a recipient's concern that he or she unknowingly infected another person, nor the other person's distress at having possibly become infected under those circumstances can, by itself, give rise to a cause of action.[19,20] Some would hold that infected recipients and uninfected third parties can be compensated for the emotional distress they endure during the "window of anxiety"—the limited period between the time the recipient is notified of his or her infection and the time that the possibility of the third-party's prenotification infection can be excluded.[21]

Duty and Breach

The two remaining elements of negligence focus primarily on the conduct of the defendant, rather than on the consequences of that conduct. With regard to the element of duty, the relationship of the defendant to the plaintiff is critical to the analysis. Because the medical treater, the blood collector and the hospital all stand in a different position *vis-a-vis* the transfusion recipient, the specific duties that each owes to a recipient differ. With regard to the requisite breach of that duty, the difference lies in the law's determination of what constitutes reasonable conduct on the part of each.

Physicians

Case law discussion of the duties that a physician owes to a patient falls primarily into two areas: the duty to obtain the patient's informed consent to treatment, and the duty to use due care in the patient's treatment, broadly defined here as including diagnosis of the patient's condition, performance of medical procedures, prescription of drugs and biologic agents, and appropriate monitoring of the patient's condition. A physician's failure to act reasonably in the discharge of either duty constitutes a breach of that duty, and such a breach can create legal liability in the event that the physician's unreasonable conduct is the proximate cause of a patient's injury.

The classic formulation of the duty to obtain a patient's informed consent requires the physician, except in limited cases of medical emergency, to advise the patient (or surrogate decision maker when the

patient cannot be advised or make a competent decision) of the material risks and likely benefits of a recommended course of treatment and of the material risks associated with the alternatives to such treatment, including the alternative of foregoing treatment.[22] Absent effective communication, the provision of such information, even in a signed consent to treatment, is not a defense to legal liability.[23] If a plaintiff can sustain his burden of establishing that he would have refused a particular course of treatment had a particular material risk been adequately disclosed, principles of proximate causation may warrant imposition of liability, even where the injury caused by the transfusion was unrelated to the inadequately disclosed risk.[24] Conversely, a plaintiff's consent to the treatment after having been adequately informed of more serious risks constitutes a formidable barrier to establishing that knowledge of the less severe risk would have changed his decision to accept the treatment, thereby preventing the injury.[25]

In the context of informed consent, a risk's materiality is a function of its severity and frequency.[26] While these components can be quantified, any number of equally reasonable patients might weigh the significance of a particular risk differently, depending on each patient's overall medical conditions, personal circumstances, general attitude toward risk, level of sophistication regarding medical issues, and other idiosyncratic factors. Focusing materiality on patients thus makes the determination of materiality much more subjective than would be the case if the focus were instead on physicians who, as a result of their training and the fact that they are not personally confronting the risks in question, tend to have a more uniform and objective view of materiality.

Because any materiality standard that focuses on what physicians consider significant may prevent patients from obtaining information that they would consider highly relevant in deciding whether to give consent, the more objective physician-based standard has been subject to attack. Although such a standard is still followed in a great many jurisdictions,[27] a great many other jurisdictions now look at materiality from the patient's perspective.[28] In most of the latter, this shift requires disclosure of those risks that would be material to a "reasonable patient" with the outlook, attitudes, concerns, and values of the very real patient who must act on the information received.[29]

In cases alleging liability for transfusion-transmitted injuries due to negligent failure to obtain informed consent, the materiality of transfusion-associated risks is often a key issue. Until the last decade, there was little authority to suggest that the risks associated with transfusion were sufficiently material to be the subject of specific informed consent. Rather, with the exception of cases involving patients, such as Jehovah's Witnesses, who refused transfusion as a matter of principle, blood transfusions were generally treated as an inseparable component of medical procedures for which no specific consent was required.[30]

It is probably no longer prudent for a physician to adhere to this view, particularly when the need for a transfusion is, at a minimum, a strong possibility.[31] In part, the desirability of informed consent for transfusion reflects real changes in the practice of transfusion medicine, specifically the availability of autologous services prior to and during surgery and other alternatives to homologous transfusion. In part, it reflects changes, not in reality, but in public perception about the safety of the blood supply and the risk of blood transfusion, relative to the other risks of treatment.

Both the reality and the perception are given effect in legislation enacted in California and a number of other states that requires physicians, where possible, to obtain specific informed consent for the administration of blood transfusions, some of which statutes even dictate the specific risks that must be disclosed and alternatives to be discussed.[32,33] Even in the majority of states, in which no similar legislation has been enacted, the existence of such laws in other jurisdictions may serve to bolster the presumption that the risks of blood transfusion are material and require separate consent.

This evolving presumption of materiality, in the face of incontrovertible evidence that the blood supply is safer than it has ever been, highlights the principal difference in the two perspectives from which risk is assessed. Under the traditional view, whether a given risk or set of risks is material is a product of professional consensus: if practitioners believe that the information should have no bearing on the decision to consent to treatment, the risk need not be disclosed. Under the more modern view, the determination of materiality is produced by the consensus of patients: if the risk might influence the decision making of the reasonable patient, it must be disclosed, even if all the facts known to the medical community establish that the reasonable patient's assessment of materiality is based on substantial misperception and misinformation.

The physician's duty to exercise due care in the treatment of her patient is one that becomes greater as the physician's training, knowledge, and experience increase. Moreover, a physician specializing in a particular field is held to a standard commensurate with the greater skill and expertise common to those engaged in similar areas of practice. Thus, a podiatrist's failure to diagnose correctly and treat a patient's foot problems may breach the standard of care, whereas the same conduct by a general practitioner might not give rise to any liability.[34] In either case, the lodestar is whether the physician's conduct in making the diagnosis deviated from what a reasonable practitioner in the same field would have done under like circumstances.[35]

Historically, this standard of care accommodated variations in resources and sophistication among different-sized communities in different parts of the country.[36] Increasingly, however, the "locality rule" is being abandoned, in part because modern technology has diminished the significance of geography in the sophistication of treatment protocols; in part because the traditional focus on community was viewed as inhibiting the adoption of new therapies by fostering parochialism; and in part because of the difficulty, particularly in small communities, of identifying expert witnesses willing to testify against colleagues, even in cases involving egregious conduct.[37]

The most significant point about the higher standard to which physicians and others in the "learned professions" are held is that the conduct of a "reasonable person"—the pertinent inquiry in most negligence actions—is not relevant. Rather, the conduct expected of other physicians with similar training, knowledge, and experience determines whether physicians have breached their duty of care. In a professional malpractice case, a jury of reasonable persons cannot rely on its own sense of appropriate conduct, but must determine, solely on the basis of testimony by qualified experts, whether the defendant's conduct so deviated from the ordinary practice in that field as to constitute a deviation from the standard of care.[38] Thus, in cases in which an injury occurs despite a physician's adherence to established practice, the higher standard of care actually provides substantial protection against a finding of legal liability.

Perhaps the best example of the significance of the higher professional standard is found in a case in which it was rejected, *Helling v. Carey,* a 1974 case decided by the Supreme Court of Washington. The case involved an ophthalmologist's failure to administer a glaucoma test to a 32-year-old woman. Undisputed evidence presented by the defendant established that the chances of a woman that age suffering from glaucoma were so remote (1 out of 25,000 under 40 years of age) that the standard practice among ophthalmologists was not to test for the disease among patients under the age of 40. Notwithstanding this evidence, the *Helling* court found that a jury, applying its own notions of what would be reasonable under the circumstances, could find the defendant's conduct negligent.[39]

Fortunately for malpractice defendants, the holding in *Helling* was not adopted by any other state. Indeed, in Washington state itself, the ruling was largely overturned by legislation that reorients the professional standard to that expected of reasonable practitioners in the same field.[40] The primary significance of *Helling* is its illustration of the distinction between the standard of care applicable in a professional malpractice action and that found in an ordinary negligence case. In the former, the "collective wisdom . . . of professionals" is accorded judicial deference; in the latter, a jury is free to substitute its own notion of reasonable conduct.[41]

With regard to a physician's liability for a transfusion-transmitted disease, it is important to keep in mind the expansive concepts of causation discussed above. Specifically, unreasonable conduct can be the basis of liability, regardless of whether it involved the decision to transfuse. A misdiagnosis or surgical error that results in a condition that requires an injury-causing transfusion at a later point in time can give rise to liability, even for physicians who are physically and temporally distant from the transfusion.

Blood Collectors

Generally stated, a blood collector's duty is to exercise reasonable care in the selection of donors and in the testing, preparation, labeling, and distribution of blood and blood components. In contrast to the relatively settled law of physician liability, the "reasonable care" standard applicable to blood collectors is unsettled, contentious, and variable from one jurisdiction to the next.

Before the HIV epidemic, the few reported cases on blood collector liability held, in essence, that the medical and scientific issues that permeate the activities of blood collectors required application of the higher professional standard of care associated with negligence actions against physicians and other professionals. Determinations about donor screening criteria or decisions about the suitability of a specific donor based on those criteria involve technical judgments by health care professionals; the same type of judgments are at the root of decisions to implement specific serologic tests and to release blood components based on results of those tests. Plaintiffs could establish negligence only if they could prove, through expert testimony, that the actions in question deviated from that which would have been taken by a reasonably prudent blood collector under the same or similar circumstances.[42] Stated simply, if a blood collector's actions conformed to applicable regulations, the standards of the American Association of Blood Banks, and the collector's own procedures, there could be no liability.[43,44]

Strict application of this standard to lawsuits alleging blood collector liability in connection with transfusion-transmitted HIV infection would, in virtually all cases, result in a finding of non-negligence "as a matter of law," that is, without need to submit the matter to trial. For example, under the professional standard, evidence that, prior to the availability of a test for HIV antibody, the hepatitis B core antibody test could have been used to identify some group of donors at risk of the causative agent for AIDS would be legally irrelevant in the face of evidence that the consensus of blood collectors, informed by both government recommendations and available data, was not to implement such a surrogate test.

Some courts have come to precisely that conclusion.[45,46] Others, more reluctant to permit blood collectors to use collective decision making as means of insulating themselves from collective liability, have held that blood collectors are not entitled to the deference traditionally accorded judgments of those who practice in a "learned profession."[47] Still others have purported to apply a professional standard of care but have created an exception whereby plaintiffs can establish negligence by demonstrating that the conduct of an entire profession was deficient.[48] The latter two views may reflect judicial skepticism about the ability of any group of professionals to make decisions that are not motivated by self-interest and, in turn, a devaluation of the legal significance of membership in any learned profession; these views may reflect an underlying belief that, while medical professionals are entitled to deference, blood collectors are not true medical professionals; they may represent some combination of those rationales. Clearly, however, the complete survival of the professional standard of care in cases involving blood collector liability is uncertain.

This issue most often surfaces in determining when compliance with the standards of the profession is conclusive evidence of non-negligence and when those standards themselves can be challenged as "deficient." If plaintiffs are required to demonstrate that the general practice within the profession was contrary to the weight of recent peer-reviewed research or the recommendations of public health agencies, liability would rarely be established. If, however, testimony from a single expert that an additional measure should have been taken will suffice to create a triable issue of fact regarding the purportedly deficient conduct of all or nearly all blood collectors—even in the absence of scholarship or practice to support that expert's views—virtually every case will offer an opportunity for judges or juries to revisit the judgment of the entire profession. In these cases, application of the professional standard of care will be indistinguishable from the ordinary standard negligence.

In addition to exercising due care in the collecting, testing, processing, and distribution of blood components and products, blood collectors also have some legal duties with regard to transmitting information to patients. While the duty to provide a patient with the information necessary to make an informed decision, as well as information subsequently derived about possible exposure from a transfusion, is one that belongs to the attending physician providing the patient's treatment, a blood collector can be held negligent for failing to communicate information that a physician would need to discharge her duties or for communicating incorrect information. The blood collector's duty in this respect is to act reasonably in providing others—the "learned intermediaries"—with the information necessary to the discharge of their duties.[49]

Hospitals

A hospital can be liable for an act of negligence relating to those things that its blood bank or transfusion service does in connection with a transfusion. Crossmatching and ensuring that patients are provided with the correct units are two potential areas of liability.[50,51] In addition, a hospital is responsible for acting appropriately with regard to the provision of information that would enable a physician to communicate with patients about blood transfusions. Such information includes the contents of the Circular of Information, additional data about risks of transfusion that it may receive from blood collectors or public health agencies, information regarding available alternatives to homologous transfusion, and notifications from blood collectors that bear on potential injuries to transfusion recipient.[52] In the absence of specific legislation, a hospital's failure to provide for or facilitate directed donations should not give rise to such liability, as donations designated for specific individuals have not been shown to be safer than nondesignated donations.[53] By contrast, a hospital blood bank's failure to inform physicians about and, where appropriate, to facilitate autologous donations, or the hospital's failure to use other autologous techniques (again, when appropriate), could give rise to liability, since these are recognized as safer than homologously donated blood.[54] A hospital can also be subject to the full range of potential liabilities associated with blood collectors if it collects blood for transfusion.

Most assertions of negligence directed toward hospitals in cases involving transfusion-transmitted disease, however, relate to acts committed by house staff physicians, nurses, and other employees for whose actions the hospital is liable under principles of *re-*

spondeat superior.[55] If a resident's diagnosis is negligent, if the resident fails to obtain the requisite informed consent, or if the resident orders the administration of an unnecessary transfusion, the hospital, as the resident's employer, can be held liable. Similarly, if a nurse fails to act reasonably in monitoring a postoperative patient, and that failure requires a subsequent transfusion that causes injury to the recipient, the hospital, as the nurse's employer, will share legal liability. Unlike cases dealing with a hospital's liability for inadequate monitoring of independent contractors, such as surgical staff with medical privileges, liability under the doctrine of *respondeat superior* is, as its English name suggests, truly "vicarious": if the employee acts negligently, no separate act of negligence by the institution is required and liability attaches, regardless of whether the institution acted reasonably in hiring, training, or supervising the employee or agent.[56]

Of particular significance to the hospital in these cases is the previously discussed issue of causation. Just as principles of legal causation can expand the range of physicians who may be liable for transfusion-transmitted disease, these principles, combined with the doctrine of vicarious liability, produce a nearly infinite number of scenarios that can lead to hospital liability.

REFERENCES

1. *Greenman v. Yuba Power Products, Inc.,* 59 Cal. 2d 57, 377 P.2d 897 (1962)
2. *Henningsen v. Bloomfield Motors, Inc.,* 32 N.J. 358, 161 A.2d 69 (1960)
3. *Perlmutter v. Beth David Hosp.,* 308 N.Y. 100, 123 N.E. 2d 792 (1954)
4. *Balkowitsch v. Minneapolis War Memorial Blood Bank,* 270 Minn. 151, 132 N.W.2d 805 (1965)
5. *Cunningham v. MacNeal Memorial Hosp.,* 46 Ill. 443, 266 N.E.2d (1970)
6. *Hoder v. Sayet,* 196 So.2d 205 (Fla. Dist. Ct. App. 1967)
7. *Whitehurst v. American Red Cross,* 1 Ariz. App. 326, 402 P.2d 584 (1965)
8. *Fisher v. Sibley Memorial Hosp.,* 403 A.2d 1130 (D.C. 1979)
9. Cal. Health & Safety Code §§ 1606 & 1603.5
10. Pa. Cons. Stat. Ann. § 8333 (1982)
11. Keeton WP, Dobbs DB, Keeton RE, Owen DG: Prosser and Keeton on the Law of Torts. 5th Ed. West, St. Paul, 1984
11a. Eystae ME, Goedert JJ, Sarngadharan MG et al: Development and early natural history of HTLV-III antibodies in persons with hemophilia. JAMA 253:2219, 1985
12. Dodd RY: The risk of transfusion-transmitted infection. N Engl J Med 327:419, 1992
13. Hepatitis Surveillance Report No. 55: Centers for Disease Control and Prevention, Atlanta, 1994
14. *Marcella v. Brandywine Hosp.,* 838 F.Supp. 1004 (E.D. Pa. 1993), *rev'd on other grounds,* 47 F.3d 618 (3d cir. 1995)
15. *Kozup v. Georgetown University,* 663 F.Supp.1048 (D.D.C. 1987) *aff'd in relevant part,* 851 F.2d 437 (D.C. Cir. 1988)
16. *Doe v. American Red Cross Blood Services S.C. Region,* 125 F.R.D. 646 (D.S.C. 1989)
17. *Murray v. Hamot Medical Center,* 633 A.2d 196 (Pa. Super. 1993)
18. *Marinari v. Asbestos Corp. Ltd.,* 612 A.2d 1021 (Pa. Super. 1992)
19. *Zaccone v. American National Red Cross,* 827 F.Supp. 457 (N.D. Ohio 1994)
20. *McKnight v. American Red Cross,* 1994 WL 323861 (E.D. Pa. 1994)
21. *Faya v. Almaraz,* 329 Md. 435, 620 A.2d 327 (1993)
22. Louisell D, Williams H: Medical Malpractice. Matthew Bender, New York, 1981
23. *Hansbrough v. Kosyak,* 141 Ill. App.3d. 538, 490 N.E.2d 181 (1986)
24. *Hook v. Rothstein,* 281 S.C. 541, 316 S.E.2d 690 (Ct. App.), *writ denied,* 283 S.C. 64, 320, S.E.2d 354 (1984)
25. *Cunningham v. United States,* 683 F.2d 847 (4th Cir. 1982)
26. *Harbeson v. Parke-Davis, Inc.,* 746 F.2d 517 (9th Cir. 1984)
27. *Guebard v. Jabaay,* 117 Ill. App.3d 1, 452 N.E.2d 751 (1983)
28. *Crain v. Allison,* 443 A.2d 558 (D.C. 1982)
29. *Truman v. Thomas,* 27 C.3d 285, 165 Cal. Rptr. 308, 611 P.2d 902 (1980)
30. *Sawyer v. Methodist Hospital,* 522 F.2d 1102 (6th Cir. 1975)
31. *Doe v. Johnston,* 476 N.W.2d 28 (Iowa 1991)
32. Cal. Health and Safety Code § 1645 (1990)
33. N.J. State: Ann. 26:2A 14 (Supp. 1992)
34. *Coye v. Cirillia,* 45 Or. App. 177, 607 P.2d 1383, *review denied,* 289 Or. 155 (1980)
35. *Sullivan v. Henry,* 160 Ga. App. 791, 287 S.E. 2d 652 (1982)
36. *Hirn v. Edgewater,* 86 Ill. App.3d 939, 408 N.E. 2d 970 (1980)
37. *King v. Williams,* 276 S.C. 478, 279 S.E.2d 618 (1981)

38. *Washington v. Washington Hospital Center*, 579 A.2d 177 (D.C. 1990)

39. *Helling v. Carey*, 83 Wash. 2d 514, 519 P.2d 981 (1974)

40. Wash. Rev. Code § 4.24.290 (1988)

41. Keeton WP: Medical negligence—the standard of care. Tex Tech L Rev 10:351, 1979

42. *Hutchins v. Blood Services of Montana*, 161 Mont.359 509 P.2d 449 (1973)

43. *Hines v. St. Joseph Hosp*, 86 N.M. 763, 527 P.2d 1075 (Ct. App.), *cert. denied*, 529 P.2d 1232 (1974)

44. *Tufaro v. Methodist Hosp*, 368 So. 2d 1219 (La. Ct. App. 1979)

45. *Doe v. American Red Cross Blood Services*, 297 S.C. 430, 377 S.E.2d 323 (1989)

46. *Valdivez v. United States*, 884 F.2d 196 (5th Cir. 1989)

47. *Vuono v. New York Blood Center*, 696 F.Supp. 743 (D. Mass. 1988)

48. *United Blood Services v. Quintana*, 827 P.2d 509 (Colo. 1992)

49. *Seley v. G.D. Searle & Co.*, 67 Ohio St. 2d 192, 423 N.E.2d 831 (1981)

50. *National Homeopathic Hospital v. Phillips*, 181 F.2d 293 (D.C. Cir. 1950)

51. *Necolayff v. Genessee Hospital*, 170 A.D. 648, 61 N.Y.S.2d 832 (App. Div. 1946) *aff'd mem*, 296 N.Y. 936, 73 N.E. 2d 117 (1947)

52. *McClaine v. Alger*, 150 Mich. App. 306, 388 N.W.2d 349 (1986)

53. Starkey Macpherson JL, Bolgiero DC, et al: Markers for transfusion-transmitted disease in different groups of blood donors. JAMA 262:3452, 1989

54. Birkmeyer JD, Goodnough LT, AuBuchon JP, et al: The cost-effectiveness of preoperative autologous blood donation for total hip and knee replacement. Transfusion 33:544, 1993

55. *Doctors Hosp. v. Bonnie*, 195 Ga. App. 152, 392 S.E.2d 897 (1990)

56. *Albain v. Flower Hosp.*, 50 Ohio St. 3d 251, 553 N.E.2d 1038 (1990)

Platelet Transfusions

Lawrence D. Petz

He who feels confident that he has a thorough understanding of platelet transfusions is confused.

A number of significant scientific questions remain unanswered regarding platelet transfusion therapy, as will be pointed out throughout this chapter. Nevertheless, some clinical guidance regarding appropriate usage can be derived from consensus conference statements[1] and from several published reviews and guidelines[2–4] developed by physicians practiced in the use of platelet transfusions.

This chapter reviews current concepts concerning various aspects of platelet transfusions including

Indications, with a specific discussion of prophylactic platelet transfusions for medical and surgical patients

Appropriate clinical and laboratory evaluation and management of thrombocytopenic patients who are bleeding

Platelet transfusion therapy in specific clinical settings including cardiopulmonary bypass, massive transfusion, splenomegaly, disseminated intravascular coagulation

Platelet transfusion therapy for patients with disorders of platelet function

Practical aspects of platelet transfusion including the use of ABO and Rh incompatible plate-

lets, appropriate dosage, and means of assessing the effectiveness of transfusions

Methods for diagnosing and managing patients refractory to platelet transfusion

Methods for prevention of alloimmunization

The risks of platelet transfusion

New concepts including the transfusion of platelet microparticles and the potential effectiveness of thrombopoietin.

INDICATIONS

Prophylactic Platelet Transfusions

Rather surprisingly, most platelets are transfused to patients who are not bleeding. In one large medical center where 17,557 random donor concentrates and 5,160 apheresis products were used during a 3-month period, 86 percent of the platelets were transfused to patients with a diagnosis of a hematologic malignancy or aplastic anemia or who were undergoing bone marrow transplantation, and 68 percent were administered prophylactically.[5] A survey conducted by the Transfusion Practices Committee of the American Association of Blood Banks[6] revealed that prophylactic platelet transfusions constituted 69.4 percent of platelet transfusions ordered by pediatric hematologists/oncologists and 58.4 percent of those ordered by internist hematologists/oncologists. Careful and continued scrutiny of policies that result in the use of such large numbers of platelet transfusions is clearly warranted.

The following discussion of prophylactic platelet transfusions pertains particularly to patients with chronic hypoproliferative thrombocytopenia (e.g., hematologic malignancies and aplastic anemia). Prophylactic transfusions before invasive procedures are considered subsequently.

The factors that must be considered in the development of a policy concerning prophylactic platelet transfusions are the risk of bleeding at various platelet counts, the effectiveness of prophylactic transfusions to prevent such bleeding, and the adverse effects of platelet transfusions, the most important of which are alloimmunization, infectious disease transmission, and expense.

The Risk of Bleeding in Patients with Thrombocytopenia

If there were a reasonably precise platelet count above which patients were safe from bleeding and below which clinically important bleeding was likely

to occur, one could more confidently develop a rational policy regarding prophylactic platelet transfusions. Unfortunately, of course, this is not the case.

Data regarding the incidence of bleeding at various platelet count levels were published in the early 1960s and still provide the basis for many clinical decisions regarding platelet transfusions.[7,8] A widely quoted early study on platelet transfusion and leukemia noted no threshold above which patients were consistently safe from spontaneous hemorrhage and below which they were at risk.[7]

Concern about bleeding and consideration of the use of prophylactic platelet transfusions when the platelet count is less than 20,000/µl has developed at least in part from data displayed in Figure 16-1.[7] The incidence of all bleeding, including skin hemorrhage and epistaxis, is not increased significantly until counts less than 20,000/µl are reached, and the incidence of grossly visible hemorrhage is only minimally increased even at counts of 5,000 to 10,000/µl. The authors also compared the data in Figure 16-1 with those regarding a group of patients who had been treated for leukemia but who had not re-

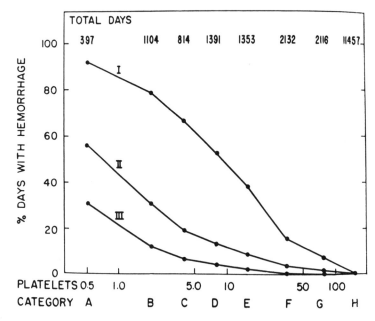

Fig. 16-1. The percentage of days with hemorrhage for the 92 patients combined is shown for each of the eight platelet count categories. (Figures across the top are the total number of patient days in each of the categories.) Curve I shows data for all hemorrhagic manifestations. In curve II, skin hemorrhage and epistaxis are excluded. Curve III refers only to grossly visible hemorrhage. (From Gaydos et al.,[7] with permission.)

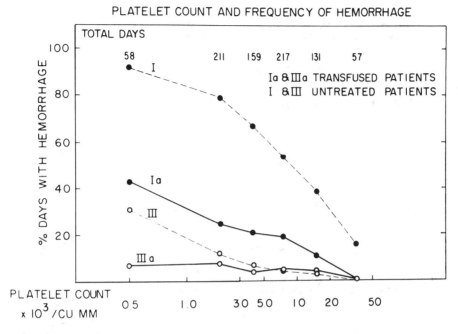

PLATELET COUNT AND FREQUENCY OF HEMORRHAGE

Fig. 16-2. The relationship between platelet count and frequency of hemorrhage. The data from the 28 patients in the present study (shown in solid lines, Ia and IIIa) are compared with a group of patients studied previously who had not received platelet transfusions (shown in broken lines, I and III). All observed hemorrhage is shown by solid circles, while gross, serious hemorrhage only is shown by open circles. (From Freireich et al.,[8] with permission.)

ceived platelet transfusions (Fig. 16-2). The incidence of "all observed hemorrhage" was higher among nontransfused patients than among transfused patients (curves I and Ia), but the incidence of gross, serious hemorrhage was not different among transfused patients versus untransfused patients until the platelet count was below 5,000/μl (curves III and IIIa). In addition, the number of days when hemorrhage was noted and the proportion of those during which grossly visible hemorrhage (hematuria, melena, and hematemesis) occurred were computed for each platelet level (Fig. 16-3). The proportion of bleeding days with serious hemorrhage was highest at platelet counts of less than 5,000/μl but was not much different in patients whose platelet counts were between 5,000 and 100,000/μl, about 4 and 8 percent, respectively.[8]

The above data were published before it was recognized that aspirin causes platelet dysfunction. Because many of the patients were undoubtedly febrile and thus receiving aspirin, the actual bleeding risk

at any given platelet level is probably less than these data indicate.[9]

In another study, published in 1973, of 62 leukemic children in whom the relationship between bleeding manifestations and platelet count was assessed, serious bleeding occurred in 26 percent of the patients with platelet counts between 0 and 10,000/μl, in 10 percent of patients with platelet counts between 10,000 and 20,000/μl, and in 4 to 5 percent of patients with platelet counts between 20,000 and 40,000/μl.[10]

Slichter and Harker[11] measured chromium-labeled stool blood loss to assess thrombocytopenic bleeding in 20 patients with aplastic anemia. At platelet counts between 5,000 and 10,000/μl, blood loss averaged 9 ± 7 ml/day, whereas at levels less than 5,000/μl blood loss was markedly elevated (Fig. 16-4).

Aderka et al.[12] retrospectively studied 64 leukemic patients and reported that there was a clear increase in bleeding risk for patients with acute nonlymphoblastic leukemia (ANLL) who had platelet counts less

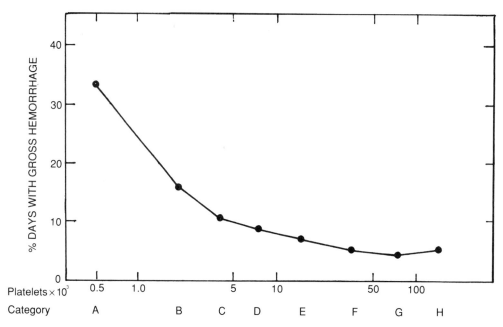

Fig. 16-3. Fraction of total bleeding days with grossly visible hemorrhage according to platelet count category. (From Gaydos et al.,[7] with permission.)

than 10,000/μl compared with patients with counts between 10,000 and 20,000/μl. In general, the risk of bleeding was increased for leukemic versus chemotherapy-induced thrombocytopenia, for patients with decreasing rather than stable or increasing platelet counts, and for febrile versus afebrile patients. This study also indicated that the bleeding risk was greater in patients under 18 years of age and in those with acute lymphoblastic leukemia versus those with ANLL.

More recent data have been supplied by Gmur et al.,[13] who noted a progressive increase in the frequency of hemorrhage with declining platelet counts as illustrated in Figure 16-5.

It is evident that a precise "threshold" type of relationship does not exist between platelet count and hemorrhage. Some patients may not demonstrate evidence of hemorrhage despite prolonged thrombocytopenia with levels as low as 5,000/μl, whereas other patients may show evidence of grossly visible hemorrhage with platelet counts above 20,000/μl.

In addition to the above information concerning the overall risk of hemorrhage, a particular concern is intracranial hemorrhage, which may result in se-

vere chronic disability or death and which may occur as the initial manifestation of bleeding in a thrombocytopenic patient. There is a paucity of published data regarding intracerebral hemorrhage in thrombocytopenic patients. A 1962 study reported the risk of intracranial hemorrhage in patients with acute leukemia who were followed for evidence of bleeding at various platelet counts, excluding patients in "blastic crisis." Eight of the 92 patients in the study had intracranial hemorrhage. Of these, only one had a platelet count of over 5,000/μl, and in none did the level exceed 10,000/μl. Intracranial hemorrhage occurred at a frequency of 0.76 percent of days on which platelet levels were below 1,000/μl.[7] Han et al.[14] reported in 1966 that there were no antecedent bleeding manifestations in 7 of 46 patients in whom intracerebral hemorrhage was found at autopsy. Also, even in patients who do manifest "warning signs," emergency platelet transfusions may not reverse bleeding acutely enough to prevent serious sequelae.

Many clinicians feel that the risk of hemorrhage at a given platelet count is higher in the presence of complicating clinical factors such as sepsis; coexis-

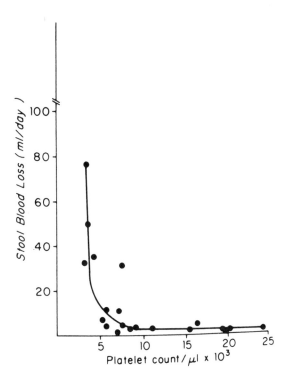

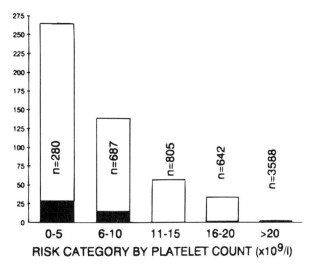

Fig. 16-4. Stool blood loss as a measure of thrombocytopenic bleeding. When stool blood loss (expressed as ml/day) was determined in 20 aplastic thrombocytopenic patients (closed circles), blood loss was less than 5 ml/day at platelet counts greater than 10,000/μl. At platelet counts between 5,000 and 10,000/μl, blood loss averaged 9 ± 7 ml/day. At levels less than 5,000/μl blood loss was markedly elevated at 50 ± 20 ml/day. (From Slichter and Harker,[11] with permission.)

Fig. 16-5. Relation of bleeding risk to blood platelet counts, computed per 1,000 days of risk. Open bars: minor bleeding complications. Solid bars: Major bleeding complications. Numbers in bars are numbers of observed days at risk in a given class. The correlation coefficient between class 1–4 and the incidence of bleeding is r = 0.963, $P < 0.01$. Risk category platelets, $20 \times 10^9/1$ not included in correlation coefficient because the few bleeding complications in this group were related to factors other than solely the platelet count, and because of the broad range of counts in this category. (From Gmur,[13] with permission.)

tent coagulation disturbances such as in disseminated intravascular coagulation (DIC), hepatic failure, or anticoagulant therapy; anatomic lesions; a rapidly falling platelet count; and high fever.[3,12,15,16]

Effectiveness

Several researchers have studied the effectiveness of strategies designed to prevent serious spontaneous hemorrhage with prophylactic platelet transfusion. Higby et al.[17] studied 12 thrombocytopenic patients who were given prophylactic platelet transfusions and compared results with 9 patients who were not transfused with platelets. They found that patients who were not transfused with platelets had a higher frequency of bleeding, "affirming the value of prophylactic platelet transfusions."

Roy et al.[10] studied 62 patients who received prophylactic platelet transfusions when the count was less than 25,000/μl and compared the prevalence of bleeding with retrospective controls consisting of patients treated approximately 20 years earlier. The differences in the frequency of bleeding between the transfused and nontransfused patients were highly significant.

Two randomized studies have compared "prophylactic" platelet transfusions with "therapeutic" platelet transfusions in which transfusions were given only when the patient had clinically significant bleeding (i.e., more than petechiae, mucous membrane bleeding, or epistaxis). One showed no difference between the prophylactic group (17 patients) and therapeutic group (12 patients) in remission induction or duration, mortality, or number of red blood cell (RBC) transfusions required. An important finding was that the patients randomized to receive prophylactic transfusions used twice as many platelets as did the therapeutic group.[18] The second study, which was done in children, showed less bleeding early in the course of patients in the prophylactic group (35 patients) compared with the therapeutic group (21 patients). However, over the entire study period the total number of days on which bleeding was present was the same in the two groups and survival was identical.[19]

Adverse Consequences

The benefits of a policy of prophylactic platelet transfusions must justify the increased risks involved with the use of increased numbers of transfusions. The major risks of platelet transfusions are alloimmunization and the transmission of infectious diseases.[1]

The effect of larger numbers of platelet transfusions on the incidence of alloimmunization was studied by Dutcher et al.[20] Using the existence of lymphocytotoxic antibodies to define immunization, these investigators state that the overall rate of immunization is independent of the number of platelet transfusions administered.[20,21] Klingeman et al.[22] were also unable to show a dose–response relationship between the number of platelet units transfused and the development of lymphocytotoxic antibodies. On this basis one would conclude that there is no reason to withhold prophylactic platelet transfusions expressly to prevent alloimmunization in patients with acute leukemia because all patients receiving intensive induction chemotherapy will require therapeutic transfusions of at least 10 to 20 units of platelets and the rate of alloimmunization does not change at this "dose" of platelets or higher.[23] Whether the severity of alloimmunization is affected by more frequent platelet transfusions was not addressed.

Published data (reviewed below) indicate that alloimmunization may be minimized by the use of leukocyte-depleted blood products and, in addition, most patients who do become alloimmunized can be managed with special platelet products. Accordingly, most investigators do not consider the possible increased frequency or severity of alloimmunization to be a strong argument against prophylactic platelet transfusions.

Safety of the Blood Supply

It is self evident that giving fewer platelet transfusions will result in less transmission of infectious disease by blood products. Since any policy must be based on an assessment of risks as compared with benefits, it is apparent that even if one could establish a "perfect" transfusion "trigger" that just balanced risks and benefits, this trigger would change as the safety of the blood supply changed. In recent years there have been major improvements in the safety of the blood supply as is reviewed in detail elsewhere in this text (section V). Therefore, the magnitude of the safety provided by minimizing platelet transfusions must be considered carefully. A policy of providing platelet transfusions only for patients with serious episodes of thrombocytopenic bleeding would probably have been optimal in 1983–1984, but not today.

Beutler[24] developed his recommendations for a stringent policy of platelet transfusion on the estimate of a shortening of life span of a 50-year-old recipient by an average of 1 day for each 2 units of blood transfused. A more recent analysis indicates that substituting autologous for allogeneic blood results in little expected health benefit, only 0.0002 to 0.00044 quality-adjusted years of life saved (1.75 to 3.85 hours) for patients 49 to 68 years of age.[25]

The significance of the safety of the blood supply is illustrated in the following example. Consider the policy of withholding prophylactic platelet transfusions when the platelet count is between 5,000/μl and 20,000/μl. Some have stated that a prophylactic transfusion policy using a platelet count of 5,000/μl in stable patients is "safe." However, one must consider this policy in light of the present risk of human immunodeficiency virus (HIV) transmission, which is estimated to occur about once in every 420,000 units of blood. If the frequency of fatal bleeding episodes (as may be caused by intracerebral hemorrhage) that could be preventable by a prophylactic transfusion is greater than once in 420,000 instances in which the platelet count is between 5,000 and 20,000/μl, it is safer from the standpoint of HIV transmission to transfuse than to withhold transfusion. Hepatitis C is the other major infectious complication of blood transfusion. It occurs about once per 5,000 donor exposures but with perhaps only

10% of patients (1/50,000 donor exposures) developing serious clinical sequelae (see section V). Indeed, Aderka et al.[12] reported that of 89 episodes of thrombocytopenia below 20,000/μl in patients with ANLL, bleeding was the cause of death in "only one patient" who had a platelet count of 5,000/μl. One death in 89 episodes of thrombocytopenia (445 days of thrombocytopenia) at a count of 5,000 to 20,000/μl is a far greater complication rate than one case of HIV transmission in 420,000 units transfused or one case of symptomatic hepatitis C disease in 50,000 units transfused.

Thus, in regard to infectious disease transmission, it is difficult to be confident that avoiding infectious disease transmission by not transfusing when the platelet count is between 5,000 and 20,000/μl is safer than transfusing. Even if it were true that a stringent prophylactic platelet transfusion policy were safer than the more generous use of prophylactic transfusions, it would probably be impossible to perform a study of sufficient magnitude to have statistical validity to document this. Certainly, such studies have not yet been performed.

The Expense of Platelet Transfusions

Platelets are expensive and it is appropriate to consider health-care costs in formulating a policy regarding prophylactic platelet transfusions. Physicians are often criticized for utilizing expensive procedures which do not provide commensurate benefit. Gmur et al.[13] reported that a more restrained use of platelets resulted in substantial health-care savings.

Present Practices

Pisciotto et al.[6] surveyed hospital institutional members of the American Association of Blood Banks concerning platelet transfusion practices in 1991. Greater than 70 percent of hospitals reported transfusing platelets primarily for prophylaxis: 60 percent of hospitals set the "threshold" platelet count for prophylactic platelet transfusion at 20,000/μl, with approximately 20 percent of hospitals transfusing either at higher or lower levels.

Numerous recommendations regarding prophylactic platelet transfusion policies have been made.[3,9,12,13,16,24,26–29]

Aderka et al.[12] provide prophylactic platelet trans-

fusions only at counts below 10,000/μl. They evaluated the effectiveness of this policy in a retrospective study of 64 patients with acute leukemia and concluded that prophylactic platelet administration can be safely postponed until the count is below 10,000/μl in patients with acute nonlymphatic leukemia, without fever, with chemotherapy-induced thrombocytopenia (as compared with leukemia-related thrombocytopenia), and in patients older than 18 years regardless of the platelet trend.

Data tending to confirm the advisability of such a comparatively restrictive prophylactic policy was provided by Gmur et al.,[13] who prospectively assessed 102 patients being treated for acute leukemia. They concluded that the threshold for prophylactic transfusions can safely be set at 5,000/μl in patients without fever or bleeding manifestations and at 10,000/μl in patients with such signs. For patients with coagulation disorders or anatomic lesions, or for those on heparin, the threshold should be at least 20,000/μl.

Simon[26] recommended a policy by which prophylactic platelet transfusions would be administered at a level below 5,000/μl, regardless of the clinical status of a leukemia patient. If the platelet count is 10,000/μl and above, the patient would be transfused if there were clinically significant bleeding (e.g., massive confluent petechiae, severe purpura or bleeding at venipuncture sites, excess mucous membrane bleeding, or continuous, severe epistaxis). The patient who seemed stable with regard to clinical bleeding risk would not be transfused. As the count falls below 10,000/μl to the level of 5,000/μl, at which an increased bleeding risk can be regularly expected, one would transfuse more quickly in early induction or septic periods than at other times.[26]

Schiffer and co-workers[3,27] recommend that attempts be made to individualize prophylactic platelet transfusion according to each patient's condition. Patients with stable clinical condition and diseases such as myelodysplasia that are expected to be associated with long-term nonreversible thrombocytopenia do not routinely receive prophylactic platelet transfusions regardless of the platelet count, unless hemorrhage or infectious episodes occur, at which time prophylactic platelet transfusion is used temporarily. On the other hand, there are patients in whom prophylactic platelet transfusions are given in an attempt to keep the platelet count well above 20,000/μl. These include patients with acute progranulocytic leukemia, patients receiving systemic anticoagulation, patients with hyperleukocytosis before and during chemotherapeutic cytoreduction, patients with severe infections, patients with severe gastrointestinal tract mucositis, and some patients with solid tumors such as malignant melanoma or renal cell carcinoma, which have a tendency to have hemorrhagic central nervous system metastasis.

Beutler[16,24] suggests that a platelet count of less than 5,000/μl as an indication for transfusion seems satisfactory based on his own experience (data not provided) but adds that a "doctrinaire insistence on a 5,000 platelet/μl trigger is not clearly justified by data. A somewhat higher level may be appropriate; there are insufficient data to allow one to decide."[16] In his view, 20,000/μl is clearly too high a platelet count to justify prophylactic transfusion for the patient without additional risk factors.

Slichter[9] states that patients with production-related thrombocytopenia and platelet counts less than 5,000/μl should be given prophylactic platelet transfusions to avoid the risk of substantial bleeding. At platelet counts between 5,000 and 20,000/μl, clinical judgment should be used to assess the severity of bleeding and the need for platelet therapy. When a patient has significant bleeding at a platelet count higher than 10,000/μl, platelet dysfunction is present, the vascular system has been disrupted, or there are additional coagulation factor deficiencies. Platelets should be given only to control significant bleeding until the underlying problem can be resolved.

A minority view has been stated by Patten,[28] who suggests that a program of therapeutic platelet transfusion should be considered as a justifiable alternative to prophylactic platelet transfusion. A therapeutic platelet transfusion program consists of transfusion for serious episodes of bleeding such as epistaxis or gingival bleeding that is not responsive to local measures, hemoptysis, hematemesis, melena, gross hematuria, profuse vaginal bleeding, headache, or retinal or central nervous system bleeding in the presence of a platelet count less than 20,000/μl. At her institution, a policy of therapeutic platelet transfusions in leukemia patients has been followed for more than a decade with the endorsement of the transfusion committee and medical staff.[29] During this period, the platelet: red cell transfusion ratio averaged 0.26 per year. This is significant in that many hospitals with active hematology/oncology units report a platelet:red cell transfusion ratio of greater than one. She states that, providing platelets are on hand and immediately available, a policy of therapeutic transfusion does not increase mortality or serious bleeding episodes and decreases the patient's donor exposure to a minimum, thereby decreasing both the risk and cost of platelet transfusion. Unfortunately, data documenting patient outcome in the therapeutic platelet transfusion program were not provided. Strauss[30] also feels that the use of truly prophylactic platelet transfusions in nonbleeding patients should be discouraged.

Appropriate Dose

If prophylactic platelet transfusions are administered, a dose of 1 unit/10 kg body mass is sufficient, and transfusion usually need not be administered more than two or three times each week, unless the patient is refractory to platelet transfusion (see below). Indeed, at University of California, Los Angeles, Medical Center, we have long had a policy of transfusing a maximum of 5 units of platelets for patients who are not bleeding. Even if the platelet count does not increase after transfusion, another transfusion is not given until the next day provided there is no evidence of significant bleeding. Unfortunately, plateletpheresis products provide less flexibility of dosage and transfusion of one such product usually provides more platelets than are necessary.

Policies

Prophylactic platelet transfusions are commonly administered to patients with hypoproliferative thrombocytopenia, usually when the platelet count is 20,000/μl or below. However, a number of investigators have suggested that a platelet count less than 20,000/μl would be a more appropriate "trigger," with some authors suggesting platelet counts of 5,000 or 10,000/μl.

Great emphasis should be placed on individualizing prophylactic platelet transfusion decisions according to each patient's condition since a number of complicating clinical factors have been recognized as causing an increased risk of bleeding. A trigger of

20,000/μl should initiate consideration of platelet transfusion, not an automatic decision to transfuse.

However, since the safety of the blood supply has improved remarkably in recent years, withholding transfusion is increasingly more difficult to justify. One must compare the risk of not transfusing (severe morbidity or mortality caused by bleeding) with the risk of transfusing (primarily the transmission of infectious diseases). Only a small risk of death from bleeding would overwhelm the present risk of transfusion-transmitted infectious diseases. On the other hand, platelet transfusions to a patient with little chance of benefit cannot be justified and waste health-care resources.

Because there are insufficient data to allow one to decide on an appropriate prophylactic transfusion policy, one must make a judgment based on a comparison of the risks of bleeding at various platelet counts in patients with various complicating clinical conditions and the risk of transfusion while also keeping in mind the high cost of this valuable blood product.

Our policy is to evaluate the patient daily and to provide a prophylactic platelet transfusion in clinically stable patients only when the platelet count is below 10,000/μl. When patients have an increased risk for bleeding, prophylactic transfusions are given if the count is less than 20,000/μl.

Prophylactic Platelet Transfusion for Invasive Procedures

Surgery in Thrombocytopenic Patients

Patients with platelet counts of 50,000/μl or greater usually tolerate surgical procedures without excessive blood loss. However, when the platelet count is below 50,000/μl, available data are insufficient to formulate a policy that one can be confident is optimal. A review of the experience of 95 thrombocytopenic (platelet count, less than 100,000/μl) patients with hematologic malignancy subjected to 167 surgical procedures provides valuable information.[31] All patients with counts below 50,000/μl received platelet transfusion before or during surgery (a median of six units). All with counts above 50,000/μl did not receive a prophylactic transfusion. After surgery, the platelet count was maintained above 50,000/μl for 3 days for major surgery and above 30,000/μl for minor procedures such as tooth extractions and Hickman catheter insertion.

Overall, in 62 percent of operations less than 20 ml of blood was lost intraoperatively. Less than 50 ml of blood was lost intraoperatively at 76 percent of operations, 50–500 ml was lost at 17 percent and more than 500 ml was lost at only 7 percent. There was no correlation between the preoperative platelet count and perioperative bleeding. Instead, intraoperative blood loss of more than 500 ml or perioperative red blood cell transfusions of more than four units were correlated with major operations, preoperative fever, and preoperative coagulation abnormalities.[31] From these data one would conclude that when the platelet count is above 50,000/μl, prophylactic platelet transfusions are not warranted.

If a decision is made to administer platelets before surgery, they should be transfused on the evening before surgery, thus allowing a determination of the post-transfusion increment and survival by evaluating post-transfusion platelet counts (see the later section on assessing the effects of platelet transfusion). Knowledge of the response to platelet transfusion before an operation allows the surgical team to plan for normal hemostasis during the surgery and the 3 to 4 postoperative days when the patient will be at risk for thrombocytopenic hemorrhage. If the patient does not respond to the presurgery transfusion, the causes of this poor response should be investigated and alternative plans made before surgery begins.

While these guidelines apply to most thoracic, abdominal, and orthopedic procedures, an important exception may occur in patients undergoing central nervous system surgery, retinal surgery, and surgery on structures such as the ureter where small organizing clots or hematomas may cause serious damage or obstruction. In this setting, the major concern is not the hazard of massive blood loss but rather the risk of damage to vital structures that may occur from even small extravasations. It may be advisable to attempt to maintain the platelet count at a higher level than that needed simply to avoid excessive bleeding in other types of surgery, but there are no pertinent studies indicating an appropriate platelet level or whether transfusion to a level greater than 50,000/μl produces significant benefit.

Lumbar Puncture

Because there are apparently no studies or careful reviews of the frequency of complications from lumbar puncture in thrombocytopenic patients, a brief survey was sent to 20 hematologists, neurologists, and blood bank specialists with the instruction to distribute the survey to other hematologists and neurologists.[32] Only 5 of 40 physicians had observed complications in thrombocytopenic patients; 35 patients with complications were cited. It was not possible to determine how many lumbar punctures without complication had been reviewed. Six of the 35 patients with complications were thrombocytopenic (less than 20,000/μl). One additional patient had chronic myelogenous leukemia with a profoundly elevated white cell count; the physician reporting this case felt infiltration from leukocytes had caused cord compression (platelet count, 85,000/μl). The other 28 patients with complications had normal platelet counts. One patient with a normal platelet count had a platelet function abnormality. Nine patients were hemophiliacs, and 14 were being treated with anticoagulants. There was no diagnosis for the other four patients with normal platelet counts and complications from lumbar puncture. Thus, of the 35 complications observed, only 7 were known to be associated with decreased platelet counts (less than 20,000 platelets/μl) or thrombocytopathy.

Three physicians indicated that they would not routinely administer platelets to patients before lumbar puncture no matter how low the platelet count unless there were other complicating features of the patient's illness that increased the likelihood of hemorrhage. The other 37 physicians indicated that they would likely administer prophylactic platelet transfusions before lumbar puncture if the patient's platelet count was less than a specific level. The level selected by three respondents was 10,000/μl, one selected 15,000/μl, 16 selected 20,000/μl, 2 selected 30,000/μl, 13 selected 50,000/μl, 1 selected 75,000/μl, and 1 selected 100,000/μl.

This informal survey seems to indicate that abnormalities in protein coagulation factors are more likely than thrombocytopenia to be associated with complications of lumbar puncture. It seems that the platelet count must be very low (less than 20,000/μl) before the risk increases. The survey does not provide information on which to make a recommendation about transfusing platelets before lumbar puncture, but it does suggest that the risk of lumbar puncture in thrombocytopenic patients is not great until the platelet count is less than 20,000/

μl, and it may not increase dramatically at counts even lower. One also gains a sense of the profound differences in practice among physicians, once again emphasizing the need for continued evaluation of platelet transfusion practice to try to develop rational guidelines.

ASSESSMENT OF BLEEDING THROMBOCYTOPENIC PATIENTS

An assessment of bleeding thrombocytopenic patients should include a clinical evaluation, laboratory tests, and consideration of the cause of the thrombocytopenia.

Clinical Assessment

The clinical assessment of a bleeding patient in regard to the appropriateness of platelet transfusion therapy should take into account the patient's diagnosis, the volume and nature of the bleeding, and the platelet count. The bleeding time has also been proposed as a useful adjunct in determining the need for platelet transfusion.

Blood loss exceeding 5 ml/kg of body mass per hour is unlikely to be caused exclusively by thrombocytopenia or thrombocytopathy, and, therefore, platelet transfusion is very unlikely to be the definitive or appropriate therapy for rapid hemorrhage. Particularly in the postsurgical setting, inadequate surgical hemostasis and mechanically correctable problems should be considered primary factors.[32] Clinical evidence of a platelet deficit consists of microvascular bleeding that results in bleeding from mucous membranes, oozing from surgical incisions and venipuncture sites that persists after application of pressure, and scattered petechiae and ecchymoses in areas not associated with trauma or a surgical incision.[33–35] Such microvascular bleeding may be referred to as "thrombocytopenic bleeding."

Platelet Count

The platelet count is the most commonly used and most practical laboratory test both for determining the need for platelet transfusions and for assessing platelet deficiency.[7,8]

Severe Thrombocytopenia

Patients with hypoproliferative thrombocytopenia and platelet counts of less than 20,000/μl are candidates for consideration of prophylactic platelet transfusions as discussed previously.

Moderate Thrombocytopenia

Patients who are clinically stable and have platelet counts in the range of 20,000 to 50,000/μl do not require prophylactic platelet transfusions when they are at bed rest or during routine daily activity. Nevertheless, if a patient in this range requires surgery or is severely injured, platelet transfusions may be beneficial after the major sites of blood loss are repaired. Elective surgical procedures in patients with platelet counts in the lower part of this range are usually not attempted without transfusion support (see the previous section on surgery in thrombocytopenic patients).

Mild Thrombocytopenia

Patients with normal platelet function and platelet counts between 50,000 and 100,000/μl rarely bleed excessively from injuries. As indicated above, these patients should not be treated routinely with platelets at the time of injury or surgery. Only rarely is surgery or injury complicated by excessive generalized hemorrhage that might be related to thrombocytopenia in this range. Platelet transfusions are indicated in such patients when there is excessive thrombocytopenic bleeding. Otherwise, an alternative explanation for the bleeding should be sought rather than increasing the patient's risk and wasting time and valuable resources by futile platelet transfusions.

Patients with 100,000/μl or more normally functioning platelets do not require platelet transfusion therapy.

The Bleeding Time

A significant limitation of the platelet count is its failure to detect acquired or congenital defects of platelet function that may cause serious hemorrhage in association with platelet counts that would be hemostatic if platelet function were normal. The bleeding time (BT) has been proposed as a means of diagnosing platelet dysfunction that could result in bleeding despite an adequate platelet count. The BT has also been proposed for use as (1) a diagnostic test for platelet-related bleeding disorders; (2) a measure of efficacy in various forms of therapy; and (3) a prognosticator of abnormal bleeding.[36]

Unfortunately, a critical reappraisal of the BT has brought its validity into serious question. A detailed meta-analytical study[37] concluded that the BT is not a specific in vivo indicator of platelet function, that there is no evidence that it is a predictor of the risk of hemorrhage, that there is no evidence that bleeding from a standardized cut in the skin reflects the risk of bleeding elsewhere in the body, that there is no evidence that the BT is a useful indicator of the efficacy of therapy, and that there is no evidence that the utility of the BT has been enhanced by recent advances in standardization of the method. Also, the previously described inverse relationship between the BT and platelet count[38] was examined and the authors found the data of most investigators indicated a broad statistical scatter,[39–46] making it impossible to predict precisely one variable given the other. A review by Lind[47] also concludes that the BT has limited value and does not predict surgical bleeding, so that its use as a routine screening test for that purpose is not warranted.

The BT can unquestionably distinguish between certain predefined populations. For example, the mean bleeding time of a large group of patients with von Willebrand disease will reliably exceed the mean bleeding time from a matched group of healthy persons. However, overlap of the distributions of results for the two populations can lead to significant misclassification if the test is used to predict which patients have the disease. Thus, one must distinguish between its application to the study of populations (an epidemiologic application of the test) and its application to the care of individuals (a clinical application of the test).[37]

The pathophysiology of an abnormal bleeding time remains poorly understood. The bleeding time is affected by a large number of diseases, drugs, physiologic factors, test conditions, and therapeutic actions, not all of them platelet-related. The test is likely to remain widely used for the diagnosis of inherited disorders of platelet function, such as von Willebrand disease, despite the lack of clear criteria for its use in this context.

There is no evidence that the BT is useful for monitoring the effects of hemodialysis or transfusion therapy.[37]

The Cause of the Thrombocytopenia

Although the clinical examination and platelet count are very helpful in deciding whether to administer platelets, one must also carefully consider other aspects of the clinical situation. The cause of the thrombocytopenia influences the potential for successful platelet support.

Low Platelet Count With Decreased Rate of Platelet Production

The most common diseases having low platelet count with decreased risk of platelet production (Table 16-1) are acute leukemia, aplastic anemia, marrow-infiltrative diseases, and bone marrow aplasia induced by intensive radio therapy/chemotherapy for malignancies. In these situations, the survival of endogenous platelets is normal or nearly normal in the absence of other complications. Normal platelet survival is generally associated with successful platelet transfusion therapy, but unfortunately, patients with these clinical conditions are at risk for serious infections, drug toxicity, alloimmunization, and other factors that may cause shortened platelet survival and make planning for platelet support very difficult.[48] Platelets should be administered to these patients as part of a carefully planned transfusion strategy to help support them through thrombocytopenic periods.

Low Platelet Count With Normal or Increased Rate of Platelet Production

In clinical situations in this category (Table 16-2), the recovery or survival of transfused platelets will be decreased as a result of immunologic or nonim-

Table 16-1. Situations Involving Low Platelet Count With Decreased Platelet Production

Leukemia
Chemotherapy
Aplastic anemia
B_{12} or folic acid deficiency[a]
Marrow infiltrative diseases

[a] Thrombocytopenia from these is rarely severe enough to require platelet transfusion.

Table 16-2. Situations Involving Low Platelet Count With Normal or Increased Platelet Production

Massive transfusion
Cardiopulmonary bypass
Splenomegaly
Infection,[a] DIC, and other nonimmunologic processes
TTP and other angiopathic processes
ITP
Drug-induced immune thrombocytopenia
Other syndromes with short platelet survival

[a] Infection also suppresses platelet production.

munologic processes, and this makes platelet transfusion therapy more difficult.

PLATELET TRANSFUSION IN SPECIFIC CLINICAL SETTINGS

Cardiopulmonary Bypass

Excessive bleeding in patients during and shortly after cardiopulmonary bypass (CPB) is unusual but can be a serious management and puzzling diagnostic problem.[49] The cause for the bleeding is often surgical, but in some instances it is associated with abnormalities in hemostasis.[50] Thrombocytopenia is commonly observed during CPB but usually not to a level thought to be clinically significant. A platelet functional abnormality seems to be regularly induced by CPB, but this defect does not consistently contribute to excessive blood loss.[51-53]

Only rarely does the platelet count drop to levels typically associated with microvascular hemorrhage (thrombocytopenic bleeding). Kestin et al.[49] suggest that CPB results in

1. Markedly deficient platelet reactivity in response to an in vivo wound
2. Normal platelet reactivity in vitro
3. No loss of platelet surface GPIb-IX and GPIIb-IIIa complexes
4. A minimal number of circulating degranulated platelets.

They suggest that the "platelet function defect" of

CPB is not a defect intrinsic to the platelet, but is an extrinsic defect such as an in vivo lack of availability of platelet agonists. The near universal use of heparin during CPB is likely to contribute substantially to this defect via its inhibition of thrombin, the preeminent platelet activator.[49]

It has been shown that the bleeding time is regularly markedly abnormal during bypass but shortens soon after terminating bypass. "Hemostatic" bleeding time levels (8.9 ± 0.6 minutes) were reached within 2 hours after bypass except in patients who had excessive postoperative bleeding.[54] However, as described previously, the significance of bleeding time determinations has been seriously questioned.

The routine administration of platelets to patients undergoing CPB is an unnecessary practice that exposes the patient to the risk of transfusion without significant hope of beneficial effect.[1,2,55-58] Goodnough et al.[56] have pointed out that the percentage of patients transfused with platelets among first-time coronary artery bypass graft (CABG) surgery patients at various institutions varies remarkably. As illustrated in Figure 16-6, 50 to 75 percent of CABG patients received platelet transfusions at some institutions, whereas at most institutions, platelets were transfused to 13 percent or fewer patients.

Indeed, it has been demonstrated that platelet transfusions are only rarely necessary during cardiac surgery.[59] In many well-controlled series, patients given platelet transfusions or fresh blood show no significant differences in blood loss after CAB when compared with patients receiving only banked blood or frozen RBCs.[60-69] There is no correlation between platelet counts, results of platelet function tests, and abnormal hemorrhage in cardiac surgery.

Although excessive bleeding in the first few hours following CPB is frequently attributed to a platelet functional defect, a lack of adequate surgical hemostasis may be more common. When excessive bleeding is thought to be due to platelet functional abnormalities or thrombocytopenia, a therapeutic platelet transfusion (1 unit/10 kg) is indicated. It is best to administer the platelet transfusion after surgery.[52,54] If the transfusion is administered during surgery while the patient is still attached to the pump, the beneficial effect will be less than if the transfusion is

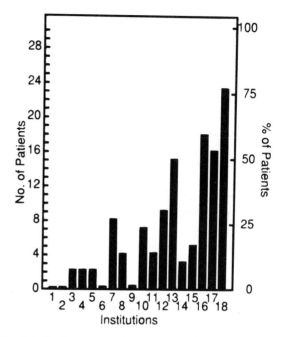

Fig. 16-6. Percentage of patients transfused with platelets among 30 first-time coronary bypass graft patients at each institution. The distribution of patients who received platelets varied among institutions. (From Goodnough et al.,[58] with permission.)

administered after major surgical bleeding is controlled and the patient's blood is no longer exposed to the bypass pump.

Fresh Blood as a Platelet Source

Some investigators have suggested that transfusion of fresh whole blood is optimal for minimizing bleeding after open heart surgery. Mohr et al.[70] compared the effectiveness of fresh blood with that of platelet transfusions in adults having CPB surgery and reported no statistical difference in postoperative blood loss after a transfusion of 1 unit of fresh whole blood compared with transfusion of 10 units of platelets. This is readily understandable as there is no evidence that either product should affect postoperative blood loss in uncomplicated CPB surgery.

Similarly, the study by Lavee et al.[71] suggested that the effect of one unit of fresh whole blood on platelet aggregation after cardiopulmonary bypass is at least equal, if not superior, to the effect of 8 to 10 platelet units. This study did not determine the relationship of these findings to blood loss following CPB.

The most detailed study to compare the hemostatic effects of fresh whole blood, stored whole blood, and components after open heart surgery was conducted by Manno and colleagues.[72] They compared postoperative blood loss in 161 children undergoing open heart surgery with CPB whose immediate postoperative transfusion requirements were met with either very fresh whole blood (VFWB), 24- to 48-hour-old whole blood, or reconstituted whole blood (packed red blood cells, fresh frozen plasma, and platelets). Comparison of mean 24-hour blood loss for the 68 children older than 2 years did not show a significant difference among the treatment groups. In the 93 children younger than 2 years of age, mean blood loss in ml/kg was significantly higher in the patients receiving reconstituted whole blood compared with the other two groups. They concluded that the lesser blood loss associated with the transfusion of VFWB and 24- to 48-hour-old blood compared to reconstituted whole blood was not explained by postoperative coagulation tests and may have been due to better functioning platelets. The authors' policy is to transfuse refrigerated 24- to 48-hour-old whole blood for early blood replacement requirements following complex open heart surgery with CPB in children.

However, Manno et al.[72] pointed out that platelet function in blood refrigerated for up to 48 hours is presumably significantly impaired. Further, they did not compare the use of fresh platelet products with the other types of blood products. In particular, their "reconstituted whole blood" contained platelets stored up to 5 days.

Optimal platelet preservation is provided by storage of platelets at room temperature rather than at 4°C and, accordingly, our policy is to provide fresh platelets (as fresh as are available and, in any case, less than 48 hours old) rather than supplying platelets from refrigerated whole blood for young children having complex open heart surgery.

Finally, the data of Manno et al. indicated that there was no benefit of fresh blood products for patients older than 2 years, and we know of no justification for the provision of fresh blood products for patients having CPB surgery after the first 2 years of life.

Massive Transfusion

Patients receiving massive RBC transfusions (more than 15 to 20 units in an adult in a few hours) may suffer a moderate degree of thrombocytopenia.[33,34,73,74] The platelet count rarely drops below 50,000/μl, and therefore bleeding on the basis of thrombocytopenia is infrequent[75,76] (see Ch. 25). The cause of the thrombocytopenia is a loss of endogenous platelets from the body through massive bleeding and replacement with banked blood, which generally contains no viable platelets. The bone marrow of a bleeding patient who requires a very rapid replacement transfusion cannot make platelets fast enough to compensate for this loss. However, there is evidence suggesting that platelets normally sequestered in the spleen might be released during a massive hemorrhage. Several groups have demonstrated that platelet counts after massive transfusion are higher than predicted from a standard washout equation.[34,77,78]

Thrombocytopenic hemorrhage occurs in only a minority of patients receiving large quantities of blood.[34,73,76–78] Indeed, thrombocytopenia is unlikely until an adult has received 15 to 20 units of blood (about 1.5 to 2.0 times the blood volume).[34] In one study, only 6 of 33 patients who received an average of 20.6 units of whole blood or modified whole blood (whole blood from which platelets had been removed) developed microvascular bleeding, and in only 1 of these 6 patients was dilutional thrombocytopenia the cause of the microvascular bleeding.[34]

Several reports have indicated that commonly used empiric replacement formulas are not likely to prevent bleeding in the massively transfused patient, because consumption of platelets and clotting factors, rather than simple dilution, is a major cause of deficiencies leading to the bleeding.[33,34,79,80] Thus, such routine prophylactic component transfusion usually overestimates the need for transfusion but, when comsumptive disorders are present, the same formulas underestimate transfusion needs. Thus, the formulas are both unnecessary and insufficient to correct consumptive disorders.[79]

Patients receiving a massive RBC transfusion should be examined periodically for signs of thrombocytopenic hemorrhage (generalized oozing, petechiae, ecchymoses). If these signs are present or if thrombocytopenia is likely (e.g., platelet count was borderline at the onset of surgery), a platelet count should be performed. If thrombocytopenic hemorrhage occurs in these patients, platelet transfusion is the proper therapy.

As long as the bleeding is uncontrolled, maximum transfusion effort should be directed at maintenance of the intravascular volume and the oxygen-carrying capacity. After the vascular damage is repaired and the major bleeding controlled, one platelet transfusion (1 unit/10 kg; see later for a complete discussion of the platelet transfusion dose) is usually sufficient to terminate the microvascular bleeding caused by thrombocytopenia.

Splenomegaly

In normal individuals, about one-third of the total body platelet mass is sequestered in the spleen.[81] As the spleen increases in size, the percentage of the body's platelets that are sequestered increases.[82] Patients with massively enlarged spleens and often decreased bone marrow function, as in myeloproliferative disease, may have moderate to severe thrombocytopenia, at least partially on the basis of increased sequestration of platelets. Some patients with myeloproliferative diseases have poor platelet function as well.[83,84]

Transfusion therapy is complicated by splenomegaly because an increased proportion of transfused platelets is sequestered. Transfused platelets survive nearly as well in patients with splenomegaly as in patients with normal spleens,[4] but the immediate post-transfusion recovery is moderately to markedly reduced to as low as 15 to 20 percent.[4,82] Because of this poor post-transfusion recovery, a larger dose of platelets (1.5 units/10 kg) is reasonable as initial therapy when platelet transfusion support is necessary. The appropriate dose for subsequent transfusions can best be determined by observing the results of prior transfusions.

Some patients with enlarged spleens are transfused frequently enough with both RBCs and platelets to become alloimmunized and refractory to random-donor platelet transfusions. After many transfusions, it is difficult to determine whether alloimmunization or splenomegaly is more important in reducing transfusion responses, and often an empiric trial of HLA-matched platelets is necessary.

Infection and DIC

In severely infected patients (especially with gram-negative organisms), even without DIC, thrombocytopenia is a frequent complication. The thrombocytopenia may be caused by decreased platelet life span, marrow suppression, or a combination.[85–87] Although there is agreement that platelet survival in thrombocytopenic septic patients is shortened, the mechanism of the thrombocytopenia is controversial. Some investigators feel that cryptantigen-bound antibody or immune complexes produce the thrombocytopenia, but other explanations are possible.[88–92] The degree of thrombocytopenia does not regularly lead to excessive bleeding, and therefore platelet transfusion is not routinely necessary in these patients.[93] Successful therapy for the infection corrects the platelet deficit. If the platelet count falls to very low levels and serious thrombocytopenic blood loss occurs, platelets should be administered, perhaps beginning with a large dose (1.5 units/10 kg).

In some patients with DIC, the platelet count may occasionally reach very low levels. In this syndrome, bleeding can be life-threatening. Appropriate therapy for patients with DIC is treatment of the underlying cause of the syndrome. If the cause of the DIC cannot be corrected, hemostatic replacement therapy is not often helpful.[94,95] Life-threatening hemorrhage in patients with DIC is not always caused by severe thrombocytopenia, but when it is, platelet transfusion therapy may be beneficial if the cause of the DIC is reversible. Frequent, large doses of platelets (1.5 units/10 kg) may be necessary to maintain the platelet count in the hemostatic range.[96] If the thrombocytopenia is contributing significantly to hemorrhage, it may be possible to reduce blood loss during the time that the basic process is being treated. Platelet transfusion should be monitored with frequent platelet counts to ensure that the desired result has been obtained and to plan for future transfusions (see section on practical aspects of transfusion therapy).

Thrombotic Thrombocytopenic Purpura

The very low platelet counts in thrombotic thrombocytopenic purpura (TTP) are probably produced by consumption of platelets in thrombotic lesions.[97] Microthrombi consisting of hyaline material are found in the microvasculature. Special staining has demonstrated that these thrombi are composed primarily of platelet components.[98] One report of three patients suggested that platelet transfusion does not increase the platelet count and is not appropriate therapy for patients with this syndrome. Other reports suggest that platelet transfusion may be associated with dramatic worsening of the signs and symptoms of the syndrome and, therefore, physicians should be very cautious about administering platelets to patients with TTP.[99–101] Blood products containing platelets probably should not be administered to patients with acute TTP unless necessary as therapy for life-threatening, platelet-related bleeding. Plasma exchange, whole blood exchange, and plasma transfusion along with splenectomy and certain drug protocols have improved survival dramatically in patients with TTP.[102–107]

Idiopathic Thrombocytopenic Purpura

Thrombocytopenia in ITP is apparently caused by an autoantibody that leads to a profound decrease in the survival of endogenously produced platelets. The specificity of the autoantibody is broad, and it reacts in in vitro systems with the platelets of most normal individuals.[108–110] Many studies of platelet transfusion in patients with ITP have demonstrated that survival of transfused platelets is also profoundly shortened.[82] Platelet transfusion, therefore, is often of no therapeutic value, but there may be a benefit from carefully planned and monitored platelet transfusions in certain patients with ITP.[111–113]

A minority of patients with ITP do have an increase in platelet count after a platelet transfusion. In one study, 13 of 31 platelet transfusions (42 percent) resulted in immediate post-transfusion count increments of 20,000/μl or more. Thus, it is reasonable to evaluate the efficacy of platelet transfusion during significant bleeding episodes occurring in ITP patients.[112] If major elective surgery is planned for a patient with ITP, the effects of platelet transfusions can be assessed before the operation. Some patients can be supported for a short period during and after the procedure if a transfusion is determined to be necessary because of the anatomic site of the surgery. Minor surgery is usually best accomplished in ITP patients without platelet transfusions.

It is appropriate to treat ITP before surgery, if possible, with corticosteroids, intravenous immunoglobulin, or immunosuppressive drugs.[114]

Drug-Induced Immune Thrombocytopenia

Drug-induced thrombocytopenia, often as a consequence of immune-mediated platelet destruction, has been documented for more than 100 low-molecular-weight compounds and therapeutic agents.[115] Drugs that have been implicated as a cause of immune-mediated thrombocytopenia include vancomycin,[116] pentamidine,[117] methicillin,[118] sulfonamides, oral diuretics, heparin, gold salts, trimethoprim/sulfamethoxazole, dipyridamole, sulfonylureas and salicylates.[119] Whenever a patient develops consistently poor responses to donor platelet transfusions without other identifiable causes, the possibility of a drug-related antibody should be considered. Unfortunately, in vitro platelet antibody assays are not readily available and it may be necessary to develop a clinical diagnosis by discontinuing possible offending drugs and then observing for greater platelet counts after transfusion.

Appropriate therapy for drug-induced immune thrombocytopenia consists of supportive care and withdrawal of the offending drug. After the drug therapy has been stopped, the platelet count generally returns to normal within 4 to 14 days.[120,121] Because in most circumstances drug-induced thrombocytopenia is associated with short platelet survival and because patients recover rapidly, platelet transfusion has little or no role in therapy for patients with this syndrome. Occasionally, severe thrombocytopenia and generalized, life-threatening hemorrhage occur in these patients; in such cases platelet transfusions might be administered.[112] Platelet transfusions should not be administered to these patients for minor bleeding or bruising.

Two particularly important drug-induced syndromes have been described relatively recently (i.e., heparin induced thrombocytopenia and a variety of abnormalities associated with quinine administration).

Heparin-Induced Thrombocytopenia

Thrombocytopenia occurs in about 5 percent of patients receiving heparin therapy.[122] Some of these patients simultaneously develop acute thromboembolic complications, including cerebral thrombosis, myocardial infarction, and peripheral arterial thrombosis resulting in limb ischemia. When it occurs, heparin-induced thrombocytopenia and thrombosis is a serious clinical problem that often leads to disastrous consequences such as limb amputation, permanent neurologic deficiencies, and death.[122] The clinical and laboratory features and approaches to the prevention and treatment of this problem have been reviewed by Warkentin and Kelton.[123]

Quinine-Associated Thrombocytopenia

Quinine has been well described as a cause of immune-mediated thrombocytopenia. More recently, a number of associated phenomena have also been reported including hemolytic uremic syndrome,[124–127] neutropenia, and renal failure,[125] and DIC.[128,129]

Other Causes of Immune Mediated Thrombocytopenia

One must be aware that platelet autoantibodies may be associated with other disorders and may contribute to shortened platelet survival of endogenous platelets as well as decreased recovery and shortened survival of transfused platelets. Platelet autoantibodies have been detected in patients with hematologic malignancies and after both autologous and allogeneic bone marrow transplantation.[4] Also, circulating immune complexes may be present in patients with autoimmune or alloimmune-mediated thrombocytopenias.[130–132] In 15 patients with leukemia, the level of circulating immune complexes correlated inversely with posttransfusion platelet increments.[131]

Disorders Associated With Platelet Dysfunction

Therapy for patients with reversible defects of platelet function differs from therapy for patients with permanent defects (Table 16-3).

With the enormous consumption of aspirin, the frequent hospital use of parenteral β-lactam antibiotics, the ability of many drugs and foods to diminish platelet function, and the occurrence of abnormal platelet function in hematologic and other systemic diseases, acquired abnormalities of platelet function are probably the most common hematologic disor-

Table 16-3. Acquired Defects of Platelet Function

Irreversible Defects	Reversible Defects
Idiopathic thrombocythemia	Drug-induced platelet functional abnormality
Polycythemia rubra vera	Uremia
Myelofibrosis	DIC
Chronic myelogenous leukemia	Scurvy
Acute leukemia	

der.[133] When significant hemorrhage occurs in these patients, it is often assumed to be related to abnormal platelet function because the bleeding time is prolonged and platelet aggregation is abnormal. However, the contribution of these abnormalities of platelet function to clinical bleeding is often uncertain.[134]

The etiology of bleeding in systemic diseases that has been postulated to result from abnormal platelet function can be more clearly understood by comparison with patients with isolated defects in platelet function (e.g., those with Glanzmann's thrombasthenia).[134] For example, patients with chronic renal failure can have bleeding suggestive of abnormal platelet function, such as purpura, epistaxis, and menorrhagia, but other bleeding complications reported in uremic patients do not occur in thrombasthenia: retroperitoneal hematomas, mediastinal hematomas, and hemorrhagic pleural and pericardial effusions.[133] Therefore, these visceral hemorrhages should be attributed to other hemostatic abnormalities, such as the mucosal lesions of uremia and complications of heparin anticoagulation used for dialysis.

Reversible Acquired Defects of Platelet Function

Aspirin Administration

Aspirin inhibits platelet function by irreversibly acetylating cyclo-oxygenase, thus preventing formation of the platelet aggregator and vasoconstrictor, thromboxane-A_2.[135] On this basis aspirin is widely prescribed to prevent thrombotic coronary artery occlusion and reduce the risk of myocardial infarction, particularly in patients with prior myocardial infarction and with unstable angina pectoris.[136] Thus, recent aspirin use is common in patients undergoing CABG, and several studies have suggested that aspirin increases blood loss, transfusion requirements, and need for reoperation for bleeding in cardiac surgery patients.[137–143]

In contrast, Rawitscher et al.[144] observed no increased blood loss or packed RBC requirements in aspirin-treated patients compared with controls in a randomized prospective study of 100 consecutive patients undergoing CABG. Similarly, Reich et al.[145] reexamined this issue in light of recent transfusion-sparing practices and autologous cell salvaging techniques. They performed a retrospective study on 197 patients who underwent reinfusion of postoperatively shed mediastinal autologous whole blood including 87 patients who received aspirin within 1 week before surgery and 110 control patients. Patients undergoing repeat cardiac operations were excluded from the study. Although significantly more mediastinal tube drainage occurred in the aspirin group (27 percent), this did not affect allogeneic blood component requirements because the shed blood was autotransfused. In addition there were no significant differences in platelet, fresh frozen plasma, and cryoprecipitate use between the groups. This suggests that it is not necessary to delay elective primary CABG because of exposure to aspirin.

Patients who may require blood transfusions during other elective major surgical procedures should be questioned about medications and be instructed to stop taking aspirin 1 week or more before surgery.[146,147] An alternative drug without platelet effect (e.g., acetaminophen) should be substituted if necessary during the time the patient is at risk. If surgery must be performed on a patient whose platelet function is inhibited by a drug, close clinical examination before and during surgery will allow an appropriate decision concerning platelet transfusion. Prophylactic platelet transfusion is not indicated. Only rarely will therapeutic platelet transfusion during surgery be necessary, but if so, 0.5 to 1 unit of platelets/10 kg is appropriate, assuming the response to platelet transfusions is normal. In aspirin-treated patients with normal platelet counts, normal function in 20 percent of the platelets will provide adequate hemostasis, and therefore large doses of platelets are not necessary.[148]

Uremia

Uremia is accompanied by variable degrees of platelet dysfunction, and serious bleeding may occur despite normal platelet count.[149–151] Peritoneal dialysis and hemodialysis are effective in correcting the hemorrhagic diathesis. Platelet transfusions are only temporarily effective in uremic patients. Some investigators recommend on the basis of anecdotal evidence that patients being prepared for nephrectomy, transplantation, renal biopsy, or other surgical procedure undergo dialysis until the bleeding time is returned to the hemostatic range.[151] However, correlations between abnormal platelet function test results and clinically significant bleeding are poor.

Several studies have demonstrated that a low hematocrit is the main determining factor of the prolonged bleeding time often encountered in uremic patients.[152,153] Livio et al.[152,153] reported that bleeding times in uremic patients are profoundly influenced by anemia, and that the platelet-mediated hemorrhagic tendency in uremia may be successfully managed by raising the hematocrit to above 30 percent. In addition to effects on the bleeding time, the authors transfused six patients with hemorrhagic complications with washed red blood cells and found that hemorrhagic manifestations "seemed to be reduced in severity" in five of the patients.

Desmopressin (DDAVP) has been used to treat bleeding in patients with mild hemophilia and von Willebrand's disease. It may also shorten the bleeding time and decrease blood loss when patients with uremia or certain thrombocytopathies or those receiving drugs affecting platelet function are subjected to surgery.[154–157] These observations have led physicians to recommend DDAVP therapy instead of blood component therapy for hemophiliacs, uremics, and patients taking aspirin if they are scheduled for surgical procedures. Although the ability of DDAVP to shorten the bleeding time has been reported in a number of disorders, the effectiveness of the drug in decreasing clinically significant bleeding has been less well documented.

Few serious side effects of DDAVP therapy have been identified although cases of hyponatremia and seizures within 24 hours after the administration of DDAVP in children under the age of 2 years have been reported by two groups of investigators.[157,158]

The drug is probably contraindicated in pseudo-von Willebrand's disease and in von Willebrand's disease, type IIB, because it may cause severe thrombocytopenia in these patients.[159] Certainly many more studies are necessary before DDAVP is administered routinely to patients with uremia, patients taking aspirin who are scheduled for surgical procedures, etc.

Abnormal platelet function has been described in patients with scoliosis. A study of the effect of DDAVP on blood loss during Harrington rod spinal fusion surgery showed a dramatic decrease in blood loss and in the need for RBC transfusion. The patients studied had normal bleeding profiles and no history of abnormal bleeding. The author did not notice any severe side effects and did not mention any thrombotic events.[160]

Irreversible Defects of Platelet Function

Myeloproliferative Disorders

Patients with myeloproliferative disease may have defects of variable severity.[83,84] Spontaneous and surgical bleeding associated with normal or elevated platelet counts but prolonged bleeding times have been described in polycythemia vera, acute myelogenous leukemia, acute monocytic leukemia, and chronic myelogenous leukemia, but there is no true correlation between the presence of laboratory abnormalities and microvascular hemorrhage. In most instances, effective treatment of the underlying disease corrects the bleeding diathesis, although platelet transfusion or DDAVP may be helpful in acute surgical situations for bleeding associated with a platelet function defect. The risk and the potential benefit must be weighed carefully. Since the consequences of sensitization to platelet antigens and refractoriness to platelet transfusions are severe, platelet transfusions should be used conservatively. Minor bleeding events, for example, nose bleeds, should be treated with local measures when possible.

Congenital Defects of Platelet Function

Some patients with congenital defects of platelet function (Table 16-4) bleed excessively from birth after even minor trauma, and others are not diagnosed until they bleed excessively at the time of major surgery as an adult. Although other therapeutic modalities have been tried, platelet transfusion is

Table 16-4. Congenital Disorders That May Be Associated With a Prolonged TBT and a Bleeding Diathesis

von Willebrand's disease
Glanzmann's thrombasthenia
Bernard-Soulier syndrome
Marfan syndrome
Ehlers-Danlos syndrome
Wiscott-Aldrich syndrome
Albinism
Storage pool disease
Defects of platelet release reactions

appropriate therapy for most of these patients.[161] The administration of an appropriate dose of normally functioning platelets provides adequate hemostasis.

Glanzmann's Thrombasthenia. The probability of alloimmunization appears to be greater in association with Glanzmann's thrombasthenia and Bernard-Soulier syndrome than with other platelet functional defects.[162,163] The platelets in these disorders have deficiencies or abnormalities of platelet glycoproteins.[134,164,165]

In patients with Glanzmann's thrombasthenia, one must be concerned about the possibility of developing alloantibodies against GP IIb-IIIa, because GP IIb-IIIa on transfused platelets is strongly immunogenic and is deficient or structurally abnormal in thrombasthenia. However, George et al.[134], in their detailed review of Glanzmann's thrombasthenia, provided information on 51 patients studied in Paris, France; they indicated that an alloantibody to GP IIa-IIIb has been found among these patients only once even though all but two patients had been transfused with either red cells or platelets. The authors noted that three other thrombasthenic patients have been reported who developed alloantibodies that reacted primarily with GP IIIa.[166–168] Two further patients may have developed similar alloantibodies.[169,170] The authors speculate that the presence of some residual platelet GP IIb-IIIa may protect many patients from alloimmunization.

Therefore, judicious use of platelet transfusions is indicated in patients with Glanzmann's thrombasthenia. Bleeding can be so unpredictable that platelet transfusions before an invasive procedure may be indicated even in patients with minimal past hemorrhagic symptoms. The risk of alloantibody formation against GP IIb-IIIa appears to be very rare and not a reason to withhold platelet transfusion.[134]

The efficacy of antifibrinolytic drugs, epsilon aminocaproic acid (EACA) and tranexamic acid, remains uncertain in thrombasthenia except that EACA has been recommended for tooth extractions as an adjunct to platelet transfusions. A dose of 40 mg/kg four times daily may be given.[134] DDAVP has been tried in some patients with Glanzmann's thrombasthenia without evidence of efficacy,[171,172] although some investigators indicate an effect on the bleeding time.[157]

von Willebrand Disease. Castillo et al.[173] studied the hemostatic effect of normal platelet transfusion in severe von Willebrand disease (vWD) patients. They examined the effect of normal platelet concentrate transfusion 1 hour after cryoprecipitate infusion in five type III vWD patients. The cryoprecipitate infusion attained normal circulating levels of ristocetin cofactor, vWD antigen, and factor VIII activity. In two patients cryoprecipitate infusion did not modify the bleeding time (more than 30 minutes), whereas in the remaining three patients the bleeding time was only partially corrected (from more than 30 minutes to 12, 18, and 21 minutes). However, the subsequent platelet transfusion completely corrected the bleeding time in four patients, and in one patient it shortened the bleeding time to near normal levels. The authors concluded that their data support the occasional addition of platelet transfusion to the cryoprecipitate infusion for the control of serious bleeding episodes resistant to cryoprecipitate in severe vWD patients.

PRACTICAL ASPECTS OF PLATELET TRANSFUSION

ABO Compatibility

Platelets carry ABH antigens on their surface; some are intrinsic to the platelet membrane, and the remainder are adsorbed from the surrounding plasma.[174,175] The relevance of ABH antigens was first reported in 1965 by Aster.[176] Radiolabeled A_1

platelets, when given to group O normal recipients, resulted in recoveries of 19 percent compared with 63 percent observed with ABO-compatible platelets. When group A_1B platelets were given to group O recipients, average recovery was only 8 percent, whereas group B platelets given to incompatible recipients averaged 57 percent recovery. ABO-incompatible platelet recovery was inversely related to the isohemagglutination titers of the transfused recipient.

A number of subsequent studies have provided more details concerning the relevance of donor-recipient ABO antigen compatibility. Duquesnoy et al.[177] reported that the mean 24-hour recovery of platelets from histocompatible donors and from donors selectively mismatched for cross-reactive HLA antigens was decreased by approximately 23 percent if there was a major ABO mismatch between donor and recipient. The authors stated, however, that such a reduction in platelet recovery associated with ABO incompatibility is not of a magnitude that would contraindicate transfusion of ABO-mismatched platelets.

Lee and Schiffer[178] studied patients with untreated acute leukemia who alternately received either ABO-matched or ABO-mismatched random-donor platelet transfusions prepared from pooled platelet concentrates stored for 1 to 3 days. Of 33 such patients who received at least four transfusions, 9 (27 percent) had substantial differences between mismatched and matched platelet transfusion. Elevated anti-A or -B isoagglutinin titers were demonstrated in patients with consistently poorer responses to ABO-mismatched platelet transfusions. They concluded that although it is not mandatory to use ABO-compatible platelets, the provision of such platelets is advisable because, in a significant percentage of patients, ABO-incompatible platelet transfusions produce inferior results.

Ellinger et al.[179] reported results of studies using anti-IgG or -IgM typing reagents in a platelet radioimmunoassay crossmatch test. They found that anti-A or anti-B antibodies could not be detected with incompatible platelets until the antibody titer was greater than 64. Group O plasma was crossmatch incompatible with group A or B platelets 52 percent and 17 percent of the time, respectively. Others studies indicated that anti-A in group B plasma rarely produced a positive crossmatch and anti-B in group A plasma never did so.[180] Furthermore, there is minimal expression of blood group A antigen on platelets from group A_2 individuals, and recipients who were refractory to group A_1 platelet donors because of high-titer anti-A were responsive to platelets from A_2 individuals.[181] It therefore seems that one should particularly try to avoid giving platelets from group A_1 donors to group O recipients.

Brand et al.[182] reported two alloimmunized patients with multispecific anti-HLA and high-titered ABH antibodies who showed transfusion failures after ABH-mismatched HLA-identical platelet transfusions, whereas ABH-matched HLA-identical platelets showed sufficient increments.

Ogasawara et al.[175] have presented data suggesting that the isoagglutinin titer of the recipient is not the only relevant factor in determining the survival of ABO-incompatible platelets. They studied a patient who received 12 transfusions of HLA-matched, ABO-incompatible platelets. Ten transfusions were successful, but two failed to increase the patient's peripheral platelet count at all. They determined that transfused platelets that were rapidly cleared from the circulation of the recipient expressed an amount of B antigen more than 20 times that expressed by the blood group B platelets that were successfully transfused to the recipient. Further studies on randomly selected donors revealed that about 7 percent of donors belonged to a high-expression phenotype of either A or B antigen and that this was genetically determined.

Heal et al.[183] reported that patients transfused with ABO-identical platelets throughout their course (25 transfusions) had a mean corrected count increment (CCI) (see below) that was significantly higher (6,600 ± 7,900) than that achieved with ABO unmatched platelets (5,200 ± 7,900; p<0.01). Also, a smaller percentage of patients in the ABO-identical group became refractory (36 percent vs 75 percent; p<0.03), possibly because of the development of circulating immune complexes involving the ABO system.[184]

Carr et al.[185] reported that transfusion of ABO-mismatched platelets leads to early platelet refractoriness. Nine of 13 (69 percent) of patients receiving mismatched platelets became refractory at a median of 2 weeks compared with only one of 13 (8 percent)

patients receiving ABO matched platelets. The induction of high-titer isoagglutinins by ABO-mismatched platelets played an important role in the development of refractoriness. In addition, there was a greater incidence of lymphocytotoxic, anti-HLA antibody formation, although this observation was considered preliminary as only a small number of patients were studied.

As a result of the above information, it appears preferable to provide ABO-matched platelets to patients with marrow failure requiring long-term support.[183,184] Also, patients who experience poor increments from ABO-mismatched platelets should be given a trial of ABO-matched platelets before the initiation of HLA-matched platelet transfusions.[178] However, ABO-matched platelets are not always available and, in that circumstance, it is appropriate medical practice to transfuse ABO-incompatible platelets.[177]

Rh Compatibility

The antigens of the Rh system are probably not on platelet surfaces.[186–187] However, since units of platelets contain some contaminating RBCs, development of red cell alloantibodies is a potential problem. Goldfinger and McGinniss[188] reviewed the transfusion records of 102 Rh-negative patients treated with platelet transfusions from Rh-positive donors and reported a 7.8 percent rate of sensitization to the Rh_o (D) antigen. All but one of the patients had diseases associated with impaired immunologic reactivity and received immunosuppressive drugs. Lichtiger et al.[189] found no instances of sensitization to the Rh_0 (D) among 30 Rh-negative oncology patients who were transfused with an average of 35.5 units of Rh-positive platelets. McLeod et al.[190] found that 3 of 16 (19 percent) Rh-negative autologous bone marrow transplant recipients developed anti-D as a result of transfusion of Rh-positive platelets. Thus, there appears to be a small but finite risk of developing anti-D antibodies as a result of transfusion of Rh-negative patients with Rh-positive platelets, even if the patients are immunosuppressed.

If platelets from an Rh-positive donor must be given to an Rh-negative woman of childbearing age, Rh immune globulin might be administered shortly after the platelet transfusion. The use of Rh immune globulin for other Rh-negative recipients should be considered on an individual basis.

Administration of Platelets

Platelet concentrates are stored, with gentle agitation, at 22°C in 50 ml or more of plasma. A seven-unit pool of random-donor concentrates stored at 22°C will approximate 400 ml. Some patients with cardiovascular disease may not tolerate large infusions of plasma. Volume overload can be prevented by an additional concentration step in the blood bank. The platelet pool may be subjected to a second "hard" centrifugation and then be resuspended in 50 to 100 ml of plasma rather than 400 ml. This allows the infusion of large doses of platelets to patients with precariously balanced cardiovascular systems. These volume-reduced products should be infused at once because platelets stored at 22°C in small volumes of plasma deteriorate rapidly.[191,192]

Platelets should be administered through routine blood filters or platelet/component filters (170 μ).[193,194] Platelets must not be administered through some microaggregate filters because some filters have been shown to remove platelets.[194–198]

Determining the Appropriate Dose of Platelets

If the platelet count of a bleeding thrombocytopenic patient can be increased by 50,000/μl, this is generally sufficient to provide hemostasis. An increment of this magnitude can be provided to an uncomplicated, nonrefractory patient by administering one unit of platelets for each 10 kg of body mass (0.1 unit/kg). Thus, a 70-kg person usually responds satisfactorily to a pool of seven platelet units. Alternatively, one plateletpheresis product, which is usually considered the equivalent of six or seven units, will produce an adequate response (see below for more precise methods of evaluating the response to platelet transfusions).

Patients with splenomegaly, infection, fever, intravascular coagulation, etc., might need platelet transfusions and, if so, can be expected to have a relatively poor post-transfusion platelet count increment. Therefore, in such patients, the starting dose may be 1.5 or even 2 units/10 kg, with subsequent doses selected on the basis of the initial response.

The dose of platelets for a prophylactic transfusion for a stable thrombocytopenic patient may be smaller. At the University of California, Los Angeles, UCLA

Medical Center, we have long had a policy of transfusing a maximum of five units in such a situation.

ASSESSING THE EFFECTIVENESS OF PLATELET TRANSFUSIONS*

Transfusions administered to prevent hemorrhage cannot be evaluated in the same way as those administered to reduce active hemorrhage. Complete evaluation of both situations requires clinical and laboratory examination. A bleeding patient must be examined to detect changes in the rate of blood loss, and the patient to whom platelets are administered prophylactically must be examined to ensure that no thrombocytopenic hemorrhage has begun. Every platelet transfusion should be followed by a clinical evaluation and platelet counts.

Although some physicians feel that a thrombocytopenic patient may benefit from platelet transfusions even if there is no increment in the platelet count, inadequate data are available to support (or refute) such a conclusion. If bleeding slows or stops after platelet transfusion that does not increase the platelet count, this does not assure that the platelet transfusion was causally associated with the cessation of hemorrhage.

The recipients of platelet transfusions should preferably have three platelet counts: one immediately before platelet transfusion, one 10 minutes to 1 hour after the transfusion (the "1-hour count"), and a third about 16 to 24 hours later. This combination of platelet counts allows the determination of the expected peak recovery and the survival of transfused platelets (Fig. 16-7).

There is a direct relationship between the patient's platelet count and the survival of transfused platelets at platelet counts of less than 100,000/μl. In clinically stable nonalloimmunized thrombocytopenic patients with average baseline platelet counts of 19,000 ± 6,000/μL, platelet survivals were only 3.4 ± 1.1 days (range, 2.3 to 5.0 days) compared with the normal autologous platelet survival of 9.6 ± 0.6 days (range, 8.5 to 10.4 days) measured in nonthrombocytopenic volunteers.[4]

* This section was written in collaboration with Elliot M. Landaw, M.D., Ph.D., Associate Professor, Department of Biomathematics, University of California, Los Angeles, UCLA School of Medicine, Los Angeles, California.

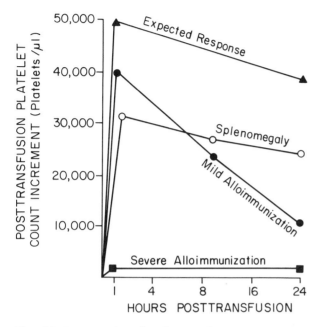

Fig. 16-7. Typical results after transfusion of 0.1 unit of platelets/kg to a severely thrombocytopenic patient in various clinical settings. The upper curve is the expected response in a nonimmunized recipient. There is a post-transfusion platelet count increment of about 45,000 to 50,000/μl with about a 20 percent decrease in 24 hours. In patients with mild alloimmunization, the 1-hour post-transfusion platelet count increment may be adequate, but there is decreased survival of the platelets in subsequent hours. In patients with splenomegaly, there may be a decreased recovery but with essentially normal subsequent survival. In patients with sepsis, DIC, or fever with a temperature greater than 38.5°C, the response is often similar to that with mild alloimmunization, although in some patients the response is similar to that with severe alloimmunization.

Knowledge of the one-hour post-transfusion increment is helpful when choosing a dose of platelets for subsequent transfusion. Knowledge of the survival allows the clinician to determine the period of protection from hemorrhage associated with each platelet transfusion. The cost of the platelet counts is minimal when compared with the risk the patient incurs without appropriate therapy. This two-part assessment is desirable whether platelets are administered therapeutically to stop acute thrombocytopenic hemorrhage or for prophylactic purposes. The platelet count is the only convenient objective measure of the success or failure of a prophylactic platelet transfusion.

Although three platelet counts, as just indicated, are generally optimal, there are some situations in which this approach may be modified. For example, if the 1-hour count indicates a very small post-transfusion increment, the 24-hour count would not add additional information. However, if one only measures the 24-hour count, the presence of a temporary but significant post-transfusion platelet count increment may be missed (Fig. 16-7).

If repeated platelet transfusions are unsuccessful, possible explanations (infection, fever, DIC, ITP, splenomegaly, drugs, etc.) should be considered, and one must consider the use of special products for subsequent transfusions. The early documentation of refractoriness to platelet transfusions can lead to a timely switch to special platelet products when random-donor platelets are no longer effective as a result of alloimmunization.

Determining the Effectiveness of Platelet Transfusions

Because the number of platelets per unit varies, precise calculation of expected post-transfusion increments is impossible unless platelet counts are performed on each concentrate.

The number of platelets in a "unit" (a suspension prepared from 450 ml of routinely donated whole blood) may be highly variable, depending on such things as method of separation and donor count. Some investigators use a figure of 5.5×10^{10} platelets as a unit since minimum standards of quality assurance require that periodic counts on randomly selected platelet preparations reveal at least 5.5×10^{10} platelets/unit in 75 percent of units tested at maximal storage time or at the time of use.[199] Average yields are generally somewhat higher than the minimum levels and are generally about 7×10^{10} platelets per concentrate.

Standards of the American Association of Blood Banks also indicate that plateletpheresis products shall contain a minimum of 3×10^{11} platelets in at least 75 percent of the units tested.[199] Plateletpheresis products may contain significantly higher numbers of platelets, depending on the collection process, and may exceed 6×10^{11} platelets/product.

Although knowing the actual number of platelets transfused is preferable, one can easily develop clinically useful estimates of expected post-transfusion platelet count increments even without this information. By far the simplest method is to recall that a transfusion of a unit of platelets in an average-sized adult can be expected to increase the platelet count by about $7,000/\mu l$. Thus, the usual dose of platelets (i.e., 1 unit/10 kg [7 units/70 kg]) or one plateletpheresis product should increase the platelet count by about $50,000/\mu l$. A post-transfusion platelet count increment of only $25,000/\mu l$ in such a situation would obviously be 50 percent of the predicted value.

Although such estimates of efficacy of a platelet transfusion are of some value, obviously these are crude estimates because of the variability of the number of platelets per product transfused and variation in the blood volume of patients.

Estimating Maximal Platelet Count Increment and Platelet Recovery

It is often preferable to use more accurate estimates for the expected post-transfusion platelet count increment (i.e., the post-transfusion count–pretransfusion count). Taking into account the dilution principle (200) for transfused platelets and the possibility of splenic pooling,[81,201] the expected maximum platelet count increment (MPI) in platelets/μl is

$$MPI = \frac{n \cdot F}{1,000 \cdot BV}$$

where BV is the blood volume (ml), the factor 1000 converts ml to μl, n is the number of transfused platelets, and F is the initial fractional recovery of transfused platelets in the general circulation. F varies somewhat in normal subjects (Figure 16-8), averaging 0.62 in those with normal-sized spleens and 0.91 in asplenic patients at 2 hours after transfusion.[81] F is generally much lower but more variable in patients with splenomegaly, averaging 0.23 in Figure 16-8. It is common practice for the "1-hour count" to use the approximation $F = 2/3$ for subjects with normal spleens.

For example, if a patient with a normal spleen and 5,000 ml blood volume is to be transfused with 4×10^{11} platelets, the predicted maximum post-transfusion count increment is

$$MPI = \frac{4 \times 10^{11} \times (2/3)}{1,000 \times 5,000} = 53,300 \text{ platelets}/\mu l$$

Formal measures for transfusion effectiveness compare the observed post-transfusion platelet count increment (PI) to the maximum increment predicted by the MPI. In particular, the percentage platelet recovery, or PPR, is based on their ratio and in its most general form is calculated by

$$PPR = \frac{PI}{MPI} \times 100\% = \frac{1000 \cdot BV \cdot PI}{n \cdot F} \times 100\%$$
$$\text{(equation 1)}$$

Continuing the previous example, if the patient's observed post-transfusion platelet count increment is only $25,000/\mu l$, then

$$PPR = \frac{1,000 \times 5,000 \times 25,000}{4 \times 10^{11} \times (2/3)} \times 100\%$$
$$= \frac{1.25 \times 10^{11}}{2.67 \times 10^{11}} \times 100\% = 47\%.$$

This agrees with the equivalent calculation using the previous value for MPI: $PPR = 25,000/53,300 \times 100\% = 47\%$.

Comparison of Methods for Estimating Blood Volume

As blood volume is not commonly measured directly in patients, it is usual to predict the BV term in the MPI or PPR formulas using one of the many published regression equations relating BV to body size, sex, age, etc.[200,202–209] The simplest and most commonly used formulas are based on either body weight or surface area, leading (as shown below) to different approximating versions of the PPR.

Among the usual measures of body size, surface area correlates best with BV. However, the predictive precision of a regression formula based on surface area is only slightly better than one based on weight. For example, in a study of 201 men and 97 women[202,203] the best fitting two-parameter linear regressions were $BV = 3,575 \cdot SA - 1.605$ for men and $BV = 3,284 \cdot SA - 1,288$ for women, where SA is surface area in square meters. In this study SA was approximated by the DuBois formula[204]: $SA = 0.007184 \cdot (\text{height cm})^{0.725} \cdot (\text{weight Kg})^{0.425}$. Also,

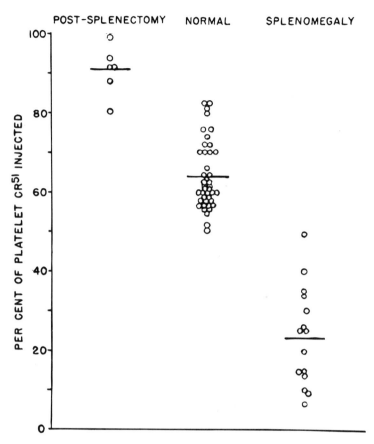

Fig. 16-8. Recovery in the general circulation of ^{51}CR-labeled platelets transfused to asplenic, normal, and splenomegalic subjects. "Recovery" is the percentage of platelets remaining in the general circulation 2 hours after injection. (From Aster et al.,[81] with permission.)

the BV regressions we summarize here have been corrected for errors introduced by hematocrit plasma trapping and the body: venous hematocrit ratio.[200,202] The prediction coefficient of variation (CV) for each regression was 8.1 percent for men and 8.6 percent for women, where CV is the residual standard deviation (SE of the estimate) divided by the mean blood volume. These CVs were not much smaller than the 8.9 percent prediction CVs found in both of the regression equations based on weight (WT) in kilograms:

$$BV = 46.7 \cdot WT + 1742 \text{ for men and}$$
$$BV = 53.7 \cdot WT + 984 \text{ for women.}$$

The above equations may be substituted for BV in equation 1 to yield good weight-based or surface-area-based approximating equations. However, simpler prediction formulas for BV tend to be favored in practice. We reanalyzed the adult blood volume data described above using one-parameter linear regression through the origin (i.e., a ratio equation) and obtained the following fits and prediction CVs:

Men	Women
BV = 2,725·SA	BV = 2,507·SA
(8.4% CV)	(8.8% CV)
BV = 70.5·WT	BV = 70.5·WT
(10.0% CV)	(9.2% CV)

These simpler regression equations are comparable to other approximations in common use,[207,209] and they have prediction CVs only moderately larger than those of the two-parameter regressions. Thus, the common approximation BV = 70 · WT may be adequate for both sexes in many cases, and substitution into equation 1 leads to the simplest weight-based approximation:

$$PPR_W = \frac{7 \times 10^4 \cdot PI \cdot WT}{n \cdot F} \times 100\% \quad \text{(equation 2)}$$

When F = 2/3, PPR_W is identical to the percent increment defined by the Milwaukee formula.[210–212]

Alternatively, substituting the one-parameter surface area regression into equation 1 leads to the simplest surface-area-based approximation for PPR:

$$PPR_S = \frac{2.725 \times 10^6 \cdot PI \cdot SA}{n \cdot F} \times 100\% \text{ for men.}$$

$$PPR_S = \frac{2.507 \times 10^6 \cdot PI \cdot SA}{n \cdot F} \times 100\% \text{ for women.}$$

$$\text{(equation 3)}$$

In the previous example, if blood volume is unknown but WT = 70 kg and SA = 1.73 m², the weight-based approximation is

$$PPR_W = \frac{7 \times 10^4 \times 25,000 \times 70}{4 \times 10^{11} \times (2/3)} \times 100\%$$

$$= \frac{1.23 \times 10^{11}}{2.67 \times 10^{11}} \times 100\% = 46\%$$

The surface-area-based approximation (assuming a male patient) is

$$PPR_S = \frac{2.725 \times 10^6 \times 25,000 \times 1.73}{4 \times 10^{11} \times (2/3)} \times 100\%$$

$$= \frac{1.18 \times 10^{11}}{2.67 \times 10^{11}} \times 100\% = 44\%$$

In this example, PPR_W and PPR_S are similar, as we expect them to be in most cases.

Recommendation

The uncertainties in F, PI, and n probably overshadow any small advantage in precision PPR_S has over PPR_W, and generally we see no strong advantage of one over the other. Either should approximate PPR adequately in most clinical situations. However, for markedly obese patients or other unusual body size features it may be advantageous to estimate BV first using one of the more detailed published regression relations and substitute this directly in equation 1 for PPR.

Comparison of PPR to CCI

A related measure of effectiveness is the widely reported corrected count increment (CCI)[2,212–218] computed by

$$CCI = \frac{PI \cdot SA \cdot 10^{11}}{n}$$

If in the previous example the patient has a body surface area of 1.73 m², the corrected count increment is

$$CCI = \frac{25,000 \times 1.73 \times 10^{11}}{4 \times 10^{11}} = 10,800$$

The CCI has qualitatively the same interpretation as the PPR: lower values imply decreased effectiveness. Also, because the CCI is a function of surface area, it is simple to convert CCI to the surface-area-based approximation for percent recovery:

$$PPR_S = 0.002725 \times (CCI/F) \text{ (\%) for men}$$

$$PPR_S = 0.002507 \times (CCI/F) \text{ (\%) for women}$$

$$\text{(equation 4)}$$

When a patient's sex is unspecified, a reasonable compromise is $PPR_S = 0.0026 \times (CCI/F)$ (percent). Table 16-5 presents these conversions for F = 2/3. For a given CCI, larger values of F (e.g., an asplenic patient) correspond to smaller values of PPR_S. For example, in the extreme case F = 1, the PPR_S values in Table 16-5 should be multiplied by 2/3.

As a rule of thumb, using BV = 2,600 × SA for either sex and assuming F = 2/3 for a patient with

Table 16-5 Relationship Between CCI and PPR_S[a]

CCI	PPRS		
	Sex Unspecified	Men	Women
1,000	3.9	4.1	3.8
2,000	7.8	8.2	7.5
3,000	11.7	12.3	11.3
4,000	16	16	15
5,000	20	20	19
6,000	23	25	23
7,000	27	29	26
7,500	29	31	28
8,000	31	33	30
9,000	35	37	34
10,000	39	41	38
11,000	43	45	41
12,000	47	49	45
13,000	51	53	49
14,000	55	57	53
15,000	59	61	56
16,000	62	65	60
17,000	66	69	64
18,000	70	74	68
19,000	74	78	71
20,000	78	82	75
22,000	86	90	83
24,000	94	98	90
26,000	(101)	(106)	98
28,000	(109)	(114)	(105)
30,000	(117)	(123)	(113)
35,000	(137)	(143)	(132)
40,000	(156)	(164)	(150)

[a] Approximation assuming platelet recovery $F = 2/3$ (normal spleen) and blood volume 2,600 ml/m² when patient's sex is unspecified, 2,725 ml/m² for men, or 2507 ml/m² for women.

a normal spleen, we may use the simple relation $PPR_S = 0.0039 \times CCI$ (percent). Thus, in our previous example, a CCI of 10,800 corresponds roughly to a PPR_S of $0.0039 \times 10,800 = 42\%$. We also note that if $F = 2/3$, PPR_S reaches its theoretical maximum value of 100 percent when CCI equals 24,500 for men and 26,600 for women.[218] Thus, larger values for CCI should alert one to the possibility of an underestimate of n or F or a regression-based overestimate of the true blood volume.

Recommendation

CCI has a slight advantage over the weight-based approximation PPR_W only to the extent that surface area is better than body weight as a predictor of blood volume. CCI has no intrinsic advantage over PPR_S, and the general PPR formulation has the educational advantage of explicitly representing the dependence of recovery on splenic pooling. Moreover, CCI units are easily misunderstood or incorrectly reported,[217,218] contributing in part to a fair amount of confusion over its precise interpretation and use. Our view is that it is preferable to use a readily understandable indication of the efficacy of a platelet transfusion. Since the percent recovery expresses the same result as the CCI but in a manner that is immediately comprehensible, we suggest use of the PPR. For ease of clinical reference, we summarize below simplified versions of the weight-based and surface-area-based formulas (when patient's sex is unspecified) after substitution of $F = 2/3$:

$$PPR_W = \frac{1.05 \times 10^5 \cdot PI \cdot WT}{n} \times 100\%$$

$$PPR_S = \frac{3.9 \times 10^6 \cdot PI \cdot SA}{n} \times 100\%$$

Alternatively, if CCI has already been computed, equation 4 or Table 16-5 can be used to convert CCI to PPR_S.

THE DIAGNOSIS OF REFRACTORINESS AND ALLOIMMUNIZATION

Refractoriness to platelet transfusions may be defined as a consistently inadequate response to platelet transfusions. Various criteria have been used to satisfy this definition (see below). *Alloimmunization*, in reference to platelet transfusion, is defined as the development of alloantibodies that have the potential to produce an inadequate response to platelet transfusion (e.g., antibodies to HLA or platelet-specific antigens). It is erroneous to use these terms interchangeably; patients who are refractory to platelet transfusion are not necessarily alloimmunized and patients who are alloimmunized may respond well to platelet transfusions.

McFarland et al.[219] reported that only about half

of the patients who demonstrate very poor increments to random-donor platelets have any evidence of platelet or lymphocytotoxic antibodies. Similarly, Moroff et al.[220] reported that lymphocytotoxic antibodies could be demonstrated in only 55 percent of patients refractory to platelet transfusions.

Sintnicolaas et al.[221] reported that anti-HLA antibodies were detected in 11 of 35 (31 percent) nonrefractory patients.

Criteria for the Diagnosis of Refractoriness

The definition of an appropriate response to platelet transfusion varies significantly among different investigators. One must have criteria by which to determine whether a platelet transfusion has produced an adequate post-transfusion platelet count increment. Various criteria have been proposed by which to diagnose refractoriness.[215]

The purpose of diagnosing refractoriness is to determine the need for the use of special platelet products (e.g., HLA-matched, crossmatched, or "HLA-antigen-negative platelets" [see below]). The optimal criterion of refractoriness is one that will indicate the need for the use of special platelet products when they are appropriate but will not suggest their need when random platelets are adequate. For example, if post-transfusion platelet count increments are less than optimal but still about 50 percent of expected, the additional increment that may be obtained may not warrant the extra expense of special

products. On the other hand, if one waits until the post-transfusion platelet count increments are consistently less than 5,000/μl after a transfusion of seven units of platelets to a 70-kg person, one is probably waiting too long to switch to special platelet products. Daly et al.[214] found that when the CCI was less than 10,000/μl, significantly improved increments were obtained using HLA-matched platelet products.

Commonly used criteria that have been established rather empirically are a CCI of 7,500 at one hour, or a CCI of 5,000 at 20 hours. As can be seen from Table 16-5, these values correspond to the percentage recovery of transfused platelets of about 30 percent and 20 percent, respectively.

Clinical Factors Affecting Post-Transfusion Increments

Patients may be refractory to platelet transfusions but not be alloimmunized or may have a combination of immune and nonimmune factors causing poor post-transfusion increments. Many nonimmune clinical factors influence the recovery of transfused platelets and their intravascular survival time.[48,216,219,222] Bishop et al.,[48,216] using multiple linear regression analyses, evaluated the significance of immune (antibodies to HLA and platelet-specific antigens) and nonimmune factors resulting in refractoriness to platelet transfusion. They identified the major factors influencing the 1-hour and 20-hour post-transfusion increments as prior splenec-

Table 16-6. Major Factors Influencing CIs Identified on Multiple Linear Regression Analyses

Factor	Coefficients	SE	95% Confidence Interval
Splenectomy	+7.7	3.5	0.8 to 15.2
Bone marrow transplantation	−6.2	1.3	−8.7 to −3.1
DIC	−4.1	2.4	−7.9 to 2.5
Amphotericin	−4.1	0.3	−6.2 to −3.0
Palpable spleen	−3.5	1.6	−6.7 to −0.8
HLA antibody grade	−3.1	0.6	−4.3 to −1.6
Platelet-specific antibody score	−0.9	1.1	−2.6 to 1.5
Number of antibacterial antibiotics	−0.7	0.4	−1.4 to 0.2
Clinical bleeding	+0.4	1.1	−2.0 to 1.9
Temperature	−0.3	0.3	−1.2 to 0.6

Only one transfusion was used per patient.
(From Bishop et al.,[48] with permission.)

tomy (which improved post-transfusion platelet count increments), bone marrow transplantation, disseminated intravascular coagulation, concurrent intravenous amphotericin B, splenomegaly, and HLA antibody grade, the latter determined by the percentage of positive cells using a standard microlymphocytotoxicity assay (Table 16-6). They also determined the relative importance of major factors influencing the CCI by calculating unbiased estimates of the regression coefficients of these factors. These estimates and the standard error (SE), given in Table 16-6, indicate the relative importance of each factor. There was no evidence that any factor has more influence at 20 hours after transfusion than at 1 hour.[216] Platelet-specific antibodies, number of concurrent antibiotics, clinical bleeding, and temperature did not significantly influence the CCI. They also pointed out that their data clearly indicate that other important but unexplained factors influence the CCI.[216]

McFarland et al.[219] concluded that fever and splenomegaly markedly reduced 1-hour CCI, while sepsis compromised the 24-hour platelet recovery. They found no correlation between HLA-match grade and transfusion response in patients without significant alloimmunization. Neither bleeding, positive lymphocytotoxic antibody tests against random-donor lymphocytes, nor ABO incompatibility between platelet donor and recipient affected the transfusion outcome.

Friedberg et al.[222] studied 71 patients and reported that fever, bleeding, neutropenia, DIC, and sepsis were each identified in at least one patient as a significant independent predictor of the CCI. Recent bone marrow transplantation, gender, and circulating IV immune globulin (IVIG) were not independent predictors of post-transfusion increment.

Although many studies list bleeding at the time of transfusion as an adverse event, there are no data to substantiate this conclusion. In one of the earliest studies on platelet therapy, there was no effect of bleeding on platelet yield in 23 patients.[223] Furthermore, none of several more recent studies using multifactorial analysis showed this as a factor associated with platelet refractoriness.[48,219,224]

As discussed previously, several investigators have indicated that ABO incompatibility adversely affects the CCI, possibly as a result of circulating immune complexes involving the ABO blood group system.[183,184]

In addition, one must keep in mind that immune mechanisms other than platelet-reactive alloantibodies may result in shortened platelet survival, including drug-induced antibodies, autoantibodies, immune complexes[4] and antibodies to plasma proteins.[225]

Doughty et al.[226] reported that immune mechanisms were not the predominant cause of platelet refractoriness in their patient population and that nonimmune factors were often multiple, most frequently a combination of fever, infection, and antibiotic therapy. They suggested, therefore, that measures for the prevention of HLA alloimmunization, such as leukocyte depletion, may have a limited impact in reducing the incidence of refractoriness to platelet transfusions.

MANAGEMENT OF PATIENTS REFRACTORY TO PLATELET TRANSFUSIONS

When patients are refractory to platelet transfusion, one should determine whether antibodies capable of causing platelet destruction are present. This is generally accomplished by lymphocytotoxicity tests using random or HLA-antigen-selected lymphocyte panels.

Although the presence of an alloantibody does not necessarily mean that a poor response to platelet therapy is due to immunization, detection of alloimmunization in a patient refractory to platelet transfusions indicates a probability that that patient will have an improved response to special platelet products. Some studies indicate that only about half of patients who are refractory to random-donor platelets have evidence of platelet or lymphocytotoxic antibodies,[219,220] although methods with increased sensitivity may indicate a higher percentage.

In general, patients who are not alloimmunized derive no benefit from special platelet products.[219,222] Accordingly, these products should be obtained for patients only when they are refractory and alloimmunized.[4,227] When a patient has both immunologic and nonimmunologic causes of poor platelet response, a trial of special platelet products is warranted.

Platelet-Specific Antibodies

In addition to tests for HLA antibodies, it is optimal to determine also if platelet-specific antibodies are present. However, such antibody tests are not as readily available and the practical value of the results is uncertain. Indeed, von dem Borne et al.[228] reviewed the fact that some investigators have suggested that antibodies against platelet-specific antigens may frequently contribute to transfusion refractoriness. However, the evidence put forward in the literature is indirect and has been rarely substantiated by detailed serologic studies. Most platelet-specific alloantigen systems are biallelic systems with a high-frequency antigen occurring in 96 percent to greater than 99 percent of the population and homozygosity for the low-frequency antigen occurring in 4 percent to less than 1 percent. Thus, refractoriness caused by alloimmunization against the high-frequency antigens is expected to occur in few patients. Alloimmunization against the low-frequency antigens is expected to occur much more often. However, this will remain undetected in transfusion of random donor platelets, because only a minority (27 percent to less than 1 percent) of the platelets in the transfused mixtures will be destroyed by the alloantibodies.[228]

Further, Slichter[4] pointed out that there are not enough platelet-specific antisera available to type community donor platelet apheresis panels for platelet-specific antigens. Also, patients with platelet-specific alloantibodies are most often found among patients who are highly refractory to all platelet donors, even those who are well matched. Therefore, the best approach to finding compatible donors for such patients is finding a platelet donor within their family. Such donors may also have to be HLA-compatible to obtain a good platelet increment.

Fresh Platelets and ABO-Matched Platelets

Although the response to transfusions of fresh or stored platelets does not differ greatly in clinically stable patients, Slichter[4] has reviewed studies indicating that stored platelets survive less well than fresh platelets in clinically unstable patients. Similarly, Norol et al.[229] reported that storage of platelets induces an impressive decrease in the in vivo platelet recovery and survival in patients with certain clinical conditions such as bacterial infections, graft-versus-host disease, splenomegaly, veno-occlusive disease, and amphotericin B therapy. Skodlar et al.[230] reported that antibody-negative patients who were refractory to platelet transfusions were refractory only to stored platelets. Accordingly, in patients who are refractory to platelet transfusions, a trial of fresh platelets may be warranted.

Similarly, one must determine that ABO-incompatibility was not the cause of the patient's refractoriness by providing ABO-compatible platelets.

These procedures may prevent the unnecessary use of HLA-matched or crossmatched platelets.

HLA-Matched Platelets

HLA-A and HLA-B antigens are the major immunogens expressed on the surface of platelets. HLA-C, HLA-D, and HLA-DR antigens are either not present or only weakly expressed on the platelet surface; incompatibility for these antigens has not been documented to cause refractoriness to platelet transfusions.[9]

Most patients who are refractory to random-donor platelets and who have HLA antibodies respond to donors selected on the basis of HLA match[211,220,231] (Figure 16-9). As indicated, a system of grading the match categories between the donor and the patient has been developed.

In seven studies in which the failure rate of HLA-A matched platelets from either family members or unrelated donors were reported, the failure rate varied between 6 percent and 39 percent, with the average being 19 percent.[231] However, for many transfusion recipients who require numerous platelet transfusions, it is not possible to find enough perfectly matched donors.

Also, a system of cross-reacting antigens is available as part of the donor and patient matching system. Cross-reactivity, as defined in HLA serology, is based on the in vitro observation that one monospecific serum may react with a single antigen and also may react consistently with additional antigens of the same locus. The original and the additional antigens become known as a cross-reactive group. Such cross-reactive groups are now known to define HLA public determinants that are on the heavy chain of the HLA molecule, and they are distinct from the allelic determinant.[4] These serologic observations were the basis of the policy of selecting platelet donors mismatched

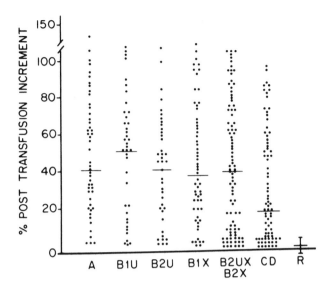

Fig. 16-9. Platelet recoveries in alloimmunized thrombocytopenic patients 24 hours after the transfusion of platelets from donors of varying degrees of HLA compatibility. The classification of donor-recipient pairs on the basis of HLA match is as follows: A, four-antigen match; B1, three-antigen match, fourth donor antigen is unknown (B1U) or cross-reactive (B1X); B2, two-antigen match, third and fourth donor antigens are unknown (B2U), cross-reactive (B2X), or both (B2UX); C, one donor antigen major mismatch; D, two or more antigen major mismatch; R, random donor. Median values are shown by horizontal bars. (From Duquesnoy et al.,[211] with permission.)

for cross-reactive HLA antigens for the transfusion support of refractory patients. Using cross-reacting antigens reduces the size of the donor pool necessary to provide "HLA-matched" platelets.[211,232–243] Most regional blood centers now have large pools of HLA-typed volunteers who are available to donate platelets by apheresis. With the development of these large pools of donors and the use of platelets selected on the basis of crossreacting antigens, "HLA-matched" platelets are widely available. Patients with common HLA types have more well-matched donors than do patients with rare HLA types, and therefore it is easier to provide platelets for patients with common HLA types.

It is generally agreed that platelets selected on the basis of cross-reactive antigens have a survival intermediate between fully matched platelets (A or BU

matches, see Fig. 16-9) and randomly selected platelets. Moroff et al.[220] reported that platelets selected on the basis of cross-reactive antigens (grade Bx) provided a 1-hour CCI of greater than 7,500 in only 11 of 30 (37 percent) of transfusions, whereas A- and BU-matched platelets provided such an increment in 16 of 22 (73 percent) of transfusions. Dahlke and Weiss[232] provided data regarding the frequency with which specific cross-reactive antigens produce an adequate transfusion response (Table 16-7). More studies are needed to provide better information on the value of public antigen matching to select compatible donors and also to determine which HLA antigens should be included within cross-reactive groups for transfusion purposes.[4]

HLA-matched transfusions to refractory patients are not always successful. After an unsuccessful platelet transfusion, it may be possible to provide platelets from another HLA-matched donor that are effective. By observing the pattern of responses to platelets from donors of various HLA types and various cross-reactive HLA antigens (Table 16-7), it may be possible to identify certain donor antigens that must be avoided and certain donor HLA types that produce good increments.[4,231,235,236]

One note of caution regarding the ordering of HLA-matched platelets is warranted. As pointed out by Friedberg et al.,[237] simply ordering platelets as HLA-matched does not necessarily lead to receiving HLA-identical or even well-matched platelets. Platelets received following a request for HLA-matched platelets are typically the closest match obtainable within the constraints of time and donor availability. In their study, 43 percent of platelets ordered as HLA-matched were relatively poor grade BX and C matches. Most of the benefit of ordering HLA-matched platelets derived from those patients who received good HLA matched platelets. Moroff et al.[214] reached a similar conclusion. Thus, if HLA-A- or BU-matched platelets are not available, other means of selecting special platelet products for alloimmunized patients may be preferable.

Platelet Compatibility Tests

A significant proportion, perhaps 25 to 40 percent, of the most closely HLA-matched platelet transfusions administered to alloimmunized patients are failures even in the absence of nonimmunologic

Table 16-7. HLA Cross-Reactive Specificities and Response to Platelet Transfusions

Poor Platelet Increments		Good Platelet Increments	
Recipient Type	Donor Type	Recipient Type	Donor Type
A3	A1, A11	A1	A11
A1	A3	A11	A1
A11	A3	A2	A28[a]
B5 Cross-reactive group	B17, Bw21	B5 Cross-reactive group	B18, Bw16
B15	B5	B18	B5
B17	B5		
B7 Cross-reactive group	B27	B7 Cross-reactive group	B7, Bw22
B8	B14		
B14	B8		
B12	Bw21		
Bw21	B12		

[a] Reverse not tried as all A28 recipients had anti-A2 antibodies.
(From Dahllse and Weiss,[232] with permission.)

causes.[4] Therefore, a reliable test for platelet-reactive antibodies that can be performed in a manner analogous to RBC crossmatching has potential value in selecting appropriate platelet donors.

Indeed, numerous investigators have reported that platelet crossmatch tests are of value in selecting donors for alloimmunized patients.[238–250] A variety of methods that measure platelet-associated immunoglobulin have been reported to yield results with a high predictive value[238,240–242,244,251–253] (Figs. 16-10, 16-11, 16-12, and 16-13). These methods include the use of radiolabeled staphylococcal protein A, radiolabeled antiglobulin reagents, enzyme-linked immunoassay, or fluorescence. Solid-phase methodology is also applicable.[249]

The crossmatch test has most often been suggested as an adjunct to HLA matching for the selection of platelets for transfusion to alloimmunized patients, although a number of studies have indicated high predictive value even when the donor and recipient are not HLA matched.[237,238,240,241,244,249,250,252–254] Available data suggest that the platelet crossmatch test is underutilized and its wider application is to be encouraged.[253] Some studies have compared the use of platelet crossmatching with HLA-based donor selection to treat refractory patients in the most effective and efficient fashion.[220,227,237,239,252,255]

von dem Borne et al.[228] reviewed the theoretical and practical aspects of platelet crossmatching. They pointed out that some HLA antigens may show a wide variability in expression on platelets and that donor platelets with low levels of certain HLA antigens may survive normally in patients with HLA antibodies directed against these antigens. They concluded that platelet crossmatching should be widely implemented in the selection of compatible platelets for alloimmunized patients, in part because of its cost-effectiveness.

HLA-Antigen-Negative Platelets

An additional method for support of refractory patients who have anti-HLA antibodies is to determine the specificity of the antibody(ies) and to supply platelets for transfusion that lack the pertinent antigen(s).[3,4] This is analogous to RBC crossmatching in that when one detects a red cell alloantibody in a patient's serum, red cells negative for that antigen are supplied but one does not ordinarily supply red cells that match the patient's extended phenotype.

Significant information can often be gained by testing patients' sera for antibody reactivity with selected lymphocyte panels. If HLA antibody specificity is determined, then HLA-typed donors can be selected to avoid the offending antigen. Avoiding a limited number of incompatible antigens rather

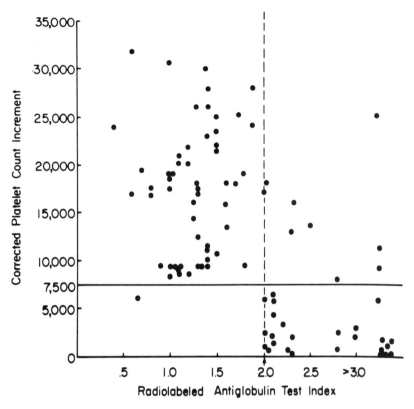

Fig. 16-10. Corrected platelet count increment 1 hour after transfusion as compared with the crossmatch index. A CCI of 7,500 was used as the criterion of an adequate increment at 1-hour post-transfusion. The radiolabeled antiglobulin test index of 2 was considered a positive result. Only nine transfusions with a positive test index of greater than 2 resulted in an adequate post-transfusion CCI at 1 hour ("false-positive" crossmatch results). Of the 26 transfusion failures, only 1 was not correctly predicted ("false-negative" crossmatch result). (From Kickler et al.,[244] with permission.)

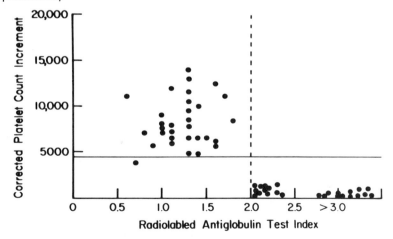

Fig. 16-11. Platelet CCI 20 hours after transfusion as compared with the crossmatch index. A CCI of 4,500 was used as the criterion of an adequate increment 20 hours after transfusion. All nine patients who had "false-positive" crossmatch results had a poor 20-hour increment. (From Kickler et al.,[244] with permission.)

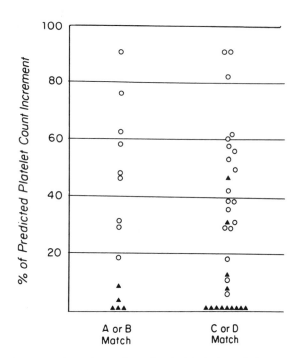

Fig. 16-12. Relationship of radiolabeled staphylococcal protein A crossmatch results, post-transfusion platelet count increment, and grade of donor-recipient HLA compatibility. There were 48 transfusion episodes in 18 alloimmunized patients. Triangles represent positive crossmatch tests, and circles represent negative results. An inadequate post-transfusion platelet count increment was defined as less than 20 percent of the predicted value. (From Yam et al.,[241] with permission.)

than matching for antigens will greatly expand the available donor pool for patients with HLA antibodies of identifiable specificity.[4]

This method has not been evaluated extensively although Bryant et al.[256] state that one-third of multiply transfused patients refractory to platelet transfusions show definable HLA antibodies using an antibody detection method that uses a double addition of serum. They illustrated the effectiveness of this technique in three patients and concluded that by using platelets compatible with recipient antibodies rather than searching for the rare individuals who are matched with the recipient's phenotype, many effective donors can easily be found for most alloimmunized patients. This method deserves more extensive evaluation.

Intravenous Immune Globulin

Alloimmunized patients have been treated with IVIG to improve the response to platelet transfusions.[257–263] A number of anecdotal reports have indicated success of IVIG in this setting[257,259–264] although reports of failures have also been recorded.[257,258,260,263]

One study[263] of three alloimmunized persons with acute leukemia reported increased platelet count increments after transfusion when these patients received IVIG before transfusion. Schiffer et al.[258] treated 11 adult acute leukemia patients with either 0.4 g IgG/kg/day for 5 days (4 patients) or 0.6 g/kg/day for 5 days (7 patients), and no patient improved in 1-hour post-transfusion platelet count increments. On this basis, they concluded that this treatment cannot be recommended for alloimmunized adults with leukemia.[258]

Studies in four patients with severe aplastic anemia who received intravenous immunoglobulin and platelet transfusions reported improved responses to transfused platelets.[265,266] In a placebo-controlled study[267] 12 persons refractory to platelet transfusions who received IVIG showed improved 1-hour post-transfusion platelet count increments, but levels at 24 hours were unchanged. A similar study[268] found that 6 of 10 patients had improved responses to selected single-donor platelets after IVIG administration.

These data indicate that IVIG is modestly effective in managing patients refractory to platelet transfusion. Considering the high cost of IVIG and the transient improvement as a result of its administration, Slichter[9] recommends that it be given only to patients who are refractory to all forms of platelet therapy and who have severe bleeding problems.

Protein A Column Therapy

Christie et al.[269] evaluated the use of protein A column therapy for the management of 10 thrombocytopenic patients who were refractory to platelet transfusion. Nine patients had previously been treated with steroids, intravenous immune globulin, and/or other forms of immunosuppressive therapy without improvement in their transfusion response. Eight patients had antibodies directed against HLA class I antigens, ABO antigens, and/or platelet-specific alloantigens. Plasma (500–2,000 ml) from each patient was passed over a protein A silica gel column

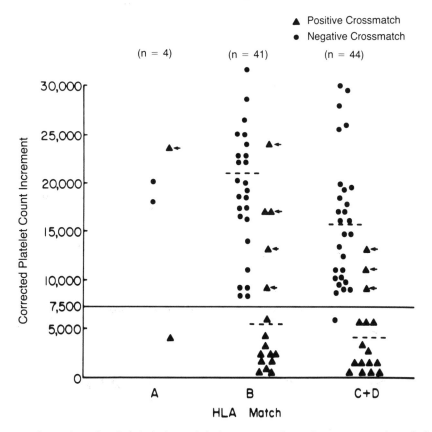

Fig. 16-13. Relationship of radiolabeled antiglobulin crossmatch results to HLA match and platelet increment at 1 hour. Arrows indicate poor survival at 20 hours. (From Kickler et al.,[244] with permission.)

and response was defined as at least a doubling of the pretreatment platelet count and/or two successive 10- to 120-minute post-transfusion CCIs ±7,500. Six of the 10 patients responded with daily platelet counts that averaged 48,000/μl as compared with counts of 16,000/μl before treatment. Post-transfusion CCI values determined in four of these patients averaged 2,480 ±810 and 10,010 ±3540 before and after treatment, respectively. They concluded that protein A column treatments may increase platelet counts and responsiveness to platelet transfusion in some patients.

However, Lopez-Plaza et al.[270] failed to demonstrate any effectiveness of protein A absorption in the treatment of platelet refractoriness. Moreover,

significant side effects of protein A columns, which can be life threatening, are of considerable concern.[271] Although this method is of interest, any benefits are derived via a mechanism that is not understood and for which there is very little, if any, evidence to indicate that the various hypotheses for effect are applicable. A standardized well-controlled study is needed.[271]

Other Methods of Managing Alloimmunized Patients

Other methods that have been tried in a limited number of cases are the use of plasma exchange, the administration of cyclosporin A[272] and the use of antithymocyte globulin. Anecdotal data suggest limited applicability of these methods.[4]

The Use of Frozen Autologous Platelets in Refractory Patients

Cryopreservation of platelets for prolonged periods makes autologous platelet therapy feasible and effective.[273-276] This is especially beneficial for highly sensitized patients with acute leukemia. Both autologous and allogeneic platelets from HLA-typed donors have been frozen.[275] Platelets collected by apheresis during remission are frozen and become available for infusion during subsequent thrombocytopenic episodes. In patients refractory even to HLA-matched platelets, frozen autologous platelets may be the only effective and reliable therapy. Platelets have been protected in dimethyl sulfoxide (DMSO)[273] and in glycerol,[277] but DMSO appears to produce adequate recovery and preserve platelet function more consistently.[273]

Epsilon-Aminocaproic Acid

In uncontrolled clinical studies, bleeding in patients with thrombocytopenia has been controlled with epsilon-aminocaproic acid (EACA). However, the only controlled prospective clinical trial randomized to receive either platelet therapy or platelet therapy plus EACA showed no difference in capillary bleeding, major vessel bleeding, or the number of platelet transfusions required per day.[4] Thus, the efficacy of this therapy remains unproven. Furthermore, there is the potential to enhance clotting in patients with DIC.[4]

MANAGEMENT OF REFRACTORY PATIENTS NONRESPONSIVE TO THE ABOVE MEASURES

There are occasional patients who are refractory to platelet transfusion and who do not respond to any of the above cited means of management. Some of these patients are highly alloimmunized, having broadly reactive HLA antibodies. Our own policy is to abandon the use of HLA-matched, cross-matched, or "HLA-antigen-negative" platelets after failure of about three transfusions of each type of product.

Patients who are not alloimmunized may also be refractory to platelet transfusions. Whether or not the patient is alloimmunized, efforts should be made to improve the patient's clinical condition (e.g., resolution of fever, sepsis, or DIC) as this may result in improved results of transfusion.

For the nonalloimmunized patient, one may nevertheless try transfusion of HLA-matched platelets that are also ABO-matched and are as fresh as is practical.[4] As with our policy for alloimmunized patients, we abandon the use of platelets selected on the basis of HLA type in nonalloimmunized patients after a maximum of three unsuccessful transfusions and revert to the use of randomly selected platelets.

If transfusions of special platelet products and the use of other measures indicated previously still fail to result in a significant post-transfusion platelet count increment, some authorities recommend that attempts to provide prophylactic platelet support should be discontinued.[2]

If hemorrhage occurs, many practitioners provide larger than usual doses of platelets.[2,4,278] Other steps that have been suggested,[278] although with modest probability of marked success, include the reversal of anemia to improve delivery of the platelets to the periphery of the flowing blood, using leukocyte-depleted red cells to avoid additional platelet consumption, and the use of leukocyte-depleted platelets to avoid a febrile response and platelet consumption. Murphy et al.[278] reported that the provision of platelets stored fewer than 2 days were not more successful than platelets stored more than 3 days in bleeding refractory patients.

One may be left only with the option of providing larger doses of platelets. There are few, if any, published specific recommendations regarding an optimal dose of platelets in this setting. Our own empirically developed policy for a bleeding adult who is refractory to platelet transfusion is to provide a maximum of about three plateletpheresis products per day (or about 1 unit/10 kg three times per day in a child) in an attempt to produce a post-transfusion increment and provide hemostasis. There is evidence that an increment of greater than $19,000/\mu l$ lasting at least 20 hours is associated with a greater chance of stopping significant bleeding than failure to achieve such an increment.[278] However, even with a post-transfusion increment of less than $5,000/\mu l$ hemostasis is achieved in about 30 percent of bleeding patients, although there may not always be a causal relationship between the platelet transfusion and the cessation of bleeding.

PREVENTION OF ALLOIMMUNIZATION

Since a significant proportion of patients receiving platelet transfusions become alloimmunized, convenient, affordable methods to prevent alloimmunization would be highly desirable. Several approaches have been suggested.

Single-Donor Platelets

One approach that has been tried is transfusing platelets from a single donor rather than using pooled platelets from multiple donors, thus decreasing the number of donor exposures. In two studies,[279,280] the incidence of alloimmunization in recipients of single random-donor apheresis platelet transfusions was reduced compared with that found in patients receiving pooled random-donor platelet transfusions. However, the patients in these studies received very few platelet transfusions. In a study in which the patients were exposed to 10 ± 9 donors in the single-donor apheresis group and 78 ± 55 donors in the pooled random-donor group, the rate of immunization in both groups was the same.[281] In another study, the alloimmunization rate in recipients of single-donor apheresis platelets did not differ from historic controls who received pooled random-donor platelet concentrates.[282] On the basis of these data, it is not common practice in the United States to routinely provide single-donor platelets to prevent alloimmunization.

Leukocyte-Poor Platelet Products

Another approach to prevention of alloimmunization has been the use of leukocyte-poor platelet products, as there is evidence that HLA alloimmunization caused by platelet transfusions is induced by contaminating lymphocytes.[282,283] A number of very efficient leukocyte reduction filters are now available requiring new techniques to count accurately the very low number of WBCs remaining in the filtered products.

Slichter[9] has reviewed the results of six prospective randomized clinical trials involving 299 patients evaluating the efficacy of leukocyte-poor RBCs and platelets compared with unmodified RBCs and platelets in preventing platelet alloimmunization.[282,284–288] There was substantial variability in patient selection, methods of leukocyte reduction,

endpoint criteria, leukocyte concentration of control and leukocyte-poor blood products, and trial results. Four of the six studies showed significant reductions in development of lymphocytotoxic antibodies in patients given leukocyte-poor products.[282,285,286,288] However, in the three studies that tested for platelet-specific alloantibodies, there were no differences between the control and the leukocyte-poor arms.[282,285,287] The incidence of clinical platelet refractoriness was reduced by leukocyte-poor blood products in only three of the trials.[285,286,288]

Williamson et al.[289] performed a prospective randomized study of the efficacy of poststorage bedside leucodepletion of blood products in the prevention of primary HLA alloimmunization and its clinical sequelae in 123 evaluable patients with hematologic malignancies. HLA antibodies developed in 21 of 56 (37.5 percent) patients receiving nonfiltered products and in 15 of 67 (22 percent) patients receiving filtered products ($P = .07$). Bedside filtration did not affect the overall incidence of febrile transfusion reactions or of platelet refractoriness. They concluded that their study failed to show clear clinical benefit.

Three editorials have suggested caution in interpreting the available data.[21,290,291] Heddle and Blajchman[291] concluded that the necessary information on which to make a policy decision regarding the routine use of leukodepletion for cellular blood products to prevent HLA-alloimmunization and/or platelet refractoriness is still lacking. Properly designed prospective studies are still needed.[291] Nevertheless, leukocyte-depleted products are being routinely used in a number of medical centers for patients who can be expected to need chronic platelet transfusion therapy in an attempt to prevent alloimmunization.

Sintnicolaas et al.[221] reported that in patients with previous pregnancies, leukocyte depletion of random single-donor platelet transfusions to less than 5×10^6 leukocytes per transfusion does not reduce the incidence of platelet refractoriness and anti-HLA alloimmunization nor the time required to become refractory or develop HLA-alloimmunization. It appears that platelets per se, soluble HLA-antigens, or microparticles escaping leukocyte filtration may result in a secondary immune response. These results are consistent with those of a similar previous study in which leukocyte-depletion of cellular blood products was not as stringent.[292]

In considering the cost effectiveness of any approach to preventing alloimmunization to platelets in, for example, patients with acute leukemia, one must consider that only about 15 percent of this population would stand to derive long-term benefit.[21,293] This is true because only about 40 to 50 percent of patients become alloimmunized after multiple platelet transfusions, some patients will die of their disease before alloimmunization can occur, alloimmunization will not be prevented by leukocyte-poor blood products in 100 percent of the patients, etc. Furthermore, many alloimmunized patients can be managed effectively by using HLA-matched or crossmatched platelets. A very significant effect on bleeding, longevity, and quality of life must be demonstrated before a costly procedure to prevent alloimmunization can be recommended. The use of pools of random platelets until the patient becomes refractory and then the use of HLA matched and/or crossmatched single-donor platelets is generally the recommended course for patients requiring long-term platelet support. However, with the availability of filtration or other methods of inexpensive and effective means of leukocyte depletion, the use of leukocyte-poor RBCs and platelet products may become the strategy of choice for patients who can be expected to require long-term platelet transfusions. It is hoped that multicenter prospective clinical trials will provide adequate information on which to make such a judgment.[4,21,290]

Ultraviolet Irradiation

Recent studies have suggested that a major route of alloimmunization is by means of antigen-presenting cells (APCs).[4] Donor APCs interact with T-helper cells of the transfused recipient to induce the recipient's plasma cells to produce alloantibodies. Ultraviolet (UV) irradiation has been documented to interfere with the function of APCs, and clinical trials have been initiated to evaluate the effectiveness of UV-irradiation of platelets as a means of prevention of platelet alloimmunization. One report by Grijzenhout et al.[294] indicated that UV-irradiation of pooled platelets failed to prevent alloimmunization.

Splenectomy

There has been an effort to detect an effect of splenectomy on the development of alloimmunization, but currently there is no convincing evidence that this therapy will delay or prevent alloimmunization.[295,296]

Spontaneous Loss of HLA Antibodies

HLA antibodies spontaneously disappear over time in some patients, often despite continued transfusions. A compilation of data from such reports indicated that antibody loss occurred in 165 of 392 patients (42 percent).[4] Once antibodies disappear, patients may regain their responsiveness to random-donor platelet transfusions. These data clearly suggest that a prudent strategy is to serially measure antibodies over time in platelet-refractory patients, with the goal of returning patients who have lost their antibodies to random-donor platelet therapy.

RISKS OF PLATELET TRANSFUSION

In addition to alloimmunization, there are numerous additional adverse effects of platelet transfusion (Table 16-8).

Febrile and Allergic Transfusion Reactions

Febrile and allergic transfusion reactions following platelet transfusion can be due to sensitization to platelet, histocompatibility, RBC, or plasma antigens.[297,298] Transfusion reactions most commonly occur during or shortly after the infusion and are usually mild, consisting of chilliness and, rarely, shaking, chills or, occasionally, rises in temperature with or without urticaria. Premedication with acet-

Table 16-8 Hazards of Platelet Transfusion

Febrile- and allergic-type transfusion reactions
Circulatory overload
Transmission of blood-borne infectious diseases
Graft-versus-host disease
Transfusion of RBC alloantibodies
Sensitization to RBC antigens
Granulocytopenia with (?) marrow suppression (alloimmunized patients)
Alloimmunization

aminophen can ameliorate these reactions but need not be administered before transfusion to most patients. Rarely, very severe reactions associated with pulmonary symptomatology are observed. In some patients, reactions can be prevented by removal of leukocytes by filtration. If the patient is alloimmunized and refractory to platelet transfusions, the post-transfusion platelet count increment may not improve after leukodepletion even though the febrile reaction may be diminished.[4]

More recent reports suggest that bioreactive substances in the plasma supernatant of the platelet product cause most febrile reactions associated with platelet transfusion.[299] Increasing levels of a number of cytokines have been found during storage of platelets, including tumor necrosis factor alpha, interleukin 1, and interleukin 6.[299,300] Since these cytokines are known as endogenous pyrogens, it may be true that the intravenous administration of plasma with high cytokine levels rather than antigen-antibody reactions are the major cause of febrile transfusion reactions.

Circulatory Overload

Circulatory overload, particularly in children or elderly recipients, can occur because a pool of 4 to 6 units represents a volume load of 200 to 300 ml of plasma. If necessary, the volume of plasma can be reduced before infusion by centrifugation of the pooled concentrates and resuspension of the platelet button in a smaller volume. These concentrated transfusions should be administered shortly after preparation because of the decreased platelet viability after storage at higher platelet concentrations. In addition, the platelets will no longer be in a totally closed system after these manipulations.[191,192]

Transmission of Infectious Diseases

Transmission of infectious diseases is a serious complication of blood transfusion and is reviewed in Section V of this text. A particular problem regarding platelet transfusion is that bacteria that have proliferated in platelet concentrates stored at room temperature can be transfused.[301–307] The clinical clue to this complication is the occurrence of a severe febrile reaction with an average temperature elevation of 2°C[300] shortly after the infusion is begun. Such a reaction mandates cessation of the infusion,

culture of the platelet bag, blood culture on the patient, and strong consideration for institution of antibiotic therapy in granulocytopenic recipients. (This topic is discussed in more detail in Chapter 40.)

Graft-Versus-Host Disease

Transfusion-associated graft-versus-host disease (TA-GVHD) can occur as a result of transfusion of cellular blood products, particularly in patients with immune deficiencies. Another critical factor in the development of TA-GVHD is a close HLA match between donor and recipient. This has led to the policy of irradiating all cellular blood components that are to be transfused to immunocompromised patients and/or that have been donated by blood relatives of the patient.[199] Also, a number of investigators have suggested that it is prudent to irradiate HLA-matched platelet products, although this is not mandated by American Association of Blood Banks standards. TA-GVHD is reviewed in detail in Chapter 42.

Hemolysis of Recipient Red Blood Cells

Passive transfer of antibody may occur as a result of transfusion of minor ABO-incompatible platelets because each platelet concentrate obtained from a unit of whole blood contains about 50 to 70 ml of plasma and plateletpheresis products may contain about 350 ml of plasma. The use of incompatible platelets is sometimes unavoidable (e.g., when inventories are inadequate or when HLA or platelet-specific antibodies are causing refractoriness and the only HLA-matched or cross-match-compatible platelet donors are ABO incompatible).[308] Several cases of severe hemolysis after transfusion of platelets with ABO-incompatible plasma have been reported.[308–315]

Hemolysis occurs when the donors have high titers of antibodies against recipient ABO blood groups. For example, Pierce et al.[312] reported two instances of severe immune hemolysis after transfusion of ABO-incompatible platelet concentrates. One of the reactions resulted in disseminated intravascular hemolysis and proved fatal and the other resulted in hemolysis of an estimated 40 percent of the patient's red cell mass. They found that the IgG anti-A titer of one donor was 32,000 and the anti-B titer of the other donor was 16,000.

In the case reported by Reis and Coovadia,[314] the plateletpheresis donor's plasma had an anti-B titer of 4,096 by indirect antiglobulin testing. In the patient reported by Conway and Scott,[311] the donor's saline anti-A titer was 8,192 and the titer of dithiothreitol-treated serum was 4,096. Transfusion of a plateletpheresis product with a volume of 200 ml resulted in severe hemolysis, disseminated intravascular hemolysis, and renal failure requiring dialysis.

The patient reported by Murphy et al.[308] received two transfusions of plateletpheresis products 25 days apart from the same donor. Stored serum from the donor, taken at the time of the first transfusion, had an anti-A titer of 512 by saline agglutination and 2,048 by indirect antiglobulin test. The patient received 155 ml of plasma with the first platelet product and 448 ml with the second. Hemolysis occurred after both transfusions and, after the second transfusion, the patient's hemoglobin dropped from 11.4 to 6.0 g/dl in one day. She developed renal failure although dialysis was not required and her renal function returned to normal.

The patient reported by McLeod et al.[310] is particularly interesting in that the patient developed hemolysis after receiving only four platelet concentrates, each containing about 50 ml of plasma. The patient developed serious hemolysis with hemoglobinuria, a drop in hemoglobin from 14.0 to 8.0 g/dl, and renal insufficiency with a rise in creatinine from 1.6 to 6.0 mg/dl. Two of the platelet donors were found to have anti-A antibody to a titer of 10,240 by indirect antiglobulin test.

Despite the above case reports, one must keep in mind that hemolysis following ABO-incompatible platelet transfusion is not common. Shanwell et al.[315] reported that bone marrow transplant recipients at their institution routinely received single-donor plateletpheresis products containing about 350 ml of plasma concentrates from blood group O donors for 5 years during which time about 1,000 concentrates with ABO-incompatible plasma were transfused. Although they have noted positive direct antiglobulin tests caused by passively adsorbed anti-A and/or anti-B from the donor plasma, they have found no cases of hemolysis. They studied 11 group A patients in detail and found that nine developed a positive DAT, and anti-A could be eluted from the patients' red cells in these cases. However, in no case

was there any clinical sign of hemolysis. Also, patients of groups A, B or AB (n = 34) required no more RBC or platelet transfusions than did patients who were group O (n = 47).

Plasma Reduction of Minor ABO Incompatible Products

One may reduce the volume of platelet concentrates,[316,317] plateletpheresis products, or bone marrow products to minimize risks related to the volume of plasma transfused. Volume reduction has generally been recommended for prevention of volume overload in infants, patients in danger of overload from intravenous fluids, patients with respiratory distress syndrome, and patients with congestive heart failure.[317] Volume reduction may also be appropriate as a means of diminishing the amount of antibody that would be transfused.

The degree of volume reduction that would prevent hemolysis by a given antibody is difficult to determine, but some published information is pertinent to this point. Inwood and Zuliani,[318] in reviewing a case of hemolysis resulting from transfusion of a unit of group O packed RBC to a group A person, determined that the group O unit contained anti-A_1 activity to a titer of 1:8,192. They estimated that the titer of the donor anti-A in the patient's circulation after transfusion was 1:164. This resulted in intravascular hemolysis and a drop in hemoglobin of 2.4 g/dl.

Studies in bone marrow transplant recipients have indicated that transfusion of ABO incompatible red cells to patients with isohemagglutinin titers of 1:16 produced no evident hemolysis.[319] Thus, in calculating the amount of plasma reduction that might be appropriate for a given product, if one reduces the volume of plasma to be transfused so that the post-transfusion isohemagglutinin titer will be less than or equal to 1:16, serious hemolysis will probably not occur.

However, measuring the isohemagglutinin titers in all minor ABO incompatible platelet products seems unnecessary since episodes of severe hemolysis caused by platelet transfusions are rare. Thus, the most practical policy is to try to avoid minor ABO incompatible platelet transfusions, especially for patients who will receive large volumes of plasma as a result of multiple transfusions. One must be cognizant of the possible consequences of passively transfused antibody, which can affect compatibility testing and occasionally cause significant hemolysis.

Sensitization to Rh$_o$ (D) and Other RBC Antigens

Sensitization to Rh$_o$ (D) and other RBC antigens can occur in recipients of multiple transfusions because some RBCs are present in most platelet preparations (see the previous section on the practical aspects of platelet transfusion).

Granulocytopenia

Granulocytopenia, lasting for a few days and, therefore, suggesting possible bone marrow suppression, has been described following the transfusion of mismatched platelets to alloimmunized patients with otherwise stable aplastic anemia.[320] The suggested mechanism is "innocent bystander" destruction of host granulocytes in association with immune lysis of transfused platelets. This is potentially an important complication of platelet transfusion because of the possibility of an acquired infection increasing the likelihood of hemorrhage. However, this complication is probably very rare and should never deter a physician from administering platelets to a patient in need.[321]

NEW CONCEPTS REGARDING PLATELET TRANSFUSION

Platelet Injury and Microparticle Formation In Vitro

Any manipulation of platelets in vitro appears to result in some degree of damage and possible impairment of function as judged by in vitro tests and/or subsequent in vivo recovery and survival after transfusion. It is important to recognize that direct evaluation of hemostatic efficacy of any platelet preparation is very difficult. The changes in vitro characteristics and in recovery and survival probably correlate sufficiently highly with hemostatic efficacy that these measurements are useful for purposes of quality control and evaluation of platelet preservation technics. A simple method of direct evaluation of hemostatic efficacy would be of great value.

The injury to platelets caused by their collection, pooling, and storage for transfusion has been called the "storage lesion." The nature and severity of this damage is highly influenced by the conditions of storage such as temperature, nature of the plastic container, and type of agitation mixing.[322] Although most of the investigation of this problem has been directed toward platelets recovered from routinely collected donor units, at least some of the same types of damage are probably sustained by the process of plateletpheresis.

The most prominent change in the composition of platelets stored in vitro is a decrease in the membrane glycoprotein GPIb. A 45 percent loss of this protein after 7 days storage has been reported. This contrasts with the relative stability of the proteins GPIIb/IIIa and GPIX. PF3 is also released into the plasma during storage.[323]

Although the mechanism of these changes is not fully known, there is increasing evidence that the formation of platelet microparticles during collection and storage is related to the biochemical alterations and to functional impairment. There have been many studies of this phenomenon, which seems to be the result of breaking off of filamentous structures of the platelet membrane. This can be induced by many mechanisms including shear stresses, the effects of complement protein complexes, and any process that stimulates platelet activation. Microparticles are concentrated in platelets for transfusion and in cryoprecipitate. They are also found in FFP. The number of microparticles increases with duration of storage. George et al.[324] have concluded that most microparticles are generated as the result of in vitro processing.

There is some evidence to suggest that platelet microparticles may have a hemostatic effect, or that the hemostatic effect of platelet transfusion might at least partly be due to microparticle formation. Large numbers of microparticles are infused with every platelet transfusion and with most blood components. They seem to cause no adverse effects in this situation. This topic, which has recently been reviewed by Owen,[323] should be studied further.

The Potential Significance of Thrombopoietin in Platelet Transfusion

One possible alternative to platelet transfusion that has been considered is the administration of hematopoietic growth factors to stimulate platelet production in vivo. Whereas the roles of erythropoietin and granulocyte-colony stimulating factor in stimulating the differentiation of RBCs and granulocytes, respectively, are well established and used successfully in clinical medicine, the factor responsible for the development of platelets is more elusive.

The murine myeloproliferative leukemia virus contains a truncated form (*v-mpl*) of the coding region of the *c-mpl* gene that is a member of the hematopoietin receptor superfamily. Several lines of evidence indicate that the *c-mpl* product is the receptor of a cytokine specifically involved in the regulation of the megakaryocytic lineage. Biologic and molecular characterization of the Mpl ligand (Mpl-L) have been performed.[325–329] Reports indicate that the ligand for c-Mpl is thrombopoietin.[322,324] Accordingly, it has been suggested that the c-Mpl ligand be officially designated thrombopoietin (TPO) or megakaryocyte growth and development factor (MGDF).[330]

The administration of recombinant thrombopoietin to normal mice has been shown to stimulate a fourfold increase in the number of circulating platelets after only 5 days. Thus the therapeutic potential of thrombopoietin in the treatment of theombocytopenia can be viewed as analogous to the use of erythropoietin in the treatment of anemia (i.e., chronic rather than acute). As a consequence, it is envisaged that the primary indications for recombinant thrombopoietin could be in the treatment of thrombocytopenia resulting from cancer chemotherapy, radiotherapy, and bone marrow transplantation. Some estimates indicate that in excess of 70 percent of all platelet units are used for these indications.

Assuming it is efficacious in humans, the potential effect on platelet transfusion practices is enormous. However, the development of thrombopoietin is at an early stage and without extensive safety and efficacy data. The next developments in this story are awaited with great interest.

ADDENDUM

To justify the opening statement in this chapter, we offer the following addendum, which is a compilation of some unresolved questions with my proposed answers.

Question: If a patient does not have an adequate response to a platelet transfusion, how can the cause of this poor response be determined?

Answer: Simple! Just consider the following: HLA antibodies, platelet antibodies, ABO incompatibility, splenomegaly, DIC, fever, infection, cardiopulmonary bypass, platelet autoantibodies, drug-induced platelet-reactive antibodies, immune complexes, antibodies to plasma protein antigens, stored platelets, bone marrow transplantation, GVHD, administration of drugs such as amphotericin B, antibiotic therapy, brisk bleeding, any combination of the above, or "other important but unexplained factors."[216] If this seems too easy, keep in mind that each of the above factors may be present without an effect on post-transfusion platelet count increment, including the presence of HLA antibodies, which have been reported to be present in 31 percent of nonrefractory patients.[221]

Question: What are the correct units for the CCI?

Answer: The correct units are probably among those that have been used in published articles, including the following[217,218]: platelets/μL (e.g., 10,000/μL) (which is actually the calculated index/μL and does not correspond to the post-transfusion increment/μL), platelets/m^2 (e.g., 10,000/m^2), platelets per 10^{11} platelets transfused per m^2 (e.g., 10,000/10^{11}/m^2), platelets/μL/10^{11}/m^2, platelets/μL/unit transfused/m^2, or (rather commonly) no units whatsoever.

Question: Who cares about the appropriate units for the CCI?

Answer: Dr. Daniel Brubaker.[217]

Question: Who does not care about the appropriate units for the CCI?

Answer: Apparently, almost everyone else concerned with publishing articles, including authors, reviewers of articles, and the editors of journals.

Question: If the CCI is 6,000 (supply your own units) following a platelet transfusion, what percent of platelets were recovered?

Answer: If you do not know the answer to this question, it suggests that you should think in terms of percent recovery rather than the CCI. For the answer, see Table 16-5.

Question: Why is the CCI used more frequently than the percent recovery even though the latter gives a more readily understandable indication of the effectiveness of a transfusion?

Answer: Possibly because of an erroneous impression that surface area is a significantly better predictor of blood volume than body weight (see discussion, pp. 382–385).

Question: Does bone marrow transplantation affect the post-transfusion platelet count increment?

Answer: Bone marrow transplantation profoundly affects post-transfusion platelet count increments[216], OR bone marrow transplantation does not affect post-transfusion platelet count increments.[222]

Question: Does fever affect the post-transfusion platelet count increment?

Answer: Yes[222] and no.[216]

Question: Do fresh platelets provide significantly better increments than stored platelets?

Answer: Yes, in refractory patients[230]; yes, in clinically unstable patients[4,229,] and no,[278].

Question: Does the use of leukocyte-depleted blood products reduce the incidence of HLA alloimmunization?

Answer: There is firm evidence that leukocyte-depletion of cellular blood products reduces HLA alloimmunization,[221] OR necessary information on which to make a policy decision regarding the routine use of leukodepletion for cellular blood products to prevent HLA-alloimmunization and/or platelet refractoriness is still lacking—properly designed prospective studies are still needed.[290]

REFERENCES

1. Consensus conference: Platelet transfusion therapy. JAMA 257:1777, 1987
2. British Committee for Standards in Heamatology: Guidelines for platelet transfusions. Transfusion Med 2:311, 1992
3. Heyman MR, Schiffer CA: Platelet transfusion therapy for the cancer patient. [Review]. Semin Oncol 17: 198, 1990
4. Slichter SJ: Mechanisms and management of platelet refractoriness. p. 95. In Nance SJ (ed): Transfusion Medicine in the 1990's. American Association of Blood Banks, Arlington, VA, 1990
5. McCullough J, Steeper TA, Connelly DP et al: Platelet utilization in a university hospital. JAMA 259: 2414, 1988
6. Pisciotto PT, Benson K, Hume H et al: Prophylactic versus therapeutic platelet transfusion practice in hematology/oncology patients. Transfusion 1995 (In Press)
7. Gaydos LA, Freireich EJ, Mantel N: The quantitative relation between platelet count and hemorrhage in patients with acute leukemia. N Engl J Med 266:905, 1962
8. Freireich EJ, Kliman A, Gaydos LA et al: Response to repeated platelet transfusions from the same donor. Ann Intern Med 59:277, 1963
9. Slichter SJ: Principles of transfusion support before and after bone marrow transplantation. p. 273. In Forman SJ, Blume KG, Donnall TE: (eds): Bone Marrow Transplantation. Blackwell Scientific Publications, Boston, 1994
10. Roy AJ, Jaffe N, Djerassi I: Prophylactic platelet transfusions in children with acute leukemia: a dose response study. Transfusion 13:283, 1973
11. Slichter SJ, Harker LA: Thrombocytopenia: mechanisms and management of defects in platelet production. Clin Haematol 7:523, 1978
12. Aderka D, Praff G, Santo M et al: Bleeding due to thrombocytopenia in acute leukemias and reevaluation of the prophylactic platelet transfusion policy. Am J Med Sci 291:147, 1986
13. Gmur J, Burger J, Schanz U et al: Safety of stringent prophylactic platelet transfusion policy for patients with acute leukemia. Lancet 338:1223, 1991
14. Han T, Stutzman L, Cohen E, Kim U: Effect of platelet transfusion on hemorrhage in patients with acute leukemia. An autopsy study. Cancer 19:1937, 1966
15. Freireich EJ: When to give platelet transfusions. Blood 82:682, 1993
16. Beutler E: When to give platelet transfusions. Blood 82:683, 1993
17. Higby DJ, Cohen E, Holland JF, Sinks L: The prophylactic treatment of thrombocytopenic leukemic patients with platelets: a double blind study. Transfusion 14:440, 1974
18. Solomon J, Bofenkamp T, Fahey JL et al: Platelet prophylaxis in acute nonlymphoblastic leukemia. Lancet 1:267, 1978
19. Murphy S, Litwin S, Herring LM et al: Indications for platelet transfusions in children with acute leukemia. Am J Hematol 12:347, 1982
20. Dutcher JP, Schiffer CA, Aisner J, Wiernik PH: Alloimmunization following platelet transfusion: the absence of a dose-response relationship. Blood 57:395, 1981
21. Schiffer CA: Prevention of alloimmunization against platelets (editorial). Blood 77:1, 1991
22. Klingemann HG, Self S, Banaji M et al: Refractori-

ness to random donor platelet transfusions in patients with aplastic anaemia: a multivariate analysis of data from 264 cases. Br J Haematol 66:115, 1987

23. Dutcher JP, Schiffer CA, Aisner J, Wiernik PH: Long-term follow-up patients with leukemia receiving platelet transfusions: identification of a large group of patients who do not become alloimmunized. Blood 58:1007, 1981

24. Beutler E: Platelet transfusions: the 20,000/microL trigger. [Review]. Blood 81:1411, 1993

25. Etchason J, Petz LD, Keeler E et al: The cost-effectiveness of preoperative autologous blood donations. N Engl J Med 332:719, 1995

26. Simon TL: Platelets: uses, abuses and indications. In Kolins JL, McCarthy LJ (eds): Contemporary transfusion practice. American Association of Blood Banks, Arlington, VA, 1987

27. Schiffer CA: Prophylactic platelet transfusion [editorial]. Transfusion 32:295, 1992

28. Patten E: Controversies in transfusion medicine. Prophylactic platelet transfusion revisited after 25 years: con. Transfusion 32:381, 1992

29. Patten E: Blood component therapy for cancer patients. Tex Med 81:31, 1985

30. Strauss RG: The risks of thrombocytopenia and the standard uses of platelet transfusions. Plasma Ther Transfus Technol 7:279, 1986

31. Bishop JF, Schiffer CA, Aisner J, Matthews JP, Wiernik PH: Surgery in acute leukemia. A review of 167 operations in thrombocytopenic patients. Am J Hematol 26:147–155, 1987

32. Simpson MB: Platelet function and transfusion therapy in the surgical patient. p. 51. In Schiffer CA (ed): Platelet Physiology and Transfusion. American Association of Blood Banks, Washington, DC, 1978

33. Counts RB, Haisch C, Simon TL et al: Hemostasis in massively transfused trauma patients. Ann Surg 190:91, 1979

34. Reed RL, Ciavarella D, Heimbach DM et al: Prophylactic platelet administration during massive transfusion. Ann Surg 203:40, 1986

35. Ciavarella D, Reed RL, Counts RB et al: Clotting factor levels and the risk of diffuse microvascular bleeding in the massively transfused patient. Br J Haematol 67:365, 1987

36. Day HJ, Rao AK: Evaluation of platelet function. Semin Hematol 23:89, 1986

37. Rodgers RPC, Levin J: A critical reappraisal of the bleeding time. Semin Thromb Hemost 16:1, 1990

38. Harker LA, Slichter SJ: The bleeding time as a screening test for evaluation of platelet function. N Engl J Med 287:155, 1972

39. Kahn RA, Meryman MT: Storage of platelet concentrates. Transfusion 16:13, 1976

40. Shulman NR, Watkins SP, Itscoitz SB, Student AB: Evidence that the spleen retains the youngest and hemostatically most effective platelets. Trans Assoc Am Physicians 81:302, 1968

41. Slichter SJ, Harker LA: Preparation and storage of platelet concentrates. II. Storage variables influencing platelet viability and function. Br J Haematol 34:403, 1976

42. Eknoyan G, Wacksman SJ, Glueck HI, Will JJ: Platelet function in renal failure. N Engl J Med 280:677, 1969

43. McKenna R, Bachmann F, Whittaker B, Gilson JR, Weinberg M: The hemostatic mechanism after open-heart surgery. II. Frequency of abnormal platelet functions during and after extracorporeal circulation. J Thorac Cardiovasc Surg 70:298, 1975

44. Murphy S, Davis JL, Walsh PN, Gardner FH: Template bleeding time and clinical hemorrhage in myeloproliferative disease. Arch Intern Med 138:1251, 1978

45. Feusner JH: Normal and abnormal bleeding times in neonates and young children utilizing a fully standardized template technic. Am J Clin Pathol 74:73, 1980

46. Ewe K: Bleeding after liver biopsy does not correlate with indices of peripheral coagulation. Dig Dis Sci 26:388, 1981

47. Lind SE: The bleeding time does not predict surgical bleeding. Blood 77:2547, 1991

48. Bishop JF, McGrath K, Wolf MM et al: Clinical factors influencing the efficacy of pooled platelet transfusions. Blood 71:383, 1988

49. Kestin AS, Valeri CR, Khuri SF et al: The platelet function defect of cardiopulmonary bypass. Blood 82:107, 1993

50. Bachmann F, McKenna R, Cole ER, Najafi H: The hemostatic mechanism after open-heart surgery. I. Studies on plasma coagulation factors and fibrinolysis in 512 patients after extracorporeal circulation. J Thorac Cardiovasc Surg 70:76, 1975

51. Pike OM, Marquiss JE, Weiner RS, Breckenridge RT: A study of platelet counts during cardiopulmonary bypass. Transfusion 12:119, 1972

52. Bick RL: Alterations of hemostasis associated with cardiopulmonary bypass: Pathophysiology, prevention, diagnosis, and management. Semin Thromb Hemost 3:59, 1976

53. Salzman EW, Weinstein MT, Weintraub RM et al: Treatment with desmopressin acetate to reduce blood loss after cardiac surgery. N Engl J Med 314:1402, 1986

54. Harker LA, Malpass TW, Branson HE et al: Mechanism of abnormal bleeding in patients undergoing cardiopulmonary bypass: acquired transient platelet dysfunction associated with selective alpha granule release. Blood 56:824, 1980
55. Simon TL, Akl BF, Murphy W: Controlled trial of routine administration of platelet concentrates in cardiopulmonary bypass surgery. Ann Thorac Surg 37:359, 1984
56. Goodnough LT, Johnston MF, Ramsey G et al: Guidelines for transfusion support in patients undergoing coronary artery bypass grafting. Transfusion Practices Committee of the American Association of Blood Banks. Ann Thorac Surg 50:675, 1990
57. Ovrum E, Holen EA, Abdelnoor M, Oystese R: Conventional blood conservation techniques in 500 consecutive coronary artery bypass operations. Ann Thorac Surg 52:500, 1991
58. Goodnough LT, Johnston MF, Toy PT: The variability of transfusion practice in coronary artery bypass surgery. Transfusion Medicine Academic Award Group. JAMA 265:86, 1991
59. Thurer RL, Lytle BW, Cosgrove DM, Loop FD: Autotransfusion following cardiac operations: a randomized prospective study. Ann Thorac Surg 27:500, 1979
60. Umlas J: In vivo platelet function following cardiopulmonary bypass. Transfusion 15:596, 1975
61. Harding SA, Shakoor MA, Grindon AJ: Platelet support for cardiopulmonary bypass surgery. J Thorac Cardiovasc Surg 70:350, 1975
62. Hardesty RL, Bayer WL, Bahnson HT: A technique for the use of autologous fresh blood during open-heart surgery. J Thorac Cardiovasc Surg 56:683, 1968
63. Schmidt PJ, Peden JC, Jr., Brecher G, et al: Thrombocytopenia and bleeding tendency after extracorporeal circulation. N Engl J Med 265:1181, 1961
64. Umlas J, Sakhuja R: The effect on blood coagulation of the exclusive use of transfusions of frozen red cells during and after cardiopulmonary bypass. J Thorac Cardiovasc Surg 70:519, 1975
65. Woods JE, Taswell HF, Kirklin JW et al: The transfusion of platelet concentrates in patients undergoing heart surgery. Mayo Clin Proc 42:318, 1987
66. Grindon AJ, Schmidt PJ: Platelet-poor blood in open heart surgery. N Engl J Med 280:1337, 1969
67. Hallowell P, Bland JHL, Buckley MJ et al: Transfusion of fresh autologous blood in open heart surgery. J Thorac Cardiovasc Surg 64:941, 1972
68. Litwak RS, Jurado RA, Lukban SB et al: Perfusion without donor blood. J Thorac Cardiovasc Surg 64:714, 1972
69. O'Brien TG, Haynes LL, Hering AC et al: The use of glycerolized frozen blood in vascular surgery and extracorporeal circulation. Surgery 49:109, 1961
70. Mohr R, Martinowitz U, Lavee J et al: The hemostatic effect of transfusing fresh whole blood versus platelet concentrates after cardiac operations. J Thorac Cardiovasc Surg 96:530, 1988
71. Lavee J, Martinowitz U, Mohr R et al: The effect of transfusion of fresh whole blood versus platelet concentrates after cardiac operations. A scanning electron microscope study of platelet aggregation on extracellular matrix. J Thorac Cardiovasc Surg 97:204, 1989
72. Manno CS, Hedberg KW, Kim HC et al: Comparison of the hemostatic effects of fresh whole blood, stored whole blood, and components after open heart surgery in children. Blood 77:930, 1991
73. Krevans JR, Jackson DP: Hemorrhagic disorder following massive whole blood transfusions. JAMA 159:171, 1955
74. Lim RC Jr, Olcott C IV, Robinson AJ, Blaisdell FW: Platelet response and coagulation changes following massive blood replacement. J Trauma 13:577, 1973
75. Simmons RL, Collins JA, Heisterkamp CA et al: Coagulation disorders in combat casualties: I. Acute changes after wounding. II. Effects of massive transfusion. III. Post-resuscitative changes. Ann Surg 169:455, 1969
76. Collins JA: Problems associated with the massive transfusion of stored blood. Surgery 75:274, 1974
77. Miller RD, Robbins TO, Tong MJ, Barton SL: Coagulation defects associated with massive blood transfusion. Ann Surg 174:794, 1971
78. Cote CJ, Lui LMP, Szyfelbein SK et al: Changes in serial platelet counts following massive blood transfusion in pediatric patients. Anesthesiology 62:197, 1985
79. Ciavarella D, Reed RL, Counts RB et al: Clotting factor levels and the risk of diffuse microvascular bleeding in the massively transfused patient. Br J Haematol 67:365, 1987
80. Mannucci PM, Federici AB, Sirchia G: Hemostasis testing during massive blood replacement. A study of 172 cases. Vox Sang 42:113, 1982
81. Aster RH: Pooling of platelets in the spleen: role in the pathogenesis of "hypersplenic" thrombocytopenia. J Clin Invest 45:645, 1966
82. Aster RH, Jandi JH: Platelet sequestration in man. II. Immunological and clinical studies. J Clin Invest 43:856, 1964

83. Inceman S, Tangun Y: Platelet defects in the myelo-proliferative disorders. Ann NY Acad Sci 201:251, 1972

84. Adams T, Schutz L, Goldberg L: Platelet function abnormalities in the myeloproliferative disorders. Scand J Haematol 13:215, 1974

85. Levin J: Bleeding with infectious diseases. p. 367. In Ratnoff OD, Forbes D (eds): Disorders of Hemostasis. Grune & Stratton, Orlando, FL, 1984

86. Cohen P, Gardner FH: Thrombocytopenia as a laboratory sign and complication of gram-negative bacteremic infection. Arch Intern Med 117:113, 1966

87. Levin J, Poore TE, Young NS et al: Gram-negative sepsis: detection of endotoxemia with the limulus test. Ann Intern Med 76:1, 1972

88. Oppenheimer L, Hryniuk WM, Bishop AJ: Thrombocytopenia in severe bacterial infections. J Surg Res 20:211, 1976

89. Kelton JG, Neame PB, Gauldie J, Hirsch J: Elevated platelet-associated IgG in the thrombocytopenia of septicemia. N Engl J Med 300:760, 1979

90. van der Lelie J, van der Plas-Van Dalen CM, von dem Borne AEGKr: Platelet autoantibodies in septicaemia. Br J Haematol 58:755, 1984

91. Paskitt TR, Paskitt PKF: Thrombocytopenia of sepsis. Arch Intern Med 145:891, 1985

92. Bessman JD, Gardner FM: Platelet size in thrombocytopenia due to sepsis. Surg Gynecol Obst 156:122, 1983

93. Emerson WA, Zieve PD, Krevans JR: Hematologic changes in septicemia. Johns Hopkins Med J 126:69, 1970

94. Sharp AA: Diagnosis and management of disseminated intravascular coagulation. Br Med Bull 33:265, 1977

95. Mant MJ, King EG: Severe acute disseminated intravascular coagulation. Am J Med 67:557, 1979

96. Hattersley PG, Kunkel M: Cryoprecipitates as a source of fibrinogen in treatment of disseminated intravascular coagulation (DIC). Transfusion 16:641, 1976

97. Lerner RG, Rapaport SI, Meltzer J: Thrombotic thrombocytopenic purpura. Serial clotting studies relation to the generalized Shwartzman reaction and remission after adrenal steroid and dextran therapy. Ann Intern Med 66:1180, 1967

98. Berkowitz LR, Dalldorf FG, Blatt PM: Thrombotic thrombocytopenic purpura. A pathology review. JAMA 241:1709, 1979

99. Berberich FR, Cuene SA, Chard RL, Hartmann JR: Thrombotic thrombocytopenic purpura. Three cases with platelet and fibrinogen survival studies. J Pediatr 84:503, 1974

100. Gottschall JL, Pisciotta AV, Darin J et al: Thrombotic thrombocytopenic purpura: experience with whole blood exchange transfusion. Semin Thromb Hemost 7:25, 1981

101. Harkness DR, Byrnes JJ, Lian ELY et al: Hazard of platelet transfusion in thrombotic thrombocytopenic purpura. JAMA 246:1931, 1981

102. Shepard KV, Bukowski RM: The treatment of thrombotic thrombocytopenic purpura with exchange transfusions, plasma infusions, and plasma exchange. [Review]. Semin Hematol 24:178, 1987

103. Byrnes JJ, Moake JL, Klug P, Periman P: Effectiveness of the cryosupernatant fraction of plasma in the treatment of refractory thrombotic thrombocytopenic purpura. Am J Hematol 34:169, 1990

104. Bell WR, Braine HG, Ness PM, Kickler TS: Improved survival in thrombotic thrombocytopenic purpura-hemolytic uremic syndrome. Clinical experience in 108 patients. N Engl J Med 325:398, 1991

105. Rock GA, Shumak KH, Buskard NA et al: Comparison of plasma exchange with plasma infusion in the treatment of thrombotic thrombocytopenic purpura. Canadian Apheresis Study Group. N Engl J Med 325:393, 1991

106. Obrador GT, Zeigler ZR, Shadduck RK, Rosenfeld CS, Hanrahan JB: Effectiveness of cryosupernatant therapy in refractory and chronic relapsing thrombotic thrombocytopenic purpura. Am J Hematol 42:217, 1993

107. Hayward CPM, Sutton DMC, Carter Jr et al: Treatment outcomes in patients with adult thrombotic thrombocytopenic purpura—Hemolytic uremic syndrome. Arch Intern Med 154:982, 1994

108. Shulman NR, Marder VJ, Weinrach RS: Comparison of immunologic and idiopathic thrombocytopenia. Trans Assoc Am Physicians 77:65, 1964

109. Shulman NR, Marder VJ, Weinrach RS: Similarities between known antiplatelet antibodies and the factor responsible for thrombocytopenia in idiopathic purpura. Physiologic, serologic and isotopic studies. Ann NY Acad Sci 124:499, 1965

110. Donnell RL, McMillan R, Yelenosky RJ et al: Different antiplatelet antibody speficities in immune thrombocytopenic purpura. Br J Haematol 34:147, 1976

111. Aisner J: Platelet transfusion therapy. Med Clin North Am 61:1133, 1977

112. Carr JM, Kruskall MS, Kage JA, Robinson SH: Efficacy of platelet transfusions in immune thrombocytopenia. Am J Med 80:1051, 1986

113. Stohl D, Cines DB, Aster RH et al: Platelet kinetics in patients with idiopathic thrombocytopenic purpura and moderate thrombocytopenia. Blood 65:584, 1985

114. Baumann MA, Menitove JE, Aster RH, Anderson T: Urgent treatment of idiopathic thrombocytopenic purpura with single-dose gammaglobulin infusion followed by platelet transfusion. Ann Intern Med 104: 808, 1986

115. Aster RH, George JN: Thrombocytopenia due to enhanced platelet destruction by immunologic mechanisms. p. 1370. In Williams WJ, Beutler E, Erslev AJ, Lichtman MA (eds): Hematology. McGraw-Hill, New York, 1990

116. Christie DJ, van Buren N, Lennon SS, Putnam JL: Vancomycin-dependent antibodies associated with thrombocytopenia and refractoriness to platelet transfusion in patients with leukemia. Blood 75:518, 1990

117. Christie DJ, Sauro SC, Cavanaugh AL, Kaplan ME: Severe thrombocytopenia in an acquired immunodeficiency syndrome patient associated with pentamidine-dependent antibodies specific for glycoprotein IIb/IIIa. Blood 82:3075, 1993

118. Schiffer CA, Weinstein HJ, Wiernik PH: Letter: Methicillin-associated thrombocytopenia. Ann Intern Med 85:338, 1976

119. Kaufman DW, Kelly JP, Johannes CB et al: Acute thrombocytopenic purpura in relation to the use of drugs. Blood 82:2714, 1993

120. Gynn TN, Messmore HL, Friedman IA: Drug-induced thrombocytopenia. Med Clin North Am 56: 65, 1972

121. Miescher PA: Drug-induced thrombocytopenia. Semin Hematol 10:311, 1973

122. Chong BH, Fawaz I, Chesterman CN, Berndt MC: Heparin-induced thrombocytopenia: mechanism of interaction of the heparin-dependent antibody with platelets. Br J Haematol 73:235, 1989

123. Warkentin TE, Kelton JG: Heparin-induced thrombocytopenia. [Review]. Prog Hemost Thromb 10:1, 1991

124. Gottschall JL, Elliot W, Lianos E et al: Quinine-induced immune thrombocytopenia associated with hemolytic uremic syndrome: a new clinical entity. Blood 77:306, 1991

125. Blayney DW: Quinine-associated immune thrombopenia, neutropenia, and renal failure in a patient with Klinefelter's syndrome. Blood 80:2686, 1992

126. Stroncek DF, Vercellotti GM, Hammerschmidt DE et al: Characterization of multiple quinine-dependent antibodies in a patient with episodic hemolytic uremic syndrome and immune agranulocytosis. Blood 80:241, 1992

127. Wu GG, Curtis BR, Shao YL, Aster RH: Analysis of quinine-dependent neutrophil-reactive antibodies in patients with quinine-induced hemolytic uremic syndrome (HUS) and quinine-induced thrombocytopenia (QITP) by flow cytometry and immunoprecipitation. Transfusion 33:77s, 1993

128. Spearing RL, Hickton CM, Sizeland P, Hannah A, Bailey RR: Quinine-induced disseminated intravascular coagulation. Lancet 336:1535, 1990

129. Schmitt SK, Tomford JW: Quinine-induced pancytopenia and coagulopathy. Ann Intern Med 120:90, 1994

130. Trent RJ, Clancy RL, Danis V, Basten A: Immune complexes in thrombocytopenic patients: cause or effect? Br J Haematol 44:645, 1980

131. Kutti J, Zaroulis CG, Safai-Kutti S et al: Evidence that circulating immune complexes remove transfused platelets from the circulation. Am J Hematol 11:255, 1981

132. Safai-Kutti S, Zaroulis CG, Day NK, Good RA, Kutti J: Platelet transfusion therapy and circulating immune complexes. Vox Sang 39:22, 1980

133. George JN, Shattil SJ: Acquired disorders of platelet function. p. 1528. In Hoffman R, Benz EJ, Shattil SJ et al (eds): Hematology: Basic Principles and Practice. Churchill Livingstone, New York, 1991

134. George JN, Caen JP, Nurden AT: Glanzmann's thrombasthenia: the spectrum of clinical disease. (Review). Blood 75:1383, 1990

135. Woodman RC, Harker LA: Bleeding complications associated with cardiopulmonary bypass. (Review). Blood 76:1680, 1990

136. Willard JE, Lange RA, Hillis LD: The use of aspirin in ischemic heart disease. (Review). N Engl J Med 327:175, 1992

137. Levy JH: Aspirin and bleeding after coronary artery bypass grafting [editorial]. Anesth Anal 79:1, 1994

138. Becker RC, Alpert JS: The impact of medical therapy on hemorrhagic complications following coronary artery bypass grafting. (Review). Arch Intern Med 150: 2016, 1990

139. Taggart DP, Siddiqui A, Wheatley DJ: Low-dose preoperative aspirin therapy, postoperative blood loss, and transfusion requirements. Ann Thorac Surg 50: 424, 1990

140. Sethi GK, Copeland JG, Goldman S et al: Implications of preoperative administration of aspirin in patients undergoing coronary artery bypass grafting. Department of Veterans Affairs Cooperative Study

on Antiplatelet Therapy. J Am Coll Cardiol 15:15, 1990

141. Bashein G, Nessly ML, Rice AL, Counts RB, Misbach GA: Preoperative aspirin therapy and reoperation for bleeding after coronary artery bypass surgery. Arch Intern Med 151:89, 1991

142. Michelson EL, Morganroth J, Torosian M, Mac Vaugh H III: Relation of preoperative use of aspirin to increased mediastinal blood loss after coronary artery bypass graft surgery. J Thorac Cardiovasc Surg 76:694, 1978

143. Ferraris VA, Ferraris SP, Lough FC, Berry WR: Preoperative aspirin ingestion increases operative blood loss after coronary artery bypass grafting. Ann Thorac Surg 45:71, 1988

144. Rawitscher RE, Jones JW, McCoy TA, Lindsley DA: A prospective study of aspirin's effect on red blood cell loss in cardiac surgery. J Cardiovasc Surg 32:1, 1991

145. Reich DL, Patel GC, Vela-Cantos F, Bodian C, Lansman S: Aspirin does not increase homologous blood requirements in elective coronary bypass surgery. Anesth Anal 79:4, 1994

146. Torosian M, Michelson EL, Morganroth J, MacVaugh H III: Aspirin- and Coumadin-related bleeding after coronary-artery bypass graft surgery. Ann Intern Med 89:325, 1978

147. Rubin RN: Aspirin and postsurgery bleeding. Ann Intern Med 89:1006, 1978

148. Stuart MJ, Murphy S, Oski FA et al: Platelet function in recipients of platelets from donors ingesting aspirin. N Engl J Med 287:1105, 1972

149. Eknoyan G, Wacksman SJ, Glueck HI, Will JJ: Platelet function in renal failure. N Engl J Med 280:677, 1969

150. Weiss HJ: Platelet physiology and abnormalities of platelet function. N Engl J Med 293:531, 580, 1975

151. Rabiner SF: Uremic bleeding. Prog Thromb Hemost 1:233, 1972

152. Fernandez F, Goudable C, Sie P et al: Low haematocrit and prolonged bleeding time in uraemic patients: effect of red cell transfusions. Br J Haematol 59:139, 1985

153. Livio M, Gotti E, Marchesi D et al: Uraemic bleeding: role of anaemia and beneficial effect of red cell transfusions. Lancet 2:1013, 1982

154. Mannucci PM, Canciani MT, Rota L, Donovan BS: Response of factor VIII/von Willebrand factor to DDAVP in healthy subjects and patients with haemophilia A and von Willebrand's disease. Br J Haematol 47:283, 1981

155. Mannucci PM, Remuzzi G, Pusineri F et al: Dea-

mino-8-D-arginine vasopressin shortens the bleeding time in uremia. N Engl J Med 308:8, 1983

156. Kobrinsky NL, Israels ED, Gerrard JM et al: Shortening of bleeding time by 1-deamino-8-D-arginine vasopressin in various bleeding disorders. Lancet 1:1145, 1984

157. DiMichele DM, Hathaway WE: Use of DDAVP in inherited and acquired platelet dysfunction. Am J Hematol 33:39, 1990

158. Shepherd LL, Hutchinson RJ, Worden EK, Koopmann CF, Coran A: Hyponatremia and seizures after intravenous administration of desmopressin acetate for surgical hemostasis. J Pediatr 114:470, 1989

159. Holmberg L, Nilsson IM, Borge L et al: Platelet aggregation induced by 1-desamino-8-D-arginine vasopressin (DDAVP) in type IIB von Willebrand's disease. N Engl J Med 309:816, 1983

160. Kobrinsky NL, Letts RM, Patel LR et al: 1-Desamino-8-D-arginine vasopressin (desmopressin) decreases operative blood loss in patients having Harrington rod spinal fusion surgery. Ann Intern Med 107:446, 1987

161. Gerritsen SW, Akkerman JWN, Sixman JJ: Correction of the bleeding time in patients with storage pool deficiency by infusion of cryoprecipitate. Br J Haematol 40:153, 1978

162. Bucher U, de Weck A, Spengler H et al: Platelet transfusions: shortened survival of HLA-identical platelets and failure of in vitro detection of antiplatelet antibodies after multiple transfusions. Vox Sang 25:187, 1973

163. Tobelem G, Levy-Toledano S, Nurden AT et al: Further studies on a specific platelet antibody found in Bernard-Soulier syndrome and its effects on normal platelet function. Br J Haematol 41:427, 1979

164. Clemetson KJ, McGregor JL, James E, Dechavanne M, Luscher EF: Characterization of the platelet membrane glycoprotein abnormalities in Bernard-Soulier syndrome and comparison with normal by surface-labeling techniques and high-resolution two-dimensional gel electrophoresis. J Clin Invest 70:304, 1982

165. Berndt MC, Gregory C, Chong BH, Zola H, Castaldi PA: Additional glycoprotein defects in Bernard-Soulier's syndrome: confirmation of genetic basis by parental analysis. Blood 62:800, 1983

166. Kunicki TJ, Furihata K, Bull B, Nugent DJ: The immunogenicity of platelet membrane glycoproteins. Transfus Med Rev 1:21, 1987

167. Bierling P, Fromont P, Elbez A, Duedari N, Kieffer N: Early immunization against platelet glycoprotein IIIa in a newborn Glanzmann type I patient. Vox Sang 55:109, 1988

168. Nurden AT, Jallu V, Hourdille P et al: Evidence for multiple antibodies in the sera of two patients with immune thrombocytopenia of different origins. Thromb Haemost 62:565, 1989

169. Muller JY, Patereau C, Soulier JP: [Glanzmann thrombasthenia, PLA1 antigen and anti-Glanzmann antibody]. [French]. Revue Francaise de Transfusion et Immuno-Hematologie 21:1069, 1978

170. Coller BS, Peerschke EI, Seligsohn U et al: Studies on the binding of an alloimmune and two murine monoclonal antibodies to the platelet glycoprotein IIb-IIIa complex receptor. J Lab Clin Med 107:384, 1986

171. Mannucci PM: Desmopressin (DDAVP) for treatment of disorders of hemostasis. [Review]. Prog Hemost Thromb 8:19, 1986

172. Mannucci PM: Desmopressin: a nontransfusional form of treatment for congenital and acquired bleeding disorders. (Review). Blood 72:1449, 1988

173. Castillo R, Monteagudo J, Escolar G et al: Hemostatic effect of normal platelet transfusion in severe von Willebrand disease patients. Blood 77:1901, 1991

174. Dunstan RA, Simpson MB, Knowles RW, Rosse WF: The origin of ABH antigens on human platelets. Blood 65:615, 1985

175. Ogasawara K, Ueki J, Takenaka M, Furihata K: Study on the expression of ABH antigens on platelets. Blood 82:993, 1993

176. Aster RH: Effect of anticoagulant and ABO incompatibility on recovery of transfused human platelets. Blood 26:732, 1965

177. Duquesnoy RJ, Anderson AJ, Tomasulo PA, Aster RH: ABO compatibility and single-donor platelet transfusion therapy of alloimmunized thrombocytopenic patients. Blood 54:595, 1979

178. Lee EJ, Schiffer CA: ABO compatibility can influence the results of platelet transfusion. Results of a randomized trial. Transfusion 29:384, 1989

179. Ellinger PJ, Morgan LK, Malecek AC, Chaplin H: Effect of ABO mismatching on a radioimmunoassay for platelet compatibility. Successful absorption of ABO alloantibodies with synthetic A and B substance. Transfusion 29:134, 1989

180. Heal JM, Mullin A, Blumberg N: The importance of ABH antigens in platelet crossmatching. Transfusion 29:514, 1989

181. Tosato G, Applebaum FR, Deisseroth AB: HLA-matched platelet transfusion therapy of severe aplastic anemia. Blood 52:846, 1978

182. Brand A, Sintnicolaas K, Claas FH, Eernisse JG: ABH antibodies causing platelet transfusion refractoriness. Transfusion 26:463, 1986

183. Heal JM, Rowe JM, McMican A, Masel D, Finke C, Blumberg N: The role of ABO matching in platelet transfusion. Eur J Haematol 50:110, 1993

184. Heal JM, Masel D, Rowe JM, Blumberg N: Circulating immune complexes involving the ABO system after platelet transfusion. Br J Haematol 85:566, 1993

185. Carr R, Hutton JL, Jenkins JA, Lucas GF, Amphlett NW: Transfusion of ABO-mismatched platelets leads to early platelet refractoriness. Br J Haematol 75:408, 1990

186. Gurevitch J, Nelken D: Studies on platelet antigens. III. Rh-Hr antigens in platelets. Vox Sang 2:342, 1957

187. Lawler SD, Shatwell HS: Are Rh antigens restricted to red cells? Vox Sang 7:488, 1962

188. Goldfinger D, McGinniss MH: Rh-incompatible platelet transfusions—risks and consequences of sensitizing immunosuppressed patients. N Engl J Med 284:942, 1971

189. Lichtiger B, Surgeon J, Rhorer S: Rh-incompatible platelet transfusion therapy in cancer patients. A study of 30 cases. Vox Sang 45:139, 1983

190. McLeod BC, Piehl MR, Sassetti RJ: Alloimmunization to RhD by platelet transfusions in autologous bone marrow transplant recipients. Vox Sang 59:185, 1990

191. Simon TL, Siena ER: Concentration of platelets into small volumes. Transfusion 24:173, 1984

192. Moroff G, Friedman A, Robkin-Kline L et al: Reduction of the volume of stored platelet concentrates for use in neonatal patients. Transfusion 24:144, 1984

193. Morrison FS: The effect of filters on the efficiency of platelet transfusion. Transfusion 6:493, 1966

194. Arora SN, Morse EE: Platelet filters—an evaluation. Transfusion 12:208, 1972

195. Cullen DJ, Ferrara L: Comparative evaluation of blood filters: a study in vitro. Anesthesiology 41:568, 1974

196. Mason KG, Hall LE, Lamoy RE, Wright CB: Evaluation of blood filters: dynamics of platelets and platelet aggregates. Surgery 77:235, 1975

197. Marshall BE, Wurzel HA, Neufeld GR, Klineberg PL: Effects of intersept micropore filtration of blood on microaggregates and other constituents. Anesthesiology 44:525, 1976

198. Snyder EL, Hezzey A, Cooper-Smith M, James R: Effect of microaggregate filtration on platelet concentrates in vitro. Transfusion 21:427, 1981

199. Klein HG (ed). Standards for Blood Banks and Transfusion Services. 16th Ed. American Association of Blood Banks, Bethesda, MD, 1994

200. Albert SN: Blood Volume and Extracellular Fluid Volume. Charles C Thomas, Springfield, IL, 1971
201. Toghill PJ, Green S, Ferguson F: Platelet dynamics in chronic liver disease with special reference to the role of the spleen. J Clin Pathol 30:367, 1977
202. Wennesland R, Brown E, Hopper J Jr et al: Red cell, plasma and blood volume in healthy men measured by radiochromium (Cr-51) cell tagging and hematocrit: influence of age, somatotype and habits of physical activity on the variance after regression of volumes to height and weight combined. J Clin Invest 38:1065, 1959
203. Brown E, Hopper Jr, Hodges Jr et al: Red cell, plasma, and blood volume in healthy women measured by radiochromium cell-labeling and hematocrit. J Clin Invest 41:2182, 1962
204. DuBois D, Dubois EF: A formula to estimate the approximate surface area if height and weight be known. Arch Intern Med 17:863, 1916
205. Nadler SB, Hidalgo JU, Bloch T: Prediction of blood volume in normal human adults. Surgery 51:224, 1962
206. Moore FD, Olesen KH, McMurrey JD et al: The Body Cell Mass and Its Supporting Environment: Body Composition in Health and Disease. WB Saunders, Philadelphia, 1963
207. Dagher FJ, Lyons JH, Finlayson DC, Shamsai J, Moore FD: Blood volume measurement: a critical study. Prediction of normal values: controlled measurement of sequential changes: choice of a bedside method. Adv Surg 1:69, 1965
208. Retzlaff JA, Tauxe WN, Kiely JM, Stroebel CF: Erythrocyte volume, plasma volume, and lean body mass in adult men and women. Blood 33:649, 1969
209. Shoemaker WC, Walker WF: Fluid-Electrolyte Therapy in Acute Illness. Year Book Medical Publishers, Chicago, 1970
210. Filip DJ, Duquesnoy RJ, Aster RH: Predictive value of cross-matching for transfusion of platelet concentrates to alloimmunized recipients. Am J Hematol 1:471, 1976
211. Duquesnoy RJ, Filip DJ, Rodey GE, Rimm AA, Aster RH: Successful transfusion of platelets "mismatched" for HLA antigens to alloimmunized thrombocytopenic patients. Am J Hematol 2:219, 1977
212. Rebulla P: Formulae for the definition of refractoriness to platelet transfusion (letter; comment). Transfus Med 3:91, 1993
213. Yankee RA, Grumet FC, Rogentine GN: Platelet transfusion. The selection of compatible platelet donors for refractory patients by lymphocyte HL-A typing. N Engl J Med 281:1208, 1969
214. Daly PA, Schiffer CA, Aisner J, Wiernik PH: Platelet transfusion therapy. One-hour post-transfusion increments are valuable in predicting the need for HLA-matched preparations. JAMA 243:435, 1980
215. Bishop JF, Matthews JP, Yuen K et al: The definition of refractoriness to platelet transfusions. Transfus Med 2:35, 1992
216. Bishop JF, Matthews JP, McGrath K et al: Factors influencing 20-hour increments after platelet transfusion. Transfusion 31:392, 1991
217. Brubaker DB: Correction of the corrected count increment units. Transfusion 33:358, 1993
218. Murphy S: Correction of the corrected count increment units. Transfusion 33:358, 1993
219. McFarland JG, Anderson AJ, Slichter SJ: Factors influencing the transfusion response to HLA-selected apheresis donor platelets in patients refractory to random platelet concentrates. Br J Haematol 73:380, 1989
220. Moroff G, Garratty G, Heal JM et al: Selection of platelets for refractory patients by HLA matching and prospective cross-matching. Transfusion 32:633, 1992
221. Sintnicolaas K, van Marwijk Kooij M, van Prooijen HC et al: Leukocyte depletion of random single-donor platelet transfusions does not prevent secondary human leukocyte antigen-alloimmunization and refractoriness: a randomized prospective study. Blood 85:824, 1995
222. Friedberg RC, Donnelly SF, Boyd JC, Gray LS, Mintz PD: Clinical and blood bank factors in the management of platelet refractoriness and alloimmunization. Blood 81:3428, 1993
223. Hirsch EO, Gardner FH: The transfusion of human blood platelets. J Lab Clin Med 39:556, 1952
224. Parker RD, Yamamoto LA, Miller WR: Interaction effects analysis of platelet transfusion data. Transfusion 14:567, 1974
225. Heal JM, Cowles J, Masel D, Rowe JM, Blumberg N: Antibodies to plasma proteins: an association with platelet transfusion refractoriness. Br J Haematol 80:83, 1992
226. Doughty HA, Murphy MF, Metcalfe P et al: Relative importance of immune and non-immune causes of platelet refractoriness. Vox Sang 66:200, 1994
227. Welch HG, Larson EB, Slichter SJ: Providing platelets for refractory patients. Prudent strategies. (Review). Transfusion 29:193, 1989
228. Von dem Borne AE, Ouwehand WH, Kuijpers RW: Theoretic and practical aspects of platelet cross-matching. (Review). Transfu Med Rev 4:265, 1990
229. Norol F, Kuentz M, Cordonnier C et al: Influence

of clinical status on the efficiency of stored platelet transfusion. Br J Haematol 86:125, 1994

230. Skodlar J, Bolglano D, Teramura G, Slichter SJ: Distinguishing between mechanisms of platelet refractoriness: abnormal post-storage platelet viability vs. immune destruction. Blood 80:260a, 1992

231. Schiffer CA: Management of patients refractory to platelet transfusion—an evaluation of methods of donor selection (review). Prog Hematol 15:91, 1987

232. Dahlke MB, Weiss KL: Platelet transfusion from donors mismatched for crossreactive HLA antigens. Transfusion 24:299, 1984

233. Tosato G, Applebaum FR, Deisseroth AB: HLA-matched platelet transfusion therapy of severe aplastic anemia. Blood 52:846, 1978

234. Schiffer CA, Keller C, Dutcher JP et al: Potential HLA matched platelet donor availability for alloimmunized patients. Transfusion 23:286, 1983

235. Influence of HLA-A2 on the effectiveness of platelet transfusions in alloimmunized thrombocytopenic patients. Blood 50:407, 1977

236. McElligott MC, Menitove JE, Duquesnoy RJ et al: Effect of HLA Bw4/Bw6 compatibility on platelet transfusion responses of refractory thrombocytopenic patients. Blood 59:971, 1982

237. Friedberg RC, Donnelly SF, Mintz PD: Independent roles for platelet crossmatching and HLA in the selection of platelets for alloimmunized patients. Transfusion 34:215, 1994

238. Kickler TS, Braine H, Ness PM: The predictive value of crossmatching platelet transfusion for alloimmunized patients. Transfusion 25:385, 1985

239. Heal JM, Blumberg N, Masel D: An evaluation of crossmatching, HLA and ABO matching for platelet transfusion to refractory patients. Blood 70:23, 1987

240. Kickler TS, Braine HG, Ness PM et al: A radiolabeled antiglobulin test for crossmatching platelet transfusions. Blood 61:238, 1983

241. Yam P, Petz LD, Scott E, Santos S: Platelet crossmatch tests using radiolabelled staphylococcal protein A or peroxidase anti-peroxidase in alloimmunized patients. Br J Haematol 57:337, 1984

242. Brand A, van Leeuwen A, Eernisse JG, van Rood JJ: Platelet transfusion therapy. Optimal donor selection with a combination of lymphocytotoxicity and platelet fluorescence tests. Blood 51:781, 1978

243. Myers TJ, Kim BK, Steiner M, Baldini MG: Selection of donor platelets for alloimmunized patients using a platelet associated IgG assay. Blood 58:444, 1981

244. Kickler TS, Braine HG, Ness PM et al: A radiolabeled antiglobulin test for crossmatching platelet transfusions. Blood 61:238, 1983

245. Herzig RH, Terasaki PI, Trapani RJ et al: The relationship between donor-recipient lymphocytotoxicity in the transfusion response using HLA-matched platelet concentrates. Transfusion 17:657, 1977

246. Waters AH, Minchinton RM, Bell R et al: A crossmatching procedure for the selection of platelet donors for alloimmunized patients. Br J Haematol 48:59, 1981

247. Kakaiya RM, Gudino MD, Miller WV et al: Four crossmatch methods to select platelet donors. Transfusion 24:35, 1984

248. Freedman J, Hooi C, Garvey MB: Prospective platelet crossmatching for selection of compatible random donors. Br J Haematol 56:9, 1984

249. Rachel JM, Summers TC, Sinor LT et al: Use of a solid phase red blood cell adherence method for pretransfusion platelet compatibility testing. Am J Clin Pathol 90:63, 1988

250. McFarland JG, Aster RH: Evaluation of four methods for platelet compatibility testing. Blood 69:1425, 1987

251. Freedman J, Garvey MB, Salomon de Friedberg Z et al: Random donor platelet crossmatching: Comparison of four platelet antibody detection methods. Am J Hematol 28:1, 1988

252. Kickler TS, Ness PM, Braine HG: A direct approach to the selection of platelet transfusions for the alloimmunized thrombocytopenic patient. Am J Clin Pathol 90:69, 1988

253. Petz LD: Platelet crossmatching (editorial). Am J Clin Pathol 90:114, 1988

254. O'Connell BA, Lee EJ, Rothko K, Hussein MA, Schiffer CA: Selection of histocompatible apheresis platelet donors by cross-matching random donor platelet concentrates. Blood 79:527, 1992

255. Freedman J, Gafni A, Garvey MB, Blanchette V: A cost-effectiveness evaluation of platelet crossmatching and HLA matching in the management of alloimmunized thrombocytopenic patients. Transfusion 29:201, 1989

256. Bryant PC, Vayntrub TA, Schrandt HA, Kalil JE, Grumet FC: HLA antibody enhancement by double addition of serum: use in platelet donor selection. Transfusion 32:839, 1992

257. Lee EJ, Norris D, Schiffer CA: Intravenous immune globulin for patients alloimmunized to random donor platelet transfusion. Transfusion 27:245, 1987

258. Schiffer CA, Hogge DE, Aisner J et al: High-dose intravenous gamma-globulin in alloimmunized platelet transfusion recipients. Blood 64:937, 1984

259. Becton DL, Kinney TR, Chaffee S et al: High dose

intravenous immunoglobulin for severe platelet allo-immunization. Pediatrics 74:1120, 1984

260. Bierling D, Cordonnier C, Rodet M et al: High dose intravenous gammaglobulin and platelet transfusions in leukemic HLA-immunized patients. Scand J Haematol 33:215, 1984

261. Junghaus RP, Ahn YS: High dose intravenous gammaglobulin to suppress alloimmune destruction of donor platelets. Am J Med 76:204, 1984

262. Atrah HI, Sheehan T, Gribben J et al: Improvement of postplatelet transfusion increments following intravenous immunoglobulin therapy for leukaemic HLA-immunized patients. Scand J Haematol 36:160, 1986

263. Kekomake R, Elfenbein G, Gardner R et al: Improved response of patients refractory to random-donor platelet transfusions by intravenous gamma globulin. Am J Med 76:199, 1984

264. Purucker ME, Cottler-Fox M: Good response to high-dose intravenous immunoglobulin in patients with alveolar hemorrhage refractory to platelet transfusion. Am J Hematol 45:269, 1994

265. Kurtzberg J, Friedman HS, Kinney TR, Chaffee S, Falletta JM: Treatment of platelet alloimmunization with intravenous immunoglobulin. Two case reports and review of the literature. Am J Med 83:30, 1987

266. Becton DL, Kinney TR, Chaffee S et al: High-dose intravenous immunoglobulin for severe platelet allo-immunization. Pediatrics 74:1120, 1984

267. Kickler TS, Braine HG, Ness PM et al: A randomized placebo controlled trial of high dose intravenous gammaglobulin in ameliorating alloantibody mediated platelet destruction. Blood 72:280a, 1988

268. Zeigler ZR, Shadduck RK, Rosenfeld CS et al: High-dose intravenous gamma globulin improves responses to single-donor platelets in patients refractory to platelet transfusion. Blood 70:1433, 1987

269. Christie DJ, Howe RB, Lennon SS, Sauro SC: Treatment of refractoriness to platelet transfusion by protein A column therapy. Transfusion 33:234, 1993

270. Lopez-Plaza I, Miller K, Leitman SF: Ineffectiveness of protein-A adsorption in the treatment of refractoriness. J Clin Apheresis 7:33, 1992

271. Rock G: The application of protein A immunoadsorption to remove platelet alloantibodies. Transfusion 33:192, 1993

272. Yamamoto M, Ideguchi H, Nishimura J et al: Treatment of platelet-alloimmunization with cyclosporin A in a patient with aplastic anemia. Am J Hematol 33:220, 1990

273. Melaragno AJ, Carciero R, Feingold H et al: Cryopreservation of human platelets using 6 percent di-methyl sulfoxide and storage at −80 degrees C. Effects of 2 years of frozen storage at −80 degrees C and transportation in dry ice. Vox Sang 49:245, 1985

274. Schiffer CA, Aisner J, Wiernik PH: Frozen autologous platelet transfusion for patients with leukemia. N Engl J Med 299:7, 1978

275. Schiffer CA, Buchholz DH, Aisner J, Wolff JH, Wiernik PH: Frozen autologous platelets in the supportive care of patients with leukemia. Transfusion 16:321, 1976

276. van Imhoff GW, Arnaud F, Postmus PE et al: Autologous cryopreserved platelets and prophylaxis of bleeding in autologous bone marrow transplantation. Blut 47:203, 1983

277. Kotelba-Witkowska B, Schiffer CA: Cryopreservation of platelet concentrates using glycerol-glucose. Transfusion 22:121, 1982

278. Murphy WG, Palmer JP, Green RH: The management of haemorrhage in the refractory non-alloimmunized thrombocytopenic patient. (Review). Vox Sang 67(Suppl 3):99, 1994

279. Gmur J, von Felten A, Osterwalder B et al: Delayed alloimmunization using random single donor platelet transfusions: a prospective study in thrombocytopenic patients with acute leukemia. Blood 62:473, 1983

280. Sintnicolaas K, Sizoo W, Haije WG et al: Delayed alloimmunization by random single donor platelet transfusions: a randomized study to compare single donor and multiple donor platelet transfusions in cancer patients with severe thrombocytopenia. Lancet 1:750, 1981

281. Kakaiya RM, Hezzey AJ, Bove JR et al: Alloimmunization following apheresis platelets vs. pooled platelet concentrates transfusion: a prospective randomized study. Transfusion 21:600, 1981

282. Murphy MF, Metcalfe P, Thomas H et al: Use of leucocyte-poor blood components and HLA-matched-platelet donors to prevent HLA alloimmunization. Br J Haematol 62:529, 1986

283. Claas FHJ, Smeenk RJJ, Schmidt R et al: Alloimmunization against the MHC antigens after platelet transfusion is due to contaminating leucocytes in the platelet suspension. Exp Hematol 9:84, 1981

284. Schiffer CA, Dutcher JP, Aisner J et al: A randomized trial of leukocyte-depleted platelet transfusion to modify alloimmunization in patients with leukemia. Blood 62:815, 1983

285. Sniecinski I, O'Donnell MR, Nowicki B, Hill LR: Prevention of refractoriness and HLA-alloimmunization using filtered blood products. Blood 71:1402, 1988

286. Andreu G, Dewailly J, Leberre C et al: Prevention of

HLA immunization with leukocyte-poor packed red cells and platelet concentrates obtained by filtration. Blood 72:964, 1988

287. Oksanen K, Kekomaki R, Ruutu T, Koskimies S, Myllyla G: Prevention of alloimmunization in patients with acute leukemia by use of white cell-reduced blood components—a randomized trial. Transfusion 31:588, 1991

288. van Marwijk Kooy M, van Prooijen HC et al: Use of leukocyte-depleted platelet concentrates for the prevention of refractoriness and primary HLA alloimmunization: a prospective, randomized trial. Blood 77:201, 1991

289. Williamson LM, Wimperis JZ, Williamson P et al: Bedside filtration of blood products in the prevention of HLA alloimmunization—a prospective study. Blood 83:3028, 1994

290. Snyder EL: Clinical use of white cell-poor blood components. (Review). Transfusion 29:568, 1989

291. Heddle NM, Blajchman MA: The leukodepletion of cellular blood products in the prevention of HLA-alloimmunization and refractoriness to allogeneic platelet transfusions. Blood 85:603, 1995

292. Brand A, Class FH, Voogt PJ, Wasser MN, Eernisse JG: Alloimmunization after leukocyte-depleted multiple random donor platelet transfusions. Vox Sang 54:160, 1988

293. Schiffer CA, Dutcher JP, Aisner J et al: A randomized trial of leukocyte-depleted platelet transfusion to modify alloimmunization in patients with leukemia. Blood 62:815, 1983

294. Grijzenhout MA, Aarts-Riemens MI, de Gruijl FR, van Weelden H, van Prooijen HC: UVB irradiation of human platelet concentrates does not prevent HLA alloimmunization in recipients. Blood 84:3524, 1994

295. Hogge DE, Dutcher JP, Aisner J et al: The ineffectiveness of random donor platelet transfusion in splenectomized, alloimmunized recipients. Blood 64:253, 1984

296. Banaji M, Bearman S, Buckner CD et al: The effects of splenectomy on engraftment and platelet transfusion requirements in patients with chronic myelogenous leukemia undergoing marrow transplantation. Am J Hematol 22:275, 1986

297. Kevy SV, Schmidt PJ, McGinness MH, Workman WG: Febrile, nonhemolytic transfusion reactions and the limited role of leukoagglutinins in their etiology. Transfusion 2:7, 1962

298. Thulstrup H: The influence of leukocyte and thrombocyte incompatibility on nonhaemolytic transfusion reactions. I. A retrospective study. Vox Sang 21:233, 1971

299. Heddle NM, Klama L, Singer J et al: The role of the plasma from platelet concentrates in transfusion reactions. N Engl J Med 331:625, 1994

300. Muylle L, Joos M, Wouters E, De Bock R, Peetermans ME: Increased tumor necrosis factor alpha (TNF alpha), interleukin 1, and interleukin 6 (IL-6) levels in the plasma of stored platelet concentrates: relationship between TNF alpha and IL-6 levels and febrile transfusion reactions. Transfusion 33:195, 1993

301. Wagner SJ, Friedman LI, Dodd RY: Transfusion-associated bacterial sepsis. [Review]. Clin Microbiol Rev 7:290, 1994

302. Blajchman MA: Transfusion-associated bacterial sepsis: the phoenix rises yet again. Transfusion 34:940, 1994

303. Chiu EK, Yuen KY, Lie AK et al: A prospective study of symptomatic bacteremia following platelet transfusion and of its management. Transfusion 34:950, 1994

304. Anderson KC, Lew MA, Gorgone BC et al: Transfusion-related sepsis after prolonged platelet storage. Am J Med 81:405, 1986

305. Punsalang A, Heal JM, Murphy PJ: Growth of gram-positive and gram-negative bacteria in platelet concentrates. Transfusion 29:596, 1989

306. Morrow JF, Braine HG, Kickler TS et al: Septic reactions to platelet transfusions. A persistent problem. JAMA 266:555, 1991

307. Yomtovian R, Lazarus HM, Goodnough LT et al: A prospective microbiologic surveillance program to detect and prevent the transfusion of bacterially contaminated platelets. Transfusion 33:902, 1993

308. Murphy MF, Hook S, Waters AH et al: Acute haemolysis after ABO-incompatible platelet transfusions. Lancet 335:974, 1990

309. Zoes C, Dube VE, Miller HJ, Vye MV: Anti-A1 in the plasma of platelet concentrates causing a hemolytic reaction. Transfusion 17:29, 1977

310. McLeod BC, Sassetti RJ, Weens JH, Vaithianathan T: Haemolytic transfusion reaction due to ABO incompatible plasma in a platelet concentrate. Scand J Haematol 28:193, 1982

311. Conway LT, Scott EP: Acute hemolytic transfusion reaction due to ABO incompatible plasma in a plateletapheresis concentrate. Transfusion 24:413, 1984

312. Pierce RN, Reich LM, Mayer K: Hemolysis following platelet transfusions from ABO-incompatible donors. Transfusion 25:60, 1985

313. Ferguson DJ: Acute intravascular hemolysis after a platelet transfusion. Can Med Assoc J 138:523, 1988

314. Reis MD, Coovadia AS: Transfusion of ABO-incompatible platelets causing severe haemolytic reaction. Clin Lab Haematol 11:237, 1989

315. Shanwell A, Ringden O, Wiechel B, Rumin S, Akerblom O: A study of the effect of ABO incompatible plasma in platelet concentrates transfused to bone marrow transplant recipients. Vox Sang 60:23, 1991

316. Moroff G, Friedman A, Robkin Kline L, Gautier G, Luban NL: Reduction of the volume of stored platelet concentrates for use in neonatal patients. Transfusion 1984

317. Simon TL, Sierra ER: Concentration of platelet units into small volumes. Transfusion 1984

318. Inwood MJ, Zuliani B: Anti-A hemolytic transfusion with packed O cells. Ann Intern Med 1978

319. Bensinger WI, Buckner CD, Thomas ED, Clift RA: ABO-incompatible marrow transplants. Transplantation 33:427, 1982

320. Tomasulo PA, Lenes BA: A plea for critical thought. Transfusion 25:441, 1985

321. Herzig RH, Poplack DG, Yankee RA: Prolonged granulocytopenia from incompatible platelet transfusions. N Engl J Med 290:1220, 1974

322. George JN, Pickett EB, Heinz R: Platelet membrane glycoprotein changes during the preparation and storage of platelet concentrates. Transfusion 28:123, 1988

323. Owen MR: The role of platelet microparticles in hemostasis. Transfus Med Rev 8:37, 1994

324. George JN, Pickett EB, Heinz R: Platelet membrane microparticles in blood bank fresh frozen plasma and cryoprecipitate. Blood 68:307, 1986

325. Bartley TD, Bogenberger J, Hunt P et al: Identification and cloning of a megakaryocyte growth and development factor that is a ligand for the cytokine receptor Mpl. Cell 77:1117, 1994

326. de Sauvage FJ, Hass PE, Spencer SD et al: Stimulation of megakaryocytopoiesis and thrombopoiesis by the c-Mpl ligand. Nature 369:533, 1994

327. Kaushansky K, Lok S, Holly RD et al: Promotion of megakaryocyte progenitor expansion and differentiation by the c-Mpl ligand thrombopoietin. Nature 369:568, 1994

328. Lok S, Kaushansky K, Holly RD et al: Cloning and expression of murine thrombopoietin cDNA and stimulation of platelet production in vivo. Nature 369:565, 1994

329. Wendling F, Maraskovsky E, Debili N et al: cMpl ligand is a humoral regulator of megakaryocytopoiesis. Nature 369:571, 1994

330. Aster RH: What makes platelets go? The cloning of thrombopoietin (editorial). Transfusion 35:1, 1995

Granulocyte Transfusion

Jeffrey McCullough

Neutropenic patients are at increased risk of infection.[1-3] The risk increases when the neutrophil count is less than 1,000/μl and becomes severe when the neutrophil level falls below 250/μl.[2] Thus, treatment of infected neutropenic patients with granulocyte replacement therapy is theoretically appealing. However, granulocyte transfusions are not used extensively, in part because the number of granulocytes in the circulation makes it difficult to obtain a large dose for transfusion.

The daily production of neutrophils is approximately 1×10^{11} in an average-size adult.[3] However, neutrophils differ from other blood cells by spending only a small portion of their mature life in the circulation; instead, they carry out their function in tissues. There are about 2×10^{10} circulating neutrophils or about 20 percent of the total daily production. During severe infection, neutrophil consumption may increase severalfold, so that even the entire circulating neutrophil pool of a normal donor might represent much less than 20 percent of the daily need of an infected patient. This problem has been, and continues to be, the central issue in granulocyte transfusion therapy.

The potential value of neutrophil replacement therapy was recognized more than 50 years ago, when injections of leukocytes were given. More than 30 years ago, elevations in leukocyte count and migration of neutrophils to sites of infection were achieved in

neutropenic dogs following leukocyte transfusion. Infection in neutropenic patients was treated experimentally by transfusion from chronic myeloid leukemia (CML) patients as a method of elevating the neutrophil count. Several pioneering studies established that white blood cells from such transfusions (1) caused an increase in granulocyte count, and (2) appeared in inflammatory lesions. A dose-response relationship indicated that the likelihood of clinical improvement and reduction in the patient's temperature following transfusion was directly related to the number of cells transfused. As a result of this experience, enthusiasm for granulocyte transfusion developed. However, during the early 1970s, the source of granulocytes shifted from CML patients to normal donors. This necessitated a reduced dose of granulocytes transfused to approximately 1×10^{10}, or less than 10 percent of that used in early studies. As a result, it became increasingly difficult to achieve substantial clinical benefits from transfusions, and controversy regarding the value of granulocyte transfusion developed. This chapter presents relevant clinical studies that provide a framework for a practical approach to the current use of granulocytes and will describe the methods used to obtain granulocytes for transfusion and information about the laboratory testing of granulocytes for transfusion. More recent developments are described that may improve granulocyte yields and lead to a new series of clinical trials of granulocyte transfusion therapy.

CLINICAL TRIALS AND STUDIES

Early studies of granulocyte transfusion involved cells collected from CML donors. Most patients received one or two transfusions of a large number of cells (up to 5×10^{11}), and a clinical effect could be observed shortly after transfusion.[4-7] In 1965, Freireich et al.[5] reported that 54 percent of recipients of 80 transfusions of CML cells experienced a disappearance of fever. There was a dose-response relationship between the number of cells transfused and the likelihood of the temperature returning to normal. With these large doses of granulocytes, an increase in the peripheral granulocyte count was observed, and this was related to the number of cells transfused. A dose-response relationship was established that showed that at least 1×10^{10} CML granulocytes were required to reduce fever. Schwarzenberg et al.[6,7] reported the successful transfusion of CML granulocytes that involved the disappearance of fever in 52 percent of their patients and an increased leukocyte count in 44 percent of patients. These changes were associated with recovery from sepsis and healing of infected lesions. In some patients, the leukocyte count remained elevated for up to 7 days following transfusion, suggesting that transient engraftment of transfused CML cells might have occurred. Mathe et al.[8] gave 165 patients transfusions from CML donors and reported a "good effect" following 52 percent of the transfusions and an elevation of the leukocyte count to greater than 1,000 following 38 percent of transfusions. These investigators also observed better clinical results following larger doses of cells.

Rather extensive experience (Table 17-1) with the use of CML cells led to the general feeling that patients with pneumonia, cellulitis, upper respiratory infections, urinary tract infections, and gram-negative sepsis benefited by transfusion. In particular, organisms of *Klebsiella* sp. and *Candida* sp. were responsive, and there was improvement in the previously very poor outlook for patients with gram-negative sepsis.

Although the CML donors used in these studies provided very large numbers of granulocytes for transfusion, there were the obvious problems of the use of abnormal or malignant cells and the limited number of CML patients available to donate. The development of blood cell separators allowed the source of granulocytes to be shifted from CML patients to normal donors. However, this resulted in a decrease in the number of cells collected and, thus, in the dose of granulocytes given for therapy. Because of the impressive clinical responses observed from the use of large doses of CML cells, there was

Table 17-1. Summary of Some Clinical Studies of the Transfusion of Granulocytes from Donors With CML or from Normal Donors

Investigators	Donor	No. of Patients	No. of Transfusions	Range of Cell Dose $\times$ 10^{10}	Clinical Improvement (%)	Fever Improvement (%)	Organisms	Diagnosis
Freireich et al.[5]	CML	40	118	0.26–18	43	54	—	Gram-negative sepsis
Vallejos et al.[9]	CML	128	454	13	49	—	*Klebsiella, Escherichia coli, Candida*	Septicemia, pneumonia
McCredie et al.[10]	NL	130	716	1.1	66	—	*Klebsiella, Candida*	Sepsis
Lowenthal et al.[11]	CML	87	78	0.2–5.6	40	41	—	Septicemia, pneumonia, cellulitis
Schwarzenberg et al.[6,7]	CML	52	—	1–120	—	52	—	—

Abbreviations: NL, normal; CML, chronic myeloid leukemia.

Table 17-2.   Summary of Some Controlled Trials of Granulocyte Transfusion

Investigators	Travel		Control	
	N	Survival (%)	N	Survival (%)
Graw et al.[12]				
All	39	46	38	30
− >4 transfused	12	100	19	26
Higby et al.[13]	17	88	19	26
Alavi[14]				
All	14	79	19	53
FUO	8	88	19	79
>21 days granulocytopenia	8	75	10	20
Vogler and Winton[15]	17	58	13	15
Fortuny et al.[16]	23	71	35	76
Winston et al.[17]	48	63	47	72
Herzig and Graw[18]				
All	53	55	48	36
Neutropenic	15	53	30	3
Herzig et al.[19]				
All	16	100	14	83
Neutropenic	12	67	8	0

Abbreviation: FUO, fever of unknown origin.

reluctance on the part of some to carry out controlled clinical trials of transfusion of normal granulocytes. Some studies showed that the clinical effect of transfusion of normal granulocytes was similar to that of CML cells, but nontransfused control patients were not included. The clinical studies carried out with normal donor granulocytes form the basis for present-day use of granulocytes; thus, it is appropriate to summarize them here.

Several controlled trials have been conducted (Table 17-2). The first was a prospectively randomized controlled trial at the National Institutes of Health (NIH),[12] in which 76 patients with gram-negative sepsis and less than 500 granulocytes/µl were studied. One group received antibiotics, and the other received antibiotics plus granulocytes. There was no significant difference in survival between the two groups; however, patients who received four or more transfusions had a 100 percent survival rate, compared with a 26 percent survival rate in comparable nontransfused patients. This is the basis for the recommendation that patients receive a course of at least four transfusions. Higby et al.[13] randomized patients prospectively to receive or not to receive granulocyte transfusions if they had hematologic malignancy, less than 500 granulocytes/µl, clinical evidence of infection, and a temperature of greater than 38°C. After 20 days, only 26 percent of the non-transfused controls were alive as compared with 88 percent of those who received granulocyte transfusions. Alavi[14] randomized patients with fever and less than 250 granulocytes/µl to receive or not to receive granulocyte transfusions. In those who remained granulocytopenic 21 days later, there was a clear benefit to transfusion (75 percent versus 20 percent survival rates). In patients in whom infection was never documented, there was no benefit from transfusion, because both controls and transfused patients had high survival rates. Vogler and Winton[15] carried out a controlled trial in patients with culture-proven infection and less than 300 granulocytes/µl, who had failed to improve after 72 hours of antibiotic therapy. Only 15 percent of nontransfused controls survived, as compared with 58 percent of the transfused patients.

Although these studies are impressive in their support of the value of granulocyte transfusion, the survival rates in the control patients were lower than those reported by other centers at about the same time. One possible explanation was differences in the use of antibiotics among different centers; this was illustrated in two studies. We were unable to demonstrate a benefit of granulocyte transfusions in infected patients with hematologic malignancies and granulocyte counts less than 1,000/µl.[16] Seventy-one percent of our transfused patients survived, as compared with 76 percent of the nontransfused controls. The major differences between our study and others published at that time were a shorter duration of neutropenia and the early use of empirical antibiotic therapy in our patients. Thus, the nontransfused patients had much higher survival rates than those of patients in other studies, and granulocyte transfusion did not add any benefit. Winston et al.[17] randomized 95 patients with infection and less than 500 granulocytes/µl to receive antibiotics or antibiotics plus granulocyte transfusion. There was no significant difference in survival between these groups; however, the survival rate of 72 percent in the nontransfused patients was much higher than that in previous studies.

Several studies brought out the importance of the duration of neutropenia and the return of the granulocyte count to greater than 1,000/µl. When the entire granulocyte transfusion experience of the National Cancer Institute (NCI) from 1969 to 1974 was analyzed, it confirmed that transfusions were effective in improving survival from gram-negative sepsis.[18] Of 53 patients who received transfusions, 55 percent survived as compared with 36 percent of the controls (P > 0.05). However, when patients who remained neutropenic throughout the study were analyzed, 53 percent of the transfused patients recovered from gram-negative sepsis, as compared with only 3 percent of the controls. This experience was confirmed in a subsequent study from the same group.[19] In patients whose neutrophil count rose to greater than 1,000/µl during the study, survival from gram-negative sepsis was 83 percent in controls and 100 percent in transfused patients. Those patients who remained neutropenic showed a statistically significant improvement in survival, among those receiving granulocyte transfusions (67 percent versus 0 percent).

The experience with the use of CML cells and the controlled trials described earlier represent considerable effort and data. The results are probably about as good as can be expected, given the complex clinical condition of infected neutropenic patients. The general conclusion to be drawn is that granulocyte transfusions were helpful for patients with gram-negative sepsis who had prolonged neutropenia of probably 10 days or more. It was at about this time that new antimicrobials became available and new approaches to the recognition and management of infection in neutropenic patients occurred. As a result, the outcome of infection managed without transfusion improved. Very few data describing granulocyte use with newer antibiotic regimens have been obtained under carefully controlled conditions. Despite this, it is appropriate to continue to consider granulocyte transfusion therapy in the management of infected neutropenic patients because the mortality from gram-negative sepsis and fungal infections remains high[20] and infection accounts for 20 to 30 percent of deaths in patients with acute leukemia.[21]

The specific approach to the use of granulocyte transfusions is described later in this chapter.

RECOGNITION AND MANAGEMENT OF INFECTION IN GRANULOCYTOPENIC PATIENTS

Risk factors for infection in neutropenic patients are the severity of neutropenia[1], duration of neutropenia,[18,19,22] and the rate of fall of the neutrophil count.[23] The likelihood of infection increases as the neutrophil count falls below 1,000/µl, becomes greater at less than 500/µl, and in patients with fewer than 100 granulocytes/µl who have a temperature greater than 101°F, there is a 70 percent likelihood of infection.[24] If the patient remains neutropenic long enough, fever almost always develops (94 percent after 18 days).[2] If granulocytopenia lasts less than 10 days, recovery from infection is likely, and granulocyte transfusions are unnecessary.[18,19] Part of the initial decision regarding the use of granulocyte transfusion is evaluating the expected duration of granulocytopenia. This can be done by considering the myelosuppressive agent used and the time of last therapy or it can be done by a bone marrow examination.

The first indication of infection in a granulocytopenic patient is usually fever. Since fever may be the only sign of infection, its significance in these patients must be recognized. The infections are potentially serious since most are bacterial and almost one-fourth involve bacteremia. If aggressive efforts are used, infection can be identified in 60 to 90 percent of febrile granulocytopenic patients.[2] The inability of a neutropenic patient to mount the usual inflammatory response must be considered in evaluating these patients for possible infection.[20,25] For example, there may be no pulmonary infiltrates on chest radiography; no sputum production in patients with pneumonia; no pyuria in patients with urinary tract infection; and no localized erythema, edema, or pain at a skin or mucosal infection site. In fact, the diagnostic yield of a chest radiograph in these patients may be so low as to make it unnecessary.[26]

Infections in granulocytopenic patients are usually caused by gram-negative organisms, *Staphylococcus aureus,* or fungi.[20] The incidence of bacteremia due to *Staphylococcus epidermis* is increasing, possibly due to the use of long-term indwelling catheters or oral nonabsorbable antibiotics, or both.[27] Fungal infections are primarily due to *Candida* sp. and *Aspergillus* sp.[28] However, the spectrum of organisms responsible for infection in granulocytopenic patients is continuously changing, probably because of changes in the treatment of malignancies and changes in antibiotic therapy. Since most endogenous pathogens are from the gastrointestinal or respiratory tract, surveillance cultures may be obtained periodically from these sites. There is disagreement, however, about the value of a surveillance culture program, and many institutions do not use them.

Other than attaining a normal granulocyte count, the most important determinant of the outcome of infection in granulocytopenic patients is the antibiotic regimen. The usual practice involves the administration of combinations of antibiotics.[20] It is not within the scope of this chapter to review the extensive literature on the optimal use of antibiotics. This is usually based on local experience, which defines the common pathogens and their antibiotic susceptibility. The proportion of granulocytopenic patients who respond is based on the adequacy of the antibiotic therapy.[22] Response rates of up to 80 percent or more may be achieved. Patients who respond to antibiotics would not be candidates for granulocyte transfusion therapy; however, it is difficult to predict which patients will not respond and thus might benefit from the addition of granulocyte transfusion therapy.

Granulocyte-colony-stimulating factor and granulocyte-macrophage-colony-stimulating factor (G-CSF and GM-SCF) appear to be effective in shortening the period of neutropenia following chemotherapy or bone marrow transplantation and thus reducing the likelihood or severity of infection. In one small study, the prophylactic use of G-CSF in children with cancer undergoing chemotherapy reduced the number of days of neutropenia to <250/μl but did not decrease the frequency of fever or bacteriologically proven infection.[29] In other studies, the prophylactic use of G- or GM-CSF has elevated the neutrophil nadir following chemotherapy and reduced the time of neutropenia, the number of febrile days, and the number of days during which patients received parenteral antibiotics.[30] However, the value of these hematopoietic growth factors in treating established infection in patients who are

neutropenic due to marrow failure has not been established. It is not customary to add growth factors to the treatment of infected neutropenic patients, unless the patient is expected to have unusually prolonged neutropenia. In those situations, growth factors are usually used because of the anticipated duration of neutropenia regardless of the presence of evidence of infection. Thus, the availability of growth factors does not alter the approach to considering the use of granulocyte transfusion.

The value of prophylactic intravenous immunoglobulin (IVIg) is debated,[31,32] but many patients who are neutropenic and infected are receiving IVIg as part of general treatment protocols. The IVIg is given to reduce the likelihood of post-transplant graft-versus-host disease (GVHD) and infection with cytomegalovirus (CMV) or bacteria or fungi and to reduce the likelihood of interstitial pneumonia. For neutropenic patients not receiving prophylactic IVIg, it is not customary to add IVIg to their therapy along with antibiotics when they become febrile and exhibit signs of infection.

Based on the approach to managing infection described above, the following steps are recommended when the physician is presented with the possibility of infection in a granulocytopenic patient[23,24,33]:

1. Take a history and perform a physical examination, seeking signs and symptoms of infection, especially in the oropharynx, axilla, groin, perineum, including anus, vascular catheter sites, and bone marrow aspiration sites.
2. Obtain a chest radiograph of the patient.
3. Obtain a urinalysis, including a microscopic examination for bacteria.
4. Obtain at least two blood cultures.
5. Culture of the tip of any indwelling catheter and obtain a culture from each lumin.
6. Consider obtaining a set of surveillance cultures from the nose, gingiva, and rectum.
7. Initiate empirical antibiotic therapy immediately after the history, physical examination, and laboratory studies are completed.
8. Use a broad-spectrum and bactericidal antibiotic regimen. The antibiotics should be given at their full dosage and the dosage should be adjusted on the basis of the drug blood levels. Select antibiotics on the basis of a knowledge of the antibi-

otic sensitivity patterns of the microorganisms currently present in the particular hospital.

9. Administer more than one antibiotic, in order to take advantage of drug synergism. This practice may be changing, however, with the availability of new antibiotics.[34]

10. In patients with documented infection, continue antibiotic therapy for a minimum of 10 to 14 days, and longer if necessary.

11. In patients in whom the subsequent clinical course and laboratory data indicate that bacterial infection is doubtful, antibiotic therapy may be discontinued, although some physicians prefer to continue antibiotic treatment until the neutrophil count begins to increase.[35]

12. Consider beginning the administration of G-CSF or GM-CSF if unusually prolonged neutropenia is expected.

13. Consider adding granulocyte transfusion to the management of patients who do not respond to initial antibiotic therapy. This decision can usually be made in approximately 48 hours, as most of the laboratory data are then available, including the preliminary results of blood cultures, and the patient will have been re-examined several times to determine whether clinical signs and symptoms are infection are present. Patients who continue to have severe, persistent symptoms, such as specific signs of infection or a temperature greater than 101°F, and particularly those with granulocyte levels below 100/μl are candidates for granulocyte transfusion. "It seems reasonable to initiate therapy with antibiotics and recombinant growth factors and to consider adding granulocyte transfusions to treat patients with severe bacterial, yeast, or fungal infections that continue to progress despite initial measures."[36] This is consistent with the recommendations that have been in place for the past several years.

RECOMMENDATIONS FOR THE USE OF GRANULOCYTE TRANSFUSION
Specific Clinical Situations
Sepsis

Most controlled trials of granulocyte transfusions involved gram-negative sepsis. Transfusion was clearly beneficial and caused a statistically significant im-

provement in survival.[12,18,19] The data regarding gram-positive sepsis are insufficient to allow a conclusion about the efficacy of granulocyte transfusion.[37] However, granulocytes readily phagocytize and kill the gram-positive organisms responsible for most cases of sepsis, and it is reasonable to expect that the clinical effects of transfusion are similar to gram-negative sepsis.

Pneumonia

Strauss[37] was able to find a description of only 18 such patients in whom the effect of granulocyte transfusion could be determined. Although the outcome was good (72 percent survival rate), no control data were available for comparison. Some studies in which a large dose of CML granulocytes was given to patients with pneumonia reported severe respiratory distress when transfused cells localized in the lungs. Thus, Bodey[20] recommends that granulocyte transfusion be used cautiously, if at all, in patients with pneumonia. We would use granulocyte transfusion in these patients, but cautiously and closely observing the patient and administering the transfusion slowly.

Urinary Tract Infection

Very few cases of urinary tract infection treated with granulocyte transfusion have been reported in enough detail to allow conclusion. This has not been a common indication for granulocyte transfusion, although there is no reason to withhold transfusion in patients with severe infection unresponsive to antibiotics.

Cellulitis or Abscess

The number of these cases reported in detail also does not allow generalization as to the value of granulocyte transfusion. When large doses of CML cells were used for granulocyte transfusion, it was possible to observe the development of erythema and induration, and patients would report the development of pain at a previously unknown abscess or cellulitis site. These conditions have been an indication for use of granulocyte transfusion in patients who are unresponsive to appropriate antibiotics.

Fungal Infections

Increasingly, a side effect of medical therapy involves some compromise in the immune system. When this occurs, innocuous microbes may become dangerous pathogens. Fungal infections account for up to 30 percent of fatal infections in patients with acute leukemia and 15 percent in patients with lymphoma.[20] The fungal infections most likely to occur in neutropenic patients are *Candida, Aspergillus,* and *Mucorales.*[38] The most critical factor in survival from fungal infection is recovery from neutropenia.[20] Granulocytes phagocytize and kill *Candida* sp. and might therefore be of value in treating fungal infections. In one study, the diagnosis of invasive fungal infection was established premorten in only one-third of patients, which led the investigators to propose criteria for empirical antifungal therapy.[28] There are some individual reports of the use of granulocyte transfusion in patients with fungal infections,[39,40] but the human data are insufficient. In granulocytopenic dogs given intravenous *Candida albicans* and treated with granulocyte transfusion, there was a reduction in the number of *Candida* organisms in several organs.[41] In one retrospective study, no benefit was observed from the use of granulocyte transfusion to treat fungal infections following bone marrow transplantation in 87 patients.[42] This was true for *Candida* sepsis and invasive noncandidal infections and in patients with delayed marrow recovery. This study suffered from the shortcomings of many clinical trials of granulocyte transfusion, including its retrospective nature, the low dose of cells transfused, and the lack of matching of donor and recipient. Careful controlled randomized trials are necessary to establish the value of granulocyte transfusions in fungal infections, but granulocyte transfusions should be considered as part of the treatment for disseminated yeast and fungal infections.[36]

Fever of Unknown Origin

Patients with no documented source of infection do well without granulocyte transfusions.[11,14,20,43] Survival rates range up to 98 or 99 percent. Since it is not possible to know at the onset of symptoms which patients have fever of unknown origin (FUO), decisions regarding the use of granulocytes in these patients are different. The management of transfusion in these patients is discussed later.

Septic Neonates

Neutropenia in the newborn may be due to maternal hypertension, bacterial sepsis, immune mechanisms, Kostmann syndrome, or other more rare circum-

stances (see Ch. 31). Most neonatal neutropenia is not due to infection but more severe and/or prolonged neutropenia carries a high risk of infection,[44,45] especially in premature infants. Bacterial sepsis occurs in 1 to 10 in 1,000 births and is associated with a mortality of 20 percent.[46] This may reach 100 percent, however, in extremely premature infants with group B streptococcal sepsis. Thus, early diagnoses and aggressive therapy, possibly involving granulocyte transfusion, is important. Neonate granulocytes have a reduced chemotactic and bactericidal response to stress or infection, compared with the heightened response seen in older children and adults. In addition, severe infection causes neutropenia and depletion of granulocyte stores in neonates. Several clinical trials have, to different degrees, shown a significant role of granulocyte transfusion in reducing the mortality from infections.[46–48] However, Baley et al.[49] could demonstrate no improvement in survival of neutropenic neonates as a result of buffy coat granulocyte transfusions at a mean dose of 0.35×10^9 polymorphonuclear leukocytes (PMN) in a small, prospective randomized trial. At the same time, most of the neonates enrolled in their study did have rapid and spontaneous resolution of neutropenia, with only five infants requiring more than one transfusion. Thus, the possible benefit of granulocyte transfusions was not extensively tested.

Cairo et al.[50,51] conducted two prospective and randomized trials to evaluate the potential role of granulocyte transfusion in the setting of human neonatal sepsis. Infants were eligible for each study if they met the following criteria: weight greater than 1,000 g, age less than 28 days, and admittance to the neonatal intensive care unit (ICU) with signs and symptoms of an overwhelming neonatal sepsis. In the first study, 35 newborn infants with at least one criterion of neonatal sepsis were randomized to receive either granulocyte transfusion or no other adjuvant therapy in addition to standard antimicrobial therapy. Twenty-one septic infants received leukapheresed granulocytes obtained by continuous flow centrifugation leukapheresis ($0.5–1 \times 10^9$), and 14 infants were randomized to the control group. Survival rate was 20 of 21 (95 percent) and 9 of 14 (64 percent) in the treatment and control groups, respectively ($P < 0.05$). In the second study,

35 patients were randomized to receive either granulocyte transfusion or IVIg as adjuvant therapy to antibiotics. There was a significantly different survival rate in the group receiving granulocyte transfusion (100 percent, 21/21) compared with the group receiving IVIg (64 percent, 9/14; $P < 0.03$).

The neonates most likely to benefit from granulocyte transfusion are those who are neutropenic with depleted granulocyte bone marrow stores.[48] These patients can often be identified simply by finding greater than 75 percent immature neutrophils on a peripheral blood differential count.[52] Other investigators suggest that patients likely to benefit are those with bacterial sepsis, a neutrophil count below 3,000/μl (3.0×10^9/L), and evidence of neutrophil storage pool depletion (less than 10 percent of nucleated marrow cells being postmitotic neutrophils).[53] Another group of neonates shown to benefit from granulocyte transfusion are those with antibiotic-resistant gram-negative sepsis.[47] Thus, granulocyte transfusions may be indicated for neonates or premature infants with evidence suggestive of bacterial sepsis who have neutropenia and diminished marrow granulocyte stores or those with documented antibiotic-resistant gram-negative sepsis.

One problem is the method of providing the granulocytes for transfusion. Infected neonates require transfusion urgently because some forms of neonatal sepsis may be fatal within 24 to 48 hours. Because of limitations on the ability to store granulocytes, it is not customary to maintain a stock or bank supply. Clinical trials have used granulocyte doses of up to 1.0×10^9/kg/day in a volume of approximately 15 ml.[47,48] This dose is easily attainable by standard leukapheresis techniques by merely removing 15 ml from the usual adult granulocyte concentrate (Table 17-3). To obtain granulocytes at other times, the buffy coat can be removed from units of fresh whole blood.[46] However, this approach often does not produce an adequate number of granulocytes.

Granulocytes can also be provided by exchange transfusion. Christensen et al.[54] gave six septic neonates a double-volume exchange using whole blood stored at room temperature for an unspecified time. This provided 0.3 to 0.7×10^9 granulocytes/kg. By having the donors exercise for 2 minutes, a 30 percent increase in the granulocyte count was obtained, although their patients were not treated with blood obtained in this manner.

Granulocyte function deteriorates within a few hours after collection.[55] Thus, during the night or early morning hours, suitable whole blood units probably would not be available in most blood banks for preparation of buffy coats for transfusion or for exchange transfusion. In addition, it is unlikely that the blood can be tested for syphilis, hepatitis B surface antigen, hepatitis B core antibody, alanine transaminase (ALT), and human immunodeficiency virus (HIV). Thus, there is no easy solution to the problem of providing an adequate number of suitably functional granulocytes for neonatal transfusion.[45] Some hospitals or regional blood centers that support an active neonatal ICU routinely prepare a pediatric-size group O granulocyte concentrate,

Table 17-3. General Description of Leukapheresis and Granulocyte Concentrates Prepared Using Different Techniques

Parameter	CFC	IFC With HES	CFC or IFC With HES	CFC or IFC With HES + CS
Blood volume processed (L)	8	4.5	8	8
Blood flow rate	40	60–80	40	40
Time required	3.5	3	3.5	3
Granulocytes extracted (%)	20	40	20	20
Content of concentrate				
Leukocytes $\times 10^9$	10	8	17	26
Granulocytes $\times 10^9$	4	5	9	15
RBCs (ml)	60	50	40	—
Platelets $\times 10''$	1	6	—	—

Abbreviations: CFC, continuous flow centrifugation; IFC, intermittent flow centrifugation; HES, hydroxyethyl starch; CS, corticosteroids.

either from an adult granulocyte concentrate or from a unit of fresh whole blood, and store this overnight while recognizing that these will be needed only occasionally. Each neonatology and blood bank staff should develop some system that is a realistic compromise approach but workable for their specific situation.

Disorders of Granulocyte Function

Granulocyte transfusion has been used infrequently in patients with normal granulocyte counts but defective function. Several patients with chronic granulomatous disease (CGD) who received granulocyte transfusions have been reported.[56,57] These patients have been infected with *S. aureus, Aspergillus nidulans, Pneumocystis carinii,* and *Aspergillus* sp. Granulocyte transfusions usually seemed to be helpful. Thus, severe infection unresponsive to appropriate antibiotics in patients with congenital granulocyte function defects can be considered an appropriate indication for granulocyte transfusion. However, transfusions should be reserved for patients with severe infections, due to the likelihood of subsequent immunization to the granulocytes.

AIDS Patients

Hematologic abnormalities including neutropenia occur frequently in acquired immunodeficiency syndrome (AIDS) patients, especially as the disease progresses. The neutropenia appears to have many causes and the strategies for management are not as well defined and structured as for the management of neutropenia in patients with hematologic malignancies or who are undergoing bone marrow transplantation.

Generally, neutropenic AIDS patients have more moderate neutropenia and do not appear to be at increased risk of infection during their neutropenia compared with their non-neutropenic phase.[58] In fact, they have fewer infections than do patients with hematologic malignancies and, when infections do occur, they are less likely to be due to gram-negative organisms.[58] These differences are probably due to the severe T-cell dysfunction present in AIDS patients. Because of the different character of infections in AIDS patients and the more moderate neutropenia that occurs, granulocyte transfusions are rarely used.

Prophylactic Granulocyte Transfusions

Since granulocyte concentrates contain a relatively small dose of cells in relation to the total body production, transfusions might be more effective if used prophylactically when the number of microorganisms would be small. Two studies of prophylactic granulocyte transfusions reported a statistically significant reduction in the incidence of infections, but not deaths.[59,60] One study found no benefit,[61] and one study[62] was stopped prematurely because of the severity of the side effects of the transfusions. The largest study of prophylactic granulocyte transfusions involved patients with acute nonlymphoid leukemia in a blinded, prospectively randomized, controlled trial[63] carried out at four centers. There was a statistically significant reduction in the incidence of infection, but the study was stopped prematurely because of an excess of pulmonary complications and deaths in the transfused patients. As a result of the overall experience, prophylactic granulocyte transfusions are not recommended.

Specific Approach

In using granulocyte transfusion therapy, several specific issues must be considered. These are described in the following sections.

Timing of Starting the Transfusion

It may be important to begin the transfusion promptly after the appearance of signs or symptoms of infection and before the infection becomes widespread.[64] However, most patients respond to antibiotics,[20] and many would receive unnecessary transfusions if these were begun early. However, any advantage of early transfusion is lost by waiting for culture results and response to antibiotics. Two studies are informative on this point. Vogler and Winton[15] entered patients into a granulocyte transfusion study if they failed a 72-hour trial of antibiotics, whereas Alavi[14] entered patients when they became febrile. Alavi found a 53 percent survival rate in the control group and could not show a benefit from the transfusions. By waiting 72 hours, Vogler and Winton may have selected a more severely affected group to study. Only 15 percent of their controls survived, and the transfused patients had a significantly improved survival rate of 58 percent. In addition, 25 percent of their patients were spared transfusions because they responded to antibiotics. In retrospect, about one-half of Alavi's[14] patients responded to antibiotics and could have avoided transfusion. Thus, it seems appropriate to carry out a 72- to 96-hour trial of appropriate antibiotics before initiating granulocyte transfusion.

Dose of Granulocytes

Early studies showed improvement following very large doses (up to 1×10^{12}) of CML cells,[5,6] and clinical responses were not seen with fewer than 1×10^{10} CML cells.[5] There was a dose-response relationship when either CML[5] or normal cells were used,[11,15,65,66] but it was difficult to define a minimum therapeutic dose of normal granulocytes. The usual granulocyte concentrate contains approximately 1×10^{10} granulocytes, which represents only 10 percent of the normal daily production, or much less during infection when granulocyte production is increased. Higby et al.[67] have advocated using very large doses of granulocytes (4 to $31 \times 10^{10}/m^2$), and Bodey[20] recommends a dose of 10×10^{10} cells. It would be necessary to administer several granulocyte concentrates to achieve these doses. Although clinical improvement has been documented when using doses of less than 1×10^{10},[12,19] it seems advisable to use the largest dose that is practical. At least 1×10^{10} granulocytes should be given, and efforts should be made to either increase the cell content of each granulocyte concentrate or give more than one transfusion daily.

Number of Transfusions

Granulocyte transfusions should be used as a course of therapy, just as antibiotics are used. Although the patient should be evaluated at least daily, this information should not be used to make daily decisions regarding granulocyte transfusion. Graw et al.[12] showed that at least four transfusions were necessary to obtain improvement from gram-negative sepsis, and in a later study, those investigators continued the transfusions until all signs and symptoms of infection cleared.[19] When the decision is made to institute granulocyte transfusion, the course of therapy should be determined. At least four transfusions are recommended, and seven might be preferable. After that, the patient's course can be evaluated and a deci-

sion made whether to continue. Of course, clinical judgment should prevail. If the patient experiences severe complications of transfusions, they can be discontinued, and if the patient shows a sustained marked clinical improvement, transfusions can be stopped before the end of the planned therapy period.

EVALUATING THE EFFECTIVENESS OF GRANULOCYTE TRANSFUSION

Each blood bank that produces granulocyte concentrates must carry out a quality assurance program to determine that the expected number of cells is being obtained.[68] As is the case for other blood components, these quality assurance programs do not include functional testing, although the procedures used for neutrophil collection should result in cells with normal function.[69] The methods that have been suggested for evaluating granulocyte transfusion include (1) change in peripheral blood granulocyte count, (2) clinical improvement in the patient, (3) appearance of granulocytes in the mouth or sputum, and (4) injection of isotopically labeled granulocytes. None of these is very effective or widely used, and in practice most granulocyte transfusions are not evaluated.

The change in granulocyte count following transfusion is too small to be meaningful. The usual granulocyte concentrate containing approximately 1×10^{10} granulocytes would be expected to raise the count approximately $200/\mu l$ in a 70-kg patient. Given the error of leukocyte counting and the complex clinical status of these patients (e.g., fever, disseminated intravascular coagulation [DIC], sepsis, bleeding), changes of this magnitude are too small to be meaningful. Clinical improvement is not expected following a single transfusion because of the small dose of cells. Therefore, this cannot be used as a way of determining the effectiveness of an individual transfusion.

The analysis of granulocytes in the mouth or sputum provides an interesting opportunity to determine the transfused cells' ability to migrate in vivo. Following granulocyte transfusion to a patient with CGD, Beuscher and Gallin[57] demonstrated that 18 percent of all leukocytes in sputum that was obtained 42 hours after transfusion were positive for nitroblue tetrazolium (NBT). However, this approach to monitoring would only be possible in patients with CGD whose granulocytes were abnormal. We carried out a similar monitoring study in a patient with CGD.[70] Following transfusion, the intravascular recovery and survival of granulocytes was determined by measuring blood NBT reduction, chemiluminescence, and ^{111}In activity. Since the transfused cells were from a normal donor and labeled with ^{111}In, the concurrence of all three measurements indicated that the donor cells survived in vivo satisfactorily.

Granulocytes are normally present in the oral cavity, and their number is related to the number in the peripheral blood.[71] Arnold et al.[71] described a technique for quantitating the granulocytes from mouth washings and used this as a way of determining migration in vivo of transfused cells. Most patients had an increase in oral granulocytes following transfusion. This is probably the only practical way reported thus far to obtain some in vivo assessment of granulocytes in vivo.

Granulocytes can be labeled with ^{51}Cr, DF[32]P, or ^{111}In and the intravascular kinetics determined. Since ^{111}In allows body scanning, it is also possible to observe failure of transfused cells to localize at sites of inflammation or the sequestration of granulocytes at abnormal sites. Thus, the method can be used to study the effects of storage on granulocytes or to compare different leukocyte crossmatch techniques.[72] However, the technique is complex and not suitable as part of a routine quality assurance program. It seems that the only practical parts of quality assurance for granulocyte transfusion are to ensure that an adequate number of cells is collected and that these are stored properly.

COMPLICATIONS OF GRANULOCYTE TRANSFUSION

Transfusion Reactions

Reactions to granulocyte transfusions are common; these usually consist of chills and fever. More severe reactions involving hypotension and respiratory distress can occur. Precise incidence figures are difficult to obtain because of the clinical variables involved. Mild to moderate reactions probably occur following 25 to 50 percent of transfusions, and severe reactions probably follow about 1 percent of transfusions. Re-

actions can be reduced in incidence and severity by transfusing granulocytes slowly, at a rate of not more than 1×10^{10}/h. Generally a granulocyte concentrate should be transfused over 1 to 2 hours. Routine premedication of the patients is not recommended. Reactions can be treated with acetaminophen (650 mg) and, if more severe, with intravenous hydrocortisone (50 to 100 mg). In patients who have a severe reaction, subsequent transfusions should be given cautiously because of the danger of severe pulmonary reactions caused by sequestration of cells in the pulmonary vascular system. This is one of the most serious complications of granulocyte transfusion.[63,73,74] The cause is usually difficult to identify but may involve localization of granulocytes at a clinically inapparent site of inflammation, complement activation, transfusion of aggregated granulocytes, or fluid overload.[75] Thus, patients known to have pneumonia are candidates for pulmonary reactions due to localization of transfused cells. There is no effective way of identifying other patients who might have severe pulmonary reactions.

It has been suggested that the combination of granulocyte transfusion and amphotericin B therapy was associated with severe pulmonary reactions[76]; however, this has not been substantiated in later studies.[73,77] Patients can receive both granulocyte transfusions and amphotericin B when indicated, but these should not be administered simultaneously, and the transfusion should be given slowly.

Transmission of Diseases

Granulocyte concentrates can transmit the diseases associated with blood transfusion, although syphilis and AIDS have not specifically been attributed to granulocyte transfusion. Transmission of cytomegalovirus (CMV) by granulocytes has been a particular concern.[78] It is important to focus on the characteristics of the recipient so that patients in whom the development of CMV is a potentially serious problem are managed in a way to prevent this. In patients who are not severely immunosuppressed, the risk of marked morbidity or mortality from CMV infection is low. For example, in the study by Winston et al.,[78] mortality from CMV infection was observed in bone marrow transplant patients, but not in patients with acute leukemia treated with chemotherapy.

Rather than an isolated concern about CMV transmission from granulocyte transfusion, an overall program including appropriate transfusion support should be arranged to suit the clinical situation. For example, when both a marrow transplant recipient and the donor are seronegative for CMV, the patient should receive only seronegative blood products.[79] Other means of modifying CMV infection that have been investigated but not adopted for routine use are CMV hyperimmunoglobulin or plasma and vaccination of the marrow transplant recipient, or possibly the donor, since the transfer of humoral immunity by marrow transplantation has been demonstrated. New filters that remove approximately 3 $\log_{10}$ leukocytes from blood components may be equally as effective as CMV antibody negative blood components in preventing CMV infection.[80] However, since the filters prevent CMV by removing leukocytes, including granulocytes, this is not an effective strategy for providing CMV "safe" granulocyte transfusions.

Graft-Versus-Host Disease

Graft-versus-host disease (GVHD) is a known complication of transfusion of viable lymphocytes to severely immunodeficient patients (see also Ch. 42). The degree of immunodeficiency in relation to the dose of lymphocytes necessary to elicit GVHD is unknown. Since granulocyte concentrates contain lymphocytes, the development of GVHD is possible. This was particularly true of the early trials of granulocyte transfusion, in which CML cells were used,[81] but it was believed to be of benefit in some patients.[7] Four other patients who received normal donor granulocyte transfusion have developed GVHD.[82–85] Two were adults with acute leukemia, and two were children with lymphoma and acute leukemia. Patients with severe congenital immunodeficiency or those undergoing bone marrow transplantation are at such risk of GVHD that all blood components are irradiated. The risk of GVHD from the transfusion of normal donor granulocyte concentrates into patients with hematologic malignancies receiving chemotherapy is unknown. Routine irradiation of granulocyte concentrates is not recommended. Instead, it seems more appropriate to focus on the patient. If the clinical situation involves severe immunosuppression, then all blood components should be irradiated (see Ch. 42).

COLLECTION OF GRANULOCYTES FOR TRANSFUSION

Donor Screening

Granulocytes for transfusion are usually collected by leukapheresis using blood cell separators. Isolating granulocytes from standard units of whole blood and pooling them is not recommended. Because of the nature of the leukapheresis procedure, the attachment of the donor to an instrument, the extracorporeal processing of blood, and the administration of additives or stimulants to the donor, the medical screening of donors is different from that used for whole blood donation.[86] In general, the standards that apply to whole blood donation apply to the selection and care of cytapheresis donors as well. The major additional requirements are that an interval of at least 48 hours should elapse between procedures and that not more than 1,000 ml of plasma should be removed each week or 200 ml of red cells for a period of 8 weeks. The donor must be monitored, to avoid the development of cytopenia or a low albumin or immunoglobulin level. The maximum amount of blood that can be extracorporeal is limited, and the donor's medical history must be reviewed to ensure that the administration of corticosteroids, hydroxyethyl starch (HES), or other additives is not potentially harmful.

Collection Techniques

During leukapheresis, the donor undergoes venipunctures in each arm, and blood is pumped out of one vein through the blood cell separator where the granulocytes are removed, and the remaining blood is returned to the other arm.[87] There are differences in the design and operation of these instruments, but they extract approximately 20 to 40 percent of the granulocytes that pass through the instrument. Therefore, it is necessary to process a large volume of blood to obtain a usable dose of granulocytes. Without additional modification, leukapheresis does not yield a large enough dose of granulocytes to be clinically useful. It is customary to use a red cell sedimenting agent to improve the yield. The agent most commonly used is HES. Such procedures usually produce a concentrate containing approximately 5 $\times 10^9$ granulocytes (Table 17-3). Since this is probably not a clinically effective dose (see under the earlier section on approaches to granulocyte transfusion), most centers administer corticosteroids to elevate the donor's granulocyte count and, thus, improve the yield (Table 17-3). There is no defined minimum number of granulocytes that must be obtained, because the Food and Drug Administration (FDA) has not licensed granulocytes, although the American Association of Blood Banks (AABB) standards require at least 1×10^{10} granulocytes in 75 percent of the concentrates.[68] Thus, the content of granulocyte concentrates prepared by different blood banks may vary, depending on the method used. The composition of the final product should be based on local needs and attitudes; however, a content of at least 1×10^{10} granulocytes is recommended.

For several years, granulocytes were also obtained by passing whole blood over nylon wool columns to which the granulocytes selectively adhere. After leukapheresis, the granulocytes were released from the fibers and concentrated for transfusion. This yielded a larger number of cells than was achieved with the centrifuge procedures, but some damage to the granulocytes resulted from their adhesion to the fibers. More importantly, there were serious complications in donors, including complement activation, pulmonary leukostasis, perineal pain in women, and priapism in men. As a result of these donor effects, filtration leukapheresis is no longer used.

Function of Granulocytes Collected by Leukapheresis

Granulocytes collected by centrifuge leukapheresis techniques function normally in vitro and have normal circulating and migration characteristics in vivo.[87] In vitro bacterial killing is normal, as are functions related to the metabolic activity associated with phagocytosis, including NBT reduction, chemiluminescence, and superoxide production. In vitro chemotaxis is normal.[88] Thus, there is no evidence that the collection procedure damages the granulocytes. Studies of granulocytes in vivo are more difficult. These usually involve the use of isotope-labeled cells. Several studies have shown that granulocytes obtained by leukapheresis, isotope labeled, and transfused to the cell donor (autologous) have a normal intravascular recovery and survival.[87–89] These cells also migrate to sites of inflammation.[89–93] The use of corticosteroids in donors to improve the granulocyte

yields does not adversely affect function of the cells in vitro or in vivo.[89–94]

Storage of Granulocytes for Transfusion

Granulocytes retain bactericidal capacity and metabolic activity related to phagocytosis and bacterial killing for 1 to 3 days of storage at refrigerator temperatures.[95,96] However, there is a 30 to 50 percent decline in chemotactic response after 24 hours. The loss of chemotaxis is less severe if the cells are maintained at room temperature but still approaches 30 percent after the first day of storage.[92,96] Storage of granulocytes at 1 to 6°C for 24 hours is associated with a reduction in the percentage of transfused cells that circulate and about a 75 percent reduction in migration into a skin window.[89] Using ^{111}In-labeled granulocytes, we have shown that storage at room temperature for 8 hours does not reduce the intravascular recovery, survival, or migration into a skin chamber.[52] These in vivo functions were reduced when granulocytes were stored longer than 8 hours at room temperature or for even 8 hours at 1 to 6°C. It appears that granulocytes can be stored for up to 8 hours at room temperature before transfusion; however, for optimum results, transfusion should be given as soon as possible after collection.

DONOR–RECIPIENT MATCHING FOR GRANULOCYTE TRANSFUSION

Role of ABO Blood Groups

Granulocyte concentrates being used for transfusion must be ABO compatible with the recipient because of the red cell content of the concentrates (Table 17-3). ABO antigens were believed to be present on granulocytes; however, recent work using more modern techniques indicates that this is not so. Therefore, we determined the effect of ABO incompatibility on the fate of granulocytes in vivo that were ABO incompatible with the patients.[97] A small number of ^{111}In-labeled granulocytes free of red blood cells were injected into ABO-incompatible recipients. The intravascular recovery, survival, or tissue localization of the cells was not different from that seen when similar injections were given to ABO-compatible subjects. This finding is not meant to encourage the use of ABO-incompatible granulocyte transfusions, but it could be considered if, in the future, granulocyte concentrates can be prepared that are depleted of red blood cells.

Histocompatibility Testing and the Role of the HLA System in Granulocyte Transfusion

Studies using CML cells showed that incompatibility by leukoagglutination or lymphocytotoxicity (LC) was associated with the failure of transfused cells to circulate or localize at sites of inflammation.[98,99] Subsequently, studies of the importance of HLA matching and crossmatching of normal donor granulocytes gave mixed results of the value of these tests.[76] One problem is that, with the number of normal donor granulocytes transfused, changes in the recipient's granulocyte count are so small that this is not a satisfactory measurement of the effect of matching. Studies in dogs clearly showed that immunization to granulocytes interfered with the outcome of transfusion.[100,101] However, the sera of most animals reacted in several different leukocyte antibody assays, so the optimum technique could not be specified.

We have used ^{111}In to determine the fate in vivo of individual granulocyte transfusions. Granulocyte agglutinating (GA) antibodies were associated with decreased intravascular recovery, survival, and a failure of the cells to localize at known sites of inflammation.[72] Dutcher and colleagues[91,102] also found that ^{111}In-labeled granulocytes failed to localize at sites of inflammation and were sequestered in the pulmonary vasculature when the patients were immunized. Their serologic studies involved only LC testing, whereas our results comparing LC and GA showed the importance of GA, and not of LC. We were unable to show that sera reactivity by granulocyte immunofluorescence (GIF) only was associated with altered in vivo granulocyte circulation or localization. However, GIF is effective in selecting granulocytes that will provide a greater increase in peripheral blood leukocyte count in dogs[102] and a higher incidence of recovery from infection in humans.[103] Despite the apparently ambiguous information supporting the value of GIF, LC, or GA, some general conclusions can be drawn. Most highly immunized patients' sera react in all three of these assays. The sensitivity and specificity of the assays differ. GIF detects both HLA and neutrophil-specific antigens, LC detects primarily HLA, and GA detects primarily neutrophil specific and some strongly reactive HLA antibodies. If the interpretation of the LC or GIF tests were made more stringent, they possibly would provide information similar to that for GA.[72]

Applying these research data to the practical operation of a blood bank and granulocyte transfusion service is difficult. Granulocytes can be stored for only a few hours, so cells are not usually available for crossmatching to allow selection of compatible donors. Presently, the only practical approach is to screen the patients' serum against a panel of cells periodically (i.e., two or three times weekly) to determine whether the patient is immunized. If so, HLA-matched unrelated donors or family members can be selected for leukapheresis. Either GA, GIF, or LC can be used for this testing if the interpretation of the GIF or LC reactions is stringent.

Role of Hematopoietic Growth Factors

Improved understanding of hematopoiesis and the identification, gene cloning, and production of hematopoietic growth factors by recombinant DNA technology may lead to a new phase of granulocyte transfusion therapy using large doses or properly matched cells (see Chs. 17 and 31). Some experience with the potential role of G-CSF in granulocyte transfusion is already available and is summarized here.

Granulocyte-Colony-Stimulating Factor

G-CSF is a protein of 175 amino acids that binds to specific receptors on the surface of hematopoietic cells, causing a complex response, including an increase in the number of circulating hematopoietic stem cells and proliferation and differentiation of myeloid progenitors, especially myeloblasts and promyelocytes. This results in a substantial increase in the circulating leukocyte and granulocyte count. The response to injected G-CSF can be divided into four phases.[104] Within 30 minutes, there is a decrease in circulating neutrophils, probably due to neutrophil adhesion to vascular endothelium due to activation and expression of activation surface molecules. During the next 12 hours, there is a gradual increase in neutrophil count, probably due to the release of stored pool neutrophils. Because G-CSF reduces the marrow transit time, but causes an increase in the number of amplification divisions, there may be an increased level of circulating mature neutrophils 24 hours or more after injection. The fourth phase of effect of G-CSF occurs after several days, when the neutrophils produced in response to G-CSF are in the tissue.

Use of G-CSF in Granulocyte Collection

G-CSF may be administered either intravenously or subcutaneously. Maximum serum levels occur 3 to 6 hours after intravenous administration of G-CSF and persist for 10 to 16 hours.[105,106] The timing, degree, and duration of increase in granulocyte counts differ somewhat, depending on the dose and route of administration of G-CSF. Bensinger et al.[107] administered 3.6 to 6.0 µg/kg/day to normal subjects for 9 to 14 days. The subject's granulocyte counts increased to an average of about 42,000/µl. Granulocytes were collected each day by leukapheresis, so the preapheresis granulocyte count varied based on the duration of G-CSF treatment. Overall, the number of granulocytes collected by apheresis from these stimulated donors was 41.6×10^9 or six times higher than historical controls not treated with G-CSF. On the last day of G-CSF administration, when granulocyte counts were highest, the average number of granulocytes collected was about 90×10^9. Caspar et al.[105] gave a single subcutaneous injection of G-CSF to 22 normal subjects and collected granulocytes by leukapheresis 12 to 16 hours later. The circulating leukocyte count increased to approximately 23,000/µl and the granulocyte count to 20,000/µl. This resulted in a average granulocyte yield of 44.3 $\times 10^9$ when 5 to 7 L of blood was processed. As part of a study to determine the optimum dose of G-CSF needed to mobilize peripheral blood stem cells, we have administered doses of 2, 5, 7.5, or 10 µg/kg of G-CSF SC each day for 5 days to normal volunteers. We have observed granulocyte counts in our apheresis products of 20 to 60×10^9, depending on the dose. Thus, it seems clear that G-CSF administration to normal donors can substantially increase their circulating granulocyte level and the number of granulocytes collected for transfusion.

Adverse Effects of G-CSF

There is considerable experience with the use of G-CSF to speed marrow recovery and shorten the duration of neutropenia following chemotherapy or bone marrow transplantation. The most serious adverse effects of G-CSF in cancer patients has been bone pain.[106] Up to 25 percent of patients have reported this and it has been reported more frequently in patients who receive 20 to 100 µg/kg/day IV, a dose much larger than that given to normal donors. In most cases, the pain could be effectively treated by non-narcotic analgesics. During chronic administration, skin rashes, alopecia, thrombocytopenia, osteoporosis, hematuria, and proteinuria have been reported, but rarely.[106] Some patients have reported exacerbation of pre-existing skin conditions such as psoriasis or eczema. Transiently mild elevations of serum alkaline phosphatase, lactate dehydrogenase (LDH), and uric acid have been reported. These return quickly and spontaneously to normal following discontinuation of G-CSF. Rare allergic reactions have been reported in patients receiving G-CSF, including dyspnea, hypotension, and urticaria. The estimated incidence of these reactions is less than 1 in 100,000.[106] The use of the drug is contraindicated in patients with angina, cardiac dysrhythmia, or hypersensitivity to *Escherichia coli*-derived drugs.

In normal donors, Bensinger et al.[107] reported that two of nine donors receiving an average of 5 µg/kg/day experienced bone pain that was controlled with acetaminophen. No donors had to discontinue receiving G-CSF because of adverse reactions. Caspar et al.[105] reported that 300 µg of G-CSF administered subcutaneously was generally well tolerated by the donors.

Function of Granulocytes Produced Following Stimulation With G-CSF

Another issue is whether granulocytes obtained from normal subjects stimulated with G-CSF function normally. Granulocytes collected 12 to 16 hours after a single subcutaneous dose of 300 µg of G-CSF had normal chemotaxis and phagocytosis and increased chemiluminescence and superoxide formation.[105] In other studies, G-CSF enhanced phagocytosis, antibody-dependent cellular cytotoxicity, and chemotaxis, and neutrophil production of superoxide and hydrogen peroxide–important parts of the bacterial killing system were normal.[108–110] In addition, the surface expression of β_2 integrins, and possibly leukocyte adhesion molecule-1, was increased.[111] In addition, there was increased expression of C3bi receptor, the appearance of the high-affinity IgG receptor FcRI, no change in FcRII, and a decreased expression of FcRIII.[104] Thus, it appears that after G-CSF administration, granulocyte function is enhanced, and adhesiveness may also be increased. Whether these functional alterations will prove clinically important remains to be established.

Ex Vivo Culture to Produce Granulocytes for Transfusion

Another approach that may provide granulocytes for transfusion is to produce them in the laboratory using culture techniques. Bone marrow or peripheral blood stem cells can be expanded 21 to 66-fold by culture with hematopoietic growth factors.[112,113] This could be developed into a method designed to make large numbers of myeloid cells for transfusion. Additional work will be necessary to establish that such cells function and circulate normally before this approach is put into clinical use.

CONCLUSION

Granulocyte transfusions continue to have a role in the management of infection in neutropenic patients. Their role is limited because most of the infections are responsive to antibiotics. In addition, the dose of granulocytes contained in most transfusions is small, and histocompatibility testing between donor and recipient is difficult. The availability of hematopoietic growth factors is promising, and it seems likely that new efforts to collect and administer granulocytes to treat infections in neutropenic patients may be imminent.

REFERENCES

1. Bodey GP, Buckley M, Sath YS, Freireich EJ: Quantitative relationships between circulating leukocytes and infection in patients with acute leukemia. Ann Intern Med 64:328, 1966
2. Gurwith MJ, Brunton JL, Lank BA et al: Granulocytopenia in hospitalized patients. I. Prognostic factors and etiology of fever. Am J Med 64:121, 1978
3. Cline MJ: The White Cell. Harvard University Press, Cambridge, MA, 1975
4. Morse EE, Freireich EM, Carbone PP et al: The transfusion of leukocytes from donors with chronic myelocytic leukemia to patients with leukopenia. Transfusion 6:183, 1966
5. Freireich EJ, Levin RH, Wang J et al: The function and fate of transfused leukocytes from donors with chronic myelocytic leukemia in leukopenic recipients. Ann NY Acad Sci 113:1081, 1965
6. Schwarzenberg L, Mathe G, Amiel JL et al: Study of factors determining the usefulness and complications of leukocyte transfusions. Am J Med 43:206, 1967
7. Schwarzenberg L, Mathe G, De Grouchy J et al: White blood cell transfusions. Israel J Med 1:925, 1965
8. Mathe G, Amiel JL, Schwarzenberg L: Leucocyte transfusions. p. 104. In: Bone Marrow Transplantation and Leukocyte Transfusion. Charles C. Thomas, Springfield, IL, 1971
9. Vallejos C, McCredie KB, Bodey GP et al: White blood cell transfusions for control of infections in neutropenic patients. Transfusion 15:28, 1975
10. McCredie KB, Hester JP, Vallejos CS, Freireich EJ: Clinical results of granulocyte transfusions using normal donors. p. 287. In Goldman JM, Lowenthal RM (eds): Leucocytes: Separation, Collection and Transfusion, Academic Press, London, 1975
11. Lowenthal RM, Goldman JM, Buskard NA et al: Granulocyte transfusions in treatment of infections in patients with acute leukemia and aplastic anemia. Lancet 1:353, 1975
12. Graw RG Jr, Herzig G, Perry S, Henderson ES: Normal granulocyte transfusion therapy. Treatment of septicemia due to gram-negative bacteria. N Engl J Med 287:367, 1972
13. Higby DJ, Yates JW, Henderson ES, Holland JF: Filtration leukapheresis for granulocyte transfusion therapy—clinical laboratory studies. N Engl J Med 1292:761, 1975
14. Alavi JB: A randomized clinical trial of granulocyte transfusions for infection in acute leukemia. N Engl J Med 296:706, 1977
15. Volger WR, Winton EF: A controlled study of the efficacy of granulocyte transfusions in patients with neutropenia. Am J Med 63:548, 1977
16. Fortuny IE, Bloomfield CD, Hadlock DC et al: Granulocyte transfusions: a controlled study in patients with acute nonlymphocytic leukemia. Transfusion 15:548, 1975
17. Winston DJ, Ho WG, Gale RP: Therapeutic granulocyte transfusions for documented infections. Ann Intern Med 97:509, 1982
18. Herzig GP, Graw RG Jr: Granulocyte transfusions for bacterial infections. p. 209. In Brown EB (ed): Progress in Hematology. Vol. 9. Grune & Stratton, Orlando, FL, 1975
19. Herzig RH, Herzig GP, Graw RG Jr et al: Successful granulocyte transfusion therapy for gram-negative

septicemia. A prospective randomized controlled study. N Engl J Med 296:701, 1977

20. Bodey GP: Infection in cancer patients. A continuing association. Am J Med 81:11, 1986

21. Foon KA, Gale RP: Controversies in the therapy of acute myelogenous leukemia. Am J Med 72:963, 1982

22. Love LJ, Schimpff SC, Schiffer CA, Wiernik PH: Improved prognosis for granulocytopenic patients with gram-negative bacteremia. Am J Med 68:643, 1980

23. Hughes WT, Armstrong D, Bodey GP et al: Guidelines for the use of antimicrobial agents in neutropenic patients with unexplained fever. J Infect Dis 171:381, 1990

24. Wiernik PH: The management of infection in the cancer patient. JAMA 244:185, 1980

25. Sickles EA, Greene WH, Wiernik PH: Clinical presentation of infection in granulocytopenic patients. Arch Intern Med 135:715, 1975

26. Jochelson MS, Altschuler J, Storeper PC: The yield of chest radiograph in febrile and neutropenic patients. Ann Intern Med 104:708, 1986

27. Wade JC, Schimpff SC, Newman KA, Wiernik PH: *Staphylococcus epidermidis:* an increasing cause of infection in patients with granulocytopenia. Ann Intern Med 97:503, 1982

28. Degregorio MW, Lee WMF, Linker CA et al: Fungal infections in patients with acute leukemia. Am J Med 73:543, 1982

29. Adachi N, Hashiyama M, Matsuda I: rhG-CSF and aztreonam as prophylaxis against infection in neutropenic children. Lancet 337:1174, 1991

30. Herrmann F, Schulz G, Wieser M et al: Effect of granulocyte-macrophage colony-stimulating factor on neutropenia and related morbidity induced by myelotoxic chemotherapy. Am J Med 88:619, 1990

31. Wolff SN, Fay JW, Herzig H et al: High-dose weekly intravenous immunoglobulin to prevent infections in patients undergoing autologous bone marrow transplantation or severe myelosuppressive therapy. Ann Intern Med 118:937, 1993

32. Sullivan KM, Kopeck KJ, Jocom J et al: Immunomodulatory and antimicrobial efficacy of intravenous immunoglobulin in bone marrow transplantation. N Engl J Med 232:705, 1990

33. Donelly JP: Assessment and reporting of clinical trials of empirical therapy in neutropenic patients. J Antimicrob Chemother 27:377, 1991

34. Verhoef J: Prevention of infections in the neutropenic patient. Clin Infect Dis 17:S359, 1993

35. Pizzo PA, Robichaud KJ, Gill FA et al: Duration of empiric antibiotic therapy in granulocytopenic patients with cancer. Am J Med 67:194, 1979

36. Strauss RG: Therapeutic granulocyte transfusions in 1993. Blood 81:1675, 1993

37. Strauss RG: Therapeutic neutrophil transfusions. Are controlled studies no longer appropriate? Am J Med 65:1001, 1978

38. Armstrong D: Problems in management of opportunistic fungal disease. Rev Infect Dis II:S1591, 1989

39. Bujak JS, Kwong-chung KJ, Chusid MJ: Osteomyelitis and pneumonia in a boy with chronic granulomatous disease of childhood caused by a mutant strain of *Aspergillus nidulans.* Am J Clin Pathol 61:631, 1974

40. Raubitschek AA, Levin AS, Stites DP et al: Normal granulocyte infusion therapy for aspergillosis in chronic granulomatous disease. Pediatrics 51:230, 1973

41. Ruthe RC, Andersen BR, Cunningham BL, Epstein RB: Efficacy of granulocyte transfusions in the control of systemic candidiasis in leukopenic host. Blood 52:493, 1978

42. Bhatia S, McCullough J, Perry EH et al: Granulocyte transfusions: efficacy in treating fungal infections in neutropenic patients following bone marrow transplantation. Transfusion 34:226, 1994

43. Hershko C, Naparstek E, Eldor A, Izak G: Granulocyte transfusion therapy, a clinical trial in patients with acute leukemia and sepsis. Vox Sang 34:129, 1978

44. Koenig JM, Christensen RD: Incidence, neutrophil kinetics, and natural history of neonatal neutropenia associated with maternal hypertension. N Engl J Med 321:557, 1989

45. Christensen RD: Granulocytopoiesis in the fetus and neonate. Transfus Med Rev 4:8, 1990

46. Strauss RG: Current issues in neonatal transfusions. Vox Sang 51:1, 1986

47. Laurenti F, Ferro R, Isacchi G et al: Polymorphonuclear leukocyte transfusion for the treatment of sepsis in the newborn infant. J Pediatr 98:118, 1981

48. Christensen RD, Rothstein G, Anstall HB, Bybee B: Granulocyte transfusions in neonates with bacterial infection, neutropenia, and depletion of mature marrow neutrophils. Pediatrics 70:1, 1982

49. Baley JE, Stork EK, Warkentin PI, Shurin SB: Buffy coat transfusions in neutropenic neonates with presumed sepsis: a prospective, randomized trial. Pediatrics 80:712, 1987

50. Cairo M: Granulocyte transfusions in neonates with presumed sepsis. Pediatrics 80:712, 1987

51. Cairo M, Worcester C, Rucker R et al: Randomized trial of granulocyte transfusions versus intravenous immune globulin therapy for neonatal neutropenia and sepsis. J Pediatr 120:281, 1992

52. Christensen RD, Bradley PP, Rothstein G: The leukocytc left shift in clinical and experimental neonatal sepsis. J Pediatr 98:101, 1981

53. Huestis DW, Glasser L: The neutrophil in transfusion medicine. Transfusion 34:630, 1994

54. Christensen RD, Hill HR, Anstall HB, Rothstein G: Exchange transfusion as an alternative to granulocyte concentrate administration in neonates with bacterial sepsis and profound neutropenia. J Clin Apheresis 2:177, 1984

55. McCullough J, Weiblen JB, Fine D: Effects of storage of granulocytes on their fate in vivo. Transfusion 23:20, 1983

56. Yomtovian R, Abramson J, Quie P, McCullough J: Granulocyte transfusion in chronic granulomatous disease. Transfusion 21:739, 1981

57. Beuscher ES, Gallin JI: Leukocyte transfusions in chronic granulomatous disease. N Engl J Med 307:800, 1982

58. Farber BF, Lesser M, Kaplan M et al: Clinical significance of neutropenia in patients with human immunodeficiency virus infection. Infect Control Hosp Epidemiol 12:429, 1991

59. Mannoni P, Rodet M, Vernant JP: Efficacy of prophylactic granulocyte transfusion in preventing infections in acute leukemia. Blood Transf Immunohematol 22:503, 1979

60. Clift RA, Sanders JE, Thomas ED et al: Granulocyte transfusions for the prevention of infection in patients receiving bone marrow transplants. N Engl J Med 298:1052, 1978

61. Ford JM, Cullen MH: Prophylactic granulocyte transfusions. Exp Hematol 5:65, 1977

62. Schiffer CA, Aisner J, Daly PA et al: Alloimmunization following prophylactic granulocyte transfusions. Blood 54:766, 1979

63. Strauss RG, Connett JE, Gale RP et al: A control trial of prophylactic granulocyte transfusions during initial induction chemotherapy for acute myelogenous leukemia. N Engl J Med 305:597, 1981

64. Schiller CA, Buchholz DH, Aisner J et al: Experience with transfusion of granulocytes obtained by continuous flow filtration leukopheresis. Am J Med 58:373, 1975

65. Aisner J, Schiffer CA, Wiernik PH: Granulocyte transfusions: evaluation of factors influencing results and a comparison of filtration and intermittent centrifugation leukapheresis. Br J Haematol 38:121, 1978

66. Berkman EM, Eisenstaedt RS, Caplan SN: Supportive granulocyte transfusion in the infected severely neutropenic host. Blood 52:493, 1978

67. Higby D, Freeman A, Henderson ES et al: Granulocyte transfusions in children using filter-collected cells. Cancer 38:1407, 1976

68. Holland PV, Schmidt PJ: Standards for Blood Banks and Transfusion Services. 15th Ed. p. 13. American Association of Blood Banks. Arlington, VA, 1993

69. Glasser L, Lane TA, McCullough J, Price TH: Panel VII: Neutrophil concentrates: functional considerations, storage, and quality control. J Clin Apheresis 1:179, 1983

70. Elliott GR, Clay ME, Mills EL, et al: Neutrophil transfusion kinetics measured by chemiluminescence, nitroblue tetrazolium reduction, and recovery of Indium-111-labeled granulocytes. Transfusion 27:23, 1987

71. Arnold R, Pflieger H, Dietrich M, Heimpel H: The clinical efficacy of granulocyte transfusions: studies on the oral cavity. Blut 35:405, 1977

72. McCullough J, Clay M, Hurd D et al: Effect of leukocyte antibodies and HLA matching on the intravascular recovery, survival, and tissue localization of 111-Indium granulocytes. Blood 67:522, 1986

73. Karp DD, Ervin TJ, Turtle S et al: Pulmonary complications during granulocyte transfusions: incidence and clinical features. Vox Sang 42:57, 1982

74. Schiffer CA, Aisner J, Daly PA et al: Alloimmunization following prophylactic granulocyte transfusions. Blood 54:766, 1979

75. Higby DJ, Burnett D: Granulocyte transfusions: current status. Blood 55:2, 1980

76. Wright DG, Robichaud KJ, Pizzo PS, Deisseroth AB: Lethal pulmonary reactions associated with the combined use of amphotericin B and leukocyte transfusions. N Engl J Med 304:1185, 1981

77. Dana BW, Durie BGM, White RF, Huestis DW: Concomitant administration of granulocyte transfusion and amphotericin B in neutropenic patients: absence of significant pulmonary toxicity. Blood 57:90, 1981

78. Winston DJ, Ho WG, Howell CL et al: Cytomegalovirus infections associated with leukocyte transfusions. Ann Intern Med 93:671, 1980

79. Bowden RA, Sayers M, Flournoy N et al: Cytomegalovirus immune globulin and seronegative blood products to prevent primary cytomegalovirus infection after marrow transplantation. N Engl J Med 314:1006, 1986

80. Hillyer CD, Emmens RK, Zago-Novaretti M, Berkman EM: Methods for the reduction of transfusion-transmitted cytomegalovirus infection: filtration versus the use of seronegative donor units. Transfusion 34:929, 1994

81. Graw RG, Buckner CD, Whang-Peng J et al: Complication of bone-marrow transplantation. Graft-versus-

host disease resulting from chronic-myelogenous-leukemia leucocyte transfusions. Lancet 2:338, 1970

82. Ford JM, Lucey JJ, Cullen MH, Tobias JS: Fatal graft-versus-host disease following transfusion of granulocytes from normal donors. Lancet 2:1167, 1976

83. Rosen RC, Huestis DW, Corrigan JJ: Acute leukemia and granulocyte transfusion: fatal graft-versus-host reaction following transfusion of cells obtained from normal donors. J Pediatr 93:268, 1978

84. Betzhold JB, Hong R: Fatal graft-versus-host disease after a small leukocyte transfusion in a patient with lymphoma and varicella. Pediatrics 62:63, 1978

85. Weiden PL, Zuckerman N, Hansen JA et al: Fatal graft-versus-host disease in a patient with lymphoblastic leukemia following normal granulocyte transfusion. Blood 57:328, 1981

86. Holland PV, Schmidt PJ: Standards for Blood Banks and Transfusion Services. 15th Ed. p. 24. American Association of Blood Banks, Arlington, VA, 1993

87. McCullough J: Leukapheresis and granulocyte transfusion. CRC Crit Rev Clin Lab Sci 10:275, 1979

88. McCullough J, Weiblen BJ, Deinard AS, et al: In vitro function and post-transfusion survival of granulocytes collected by continuous-flow centrifugation and by filtration leukapheresis. Blood 48:315, 1976

89. Price TH, Dale DC: Blood kinetics and in vivo chemotaxis of transfused neutrophils: effect of collection method, donor corticosteroid treatment, and short term storage. Blood 54:977, 1979

90. McCullough J, Weiblen BJ, Fine D: Effects of storage of granulocytes on their fate in vivo. Transfusion 23:20, 1983

91. Dutcher JP, Schiller CA, Johston GS et al: The effect of histocompatibility factors on the migration of transfused [111]Indium-labeled granulocytes, abstracted. Blood 58:181, 1982

92. Glasser L: Functional considerations of granulocyte concentrates used for clinical transfusions. Transfusion 19:1, 1979

93. Strauss RG, Maguire LC, Koepke JA, Thompson JS: Properties of neutrophils collected by discontinuous flow centrifugation leukapheresis employing hydroxyethyl starch. Transfusion 19:192, 1979

94. Glasser L, Huestis DW, Jones JF: Functional capabilities of steroid-recruited neutrophils harvested for clinical transfusion. N Engl J Med 297:1033, 1977

95. Glasser L: Effect of storage on normal neutrophils collected by discontinuous-flow centrifugation leukapheresis. Blood 50:1145, 1977

96. McCullough J: Liquid preservation of granulocytes. Transfusion 20:129, 1980

97. McCullough J, Clay ME, Loken MK, Hurd JJ: Effect of ABO incompatibility on fate in vivo of [111]Indium granulocytes. Transfusion 28:358, 1988

98. Eyre HJ, Goldstein IM, Perry S, Graw RG Jr: Leukocyte transfusions: function of transfused granulocytes from donors with chronic myelocytic leukemia. Blood 36:432, 1970

99. Applebaum FR, Trapani RJ, Graw RG: Consequences of prior alloimmunization during granulocyte transfusion. Transfusion 17:460, 1977

100. Westrick MA, Debelak-Fehir KM, Epstein RB: The effect of prior whole blood transfusion on subsequent granulocyte support in leukopenic dogs. Transfusion 17:611, 1977

101. Chow HS, Alexander DL, Epstein RB: Detection and significance of granulocyte alloimmunization in leukocyte transfusion therapy on neutropenic dogs. Transfusion 23:45, 1983

102. Dutcher JP, Fox JJ, Riggs C et al: Pulmonary retention of Indium-111-labeled granulocytes in alloimmunized patients, abstracted. Blood 58:171, 1982

103. Dahlke MB, Keashen M, Alavi JB et al: Granulocyte transfusions and outcome of alloimmunized patients with gram-negative sepsis. Transfusion 22:374, 1982

104. Kerst JM, de Haas M, van der Schoot CE: Recombinant granulocyte colony-stimulating factor administration to health volunteers: induction of immunophenotypically and functionally altered neutrophils via an effect on myeloid progenitor cells. Blood 82:3265, 1993

105. Caspar CB, Seger RA, Burger J, Gmur J: Effective stimulation of donors for granulocyte transfusions with recombinant methionyl granulocyte colony-stimulating factor. Blood 81:2866, 1993

106. Hollingshead LM, Goa KL: Recombinant granulocyte colony-stimulating factor (rG-CSF). A review of its pharmacological properties and prospective role in neutropenic conditions. Drugs 42:300, 1991

107. Bensinger WI, Price TH, Dale DC et al: The effects of daily recombinant human granulocyte colony-stimulating factor administration on normal granulocyte donors undergoing leukapheresis. Blood 81:1883, 1993

108. Khwaja A, Carver JE, Linch DC: Interactions of granulocyte-macrophage colony-stimulating factor (CSF), granulocyte CSF, and tumor necrosis factor α in the priming of the neutrophil respiratory burst. Blood 79:745, 1992

109. Ohsaka A, Kitagawa S, Sakamoto S et al: In vivo activation of human neutrophil functions by administration of recombinant human granulocyte colony-stimulating factor in patients with malignant lymphoma. Blood 74:2743, 1989

110. Lindemann A, Herrmann F, Oster W et al: Hematologic effects of recombinant human granulocyte colony-stimulating factor in patients with malignancy. Blood 74:2644, 1989

111. Yong KL, Linch DC: Differential effects of granulocyte- and granulocyte-macrophage colony-stimulating factors (G- and GM-CSF) on neutrophil adhesion in vitro and in vivo. Eur J Haematol 49:251, 1992

112. Haylock DN, To LB, Dowse TL et al: Ex vivo expansion and maturation of peripheral blood CD34+ cells into the myeloid lineage. Blood 80:1405, 1992

113. Koller MR, Emerson SG, Palsson BO: Large-scale expansion of human stem and progenitor cells from bone marrow mononuclear cells in continuous perfusion cultures. Blood 82:378, 1993

Chapter 18

Coagulation Factor Replacement for Patients With Acquired Coagulation Disorders

Sanford R. Kurtz

Acquired coagulopathies are a ubiquitous group of disorders that include the coagulation abnormalities of liver disease, those of acquired circulating anticoagulants, disseminated intravascular coagulation (DIC), antiphospholipid-dependent antibody bleeding and thrombotic syndromes, drug-induced alterations of hemostasis, and hypercoagulable states. In addition, hemostatic abnormalities are commonly found in patients with surgical bleeding, plasma cell dyscrasia associated with monoclonal proteins, and cancer. Despite the prevalence of hemorrhagic and thrombotic complications in patients treated by both the medical and surgical disciplines, the diagnosis, management, and treatment of these disorders in individual patients represents a complex confusing process. In addition, the high incidence of morbidity and death in these conditions adds to the importance of clinicians having a clear understanding of the cause and pathophysiology to make rapid diagnostic and therapeutic decisions.

Transfusion medicine services are commonly asked to provide red cells and other blood components early in the course of these disorders, frequently before coagulation specialists are consulted. Perhaps the most important step in the process of transfusion support for these patients, is the prospective review of component orders. At this point in the process the diagnosis, management plan and adequacy of laboratory analysis can be assessed. The

transfusion medicine specialist can assess the relationship of laboratory abnormalities to clinical evidence of thrombosis and/or bleeding because abnormal coagulation parameters are not always associated with bleeding, even when invasive procedures have been or will be performed. Unfortunately, this type of analysis is frequently not made before blood component replacement is instituted.

In this chapter, the acquired coagulopathies associated with liver disease, DIC, and more common hypercoagulable states are described to elucidate the role of soluble clotting factor replacement (Table 18-1). Because teaching in this area can focus on either the use of therapeutic agents or on treatment by clinical condition, a description of relevant blood components and derivatives is presented first, followed by a discussion of the clinical disorders.

FRESH FROZEN PLASMA

Historical Overview

The 1978 Annual Report of the American Association of Blood Banks indicates that 600,000 units of fresh frozen plasma (FFP) were transfused. This figure jumped to greater than 1.6 million units in 1984, representing an increase of 266 percent.[1] Approximately 2 million units were transfused in 1990.[2] The 25 percent increase over the latter 6-year interval is

Table 18-1. Acquired Coagulopathies

Liver disease (liver biopsy and liver resection)
Vitamin K deficiency
Disseminated intravascular coagulation (severe or mild)
Antithrombin III deficiency
Protein C deficiency
Protein S deficiency
Activated protein C deficiency
Antiphospholipid antibody
Thrombotic thrombocytopenic pupura

impressive but is dramatically lower than the increase in the previous 6-year period of 1978 to 1984. It seems reasonable to attribute this slowdown in the transfusion of FFP to the National Institutes of Health Consensus Development Conference on FFP convened in 1984.[3] The recommendations of this conference provided a foundation for aggressive educational efforts by blood bank directors to modify the transfusion practice of this component. The recognition of transfusion-transmitted acquired immunodeficiency syndrome probably also had a dramatic impact on the decreasing transfusion rates of FFP.[4] Furthermore, the concern over transfusion-transmitted disease has more recently led to the development of solvent-detergent FFP (SD FFP), which is discussed later in this chapter.[5]

Amberson's[6] review in 1937 chronicles early work on serum and plasma transfusion. The first extensive clinical use of plasma was begun by Max Strumia in 1927 at the Bryn Mawr Hospital in Pennsylvania.[7] By 1931, it was used there routinely in place of whole blood for the treatment of certain hemorrhagic diseases and streptococcal and pneumococcal infections. The preparation process involved fresh blood, and the final product was diluted with an equal part of saline or saline glucose solution to dilute isoagglutinins and administered within 24 hours. Although it was safe, it was not a practical system because plasma was not immediately available for use in emergencies and bacterial contamination occurred. The first method of preservation was storage of liquid plasma in the refrigerator. However, this was accompanied by progressive flocculation, with the consequent necessity for filtration. In retrospect, this fibrin-like material was cryoprecipitate. At least one

death was reported as a result of the transfusion of citrated plasma preserved in the refrigerator without filtration before transfusion.[7]

Dried plasma was transfused to humans for the treatment of shock and hypoproteinemia in 1938 at Bryn Mawr Hospital by Strumia. However, as Strumia and McGraw[7] noted, "it is rather useless to remove water from plasma only to add it a few days later" when a better method of preservation is available. That method was freezing plasma. Interestingly, Strumia observed that frozen plasma thawed rapidly in a water bath at 37°C and, allowed to warm to room temperature before being removed from the water bath, remained clear; precipitation occurred if the plasma was removed before it had a chance to warm to room temperature. This is probably the basis for instructions on thawing FFP today. By the beginning of World War II, plasma was regularly transfused to restore volume as part of the treatment of hemorrhagic shock. Until the 1960s, FFP was used to treat hemophilia A based on the pioneering work of Brinkhous who established that plasma was a source for factor VIII and FFP was an effective vehicle to deliver it.[8]

Paradoxically, during the 1970s and 1980s, when FFP usage was exploding, albumin was available to treat hypoalbuminemia without infectious disease transmission, and both cryoprecipitate and factor VIII concentrates had replaced FFP as the treatment of choice for hemophilia A. No theories have satisfactorily explained this phenomenon. Crowley et al.[9] provided the most practical explanation. They postulated that the dramatic increase in FFP transfusion in the late 1970s and early 1980s was the result of increased availability (i.e., increased to meet available supplies), increased numbers of open heart operations, and an increased severity of illness in patients in addition to intensified coagulation testing. Schmidt[10] in 1978 and Head[11] in 1985 expressed concern over a blood system that lack of the availability of whole blood. This led to several subsequent studies to establish whether FFP was being transfused to reconstitute packed red cells as whole blood.[12–16] Snyder et al.[14] studied FFP utilization in nine Wisconsin hospitals over a 1-month period. Forty-two percent of the FFP transfused was into patients undergoing open heart surgery. This figure was 39 and 27 percent in 1983 and 1985, respectively, in one hospital from Rhode Island.[8] Silbert et al.[15] found that, in 1981, 52 percent of FFP usage by surgical services was for volume replacement; this percentage had dropped to 24 percent for surgery by 1986 in one study[13] and a combined 31 percent in medicine, pediatrics, and surgical services in the 1986 study by Blumberg et al.[16] Although geographic usage patterns might explain these differences, it is also possible they represent better availability of albumin and hydroxyethyl starch and a better understanding during the intervening years that FFP was contraindicated for volume expansion. In all these reports, FFP was most commonly transfused for excessive bleeding or abnormal coagulation test results. Snyder et al.[14] insightfully concluded that "the general acceptance of FFP efficacy" and the "logical expectation" by physicians that FFP can treat or prevent bleeding indicates that changes in ordering practices will be difficult to achieve."

Unfortunately, these studies suffer from being at least 7 years old, and there have been no recent investigations of FFP utilization. FFP is not routinely necessary for cardiac surgery, and experience suggests that only a small fraction of FFP orders secondary to cardiovascular surgery are for volume expansion today. At Lahey Clinic, only 8 percent of patients undergoing cardiac surgery receive FFP during their hospitalizations. Instead, most FFP appears to be prophylactically transfused in patients with various diagnoses who have abnormal coagulation study findings before or after procedures with the potential for hemorrhage.

Blood Component

FFP is plasma separated and frozen within 8 hours after collection of 1 unit of whole blood. It contains all coagulation factors and plasma proteins. With the exception of factors V and VIII, the other coagulation factors are remarkably stable during red cell and platelet concentrate storage, and despite a decline in levels, clinically important levels of factor V and VIII activity are still present in FFP. Factor VIII loss is biphasic, with a rapid decrease within the first several days of storage; nonetheless, as much as 50 percent of factor VIII and 36 percent of factor V activities have been found after 21 days of red cell storage in acid-citrate-dextrose solution.[17] In addition, 68 percent of factor VIII and 47 percent of factor V

activities have been noted in platelet concentrates stored for 72 hours at 22°C.[18] This information is useful to assess the need for FFP as a source of clotting factors in congenital or acquired factor deficiency states in situations such as massive transfusion when other blood components are also being simultaneously transfused.

General Contraindications

In 1984, Braunstein and Oberman[19] published their review of FFP to establish guidelines for its transfusion. That same year, the National Institutes of Health Consensus Development Conference recommendations for FFP were published (Table 18-2). Since then, cardiopulmonary bypass procedures and the approach to massive transfusion have been refined, liver transplantation has become well established, and new pharmacologic agents such as intravenous immunoglobulin, desmopressin, and aprotinin have been developed to improve immunotherapy and hemostasis. Acceptable indications for FFP transfusion have become exceptionally narrow. FFP is contraindicated for volume expansion, nutritional supplementation, prophylactic use in the set-

Table 18-2. National Institutes of Health Consensus Conference Indications for the Use of Fresh Frozen Plasma

---

Replacement of isolated deficiencies of factors II, V, VII, IX, X, and XI when specific component therapy is neither available nor appropriate

Replacement of the functional vitamin K-dependent coagulation factors II, VII, IX, and X and proteins C and S in patients who are anticoagulated with warfarin and are actively bleeding or require emergency surgery

Reversal of hemostatic disorders in patients who have received massive blood transfusion (greater than one blood volume within several hours) and in whom factor deficiencies are presumed to be the sole or principal derangement

Replacement of antithrombin III in patients who are deficient in this inhibitor and are undergoing surgery or who require heparin for treatment of thrombosis

Replacement of immunoglobulins in infants with immunodeficiency secondary to severe protein-losing enteropathy in whom total parenteral nutrition is ineffectual and in children and adults with humoral immunodeficiency

In conjunction with therapeutic plasma exchange for the treatment of thrombotic thrombocytopenic purpura

ting of cardiopulmonary bypass, and massive transfusion.[3] Massively transfused patients do not demonstrate a correlation between the number of red cell units transfused and coagulation test results and also show unpredictable amounts of coagulation factor dilution.[20,21] FFP is also contraindicated to neutralize heparin. Although this should be obvious, the Lahey Clinic Blood Bank receives several FFP requests from house staff each year to treat overheparinized patients. Because FFP is a source of antithrombin III (AT III), transfusion could instead potentiate the action of heparin.

General Indications

Specific blood components, derivatives, and pharmacologic agents have relegated FFP use in patients to a few diseases, such as congenital deficiencies of factor V, factor VII, factor XI, protein C, protein S, and AT III, if AT III concentrates are unavailable. The percent factor concentrations needed for normal coagulation are between 20 and 40 percent,[22] which are easily achievable with FFP administration. FFP is rarely indicated in massively transfused patients because factor VIII is an acute-phase reactant and there is residual factor activity present in stored red cells and platelets. In fact, hemostasis is best accomplished in such patients by maintaining the platelet count above 50,000/μl because (1) there is a greater reserve of coagulation factors than circulating platelets; (2) the platelet membrane serves as a required physical surface in coagulation; and (3) the platelet is subject to injury and dysfunction, which can amplify the bleeding tendency associated with thrombocytopenia.[23]

SOLVENT-DETERGENT FRESH FROZEN PLASMA

Blood Component

SD FFP is not yet a licensed blood component. It consists of FFP that has undergone an SD method of viral inactivation. Thawed units of FFP are pooled into batch sizes of 2,000 to 5,000 donors per batch. The plasma pool is pasteurized for 10 hours at 60°C and incubated with tri-n-butyl phosphate (solvent) and Triton X-100 (detergent). The chemicals are removed by chromatography. The product is filtered and frozen in 200-ml aliquots. Each unit is ABO specific and may be stored for up to 2 years at −18°C.

Virus kill studies on treated plasma indicate that the SD method removes a minimum of 10^5 tissue culture infectious doses of the human immunodeficiency virus (HIV), hepatitis B virus (HBV), hepatitis C virus (HCV), Sindbis, and vesicular stomatitis virus (VSV). This is equal to or superior to other viral inactivation methods. From 13 studies involving almost 11 million units of coagulation factors infused, there is no evidence of any individual who has developed serologic or clinical evidence of HCV or HIV.[24] The coagulation characteristics of SD plasma are comparable but not identical to FFP. The final concentrations of the coagulation factors are within the normal range, with the exception of protein S, high-molecular-weight von Willebrand factor (vWF) multimers, and fibrinogen, which are lower. The reason for the loss of this material is not known. With regard to low-molecular-weight vWF, there is no change in vWF antigen or ristocetin cofactor activity. Toxicity studies suggest that SD plasma is comparable to FFP with a 4 percent reaction rate composed of mild reactions such as hives and occasionally fever.

Efficacy studies coordinated by the New York Blood Center have shown the product to be therapeutically beneficial. In 52 treatments of 39 patients with congenital single-factor deficiencies, SD plasma was 100 percent effective in achieving or maintaining hemostasis, as evidenced by cessation of bleeding or prevention of abnormal bleeding during or after an invasive procedure. In European studies that assessed the ability of SD to reverse coumarin-induced anticoagulation, nine patients had the drug effect successfully reversed. SD plasma has also been reported to be as successful as FFP in increasing or maintaining platelet counts in patients with acute or chronic relapsing thrombotic thrombocytopenic purpura (TTP).[25] As reported in a Food and Drug Administration FDA-sponsored conference on virus-inactivated plasma, 128 patients with a variety of diagnoses had received 384 treatment episodes involving 2,492 units of SD plasma with the same therapeutic effect as FFP.[24]

There are, however, several outstanding issues associated with this product. The first is that nonenveloped viruses, including hepatitis A virus (HAV) and parvovirus, are not eliminated by the SD method. The concern with both of these viruses is the multiplier effect of infection of a pooled product that would be transfused to many patients. This concern also applies to unknown pathogens. If an unknown pathogen entered the donor pool and the SD method of viral inactivation was ineffective, many recipients would potentially be exposed to that virus. There are also issues of cost and cost-effectiveness.[26] It is unknown whether the benefit of the marginal increase in safety outweighs the likely increased cost of this product.

ANTITHROMBIN III CONCENTRATE

Blood Derivative

The source material for the production of AT III concentrate is large pools of human plasma or plasma fractions prepared by Cohn ethanol fractionation. The major purification steps use heparin as the affinity ligand bound to a solid matrix. The AT III is eluted with a high-salt-concentration solution. Protein impurities are removed using precipitation and ion-exchange techniques.[27] Viral inactivation takes place through heat treatment in solution during the manufacturing process. No cases of HBV, HCV, or HIV have been reported to date with the use of this derivative.

AT III concentrates are supplied as a freeze-dried concentrate with water for reconstitution. The dating period ranges from 2 to 3 years when they are stored at 2 to 8°C. The half-life, based on either antigen or activity units, is 43 to 77 hours. AT III concentration measured as heparin cofactor activity is 50 to 100 international units/ml of reconstituted material. Like most factor concentrates, it is an expensive product, $0.80 to $1.00/unit, with several thousand units being given daily for usually 5 days.

General Indications

This product is FDA approved only for replacement of AT III in patients with hereditary deficiency. As discussed later in this chapter, widespread availability is prompting studies of the efficacy of AT III replacement in acquired coagulopathies with documented reduced levels of AT III.

LIVER DISEASE

The magnitude of hemostatic abnormalities in liver disease correlates with the degree of parenchymal cell damage. Impaired coagulation can be the result of decreased factor synthesis, production of dysfunctional soluble coagulation proteins, increased consumption, and/or abnormal clearance of activated factors.[28,29] The liver is the site of synthesis for all of the factors of the clotting system except for vWF, which is produced by endothelial cells. The liver is also the source of the proteins of the fibrinolytic system other than plasminogen activators, both tissue and urokinase types, which are produced by the endothelial cells and kidneys, respectively.

When destruction of parenchymal cells reaches a critical mass, no matter what the cause of the liver disease, decreased synthesis of the vitamin K-dependent proteins; factors II, VII, IX, and X, and anticoagulant proteins C and S occurs. The prothrombin time (PT) represents a sensitive indicator of liver damage because, as shown in Table 18-3, factor VII and protein C are the most sensitive coagulation factors to parenchymal cell damage because of their shorter half-life. Subsequently, sequential declines occur in factor II and X levels followed by factor IX and protein S. As liver cell damage progresses, abnormal vitamin K-dependent factor and dysfunctional fibrinogen synthesis have been described.[30,31] Finally, with severe liver disease, increased consumption caused by either primary fibrinolysis or fibrinolysis secondary to DIC with clinical bleeding can ensue.[32,33] In addition, in the setting of DIC,

Table 18-3. Coagulation Factor Synonym and Half-Life

Factor	Synonym	In Vivo Half-Life (hr)
I	Fibrinogen	3–5 days
II	Prothrombin	72
V	AL-globulin	5–15
VII	Prothrombin conversion accelerator	2–5
VIII:c	Antihemophilic factor	8–12
IX	Christmas factor	24
X	Stuart-Power factor	24–56
XI	Thromboplastin Antecedent	60–80
Protein C		2–8
Protein S		7–72
Antithrombin III		24

both thrombocytopenia and thrombocytopathy frequently contribute to the bleeding diathesis.[34]

An abnormal PT in association with liver disease broadly describes the most common clinical setting for FFP requests. Oberman,[35] who has published extensively on this subject, gets to the heart of the issue when he states, "unfortunately, there is little information in the literature to guide us (blood bankers) in responding to requests for FFP for patients with severe liver disease." The Consensus Development Conference also did not address this issue. Although, the panel mentions FFP transfusion in patients with multiple coagulation defects including those with liver disease, it does not list this as an indication for transfusion in their recommendations.

Several studies have attempted to explore the relationship between abnormal PTs, liver disease, and prophylactic FFP transfusion in the setting of liver biopsy. Mannucci et al.[36] studied the effect of infu-

Table 18-4. Effect of Plasma Transfusions on Prothrombin Time in Patients with Liver Disease[a,b]

Patient Number	Plasma Infused (ml)	PT (%) Before	PT (%) 0.3–1 hr	PT (%) 2–4 hr
1	1,200	29	77	64
2	1,400[a]	23	41	35
3	600	41	7	77
4	800	41	64	56
5	1,200[c]	25	52	35
6	1,000	52	64	58
7	1,600	35	60	66
8	1,600	40	93	72
9	1,600[c]	40	49	—
10	1,800	21	67	—
11	1,200	40	72	60

Abbreviation: PT, prothrombin time.
[a] PT 100% = normal PT.
[b] PT 60% = within 3 seconds of control.
[c] No change in PT > 60%.
(From Spector et al.,[37] with permission.)

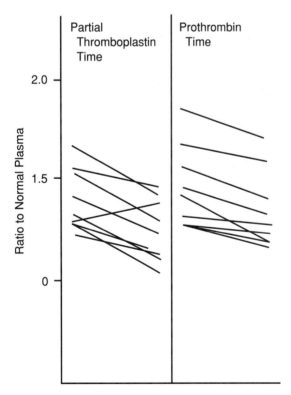

Fig. 18-1. Tests performed before and 15 minutes after administration of FFP (12 ml/kg). (Modified from Mannucci et al.,[36] with permission.)

sions of FFP, prothrombin complex concentrates, and a combination of these treatments on 30 patients with chronic liver disease (8 with cirrhosis and 22 with chronic active hepatitis) undergoing needle biopsy (Fig. 18-1). Patients with abnormal PT and partial thromboplastin time (PTT) coagulation tests and a normal bleeding time were included. In their analysis, patients with abnormal bleeding times were excluded regardless of the results of clotting assays, and all patients were stable and not bleeding at the time of the study. FFP (12 ml/kg) was administered by continuous intravenous infusion for 45 to 60 minutes and coagulation studies were obtained before and 15 minutes after the infusion. Although the PT normalized in only 4 of 11 patients, no patients had any clinical or laboratory evidence of bleeding after liver biopsy.

Spector et al.[37] studied 13 patients with liver disease and an abnormal PT refractory to vitamin K therapy (Table 18-4). None of the patients were actively bleeding or had received blood transfusions within 48 hours. Eleven patients, (10 with cirrhosis and 1 with hepatitis) received FFP prophylactically in preparation for liver biopsy. PT values ranged from 19 to 26 seconds, with the upper limit of normal at 14 seconds. The goal of the study was to lower the PT to within 3 seconds of the control value (PT more than 60 percent). Repeat PTs were performed at 20 minutes to 1 hour, 2 to 4 hours, and 24 hours after infusion; 600 to 1800 ml (3 to 9 units) of FFP were infused. Eight of 11 patients initially corrected the PT to within 3 seconds, but 3 patients had only minimal improvement in their PT despite receiving 6, 7, and 8 units of FFP, respectively. Only 5 of the 9 patients with completely evaluated data achieved the desired PT level 2 to 4 hours after infusion, and only 1 of 11 had a PT at the desired level after 24 hours. These investigators concluded that there are distinct limitations to the use of FFP in this setting because large volumes of plasma were required to produce significant improvement, the effect lasted for only a short period of time, and some patients were unable to correct the PT to within 3 seconds of normal despite large-volume FFP infusion. This study is limited by the small number of patients and the fact that no mention is made whether spontaneous hemorrhage occurred after liver biopsy in the three patients whose PTs were not corrected or whether these patients had clinical predictors to help identify in advance who would not respond to FFP infusion.

Similar findings were reported by Gazzard et al.[38] who examined 30 patients with various types of chronic liver disease who required needle liver biopsy and had PT values prolonged by 4 or more seconds (Fig. 18-2). Of the 15 patients given FFP, 5 had active chronic hepatitis, 2 had subacute hepatic necrosis, 6 had alcoholic cirrhosis, and 1 each had sarcoidosis and congenital erythrocytic protoporphyria. Each patient was given 600 ml of FFP intravenously over 30 minutes, followed by liver biopsy, followed by a further 300 ml of FFP 6 hours after the initial infusion. Patients were observed for clinical evidence of bleeding, pain, or tenderness and drop in hematocrit. Only 3 of 15 patients had the PT returned to within 3 seconds or less of the upper limit of normal. Most of the remaining 12 patients had PT values prolonged by 8 to 13 seconds above normal 30 minutes after FFP transfusion; however, no clinical evidence of bleeding was observed in any patient postbiopsy, and no patient required blood transfusion. These authors therefore questioned whether replacing clotting factors is worthwhile in this type of patient and concluded that many other factors,

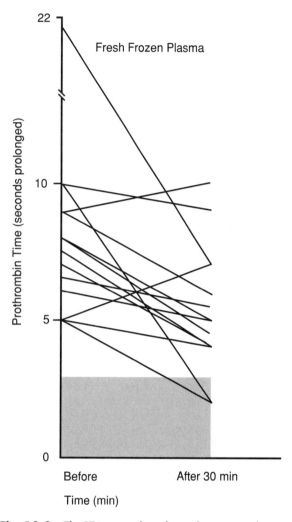

Fig. 18-2. The PT in seconds prolonged over control immediately before biopsy and 30 minutes after FFP. (Modified from Gazzard et al.,[38] with permission.)

including platelet number, platelet function, and vascular integrity, are important in hemostasis.

In an attempt to define indicators for the risk of bleeding from liver biopsy, Ewe[39] performed a prospective study on 200 consecutive patients undergoing liver biopsy using a Menghini needle. The patients had various liver diseases, and no patients were excluded because of abnormal clotting study results. A whole blood clotting time and PT were performed. Ewe developed a liver bleeding time (LBT) index, defined as the time elapsing between the moment of the biopsy and the termination of hemorrhage, as determined by irrigation of the liver surface studied by laparoscopy. After the biopsy, a thin needle was inserted through the abdominal wall using the puncture site to drip saline on the liver surface, inferior to the puncture. Bleeding from the biopsy site turned the saline pink. The time required for the saline to become clear was called the LBT. No correlation was found between the LBT and PT abnormalities (Fig. 18-3). The average LBT was approximately 4 minutes. Ten patients with an LBT more than 12 minutes had PT values that were no different from those of the other patients in this study. This author speculates that other factors, including clotting mechanisms operating directly at the biopsy site, influence the likelihood of bleeding and that punctures directed through a medium-sized or large vessel could account for some of the

rare clinically significant bleeds that occur after biopsy. The strengths of the Ewe study are its prospective design, objective evaluation of bleeding, and standard clotting studies. Unfortunately, 52 percent of the patients in the study had fatty liver or nonspecific histologic changes, rather than severe liver disease. Also, the results of a laparoscopic approach may not be applicable to percutaneous biopsy. For example, in four patients, the instrument was used to promote hemostasis by compressing the biopsy site. It is unclear whether significant bleeding would have occurred otherwise in these patients.

All four of these studies provide some guidance in determining the value of prophylactic FFP transfusions in patients with liver disease who require liver biopsy. These studies all accept the premise that it is only necessary to reduce the PT to within 3 seconds of the upper limit of normal, implying that PT

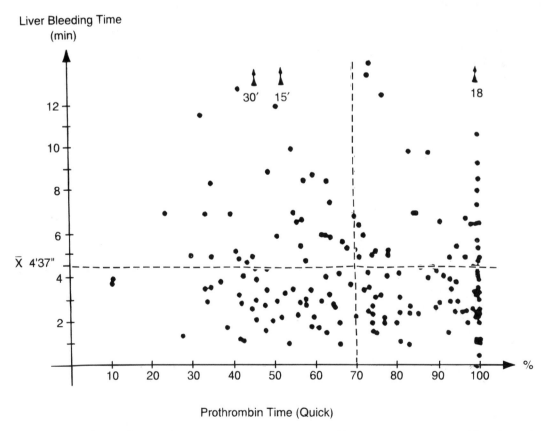

Fig. 18-3. Correlation of LBT and PT (′ = min; ″ = sec). Horizontal line: average LBT; vertical line: lower limit of normal (70%). (From Ewe,[39] with permission.)

results within 3 seconds of the upper limit of normal should not cause clinical concern about hemorrhage. Indeed, Sherlock,[40] for decades in her classic book on liver disease, stated that the "one stage prothrombin time should not be more than three seconds prolonged over controlled values." Even large volumes of FFP on the order of 5 to 10 units are incapable of reversing PT results to the normal range in many patients. The ability of FFP to lower PT values significantly is variable, unpredictable, and independent of the volume of FFP transfused. Bleeding after liver biopsy is a random event, which cannot be predicted by coagulation studies, and the presence of an abnormal PT does not necessarily imply spontaneous hemorrhage will occur.

In another study, McVay and Toy[41] retrospectively investigated the records of inpatients between 1983 and 1987 who underwent liver biopsy to determine the relationship between mild hemostatic abnormalities and the risk of increased bleeding. All patients had PT and PTT values between 1.1 and 1.5 times the midpoint of the normal range and platelet counts of 50 to 99 $\times$ 10^9/L. A hemoglobin value had to be available either 48 hours prebiopsy or within 48 hours postbiopsy, and patients were excluded if they received prophylactic FFP or had active bleeding during the study interval. A major bleeding complication after biopsy was defined as a hemoglobin drop of 2 g/dl. Study criteria were fulfilled in 177 procedures (155 standard-needle and 22 fine-needle procedures) in 169 patients. Overall, 4.5 percent of patients had either major or probable bleeding complications. No differences in the proportion of patients with bleeding complications or in the average hemoglobin decrease postbiopsy were observed in patients with normal or mildly abnormal PTs. Eight patients had bleeding complications (Table 18-5). Four had a normal PT, and four had a PT value between 11.6 and 13.5 seconds (normal range 9.5 to 11.5 seconds). Three of these eight patients had platelet counts less than 70,000/μl. Eleven patients with PT values of 13.6 to 15.7 had no bleeding complications. McVay and Toy found that pain and liver malignancy were associated with an increased risk of bleeding. In light of their findings, the authors speculated that it is not necessary to transfuse FFP prophylactically in liver biopsy procedures. The validity of their conclusion is limited by the small number of patients and the retrospective nature of their study.

Table 18-5. Bleeding Complications and Average Hemoglobin Difference by Prothrombin Time in Patients Undergoing Liver Biopsy

PT Range (seconds)	Total Events (%)	No. of Bleeding Complications (% of events)	Average Hemoblogin Difference ± SD (g/L)[a]
Normal			
<11.5	100 (57)	4 (4.0)	−2.7 ± 8.9
Mildly prolonged			
11.6–13.5	65 (37)	4 (6.2)	−2.6 ± 9.8
13.6–15.7	11 (6)	0	
Total	176 (100)	8 (4.5)	−2.2 ± 6.2

Abbreviations: PT, prothrombin time; SD, standard deviation.
[a] 10 × g/dL (e.g., −2.7 g/L = −0.27 g/dL).
(From McVay and Toy,[41] with permission.)

Additional studies on the ability of the PT to predict surgical hemorrhage requiring red cell transfusion in other groups of patients also support the conclusion that less than a 3-second elevation of the PT above the upper limit of normal (or PT values 1.5 times the midpoint of the normal range) does not require prophylactic FFP transfusion. Aghajanian et al.[42] evaluated the usefulness of screening PT tests before elective gynecologic operations. Only 30 of 1,859 (1.9 percent) patients had PT results greater than 3 seconds above the upper limit of normal. Twenty patients had no indications in the history or physical examination to explain the abnormal PT. Despite the abnormality, no change in perioperative management and no bleeding complications occurred. In 1955, Littman and Brodman[43] compared 15 patients with PT values of 21 to 51 seconds (control 14.5 to 15 seconds) with 45 patients with normal PT values undergoing vascular surgery. The group of patients with abnormal PT results had either received dicumarol before or at the time of surgery. The surgical operations included femoral and inferior vena cava vein ligations, lower limb amputations, and lumbar sympathectomies. Morbidity, mortality, and bleeding complications were similar in both groups. The authors concluded that certain types of surgery can be performed safely on patients with prolonged PTs.

Liver Resection and Peritoneovenous Shunts

During liver resection, a large vascular-rich surface is traumatized; this factor seems to be the main cause for bleeding during surgery and in the 24-hour postsurgical period. However, DIC and decreased concentrations of vitamin K-dependent factors have been observed in patients after liver resection.[44,45] Tsuzuki et al.[45] reported on their experience with DIC after hepatic resection in 192 patients 18 to 78 years of age. The overall incidence of DIC was 9.4 percent, and there was no statistically significant difference in incidence between resection for benign or malignant conditions. The most important variable was the extent of hepatic resection. Seventeen percent of patients who underwent resection of two or more segments of the liver had DIC, whereas only 2 percent who underwent resection of one segment or partial resection had DIC. In another study of bleeding after liver resection, Iwatsuki et al.[46] emphasized that complete hemostasis is considered the most important factor in preventing postoperative complications. The cause of death in the 4 percent of 150 patients reported in their series was irreversible liver failure rather than a coagulopathy such as DIC. Clearly, the extent of liver damage before surgery, whether the resection is related to trauma or malignancy, and extent of resection affect the likelihood of postsurgical coagulopathy. Thus, the need for FFP in patients undergoing liver surgery and in the immediate postsurgical period must be individualized. Furthermore, FFP should not be given prophylactically without laboratory studies. In general, patients should not receive FFP postoperatively unless the PT is greater than 3 seconds above the upper limit of normal and/or there is clinically active bleeding or coagulopathy.

Ascitic fluid is rich in material and factors that activate the clotting and fibrinolytic systems.[47] DIC with fibrinolysis has been reported in patients with peritoneovenous and LeVeen shunts.[48]

VITAMIN K DEFICIENCY

Historically, the source of most of the vitamin K required for the hepatic production of coagulation factors was presumed to be the intestinal microbial flora. However, dietary sources of vitamin K are also crucial to maintain an adequate coagulation factor supply.[49,50] Deficiencies in vitamin K can be seen in patients with obstructive jaundice, malabsorbtion, and other short gut syndromes. A group of antibiotics that contain the methyltetrazolethiol (MTT) side chain, including cefamandole, moxalactam, and cefoperazone, are associated with prolonged PTs. The MTT moiety has been shown to inhibit both the vitamin K-dependent carboxylase enzyme and the vitamin K epoxide reductase.[51] Hypoprothrombinemia does not develop in healthy persons who receive these antibiotics; risk factors for the development of a vitamin K-dependent coagulation deficiency include renal failure, lack of oral intake of food, and cancer.[52] A relative deficiency of vitamin K secondary to malnutrition, inadequate hyperalimentation, or any of the above reasons may also predispose patients who receive these antibiotics to hypoprothrombinemia.[53] Replacement of vitamin K is the treatment of choice. Transfusion of FFP is not necessary.

One of the most effective and clearly documented indications for FFP is the need for immediate correction of the coagulopathy of oral anticoagulant drugs such as warfarin in the patient who is actively bleeding. These drugs interfere with the interconversion of vitamin K by inhibiting vitamin K epoxide reductase and, possibly, vitamin K reductase. Vitamin K epoxide accumulates, which limits carboxylation of the vitamin K-dependent proteins, impairing their biologic function.[54] Bleeding is a major complication in a small but significant percentage of patients therapeutically anticoagulated or who become overanticoagulated. Anticoagulated patients who are bleeding, who need surgery, or who must undergo emergency procedures that have the potential for hemorrhage require rapid correction of hemostasis. Intravenously infused vitamin K requires 6 to 12 hours for effectiveness because new factors must be synthesized by the liver.[52] In contrast, FFP restores these factors instantly.

DOSAGE

The impetus for educational efforts in FFP transfusion have focused on the unnecessary transfusion of this component. Paradoxically, when transfusion of FFP is indicated, it is frequently the case that not enough is transfused. For example, emergency transfusion of FFP to reverse the effect of warfarin frequently requires 3 or more units of FFP. Similar doses are required in bleeding patients with severe liver disease and PT values 3 to 5 seconds or greater than the upper limit of normal. The lack of documentation in the literature on the inadequacy of 2-unit FFP transfusions, which are frequently ordered, probably indicates that most of these transfusions are given prophylactically in patients with PT values within 3 seconds of the upper limit of normal. These same patients are also judged unlikely to bleed, making transfusion unnecessary.

DISSEMINATED INTRAVASCULAR COAGULATION

A number of inciting factors can trigger DIC. Increased coagulation system activation and secondary fibrinolysis are important features of this disorder.

Although transfusion of blood products in this condition is largely supportive in nature, the recent availability of AT III concentrates and new laboratory assays warrant review of the subject.

Figure 18-4 represents a cartoon characterization of some laboratory tests and protein and molecular activation markers associated with the procoagulant, the fibrinolytic, and the inhibitor systems. The exposure of subendothelial components such as collagen as a result of damage of the endothelium initiates the intrinsic clotting system through contact factor XII, prekallikrein, high-molecular-weight kininogen, and factor XI, leading to activation of factor IX and VIII.[55] The extrinsic pathway is initiated when factor VII binds to tissue factor, a membrane glycoprotein expressed by the subendothelium of the vessel wall. It is important to note that the factor VII-tissue factor mechanism is an important physiologic activator of factors IX and X. Factor X activation can

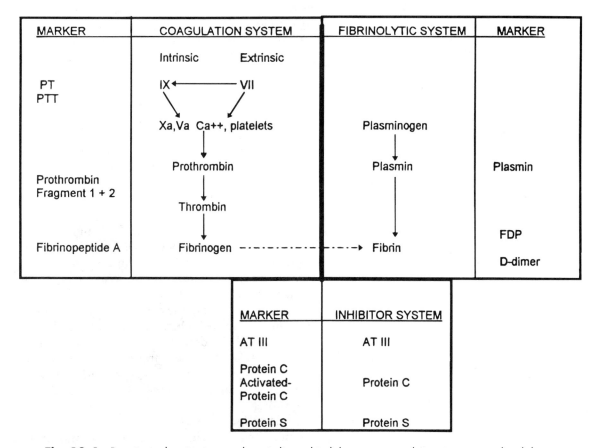

Fig. 18-4. Protein and activation markers indicated in laboratory tests that are associated with hemostasis.

be monitored by measuring the factor Xa activation peptide.[56]

Thrombin generation occurs only in the presence of factors Xa and Va, calcium ions, and activated platelets. Activation of prothrombin can be measured through the release of prothrombin fragments 1 and 2 or the release of fibrinopeptide A from fibrinogen in the conversion to fibrin.[56,57]

The fibrinolytic system is responsible for the destruction of a fibrin clot. It consists of a proenzyme, plasminogen, which is converted by many mechanisms into the active enzyme, plasmin, a nonspecific serine protease. Evidence for activation of the fibrinolytic system includes elevated fibrin degradation products (FDP), D-dimer, and plasmin levels.

The most important inhibitors of hemostasis are AT III, protein S, and protein C. In addition to the generation of fibrin, thrombin also rapidly activates protein C by binding to thrombomodulin on vascular endothelial cells. Assays have been developed to monitor activation of inhibitor proteins, including increased concentrations of protein C activation peptide and decreased AT III, protein C, and protein S levels.

The general clinical settings in which DIC occurs are summarized in Table 18-6. Once the coagulation system is activated, hemorrhage, microvascular thrombosis, and sometimes large-vessel thrombosis occur, leading to impairment of blood flow, ischemia, and associated organ damage. The deposition of fibrin in the microcirculation as a result of circulating thrombin is largely responsible for thrombosis; the production of FDP, which interfere with fibrin monomer polymerization as a result of circulating plasmin, account for hemorrhage. Clinical signs of bleeding are oozing from venipuncture sites, line placements, surgical wounds, and large hematomas. Fever, hypotension, acidosis, and hypoxia

are usually present. Laboratory tests reflect abnormalities of the coagulation, fibrinolytic, and inhibitor systems in addition to prolongation of the PT and activated PTT and thrombocytopenia (Fig. 18-4).

Therapeutic management is frequently confusing and dependent on the underlying condition, severity of hemorrhage or thrombosis, age of the patient, and other individual factors. The most effective approach is to eliminate the underlying process responsible for DIC along with aggressive supportive care. If bleeding or thrombosis remains significant after the institution of supportive care, treatment of the intravascular clotting process is required. Usually, subcutaneous heparin at approximately 100 units/kg every 4 to 6 hours or intravenous heparin at approximately 30,000 units/24 hr by constant infusion is given. Investigators have successfully treated severe DIC with AT III concentrates in small groups of patients.[58,59] Bick and Baker[60] believe that the level should always be 125 percent or greater and the concentrate should be delivered every 8 hours. Low patient levels of AT III must be documented before using this concentrate. These uncontrolled studies included a mixture of patients with septicemia, trauma-related conditions, carcinoma, and liver diseases, who often received multiple transfusions of different blood components. Evidence for the efficacy of AT III has been based largely on a more rapid normalization of abnormal coagulation values rather than on morbidity or mortality data. No randomized control studies using AT III have been performed.

Transfusion of red blood cells, FFP, and platelets frequently occur during severe DIC. When bleeding continues but laboratory and clinical signs of improvement and resolution are present, the rationale for transfusion is based on replacement of soluble clotting factors or cells the depletion of which is contributing to continued bleeding. Conversely, bleeding associated with deterioration of clinical and laboratory status suggests transfusion of blood components will unfortunately provide both substrate for DIC and replacement of diminished clotting proteins.

Therapy for patients with mild DIC focuses on treating the underlying disease process. Anticoagulant therapy is rarely required because of the low

Table 18-6. Clinical Disorders Associated with Disseminated Intravascular Coagulation

Obstetric	Liver disease
Septicemia	Burns
Solid tumors	Trauma
Leukemia	Peritoneal shunts
Intravascular hemolysis	Vascular conditions

frequency of catastrophic hemorrhage or thrombosis. Anticoagulant therapy may be indicated if progression to severe DIC is suspected. However, this must be balanced against bleeding complications as a result of the anticoagulant treatment. Blood product replacement therapy is rarely indicated in mild DIC.

HYPERCOAGULABILITY

Antithrombin III, Protein C, and Protein S

Hypercoagulability represents a tendency toward thromboembolic events. Most patients with these disorders have been shown to be deficient in natural anticoagulant proteins, AT III, protein C, protein S, or resistant activated protein C (APC) through hereditary or acquired defects. These disorders were reviewed recently.[61] Knowledge about acquired deficiencies of these protein inhibitors of coagulation is useful because new therapeutic concentrates may be developed in the future for specific indications associated with hypercoagulable states.

The most common and frequently most severe acquired deficiencies of AT III occur in consumptive coagulopathies associated with major surgery, DIC, and leukemia.[62] AT III is a plasma glycoprotein with a molecular weight of 58,000. A small fraction of this protease inhibitor is normally bound to a specific population of heparan sulfate proteoglycans synthesized by endothelial cells, which permits it to be selectively activated at blood surface interfaces. AT III is the major inhibitor of thrombin and factor Xa and, to a lesser extent, other serine proteases generated during the coagulation process, including IXa, XIa, and XIIa. The thrombophilic tendency of patients with hereditary AT III deficiency is believed to be the result of excess concentrations of factor Xa. The narrow reference range for AT III in adults is 0.8 to 1.2 international units/ml. A moderate decrease in concentration to 55 percent of normal has been associated with an increased risk of thrombosis.

Low levels of AT III have been documented in a variety of disorders. Failure to synthesize adequate amounts of AT III has been reported in patients with cirrhosis and malnutrition.[63,64] Protein loss states such as nephrotic syndrome and inflammatory bowel disease are also associated with low AT III levels.[65] Approximately 70 percent of individuals with deep venous thrombosis or pulmonary embolus have decreased levels of AT III before the initiation of anticoagulation therapy. Usually, this is related to consumption at the time of thrombosis development, with levels correlating with the severity of the intravascular event. Low levels of AT III in association with thrombotic episodes have and have not been reported in chronic use of oral contraceptive agents, but the studies are too disparate to draw any firm conclusions.[66]

AT III has been reported to be of therapeutic benefit in some coagulopathies. For example, thrombotic events were reported in patients with acute lymphoblastic leukemia, especially during or after L-asparaginase administration; laboratory tests documented a hypercoagulable state. A recent uncontrolled study concluded that AT III concentrates reduce the coagulopathy associated with L-asparaginase therapy.[67] The authors administered AT III concentrates daily at a dose of 50 international units/kg for 10 consecutive days from the beginning of L-asparaginase therapy in 25 adult patients with acute lymphoblastic leukemia. A marked increase in AT III levels with no change in levels of protein C, protein S, plasminogen, α_2-antiplasmin, factor VII, and platelet count were observed. There was no evidence of DIC in the treated group. Francis et al.[68] showed a reduced incidence of venous thrombosis after total hip and knee replacement by using AT III given 2 hours preoperatively and daily for 5 days. However, AT III therapy is expensive, approaching $0.80 to $1.00/unit. The dose used in this study was 2,000 to 3,000 units/day. As previously discussed, AT III has been given as part of the therapy for DIC, apparently resulting in amelioration of symptoms and improvement in hemostasis. However, in a group of patients with DIC associated with liver disease and peritoneovenous shunts, no benefit of AT III replacement was found.[69] Two randomized but uncontrolled studies of AT III treatment of DIC have been performed. Blauhut et al.[70] studied 51 patients with DIC and shock who were randomly assigned to treatment regimens of heparin, heparin combined with AT III concentrate, or AT III concentrate alone. The time required for an increase in AT III, fibrinogen, and/or platelets levels was used as the end point. Restoration of AT III levels occurred most rapidly with infusion of AT III concentrate alone. Increased blood loss was observed in the heparin and AT III concentrate group. In the other study, Maki et al.[71] studied 77 patients with DIC and obstetric diseases. Bleeding ended more quickly in the patients who received AT III concentrate compared with those who received a synthetic protease inhibitor FOY. Other successful reports of AT III concentrates associated with acquired AT III deficiency include hemolytic uremic syndrome, fatty liver of pregnancy, and chronic leg ulcers caused by sickle cell β-thalessemia. Only small numbers of patients have been included in these studies.[72–74]

AT III was not beneficial in a few clinical situations. Older observations suggested that heparin administration may cause adverse clinical effects in patients with AT III deficiency by reducing existing AT III levels and aggravating the hypercoagulable state. However, there is no apparent increased risk of thrombosis and no need for AT III replacement. A recent controlled trial of AT III supplementation in fulminant hepatic failure did not demonstrate improvement in laboratory markers of intravascular coagulation or survival.[75] Twenty-five patients in grade III or IV coma were selected based on evidence of sepsis and intravascular coagulation. Thirteen patients received AT III. The authors suggest that AT III be studied at an earlier stage of liver disease.

Acquired protein C and protein S deficiency are also seen in DIC, extensive deep vein thrombosis, severe liver disease, malignancy, after L-asparaginase therapy in leukemia.[76,77] In 1993, Dahlback et al.[78] characterized a hereditary defect in the plasma samples of three thrombophilic patients who gave a poor anticoagulant response to APC, an anticoagulant serine protease known to inactivate factors Va and VIIIa in plasma. This new defect may be present in 50 to 60 percent of thrombophilic patients previously undiagnosed. It is unknown whether an acquired deficiency of the new APC cofactor could be associated with an acquired risk of thrombosis in a variety of clinical settings.[79]

ANTIPHOSPHOLIPID SYNDROME

Lupus anticoagulants, anticardiolipin antibodies, the antiphospholipid syndrome, and the associated predisposition to thrombosis create difficulties in diagnosis and management. Recent evidence suggests that "antiphospholipid" autoantibodies are not directed against anionic phospholipids, as was previously thought, but are a part of a larger group of autoantibodies against certain phospholipid-binding proteins.[80] Thrombotic disease in these patients, as in all of the hypercoagulable states, should be managed with anticoagulant agents. Plasmapheresis and intravenous immunoglobulin have been used in patients with high titers of cardiolipin antibodies who present with diffuse acute noninflammatory visceral and peripheral vascular occlusion.[61]

THROMBOTIC THROMBOCYTOPENIC PURPURA

TTP is a multisystem disorder characterized by consumptive thrombocytopenia, microangiopathic hemolytic anemia, neurologic signs, and renal dysfunction. Two circulating platelet-aggregating activities have been described in patients. Murphy et al.[81] observed calpain (calcium-dependent cysteine protease) in sera from patients with TTP. Lian et al.[82] described another enzyme activity with different in vitro characteristics similar to a lysosomal cathepsin. Despite the uncertainty about the cause of TTP, the mortality and morbidity rates in this condition have improved dramatically in the past decade as a result of therapy with corticosteroids, plasma infusion, or a combination of plasma exchange with plasma infusion.[83,84] First-line treatment is now plasma exchange with large-volume FFP infusion. In some cases, cryoprecipitate-poor plasma is more effective than FFP.[85] A recent article showed no significant difference in response rate or survival between plasma infusion or plasma exchange, once again reviving this controversy.[86]

SUMMARY AND RECOMMENDATIONS

The inappropriate use of FFP has declined markedly over the past 5 years. Most transfusion medicine specialists still feel a stronger obligation to monitor FFP, factor concentrates, cryoprecipitate, and platelet usage compared with red blood cells.[87–91] It is comforting to know that studies have promulgated screening criteria to monitor FFP orders and documented the effectiveness of these programs in reducing unnecessary FFP transfusions.[92,93] FFP use

Table 18-7. Guidelines and Recommendations for Transfusion of Fresh Frozen Plasma and Other Blood Products

FFP is not indicated prophylactically in massive transfusion and cardiopulmonary bypass, to reverse heparin, for volume expansion, or as a nutritional supplement

FFP cannot correct the coagulation abnormalities associated with severe liver disease

One-unit FFP orders in adult patients are homeopathic and inappropriate.

For patients with factors XI, VII, V, protein C, protein S, and AT III deficiencies, transfuse FFP to maintain coagulation tests in the normal range.

To reverse the effect of warfarin immediately, transfuse FFP to normalize the PT; may require 3 or more units of FFP

To treat thrombotic thrombocytopenic purpura with plasma exchange, replace with FFP

FFP is not indicated prophylactically in patients without clinical evidence of active bleeding who have mild elevations of PT to 3 seconds above the upper limit of normal for line placements, removal of chest tubes, and other "open" procedures or surgery

FFP transfusion is probably not indicated prophylactically in patients with mild elevations of PT within 3 seconds of the upper limit of normal before liver biopsy.

There is no correlation between abnormal PTs and which patients will bleed after liver biopsy

The value of FFP in patients with active bleeding and severe liver disease is uncertain. If used, large volumes of FFP in excess of 5 units are probably necessary. A reasonable end point is to have the PT within 3 seconds of the upper limit of normal. Normalization of the PT is almost certainly not possible, and any improvement in PT will be reversed within hours.

The role of FFP transfusion in patients with liver disease undergoing liver surgery in the postsurgical period is uncertain. FFP should not be given prophylactically without laboratory studies. In general, patients should not receive FFP postoperatively unless the PT is greater than 3 seconds above the upper limit of normal or unless there is clinically active bleeding.

The only approved indication for AT III concentrates is hereditary deficiency of AT III.

AT III replacement may be valuable in severe DIC associated with low levels of AT III, but no controlled trials have proved its efficacy.

AT III replacement appears to be valuable in the coagulopathy associated with L-asparaginase therapy.

Abbreviations: FFP, fresh frozen plasma; PT, prothrombin time; AT III, antithrombin III; DIC, disseminated intravascular coagulation.

should be reviewed prospectively before issue of the blood component. Criteria should be developed by the transfusion committee for the blood bank physician to utilize in reviewing orders. When requests are received in the blood bank, personnel should review the patient's laboratory data and the request. If the request is within established criteria, the order can be processed immediately. If the criteria are not met, a blood bank physician should be asked to review the order, and a decision should be made based on consultation with the physician treating the patient. These procedures should apply to all clinical areas, including the operating room. If trends are established regarding inappropriate usage, the issue should be brought to the transfusion committee for discussion and the development of a plan of corrective action.

Despite the recent interest in clinical guidelines, clinical judgment remains an important aspect of medical care. Physicians must understand the risk of bleeding and feel comfortable not transfusing blood products. A reasonable set of recommendations is presented in Table 18-7.

REFERENCES

1. American Association of Blood Banks: Annual Reports 1979–1985. American Association of Blood Banks, Arlington, VA, 1986
2. American Association of Blood Banks: Annual Report 1991. American Association of Blood Banks, Arlington, VA, 1992
3. NIH Consensus Conference: Fresh frozen plasma. Indications and risks. JAMA 253:551, 1985
4. Surgenor DM, Wallace EL, Hale SG et al: Changing patterns of blood transfusions in four sets of United States hospitals 1980–1985. Transfusion 28:513, 1988
5. Horowitz B, Bonomo R, Prince AM et al: Solvent/de-

tergent-treated plasma: a virus-inactivated substitute for fresh frozen plasma. Blood 79:826, 1992

6. Amberson W: Blood substitutes. Biol Rev 12:48, 1937
7. Strumia MM, McGraw JJ: The development of plasma preparations for transfusions. Ann Intern Med 80:80, 1941
8. Graham J, Buckwalter J, Hartley L et al: Canine hemophilia: observations on the course, the clotting anomaly, and the effect of blood transfusions. J Exp Med 90:97, 1949
9. Crowley JP, Guadagnoli E, Pezzullo J et al: Changes in hospital component therapy in response to reduced availability of whole blood. Transfusion 28:4, 1988
10. Schmidt PJ: Red cells for transfusion. N Engl J Med 299:1411, 1978
11. Head DR: Whole blood versus packed cells. Transfusion 25:591, 1985
12. Kahn RA, Staggs SD, Miller WV et al: Use of plasma products with whole blood and packed RBCs. JAMA 242:2087, 1979
13. Shaikh BS, Wagar D, Lau PM et al: Transfusion pattern of fresh frozen plasma in a medical school hospital. Vox Sang 48:366, 1985
14. Snyder AJ, Gottschall JL, Menitoue JE: Why is fresh-frozen plasma transfused? Transfusion 26:107, 1986
15. Silbert JA, Bove JR, Dubin S et al: Patterns of fresh frozen plasma use. Conn Med 45:507, 1981
16. Blumberg N, Laczin J, McMican A et al: A critical survey of fresh-frozen plasma use. Transfusion 26:511, 1986
17. Bowie EJW, Thompson JH, Owen CA: The stability of antihemophilic globulin and labile factor in human blood. Mayo Clin Proc 39:144, 1964
18. Henderson R, Simon TL: Coagulation factor activity in platelet concentrates. Transfusion 19:186, 1979
19. Braunstein AH, Oberman HA: Transfusion of plasma components. Transfusion 24:281, 1984
20. Harke H, Rahman S: Coagulation disorders in massively injured patients. p. 213. In Collins JA, Murawski K, Shafer AW (eds): Massive Transfusion in Surgery and Trauma. Alan R. Liss, New York, 1982
21. Mannucci PM, Federici AB, Sirchia G: Hemostasis testing during massive blood replacement: a study of 172 cases. Vox Sang 42:113, 1982
22. Suchman AL, Griner PF: Diagnostic uses of the activated partial thromboplastin time and prothrombin time. Ann Intern Med 104:810, 1986
23. Dzik WH: Massive transfusion. p. 211. In Churchill WH, Kurtz SR (eds): Transfusion Medicine. Blackwell Scientific Publications, Oxford, 1988
24. Food and Drug Administration: FDA-Sponsored Conference on Viral Inactivation of Plasma. Washington, DC, March 29, 1994
25. Moake J, Chintagumpala M, Turner P et al: Solvent/detergent treated plasma suppresses shear-induced platelet aggregation and prevents episodes of thrombotic thrombocytopenia purpura. Blood 84:490, 1994
26. AuBuchon JP, Birkmeyer JD: Safety and cost-effectiveness of solvent-detergent-treated plasma: in search of a zero risk blood supply. JAMA 272:1210, 1994
27. Hoffman DL: Purification and large-scale preparation of antithrombin III. Am J Med, suppl 3B., 87:3B, 1989
28. Lechner K, Niessner H, Thaler E: Coagulation abnormalities in liver disease. Semin Thromb Hemost 4:40, 1977
29. Joist JH: Hemostatic abnormalities in liver disease. p. 861. In Coleman RW, Hirsh J, Marder VJ, Salzman EW (eds): Hemostasis and Thrombosis: Basic Principles and Clinical Practice. 2nd ed. JB Lippincott, Philadelphia, 1987
30. Blanchard RA, Furie BC, Jorgensen M et al: Acquired vitamin K-dependent carboxylation deficiency in liver disease. N Engl J Med 305:242, 1981
31. Soria J, Soria C, Samana M et al: Study of acquired dysfibrinogeniemia in liver disease. Thromb Res 19:29, 1980
32. Kemkes-Matthes B, Bleyl H, Matthes KS: Coagulation activation in liver disease. Thromb Res 64:25, 1991
33. Kario K, Matsuo T, Kodama K et al: Imbalance between thrombin and plasmin activity, disseminated intravascular coagulation. Hemostasis 22:179, 1992
34. Thomas DP, Ream VJ, Stuart RK: Platelet aggregation in patients with Laennec's cirrhosis of the liver. N Engl J Med 276:1344, 1967
35. Oberman HA: Appropriate use of plasma and plasma derivatives. p. 53. In Summers SH, Smith DM, Agranenko VA (eds): Transfusion Therapy: Guidelines for Practice. American Association of Blood Banks, Arlington, 1990
36. Mannucci PM, Franchi F, Dioguardi N: Correction of abnormal coagulation in chronic liver disease by combined use of fresh-frozen plasma and prothrombin complex concentrates. Lancet 2:542, 1976
37. Spector I, Corn M, Ticktin HE: Effect of plasma transfusion on the prothrombin time and clotting factors in liver disease. N Engl J Med 275:1032, 1966
38. Gazzard BG, Henderson JM, Williams R: The use of fresh frozen plasma or a concentrate of factor IX as replacement therapy before liver biopsy. Gut 16:621, 1975
39. Ewe K: Bleeding after liver biopsy does not correlate with indices of peripheral coagulation. Dig Dis Sci 26:388, 1981

40. Sherlock S: Needle biopsy of the liver. p. 36. In Sherlock S (ed): Diseases of the Liver and Biliary System. Blackwell Scientific Publications, Oxford, 1989

41. McVay PA, Toy PTCY: Lack of increased bleeding after liver biopsy in patients with mild hemostatic abnormalities. Am J Clin Pathol 94:747, 1990

42. Aghajanian A, Grimes DA: Routine prothrombin time determination before elective gynecologic operations. Obstet Gynecol 78:837, 1971

43. Littman JK, Brodman HR: Surgery in the presence of the therapeutic effect of dicumarol. Surg Gynecol Obstet 101:709, 1955

44. Ro JS: Hemostatic problems in liver surgery. Scand J Gastroenterol, suppl. 19, 8:71, 1973

45. Tsuzuki T, Toyama K, Nakaysu K et al: Disseminated intravascular coagulation after hepatic resection. Surgery 107:172, 1990

46. Iwatsuki S, Shaw BW, Starzl TE: Experience with 150 liver resections. Ann Surg 197:247, 1983

47. Scholmerich P, Zimmermann U, Kottgen E et al: Proteases and antiproteases related to the coagulation system in plasma and ascites. Prediction of coagulation disorders in ascites retransfusion. J Hepatol 6:359, 1988

48. Salem HH, Koutts J, Handley C et al: The aggregation of human platelets by ascitic fluid: a possible mechanism for disseminated intravascular coagulation complicating LeVeen shunts. Am J Hematol 11:153, 1981

49. Lipsky JJ: Nutritional sources of vitamin K. Mayo Clinic Proc 69:462, 1994

50. Suttie JW, Mumah-Schendel LL, Shah DV et al: Vitamin K deficiency from vitamin K restriction in humans. Am J Clin Nutr 47:475, 1988

51. Shearer MJ, Bechtold H, Andrassy K et al: Mechanism of cephalosporin-induced hypoprothrombinemia: relation to cephalosporin side chain vitamin K metabolism and vitamin K status. J Clin Pharmacol 28:88, 1988

52. Alperin JB: Coagulopathy caused by vitamin K deficiency in critically ill, hospital patients. JAMA 258:1916, 1987

53. Lipsky JJ: Antibiotic-associated hypothrombinemia. J Antimicrob Chemother 21:281, 1988

54. Hirsh J: Oral anticoagulant drugs. N Engl J Med 324:1865, 1991

55. Furie B, Furie BC: Molecular and cellular biology of blood coagulation. N Engl J Med 326:800, 1992

56. Pelzer H, Schwartz A, Stuber W: Determination of human prothrombin activation fragment 1 + 2 in plasma with an antibody against a synthetic polypeptide. Thromb Haemost 65:153, 1991

57. Nossel HL, Yudelman I, Canfield RE et al: Measure-ment of fibrinopeptide A in human blood. J Clin Invest 54:43, 1974

58. Bick RL, Baker WF: Disseminated intravascular coagulation. Hematol Pathol 6:1, 1992

59. Hoak HL, Stolk JC, Graatama JW et al: Use of antithrombin III concentrate in stable diffuse intravascular coagulation. Acta Haematol 68:28, 1992

60. Bick RL: Disseminated intravascular coagulation. Hematol Oncol Clin North Am 6:1259, 1992

61. Nachman RL, Silverstein R: Hypercoagulable states. Ann Intern Med 119:819, 1993

62. Tornebohm E, Blomback M, Lockner D: Bleeding complications and coagulopathy in acute leukemia. Leuk Res 16:1041, 1992

63. Zurborn KH, Kirch W, Bruhn HD: Immunological and functional determination of the protease inhibitors, protein C and antithrombin III in liver cirrhosis and in neoplasia. Thromb Res 52:325, 1988

64. Jimenez RA, Jimenez E, Ingram GIC et al: Antithrombin activities in childhood malnutrition. J Clin Pathol 32:1025, 1979

65. Elidrissy ATH, Gader AMA: Antithrombin III (AT III) and fibrinogen levels in nephrotic syndrome in children. Haemostasis 15:388, 1985

66. Mammen E: Oral contraceptives and blood coagulation. A critical review. Am J Obstet Gynecol 142:781, 1992

67. Mazzucconi MG, Gugliotta L, Leone G et al: Antithrombin III infusion suppresses the hypercoagulable state in adult patients treated with a low dose of Escherichia coli L-asparaginase. A GIMEMA study. Blood Coagul Fibrinolysis 5:23, 1994

68. Francis CW, Pelleginini VD, Harris CM: Prophylaxis of venous thrombosis following total hip and total knee replacement using antithrombin III and heparin. Semin Hematol 28:39, 1991

69. Buller HR, ten Cate JW: Antithrombin III infusion in patients undergoing peritoneovenous shunt operation: failure in the prevention of disseminated intravascular coagulation. Thromb Haemost 49:128, 1983

70. Blauhut B, Necek S, Vinazzer H et al: Substitution therapy with an antithrombin III concentrate in shock and DIC. Thromb Res 27:271, 1982

71. Maki M, Terao T, Ikenoue T et al: Clinical evaluation of antithrombin III concentrate (BI 6.013) for disseminated intravascular coagulation in obstetrics. Gynecol Invest 23:230, 1987

72. Brandt P, Jespersen J, Gregersen G: Postpartum haemolytic-uraemic syndrome successfully treated with antithrombin III. BMJ 1:449, 1980

73. Laursen B, Mortensen JZ, Frost L et al: Disseminated

intravascular coagulation in hepatic failure treated with antithrombin III. Thromb Res 22:701, 1981

74. Cacciola E, Giustolisi R, Musso R et al: Antithrombin III concentrate for treatment of chronic leg ulcers in sickle cell-beta thalassemia: a pilot study. Ann Intern Med 111:534, 1989

75. Langley PG, Hughes RA, Keays R: Controlled trial of antithrombin III supplementation in fulminant hepatic failure. J Hepatol 17:326, 1993

76. D'Angelo A, Vigano S, Esman CT et al: Acquired deficiencies of protein S. J Clin Invest 81:1445, 1988

77. Griffin JH, Mosher DF, Zimmerman TS et al: Protein C, an antithrombotic protein, is reduced in hospitalized patients with intravascular coagulation. Blood 60:261, 1982

78. Dahlback B, Carlsson M, Svensson PJ: Familial thrombophilia due to a previously unrecognized mechanism characterized by poor anticoagulant response to activated protein C: predication of a cofactor to activated protein C. Proc Natl Acad Sci U S A 90:1004, 1993

79. Griffin JH, Evatt B, Wideman C et al: Anticoagulant protein C pathway defective in majority of thrombophilic patients. Blood 82:1989, 1993

80. Roubey RAS: Autoantibodies to phospholipid-binding plasma proteins: a new view of lupus anticoagulants and other "antiphospholipid" autoantibodies. Blood 84:2854, 1994

81. Murphy WG, Moore JC, Kelton JG: Calcium dependent cystein protease activity in the sera of patients with thrombotic thrombocytopenic purpura. Blood 70:1603, 1987

82. Lian ECY, Harkness DR, Byrnes JJ et al: Presence of a platelet aggregating factor in the plasma of patients with thrombocytopenic purpura (TTP) and its inhibition by normal plasma. Blood 53:333, 1979

83. Rock GA, Shumak KH, Buskard NA et al: Comparison of plasma exchange with plasma infusion in the treatment of thrombotic thrombocytopenic purpura. N Engl J Med 325:393, 1991

84. Bell WR, Braine HG, Ness PM, Kickler TS: Improved survival in thrombotic thrombocytopenic purpura-hemolytic uremic syndrome. N Engl J Med 325:398, 1991

85. Byrnes JJ, Moake JL, Klug P, Periman P: Effectiveness of the cryosupernatant fraction of plasma in the treatment of refractory thrombotic thrombocytopenic purpura. Am J Hematol 34:169, 1990

86. Novitzky N, Jacobs P, Rosenstrauch W: The treatment of thrombocytopenic purpura: plasma infusion or exchange. Br J Haemol 87:317, 1994

87. Kurtz SR, Summers SH, Kruskall MS (eds): Improving Transfusion Practice: The Role of Quality Assurance. American Association of Blood Banks, Arlington, 1989

88. Coffin C, Matz K, Rich E: Algorithms for evaluating the appropriateness of blood transfusion. Transfusion 29:298, 1989

89. Mozes B, Epstein M, Ben-Bassat I et al: Evaluation of the appropriateness of blood and blood product transfusion using preset criteria. Transfusion 29:473, 1989

90. Giovanetti AM, Parravicini A, Baroni L et al: Quality assessment of transfusion practice in elective surgery. 28:166, 1988

91. American College of Physicians: Practice strategies for elective red blood cell transfusions. Ann Intern Med 116:403, 1992

92. Solomon RR, Clifford JS, Gutman SI: The role of laboratory intervention to stem the flow of fresh-frozen plasma. Am J Clin Pathol 89:518, 1988

93. Shanberge JN: Reduction of fresh-frozen plasma use through a daily survey and education program. Transfusion 27:226, 1987

Chapter 19

Transfusion Therapy for Chronic Anemic States

Scott N. Swisher and Lawrence D. Petz

Chronic anemia of variable severity is associated with a wide range of illnesses; it is therefore a problem that frequently confronts the clinician. In many instances, the associated anemia is insignificant because of adequate compensatory physiologic adjustments. In these situations, it is more important to understand the pathogenesis of the anemic state than it is to correct it per se; clarification of the cause of the anemia may disclose the presence of a serious and potentially treatable underlying disorder, such as an occult tumor or chronic infection. Anemia is no longer an acceptable diagnosis. It is the cause of the anemia that is important for the rational management of the anemic patient.

Similarly, the appropriate treatment of chronically anemic patients varies widely; elimination or control of an underlying disease leads all strategies in importance and effectiveness. Where this is not possible, replacement of substances necessary for hematopoiesis, such as vitamin B_{12}, folic acid, and iron or of blood itself by transfusion, is a secondary strategy of therapy, again of variable effectiveness. Replacement of vitamin B_{12}, folic acid, or iron deficiencies is effective only if there is significant lack of the specific substance and in the absence of other mechanisms that will suppress normal hematopoiesis. Transfusion, particularly chronic transfusion, then becomes a strategy of final resort in the management of patients with chronic anemia.

Chronic transfusion may be a lifelong commitment in many patients. It frequently leads to a number of hazardous complications, including some that are life-threatening. At times, these patients become effectively untransfusable. The decision to transfuse chronically is therefore of great importance. It is usually much to be preferred to have the patient somewhat limited and symptomatic than exposed to the risks of chronic transfusion.

This chapter deals with a broad group of disorders, listed in Table 19-1, that share a number of common problems related to transfusion therapy. It is important to integrate transfusion therapy in a thoughtful way into the program of management of patients with these disorders. The discussion here is based on some general principles, pertinent to all these disorders, followed by comments on the transfusion problems encountered in the specific diseases listed in Tables 19-1 and 19-2.

ASSESSMENT OF THE ANEMIC PATIENT

Three kinds of information are usually available for assessment of the anemic patient: (1) laboratory measurements of levels of hemoglobin and/or hematocrit, (2) evaluation of the patient's symptoms, and (3) physiologic assessments of the patient's functional capacities. The first of these is clearly the most objective, but it may not be the most informative

Table 19-1. Chronic Anemic States That May Require Chronic Transfusion Therapy[a]

Hypoproliferative anemias
    Hypoplastic or aplastic states of unknown cause
        With pancytopenia
        Pure red cell aplasia
    Drug- or chemical-induced hypoplastic or aplastic disorders
    Radiation-induced marrow destruction
    Marrow destruction secondary to myelofibrosis or myelophthisic processes
    Aplastic or hypoplastic phase of paroxysmal nocturnal hemolytic anemia
Chronic dysplastic disorders of the bone marrow
    Preleukemic-states
    Sideroblastic anemias not due to pyridoxine deficiency
    Congenital dyserythropoietic anemias
    Congenital hyporegenerative disorders of bone marrow
        Fanconi syndrome ("constitutional aplastic anemia")
        Diamond-Blackfan syndrome of congenital red cell aplasia
Anemias of chronic disease; anemia associated with
    Renal failure unresponsive to erythropoietin, or when this therapy is unavailable
    Chronic inflammation
    Hepatic failure
    Malignant tumors
    Endocrine failures
Anemia due to chronic blood loss uncontrolled by iron therapy
    Hereditary hemorrhagic telangiectasia
    Chronic gastrointestinal blood loss of multiple causes
    Chronic uterine blood loss of multiple causes
    Iron deficiency with associated marrow hyporegeneration

[a] Not included are the major congenital and acquired hemolytic disorders or anemias associated with malignant diseases, which are dealt with elsewhere in this book.

Table 19-2. Other Acute or Chronic Anemic States in Which Transfusion Therapy is Required Only Under Exceptional Circumstances

Anemias of nutritional deficiency
    Megaloblastic anemias
        Vitamin B_{12} deficiency
        Folic acid deficiency
    Chronic severe malnutrition
Hemolytic anemias[a]
    Microangiopathic hemolytic disorders
    Hemolytic-uremic syndrome
    Traumatic cardiac hemolytic anemia
    Hemolytic anemia due to chemical or physical agents
    Hemolytic anemia secondary to infection
    Hemolytic anemia associated with hypersplenism
Anemia associated with pregnancy and delivery
    Megaloblastic anemia of pregnancy
    Postpartum anemia

[a] Not included are major congenital and acquired hemolytic states, anemia associated with malignant disease, or acute blood loss dealt with elsewhere in this book.

for making decisions about the need for transfusion. The latter two are less objective and are more likely to be influenced by such factors as the rapidity of onset of anemia, the presence of other physiologic abnormalities (e.g., fever or cardiovascular or pulmonary disease), and the nature of the patient's underlying illness. Nevertheless, these data are probably of greater value in determining the need for red cell transfusion than are the measurements of hemoglobin and hematocrit. Once an unacceptable level of physiologic impairment due to anemia has been associated with a specific level of hemoglobin or hematocrit, the value of these laboratory measurements increases as guidelines for the management of future transfusion schedules. Evaluation of the need for transfusion in a given patient is therefore a sophisticated, clinically based process of decision that requires skilled interviewing, refined physical examination, and, at times, physiologic testing. It should rarely be based upon measurements of hemoglobin and hematocrit alone.

Hemoglobin and Hematocrit Levels and Red Cell Mass

Hemoglobin and hematocrit levels nevertheless do provide a general indication of the probability of significant physiologic impairment of a patient. A physician conservative in the use of transfusion might employ the guidelines shown in Table 19-3. These guidelines are consistent with recommendations for elective red blood cell transfusion that have been published by others.[1-3]

Although hemoglobin and hematocrit are the usually available laboratory measurements for the assessment of anemia, they are useful because they are relatively highly correlated with the patient's red cell mass.[4] It is red cell mass that is of greater physiologic significance rather than the blood's concentration of

Table 19-3.   Guidelines for Assessing Physiological Impairment of the Anemic Patient and Prescribing Transfusion Strategy

Average Hemoglobin Level (g/dl)	Probability of Significant Impairment	Transfusion Strategy
≥10	Very low	Avoid
8–10	Low	Avoid; transfuse only if demonstrably better after transfusion trial
6–8	Moderate	Try to avoid by decreased activity; if impossible, transfuse
≤6	High	Frequently requires transfusion

hemoglobin. Situations in which the red cell mass is lower or higher than would be indicated by the hematocrit are usually recognizable clinically. These are situations in which the plasma volume is reduced as in "stress" polycythemia or excessive diuresis or dehydration, in which case the hematocrit will be higher in relation to red cell mass than is normal. Conversely, states of hydremia associated with intravascular fluid retention, as in the last trimester of pregnancy, will have a lower hematocrit, even in the presence of a normal red cell mass.

Red blood cell mass or plasma volume can be measured by radioisotopic methods employing ^{51}Cr-labeled red cells or radio-iodinated serum albumin.[5] These measurements are rarely necessary in the clinical setting where transfusion is under consideration. Even in marked states of hydremia of pregnancy, the normal red cell mass is infrequently diluted to a hematocrit of less than 30 percent. In situations in which a patient's red cell mass is in fact reduced, hydremia or loss of plasma volume will confuse the evaluation of the severity of anemia by the hematocrit. This may be a significant difficulty. A comprehensive evaluation of the patient will usually provide the information needed to estimate the true state of the red cell mass. In rare instances, direct measurements of red cell mass may be of value.[5]

In situations of acute blood loss, the hemoglobin concentration and hematocrit are recognized to be unreliable guides to the size of the red cell mass. The correlation between these measurements and

red cell mass will not be reestablished until the blood volume has again stabilized and the red cell mass deficit has been replaced by additional plasma. This may require 24 to 48 hours or more after an acute blood loss, depending on the availability of fluid and other physiologic factors.

Virtually by definition, this problem does not occur in chronic anemic states in which a relatively stable blood volume is usually present, and the hemoglobin concentration and hematocrit reasonably and usefully reflect the size of the red cell mass. Wiesen et al.[6] have pointed out that there are scant data supporting the concept that equilibration of hemoglobin concentration requires 24 hours after red cell transfusion in stable medical patients. These investigators studied 46 adult patients who received a 2-unit transfusion and determined the subsequent hemoglobin concentration at 15 minutes, 2 hours, and 24 hours after the end of the transfusion. These workers found that the hemoglobin level 15 minutes after transfusion was nearly identical to the 24-hour level in patients not actively bleeding. It was concluded that each unit of packed erythrocytes increases the hemoglobin level an average of 1 g/dl and that hemoglobin measurements made 15 minutes after transfusion reflect steady-state values. These conclusions are consistent with the data of Greenfield et al.,[7] who showed that after large-volume saline infusions, most excess fluid is eliminated from the intravascular space in minutes.

The need for chronic transfusion and the level of hemoglobin that should be maintained are greatly influenced by the level of the patient's activity. Younger people who are strenuously active in daily living or employment may require higher levels of hemoglobin if they are unable or unwilling to reduce this level of activity; conversely, they usually have the greatest capacity for physiologic compensation of anemia in the absence of significant cardiovascular or pulmonary disease. Sedentary people may require less transfusion, but there is substantial patient-to-patient variation. These factors strongly influence the decision to transfuse or not and the level of hemoglobin that should be maintained in the patients who are given blood.

The first step in the decision process is to determine the minimum level of hemoglobin at which the patient can function satisfactorily. This decision should not be made by the physician alone. The various risks, costs, and inconveniences of transfusion and its avoidance should be explained. The patient's feelings should strongly influence the physician's ultimate recommendations for a program of management. Availability of transfusion facilities, blood, and costs involved are other important but secondary factors in the decision.

Evaluation of Symptoms

The most important pieces of historical information from the anemic patient are those related to the level of activity that can be sustained and what happens when this level is exceeded. If other factors that limit functional capacity coexist, it may be difficult or impossible to untangle those symptoms due primarily to anemia. In general, the most informative data are those that demonstrate the level of cardiorespiratory compensation evoked by exertion in the anemic state.

It is important that these questions be asked in an open-ended, nonleading way. Initial questions, such as "What are your physical activities at present?," "What happens if you climb two flights of stairs rapidly?," or "What happens when you exert yourself?," do not lead the patient into an expected answer or focus attention on a specific system. An initial question, such as "Do you become short of breath and have to stop when you try to climb two flights of stairs rapidly?," suggests that these are the symptoms of interest to the physician. The patient then might or might not reveal personal observations about a pounding heart or chest pain caused by the exertion. More specific questions such as the latter can be asked appropriately after such patients have had an opportunity to tell of their own observations as they see and evaluate them.[8]

Specificity of Symptoms

A number of other symptoms are traditionally associated with anemia both by physicians and by the public. They are very much less specific for anemia and may not be statistically associated with anemia in large populations until levels of hemoglobin lower than 7 to 8 g/dl have developed. At this point, significant cardiovascular changes may be evoked. Elwood et al.[9] studied the symptoms of irritability, palpitation, dizziness, breathlessness, fatigue, and head-

ache in a population of iron-deficient women in England with hemoglobin levels of 8 to 12 g/dl after effective iron therapy and placebo treatment. No evidence was found to support a significant relationship of these symptoms to iron deficiency or the associated anemia. Other studies have reached similar conclusions.[10,11]

These results corroborate the views of experienced clinicians who recognize the nonspecific nature of many of these symptoms because of their daily contacts with patients. The frequency of a symptom such as fatigue alone, estimated to be present in more than 90 percent of patients consulting a general internist for all causes in one study, documents its lack of specificity (L.A. Kohn, unpublished observations). Psychological mechanisms may be responsible for many of these symptoms. Elwood obtained some data to suggest that the six symptoms they evaluated were more clearly related to "neurotic" phenomena than to hemoglobin level.[9] These data and common experience indicate that it is no simple task to evaluate the symptoms presented by the anemic patient in terms of the need for transfusion. Nevertheless, these data are among the most important in making the required decisions.

Physiologic Compensations for Anemia and Their Evaluation

The physiologic adjustments caused by acute blood loss (i.e., acute anemia) are mainly due to an acutely decreased blood volume. By contrast, the blood volume of the chronically anemic patient is normal or only moderately and slowly decreased in most instances. These two circumstances evoke different physiologic adjustments. Three principal adjustments are caused by chronic anemia: (1) shift of the hemoglobin–oxygen dissociation curve, (2) cardiovascular compensations, and (3) respiratory compensations.

Shift of the Hemoglobin–Oxygen Dissociation Curve

In order to transport an equivalent volume of oxygen, the cardiac index (cardiac output in liters per minute per meter squared [$L/m/m^2$] of body surface area) would have to rise in inverse proportion to the level of blood hemoglobin if no other compensations occurred. In most states of chronic anemia, however, there is an increase in oxygen abstraction from the

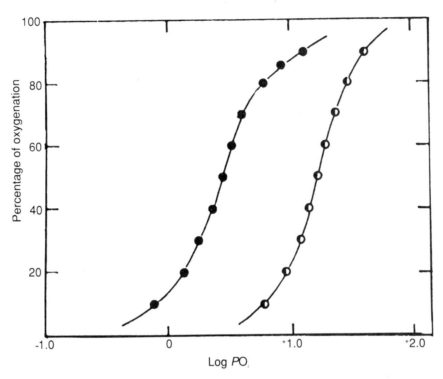

Fig. 19-1. Comparison of oxygenation curves of hemoglobin and whole blood: ●, 0.3 percent "stripped" hemoglobin in 0.01 M NaCl at 30°C, pH 7.0 (before deoxygenation); ○, whole blood at 30°C. (From Harris and Kellermeyer,[12] with permission.)

blood as it passes through the low-oxygen tension areas of the systemic microcirculation. That is, a larger proportion of the oxygen being transported bound to hemoglobin is released in these areas. This is accomplished by shifting the oxygen dissociation curve (oxygen tension plotted against hemoglobin saturation) to the right[12] (Fig. 19-1). This means that, at a given level of oxygen tension in the tissue that is lower than that in the lung capillaries and pulmonary arteries, more oxygen is removed from 1 g of hemoglobin in chronically anemic blood than would be the case with 1 g of hemoglobin from normal blood. This remarkable effect is due to the role of intracellular erythrocyte 2,3-diphosphoglycerate (2,3-DPG), an intermediate of red cell glucose metabolism, in controlling the position of the oxygen dissociation curve. Binding of oxygen to hemoglobin within the red cell involves the formation of a complex of oxygen, hemoglobin, and 2,3-DPG, with the latter having the effect of decreasing the hemoglobin

affinity for oxygen; the affinity of hemoglobin for oxygen is thus inversely related to the red cell concentration of 2,3-DPG. The precise mechanism by which the compensatory rise in 2,3-DPG occurs is unclear; it may be due to intracellular alkalosis.[13–18] The effect may be responsible for a substantial part of the overall adjustment in oxygen transport that results in a major saving of cardiac work.[19,20] Metabolic disorders such as diabetic ketoacidosis reduce the red cell 2,3-DPG concentration and may influence oxygen transport unfavorably in the patient who is also chronically anemic. Other disorders characterized by hypoxemia, such as high-altitude adaptation and anoxia due to lung or heart disease, also result in a rise in red cell 2,3-DPG concentration. Blood pH also influences the position of the oxygen dissociation curve by the Bohr effect (Fig. 19-2). Lower pH decreases oxygen affinity, whereas a higher pH within the physiologic range increases oxygen binding. These changes partially offset the in-

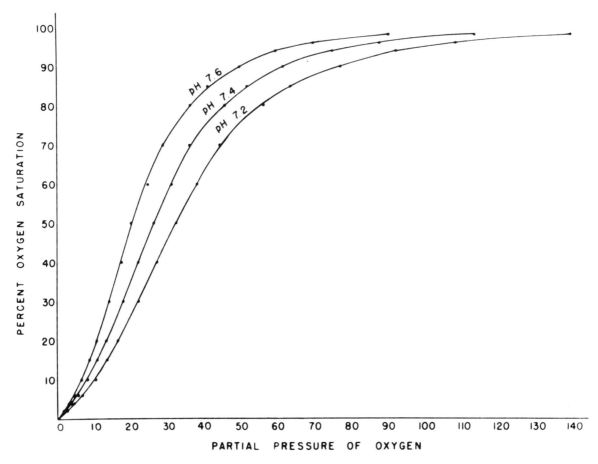

Fig. 19-2. Oxygen dissociation curves of human hemoglobin at various pH values. (From Harris and Kellermeyer,[12] with permission.)

creased oxygen affinity associated with 2,3-DPG depletion in the presence of ketoacidosis.[21]

In spite of an apparently important role in adapting certain patients to states of chronic anemia, the value of transfusing red cells with high 2,3-DPG (as compared with stored erythrocytes, in which this compound has been depleted) has not been convincingly demonstrated. Some 2,3-DPG is regenerated within hours of transfusing stored depleted red cells, and it is virtually normal in concentration after 24 hours. It is clear that the concentration of blood hemoglobin, and thus oxygen-carrying capacity is of greater physiologic importance than is 2,3-DPG level in correcting the oxygen transport deficits of anemic patients. Thus, it is rarely justified to use

fresh blood with high 2,3-DPG levels for transfusing anemic patients.

Cardiovascular Compensations

Increased cardiac output is the other major mechanism of compensation for severe anemia. Both stroke volume and cardiac rate increase, with the former predominating.[22,23] Significant cardiovascular compensation is not evoked until the hemoglobin level has decreased about one-half that in otherwise normal persons. Exercise increases cardiovascular compensations that may be minimal in the resting state.

If symptoms and findings of congestive heart failure occur with levels of hemoglobin of around 7 g/

dl or higher, it is almost always due to associated intrinsic heart disease—most frequently coronary artery disease or hypertensive heart disease.[24–28] Coronary circulation is increased in the normal heart as the left ventricular work load rises. In severe anemia, however, with hemoglobin levels of less than 5 g/dl, coronary blood flow may become relatively inadequate, and ventricular function is decreased. This may lead to congestive heart failure with decreased renal blood flow and sodium retention.[29]

Clinical assessment of the adequacy of cardiovascular compensations for anemia rarely needs to go beyond standard clinical techniques. Careful evaluation of the patient's history regarding exercise tolerance, anginal pain, or other chest discomfort, edema, dyspnea, and orthopnea, is of great importance. The main observations of importance in the physical examination are heart rate, cardiac rhythm, precordial activity, heart size, venous pressure, presence or absence of hepatojugular reflux, pulmonary rales, and peripheral edema. Systolic flow murmurs are not uncommon in anemic patients; their importance lies in differentiating them from murmurs of valvular or other origin. Gallop rhythms of the S_3 or S_4 type may be heard and raise the question of early onset of cardiac decompensation. The blood pressure may show a wide pulse pressure, and the pulse may be bounding; peripheral resistance is usually decreased in chronic anemia in contrast to its increase in acute blood loss.[30]

At times, electrocardiography (ECG), including stress tests, may be useful in evaluating these patients. Chest radiographs may also be useful, and a wide range of the present-day noninvasive diagnostic technology will be useful on occasion. These procedures are usually directed toward assessment of the nature and extent of underlying heart disease, rather than the effects of anemia itself on the heart.

The importance of detecting early cardiac failure is twofold: a transfusion may increase blood volume rapidly and precipitate acute pulmonary edema[27]; if the patient is severely anemic, heart failure may signal the need for increased amounts of transfusion to reduce the need for cardiac work and improve the patient's state of compensation. Other appropriate measures for control of congestive failure should also be employed. The anemic patient in congestive heart failure requires transfusion with sedimented red cells at very slow rates.

Studies of the cardiovascular status of anemic surgical patients may be relevant in indicating the risk of anemia in medical patients with cardiovascular disease. Nelson et al.[31] reported that morbid cardiac events (cardiac death, myocardial infaction, unstable angina, and ischemic pulmonary edema) occurred more frequently in patients having surgery with a hematocrit of less than 28 percent than in those with a hematocrit above this level. Ten of 13 high-risk patients undergoing infrainguinal arterial bypass procedures with a hematocrit of less than 28 percent sustained a morbid cardiac event, whereas only 2 of 14 did so with a hematocrit of greater than 28 percent. Similarly, Christopherson et al.[32] reported that when the incidence of cardiac ischemia in a 3-day postoperative period was plotted as a function of the hematocrit on postoperative day 2, those with hematocrits of less than 29 percent had a high incidence of cardiac ischemia (55 percent), while those with hematocrits of greater than 29 percent had a much lower incidence (16 percent, $P = 0.01$).

These findings emphasize that severe anemia may result in significant risk in patients with cardiovascular disease. Optimal management of patients' transfusion needs involves therapeutic intervention prior to evidence of physiologic decompensation, not afterward. Thus, some margin of safety is desirable in planning transfusion needs.[33] Clinical judgment must prevail, as the remarkable safety of the blood supply makes it unlikely that a statistically valid study could be designed to demonstrate the comparative safety of transfusing versus not transfusing in a variety of clinical settings[34] (see Ch. 7).

Respiratory Compensation

Changes in pulmonary function generally occur in parallel with those of the cardiovascular system. The respiratory rate and depth may be increased with a rise in minute volume. The arterial oxygen tension may be reduced with an increased oxygen gradient to alveolar air. There is usually decreased maximal oxygen uptake, but this does not reflect abnormal lung function. Anemic subjects incur a higher oxygen debt at a given work load as compared with nonanemic persons.[18,35,36] These observations indicate that all compensations available for anemia are unable to transport the oxygen required for work loads above a certain level and that the compensations themselves impose a significant work load.[37]

Any limitation of respiratory function—particularly those disorders that decrease maximum ventilation or decrease gas diffusion between alveoli and lung capillaries—will limit the effectiveness of the integrated compensations for anemia. Again, clinical techniques of evaluation of respiratory function are usually adequate for assessment of the average anemic patient. Arterial blood gas measurements along with spirometry may be useful when there is some uncertainty about a patient's pulmonary function. When there are clear-cut abnormalities, a more complete pulmonary function study may be in order (see Ch. 21).

STRATEGY OF CHRONIC TRANSFUSION THERAPY

Accurate periodic assessments of chronically anemic patients are critical in making the decision to transfuse them and deciding how much blood to administer. One must differentiate between tolerable levels of physiologic compensation, particularly those of the cardiovascular system, and excessive requirements for compensation that the patient is unable to maintain within reasonable physiologic costs. The existence of intrinsic cardiovascular or pulmonary disease frequently limits these compensations. Such patients usually require institution of chronic transfusion therapy at higher levels of hemoglobin than do patients without these limitations for a given level of activity. Requirements for transfusion may be increased by lifestyles that involve high levels of exertion if the level of activity cannot be reduced. The coexistence of many other diseases may also limit the effectiveness of the compensatory mechanisms; these diseases must be factored into the decisions about transfusion. The aim of a transfusion program should be to reduce the requirement for compensation to a tolerable point, not to remove the need for all compensation. The least amount of blood required to accomplish this is the proper amount.

There is an unfortunate tendency to overtransfuse many chronically anemic patients who do require blood and to transfuse patients who are adequately adjusted to living with a low hematocrit. This is often done with the laudable goal of "making the patient feel better" and with inadequate recognition of the hazards and inconvenience of long-term transfusion. It is important that transfusions meet the patient's real needs, not the physician's concepts of what those needs should be. It is usually better for the patient to live with even significant symptoms or limitations than to face the hazards of lifelong transfusion.

Transfusion Schedules

If the decision has been made to institute chronic transfusion, the initial several months of this program should be regarded as a therapeutic trial. The patient should be evaluated carefully and frequently to determine whether the desired effects are being obtained. The level of hemoglobin or hematocrit that adequately reduces the undesirable effects of chronic anemia can usually be determined within 3 months, and the amount of blood required to maintain this level can be approximated. The goal is to minimize variations in the hematocrit around a target level while administering the least amount of blood needed to do this.

After these factors have been determined, it is nearly always better long-term strategy to schedule transfusion at regular intervals than to follow the hematocrit with transfusion after it reaches a predetermined level. Scheduled transfusions usually result in a higher average hematocrit with less administered blood and avoid the oscillations frequently encountered when the hematocrit is being "chased." Regular scheduled transfusions are generally better integrated into the patient's pattern of daily living, as they can be planned in advance. They reduce the need for medical or laboratory visits. When the patient is transfused on indication of a low hematocrit, visits to the laboratory and then to the physician are required if the decision to give blood is to be made. Often a second visit to a transfusion facility must be made to receive the transfusion.

Transfusion of the patient on the basis of the recurrence of symptoms is usually quite unsuccessful. Wide swings of hematocrit values usually occur. The hematocrit is usually well below the target level when unacceptable symptoms occur, and a number of transfusions may be required over several days to restore an adequate red cell mass. This strategy has little to be said for it, except possibly in those few patients whose need for transfusion is relatively unpredictable. Even in these patients, periodic surveillance of the hematocrit level may be preferable, with transfusion at a predetermined low level.

Two variables can be manipulated to achieve the best results of chronic transfusion: the amount of blood administered, and the interval between transfusions. Most patients are able to receive 2 units of red blood cells at one sitting. The circulatory volume increase is usually tolerable, and the time required for infusion is not excessive. As a reference point and general rule of thumb, it can be calculated that a requirement for 2 units of red cells every 2 weeks in an average adult reflects the situation encountered with essentially total failure of red cell production. More frequent weekly transfusions of 1 unit might result in a reduction in the variations of the hematocrit value but at the cost of greater inconvenience for the patient. Thus, it is reasonable policy to transfuse 2 units at a time to most patients and to determine the interval between transfusion on the basis of the total need for blood. In the absence of blood loss, alloimmunization, or other causes of inefficient transfusion, this usually results in an interval of 2 to 4 weeks between transfusions.

Inefficient Transfusions

Transfusion requirements above the level of about 2 units every 2 weeks in an adult suggest inefficiency of the transfusion for one or more reasons. The expected rise in hematocrit value following a transfusion should be calculated; if it is not met, further evidence of inefficient transfusion is present. Does the patient have an occult alloimmunization to a red cell antigen, with destruction of the transfused erythrocytes at an increased rate, but not so rapidly as to result in an overt hemolytic transfusion reaction? Unfortunately, in some instances, donor red cells are destroyed without serologic evidences of donor–recipient incompatibility (see Ch. 9). Investigations of this type are in the domain of a sophisticated transfusion service and laboratory, but the clinician caring for the patient is responsible for determining that a problem may be present and for obtaining the necessary consultative help.

Before beginning a program of chronic transfusion, one should consider extended phenotyping of the patient's red cells. These data may be useful in

the search for suspected alloimmunization in that they limit to some extent the possibilities to be looked for and may suggest the most probable antigenic responses.[38] Extended typing is more difficult after transfusion has begun because donor and recipient cells are then admixed. Storage of a pretransfusion specimen of the donor's red cells in the frozen state should be considered where possible.

Since at least 70 percent of patients who are chronically transfused do not develop clinically significant red cell alloantibodies, prophylactic extended antigen matching prior to any evidence of alloantibody production may not the the optimal transfusion policy. A reasonable alternative approach is the provision of blood selected to match the patient's phenotype only after an initial antibody becomes detectable[39] (see Ch. 32).

The presence of autoimmune acquired hemolytic anemia of the warm autoantibody type may also account for increased blood requirements and inefficient transfusion. This disorder may develop insidiously, particularly in patients with an underlying neoplastic disease of the lymphoreticular system or another autoimmune disorder. Usually, but not in all instances, the direct red cell antiglobulin test will be positive for either IgG or complement components, or both. Again, the assistance of a sophisticated transfusion service, transfusion reference laboratory, or general immunodiagnostic laboratory will frequently be needed to define this problem adequately before further transfusion therapy can proceed (see Ch. 20).

Occult or overt blood loss from the gastrointestinal tract or other sources may be another cause of an apparently inefficient transfusion and may result in an increased requirement for blood. Appropriate investigation of these possibilities should be carried out, particularly if the requirement for blood increases suddenly. This is most likely to occur in patients who also have thrombocytopenia in association with generalized bone marrow failure.

Nonimmunologic mechanisms of hemolysis secondary to splenic enlargement, so-called hypersplenism, may be responsible for high transfusion requirements. This can usually be evaluated on clinical grounds alone. The existence of portal hypertension or substantial splenomegaly of any cause may be a diagnostic clue in this direction. Preferential localization of ^{51}Cr-labeled red cells in the spleen may corroborate this diagnostic suspicion. Hypersplenic destruction of red cells rarely occurs in the absence of significantly enlarged and easily palpable spleen.

Coincident blood loss or hemolysis should be suspected, particularly if the patient has some evidence of blood regeneration, even though this is inadequate to meet red cell needs. Some degree of persistent or increasing reticulocytosis in the face of a requirement for transfusion that is compatible with total red cell aplasia may suggest one or more of these possibilities.

RISKS AND BENEFITS OF CHRONIC TRANSFUSION THERAPY

Categorical statements of risks and benefits cannot be made for groups of patients in various diagnostic categories. These assessments must be made for each patient in whom chronic transfusion therapy is considered. The policies of individual physicians seem to vary widely in these respects. There is little doubt that many chronically anemic patients are transfused beyond their real requirements. Since the risks of transfusion are largely linearly related to the amount of blood given, these patients face an unnecessary risk for little or no added benefit. Other patients would receive higher benefits from the same amount of transfusion if a more effective scheduling strategy were employed. In our experience, only a small number of chronically anemic patients are significantly undertransfused; however, when this occurs, it usually presents a significant clinical problem.

The patient's overall prognosis, based on the nature of the underlying disease or process causing the anemia, is a major determinant of a rational transfusion policy. If the patient has a relatively short life expectancy, a year or less, those longer-term problems of chronic transfusion—such as iron overloading, recurrent severe febrile transfusion reactions, and multiple red cell alloimmunizations—are of less importance. Taking the prognosis into account may result in a somewhat more liberal administration of blood in an effort to maximize the functional capacity of lethally ill patients for the remainder of their lives. However, this consideration still does not justify transfusion beyond the patient's real physiologic needs.

When the patient's prognosis for longer survival is more favorable, the physician formulating the transfusion policy must consider the long-term hazards of transfusion, as well as the short-term risks now aggregated over a longer time span with increased probability of their occurrence. This should lead to efforts to administer the least amount of blood compatible with an acceptable, although reduced, functional capacity. Where the prognosis is uncertain, a conservative position of planning for the longest possible period of survival would seem reasonable.

There will certainly remain reasonable differences of opinion and practice in these decisions among competent physicians. Similarly, patients will vary in their decisions if the issues of risks and benefits of transfusion are clearly and accurately presented to them. While we urge a generally conservative policy of transfusion for all patients, it can be said that the decision to be conservative, like all therapeutic decisions, should also be subjected to careful and informed scrutiny of both patient and physician. Consultation may be helpful in doubtful situations. Decisions made on the basis of hemoglobin levels alone are too frequently wrong, as are fixed policies applied to groups of patients in various diagnostic categories. The decision to transfuse patients chronically should include a plan for blood administration and for evaluation of its efficacy and safety. Only in this way does the patient receive maximal benefit from the use of a precious and limited human resource.

CLINICAL ASPECTS OF TRANSFUSION IN CHRONIC ANEMIC STATES

Transfusion therapy is employed in a wide range of hematologic disorders characterized by anemia. It is beyond the scope of this chapter to discuss in detail the many complexities of management of these anemic disorders. The reader may refer to any of the several excellent modern textbooks of hematology, for more detailed discussions of the overall management problems posed by these disorders. Nevertheless, some comments with regard to specific aspects of transfusion therapy in certain of these anemic states may be of value. They are listed in Tables 19-1 and 19-2.

Hypoproliferative Anemias

There are two major determinants of the strategy of transfusion of this very large and heterogeneous group of patients:

1. Does the patient have primarily a deficit of red cells of clinically significant magnitude, or is the patient pancytopenic to a degree where significant thrombocytopenia and/or leukopenia are also present?
2. Is the prognosis of the patient's disorder favorable or unfavorable in the long term?

If the patient's only significant cytopenia is reflected by chronic anemia of clinically significant severity, the problem is manageable in a relatively straightforward fashion; the patient can be given transfusions on previously discussed indications for whatever period they are required. In some instances, this involves a lifelong commitment to transfusion. By contrast, the patient with a pancytopenic state in which clinically significant thrombocytopenia and/or leukopenia is also present may require a very different strategy of management. Here, prevention and/or control of bleeding using platelet transfusions (see Ch. 16) and management of infections, possibly using granulocyte transfusions (see Ch. 17), may be of the greatest importance.

It is now quite clear that patients with severe aplastic anemia have a poor prognosis with virtually all forms of medical therapy and that early marrow transplantation seems to offer the best outlook in this situation. Unfortunately, not all patients are candidates for transplantation, and suitable donors may not be available in many cases. Here, standard medical therapy using transfusion as necessary seems reasonable, although it may become ineffective in the long term.

Hyporegeneration With Normal or Increased Marrow Cellularity

A number of patients clinically categorized as having hyporegenerative bone marrow disorders do, in fact, have normally cellular or somewhat hypercellular marrows. Although the clinical problem presented by such patients may look very much like that associated with hypoplastic bone marrows, the long-term outlook is generally quite different. Many of these patients may need a variable amount of support by transfusion from time to time, although many also can be stabilized in a satisfactory functional condition without transfusion. Frequently, these patients, who also have some evidence of dysplastic hematopoiesis along with the hyporegeneration of cellular elements, will undergo transformation to a neoplastic disorder, commonly an acute leukemia. The need for increasing amounts of transfusion may herald this when it occurs in a patient who otherwise has been stable for some length of time. Careful re-examination of the blood, and possibly the bone marrow, in the face of an increasing requirement for transfusion may establish the diagnosis of a malignant blood dyscrasia at an earlier point than would otherwise occur.

Myelofibrosis

The problem of transfusion therapy in patients with myelofibrosis of the type now recognized as a myeloproliferative disorder may also reflect significant changes in the character and clinical course of the underlying disorder. Relatively few of these patients will require chronic transfusion therapy, although they may require transfusion from time to time, when hematopoiesis is suppressed by infection or other similar causes. These patients are also subject to transformation to a fully neoplastic disorder, particularly acute myeloid leukemia, myelomonocytic leukemia, and on occasion a wide variety of other leukemic and malignant reticuloendothelial disorders. This may be heralded by an increasing transfusion requirement, increasingly severe thrombocytopenia or a rising or falling white blood cell count.

More commonly, as the spleen enlarges in patients with myeloid metaplasia, there may be increasing severity of anemia and a requirement for increasing amounts of transfusion. When the amount of transfusion required by such patients exceeds that required by total red cell aplasia (i.e., more than about 2 units of sedimented red cells every 2 weeks in the average adult), it is appropriate to suspect that the massive splenomegaly has induced a hypersplenic type of hemolysis. These patients may benefit from splenectomy.

Patients with myeloid metaplasia who have increasing transfusion requirements should also be investigated for the presence of alloimmunization, as discussed earlier where inefficient transfusions are considered. These patients also develop esophageal varices that may bleed chronically, rather than massively.[40] These patients should also be investigated carefully for gastrointestinal blood loss.

Chronic Dysplastic Disorders of Bone Marrow

In patients with chronic dysplastic disorders of bone marrow, the marrow is usually of normal cellularity. Anemia, thrombocytopenia, and leukopenia occur as a result of ineffective cell proliferation and differentiation, at times with evidence that cells are being destroyed in the bone marrow prior to their release. As a group, they are usually very long-term disorders, at times manifested shortly after birth. Their management must be developed with full consideration of the disorder's probable time course.

These patients are generally best managed without transfusion, if at all possible. If not, it may be possible to transfuse them for relatively brief periods of severe anemia or control transient episodes of thrombocytopenic bleeding by platelet transfusion. Chronic red cell transfusion may be required in some patients. The incidence of cardiac and hepatic dysfunction secondary to iron overload does not seem to constitute the same type of serious limitation on life span that it does in disorders such as thalassemia major and sickle cell anemia. In general, it seems appropriate to transfuse these patients with the least amount of blood compatible with reasonable functional activity and normal growth and development during childhood. Transfusion requirements may change in later life, as puberty occurs in females, or as activity levels increase or decrease. The previously outlined principles of managing chronic transfusion will apply to such patients as adulthood is reached.

Virtually all the disorders in this heterogeneous group place patients at risk of the development of a fully neoplastic malignant blood dyscrasia. Again, worsening anemia, increasing thrombocytopenia, or changes in the white blood cell count and differential leukocyte count may herald this change in clinical course prior to the appearance of overt leukemic manifestations. If severe chronic thrombocytopenia is part of the picture, blood loss may add to the patient's transfusion requirement. Every effort should be made to minimize blood loss, including suppression of menstrual function in postpubertal women, if menstrual blood loss is excessively heavy.

Anemias of Chronic Disease

Most patients with anemia of chronic disease rarely require transfusion. Occasionally, additional factors in this broad category, such as blood loss, acute infection, or adverse drug effect, may result in increasing anemia, and a brief period of transfusion therapy may be useful. In general, most patients in this group have a poor long-term prognosis or are significantly limited by their primary disease, so that they do not require transfusion for the primary purpose of improving their functional state. Transfusions given under these circumstances should be carefully evaluated for their objective clinical effect. The risk involved should be balanced against the value to the patient, of whatever improvement may have been produced.

Renal Failure

As the previous edition of this text was being written, erythropoietin had not yet been introduced into clinical practice. Since then, the transfusion needs of patients with chronic renal failure have changed dramatically. As many as 25 percent of patients requiring chronic hemodialysis were transfusion dependent; the use of recombinant erythropoietin has dramatically reduced this need. This topic is discussed in more detail in Chapter 47.

Anemia Caused by Chronic Blood Loss Uncontrolled by Iron Therapy

In this group of disorders of various etiologies, the common feature is chronic blood loss of such magnitude that, even with iron therapy, the patient cannot maintain a normal hematocrit. Again, the same criteria apply as to the indications for transfusion, namely that the patient be functionally limited or seriously symptomatic in order to justify the risks of chronic transfusion. In many of these patients, blood loss is quite variable from time to time, and there may be substantial variation in the degree of anemia. In contrast to the usually preferable strategy of scheduled transfusions, these patients may be better managed, and the amount of transfusion may be minimized, by periodically determining the hematocrit and hemoglobin levels, as well as by keeping the patient under close surveillance for symptomatic anemia. Transfusions can then be administered on the basis of these indications, rather than on a scheduled basis.

It is, of course, important to attempt to control the source of the abnormal blood loss by whatever means are appropriate for the particular clinical situation presented by the patient. Control of blood loss is always a preferable strategy, and even substantial surgical risks can be accepted when contrasted with the serious cumulative risks of chronic transfusion.

If there is any degree of suppression of bone marrow responsiveness in those patients with severe and continuing blood loss, iron lack may not be the principal limitation on the regeneration of red cells. Any of the chronic diseases that cause anemia may also be present in the patient with chronic blood loss. Thus, if iron therapy has resulted in normalization of the patient's iron stores, but the anemia has not been corrected, it is well to look for other causes of limited red cell production.

Patients in whom oral iron therapy does not permit absorption of sufficient iron to compensate for iron lost by bleeding may justifiably be treated with parenteral iron. The risks of parenteral iron therapy, although not prohibitive, are nevertheless significant. Most hematologists are conservative in the use of this modality of iron administration.[41,42] Uncompensated iron deficiency anemia secondary to uncontrollable chronic blood loss does constitute one of the legitimate indications for this treatment. It is only after all these approaches to increasing the patient's own compensatory hematopoiesis have been tried that a program of transfusion therapy would appear to be justified.

OTHER DISORDERS THAT MAY REQUIRE TRANSFUSION

In a number of other disorders characterized by acute or chronic anemia, transfusion is required only under exceptional circumstances. Some of these disorders are listed in Table 19-2.

Anemias of Nutritional Deficiency

Transfusion is rarely required for anemias of nutritional deficiency. An occasional patient with severe megaloblastic anemia, usually due to vitamin B_{12} de-

ficiency in whom advanced heart failure is immediately life-threatening, may be encountered. In these patients, a program of partial exchange transfusion in which the plasma volume is reduced and partially replaced with donor red cells may be of immediate therapeutic value. The patient should be treated promptly with vitamin B_{12} or folate, as indicated by the etiologic mechanism responsible for anemia. All other necessary measures designed to control cardiac failure should be administered as well. It is of interest that transfusion does not correct the delirium associated with advanced vitamin B_{12} deficiency, even though the patient may be quite severely anemic. This manifestation of B_{12} depletion appears to depend on some direct metabolic role of vitamin B_{12} in the central nervous system.[43] It should be noted that correction of the anemia does not correct the metabolic defects associated with folate depletion; in some instances, these manifestations, rather than anemia, dominate the clinical picture.

Severe chronic malnutrition is a relatively uncommon disorder in the United States. Most patients so affected have a variety of other associated illnesses. Some have severe generalized malabsorption syndromes. Even in severely malnourished people, rarely is anemia so severe as to require transfusion. The primary problem in these patients is to re-establish a level of normal nutrition that will replete all the associated nutritional deficiencies that they manifest.

Uncommon Acquired Hemolytic Anemias

Chronic transfusion therapy is necessary in only the most severely affected of this diverse group of patients. Severe traumatic hemolytic anemia secondary to cardiac abnormalities or artificial heart valves may require a program of transfusion. One must keep in mind that transfusions that increase the patient's red cell mass may result in increased hemolysis (but not the rate of hemolysis), as the number of cells destroyed in a unit of time is a percentage of the number of cells present at the start of this interval. Patients with prosthetic cardiovascular materials who have hemolysis severe enough to require transfusion will generally require correction of the defect that is causing the hemolysis.

Transfusion is rarely justified by the phenomenon

of hypersplenism alone. In most instances of hypersplenism due to congestive splenomegaly, hemolysis of such severity that the patient becomes seriously anemic does not occur in the absence of other disorders that limit the response of the bone marrow. Patients in whom hypersplenism is secondary to chronic liver disease and portal hypertension may also have chronic or recurrent gastrointestinal blood loss to account in part for their anemia. They should be carefully investigated for this problem and managed appropriately. Occasionally, the combination of splenic hyperfunction and hemolysis with recurrent blood loss and relatively marginal capability of the marrow to respond to anemia does produce a degree of anemia sufficient to justify transfusion, even chronically.[44]

Paroxysmal Nocturnal Hemoglobinuria

The red blood cells of patients with paroxysmal nocturnal hemoglobinuria (PNH) have increased sensitivity to complement-mediated lysis. Transfusion of patients with PNH is usually uncomplicated, but Dacie[45] pointed out that some patients regularly experience exacerbations of hemolysis following transfusion of apparently compatible blood. Dacie further stated that these hemolytic episodes following transfusion are associated with increases in the rate of destruction of the patients' own cells. He suggested that the autohemolysis was brought about by transfusion of plasma along with the homologous RBCs and might be due to an antigen-antibody reaction involving leukocyte antibodies.

Sirchia et al.[46] demonstrated that when PNH red cells were incubated with leukocytes and a fresh unacidified serum containing an anti-leukocyte antibody, hemolysis was observed and the intensity of lysis varied according to the number of leukocytes used. They concluded that these findings supported the opinion that the hemolytic transfusion reactions that occur in some PNH patients may be caused by the interaction between transfused leukocytes and specific antibodies in the patients' sera. This immune reaction causes activation of components of complement, which then react with the PNH red cells, causing their lysis.

Accordingly, it has been the general practice to use only washed or frozen-deglycerolized red blood cells when transfusion is necessary in these patients.[47–49] Although there is some evidence to the contrary,[50] many investigators have reported that saline-washed RBCs are of value in patients who are sensitive to whole blood transfusions.[45]

Jenkins[51] has reviewed this problem and has adopted frozen-deglycerolized red cells as the principal transfusion product for his large group of PNH patients. This policy has been adopted with full recognition that other methods of removing leukocytes from donor blood will be adequate for many patients most of the time. Indeed, if complement activation as a result of leukocyte antibodies is responsible for the posttransfusion hemolytic episodes, filtered blood may be preferable, as filtering results in a product that has fewer leukocytes than are in washed red cells or frozen-stored red cells.

Anemias Associated With Pregnancy and Delivery

Complications of pregnancy associated with operative procedures or with excessive postpartum blood loss, while fortunately uncommon, can be dealt with in the same way that patients with other similar causes of blood loss are managed. Beyond these indications, transfusion is rarely justified or necessary in the course of even a complicated pregnancy. The megaloblastic anemia of pregnancy, a rare disorder, constitutes a bona fide emergency and requires prompt treatment with folic acid.

Unfortunately, in the past, transfusions have been used all too frequently to correct mild to moderate degrees of postpartum anemia. The theory justifying this practice was that the new mother, going home with a newborn, would not tolerate anemia. At the very least, she would not "feel well" and would be less able to cope with her responsibilities as a mother. The practice of transfusing such patients ignores an assessment of the real risks of transfusion. If there is no reason to believe that the patient will not adequately recover her red cell mass in a period of 6 weeks, there is no reason to consider transfusing the postpartum patient. If, for example, the patient's anemia is so severe that she is symptomatic and truly limited from the physiologic point of view, the probability is very high that there are other etiologic factors involved that require investigation in depth. It can now be said with confidence that transfusing the postpartum patient without greater indication than a moderate level of tolerable symptoms does not justify the risk of transfusion.

Also, in the past, before recognition of the phenomena of hydremia of pregnancy with hemodilution and a physiologic fall in hematocrit during the last trimester, some patients were transfused in anticipation of delivery. These patients were not truly anemic in that their total body red cell mass is usually within normal limits. The practice of transfusing such patients, or even treating them for "anemia" with a variety of hematinics, is unacceptable. The pregnant patient usually requires some iron supplementation in the diet, but for reasons other than anemia. She must transfer iron to the developing fetus and prepare for some iron loss during the period of lactation, as well as for a small amount of blood loss at delivery. Fortunately, the practice of transfusing the pregnant woman, either prepartum or postpartum, is now declining rapidly in the United States. Indeed, Combs et al.[52] reported that red cell transfusion was used in only 1.1 percent of 150 deliveries and that four risk factors were significantly predictive of red cell transfusion: pre-eclampsia, multiple gestation, elective cesarean, and nulliparity. These data are consistent with those of other reports.[53-55] (See Ch. 26 for a more detailed discussion of transfusion in obstetrics and gynecology.)

PREOPERATIVE TRANSFUSION OF THE ANEMIC PATIENT

Since the post-World War II era, a belief has developed that patients could not safely receive anesthesia or be operated upon unless the preoperative hemoglobin level was at least 10 g/dl. The origin of this practice, which has become a policy in most hospitals, is unclear. Certainly there are no valid scientific studies on which to base this practice. William Howland, a distinguished anesthesiologist, writing in the first edition of this book, said: "The origin of the traditional recommended requirement of 10 grams of hemoglobin in order to receive anesthesia is shrouded in obscurity, unsubstantiated by clinical investigation, and yet a standard in anesthetic practice." In the 14 years since his writing, nothing has appeared to contradict his statement. However, both information derived from research and increasing experience with anesthesia and surgery on significantly more anemic patients have accumulated. (This topic is discussed in detail in Chs. 7 and 21.)

REFERENCES

1. Welch HG, Meehan KR, Goodnough LT: Prudent strategies for elective red blood cell transfusion. Ann Intern Med 116:393, 1992
2. American College of Physicians: Practice strategies for elective red blood cell transfusion. Ann Intern Med 116:403, 1992
3. Stehling L, Luban NLC, Anderson KC et al: Guidelines for blood utilization review. Transfusion 34:438, 1994
4. Mollison PL, Engelfriet CP, Contreras M: Blood Transfusion in Clinical Medicine. 9th Ed. Blackwell Scientific, London, 1993
5. Erslev AJ: Erythrokinetics. p. 414. In Williams WJ, Beutler E, Erslev AJ, Lichtman MA (eds): Hematology. McGraw-Hill, New York, 1990
6. Wiesen AR, Hospenthal DR, Byrd JC et al: Equilibration of hemoglobin concentration after transfusion in medical inpatients not actively bleeding. Ann Intern Med 121:278, 1994
7. Greenfield RH, Bessen HA, Henneman PL: Effect of crystalloid infusion on hematocrit and intravascular volume in healthy, nonbleeding subjects. Ann Emerg Med 18:51, 1989
8. Enelow AJ, Adler LM: Basic interviewing. p. 35. In Enelow AJ, Swisher SN (eds): Interviewing and Patient Care. 2nd Ed. Oxford University Press, New York, 1979
9. Elwood PC, Waters WE, Greene WJW et al: Symptoms and circulating haemoglobin level. J Chron Dis 21:615, 1969
10. Wood MM, Elwood PC: Symptoms of iron deficiency: a community survey. Br J Prev Soc Med 20:117, 1966
11. Elwood PC, Wood MM: Effect of oral iron therapy on the symptoms of anemia. Br J Prev Soc Med 20:172, 1966
12. Harris JW, Kellermeyer RW: The Red Cell. Rev Ed. Harvard University Press, Cambridge, MA, 1970
13. Rodman T, Clare HP, Purcell MK: Oxyhemglobin dissociation curve in anemia. Ann Intern Med 52:295, 1960
14. Edwards MJ, Novy MJ, Walters CL, Metcalfe J: Improved oxygen release: an adaptation of mature red cells to hypoxia. J Clin Invest 47:1851, 1969
15. Torrance J, Jacobs P, Lenfant C, Finch CA: Intraer-

ythrocytic adaptation to anemia. Blood 34:843, 1969

16. Bellinghaus AJ, Grimes AJ: Red cell 2,3-diphosphoglycerate. Br J Haematol 25:555, 1973

17. Oski FA, Gottlieb AJ, Miller WW, Deliviria-Papadopoulas M: The effects of deoxygenation of adult and fetal hemoglobin on the synthesis of red cell 2,3-diphosphoglycerates and its in vivo consequences. J Clin Invest 49:400, 1970

18. Finch CA, Lenfant C: Oxygen transport in man. N Engl J Med 286:407, 1972

19. Oski FA, Gottlieb AJ, Deliviria-Papadapoulas M, Miller WW: Red cell 2,3-diphosphoglycerate levels in subjects with chronic hypoxemia. N Engl J Med 280:1165, 1969

20. Oski FA, Marshall BE, Cohen PJ et al: Exercise with anemia: the role of the left-shifted on right-shifted oxygen-hemoglobin equilibrium curve. Ann Intern Med 74:44, 1971

21. Riggs A: Functional properties of hemoglobins. Physiol Rev 45:619, 1965

22. Roy SB, Bhatia ML, Mathur VS, Virmani S: Hemodynamic effects of chronic severe anemia. Circulation 28:346, 1963

23. Roy SB, Bhatia ML, Joseph G: Determinants and distribution of high cardiac output in chronic severe anemia. Indian Heart J 18:325, 1966

24. Bartels EC: Anemia as the cause of severe congestive heart failure. Ann Intern Med 11:400, 1937

25. Whitaker W: Some effects of severe chronic anemia on the circulatory system. Q J Med 25:175, 1956

26. Zoll PM, Wessler S, Blumgart HL: Angina pectoris: clinical and pathological correlation. Am J Med 11:331, 1951

27. Graettinger JS, Parsons RL, Campbell JA: A correlation of clinical and hemodynamic studies in patients with mild and severe anemia with and without congestive heart failure. Ann Intern Med 58:617, 1963

28. Varat MA, Adolph RJ, Fowler NO: Cardiovascular effects of anemia. Am Heart J 83:415, 1972

29. Bradley SE, Bradley GP: Renal function during chronic anemic in man. Blood 2:192, 1947

30. Fowler NO, Franeh RH, Bloom WL: Hemodynamic effects of anemia with and without plasma volume expansion. Circ Res 4:319, 1956

31. Nelson AH, Fleisher LA, Rosenbaum SH: Relationship between postoperative anemia and cardiac morbidity in high-risk vascular patients in the intensive care unit. Crit Care Med 21:860, 1993

32. Christopherson R, Frank S, Norris E et al: Low postoperative hematocrit is associated with cardiac ischemia in high-risk patients, abstracted. Anesthesiology 75:A99, 1991

33. Stehling L, Simon TL: The red blood cell transfusion trigger: physiology and clinical studies. Arch Pathol Lab Med 118:429, 1994

34. Gillon J: Controversies in transfusion medicine. Acute normovolemic hemodilution in elective major surgery: con. Transfusion 34:269, 1994

35. Ryan JM, Mickam JB: The alveolar-arterial oxygen pressure gradient in anemia. J Clin Invest 31:188, 1952

36. Sproule BJ, Mitchell JH, Miller WF: Cardiopulmonary physiological responses to heavy exercise in patients with anemia. J Clin Invest 39:378, 1960

37. Anderson HT, Barkve H: Iron deficiency and muscular work performance. An evaluation of the cardiorespiratory function of iron deficient subjects with and without anaemia. Scand J Clin Lab Invest, suppl. 25:114, 1970

38. Arlina AR, Unger RJ, Rosky M: Post-transfusion alloimmunization in patients with sickle cell disease. Am J Hematol 5:101, 1978

39. Ness, PM: To match or not to match: the question for chronically transfused patients with sickle cell anemia. Transfusion 34:558, 1994

40. Rosenbaum DL, Murphy GW, Swisher SN: Hemodynamic studies of the portal circulation in myeloid metaplasia. Am J Med 41:360, 1966

41. Becker CE, MacGregor RR, Walker KS: Fatal anaphylaxis after intramuscular iron dextran. Ann Intern Med 65:745, 1966

42. Jacobs J: Death due to iron parenterally. South Med J 62:216, 1969

43. Samson DC, Swisher SN, Christian RM, Engel GL: Cerebral metabolic disturbance and delerium in pernicious anemia: clinical and electroencephalographic studies. Arch Intern Med 90:4, 1952

44. Petz LD, Tomasulo PA: Red cell transfusion. p. 1. In Contemporary Transfusion Practice. American Association of Blood Banks, Arlington, VA, 1987

45. Dacie JV: The Haemolytic Anaemias. Grune & Stratton, Orlando, FL, 1967, p. 1231

46. Sirchia G, Ferrone S, Mercuriali F: Leukocyte antigen-antibody reaction and lysis of paroxysmal nocturnal hemoglobinuria erythrocytes. Blood 36:334, 1970

47. Dacie JV, Lewis SM: Paroxysmal nocturnal hemoglobinuria: clinical manifestations. Haematology and nature of the disease. Semin Haematol 5:3, 1972

48. Gockerman FP, Brouillard RP: RBC transfusions in paroxysmal nocturnal hemoglobinuria. Arch Intern Med 137:536, 1977

49. Rosse WF: Transfusion in paroxysmal nocturnal hemoglobinuria. Transfusion 29:663, 1989

50. Brecher ME, Taswell HF: Paroxysmal nocturnal hemoglobinuria and the transfusion of washed red cells: a myth revisited. Transfusion 29:681, 1989

51. Jenkins DE: Paroxysmal nocturnal hemoglobinuria hemolytic systems. p. 45. In Bell C (ed): A Seminar of Laboratory Management of Hemolysis. American Association of Blood Banks, Washington, DC, 1979

52. Combs CA, Murphy EL, Laros RK: Cost-benefit analysis of autologous blood donation in obstetrics. Obstet Gynecol 80:621, 1992

53. Naef RW, Chauhan SP, Chevalier SP et al: Prediction of hemorrhage at cesarean delivery. Obstet Gynecol 83:923, 1994

54. Klapholz H: Blood transfusion in contemporary obstetric practice. Obstet Gynecol 75:940, 1990

55. Dickason LA, Dinsmoor MJ: Red blood cell transfusion and cesarean section. Am J Obstet Gynecol 167:327, 1992

Chapter 20

Blood Transfusion in Acquired Hemolytic Anemias

Lawrence D. Petz

AUTOIMMUNE HEMOLYTIC ANEMIAS

Patients with autoimmune hemolytic anemia (AIHA) frequently present with anemia of sufficient severity to suggest the possible need for blood transfusion. Indeed, when anemia of such severity is discovered, physicians frequently refer a sample of blood to the blood transfusion laboratory while simultaneously initiating diagnostic studies to determine the cause of the anemia. A diagnosis of AIHA is often first made by the blood transfusion service when autoantibodies are detected during compatibility testing.

Nowhere in the management of patients with immune hemolytic anemias is the communication between clinician and laboratory personnel more important than in regard to blood transfusion. As with all clinical decisions concerning therapy, the possible benefits must be weighed in relationship to potential risks. The advisability of blood transfusion is related to the severity of the anemia, to whether the anemia is rapidly progressive, and especially to the associated clinical findings. However, a clinical decision based on such facts must be tempered by the knowledge that blood transfusion has a greater than usual risk in patients with AIHA.

This chapter first discusses the appropriate use of blood transfusion in various clinical settings in patients with AIHA. This is followed by a description, from the point of view of practicing clinicians, of the nature and clinical significance of the unique risks encountered when transfusion is necessary in a patient with AIHA. In essence, the risks relate to two factors: (1) the autoantibody often complicates the compatibility test and may make it difficult to detect coexisting alloantibodies or to exclude their presence with confidence, thereby increasing the risk of an alloantibody-induced hemolytic transfusion reaction; and (2) the autoantibody itself may cause marked shortening of the survival of donor red cells. Despite these added risks, I emphasize that blood should never be denied a patient with a justifiable need, even though the compatibility test may be strongly incompatible. On the other hand, in discussing the difficulties faced by laboratory personnel, and adverse reactions to blood transfusion unique to patients with acquired hemolytic anemia, I hope to justify the view that frequently the course of lesser risk is to withhold blood transfusions in some settings in which the initial clinical judgment would suggest their need.

Next, the principles and methods that promote the optimal selection of blood for AIHA patients are reviewed, with emphasis on efforts to detect red cell alloantibodies in the presence of autoantibodies. Subsequent segments discuss compatibility testing in various kinds of AIHA, in vivo compatibility testing, the optimal volume of blood to be transfused (which may be of critical importance in safely treating patients with severe hemolytic anemia), the use of warm blood for patients with cold antibody AIHA, the use of washed or leukocyte-depleted red cells, and autologous transfusion for patients with AIHA. The chapter concludes with a discussion of compatibility testing and transfusion in patients with drug-induced immune hemolytic anemias.

ASSESSING THE NEED FOR TRANSFUSION IN AIHA

Acuteness of Onset and Rapidity of Progression

When a patient presents with AIHA and a moderately severe anemia, it is not possible to predict with certainty whether the anemia will rapidly become more severe. Thus, serial determinations of the hemoglobin and hematocrit should be performed at appropriate intervals, depending on the severity of the hemolysis. In particular, the physician should note whether the patient appears acutely ill with symptoms attributable to acute hemolysis, such as fever, malaise, and pain in the back, abdomen, and legs.[1] The presence or absence of hemoglobinuria and hemoglobinemia should be noted. These findings are usually manifestations of severe hemolysis.[1]

If a patient is acutely ill, has a history of an abrupt onset of the illness, or has grossly evident hemoglobinuria, the hematocrit should be tested every 2 to 4 hours initially, whereas in less acutely ill patients, initial testing may be at 12- to 24-hour intervals. The frequency of testing may soon be decreased if the severity of the anemia proves to be essentially constant. In some cases of fulminant hemolysis, a significant fall in the hematocrit may occur within hours, whereas in a majority of patients with AIHA the anemia is essentially stable or only slowly progressive over a period of days.

Severe But Stable Anemia During Initial Evaluation

Patients with an anemia that is essentially stable during the initial evaluation period generally should not be transfused at this point, even though they may have such symptoms as a marked decrease in exercise tolerance and palpitations with exertion. Even severe anemia found in AIHA is generally well tolerated, even in the elderly, if bed rest is employed.[2] Furthermore, response to therapy or spontaneous improvement may be rapid. For example, 50 percent of patients with warm antibody AIHA will respond to adequate doses of corticosteriods during the first week of therapy,[2] and acute paroxysmal cold hemoglobinuria seldom lasts longer than 7 to 10 days.[3]

Progressively Severe Anemia

Some patients do, however, have an anemia that is steadily progressive in severity, leading to the development of symptoms of hypoxemia. Indeed, as emphasized by Pirofsky,[4] progression of the severity of anemia frequently occurs in patients with warm antibody AIHA. Among 213 patients, the lowest hematocrit ranged from 7.5 to 41.5 percent, but with a median value of only 19 percent. A hematocrit of 15 percent or less was observed in 49 patients! Even in severely anemic patients, there usually is no evidence of vascular collapse, because blood volume remains near-normal, but progressively more severe angina and cardiac decompensation may occur. Extremely anemic patients (hematocrit of 12 percent or hemoglobin of 4 g/dl) may develop neurologic signs, beginning as marked lethargy and weakness, and progressing to somnolence, mental confusion, obtundation, and death. In patients with anemia of such severity (or in those whose rate of progression indicates that this point will likely be reached), red cells are urgently needed, and nothing can substitute for their use, although oxygen should also be administered. In these patients, the use of packed red cells sufficient to maintain a modest increase in hematocrit until therapy for the AIHA becomes effective is probably optimal (see the later section on the optimal volume of blood to be transfused to patients with AIHA).

In some patients, in spite of adequate therapy, hemolysis proceeds chronically at a rate greater than that of red cell production, resulting in a relentlessly progressive anemia. In this situation, chronic transfusion is necessary to sustain life, and the attendant risks, cost, and inconvenience must be accepted.

Chronic Stable Anemia

Many patients (especially those with cold agglutinin disease) are able to compensate partially for their shortened red cell survival and maintain a relatively stable (albeit occasionally quite severe) degree of anemia. In these patients, where transfusion may be considered as a means of relieving symptoms, the advantages and disadvantages of such management are similar to those with other "refractory anemias" and must be very carefully weighed (also see Ch. 19).

As in any patient with chronic anemia, transfusions should be given as packed red cells, although a leukocyte-poor red cell preparation may ultimately be required to prevent repeated febrile reactions.

Transfusions will at least partially suppress erythropoiesis. The frequency of transfusions will have to be determined arbitrarily and will depend on the rate of hemolysis. It is usually convenient to give 2 to 3 units of packed red cells at a time when necessary. It is not advisable to completely correct the anemia; transfusion to a level of hemoglobin that will prevent severe symptoms is usually optimal.

Fulminant Hemolytic Anemia

Least common among the indications for transfusion in immune hemolytic anemia is rapidly progressive anemia caused by acute massive hemolysis. Nevertheless, such fulminant hemolysis does occur, and such patients may even be hypotensive.

Patients who have AIHA of such severity can be expected to have gross evidences of hemolysis, particularly hemoglobinuria and hemoglobinemia. Diagnoses such as *Clostridium perfringens* (*welchii*) septicemia and drug-induced immune hemolytic anemia (see below) should also be quickly investigated. The onset may be so acute that a reticulocytosis may not be present, since the bone marrow may not have had time to compensate. Indeed, a maximal increase in the reticulocyte count in response to a sudden decrease in red cell mass requires 7 to 10 days.[5]

Although such cases are uncommon, transfusion is urgent. If manifestations of shock are present, the immediate aim of transfusion is improvement in vital signs, which may be temporarily restored by the use of electrolyte or colloid solutions. Simultaneously, the physician should communicate to the blood transfusion laboratory the urgency of finding optimal red cells for transfusion. Rarely will these red cells be "compatible" in the crossmatch; nevertheless, their use is mandatory in this acutely life-threatening setting.

RISKS OF TRANSFUSION IN PATIENTS WITH AIHA

In AIHA, the risks of blood transfusion beyond the usual risks relate to the presence of the patient's red cell autoantibody. Autoantibodies usually will react with all normal red cells so that transfused cells usually have a shorter-than-normal life span. This cannot be avoided, assuming that optimal therapeutic measures are being used to treat the AIHA. The red cell autoantibody may react strongly in vitro (e.g., $2+$ to $4+$ by indirect antiglobulin test) with all available donor red cells to be transfused, thus making it impossible to obtain compatible blood for transfusion. Nevertheless, acute symptomatic transfusion reactions occur only infrequently. Subsequent survival is about as good as the patient's own red cells, and the net result is that transfusion generally produces temporary benefit. Thus, the reactivity in vivo of the autoantibody causes shortened survival of transfused red cells but usually does not contribute greatly to the acute risk of transfusion.

Although this is generally true, if the patient has very severe hemolysis, the autoantibody may cause striking destruction of transfused red cells, resulting in no benefit[6] or in dangerous degrees of hemolysis with hemoglobinemia, hemoglobinuria, renal failure,[7] and clinical deterioration.[8] This is probably particularly true if relatively large volumes of blood are given (see the later section on the optimal volume of blood to be transfused).

In some patients, the autoantibody demonstrates clinically significant "relative specificity" in that it reacts stronger with red cells bearing certain common Rh antigens than with red cells lacking these antigens. Tests for determining autoantibody relative specificity should be performed since red cells lacking the more strongly reactive antigen may survive significantly better than cells containing the more reactive antigen (see under Significance of Autoantibody Specificity).

Furthermore, when the patient's serum reacts with all red cells in routine crossmatch and antibody identification tests, the blood transfusion laboratory must utilize additional techniques in an attempt to demonstrate red cell antibodies other than the autoantibody. This is a critical aspect of selection of donor blood because, if the patient has previously been transfused or has been pregnant, and has developed red cell alloantibodies (e.g., anti-Rh, anti-Kell, anti-Kidd), donor red cells lacking such antigens must be selected for transfusion or a severe alloantibody-induced hemolytic transfusion reaction may ensue.

DIFFERENTIAL DIAGNOSIS OF IMMUNE HEMOLYTIC ANEMIAS

The problems relating to blood transfusion in patients with immune hemolytic anemias vary significantly, depending on the specific diagnosis. Table 20-1 classifies AIHA. Some characteristic features of autoimmune and drug-induced immune hemolytic anemias are indicated in Table 20-2. Detailed descriptions of the laboratory tests necessary for definitive diagnosis of these disorders have been published[9–11] and are briefly summarized in Table 20-3. The method of selection of donor blood for transfusion varies, depending on the type of AIHA (i.e., warm antibody AIHA, cold agglutinin syndrome, or paroxysmal cold hemoglobinuria).[10–15]

Table 20-1. Classification of Immune Hemolytic Anemias

AIHA
  Warm antibody AIHA
    Idiopathic
    Secondary
      Chronic lymphocytic leukemia, lymphomas, systemic lupus erythematosus, etc.
  Cold agglutinin syndrome
    Idiopathic
    Secondary
      Mycoplasma pneumoniae infection, infectious mononucleosis, viral infections, lymphoreticular malignant processes
  Paroxysmal cold hemoglobinuria
    Idiopathic
    Secondary
      Viral syndromes, syphilis
  Atypical AIHA
    Antiglobulin-test-negative AIHA
    Combined cold plus warm AIHA
Drug-Induced Immune Hemolytic Anemia
Alloantibody-Induced Immune Hemolytic Anemia
  Hemolytic transfusion reactions
  Hemolytic disease of the newborn

Table 20-2. Some Characteristic Features of Autoimmune and Drug-Induced Immune Hemolytic Anemias

Warm antibody AIHA
  Clinical manifestations: variable, usually symptoms of anemia, occasionally acute hemolytic syndrome
  Prognosis; fair, with significant mortality
  Therapy: steroids; splenectomy; immunosuppressive drugs
Cold agglutinin syndrome
  Clinical manifestations: moderate chronic hemolytic anemia in middle-aged or elderly person, often with signs and symptoms exacerbated by cold
  Prognosis: good; usually a chronic and quite stable anemia
  Therapy: avoid cold exposure; chlorambucil
Paroxysmal cold hemoglobinuria
  Clinical manifestations: acute hemolytic anemia, often with hemoglobinuria, particularly in a child with history of recent viral or viral-like illness
  Prognosis; excellent after initial stormy course
  Therapy: not well defined; steroids empirically and transfusions if required
Drug-induced immune hemolytic anemia
  Clinical manifestations: variable, most commonly subacute in onset, but, occasionally, acute hemolytic syndrome
  Prognosis: excellent
  Therapy: Stop drug; occasionally, a short course of steroids empirically

(From Petz and Garratty,[9] with permission.)

SELECTION OF DONOR BLOOD FOR TRANSFUSION IN SPECIFIC TYPES OF AIHA

Warm Antibody Autoimmune Hemolytic Anemia

With the exception of ABO red blood cell grouping, the most important aspect of selection of donor blood for transfusion is detection of red cell alloantibodies that may produce a hemolytic transfusion reaction. Indeed, the purpose of routine compatibility testing for all patients requiring transfusion, regardless of diagnosis, is the detection of red cell alloantibodies. There is no justification for ignoring this aspect of compatibility testing in patients with AIHA. This is particularly true now that several serologic techniques are available for detection of alloantibodies even when a patient's autoantibody reacts with all donor red cells.[9,10,12–15] These procedures

Table 20-3. Classification and Expected Findings in Autoimmune and Drug-Induced Immune Hemolytic Anemias

Type	Direct Antiglobulin Test	Eluate	Serologic Characteristics	Antibody Specificity
Autoimmune				
Warm antibody AIHA (most common type)	IgG and/or complement (C3)	IgG antibody	IAT positive (57%), agglutinating enzyme premodified cells (90%), hemolyzing enzyme premodified cells (13%)	Usually within Rh system; other specificities include LW, U, 1^T, K, Kp^b, K13, Ge, Jk^a, En^a, Wr^b
Cold agglutinin syndrome	Complement (C3) alone	Negative	Agglutinating activity up to 30°C in albumin; high titer at 4°C (usually >1,024)	Usually anti-I; other specificities include i, Pr, Gd, Sd^x
Paroxysmal cold hemoglobinuria	Complement (C3) alone	Negative	Biphasic hemolysin (i.e., sensitizes red cells in the cold and then hemolyzes them when moved to 37°C)	Anti-P (reacts with all normal red cells except p or P^k cells)
Drug-induced				
α-Methyldopa (aldomet)	IgG alone	IgG antibody	Similar to warm antibody AIHA	Usually within Rh system
Penicillins	Usually IgG alone, but complement (C3) may also be detected	Negative unless penicillin-coated red cells are tested	Negative unless penicillin-coated red cells are tested	Reacts with penicillin-coated red cells
Other drugs (i.e., quinidine, phenacetin—usually reactive due to immune complex formation)	Usually complement (C3) alone, but IgG may also be detected	Negative unless drug + patient's eluate + red cells tested	Negative unless drug + patient's serum or eluate + red cells tested	Reacts with red cells if incubated with drug + patient's serum or eluate

(From Petz and Branch,[10] with permission.)

are quite practical and not excessively time-consuming.

The approach to selection of donor blood for transfusion to patients with warm antibody AIHA (described below) considers first the various serologic techniques that are useful for red cell typing. Next we indicate practical methods for detecting alloantibodies in the presence of autoantibodies, discuss the determination of autoantibody specificity within the Rh system, and discuss the significance of the specificity in relation to blood transfusion.

Determining the Patient's Red Cell Phenotype

A knowledge of the patient's red cell phenotype is extremely useful, particularly when repeated transfusions are required. When a patient with AIHA has persistent hemolysis and requires repeated transfusions, the question frequently arises as to whether the continued hemolysis is, at least in part, caused by alloantibodies. Although numerous serologic procedures are useful in detecting alloantibodies in the presence of panagglutinating autoantibodies (see below), results are sometimes uncertain. In this situation, knowledge of the patient's red cell phenotype is extremely important in determining which alloantibodies are potentially present and which red cell antigens in donor blood are of potential significance in alloantibody-induced hemolysis. If the patient's Rh phenotype is known, it is often feasible to select donor units of the same phenotype to avoid alloantibody-induced hemolysis. Also, if the patient is, for example, Jk^a-positive, one need not be concerned about anti-Jk^a alloantibodies; if the patient is Kell negative, the use of Kell-negative blood would eliminate concern about the possible presence of anti-Kell alloantibodies. One must keep in mind that determining the patient's red cell phenotype is more difficult after the patient has received a transfusion (see later section on red cell typing in the recently transfused patient) and in some instances may not be possible; therefore the opportunity when the patient is first examined should not be missed.

ABO Red Cell Grouping

There is usually no problem in determining the ABO group of patients with AIHA. Cells are tested in the usual fashion, with anti-A and anti-B, but a negative control of 6 percent bovine serum albumin (BSA) in saline should also be used. Testing with anti-A,B is indicated only if negative reactions are obtained using anti-A and anti-B. A positive result in the control tube using 6 percent albumin indicates either nondispersed autoagglutination or spontaneous agglutination of heavily sensitized cells in albumin, and the ABO grouping results cannot be properly interpreted. When the control is positive in a patient with warm antibody AIHA, washing the patient's cells using saline heated to 45°C in saline for 5 to 10 minutes may result in negative controls and permit reliable typing. Alternatively, the pretreatment of the patient's red cells using ZZAP reagent (Table 20-4) can eliminate the spontaneous agglutination and allow for reliable ABO grouping. Chloroquine diphosphate treatment of the red cells may also prove effective (Table 20-4). When using red cells for typing that have been treated with either of these reagents, all antisera must be standardized using red cells of known types that have been similarly treated.

In patients with cold agglutinins reactive at room temperature, washing the red cells at 37 to 45°C may be necessary to prevent cold autoagglutination. Al-

Table 20-4. Removal of Red-Cell-Bound IgG

Removal of Red-Cell-Bound IgG with Chloroquine Diphosphate

Chloroquine reagent
1. 20 g chloroquine diphosphate (Sigma Chemical, St. Louis, Mo.) is dissolved in 100 ml of 0.01 M phosphate buffered saline, pH 7.2 (200 mg/ml chloroquine diphosphate).
2. The pH is adjusted to 5.0 using 5N NaOH. The reagent is stable indefinitely at 4°C.
Procedure
1. To one volume of washed packed red cells is added 4 vol chloroquine reagent.
2. After mixing by inversion, the sample is left at room temperature for 2 hours, with periodic mixing.
3. After incubation, the chloroquine treated red cells are washed 4 times with large volumes of isotonic saline and then resuspended to 2 to 5 percent in saline for testing.
Chloroquine has its main application in antigen typings where the DAT is positive (see text).

Removal of Red-Cell-Bound IgG With ZZAP Reagent

Reagents Required
1. Stock 1 percent cysteine-activated papain; store at −20°C. (Ficin, bromelin, or trypsin may be substituted for cysteine-activated papain.)
2. Stock 0.2 M DTT (Calbiochem, La Jolla, CA); store at −20°C. (0.2 M 2-mercaptoethanol may be substituted for 0.2 M DTT.)
3. PBS, 0.01 M, pH 7.3; store at 4°C.

ZZAP Reagent (0.1 M DTT + 0.1% Cysteine-Activated Papain)
1. Mix 2.5 ml of stock 0.2 M DDT, 0.5 ml of stock 1 percent cysteine-activated papain and 2 ml PBS buffer, pH 7.3.
2. Invert several times to mix; pH should be 6.0 to 6.5. The reagent is stable for at least 5 days at 4°C.

ZZAP Treatment of Red Cells
1. Pack red cells to be treated with ZZAP reagent; remove supernate.
2. To one volume of packed red cells, add 2 vol of ZZAP reagent.
3. Incubate at 37°C for 30 min with periodic mixing.
4. Wash red cells 3–4 times with isotonic saline.
5. Resuspended ZZAP treated red cells to 2 to 5 percent in saline for testing.

Abbreviations: DAT, direct antiglobulin test; PBS, phosphate-buffered saline.
(From Petz and Branch,[10] with permission.)

ternatively, one could treat the red cells with 0.01 M dithiothreitol (DTT) for 30 minutes at 37°C before ABO typings.[10,16]

ABO Serum Grouping

When the patient's serum is tested against red cells of group A, B, and O, as well as against his own cells to confirm ABO grouping, it may be necessary to perform these tests using a prewarmed technique at 37°C if cold autoagglutination occurs.

Rh-hr Typings

Slide and rapid tube Rh-hr antisera may be used for Rh typing of patients with AIHA. It is advisable to test the patient's red cells for the Rh antigens, $Rh_o(D)$, rh'(C), rh"(E), hr'(c), and hr"(e). If the patient has been transfused within the last month, only the $Rh_o(D)$ antigen need be typed, since unreliable results may be obtained with the other Rh antisera. If the Rh-hr diluent control is positive, the patient's red cells should be treated with ZZAP reagent, and the antigen typings repeated. As typing reagents are not standardized against ZZAP-treated red cells, all antisera must be standardized by testing their specific reactivity against ZZAP-treated panel cells. Correct results should be demonstrated using red cells both positive and negative for the appropriate antigen.

It is preferable to perform Rh typing on ZZAP-treated red cells using "slide and rapid tube" typing antisera rather than saline reactive or chemically modified antisera because Rh typing cannot always be performed using saline reactive or chemically modified antisera when spontaneous agglutination is present, and it is convenient to use only one type of antisera.

Typing for Other Red Cell Antigens

When the red cells to be antigen typed have a strongly positive direct antiglobulin test (DAT) and when the antisera available for typing are reactive only in the indirect antiglobulin test (IAT), several approaches may be used.

1. Heating red cells for 5 to 30 minutes at 45°C or for 3 to 10 minutes at 50°C will sometimes dissociate enough bound antibody to allow the red cells to be typed by strongly reactive antisera. Occasion-

ally, the cells must be heated for about 3 to 5 minutes at 51 to 56°C. The main disadvantages of this method are that hemolysis often occurs and that red cell antigens may become weakened when they are heated above 37°C. This is particularly true at temperatures above 45°C. The degree of weakening depends on the antigens involved, the temperature, and the length of incubation. Heating at 45°C is not usually successful if the DAT is strongly positive; temperatures of at least 50°C must be used.

Unfortunately, many commercial typing sera react rather weakly (2+) when the IAT is used, especially against red cells heterozygous for the antigen. This makes typing virtually impossible using the heat elution methodology, unless the elution results in a negative or a very weakly positive DAT. When dealing with red cells that give a very strongly positive DAT, it is rarely possible to reduce the reactivity enough to perform reliable antigen typing with such weakly reactive typing reagents

Alternative methods, described below, are necessary.

2. ZZAP-treated red cells[17] are useful for typing red cells for ABO, Rh-hr and Kidd antigens.[10] After ZZAP treatment of red cells moderately sensitized with IgG (1+ to 3+), the antiglobulin test is usually negative. However, in the presence of very strong sensitization (4+) of red cells, ZZAP has been reported to reduce the direct antiglobulin test to negative in only 36 percent of patients tested. Since numerous red cell antigens are denatured by treatment with this reagent, including those of the Duffy, MNSs, and Kell blood group systems (Table 20-5), ZZAP-treated red cells have a limited use outside the ABO, Rh-hr, and Kidd systems. However, if ZZAP can reduce the direct antiglobulin test to very weakly reactive or negative, it is the technique of choice for Kidd-antigen typing. However, the Kidd antisera must first be shown to be specific by testing it against known Kidd-positive and -negative red cells that have been treated with the ZZAP reagent.

3. An acid solution of chloroquine diphosphate can dissociate cell-bound IgG with little or no denaturation of red cell antigens.[18] However, chloroquine does not reduce the antiglobulin test to negative in every case and the method may require incuba-

Table 20-5. Effect on ZZAP on Red Blood Cell Antigens

Antigens Unaffected		Antigens Denatured
ABH	Vel	MNS
Lewis	Lan	Duffy (Fy^a, Fy^b)
Rh-Hr	Jr^a	Kell (K, k, Kp^a, Kp^b,
Kidd (Jk^a, Jk^b, Jk:3)	Co^a	Js^a, Js^b, Ku, K:11,
Lutheran (Lu^a, Lu^b, Lu:17)	Tj^a	K:12, K:13, K:14, K:18, K:19, Gerbich)
U	Di^b	s^a
Yt^{ab}	Dy^a	Yt^{ab}

^{a} Substantially but not completely denatured.
^{b} Some examples failed to react with anti-Yt^a after ZZAP treatment while others remained reactive.
(From Branch and Petz,[17] with permission.)

Table 20-6. Jk^a-Typing of Patient With Positive Direct Antiglobulin Test Using Differential Absorption

Red Cells Used to Absorb Anti-Jk^a-Typing Serum	Dilutions of Absorbed Anti-Jk^a Tested Against Jk (a + b +) Red Cells^a						
	1	2	4	8	16	32	Score
Jk(a+b+)	2+	1+	1+	½+	0	0	16
Jk(a+b−)	1+	1+	0	0	0	0	8
Jk(a−b+)	3+	3+	2+	2+	1+	0	32
Patient's	2+	1+	0	0	0	0	10

^{a} These results indicate that the patient is probably Jk(a +).
(From Petz and Garratty,[9] with permission.)

tions as long as 2 hours to be effective. In addition, with occasional red cell samples, the chloroquine reagent may cause marked hemolysis unpredictably. Also, the typing antisera must be carefully standardized using antigen-positive and antigen-negative chloroquine diphosphate-treated red cells.

4. If ZZAP reagent and/or chloroquine diphosphate reagents fail to reduce the direct antiglobulin test sufficiently to perform reliable antigen typing, a technique employing antisera absorption can be used. Equal aliquots of a specific antiserum (usually commercial antisera used for routine antigen typings can be used) and washed packed red cells arc incubated at 37°C for 1 hour. Both heterozygous and homozygous red cells and red cells negative for the appropriate antigen are used. The activity of the supernatant absorbed serum is compared with the absorbed serum from a similar mixture of the patient's red cells and the antiserum. It is wise to titrate the absorbed serum against red cells positive for the appropriate antigen. If the patient's red cells contain the antigen, for example, Jk^a, the red cells will absorb antibody from the anti-Jk^a typing serum, leaving a lower titer. Heterozygous cells, for example, Jk(a+b+), will absorb some (or all) of the antibody and homozygous cells, for example, Jk(a+b−), will be expected to absorb the antibody even more

readily. Red cells lacking the appropriate antigen, for example, Jk(a −), will not absorb any anti-Jk^a; thus, the activity of the antibody will not be significantly changed after absorption. Titration scores of the absorbed serum from the control cells can be compared with those obtained using the patient's red cells for the absorption (Table 20-6). Although this method is tedious and time-consuming, it will yield reliable results if carefully performed.[9]

Red Cell Typing in the Recently Transfused Patient

At times it is desirable to perform red cell typing on patients who have been transfused recently. It is often possible to do so using one or another of the several techniques that have been described for this purpose. These methods depend on the separation of reticulocytes (i.e., the patient's cells) from older red cells (i.e., transfused cells) and are based on the known difference in specific gravity of young and old erythrocytes. One such method involves the use of 10 phthalate ester mixtures of varying specific gravity.[19] Another procedure uses a density gradient medium consisting of a mixture of polyvinylpyrrolidone (Percoll) and the renal contrast material Renografin-60. The method was described by Vettore et al.[20] and then further evaluated and applied in immunohematology by Conley et al.[21] and Branch et al.[22] Mean reticulocyte counts after enrichment depend on the original reticulocyte count and vary from 25 to 64 percent with a maximum reticulocyte count as high as 98 percent (Table 20-7).

With these methods, the patient's red cell type can

Table 20-7. Reticulocyte Enrichment Using a Percoll-Renografin Density Gradient

No. of Samples	Initial Reticulocyte Count (%) (Range)	Reticulocyte Count in Enriched Fraction (%) (Mean ± SD)
31	≤1.5	25 ± 18.4
15	1.6–5.0	44 ± 28.8
7	>5.0	64 ± 21.1

(From Branch et al.,[22] with permission.)

usually be determined 48 to 72 hours after transfusion. Two examples are indicated in Table 20-8 for patients who were Fy^a-negative. Patient 1 received 9 units of red cells within 12 to 24 hours; after transfusion, the circulating red cells yielded a 1+ reaction with anti-Fy^a. However, 48 hours after transfusion, the reticulocyte-enriched fraction yielded negative results with anti-Fy^a. The results in patient 2 were similar, except that a larger volume of blood was transfused, and correct typing was not possible until 72 hours after transfusion. Further examples are given by Branch and colleagues.[22] It appears that there are enough red cells of low buoyant density in transfused blood to interfere with typing for about 48 to 72 hours, but after that time transfused cells may be separated from the patient's for appropriate typing. In AIHA patients, the separated young cells may be treated with ZZAP or chloroquine diphosphate as necessary prior to typing, as described above.

Griffin et al.[23] described a dual-color cytometry method for antigen typing of recipient red cells fol-

lowing transfusion. Reticulocyte identification and antigen typing were performed on 319 samples to establish the validity of the procedure and the in vitro results were confirmed in 19 transfused patients who had received red cells antigenically different from their own, as well as cells from one chimera blood donor. The method was adaptable to an array of red cell antigens, although the S antigen produced inconsistent and unreliable results with antisera from several sources.

DETECTION OF ALLOANTIBODIES IN THE PRESENCE OF AUTOANTIBODIES

Red cell alloantibodies capable of causing a hemolytic transfusion reaction (e.g., anti-Rh, -Kell, -Kidd, -Duffy) may be present in any patient who has received a previous blood transfusion or has been pregnant. Warm autoantibodies usually react with all normal red cells, thus making more difficult the detection of alloantibodies in compatibility tests. Several serologic techniques are available for detection of "unexpected" red cell alloantibodies in patients with AIHA. The definitive methods for detection of alloantibodies in the presence of autoantibodies involve absorption of the autoantibody from the patient's serum by red cells that will not absorb the alloantibody (see the later sections on absorption techniques).

The frequency with which tests should be performed for the presence of unexpected antibodies is indicated in the Standards for Blood Banks and Transfusion Services of the American Association of Blood Banks,[24] which states, "If the patient has been

Table 20-8. Red Blood Cell Typing After Transfusion Using Reticulocyte-Enriched Blood

Patient	Time of Red Cell Typing	Anti-Fy^a Versus Patient Sample	Reticulocyte-Rich	Reticulocyte-Poor
1	Pretransfusion	0		
	24 hours post-transfusion (9 units red cells)	1½+	1+	2½+
	48 hours post-transfusion	1+	0	1+
2	Pretransfusion	0		
	24 hours post-transfusion (29 units red cells)	1½+	1+	2+
	48 hours post-transfusion	1+	1+	1+
	72 hours post-transfusion	2+	0	2+
	5 days post-transfusion	1+	0	1½+

(From Branch et al.,[22] with permission.)

transfused in the preceding 3 months with blood or a blood component containing red blood cells or has been pregnant within the preceding 3 months or if the history is uncertain or unavailable, the sample must be obtained from the patient within 3 days of the scheduled transfusion." Although not specifically commented on in the Standards, tests for "unexpected" alloantibodies should be carried out whether or not autoantibodies are present.

Comparison of Direct and Indirect Antiglobulin Tests

A comparison of the strength of reactivity of DAT and IAT sometimes affords extremely valuable information. In patients with warm antibody AIHA, the IAT caused by autoantibody is generally weaker than the DAT. Apparently, most of the antibody is absorbed to the patient's red cells in vivo. A coexisting alloantibody will not be absorbed by the patient's red cells and may produce a strongly positive IAT. Thus, if the IAT is significantly stronger than the DAT, the presence of an alloantibody is highly suspect.

If the DAT is 4 +, or if it is equal to or stronger than the IAT, no conclusion can be reached concerning the presence or absence of alloantibodies.

Testing of Patient's Serum Against a Red Cell Panel

If the screening tests for serum antibody reveal an antibody reactive at 37°C, the serum should be tested against a panel of phenotyped cells, as is routine in any blood bank determining specificities of alloantibodies. If a weakly reactive autoantibody and a strongly reactive alloantibody are present, the differences in the strength of the reaction of various cells of the panel will make this evident. For example, Table 20-9 shows a strong anti-Jk[a] together with a weak autoantibody.

However, one has no assurance that a patient's alloantibody will react more strongly than the autoantibody; thus, additional tests to detect alloantibodies are necessary.

RBC Absorption Techniques

The best techniques currently available for determining if alloantibodies are present in addition to warm autoantibodies is to absorb the autoantibody from the patient's serum at 37°C using the patient's own red cells after first eluting some of the autoantibody (warm autoabsorption technique) or by using several selected allogeneic RBC (differential absorption technique, see below). A simple elution-autoabsorption method was described in 1963 by Allen[25] and similar techniques continue to be used by numerous investigators.[26] The technique may be modified by enzyme treatment of the patient's red cells after the elution procedure.[27] After absorption of the autoantibodies, the serum can then be tested for alloantibodies, since alloantibodies will not be absorbed

Table 20-9. Serum Containing Allo Anti-Jk[a] and an Undefined Autoantibody When Reacted With a Panel of Red Cells[a]

Donor No.	Rh Phenotype	C	D	E	c	c	f	Cw	V	K	k	Kpa	Kpb
1	rr	0	0	0	+	+	+	0	0	0	+	0	0
2	rr	0	0	0	+	+	+	0	0	+	0	0	+
3	rr	+	0	0	+	+	+	0	0	+	+	0	+
4	rr	+	0	0	+	+	+	0	0	0	+	0	+
5	rr	0	0	+	+	+W	0	0	0	0		0	+
6	$R_1^wR_1$	+	+	0	0	+	0	+	0	+	+	0	+
7	R_1R_1	+	+	0	0	+	0	0	0	0	+	0	+
8	R_0	0	+	0	+	+	+	0	+	0	+	0	+
9	R_2R_2	0	+	+	+	0	0	0	0	0	+	0	+
10	R_2R_2	0	+	+	+	0	0	0	0	0	+	0	+

[a] 3 + reactions are obtained with Jk[a]-positive red cells: all other cells yield 1 + reactions.

Abbreviations: IS, immediate spin; 37°C, agglutination at 37°C; IAT, indirect antiglobulin test.

(Modified from Petz and Garratty,[9] with permission.)

onto the patient's own red cells. Since the warm autoabsorption technique is so useful, we recommend storing some of the patient's red cells obtained at the first transfusion episode so that they may be used in future autoabsorptions should continued transfusions be required. The red cells are best stored in ACD or CPD or in the frozen state if facilities are available. Details of the technique are listed in Table 20-10 and in Figure 20-1.

Most autoantibodies have IAT titers less than 16, and two autoabsorptions will remove all autoantibody, leaving any alloantibody present in the serum. If the autoantibody titer is higher than 16 by the IAT, more autoabsorptions may be necessary to remove all autoantibody. If the autoantibody titer is not high, enzyme treatment of the eluted red cells is unnecessary. Indeed, since the ratio of cells and serum is different in the in vitro absorption procedure than it is in vivo, autoabsorption without prior elution of the autoantibody (with or without enzyme treatment of the red cells) may suffice, particularly if the DAT is not strongly positive.

Following the autoabsorptions, the absorbed serum is retested. If a negative reaction is obtained, it is assumed that all the serum reactions were due to autoantibody. If a positive reaction still occurs, the absorbed serum should be tested against a panel of red cells to determine whether alloantibody or

Table 20-10. Warm Autoabsorption Technique

1. Wash patient's red cells 4 times.
2. To packed washed cells, add saline or 6 percent albumin (e.g., equal volume).
3. Incubate at 56°C for 3 to 5 minutes
4. Remove supernatant (eluate) after centrifugation.
5. Wash red cells 3 times.
6. Enzyme-treat red cells. (Papain or ficin works well.)
7. Add patient's serum to an equal volume of enzyme-treated cells.
8. Incubate at 37°C for approximately 30 min.
9. Centrifuge. Remove serum.
10. Usually steps 7 to 9 must be repeated at least once.[a]
11. Test autoabsorbed serum for activity. If negative, antibody was autoantibody. If still positive, antibody may be alloantibody or serum needs further autoabsorptions.

[a] Most autoantibodies do not have titers higher than 8; in these cases 2 autoabsorptions are usually sufficient. If the titer is higher than 16, 3 or more autoabsorptions may be necessary.

autoantibody is still present, thus requiring further warm autoabsorptions.

Morel and coworkers[27] have presented data on 20 patients who had 3+ or 4+ DATs and IATs of 1+ to 4+. Twelve patients had autoantibodies that could be completely removed by two autoabsorp-

		Duffy		Kidd		Lewis		MNS				P	Lutheran		Sex-Linked	Results		
Js^a	Js^b	Fy^a	Fy^b	Jk^a	Jk^b	Le^a	Le^b	M	N	S	s	Pl	Lu^a	Lu^b	Xg^a	IS	37°C	IAT
0	+	+	0	+	+	+	0	+	0	+	0	0	0	+	+	0	0	3+
0	+	0	+	+	0	0	+	+	0	+	+	+	0	+	+	0	0	3+
0	+	+	+	+	0	+	0	0	+	0	+	+	+	+	+	0	0	3+
0	+	0	+	+	+	0	+	0	+	0	+	+	0	+	+	0	0	3+
0	+	+	+	0	+	0	+	+	+	+	+	+	0	+	+	0	0	1+
0	+	0	+	0	+	0	+	+	0	0	+	0	0	+	+	0	0	1+
+	+	+	0	+	0	0	+	+	+	0	+	+	0	+	0	0	0	3+
0	+	+	0	+	+	0	0	+	+	+	+	+	0	+	0	0	0	3+
0	+	+	0	+	+	0	0	+	0	+	+	+	0	+	0	0	0	3+
0	+	0	+	0	+	+	0	0	+	+	0	+	0	+	0	0	0	1+

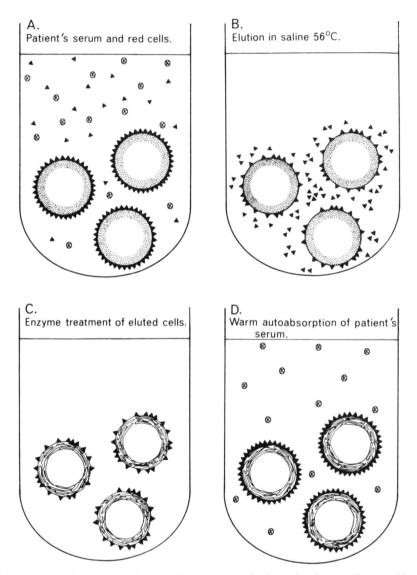

Fig. 20-1 The warm autoabsorption technique. Warm autoantibody molecules are illustrated by solid triangles and anti-Kell alloantibody molecules are indicated by the symbol K. **(A)** Kell-negative patient with warm antibody autoimmune hemolytic anemia who has formed anti-Kell as a result of previous transfusion. Autoantibody is present on the patient's red cells and the serum contains both autoantibody and anti-Kell alloantibody. **(B)** First step of the warm autoabsorption technique. An aliquot of the patient's red cells is washed and incubated in saline at 56°C for 5 minutes to elute some autoantibody. **(C)** Alteration of the red cell membrane by proteolytic enzymes, such as papain or ficin. This augments the ability of the red cells to absorb antibody. These red cells are then used to absorb the patient's serum at 37°C. **(D)** Autoantibody is removed from the serum, leaving only the alloantibody, which can then be identified by routine specificity testing against a panel of red cells. (From Petz and Garratty,[9] with permission.)

tions. Eight other patients were shown to have alloantibodies present in addition to autoantibodies. The specificities involved were anti-E (three patients), anti-V^w (one patient), anti-c + -E (two patients), anti-C^w and anti-E + -K (one patient).

Sokol et al (26) examined 3,888 samples from 2,149 patients who had red cell autoantibodies and found alloantibodies in 294 patients (13.7%). They emphasized that providing "least incompatible blood" is a practice which has little scientific basis and should be considered obsolete. Although there are clinical situations where blood must be issued before all the investigations have been carried out, convenience or external pressures must not permit short-cuts to be taken unnecessarily. Absorption studies to detect alloantibodies were considered most important since alloantibodies are frequently undetectable before absorption.

Similarly, Wallhermfechtel et al.[28] described the prevalence of alloantibodies in 125 patients who had warm autoantibodies. The sera were absorbed with red cells from three donors: R_1R_1 (CDe/CDe), R_2R_2 (cDE/cDE), and rr (cde/cde), whose phenotypes other than Rh were selected to exclude 98 percent of clinically significant alloantibodies. At least one of the three cells lacked each of the common Rh, MNSs, Kell, Duffy, and Kidd antigens. No significant alloantibodies were found in 32 patients who had no prior pregnancy or transfusion. Nineteen of 93 patients (20 percent) who had a history of pregnancy or prior transfusions had alloantibodies. Most of the antibodies showed Rh specificity. Forty-two percent of the alloantibodies were undetectable prior to the alloabsorptions. The authors concluded that patients who have previously been pregnant or transfused should be evaluated by an absorption procedure prior to the transfusion of crossmatch-incompatible red cells.

Laine and Beattie[29] tested blood samples of 109 patients with warm autoantibodies for the presence of accompanying alloantibody. Clinically significant alloantibodies were present in 41 patients (38 percent). The authors pointed out that the provision of antigen-negative donor blood to patients whose serum contains clinically significant alloantibodies but no autoantibody is standard practice. Because accelerated hemolysis of transfused cells by alloantibodies is an undesirable effect in any patient, the presence of alloantibody in patients having autoanti-

bodies should not be treated any differently from those found in patients without autoantibodies. Therefore, pretransfusion techniques to select "least incompatible" donor units cannot be condoned unless it is known with certainty that the patient has not been transfused or pregnant.[29]

Contrasting data were reported by Salama et al.,[30] who found that none of 53 multi-transfused patients with warm antibody AIHA made red blood cell alloantibodies. However, these investigators did not mention whether they used absorption techniques to define whether autoantibodies were masking the presence of alloantibodies. Garratty and Petz[31] pointed out that the inability to detect alloantibodies in multiply transfused patients with AIHA is at variance with numerous other reports (as described above) and emphasized that in patients with AIHA who have been previously transfused or pregnant, a serologic investigation that uses absorptions with autologous or allogeneic RBCs should be performed before issuing units of blood presumed to be incompatible with only autoantibodies.

The Matuhasi–Ogata phenomenon may theoretically limit the usefulness of the warm autoabsorption technique (or the differential absorption technique described later). Matuhasi and Ogata suggested that antibodies of one specificity may adhere to antigen–antibody complexes of a different specificity.[32–33] Thus, one could envision the absorption of alloantibody onto red cells that are used to absorb autoantibody from the patient's serum. Experience indicates, however, that alloantibodies are indeed detectable after absorption of autoantibodies so that the extent of absorption of the alloantibody, if any, is not sufficient to nullify the usefulness of absorption techniques.

Differential Absorption Technique

The differential absorption technique is a method of absorbing autoantibodies from serum that is rapidly gaining favor and is probably optimal in most cases. This method involves absorption of the autoantibody from the patient's serum using allogeneic red cells of varying phenotypes. For example, performing an absorption using a Jk^a-negative cell, of a serum containing a warm autoantibody and an anti-Jk^a alloantibody, will remove the autoantibody but not the anti-Jk^a. As with the warm autoabsorption technique, enzyme treatment of the red cells used for absorption will facilitate removal of the autoantibody, but it is not absolutely necessary.

The only practical limitation of the differential absorption technique is obtaining an adequate supply of red cells of the appropriate phenotypes for absorption. The most feasible approach is to obtain the red cells in advance and store them in the frozen state. It is preferable to store the red cells in aliquots of about 10 to 15 ml, so that several absorptions can be performed with each aliquot of frozen-thawed erythrocytes. Methods for freezing the red cells, thawing them, and performing the differential absorption procedure have been previously reported.[10,34]

As an alternative to using frozen stored erythrocytes for absorption, commercially available antibody detection cells and antibody identification panel cells may provide cell volumes sufficient for the performance of an abbreviated differential absorption using smaller volumes of the appropriate cell type with a concomitantly reduced volume of serum to be absorbed. The major disadvantage of using a reduced amount of serum for the differential absorption technique is that only a small volume of absorbed serum will be available for the subsequent testing for possible alloantibody specificity.

Although the differential absorption technique may seem hopelessly complicated, since hundreds of red cell alloantibodies have been identified, alloantibodies of only a few specificities are responsible for a large majority of hemolytic transfusion reactions. That is, a large percentage of hemolytic transfusion reactions are caused by ABO, Rh, Kell, Kidd, and Fy^a antibodies.[35–37]

ABO alloantibodies will present no problem, providing proper cell typing is performed. Furthermore, if the Rh phenotype of the patient is known, hemolytic transfusion reactions caused by Rh alloantibodies can be avoided by using blood of the same Rh phenotype as the patient. Thus, one may detect a large majority of potentially hemolytic alloantibodies by absorbing with several red cells, that is, Kell-negative, Jk^a-negative, Jk^b-negative, and Fy^a-negative. As a modification of this approach, one could omit the absorption with Kell-negative red cells and instead select Kell-negative donor red cells for transfusion to ensure lack of a Kell-related transfusion reaction. Although this principle could theoretically be extended to the other blood groups as

well, it is obviously unrealistic to attempt to secure donor blood that is, for example, Kell-negative, Jk^a-negative, Fy^a-negative, and of the appropriate ABO and Rh type. If the cells used for absorbing are enzyme-treated and the autoantibody titer is less than 16 by IAT, two absorptions will most likely remove all autoantibody.

In summary, then, to detect the most common clinically significant non-Rh alloantibodies, one needs only to absorb the autoantibody from the patient's serum with (enzyme-treated) Jk^a-negative, Jk^b-negative, and Fy^a-negative red cells to exclude the presence of these alloantibodies. If no alloantibodies are detected in the absorbed aliquots of the patient's serum, one may then transfuse with donor cells that are Kell-negative and of the same Rh phenotype as the patient. Although the possible presence of alloantibodies of numerous specificities is ignored, the probability of an alloantibody-induced hemolytic transfusion reaction is minimal.

If the patient's Rh phenotype is not known and cannot be determined accurately because of recent blood transfusion, differential absorptions should also be employed using R_1R_1, R_2R_2, and rr red cells, to detect Rh alloantibodies. The total number of red cells used for these absorptions can be reduced and the information gained by selecting R_1R_1, R_2R_2, and rr red cells maximized, all of which are Kell-negative and one of which is Jk^a-negative, one Jk^b-negative, and the other Fy^a-negative.[38]

Absorption with the rr cells removes anti-c and anti-e; specificities remaining in the absorbed serum are anti-C, anti-D, and anti-E. The R_1R_1 cells absorb anti-C, anti-D, and anti-e; specificities left behind are anti-E and anti-c. The R_2R_2 cells absorb anti-D, anti-E, and anti-c; remaining are anti-C and anti-e. Depending on which other antigens were absent from the red cells used for the autoabsorptions, other important alloantibodies may also be detected in the absorbed serum. For example, the aliquot of serum absorbed with Jk^a-negative red cells may contain anti-Jk^a. Secondary eluates may also be helpful in defining specificities. The choice of red cells to be used may also be influenced by knowledge of the antigenic makeup of the patient's red cells, if known. For example, one may absorb with cells of the same Rh phenotype as the patient. Furthermore, if one is confident that the patient is Jk^a-positive on the basis of the cell typing techniques described earlier, one need not absorb with Jk^a-negative red cells, as the production of an alloantibody of anti-Jk^a specificity is, of course, impossible.

Comparison of Warm Autoabsorption and Differential Absorption Techniques

The primary advantage of the warm autoabsorption technique for detection of alloantibodies over the differential absorption technique is that all alloantibodies are detectable, as a patient's own cells will only absorb autoantibody. Disadvantages are that gross hemolysis of a patient's red cells occasionally occurs, especially if heat elution is used prior to autoabsorption. More importantly, the method is not reliable if a patient has been transfused recently, because of the possibility of alloabsorption by the transfused cells.[9,38]

The differential absorption test has several significant advantages. Most importantly, the method may be used whether or not the patient has been recently transfused. Also, a supply of the appropriately phenotyped red cells adequate for numerous absorption procedures may be obtained from donor centers in anticipation of their use for this purpose. The cells should be phenotyped as completely as possible, aliquoted, and stored in a glycerol solution at $-20°C$ until needed.[10] Thus, only the simple process of deglycerolization of the red cells[10,34] need be performed prior to absorption, and the same technique may be used for each patient. Although not all clinically important alloantibodies will be detected, the procedure affords a high degree of safety. It is certainly the most reliable method for detection of alloantibodies in the presence of autoantibodies in patients who have been recently transfused. Its more widespread use should be encouraged.

Finally, if red cells are not available for perform-

ing the differential absorption procedure, a warm autoabsorption method should be performed because alloantibody may be detected. However, failure to detect alloantibodies by the warm autoabsorption technique in a recently transfused patient cannot be regarded as definitive evidence of their absence.

SIGNIFICANCE OF AUTOANTIBODY SPECIFICITY

Clinically significant Rh specificity of an autoantibody can be detected by observing the reaction of the antibody against a panel of red cells and or by performing a titer using the patient's serum or eluate against R_1R_1, R_2R_2, and rr red cells.

Autoantibodies with Rh Specificity or Relative Specificity

Serologists are frequently vague regarding the criteria used when reporting an autoantibody as having Rh specificity. Most warm autoantibodies react with all red cells of common Rh phenotypes but may fail to react with gene deletion cells such as Rh_{null} cells. Other autoantibodies will react with all red cells tested but react to a higher titer or score against red cells bearing a particular Rh antigen. In either case, the autoantibody is usually said to have Rh specificity without distinguishing such reactions from each other or from the clear cut specificity of Rh alloantibodies wherein cells lacking the appropriate antigen give strictly negative reactions. We will refer to antibodies that react with all normal red cells bearing common Rh antigens, but that consistently react to a higher titer or score against red cells containing one or another Rh antigen as having "relative specificity."

Table 20-11 shows results of an eluate that would

Table 20-11. Eluate Showing Anti-e Relative Specificity[a]

	Dilutions of Eluate							
	2	4	8	16	32	64	128	256
rr (cde/cde)	4+	3+	3+	2+	2+	1+	0	0
R_1R_1 (CDe/CDe)	4+	3+	3+	2+	2+	1+	0	0
R_2R_2 (cDE/cDE)	3+	2+	1+	0	0	0	0	0

[a] Agglutination reactions are graded as 1+ to 4+.
(From Petz and Garratty,[9] with permission.)

be interpreted as showing relative specificity against the e antigen. Such reactions should be confirmed by testing against several examples of red cells with and without the appropriate antigen before clinical decisions based on the relative specificity of the autoantibody are made.

Several investigators have studied the in vivo survival of red cells of varying Rh phenotypes in patients who have warm autoantibodies that were said to have Rh specificity. In most instances, detailed serologic data are not given and the autoantibodies are likely to have demonstrated relative specificity.

Mollison[39] described a case in which survival of the patient's own e-positive red cells was markedly shortened, whereas transfused e-negative red cells survived almost normally. The patient's serum contained an autoantibody with anti-e specificity.

Salmon[40] described two patients who had anti-e and anti-nl autoantibodies. In the first case, the T 1/2 of ^{51}Cr-labeled red cells was 23 days for -D-/-D- red cells (e−,nl−), 24 days for cDE/cDE red cells (e−,nl+), and 12.5 days for cde/cde (e+,nl+). In the second case, the T 1/2 was 14 days for cDE/cDE red cells but only 4 days for CDe/cde red cells (Table 20-12).

von dem Borne et al.[41] reported a patient who had autoanti-e and autoanti-nl antibodies. The ^{51}Cr T 1/2 of CDe/CDe red cells was 1.9 days, and that of cDE/cDE red cells was 4.0 days.

Table 20-12. Significance of Autoantibodies With Rh Relative Specificity

Case 1: Half-Life of ^{51}Cr-Labeled Red Blood Cells in a cde/cde Patient with Ante-e + nl Autoantibodies

—D—/—D—/ red cells: (e—nl—) = 23 days
cDE/cDE red cells: (e—nl+) = 24 days
cde/cde red cells: (e+nl+) = 12.5 days
cde/cde red cells: (e+nl+) = 12.5 days
The anti-e appears to be responsible for half-life diminution

Case 2: Half-Life of ^{51}Cr-Labeled Red Blood Cells in a CDe/cde Patient with Anti-e + nl Autoantibodies

cDE/cDE red cells: (e—nl+) = 14 days
CDe/cde red cells: (e+nl+) = 4 days
The anti-nl is less hemolytic in vivo than is anti-e

In Hollander's patient,[42] the autoantibodies had anti-D specificity; while cde/cde blood survived for at least 31 days, CDe/cde blood survived for only 3 days. In Crowley and Bouroncle's patient,[43] two autoantibodies, anti-D and anti-E, were present, and cde/cde cells survived normally. In the patient described by Wiener et al.,[44] the autoantibody reacted to highest titers with cells containing the rh′ (C) factor; when transfused with blood lacking this factor, the patient made a complete and lasting recovery. Previously, she had been treated with randomly selected Rh-positive donors and had failed to improve. The patient reported by Ley et al.[45] was group O cde/cde; cDE/cDE erythrocytes were demonstrated to survive normally (^{51}Cr T 1/2 = 25 days), but cde/cde cells survived even less well than the patient's own cells (^{51}Cr t1/2 = 5 days and 13 to 14 days, respectively).

The case reported by Hogman et al.[46] was of a 13-year-old child of probable genotype CDe/CDe who had formed autoanti-e as well as an apparent "nonspecific" component. The latter component did not appear to be of much importance, as cDE/cDE red cells survived normally.

Bell et al.[7] cited one patient with anti-e who tolerated 2 e-negative units with the expected rise and maintenance of hemoglobin levels. No further details were given.

Habibi[6] transfused cDE/cDE red cells to 6 patients with autoantibodies of e, ce, or Ce specificities. The blood "proved normally efficient in vivo," but two of six homozygous ee patients developed anti-E alloantibodies.

Clinical Approach Based on Autoantibody Specificity

Although the preceding data are limited, we believe that if an autoantibody demonstrates relative specificity (e.g., the titer against red cells containing an antigen is consistently two tubes higher than when tested against cells lacking that antigen), it is preferable to avoid transfusion of blood containing the antigen in question. An exception to this course is generally made if it would be necessary to give Rh-positive blood to an Rh-negative individual, especially a woman of child-bearing age. Another important although unusual exception concerns the patient who, in addition to the autoantibody, also has an alloantibody that would make it impossible to transfuse red cells simultaneously lacking antigens that the alloantibody and autoantibody are directed against. For example, if the patient has an alloanti-E and an autoanti-e, blood lacking the E antigen should be transfused.

In contrast to this approach, some immunohematologists recommend ignoring the specificity of the autoantibody. This attitude is based on two considerations. First, the evidence indicating good survival related to autoantibody relative specificity is not extensive and, in some reports, the benefit was minimal.[41] In other instances, good survival of donor blood lacking the more reactive antigen was not shown to be due to the autoantibody specificity, since survival of transfused cells containing the more reactive antigen was not studied.[6,7,43,46]

Second, if one transfuses red cells lacking an antigen with which an autoantibody reacts, one may need to use red cells containing an antigen not found on the patient's own cells, thus causing the potential for alloimmunization. This does not seem to be a critical argument, since typing for Rh antigens other than $Rh_o(D)$ is not part of routine blood transfusion practice, and we know of no data that convincingly demonstrate that patients with AIHA have an increased incidence of development of red cell alloantibodies after transfusion.

Autoantibodies Without Demonstrated Specificity

If autoantibody specificity is not demonstrable, a seemingly logical approach is to do compatibility tests using as large a number of donor units as practical (e.g., 5 to 10 units) and then select for transfusion those units that are "least incompatible" in vitro. However, when such in vitro differences in reactivity are caused by variable reactivity of the red cell autoantibody unrelated to an identified red cell antigen and not caused by the presence of alloantibody, there are no data indicating whether such comparatively weakly reactive units have better survival than more strongly reactive units.

AIHA Without Serum Autoantibody

In contrast to the above problems frequently encountered in AIHA, it should also be pointed out that in some patients with overt hemolysis the autoantibody does not interfere with compatibility testing. This is true because the autoantibody may be undetectable in the patient's serum (apparently because it is entirely absorbed onto the patient's red cells) or detectable only by techniques more sensitive than those used in routine saline and albumin crossmatch tests. Even though the donor is apparently compatible, the transfused red cells cannot be expected to survive normally because the autoantibody, although detectable only with very sensitive techniques in vitro, will react with donor cells in vivo as it has with the patient's own cells.[8] Thus, precautions concerning transfusion in patients with warm antibody AIHA apply equally, even though the routine compatibility test would tend to falsely ensure normal donor red cell survival.

When autoantibody is not detectable in the patient's serum by routine crossmatch tests, the use of more sensitive serologic techniques may be utilized (i.e., the use of enzyme-treated red cells). In addition, autoantibody is often readily detected in an eluate prepared from the patient's red cells and in this case tests for specificity against common Rh antigens may be performed by titrations against R_1R_1, R_2R_2, and rr cells as described above.

Patients who present with a positive direct antiglobulin test but who have no signs of an active hemolytic process need not receive any special consideration in the selection of donor blood.

COMPATIBILITY TESTING IN COLD ANTIBODY AIHAs

Cold Agglutinin Syndrome

Compatibility Testing at 37°C in Saline

There are several approaches to compatibility testing in patients with cold agglutinin syndrome. One method is to perform the compatibility test strictly at 37°C and use only normal saline media (i.e., without using albumin or low ionic strength solutions). Cold agglutinins from only 7 percent of patients with cold agglutinin syndrome react at 37°C in saline, although positive reactions will be obtained about 30 percent of cases in albumin media.[47] If positive reactions occur at 37°C in saline, one must first suspect faulty technique. If cells and serum are not prewarmed before mixing, if the initial washes of the cells after incubation do not use saline at 37°C, or if centrifugation is performed at a temperature lower than 37°C, reactions may occur within seconds. Even if direct agglutination is not evident, complement may be bound by the antibody reactivity and result in a positive IAT. (One molecule of IgM antibody may bind several hundred molecules of complement.) When cold agglutinins of very high thermal amplitude are present, it may be advantageous to use a monospecific anti-IgG antiglobulin serum in the antiglobulin phase of the compatibility test.

The advantages of compatibility testing at 37°C are that time consuming autoabsorptions of the patient's serum are not necessary and that the method can be utilized even if the patient has been recently transfused. The reliability of autoabsorption in the latter case is uncertain.

Several disadvantages are also apparent. First, it is obvious that red cell alloantibodies reacting at temperatures less than 37°C will not be detected. This is of little consequence since antibodies that do not react in vitro at temperatures less than 37°C are rarely, if ever, clinically significant (see Ch. 9). Giblett[36] is emphatic about this point, stating that alloantibodies that do not react at 37°C are of no concern, since she observed no in vivo hemolysis associated with a cold-reacting alloantibodies (e.g., anti-A$_1$, -P$_1$, -M, -N. -Lu^a) during a 20-year period, in which over a million units of blood were transfused. Mollison et al.[48] are somewhat more cautious in their conclusions but do state that, in view of the small amount of destruction caused by cold agglutinins that are weakly reactive at 37°C, those cold agglutinins that are active only at a temperature lower than 37°C can safely be ignored. Indeed, the Standards for Blood Banks and Transfusion Services of the American Association of Blood Banks[24] does not require a room temperature incubation phase of the crossmatch but instead states that methods for testing for unexpected antibodies "shall include 37°C incubation preceding an antiglobulin test using reagent red blood cells that are not pooled."

It is also true that antibodies reactive only in albumin or other potentiating media will be missed, but again, the risk is minimal because such antibodies are quite unusual[49] (see Ch. 9). Since compatibility testing at 37°C is quicker than other methods, can be used even if the patient has recently been transfused, and carries a very low risk of missing clinically significant alloantibodies, we find it the method of choice. However, attention to certain technical details is crucial in order to be certain that one is truly working strictly at 37°C.

A heated centrifuge or a centrifuge in a 37°C warm room may be used, a centrifuge may be placed in an incubator, or the tubes may be placed in centrifuge cups containing warm water. Samples transferred from a 37°C water bath and centrifuged immediately in a Serofuge at room temperature (20 to 25°C) drop approximately 7 to 8°C after only 1 minute of centrifugation. It is necessary to keep a Serofuge in an incubator at about 40°C, in which the samples spin at about 37°C. Similarly, saline at 40°C may be used, since it drops a few degrees when it enters a test tube and when centrifuging is in progress. Only a few simple experiments with each laboratory's equipment are required to determine the conditions that will enable all procedures to be carried out strictly at 37°C.

Facilities without heated centrifuges may use 45°C prewarmed centrifuge cups and 45°C saline for washing; this will maintain the temperature during centrifugation at about 37°C. However, there is a greater chance that the temperature will dip below the required 37°C using this technique, and 45°C saline can sometimes elute significant IgG antibody off the red cells.

Cold Autoabsorption

An alternative approach is to absorb the cold autoantibody from the patient's serum before performing the crossmatch test. This method works well for low-titer cold agglutinins. However, it is very time-consuming when high-titer antibodies causing cold agglutinin syndrome are present, requiring multiple absorptions even when using enzyme-treated red cells. This approach therefore is not optimal if blood is needed urgently. Furthermore, the reliability of autoabsorption tests in recently transfused patients is uncertain. However, the technique may be necessary in the small percentage of patients whose antibody is reactive at 37°C, even in saline. When positive reactions are obtained at 37°C, one or two autoabsorptions followed by compatibility testing at 37°C is useful. Table 20-13 shows the results of autoabsorbing a serum with a cold agglutinin titer of 2,048 in saline and 8,096 in albumin. After three

Table 20-13. Absorption of Cold Agglutinin by Patient's Own Cells at 4°C

	Titer Against Adult OI Cells					
	4°C		25°C		37°C	
	Saline	Albumin	Saline	Albumin	Saline	Albumin
Unabsorbed	2,048	8,096	1,024	8,096	0	32
Absorbed × 1	1,024	2,048	256	1,024	0	16
Absorbed × 2	256	256	128	256	0	8
Absorbed × 3	128	128	16	64	0	0

(From Petz and Garratty,[9] with permission.)

absorptions for half an hour each at 4°C, using the patient's papainized red cells, the serum still reacted strongly at 4°C and at room temperature (25°C), but no longer reacted at 37°C.

Other Methods

Still another approach to compatibility testing in cold agglutinin syndrome is to inactivate the IgM cold agglutinin with 2-mercaptoethanol[50,51] or DTT.[52]

Pirofsky and Rosner[52] described the use of DTT at a concentration of 0.01 M in a rapid 15-minute 37°C incubation test system. Dialysis was not required. They reported that this procedure caused at least a fourfold or greater decrease in IgM antibody titers, without affecting the activity of IgG antibodies.

Olson et al.[53] used DTT in a concentration of 0.01 M, added equal volumes to test sera, and incubated for 30 minutes at 37°C. Thirty sera containing red cell antibodies reactive by the IAT showed virtually no alteration in activity after DTT treatment, while 20 sera containing cold-reactive red cell antibodies showed almost total elimination of activity. However, none of the cold-reactive antibodies tested was pathologic high-titer cold agglutinins from patients with cold agglutinin syndrome.

Freedman et al.[54] reviewed the optimal conditions for use of sulphydryl compounds in dissociating red cell antibodies. They noted that incubation at 37°C with 0.2 M 2-mercaptoethanol provided the best conditions for inactivating IgM antibodies. However, it still failed to inactivate completely an extremely potent autoanti-I (titer of 1,024,000). False-positive reactions in the IAT using anti-IgG or anti-complement antiglobulin serum were consistently obtained when sera that had been treated with 2-mercaptoethanol were not subsequently dialyzed. Although dialysis for as short as 30 minutes was sufficient in many cases, in other patients, overnight dialysis was found to be necessary. Incubation of serum with DTT produced a slower effect than did 2-mercaptoethanol, and incubation for 22 hours was necessary to reduce the anti-I titer from 1,024,000 to 1,024.

Some investigators have suggested that adult i red cells be used for transfusion of patients with cold agglutinin syndrome who have anti-I autoantibodies. Van Loghem et al.[55] studied the survival of I and i red cells labeled with ^{51}Cr in one patient with chronic cold agglutinin syndrome. They demonstrated normal survival for the i donor cells, with greatly shortened survival of both the patient's I cells and donor I cells. Woll et al.[56] reported one patient with transient cold agglutinin syndrome who responded to transfusion of warmed, frozen-thawed adult i red blood cells. However, they did not test the survival of adult I red cells. Bell et al.[7] reported unfavorable experiences transfusing 2 patients with cold agglutinin syndrome with adult i red cells. Two adult i units given to a patient with strong anti-I survived for approximately the same period of time (i.e., 3 to 4 days) as several adult I units given subsequently. In a second patient with anti-I, no elevation of hematocrit was noted after transfusion of 2 units of adult i blood. The authors suggested that the minimal I antigen present on adult i erythrocytes seemed sufficient to render them biologically incompatible.

Experience indicates that transfusion of adult I

red cells to patients with chronic cold agglutinin syndrome usually results in an appropriate rise in hemoglobin. Unusual patients may fail to respond to transfusion of adult I red cells, but most available data indicate that the use of adult i cells is not a solution to the problem. In patients with chronic cold agglutinin syndrome, the repeated use of i cells is certainly not feasible because of their extreme rarity.

Paroxysmal Cold Hemoglobinuria

Transfusion of compatible blood may be possible if the rare p or p^k cells are available through a rare donor file. Although the routine crossmatch test will appear to be compatible with other red cells since the antibody reacts only in the cold (usually less than 15°C), there is evidence indicating that p or p^k red cells will survive better.[3] Patients may require transfusion before such cells are available, and transfusion of red cells of common P types should not be withheld if transfusion is urgently needed. Although there are some reports of Donath-landsteiner antibodies having other specificities, these are rare.

IN VIVO COMPATIBILITY TESTING

In vivo compatibility testing has been considered useful in AIHA by some investigators. It is based on testing the in vivo survival of an aliquot of red cells. Red cell survival may be measured crudely by means of changes in serum bilirubin[57] or plasma hemoglobin[58] or, more precisely, by using ^{51}Cr-tagged cells.[59–62] The methods have been described in detail elsewhere[62] (see Ch. 9).

There is some disagreement concerning the significance of in vivo survival studies in AIHA. We believe that in most clinical settings an in vivo survival study does not provide information that would alter AIHA patient–management decisions made on the basis of careful serologic technique and good clinical judgement. Furthermore, an in vivo compatibility test must not be considered a substitute for meticulous in vitro compatibility testing as described previously. It is pertinent to consider the potential significance of in vivo compatibility tests in various clinical settings.

Critically Ill Patients

Patients with AIHA who have progressively severe and immediately life-threatening anemia must be transfused and results of in vitro and in vivo compatibility tests must not dissuade one from this decision. For example, if a patient with overt hemolysis has a hematocrit of 20 percent on a given morning, a hematocrit of 16 percent in the early afternoon and 12 percent by late afternoon, transfusion must be given. If a careful serologic study has been done, using the techniques and principles already described, to select the best possible donor unit of blood, and an in vivo test nevertheless demonstrates a very short cell survival, there is no logical way to select a different unit of blood for transfusion. For the patient who is critically ill and is not yet responding to appropriate therapy, such as high-dose corticosteroids, this incompatible blood must still be given in the hope of obtaining temporary benefit.

Seriously Ill Patients

Many patients with AIHA are seriously ill but with hemolysis not as immediately or as definitely life-threatening as the patient described above. For example, if a 60-year-old patient has a hematocrit that is stable at 18 percent during the first several days of hospitalization, EKG evidence of an old myocardial infarct, and a persistent tachycardia, transfusion to a somewhat higher hematocrit is probably desirable. Proponents of in vivo compatibility testing feel that an acceptable in vivo 1-hour survival of ^{51}Cr-labeled cells provides an important measure of reassurance in that an acute symptomatic transfusion reaction is unlikely to occur and the transfusion will produce at least temporary benefit.[58–62] The available data support such a suggestion, the most extensive being that of Silvergleid et al.,[61] who found that if the 1-hour survival was 85 percent or greater, none of 33 patients subsequently transfused with incompatible blood had an acute symptomatic transfusion reaction. However, two additional important factors must be kept in mind.

First, even shorter in vivo survival studies do not preclude a beneficial effect of transfusion. Mollison et al.[59] reported that when the recipient's serum contains a low concentration of antibody, the survival of a large amount of incompatible red cells may be much better than the survival of a smaller amount. It is presumed that a small concentration of antibody that is able to cause the destruction of a small volume of incompatible red cells may not be capable of causing destruction of a larger volume of transfused cells. Indeed, Mayer et al.[63] reported that 11 patients with AIHA who had an in vivo survival of ^{51}Cr-labeled donor red cells of less than 70 percent at 24 hours nevertheless required transfusion. Only one of these patients had a complication directly attributable to the transfusion. Thus, short survival of an aliquot of ^{51}Cr-labeled red cells should not be interpreted to mean that transfusion is contraindicated. Data are not available to determine the rate of destruction of a test dose of red cells that would predict an acute symptomatic hemolytic reaction.

Second, even though "adequate" survival of an aliquot of ^{51}Cr-labeled cells (variably reported as greater than 70 or 85 percent at one hour[61,62] or greater than 70 percent at 24 hours[63]) apparently precludes an acute symptomatic transfusion reaction, subsequent survival is unpredictable. Indeed, dangerous degrees of hemolysis may occur in subsequent hours unless 1-hour survival is strictly normal. For example, Silvergleid et al.[61] reported one patient with warm antibody autoimmune hemolytic anemia who had a 1-hour red cell survival of 87 percent, a pretransfusion hematocrit of 10.5 percent, and a post-transfusion hematocrit of 20.6 percent, but a hematocrit of only 10 percent just 16 hours post-transfusion. Another patient, with paroxysmal cold hemoglobinuria, had a 1-hour survival of Tj(a+) red cells of 87 percent and was transfused with 0.5 units of blood; only 53 percent of the radiolabeled cells survived to 48 hours. Still another patient with an alloantibody (anti-Jk[b]) had 94-percent survival of tagged cells at 1 hour but only 10 percent survival at 24 hours.

Thus, short survival does not contraindicate transfusion, and "adequate," but subnormal survival does not ensure safety despite a high probability of temporary benefit without an immediate symptomatic hemolytic reaction. It is impossible to predict the survival of a therapeutic volume of transfused cells when survival of a small test volume of red cells is subnormal.

Clinically Insignificant Autoantibodies

Chromium survival studies of red cell life span have provided useful information regarding a relatively common cause of in vitro incompatibility that cannot be resolved, that is, the presence of autoantibodies in patients without hemolytic anemia. Silvergleid et al.[61] studied 14 patients who had positive direct antiglobulin tests and "nonspecific warm autoantibodies" in their sera. In none of these patients was there clinical evidence of hemolytic anemia. In 13 of the cases, ^{51}Cr-labeled red cell recovery at 1 hour was 99 percent with an error of ±5 percent; in the other patient, it was 92 percent. Nine of these patients were subsequently transfused; there were no clinical signs of shortened red cell survival. Three of the patients who were transfused had been taking methyldopa. On the basis of these data, it appears that autoantibodies that are not causing hemolytic anemia will not cause shortened survival of transfused red cells.

Summary

Decisions concerning the need for transfusion of patients with AIHA should be made primarily on the basis of a clinical assessment. When a decision is made that transfusion is necessary, the selection of the unit of red cells to be transfused should be made on the basis of detailed in vitro serologic studies. An in vivo survival study may provide some additional useful information in some circumstances.

If an in vivo survival study demonstrates normal survival at 1 hour, an acute symptomatic hemolytic transfusion reaction is unlikely to occur when the unit of red cells is transfused.

If a patient is seriously ill with AIHA, the survival of transfused red cells is unlikely to be normal. If an in vivo survival study demonstrates short survival, this must not be interpreted to mean that transfusion is necessarily contraindicated. If transfusion is urgently needed, the fact that the transfused red cells will not survive normally should not preclude transfusion.

If a red cell survival indicates moderate shortening of red cell survival at 1 hour, survival of a large volume of red cells is unpredictable. Brisk hemolysis may occur but, in some instances, survival of a large amount of incompatible red cells may be much better than that of a smaller amount.

OPTIMAL VOLUME OF BLOOD TO BE TRANSFUSED TO PATIENTS WITH AIHA

The optimal volume of blood to be transfused to patients with AIHA varies with the clinical setting. In patients who have severe hemolysis but may only require transfusion temporarily until therapy becomes effective, the transfusion of modest volumes of red cells just sufficient to maintain a tolerable hematocrit appears advisable. Indeed, Rosenfield and Jagathambal[64] point out that the salutary effect of just 100 ml of packed red cells may be quite remarkable when given to a patient with cardiopulmonary embarrassment from anemia. They suggest that 100 ml may be given as needed (perhaps twice daily, depending on the severity of hemolysis) and that there is no need to increase the hemoglobin, even to a level of 8 g/dl. The aim of such transfusions is to supply just enough red cells to prevent hypoxemia, while avoiding dangerous reactions resulting from overtransfusion.

Complications of Aggressive Transfusion Therapy in Patients With AIHA

Volume Overload

The dangers of overtransfusion in patients with AIHA are several. If the anemia is very severe (hematocrit of 10 to 15 percent, hemoglobin of 3.5 to 5.0 g/dl), and especially if the patient is elderly and/or if cardiac reserve may be reduced, transfusion may easily overload the circulation and precipitate cardiac failure. In such patients red cells should be administered slowly, not exceeding one ml/kg/h.[59] One must look for evidence of congestive heart failure during and following the transfusion, particularly elevated venous pressure and the presence of rales on auscultation of the chest. Although diuretics are useful and probably should be given to patients with diminished cardiac reserve, responses will vary, and their administration must not replace close clinical observation of the patient.

Patients who have a chronic hemolytic anemia that is unresponsive to therapy will, for practical purposes, require the transfusion of volumes of blood larger than 100 ml of red cells per transfusion. Patients with anemia causing signs and symptoms severe enough to require transfusion chronically may have only moderate degrees of hemolysis associated with a relatively poor marrow response (e.g., hemoglobin of 5 g/dl with less than 10 percent reticulocytes). (These patients can usually be managed as outlined in Ch. 19 for patients with chronic anemia,

that is, with several units of red cells per transfusion as required.)

Patients with chronic AIHA whose rate of hemolysis is significantly more severe and who require chronic transfusions are in greater danger of post-transfusion hemoglobinuria for reasons indicated below. Transfusion therapy will have to be individualized, with an attempt to compromise between the impracticality of repeated use of small volumes of red cells and the dangers inherent in transfusion of large volumes. Patients with marked shortening of red cell life span who require repeated frequent transfusions have a precarious outlook, at least in part because of the acute and chronic dangers of blood transfusions. Vigorous therapeutic measures for the AIHA are indicated; every attempt should be made to wean the patient off transfusion if a stable, albeit low, hematocrit can be maintained.

Some physicians recommend partial exchange transfusion, which can be conveniently carried out by starting a venesection in one arm and infusing red cells in the other, and by keeping the rates of blood administration and removal nearly equal. Since the hematocrit in the blood removed is much lower than that in the blood administered, one may rapidly increase the patient's hematocrit without changing blood volume. This can also be accomplished with cell separators by exchanging plasma for red cells. However, such measures to acutely increase the patient's red cell mass are probably contraindicated in this clinical setting.

Post-Transfusion Hemolysis and Disseminated Intravascular Coagulation

An additional danger in patients with AIHA relates to the fact that the kinetics of red cell destruction describe an exponential curve of decay, indicating that the number of cells removed in a unit of time is a percentage of the number of cells present at the start of this time interval.[64] Thus, the more cells that are present at zero time, the more cells in absolute number will be destroyed in the unit time span. Indeed, Chaplin[58] indicates that the most common cause of post-transfusion hemoglobinuria in AIHA may not be alloantibody-induced hemolysis but instead may be the quantitative effect of transfusion in increasing the red cell mass subjected to ongoing autoantibody-mediated destruction. Such marked post-transfusion hemoglobinemia and hemoglobin-uria have the potential for a significant degree of associated morbidity and, possibly, mortality. Patients undergoing severe posttransfusion intravascular hemolysis may develop disseminated intravascular coagulation (DIC), possibly as a result of procoagulant substances present in red cell lysates.[59] Such coagulation abnormalities may be fatal, again emphasizing the need for restraint in transfusion of patients with AIHA.

Case Summaries

An example of such a complication of transfusion therapy was reported by Bilgrami et al.[65] These investigators reported a patient who was infected with the human immunodeficiency virus (HIV) who had severe AIHA. His hemoglobin was 2.9 g/dl; hematocrit, 8 percent; corrected reticulocyte count, 1.2 percent; white cell count, 12,500/μl; platelet count, 101,000/μl; total bilirubin, 3 mg/dl; direct bilirubin, 0.7 mg/dl; lactate dehydrogenase (LDH), 1,902 U/L; PT, 11.8 seconds (normal 11 to 13 seconds); and PTT 20.8 seconds (normal, 25 to 35 seconds). The urine was grossly red but with no intact red cells. The peripheral smear demonstrated spherocytes, polychromasia, and nucleated red cells. The DAT was positive using polyspecific antiserum, anti-IgG, and anti-C3. Differentially absorbed serum was used to select blood for transfusion but was incompatible (w+ to 2+). Before transfusion, immune complexes were detected in the serum by several techniques.

The patient underwent aggressive transfusion, receiving 8 units of packed red cells over 24 hours, as shown in Figure 20-2. The patient was transfused to a hematocrit level of greater than 25 percent. However, signs of DIC developed, with the platelet count demonstrating a progressive decline and the PT and PTT showing an upward trend within 24 hours. One-half hour before the patient's death, the following laboratory results were obtained: PT, 16.8 seconds; PTT, 81 seconds; serum fibrinogen, 130 mg/dl (normal, 150 to 400 mg/dl); thrombin time (TT), 45 seconds (control, 16.5 seconds; fibrin degradation products (FDP) titer, greater than 40 μg/ml; and D-dimer, greater than 1 μg/ml. A diagnosis of DIC was made. The patient became hypotensive shortly thereafter and could not be resuscitated.

An autopsy demonstrated widespread multiple pulmonary thrombi. There was widespread throm-

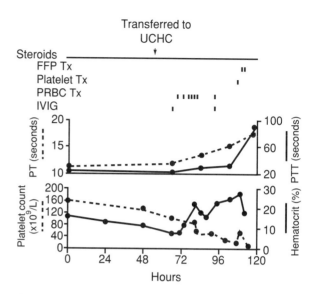

Fig. 20-2 Clinical course of AIHA and DIC in a patient with HIV infection. PT, prothrombin time; PTT, partial thromboplastin time; PRBC, packed red blood cells; FFP, fresh frozen plasma; Tx, transfusion; UCHC, University of Connecticut Health Center. (From Bilgrami et al.,[65] with permission.)

bosis of small arterioles of both lungs. Some of the thrombi had begun to organize, and others were very acute, most consistent with the formation of thrombi in situ, rather than secondary to thromboembolic disease. The extensive pulmonary thrombi resulted in acute right ventricular failure, which was the immediate cause of death.

The authors pointed out that less aggressive transfusion therapy would have sufficed to met the patient's tissue oxygen needs and concluded that the most likely etiology of the patient's DIC was the aggressive transfusion therapy.

The following two case summaries were supplied by Chaplin (Chaplin H, Jr., St. Louis, personal communication).

R.S., a 34-year-old white gravida-1, para-1, with relapsing primary AIHA for 4 months, was hospitalized with a hemoglobin of 5.0 g/dl; reticulocytes of 16 percent; direct antiglobulin test strongly positive for C3d, moderately positive for IgM, negative for IgG; and all crossmatches "incompatible." Despite high-dose corticosteroids, she required 1 to 2 units of packed red cells daily to maintain her hemoglobin at 4.5 to 6.0 g/dl. She experienced increasingly severe hemoglobinemia and hemoglobinuria associated with transfusion, clearing within a few hours. No alloantibodies were demonstrable. On the tenth hospital day, a splenectomy was performed without benefit. On the twelfth hospital day, several hours following a transfusion, she developed acute respiratory distress, followed by cardiopulmonary arrest which did not respond to resuscitative measures. Autopsy revealed a single large para-aortic lymph node diagnosed as "plasmacytoid malignant lymphoma"; death was attributed to multiple fresh small pulmonary emboli.

L.F., a 56-year-old white woman, never previously pregnant or transfused, was semistuporous at the time of admission. She had a hemoglobin of 1.6 g/dl; hematocrit 6.2 percent; reticulocytes 19 percent; DAT strongly positive for C3d, moderately positive for IgG, weakly positive for IgM; and all crossmatches "incompatible." She was given corticosteroids and 3 units of packed group O, Rh-negative red cells. She developed fever and striking hemoglobinemia and hemoglobinuria, which improved over the ensuing 3 hours. Her state of consciousness improved, and the hemoglobin rose transiently to 5.7 g/dl but was rapidly declining, when she developed severe respiratory distress, followed by cardiopulmonary arrest, which did not respond to resuscitation. At autopsy, no underlying cause for the AIHA was found; death was attributed to multiple fresh small pulmonary emboli.

These complications of transfusing patients with AIHA are not common as emphasized by Salama et al.,[30] who found no instances of a definite increase in signs of hemolysis in 53 patients with AIHA who received blood transfusion. Nevertheless, in patients with AIHA, RBCs must be transfused cautiously and for appropriate indications.[31] Aggressive transfusion therapy in patients with active hemolysis should be avoided.

USE OF WARM BLOOD IN COLD AGGLUTININ SYNDROME AND PAROXYSMAL COLD HEMOGLOBINURIA

Eminent authorities offer sharply differing opinions concerning the need for warm blood when transfusing patients with cold agglutinin syndrome. Dacie[66] states that properly crossmatched blood can proba-

bly be transfused with safety if run in at a slow drip rate, in which case there is probably no need to attempt to warm it above room temperature. By contrast, Rosenfield and Jagathambal[64] state that patients with cold agglutinin disease must receive warmed blood. Mollison et al.[59] state that blood should be prewarmed before transfusion to patients with cold agglutinin syndrome, but that it is more important to nurse the patient in a warm room. Wallace[67] comments that hemolytic reactions are unlikely, provided that the donor blood is warmed to body temperature and the recipient is kept warm. Apparently, the problem has not been studied in much depth, and no red cell survival studies comparing survival of blood transfused at various temperatures are available.

In regard to paroxysmal cold hemoglobinuria (PCH), Rawsen does report that even compatible Tj(a−) blood needs to be warmed to 37°C before transfusion.[3] Wallace,[67] however, states that even transfusion of red cells of the common P groups (either P_1 positive or negative) is unlikely to precipitate an acute hemolytic transfusion reaction in PCH, provided the donations are warmed to 37°C and the patient is maintained at a warm temperature. Johnsen et al.[68] reported that results of transfusion of 150 ml of prewarmed packed red cells (P positive) to an 18-month-old boy with PCH. The transfusion was followed by a temperature rise and passage of red urine. However, the hemoglobin improved from 4.7 g/dl to 12.4 g/dl and remained at that level.

In the absence of extensive data, logic must prevail. Our experience in cold agglutinin syndrome has been consistent with Dacie's view, although in some instances we have empirically used an "in-line" blood warmer for seriously ill patients. The use of an in-line blood warmer would appear indicated if the patient has either severe PCH or florid cold agglutinin disease. It is also logical to keep the patient warm, even if the efficacy of such a maneuver has not been proven.

If blood is to be warmed, it must be done properly. Unmonitored or uncontrolled heating of blood is extremely dangerous and should not be attempted. Warming of blood should be accomplished during its passage through the transfusion set. The warming system must be equipped with a visible thermometer and, ideally, with an audible warning system.[24] Blood must not be warmed above 42°C.[24] Red cells heated too much are rapidly destroyed in vivo and can be lethal to the patient.[64]

USE OF WASHED OR LEUKOCYTE-DEPLETED RED BLOOD CELLS

Evans et al.[69,70] reported their experience using packed red cells or washed red cells in transfusing one patient with cold agglutinin syndrome. The cold antibody of one patient agglutinated red cells to a titer of 500,000 at 4°C and caused lysis of normal red cells both at room temperature and at 37°C (maximal at room temperature). A transfusion of 2 units of packed red cells was given without subjective reaction, although hemoglobinuria occurred following completion of the transfusion. A subsequent transfusion of three units of washed red cells was given without a rise in plasma hemoglobin. The patient's serum complement was "always low." Although the data are far from conclusive, Evans et al. speculated that the small amount of plasma present in the first transfusion of red cells provided the necessary complement for the hemolysis that followed. Further studies by Evans et al.[70] indicated that transfusion of large volumes of red cells to patients with cold agglutinin syndrome caused a lowering of serum complement. ^{51}Cr-labeled normal red cells survived longer after red cell transfusions than before, and the authors suggested that the reduction in serum complement levels may have been responsible for the improved survival. In our view, the phenomenon reported by Evans remains unexplained and must be very uncommon. Serum complement is usually not reduced in patients with warm or cold antibody AIHA,[9] and we would not recommend the use of washed red cells for this rationale on the basis of the limited information available.

Some investigators recommend using washed or leukocyte-depleted red cell for patients with AIHA to avoid febrile reactions caused by factors other than red cell antibodies. This is reasonable because the interpretation of a febrile reaction in a seriously ill patient with AIHA is difficult and could lead to unnecessary cessation or delay of transfusion. The justification for the use of these products in AIHA beyond that applicable to other acutely ill patients is that the compatibility test procedures may be much more time-consuming in AIHA. Thus, unnecessary cessation of the transfusion is more costly because of the additional technical procedures, and there may be a longer delay in selecting an alternative unit.

AUTOLOGOUS BLOOD TRANSFUSION IN AIHA

Three brief reports have suggested the use of autologous red cells for transfusion of patients with AIHA. Goldfinger et al.[71] demonstrated that autologous frozen-stored red cells may be practical in some patients with AIHA. In one patient with IgM-mediated AIHA, normal in vivo recovery was demonstrated although in vitro red cell loss was 40 percent. In patients who had positive direct antiglobulin tests but not hemolytic anemia, in vitro red cell loss was only 2 to 14 percent and in vivo recovery and survival were normal. Storing red cells in the frozen state may be considered for patients who go into remission while on therapy for AIHA. In the event of later relapse, the cells may be transfused without fear of alloantibody-induced hemolysis. However, because of autoantibody in the patient's serum, red cell survival is not likely to be better than that of a homologous unit and conceivably could be worse if an antibody with a high degree of specificity for autoantigens is present.

Parr and Ballard[72] reported a patient with methyldopa-induced positive direct and indirect antiglobulin tests who required surgery. The patient had equivocal evidence of hemolysis consisting of an elevated LDH with a normal hemoglobin and hematocrit. The patient's serum antibody reacted with all normal red cells tested. Rather than wait for a fall in the autoantibody titer following cessation of the drug, 3 units of autologous blood was stored in the liquid state and utilized during surgery. A similar approach was used by Snyder and Spivack in two patients.[73] Although evidence indicates that methyldopa-induced autoantibody will not cause shortened survival of homologous blood if the patient's own red cell survival is normal, the use of autologous blood ensures that an alloantibody-induced transfusion reaction will not occur. In instances in which it is inconvenient or impossible to delay surgery until an adequate number of autologous units are collected, the warm autoabsorption technique or other serologic methods as described above for patients with warm antibody AIHA may be used to exclude the presence of alloantibody.

Table 20-14. Correlation Between Mechanism of Red Cell Sensitization and Clinical and Laboratory Features in Drug-Induced Immunohematologic Abnormalities

Mechanism	Prototype Drugs	Clinical Findings	Serologic Evaluation	
			Direct Antiglobulin Test	Antibody Identification
Immune complex formation (drug and antidrug antibody) or hapten mechanism	Quinidine, phenacetin	Small doses of drug; acute intravascular hemolysis usual; renal failure common; thrombocytopenia occasionally	Usually only complement components detected but IgG can be present	Drug + patient's serum + red cell (especially enzyme-treated) → hemolysis, agglutination or sensitization; antibody frequently IgM and capable of fixing complement; red cell eluate often nonreactive
Drug adsorbed onto red cell membrane; reacts with high-titer serum drug antibody	Penicillins, cephalosporins	Large doses of penicillin (10 million units or more daily); other manifestations of allergy not necessarily present; usually subacute extravascular hemolysis; penicillins and cephalosporins are common causes of drug-induced immune hemolysis	Strongly positive (IgG) when hemolytic anemia present; complement sensitization also in a minority of patients	Drug-coated red cells + serum → agglutination or sensitization (rarely hemolysis); higher-titer antibody associated with hemolytic anemia is usually IgG; red cell eluate reacts only with antibiotic-coated red cells
Unknown	Methyldopa, procainamide	Hemolysis in 0.8% of patients taking drug for at least 3 months; gradual onset of hemolytic anemia	Strongly positive (IgG) when hemolytic anemia present; rarely, cells are sensitized with complement as well	Antibody sensitizes normal red cells without drug; antibody in serum and eluate identical to that found in warm antibody AIHA; no in vitro relationship to drug demonstrable

(Adapted from Petz and Garratty,[9] with permission.)

DRUG-INDUCED IMMUNE HEMOLYTIC ANEMIA

During the last several decades, there has been a continuing evolution of concepts regarding the mechanisms by which the administration of drugs leads to the development of antibodies that cause hemolysis.[9,11,74-81] It is convenient to categorize drug-induced hemolytic anemias on the basis of pro-posed mechanisms as in Table 20-14, since clinical and laboratory correlations have been recognized.[81]

Mechanisms of Production of Drug-Induced Red Cell Antibodies

Drugs that are loosely bound to the red cell in vitro lead to the development of a drug-dependent anti-body that can be detected optimally by adding a solution of the drug to the patient's serum, adding red cells to the incubation mixture and observing for agglutination, sensitization to antiglobulin serum, or lysis. Such drugs frequently cause severe hemolytic anemia with manifestations of acute intravascular hemolysis, such as hemoglobinemia and hemoglobinuria; renal insufficiency is a common consequence.[9,11] Prototype drugs are stibophen, quinine, and quinidine. The pathogenesis of the immune hemolysis caused by these drugs has generally been attributed to the hapten mechanism or the immune complex mechanism.[81] Table 20-15 consists of a list of such drugs.

A number of drugs are firmly bound to the erythrocyte in which case the optimal means of detection of the drug-dependent antibody in the laboratory is with the use of drug-coated red blood cells. The antibody appears to be directed against antigenic determinants on the drug or its metabolites and this mechanism has been called the "drug-absorption" mechanism. Drugs reported to react by this mechanism include penicillins, cephalosporins, cisplatin, carbimazole, carbromal, cianidanol, erythromycin, streptomycin, and tolbutamide.[80] Clinically the hemolysis is usually, but not always, less abrupt in onset and less severe without signs of intravascular hemolysis.

Finally, there are some drugs that lead to the development of AIHA.[78] The laboratory findings in these cases is identical to that found in idiopathic autoimmune hemolytic anemia of the warm antibody type. Adding the drug to the in vitro system neither inhibits nor augments the reactions of the red cell autoantibodies and the diagnosis of drug-induced AIHA must be made clinically. The clinical diagnosis is greatly strengthened if the hemolysis subsides on cessation of the drug. Drugs that have caused AIHA are listed in Table 20-16. Proposed mechanisms for the development of the red cell autoantibodies are the altering of red cell antigens by the drugs or altering the immune system to allow for uninhibited production of autoantibodies.

Finally, a number of cases of drug-induced immune hemolytic anemias have been reported in which the antibodies showed characteristics of more than one mechanism.

Table 20–15. Drugs Reported to Cause Hemolytic Anemia by the Immune Complex Mechanism

Drug	Intravascular Hemolysis[a]	Renal Failure[a]
Acetaminophen	X	
Aminopyrine	X	
p-Aminosalicylic acid (PAS)	X	X
Antazoline	X	X
Butizide	X	X
Carbinmazole[b]	X	
Cefotaxime[b]	X	
Ceftriaxone	X	
Chlorpromazine	X	X
Chlorpropamide	X	
Cianidanol	X	X
Dipyrone[c]	X	X
Fluorouracil	X	
Hydralazine		
Hydrochlorothiazide[e]	X	X
9-Hydroxymethylellipticimium	X	X
Insulin[b]		
Isoniazid[b]	X	
Melphalan		
Methotrexate		
Nalidixic acid	X	X
Nomifensine[d]	X	X
Phenacetin[c]	X	X
Probenecid		
Quinidine[b]		
Quinine	X	
Rifampicin	X	X
Stibophen	X	X
Streptomycin[b,d]		
Sulfonamides	X	X
Teniposide (VM-26)[d]	X	X
Tolmetin[d]	X	X
Triamterene[b]	X	X
Zomax (zomepirac sodium)		

[a] An X in the column indicates that intravascular hemolysis or renal failure have been reported on at least one occasion.

[b] May also bind to red cells and hemolysis may be caused in part by drug adsorption mechanism.

[c] May also cause hemolysis by drug adsorption mechanism and has been associated with the development of autoimmune hemolytic anemia.

[d] Also caused development of red cell autoantibody.

[e] Intravascular hemolysis and renal failure occurred only with an overdose of the drug. (From Petz,[81] with permission.)

Table 20-16. Drugs Reported to Cause Autoimmune Hemolytic Anemia

---

α-Methyldopa

L-Dopa

Mefenamic acid[a]

Procainamide

Phenacetin[b,c]

Chlorpromazine[c]

Streptomycin[c]

---

[a] Other nonsteroidal antiinflammatory drugs (ibuprofen, naproxen, tolmetin, feprazone, and fenoprofen) have caused immune hemolysis, but the mechanism is unclear.

[b] Also may cause hemolysis by immune complex or drug adsorption mechanisms.

[c] Only one case associated with autoantibodies has been reported.

(From Petz,[81] with permission.)

Transfusion of Patients With Drug-Induced Immune Hemolytic Anemia

In patients with drug-induced red cell antibodies, the major compatibility test will be compatible, unless the drug causes autoantibody formation (or unless coincidental red cell alloantibodies are present). This is true, as the drug is necessary in the in vitro system in order to demonstrate the drug-related antibody (Table 20-14). However, transfused cells may not survive normally if drug administration is continued, or if the serum level of drug or drug-related immune complexes remains high.

Compatibility testing in patients with AIHA caused by methyldopa is similar to that described for warm antibody AIHA. Although no data are available, it is probable that donor red cells will survive as well as the patient's own red cells.

Other patients receiving methyldopa may have a positive DAT, but no evidence of hemolysis. In many of these patients, the indirect antiglobulin test is negative so that the major compatibility test is compatible and donor blood can be expected to survive normally.

Still other patients receiving methyldopa have both positive DAT and IAT caused by autoantibody, but have no evidence of hemolytic anemia or of compensated hemolysis.[9] In performing the compatibility test, one must search for alloantibodies that may be present, as described previously. However, even if alloantibodies do not appear to be present, all compatibility test will be incompatible. The question then arises as to whether the autoantibody will cause shortened survival of donor red cells, even though it does not lead to shortened survival of the patient's own red cells. Silvergleid et al.[61] studied the survival of radiolabeled donor cells in two such patients and demonstrated acceptable survival after one hour in each patient. Subsequent experience of our own, and in association with Drs. J. Howard and F.C. Grumet, indicates that in such circumstances, donor units appear to survive normally, and clinical evidence of transfusion reactions does not result. In 21 transfusion episodes in 19 patients who were receiving methyldopa and had positive direct and indirect antiglobulin tests caused by autoantibody, but did not have hemolytic anemia, there were no clinical manifestations of transfusion reactions; adequate post-transfusion increments in the hemoglobin and hematocrit resulted in each case. Snyder and Spivack[73] reported another similar case. Although this point merits further study, it presently appears that methyldopa-induced red cell autoantibody does not cause hemolytic transfusion reactions if the patient's own red cell survival is normal.

Although no data are available concerning compatibility testing and blood transfusion in patients with drug-induced positive antiglobulin tests and autoimmune hemolytic anemia caused by drugs other than methyldopa, one might assume that similar principles would apply.

NONIMMUNOLOGIC DRUG-INDUCED HEMOLYTIC ANEMIA

In addition to immunological mechanisms responsible for drug-induced hemolytic anemia, hemolysis may result from nonimmunological causes as a result of oxidative denaturation of hemoglobin by drugs or drug metabolites.[82–84] Although severe oxidant stress may cause hemolysis of normal red cells, intraerythrocytic metabolic abnormalities or the presence of unstable hemoglobins may predispose the red cell to the effects of oxidant drugs.

In these patients, compatibility testing presents no problem and transfused red cells may survive normally in those cases in which an intraerythrocytic defect, such as glucose 6-dehydrogenase (G6PD) deficiency, is a predisposing factor to the hemolytic anemia.

REFERENCES

1. Petz LD: The Diagnosis of Hemolytic Anemia. p.1. In Bell CA (ed): A Seminar on Laboratory Management of Hemolysis. American Association of Blood Banks, Washington, DC, 1979
2. Pirofsky B: Immune haemolytic disease: the autoimmune haemolytic anaemias. Clin Haematol 4:167, 1975
3. Rausen AF, LeVine R, Hsu TCS, Rosenfield RE: Compatible transfusion therapy for paroxysmal cold hemoglobinuria. Pediatrics 55:275, 1975
4. Pirofsky B: Clinical aspects of autoimmune hemolytic anemia. Semin Hematol 13:251, 1976
5. Hillman RS: Blood loss anemia. Postgrad Med J 64:88, 1978
6. Habibi B: Autoimmune hemolytic anemia in children. Am J Med 56:61, 1974
7. Bell CA, Zwicker H, Sacks HJ: Autoimmune hemolytic anemia: routine serologic evaluation in a general hospital population. Am J Clin Pathol 60:903, 1973
8. Leddy JP, Swisher SN: Acquired immune hemolytic disorders (including drug-induced immune hemolytic anemia). p. 1187. In Samter M (ed): Immunological Diseases. 3rd Ed. Little, Brown, Boston, 1978
9. Petz LD, Garratty G: Acquired Immune Hemolytic Anemias. Churchill Livingstone, New York, 1980
10. Petz LD, Branch DR: Serological tests for the diagnosis of immune hemolytic anemias. p. 9. In McMillan R (ed): Immune Cytopenias. Churchill Livingstone, New York, 1983
11. Petz LD, Branch DR: Drug-induced immune hemolytic anemia. p. 47. In Chaplin H Jr (ed): Immune Hemolytic Anemias. Churchill Livingstone, New York, 1985
12. Petz LD: Immunohematology: acquired immune hemolytic anemias. Curr Hematol 3:51, 1984
13. Petz LD: Red cell transfusion problems in immunohematologic disease. Annu Rev Med 33:555, 1982
14. Petz LD: Transfusing the patient with autoimmune hemolytic anemia. Clin Lab Med 2:193, 1982
15. Petz LD: Autoimmune hemolytic anemia. Human Pathol 14:251, 1983
16. Reid ME: Autoagglutination dispersal utilizing sulphydryl compounds. Transfusion 13:353, 1978
17. Branch DR, Petz LD: A new reagent (ZZAP) having multiple applications in immunohematology. Am J Clin Pathol 78:161, 1982
18. Edwards JM, Moulds JJ, Judd WJ: Chloroquine dissociation of antigen-antibody complexes: a new technique for typing red blood cells with a positive direct antiglobulin test. Transfusion 22:59, 1982
19. Wallas CH, Tanley PC, Gorrell LP: Recovery of autologous erythrocytes in transfused patients. Transfusion 20:332, 1980
20. Vettore L, De Matteis MC, Zampini P: A new density gradient system for the separation of human red blood cells. Am J Hematol 8:291, 1980
21. Conley CL, Lippman SM, Ness PM et al: Autoimmune hemolytic anemia with reticulocytopenia. A medical emergency. JAMA 244:1688, 1980
22. Branch DR, Sy Siok Hian AL, Carlson R et al: Erythrocyte age fractionation using a Percoll-Renografin density gradient. Application to autologous red cell antigen determinations in recently transfused patients. Am J Clin Pathol 80:453, 1983
23. Griffin GD, Lippert LE, Dow NS et al: A flow cytometric method for phenotyping recipient red cells following transfusion. Transfusion 34:233, 1994
24. Klein HG: Standards for Blood Banks and Transfusion Services. American Association of Blood Banks, Bethesda, MD, 1994
25. Allen NK: Hyland Reference Manual of Immunohematology. Hyland, Los Angeles, 1963
26. Sokol RJ, Hewitt S, Booker DJ, Morris BM: Patients with red cell autoantibodies: selection of blood for transfusion. Clin Lab Haemat 10:257, 1988
27. Morel PA, Bergren MO, Frank BA: A simple method for the detection of alloantibody in the presence of warm autoantibody, abstracted. Transfusion 18:388, 1978
28. Wallhermfechtel MA, Pohl BA, Chaplin H: Alloimmunization in patients with warm autoantibodies: a retrospective study employing three donor alloabsorptions to aid in antibody detection. Transfusion 24:482, 1984
29. Laine ML, Beattie KM: Frequency of alloantibodies accompanying autoantibodies. Transfusion 25:545, 1985
30. Salama A, Berghofer H, Mueller-Eckhardt C: Red blood cell transfusion in warm-type autoimmune haemolytic anaemia. Lancet 340:1515, 1992
31. Garratty G, Petz LD: Transfusing patients with autoimmune haemolytic anaemia. Lancet 341:1220, 1993
32. Bove JR, Holburn AM, Mollison PL: Non-specific binding of IgG to antibody-coated red cells (the Matuhasi–Ogata phenomenon). Immunology 25:793, 1973
33. Ogata T, Matuhasi T: Further observation of the problem of specific and cross reactivity of blood group antibodies. p. 528. In Proceedings of the Ninth Congress

of the International Society of Blood Transfusion, Mexico. S Karger, New York, 1962

34. Walker RH: Technical Manual. American Association of Blood Banks, Bethesda, MD, 1993

35. Garratty G: Mechanisms of immune red cell destruction and red cell compatibility testing. Hum Pathol 14:206, 1983

36. Giblett ER: Blood group alloantibodies: an assessment of some laboratory practices. Transfusion 17:299, 1977

37. Croucher BEE: Differential diagnosis of delayed transfusion reaction. p. 151. In Bell CA (ed): A Seminar on Laboratory Management of Hemolysis. American Association of Blood Banks, Washington, DC, 1979

38. Beattie KM: Laboratory evaluation and management of antibody specificities in warm autoimmune hemolytic anemia. p. 105. In Bell CA (ed): A Seminar on Laboratory Management of Hemolysis. American Association of Blood Banks, Washington, DC, 1979

39. Mollison PL: Measurement of survival and destruction of red cells in hemolytic syndromes. Br Med Bull 15:59, 1959

40. Salmon C: Autoimmune hemolytic anemia. p. 675. In Back JF, Sivenson RS, Schwartz RS (eds): Immunology. John Wiley & Sons, New York, 1978

41. Borne AEG Kr von dem, Engelfreit CP, Beckers DO et al: Autoimmune anaemias. Biochemical studies of red cells from patients with autoimmune haemolytic anaemia with incomplete warm antibodies. Clin Exp Immunol 8:377, 1971

42. Hollander L: Study of the erythrocyte survival time in a case of acquired haemolytic anaemia. Vox Sang 4:164, 1954

43. Crowley LV, Bouroncle BA: Studies on the specificity of autoantibodies in acquired hemolytic anemia. Blood 11:700, 1956

44. Wiener AS, Gordon EB, Russow E: Observations of the nature of the auto-antibodies in a case of acquired hemolytic anemia. Ann Intern Med 47:1, 1957

45. Ley AM, Mayer K, Harris JP: Observations of a "specific autoantibody." p. 148. In Proceedings of the Sixth International Society of Blood Transfusion, Boston, 1958

46. Hogman C, Killander J, Sjolin S: A case of idiopathic autoimmune haemolytic anaemia due to anti-e. Acta Paediatr 49:270, 1960

47. Garratty G, Petz LD, Hoops JK: The correlation of cold agglutinin titrations in saline and albumin with haemolytic anaemia. Br J Haematol 35:587, 1977

48. Mollison PL, Johnson CA, Prior DM: Dose-dependent destruction of A_1 cells by anti-A_1. Vox Sang 35:149, 1978

49. Stroup M, MacIlroy M: Evaluation of the albumin antiglobulin technic in antibody detection. Transfusion 5:184, 1965

50. Deutsch HF, Morton JI: Dissociation of human serum macroglobulins. Science 125:600, 1957

51. Grubb R, Swahn B: Destruction of some agglutinins but not of others by two sulfhydryl compounds. Acta Path Microbiol Scand 43:305, 1958

52. Pirofsky B, Rosner ER: DTT test: a new method to differentiate IgM and IgG erythrocyte antibodies. Vox Sang 27:480, 1974

53. Olson PR, Weiblen BJ, O'Leary JJ et al: A simple technique for the inactivation of IgM antibodies using dithiothreitol. Vox Sang 30:149, 1976

54. Freedman J, Masters CA, Newlands M, Mollison PL: Optimal conditions for the use of sulphydryl compound in dissociating red cell antibodies. Vox Sang 30:231, 1976

55. Van Loghem JJ, Peetom F, Van der Hart M et al: Serological and immunochemical studies in hemolytic anemia with high-titer cold agglutinins. Vox Sang 8:33, 1963

56. Woll JE, Smith CM, Nusbacher J: Treatment of acute cold agglutinin hemolytic anemia with transfusion of adult i RBCs. JAMA 229:1779, 1974

57. Walford RI, Taylor: An in vivo crossmatching procedure for selected problem cases in blood banking. Transfusion 4:372, 1964

58. Chaplin H: Special problems in transfusion management of patients with autoimmune hemolytic anemia. p. 135. In Bell CA (ed): A Seminar on Laboratory Management of Hemolysis. American Association of Blood Banks, Washington, DC, 1979

59. Mollison PL, Engelfriet CP, Contreras M: Blood Transfusion in Clinical Medicine. Oxford, Blackwell Scientific, 1993

60. Mayer K, Bettigole RE, Harris JP et al: Test in vivo to determine donor compatibility. Transfusion 8:28, 1968

61. Sivergleid AJ, Wells RP, Hafleigh EB et al: Compatibility test using ^{51}Chromium-labeled red blood cells in crossmatch positive patients. Transfusion 18:8, 1978

62. International Committee for Standardization in Haematology: Recommended method for radioisotope red cell survival studies. Br J Haematol 45:659, 1980

63. Mayer K, Chin B, Magnes J et al: Further experiences with the in vivo crossmatch and transfusion of Coombs incompatible red cells. p. 49. In The Seventeenth Congress of the International Society of Hematology and the Fifteenth Congress of the International Society of

Blood Transfusion Book of Abstracts. Paris, July 23–29, 1978

64. Rosenfield RE, Jagathambal: Transfusion therapy for autoimmune hemolytic anemia. Semin Hematol 13: 311, 1976

65. Bilgrami S, Cable R, Pisciotto P et al: Fatal disseminated intravascular coagulation and pulmonary thrombosis following blood transfusion in a patient with severe autoimmune hemolytic anemia and human immunodeficiency virus infection. Transfusion 34:248, 1994

66. Dacie J: The Haemolytic Anaemias. Vol. III: The Autoimmune Haemolytic Anaemias. 3rd Ed. Churchill Livingstone, New York, 1992

67. Wallace J: Blood Transfusion for Clinicians. Churchill Livingstone, New York, 1977

68. Johnsen HE, Brostrom K, Madsen M: Paroxysmal cold haemoglobinuria in children: 3 cases encountered within a period of 7 months. Scand J Haematol 20: 413, 1978

69. Evans RS, Bingham M, Turner E: Autoimmune hemolytic disease: observations of serological reactions and disease activity. Ann NY Acad Sci 124:422, 1965

70. Evans RS, Turner E, Bingham M, Woods R: Chronic hemolytic anemia due to cold agglutinins. II. The role of C′ in red cell destruction. J Clin Invest 47:4, 1968

71. Goldfinger D, Connelly M, Kellum S, Rosenbaum D: Transfusion of frozen autologous red blood cells in patients with positive direct antiglobulin tests. Blood, suppl 1. 54:123a, 1979

72. Parr GVS, Ballard JO: Autologous blood transfusion with methyldopa induced positive direct antiglobulin test (letter). Transfusion 20:119, 1980

73. Snyder EL, Spivack M: Clinical and serologic management of patients with methyldopa-induced positive antiglobulin tests. Transfusion 19:313, 1979

74. Petz LD, Fudenberg HH: Immunologic mechanisms in drug-induced cytopenias. p. 185. In Brown EB (ed): Progress in Hematology. Vol. 9. Grune & Stratton, Orlando, FL, 1975

75. Petz LD: Drug-induced immune haemolytic anaemia. Clin Haematol 9:455, 1980

76. Garratty G, Petz LD: Drug-induced immune hemolytic anemia. Am J Med 58:398, 1975

77. Shulman NR, Reid DM: Mechanisms of drug-induced immunologically mediated cytopenias. Transfus Med Rev 7:215, 1993

78. Petz LD: Drug-induced autoimmune hemolytic anemia. [Review]. Transfus Med Reviews 7:242, 1993

79. Garratty G: Immune cytopenia associated with antibiotics. Transfus Med Reviews 7:255, 1993

80. Garratty G: Drug-Induced Immune Hemolytic Anemia. p. 523. In Garratty G (ed): Immunobiology of Transfusion Medicine. Marcel Dekker, New York, 1994

81. Petz LD: Drug-induced immune hemolytic anemia. p. 53. In Nance SJ (ed): Immune Destruction of Red Blood Cells. American Association of Blood Banks, Arlington, VA, 1989

82. Valentine WN, Paglia DE: Erythrocyte enzymopathies, hemolytic anemia, and multisystem disease: an annotated review. Blood 64:583, 1984

83. Valentine WN, Tanaka KR, Paglia DE: Hemolytic anemias and erythrocyte enzymopathies. Ann Intern Med 103:245, 1985

84. Beutler E: G6PD deficiency. Blood 84:3613, 1994

Chapter 21

Anemia and Cardiopulmonary Disease in Surgical Transfusion Practice

Jeffrey L. Carson and Richard K. Spence

This chapter describes a framework for making surgical transfusion decisions in patients with anemia and cardiopulmonary disease. We begin by briefly describing the cardiovascular responses to acute anemia derived from a review of the data in animals and humans, followed by a discussion of the impact of cardiopulmonary disease on anemia. The discussion then focuses on perioperative anemia and transfusion. Finally, we provide recommendations on the use of red cell transfusion in patients with anemia, cardiac disease, and pulmonary disease.

CARDIOVASCULAR RESPONSE TO ANEMIA

Studies of the cardiovascular effects of acute anemia in the healthy patient have consistently demonstrated a marked increase in cardiac output and a decrease in peripheral vascular resistance.[1-29] Cardiac output begins to increase when the hemoglobin level falls below 9 to 10 g/dl,[1,2] although other data suggest that the hemoglobin level must be below 7 to 8 g/dl.[1-3] Basal cardiac output can rise fivefold to increase oxygen delivery in an anemic, but otherwise healthy, patient. Increases in cardiac output during acute anemia are produced initially by increases in heart rate, followed by increases in stroke volume and contractility, once euvolemia has been restored.[5,10,12,14,17,18] As plasma volume increases, the hematocrit decreases (in the absence of red blood

cell transfusion), resulting in a reduction in blood viscosity and, subsequently, decreased peripheral vascular resistance.[7,14,24,25]

Since the heart extracts approximately 50 percent of the oxygen delivered to it under normal conditions,[11,16] coronary blood flow must increase if the myocardium is to obtain adequate oxygen in the setting of anemia. This increase is significantly greater than the increase seen in whole-body cardiac output.[2,6-9,11,16,18] Coronary blood flow changes in the anemic patient are due, in part, to a unique ability of the coronary bed to reduce vascular hindrance. This phenomenon is a measure of resistance offered by the vessel itself and is independent of viscosity during severe anemia.[6,11]

The relative contributions of increased ventricular contraction and reduced viscosity in anemia are significant in terms of their effect on myocardial oxygen metabolism. If cardiac output rises primarily because of decreased viscosity and reduced afterload (anemia of 7 to 10 g/dl), myocardial oxygen use may not decrease significantly. Under these circumstances, myocardial oxygen consumption remains stable or may even increase,[7,11,14,16,24-26] although the loss of red cells has markedly reduced oxygen-carrying capacity of the blood. However, as hemoglobin levels drop below 7 g/dl, ventricular contractility, and consequently myocardial oxygen, demand rise.

Oxygen release during anemia is also facilitated by

a shift to the right of the oxyhemoglobin dissociation curve, which leads to decreased red cell oxygen affinity and increased tissue availability. This begins at hemoglobin levels of approximately 9 to 10 g/dl and is prominent at 6.5 g/dl.[27,28–31] This change results from increased levels of 2,3-diphosphoglycerate (2,3-DPG), and requires 12 to 36 hours to develop.[32] In a sophisticated dog model, in which oxygen consumption (VO_2) was measured directly and both cardiac output and oxygen delivery were controlled independently via an extracorporeal circuit, Cilley and colleagues[33] showed that VO_2 remained constant and independent of oxygen delivery to levels of less than 8.0 ml/kg/min during progressive decreases in hemoglobin. Adequate VO_2 was maintained primarily by changing cardiac output, and consequently oxygen delivery. Wilkerson et al.[34] have shown in the exchange-transfused baboon that VO_2 is maintained down to a hematocrit of 4 percent if left atrial pressure is held constant. These animals survived by increasing their oxygen extraction ratio significantly. The investigators detected a conversion to anaerobic metabolism at a 10 percent hematocrit level, which correlated with an oxygen extraction ratio of 50 percent, suggesting these two numbers might be useful as transfusion guidelines. Spence et al.[35] found similar results in a study of 12 nontransfused, postsurgical patients with a mean hematocrit of 7.5 percent. Oxygen extraction ratio was greater than 50 percent during the first 48 hours in nonsurvivors, a level that was significantly higher than in those who lived. The hematocrit was also lower—6.0 percent versus 9.6 percent—among those who did not survive.

There are limits to the normal heart's ability to compensate for the decreased oxygen-carrying capacity produced by acute anemia. In healthy animals undergoing acute hemodilution, this limit has been shown to be a hemoglobin level of 3 to 5 g/dl (see Ch. 7). ST-segment changes have been seen on endocardial leads at hemoglobins of less than 5 g/dl.[2] Lactate production, markedly depressed ventricular function, and deaths have been observed with a hemoglobin below 3 g/dl, although some animals survive hemoglobins as low as 1 to 2 g/dl.[18,30,36] There is also evidence in animals that prolonged anemia leads to the establishment of collateral coronary vasculature.[37]

These data are of questionable help because of interspecies variability in anatomy and physiologic response; thus, direct translation to humans is fraught with hazard. Also, artificially created laboratory hemorrhage frequently fails to mimic the same condition seen in humans, who do not bleed in isolation, that is, there usually is associated trauma or underlying disease. Consequently, this information should be used only as a guideline, and not as absolute truth, when drawing conclusions about the effect of anemia on outcome in surgical patients.

INFLUENCE OF CARDIAC AND PULMONARY DISEASE

Very few studies have examined the effect of cardiac or pulmonary disease in combination with anemia. Coronary artery disease and congestive heart failure reduce the heart's ability to compensate for anemia (Table 21-1). With coronary artery obstruction, ischemia may be precipitated by an inadequate supply of oxygen. A few small studies have examined experimental coronary stenoses varying from 50 percent to 80 percent in anemic dogs. ST-segment changes and/or locally depressed cardiac function occurred at hemoglobin levels in the range of 7 to 10 g/dl.[8,30,38] In one study, coexisting left ventricular hypertrophy led to increased sensitivity to the effects of coronary stenosis.[38]

Uren et al.[39] studied the ability of the heart to increase myocardial blood flow in patients with varying degrees of single-vessel coronary artery stenosis. Flow progressively decreased in response to the intravenous administration of the vasodilator adenosine with stenoses of 40 percent or greater. Hearts with stenoses of 80 percent were unable to elevate myocardial blood flow above baseline values.

Both cardiac function and baseline hemoglobin decline with age, producing a potentially dangerous situation for the elderly anemic patient.[40] Most parameters of cardiac function decline with increased age, including heart rate, preload, afterload, and intrinsic muscle function.[40a] Coronary atherosclerosis is common in the elderly and accounts in part for the inability of the aging heart to increase cardiac output in response to anemia.[41]

Patients with congestive heart failure may be unable to respond adequately to anemia. With anemia and normal cardiac function, cardiac output rises

Table 21-1. Pathophysiologic Consequences of Cardiac and Pulmonary Disease

Condition	Cardiac Disease Effect	Condition	Pulmonary Disease Effect
Coronary artery disease	Reduced oxygen delivery—leads to angina, myocardial infarction, arrhythmia, or sudden death Ischemia—reduces ability of heart to increase cardiac output	Acute pulmonary disease (i.e., pneumonia)	Hypoxemia—reduces oxygen delivery
Congestive heart failure	Poor left ventricular function—reduces cardiac output	Chronic pulmonary disease (i.e., chronic obstructive pulmonary disease)	Hypoxemia—reduces oxygen delivery
	Hypoxemia—reduces oxygen delivery		Respiratory acidosis—shifts oxyhemoglobin dissociation curve to the right
	Respiratory alkalosis—shifts oxyhemoglobin dissociation curve to the left		Increased red cell volume from chronic hypoxia—reduces oxygen delivery by increasing viscosity

from increased myocardial contractility and reduced afterload.[4,5] Patients with congestive heart failure are unable to augment the force of ventricular contraction; in these patients, cardiac output increases primarily by raising the heart rate, which increases myocardial oxygen demands. Furthermore, if the arterial–alveolar oxygen gradient (A-a gradient) is widened from pulmonary interstitial edema, then oxygen delivery is compromised from hypoxemia and accompanying respiratory alkalosis. Alkalosis reduces the release of oxygen, although within 1 to 2 days, rising 2,3-DPG returns the release of oxygen toward normal.

Patients with pulmonary disease also have difficulty compensating for anemia (Table 21-1). Impaired oxygen loading occurs from a ventilation-perfusion mismatch. Patients with acute defects, such as pneumonia, have a widened A-a gradient and may have hypoxemia. Moderate to severe chronic pulmonary disease is associated with hypoxemia and respiratory acidosis from carbon dioxide retention. Under these circumstances, compensatory mechanisms include an increase in the release of oxygen generated by respiratory acidosis. Chronic hypoxemia stimulates the release of erythropoietin and eventual increases in red cell mass. Unfortunately, the higher viscosity from an elevated hemoglobin level often leads to impairment in oxygen delivery by decreasing cardiac output.[1]

It is likely that compensating for severe hypoxemia and anemia simultaneously is not possible. The inability to increase myocardial blood flow will prevent the heart from increasing the cardiac output necessary to maintain oxygen delivery during anemia. Myocardial infarction, arrhythmias, and sudden death may ensue. Red cell transfusion may be necessary to maintain adequate oxygen delivery under these conditions.

PERIOPERATIVE RISKS ASSOCIATED WITH CARDIAC DISEASE

Patients with a previous myocardial infarction have a 3 to 7 percent incidence of postoperative myocardial infarction, which is approximately 10 times the rate in patients without a history of myocardial infarction.[42–45] A more recent study found a reinfarction rate of only 4 percent within 6 months.[46] The risk is greatest in patients with a history of a myocardial infarction within 6 months and levels off thereafter. The mortality from perioperative myocardial infarction is 36 to 70 percent.[42–47]

Patients with congestive heart failure are also at increased risk of perioperative congestive heart failure, pulmonary edema, and cardiac death.[46–50] The risk is greatest in those patients with clinical evidence of preoperative congestive heart failure.[42] In one study, the mortality was 57 percent in patients developing pulmonary edema. Patients undergoing coronary artery bypass with poor left ventricular function have four times the mortality of those with normal left ventricular function.[48] Patients undergoing vascular surgery have a high prevalence of coronary artery disease; cardiac disease accounts for more than 50 percent of perioperative complications.[51,52] In one study, 60 percent of patients scheduled for elective peripheral vascular surgery had at least 70 percent obstruction of one coronary artery.[51]

PERIOPERATIVE CONSEQUENCES OF CARDIAC AND PULMONARY DISEASE

Cardiac ischemia may occur with intubation and the induction of anesthesia. Of 29 patients with coronary artery disease undergoing noncardiac surgery, 11 patients had ST-segment depression.[53] In patients undergoing cardiac bypass surgery, up to 50 percent experience ischemia during induction and intubation.[54,55] A more recent report found intraoperative electrocardiographic (ECG) changes consistent with myocardial ischemia in 27 percent of patients with known cardiac disease or cardiac risk factors undergoing noncardiac surgery.[56,57] These changes appear to be related more to underlying disease than to anesthetic technique.[58]

Postoperative arterial hypoxemia occurs frequently in patients undergoing surgery.[59,60] Hyoxemia immediately after surgery may be caused by alterations in pulmonary function from the persistent effects of anaesthesia. In the subsequent days, narcotics given for analgesia may lead to depressed respiratory response and hypercapnea, hypoxia, and acidemia.[61,62] The risk is greatest in patients with thoracic and upper abdominal surgery, and in patients with underlying pulmonary disease (i.e., chronic obstructive pulmonary disease); the incidence of postoperative pulmonary complications is at least 25 percent.[62,63]

PERIOPERATIVE RISKS ASSOCIATED WITH ANEMIA

Information regarding the relationship between anemia and surgical outcome is limited and appears primarily in the form of a few studies[64–67] and anecdotal reports of surgical outcome in the Jehovah's Witness (JW) patient (see Chs. 7 and 27). Because the JW patient does not accept transfusion, it is possible to glean some information about the effect of surgical anemia on mortality and morbidity in the absence of blood transfusion. Most valuable is the information regarding what limits of hemoglobin reduction are acceptable. These studies provide no information on the effect of transfusion in improving survival and only limited help in determining the impact of various diseases in association with anemia, because the numbers in most are too limited to draw significant conclusions.

A case control study of 125 JW patients who underwent surgery showed that operative mortality was inversely proportional to preoperative hemoglobin level and was related to the amount of blood lost during the procedure.[67] To a lesser extent, the presence of cerebrovascular, renal, hepatic, or any coexisting disease was also related to poor outcome. Those patients who underwent emergency surgery or an intrathoracic, intra-abdominal, or aortic procedure had higher mortality. The effect of these confounding variables is difficult to determine, not only because of the small numbers of patients studied, but also because of the inability to stratify disease only as present or absent and not according to severity.

A subsequent study focused on those patients who underwent major elective surgery, defined as procedures that normally would result in sufficient blood loss to require transfusion.[68] This study of 107 JW patients showed that surgical mortality depended more on the amount of blood lost during surgery than the starting hemoglobin. A larger analysis of 256 similar patients has demonstrated the same results, that is, that surgical mortality is directly related to blood loss and preoperative hemoglobin.[69] The larger number of patients included in this latter analysis allowed for statifying mortality against preoperative hemoglobin level and for assessing the effect of various diseases on outcome. The former showed that preoperative hemoglobin became a risk factor for death only in the 7 to 8-g/dl range. Analysis of the effect of various pre-existing diseases—cardiac, renal, hepatic, pulmonary, diabetes—revealed that none had a significant impact on mortality.

ANEMIA, CARDIAC DISEASE, AND SURGICAL OUTCOME

Recent studies of the effect of anemia on outcome in vascular surgical patients with known atherosclerosis shed some light on the combined effect of anemia and cardiac disease. Higgins et al.[69] performed a retrospective analysis of preoperative risk factors in 5,051 patients who underwent coronary artery bypass to develop a clinical severity score as a guideline to determination of outcome. This single-institution study showed that a preoperative hematocrit of 34 percent or lower was associated with increased perioperative risk. Baxter et al.[70] studied the value of preoperative maximization of cardiopulmonary dynamics in 39 high-risk vascular surgical patients. Their results suggested that maintenance of postoperative hemoglobin levels of 10 to 12 g/dl may be necessary to maiximize oxygen delivery and prevent complications. These findings are echoed in two independent studies by Nelson et al.[71] and Christopherson et al.[72] showing increased postoperative myocardial ischemia and cardiac morbidity in high-risk vascular patients with hematocrits below 29 percent.

Several other key issues must be considered in the decision to transfuse a patient with cardiac or pulmonary disease. If the patient is elderly or has cardiac or pulmonary disease that is expected to shorten life expectancy markedly, the long-term risks from a blood transfusion are of less significance. The threshold for transfusion should be higher and focus on symptoms that might be relieved by transfusion.[73,74] If the patient is actively bleeding, it is important to anticipate how low the hemoglobin will go and to transfuse expectantly. Patients taking β-blockers are less able to compensate for anemia by increasing their stroke volume and heart rate. Patients with other forms of arteriosclerotic disease (i.e., peripheral vascular disease or cerebrovascular disease) often have asymptomatic coronary artery disease.[43,75]

CONCLUSIONS AND RECOMMENDATIONS

There are inadequate data to provide definitive transfusion guidelines in patients with anemia, cardiac disease, and pulmonary disease. No studies have been done in patients with cardiac or pulmonary disease that provide incidence rates for death and other important postoperative outcomes for anemic patients. We believe that a higher threshold for transfusion is probably appropriate in patients who have significant underlying cardiovascular or pulmonary disease with hypoxia. It seems reasonable to maintain the hemoglobin threshold around 10 g/dl to provide a margin of reserve. However, before any blood transfusion is considered in any individual patient, a careful history and physical examination must be performed to assess how the patient is tolerating the anemia. If the patient appears well compensated, careful observation may be the best action.

REFERENCES

1. Finch CA, Lenfant C: Oxygen transport in man. N Engl J Med 286:407, 1972
2. Cooper N, Brazier Maloney JV, Buckberg G: The adequacy of myocardial oxygen delivery in acute normovolemic anemia. Surgery 75:508, 1974
3. Chapler CK, Cain SM: Effects of a-adrenergic blockade during acute anemia. J Appl Physiol 52:16, 1982
4. Chapler CK, Hatcher JD, Jennings DB: Cardiovascular effects of propranolol during acute experimental anemia in dogs. Can J Physiol Pharmacol 50:1052, 1972
5. Escobar E, Jones NL, Rapaport E, Murray JF: Ventricular performance in acute normovolemic anemia and effects of beta blockade. Am J Physiol 211:877, 1966
6. Fan FC, Chen RYZ, Schuessler GB, Chien S: Effects of hematocrit variations on regional hemodynamics and oxygen transport in the dog. Am J Physiol 238: H545, 1980
7. Fowler NO, Holmes JC: Blood viscosity and cardiac output in acute experimental anemia. J Appl Physiol 39:453, 1975
8. Geha AS, Baue AE: Graded coronary stenosis and coronary flow during acute normovolemic anemia. World J Surg 2:645, 1978
9. Geha AS: Coronary and cardiovascular dynamics and oxygen availability during acute normovolemic anemia. Surgery 80:47, 1976
10. Glick G, Plauth WH, Braunwald E: Role of the autonomic nervous system in the circulatory response to acutely induced anemia in unanesthetized dogs. J Clin Invest 43:2112, 1964
11. Jan K, Shu C: Effect of hematocrit variations on coronary hemodynamics and oxygen utilization. Am J Physiol 233:H106, 1977

12. Levine E, Rosen A, Sehgal L et al: Physiologic effects of acute anemia: implications for a reduced transfusion trigger. Transfusion 30:11, 1990

13. Messmer K, Sunder-Plassman L, Jesch F et al: Oxygen supply to the tissues during limited normovolemic hemodilution. Res Exp Med 159:152, 1973

14. Murray JF, Escobar E, Rapaport E: Effects of blood viscosity on hemodynamic responses in acute normovolemic anemia. Am J Physiol 216:638, 1969

15. Murray JF, Escobar E: Circulatory effects of blood viscosity: comparison of methemoglobinemia and anemia. J Appl Physiol 25:594, 1968

16. Murray JF, Rapaport E: Coronary blood flow and myocardial metabolism in acute experimental anaemia. Cardiovasc Res 6:360, 1972

17. Rodriguez JA, Chamorro GA, Rapaport E: Effect of isovolemic anemia on ventricular performance at rest and during exercise. J Appl Physiol 36:28, 1974

18. Wilkerson DK, Rosen AL, Sehgal LR et al: Limits of cardiac compensation in anemic baboons. Surgery 103:665, 1988

19. Wright CJ: The effects of severe progressive hemodilution on regional blood flow and oxygen consumption. Surgery 79:299, 1976

20. Whitaker W: Some effects of severe chronic anemia on the circulatory system. Q J Med 25:175, 1956

21. Roy SB, Madan LB, Virender MS, Viramani S: Hemodynamic effects of chronic severe anemia. Circulation. 28:346, 1963

22. Varat MA, Adolph RJ, Fowlwer NO: Cardiovascular effects of anemia. Am Heart J 83:415, 1972

23. Brannon ES, Merrill AJ, Warren JV, Stead EA: The cardiac output in patients with chronic anemia as measured by the technique of right atrial catheterization. J Clin Invest 24:332, 1945

24. Case RB, Berglund E, Sarnoff SJ: Ventricular function. VII. Changes in coronary resistance and ventricular function resulting from acutely induced anemia and the effect theron of coronary stenosis. Am J Med 18:397, 1955

25. Vatner SF, Higgins CB, Franklin D: Regional circulatory adjustments to moderate and severe chronic anemia in conscious dogs at rest and during exercise. Circ Res 30:731, 1972

26. Nakamura Y, Takahashi M, Takei F et al: The change in coronary vascular resistance during acute induced hypoxemia. Cardiologia 54:91, 1969

27. Studzinski T, Czarnecki A, Guszak A: Effect of acute posthemorrhagic anaemia on the level of 2,3-diphosphoglycerate (2,3-DPG) in the erythrocytes of sheep. Acta Physiol Pol 31:365, 1980

28. Valeri CR, Hirsch NM: Restoration in vivo of erythrocyte adenosine triphosphate, 2,3-diphosphoglycerate, potassium ion, and sodium ion concentrations following the transfusion of acid–citrate–dextrose-stored human red cells. J Lab Clin Med 73:722, 1969

29. Duke M, Abelman WH: The hemodynamic response to chronic anemia. Circulation 39:503, 1969

30. Yoshikawa H, Powell WJ, Bland JHL, Lowenstein E: Effect of acute anemia on experimental myocardial ischemia. Am J Cardiol 32:670, 1973

31. Rodman T, Close HP, Purcell MK: The oxyhemoglobin dissociation curve in anemia. Ann Intern Med 52:295, 1960

32. Hillman RS, Finch CA: Red Cell Manual. FA Davis, Philadelphia, 1985

33. Cilley RE, Polley TZ Jr, Zwischenberger JB et al: Independent measurement of oxygen consumption and oxygen delivery. J Surg Res 47:242, 1989

34. Wilkerson DK, Rosen AL, Gould SA et al: Oxygen extraction ratio: a valid indicator of myocardial metabolism in anemia. J Surg Res 42:629, 1987

35. Spence RK, Costabile JP, Young GS et al: Is hemoglobin level alone a reliable predictor of outcome in the severely anemic patient? Am Surg 58:92, 1992

36. Hagl S, Heimisch W, Meisner H et al: The effect of hemodilution on regional myocardial function in the presence of coronary stenosis. Basic Res Cardiol 72:344, 1977

37. Beutler E, Wood L. The in vivo regeneration of red cell 2,3-diphosphoglyceric acid (DPG) after transfusion of stored blood. J Lab Clin Med 74:300, 1969

38. Anderson HT, Kessinger JM, McFarland WJ et al: Response of the hypertrophied heart to acute anemia and coronary stenosis. Surgery 84:8, 1978

39. Uren NG, Melin JA, De Bruyne B et al: Relation between myocardial blood flow and the severity of coronary artery stenosis. N Engl J Med 330:1782, 1994

40. Wei JY: Age and the cardiovascular system. N Engl J Med 327:1735, 1992

40a. Ernst E, Matral A: Hematologic data on very old people. JAMA 258:781, 1987

41. Duke M, Abelman WH: The hemodynamic response to chronic anemia. Circulation 39:503, 1969

42. Goldman L, Caldera DL, Southwick FS et al: Cardiac risk factors and complications in noncardiac surgery. Medicine (Baltimore) 57:357, 1978

43. Steen PA, Tinker JH, Tarhan S: Myocardial reinfarction after anesthesia and surgery. JAMA 239:2566, 1978

44. Tarhan S, Moffitt EA, Taylor WF, Guiliani ER: Myocardial infarction after general anesthesia. JAMA 220:1451, 1972

45. Topkins MJ, Artusio JF: Myocardial infarction and surgery. A five year study. Anesth Analg 43:716, 1964

46. Rao TLK, Jacobs KH, El-Etr AA: Reinfarction following anesthesia in patients with myocardial infarction. Anesthesiology 59:499, 1983

47. Larsen SF, Olesen KH, Jacobsen E et al: Prediction of cardiac risk in noncardiac surgery. Eur Heart J 8:179, 1987

48. Foster ED, Dans KB, Carpenter JA et al: Risk of noncardiac operation in patients with defined coronary disease: the Coronary Artery Surgery Study (CASS) registry experience. Ann Thor Surg 41:42, 1986

49. Pasternack PF, Imparato AM, Riles TS et al: The value of the radionuclide angiogram in the prediction of perioperative myocardial infarction in patients undergoing lower extremeity revascularization procedures. Circulation, suppl II. 72:11, 1985

50. Kazmers A, Cerqueria MD, Zierter RE: The role of perioperative radionuclide left ventricular ejection fraction for risk assessment in carotid surgery. Arch Surg 123:416, 1988

51. Hertzer NR, Beven EG, Young JR et al: Coronary artery disease in peripheral vascular patients. Ann Surg 199:223, 1984

52. Gersch BJ, Rihal CS, Rooke TW, Ballard DJ: Evaluation and management of patients with both peripheral vascular and coronary artery disease. J Am Coll Cardiol 18:203, 1991

53. Roy WL, Edelist G, Gilbert B: Myocardial ischemia during noncardiac surgical procedures in patients with coronary artery disease. Anesthesiology 51:393, 1972

54. Slogoff S, Keats AS: Further observations on perioperative myocardial ischemia. Anesthesiology 64:157, 1986

55. Kleinman B, Henkin RE, Glisson SN et al: Qualitative evaluation of coronary flow during anesthetic induction using thallium-201 perfusion scan. Anesthesiology 64:157, 1986

56. Mangano DT, Hollenberg M, Fegert G et al: Perioperative myocardial ischemia in patients undergoing noncardiac surgery. I. Incidence and severity during the four-day perioperative period. J Am Coll Cardiol 17:843, 1991

57. Mangano DT, Hollenberg M, Fegert G et al: Perioperative myocardial ischemia in patients undergoing noncardiac surgery. II. Incidence and severity during the first week after surgery. J Am Coll Cardiol 17:851, 1991

58. Cohen MM, Duncan PG, Tate RB: Does anesthesia contribute to operative mortality? JAMA 260:2859, 1988

59. Diament ML, Palmer KN: Postoperative changes in gas tensions of arterial blood and in ventilatory function. Lancet 2:180, 1966

60. Parfrey PS, Harte PJ, Quinlan JP et al: Postoperative hypoxemia and oxygen therapy. Br J Surg 64:390, 1977

61. Weil JV, McCullough RE, Kline JS et al: Diminished ventilatory response to hypoxia and hypercapnia after morphine in normal man. N Engl J Med 292:1103, 1975

62. Wightman JA: A prospective survey of the incidence of postioerative pulmoanry complications. Br J Surg 55:85, 1968

63. Gass GD, Olsen GN: Preoperative pulmonary function testing to predict postoperative morbidity and mortality. Chest 89:127, 1986

64. Lunn JN, Elwood PC: Anemia and surgery. BMJ 371:64, 1970 Rawstron ER: Anemia and surgery. A retrospective clinical study. Aust NZ J Surg 39:425, 1970

65. Alexiu O, Mircea N, Balaban M et al: Gastrointestinal hemorrhage from peptic ulcer. An evaluation of bloodless transfusion and early surgery. Anaesthesia 30:609, 1975

66. Carson JL, Spence RK, Poses RM: Severity of anemia and operative mortality and morbidity. Lancet 2:727, 1988

67. Spence RK, Carson JL, Poses R et al: Elective surgery without transfusion: influence of preoperative hemoglobin level and blood loss on mortality. Am J Surg 159:320, 1990

68. Spence RK, Curry C, Camishion RC et al: Influence of hemoglobin and blood loss on mortality in elective surgery in the Jehovah's Witness. In Proceedings of the Twenty-third Meeting of ISBT, 1994

69. Higgins TL, Estafanous FG, Loop FD et al: Stratification of morbidity and mortality outcome by preoperative risk factors in coronary artery bypass patients. A clinical severity score. JAMA 267:2344, 1992

70. Baxter BT, Minion DJ, McCance CL et al: Rational approach to postoperative transfusion in high-risk patients. Am J Surg 1993; 166:720, 1993 (discussion 724)

71. Nelson AH, Fleisher LA, Rosenbaum SH: The relationship between postoperative anemia and cardiac morbidity in high risk vascular patients in the ICU. Crit Care Med 21:860, 1993

72. Christopherson R, Frank S, Norris E et al: Low postoperative hematocrit is associated with cardiac ischemia in high-risk patients, abstracted. Anesthesiology 75(3A):A100, 1991

73. Canadian Erythropoietin Study Group: Association between recombinant human erythropoietin and quality of life and exercise capacity of patients receiving haemodialysis. BMJ 300:573, 1990

74. Eschbach JW, Abdulhadi MH, Browne JK et al: Recominant human erythropoietin in anemic patients with end-stage renal disease. Ann Intern Med 111:992, 1989

75. Criqui MH, Langer RD, Fronek A et al: Mortality over a period of 10 years in patients with peripheral arterial disease. N Engl J Med 326:381, 1992

Chapter 22

Surgical Blood Ordering, Blood Shortage Situations, and Emergency Transfusions

Ira A. Shulman, Richard K. Spence, and Lawrence D. Petz

Blood banks and transfusion services should develop formal standard operating procedures (SOPs) to guide their technical and patient care-related activities. Many of these SOPs have a direct impact on the services provided by the blood bank laboratory for surgical patients. This chapter reviews principles that pertain to various blood bank and transfusion service SOPs regarding routine and emergency pretransfusion testing, perioperative blood ordering, blood component selection, and transfusion strategies during times of blood shortage. Surgeons should be familiar with these SOPs because this knowledge will help them to make the most efficient use of available blood bank services.

PRETRANSFUSION TESTING

An institution's SOPs for pretransfusion compatibility testing must ensure that whole blood and red blood cell (RBC) units are compatible with transfusion recipients.[1] The SOPs must also address situations in which incompatible whole blood or RBC units are transfused. This may occur as a result of intentional transfusion of incompatible blood (i.e., when compatible RBCs are unavailable for an exsanguinating hypotensive trauma victim), as a result of an error, or after emergency transfusion of un-

crossmatched units that turn out to be incompatible after the completion of compatibility testing.

Routine Pretransfusion Testing

Routine pretransfusion patient testing consists of an ABO/Rh determination and an antibody screening test followed by a crossmatch (see Ch. 9).[1] If a patient has a negative antibody screening test result and no history of prior RBC alloantibodies, an immediate spin or electronic crossmatch may be performed.[2] However, if pretransfusion testing detects an RBC alloantibody (an "unexpected RBC antibody"), the specificity of the antibody must be determined, antigen-negative units must be selected when appropriate, and crossmatching of these units utilizing an indirect antiglobulin technique must be performed (unless the urgency of the clinical situation requires uncrossmatched blood). Depending on the number of antibodies present and their specificity(ies), compatible blood may be difficult to obtain. Thus, the turn-around time for routine pretransfusion testing may vary from less than 1 hour (if no immunohematologic problem is detected) to several days.

An institution's SOPs should define the required lead time for routine preoperative pretransfusion compatibility testing. Surgeons must understand that, if the required lead time for preoperative pretransfusion testing is not honored, compatible blood might not be available at the time of surgery. By including a request for type and screen or type and crossmatch with routine preadmission blood tests, adequate time should be available to determine whether the patient has a rare blood type, an "unexpected" RBC alloantibody, or other compatibility problem. The surgeon who waits until the day before or the day of an elective surgical procedure to order a type and screen or crossmatch runs the greatest risk of incurring a delay. This has become a more frequent problem because of the increased frequency of admitting patients to the hospital on the day of surgery.[3] Finally, there must also be a mechanism to inform a surgeon if the testing detects a problem that might cause a delay in blood availability.

Emergency Pretransfusion Testing

The timely availability of blood and components in a dire emergency should not be delayed because of incomplete compatibility testing.[1,4] However, even when blood is issued under emergency conditions before testing has been completed, SOPs must be followed by both the blood bank and clinical staff so that the risk of an incompatible transfusion is minimized. If a preplanned emergency transfusion SOP is not followed, the chance of a transfusion error is significantly increased.

The most important function of pretransfusion compatibility testing is the prevention of ABO-incompatible transfusion.[2] Transfusion reactions caused by ABO incompatibility may be fatal. Most of these occur as a result of errors committed on the "floor" or in the operating room, not in the blood bank; the most common error is the administration of the wrong unit of blood (see Ch. 9).[5]

BLOOD AVAILABILITY TIME TABLE FOR THE OPERATING ROOM

The use of group O, Rh-negative RBCs for emergency transfusion is appropriate whenever a patient requires a blood transfusion before their ABO/Rh

Table 22-1. Blood Availability Time Table for the Operating Room[a]

Time You Can Wait To Transfuse	Red Blood Cell Product Available	Risks and Comments
<5 min—immediate transfusion needed	O negative, Uncrossmatched	0.2–0.6% of population will have RBC antibody; serious hemolysis rare. Wait for group specific only if a 10–15-min wait does not cause significant risk.
15 min after clot arrives in blood bank	Group specific, uncrossmatched	Risk same or greater than O negative uncrossmatched blood. Wait for crossmatched blood if a 45-min wait does not cause significant risk.
45 min after clot arrives in blood bank (unless red cell antibody present)	Group specific, crossmatched	No RBC antibody found; blood compatible by crossmatch.
90 min to several hours; rarely, even longer	Group specific, antigen negative crossmatched in a patient with a red cell antibody	RBC antibody found; antibody identification may take 90 min to several hours. If blood is needed before compatibility testing is completed, hemolysis may occur, but transfusion should not be withheld if absolutely necessary; life-threatening morbidity is rare. Communicate with blood bank.

Abbreviation: RBC, red blood cell.

[a] In emergency settings, the type of blood product that should be used depends on how extreme the emergency is and whether or not RBC antibodies are found in screening tests. If extreme emergency exists, group O, Rh-negative RBC should be used, and hospital standard operating procedures should provide for this product being available within minutes when necessary.

Before starting the transfusion, a blood sample must be obtained for compatibility testing. If a wait of 15 minutes does not result in undue risk to the patient, group-specific uncrossmatched blood should be used. Note that this product is not safer than group O uncrossmatched blood but does conserve group O blood, which is often in short supply. Even in cases in which group O, Rh-negative uncrossmatched blood is used, a switch to group-specific uncrossmatched blood should be possible within 15 minutes.

Crossmatched blood can be supplied in about 45 minutes unless the patient has a red cell alloantibody. In this case, antibody identification, finding antigen-negative units, and crossmatching will require 90 minutes or more, depending on the antibody(ies) found.

type has been determined (Table 22-1).[6] However, once the blood bank laboratory has a specimen to test, determination of the ABO/Rh type should take no longer than 10 to 15 minutes, and un-crossmatched group-specific blood can then be made available.

Completion of antibody screening and cross-matching requires an additional 15 to 45 minutes if no RBC antibodies are found,[7] and an indeterminant amount of time if one antibody or more is present.

If actual turn-around times are longer than expected, a systems problem may be at fault, and this needs to be investigated. A careful analysis of each step in the process of emergency compatibility testing might reveal information that could shorten the turn-around time and improve patient care.[8]

STANDARD OPERATING PROCEDURES FOR ROUTINE PREOPERATIVE BLOOD ORDERS

An institution should have SOPs that address routine preoperative blood ordering.[9] The SOPs vary depending on the likelihood that blood transfusion will be required during surgery.

No Preoperative Blood Order

A surgical procedure for which minimal or no blood loss is expected does not require a preoperative blood order, that is, no specimen needs to be sent to the blood bank. If there is a possibility that transfusion will be needed, a specimen should be sent to the transfusion service where a "type and hold," "type and screen," or "type and crossmatch" can be performed. It is important for physicians to understand the difference between these various orders (Table 22-2).

Table 22-2. Type and Hold Versus Type and Screen Versus Type and Crossmatch

	Tests Performed	Significance	Comments
Type and hold	ABO group and Rh type of patient are determined, but antibody testing is not performed.	If emergency transfusion is needed, knowing the patient's blood type saves little time because typing takes but a few minutes.	Some transfusion services have abandoned the type and hold and recommend no preoperative blood order if there is little likelihood of need for transfusion, and type and screen or type and crossmatch when there is a reasonable probability that blood will be needed.
Type and screen	ABO group and Rh type of patient are determined, and a screening test is performed on the patient's serum for "unexpected" red cell alloantibodies. The screening test takes 30–40 min to complete.	If the antibody screening test result is negative, fully crossmatched blood can be made available within 10–15 min using a rapid crossmatch technique (immediate spin technique or computer crossmatch).	If there is only a modest probability of need for transfusion (e.g., ≤10% chance), the type and screen procedure is preferable to type and crossmatch because it saves blood bank resources and does not add significant risk for the patient. If the antibody screening test is positive, further compatibility testing can and should be performed to find an adequate number of compatible units in advance of surgery.
Type and crossmatch	ABO group and Rh type of the patient are performed, an antibody screening test is performed, and the needed number of units are crossmatched.	Compatible units of blood are available before surgery	If there is a reasonably high probability that blood will be needed during surgery (≥10% chance), the type and crossmatch is appropriate.

Type and Hold

The patient's ABO and Rh types are determined, but no test for RBC antibodies is performed. When crossmatched blood is needed for transfusion, time-consuming antibody detection test will still need to be performed.

Type and Screen Versus Type and Crossmatch

A procedure with a small chance of need for transfusion (i.e., 90 percent or more of the patients are not transfused or when the average RBC use is less than 0.5 units) may be managed with a type and screen order.[10]

If the antibody screening test result is negative (no RBC alloantibodies present), crossmatched blood can be available in about 15 minutes. Because RBCs can be available quickly, the blood bank will not crossmatch any donor RBC units in advance of surgery. Thus, when there is a small chance of need for transfusion, it is more practical to perform just a type and screen test before surgery rather than having crossmatched blood made available. This conserves blood bank resources and does not add significant risk for the patient. However, the SOP should require that, in the event RBC units are needed for transfusion, they be crossmatched "stat" by either an immediate spin test, an electronic crossmatch, or other rapid method to avoid any delay in providing blood for the patient. Such stat testing takes only a few minutes, and most of the time is due to clerical tasks.

If the type and screen test detects an "unexpected" RBC alloantibody, a rare blood type, or other compatibility problem, crossmatches should be done before surgery to find a sufficient number of compatible units. The surgeon should be informed if such a problem arises because delays may be encountered if more blood than was ordered initially is needed.

Preoperative Crossmatch Orders

A procedure with a 10 percent or greater chance of requiring allogeneic blood should have a type and crossmatch preoperative order; the number of units crossmatched should be sufficient to meet the anticipated total blood requirement of at least 90 percent of the patients who undergo the procedure.

MAXIMUM SURGICAL BLOOD ORDER SCHEDULE

A list of surgical procedures and their associated preoperative blood order recommendations may be referred to as a maximum surgical blood order schedule (MSBOS).[9,11,12] The MSBOS is used to determine the most appropriate preoperative blood order (i.e., no blood order, type and screen, or type and crossmatch for a certain number of units). An override mechanism must be available so that, if mitigating circumstances exist, these can be specified to the blood bank verbally or in writing to avoid having an inadequate number of crossmatched units available for a given patient's surgery.

An example of a MSBOS is presented in Table 22-3. The MSBOS should reflect local (institutional) blood usage experience and should be prepared in cooperation with the surgical staff performing these procedures. Moreover, it should be revised every few years on the basis of current blood usage. Therefore, the example in Table 22-3 should not necessarily be transposed for use into another hospital but should merely serve as a model.

It is evident that a type and screen is the appropriate order for many surgical procedures. Also, because indications for transfusion are becoming increasingly more stringent, fewer units may need be crossmatched for a number of the procedures indicated.

The Crossmatch to Transfusion Ratio

The success of a MSBOS may be measured by calculating a ratio known as the crossmatch to transfusion (C/T) ratio. The C/T ratio is well established as a useful indicator of the efficiency of physicians' blood ordering practices. The more accurately physicians predict a patient's blood needs during the perioperative period, the closer the C/T ratio will approach 1:1. Based on a study by the College of American Pathologists, more than 50 percent of hospitals have a C/T ratio of less than 2:1, and 75 percent have a C/T ratio of less than 2.2:1.[13]

Once a MSBOS is in place, it should be revised periodically if the overall C/T ratio for surgical patients exceeds 2:1. However, even if the overall C/T ratio is 2:1 or less, it may be appropriate to consult with the appropriate surgeons and consider revising

Table 22-3. Transfusion Service Guideline for Elective Surgical Procedures

General surgery		Ear, nose, and throat surgery	
Cholecystectomy	T&S[a]	Caldwell-Luc	T&S
Exploratory laparotomy (celiotomy)	T&S	Laryngectomy	T&S
Ileal bypass	T&S	Plastic surgery	
Hiatal hernia repair	T&S	Mammoplasty	T&S
Colectomy and hemicolectomy	2 U	Thoracoabdominal flap	T&S
Splenectomy	2 U	Oral surgery	
Breast biopsy	T&S	Osteotomy	T&S
Radical mastectomy	1 U	Genioplasty	T&S
Modified radical mastectomy	1 U	Bilateral subcondylar osteotomy	T&S
Simple mastectomy	1 U	Vestibuloplasty	T&S
Gastrectomy	2 U	Le Forte I osteotomy	T&S
Antrectomy and vagotomy	2 U	Anterior maxillary osteotomy	T&S
Inguinal herniorrhaphy	T&S	Neurosurgery	
Liver biopsy	T&S	Craniotomy	2 U
Vein stripping	T&S	Herniated disc	T&S
Cardiovascular surgery		Ventriculoperitoneal shunt	T&S
Saphenous vein bypass	8 U	Transphenoidal hypophysectomy	2 U
Congenital open heart surgery	8 U	Orthopaedics	
Valve replacement	8 U	Open reduction	2 U
Pleurodesis	T&S	Scoliosis fusion	3–4 U
Aortobifemoral bypass	8 U	Herniated disc	T&S
Thoracotomy	3 U	Arthroplasty	T&S
Closed mediastinal exploration	T&S	Shoulder reconstruction	T&S
Resection abdominal aortic aneurysm	8 U	Total hip replacement	2–3 U
Carotid endarterectomy	2 U	Total knee replacement	T&S
Obstetric-gynecologic surgery		Genitourinary surgery	
Total abdominal hysterectomy	T&S	Transurethral resection of prostate	T&S
Exploratory laparotomy	T&S	Radical nephrectomy	1 U
Total vaginal hysterectomy	T&S	Renal transplantation	1 U
Vaginal resuspension	T&S	Penile prosthesis insertion	T&S
Laparoscopy	T&S	Prostatectomy	2 U
Repeat cesarean section	T&S	Patch graft	T&S
Labor and delivery requests (oxytocin drips and cesarean sections)	T&S		

[a] Type and antibody screen (T&S) consists of an ABO-Rh typing and a screen for unexpected antibodies.
(From Boral et al.,[11] with permission.)

the standard blood orders for a specific procedure if the C/T ratio for that procedure exceeds 2:1.

The surgeon who routinely performs the type of surgery that results in transfusion (e.g., joint replacement or coronary artery bypass grafting) should discuss the creation of an individual MSBOS with the hospital's transfusion medicine specialist. The MSBOS carries an added advantage in its use as a guideline for ordering preoperative autologous blood collections.[14]

EMERGENCY BLOOD ORDERS

Written SOPs should be in place before a patient requires an emergency blood transfusion.[1,4] These SOPs should take into account the emergency transfusion requirements of patients who suddenly need blood during an existing hospitalization and the needs of patients who are brought to the hospital in need of acute emergency treatment. The American Association of Blood Banks (AABB) has published guidelines to assist in the development of such SOPs

Table 22-4. Guidelines for the Release of Blood Before Completion of Compatibility Testing

Protocols that avoid incorrect patient identification, inaccurate specimen labeling, and the administration of the wrong unit of blood should be strictly followed.

The blood bank records must contain the identity of the patient (either true name or alias), the unique donor number and the ABO/Rh of the donor blood or component issued, and the identity of the personnel who issued the blood or component.

A recipient whose ABO group is not known must receive group O red blood cells.

Recipients whose ABO group has been determined by the transfusing facility without reliance on previous records may receive ABO group-specific whole blood or ABO group-compatible red blood cell components.

The container tag or label must indicate in a conspicuous fashion that routine compatibility testing has not been completed at the time of issue.

Standard compatibility tests should be completed promptly. If the patient does not survive the emergency event for reasons unrelated to the transfusion, compatibility tests may be abbreviated to an extent considered appropriate by the physician who is responsible for the transfusion service.

The records must contain a statement of the requesting physician, indicating that the clinical situation was sufficiently urgent to require release of blood before completion of compatibility testing.

(Table 22-4).[1,4] If these guidelines are followed, they should prevent patient misidentification, specimen mislabeling, and administration of the wrong unit of blood and minimize undue delays in providing blood for transfusion and the risk of ABO-incompatible transfusion.

The physician requesting an emergency uncrossmatched transfusion must document in the patient's medical record the urgent need for the blood. However, it is inappropriate for blood bank staff to demand that the physician "sign" for the blood before it can be released for transfusion because such a requirement could delay blood availability.[6]

The turn-around time to respond to an emergency blood order should be short. At some institutions, particularly trauma centers, emergency blood orders can be honored at once because uncrossmatched group O RBCs are routinely stored in the emergency and operating rooms.[5] Rough estimates of the number of units to be kept on hand can be obtained from periodic review of transfusion practices and discussion with the trauma staff. In well-administered transfusion services that support trauma services and emergency rooms, type-specific blood can be made available quickly enough so that only a small number of group O, Rh-negative units are required.

However, it may take several minutes or longer to provide uncrossmatched blood in hospitals that store uncrossmatched blood only in the blood bank. According to a survey by the College of American Pathologists, only 75 of 3,655 (1.8 percent) institutions allow the routine storage of uncrossmatched group O RBC in the emergency room in case a patient requires an emergency transfusion.[15] This is a surprisingly small number, considering the lifesaving potential of such storage.

Relative Risks in Emergency Blood Ordering

Surgeons should be familiar with the relative risks of transfusing uncrossmatched RBC and whole blood before completion of compatibility testing (Table 22-1). The transfusion of uncrossmatched group O, Rh-negative RBCs carries the lowest (but not a zero) risk.[16-18] There is no risk of the transfused cells being hemolyzed by anti-A or anti-B antibodies, but the patient may have RBC alloantibodies or other blood group systems (e.g., Rhesus, Kell, Kidd, or Duffy) if they have previously been transfused or pregnant.

One should be particularly aware that uncrossmatched group-specific blood is no safer than group O uncrossmatched blood and, indeed, is less safe (see Ch. 25). This is true because laboratory error, clerical error, or patient misidentification may result in ABO-incompatible blood being transfused, whereas this is not a potential problem if only group O RBCs are used. Indeed, the transfusion of an uncrossmatched group-specific RBC or whole blood unit carries the greatest risk of any uncrossmatched transfusion.

The risk of infusing the wrong allogeneic blood or transfusing the wrong patient has been estimated to be 1 in every 12,000 RBC units.[19] When the wrong blood is given or the wrong patient is transfused, by chance, the transfused RBC will be ABO-incompatible once in three times.[20] Of these, about one-tenth are associated with a fatal outcome.[21] For this reason, many practitioners prefer to transfuse only group O RBCs in emergency situations, even after group-specific units can be made available. However, such an approach is generally not feasible in the United States because of an insufficient supply of group O blood.

Group O Rh-Positive Versus Group O Rh-Negative Red Blood Cells

The transfusion of uncrossmatched group O, Rh-positive RBCs carry a risk that is intermediate between that of uncrossmatched group-specific RBCs and group O negative RBCs (because of the absence of a risk of ABO incompatibility, but the presence of a risk of rhesus incompatibility). According to a 1993 survey of more than 4,500 laboratories by the College of American Pathologists, anti-D antibody is one of the most commonly detected significant unexpected RBC alloantibody present in the serum of potential transfusion recipients.[22] Various estimates indicate that the prevalence of anti-D antibody in transfusion recipients is 0.27 to 0.56 percent.[20]

STANDARD OPERATING PROCEDURE FOR EMERGENCY TRANSFUSION

The following is an SOP for providing uncrossmatched blood in emergency situations at the Los Angeles County, University of Southern California Medical Center.

Uncrossmatched group O RBCs preserved in additive solution-1 are stored in monitored refrigerators that are located in key emergency and surgical department areas. Each refrigerator is stocked with 6 to 8 units of group O Rh-negative RBCs (Rh-positive RBCs are stocked during shortage periods). Each RBC unit is conspicuously labeled to indicate that it has not had compatibility testing completed. Each refrigerator is designed to sound an alarm in the blood bank whenever the refrigerator door is opened. Once the alarm has sounded, a technologist in the blood bank calls to a telephone that is located adjacent to the refrigerator that was opened. The person who opened the refrigerator answers the telephone and provides the blood bank with the name and medical record number of the patient in need of the blood, the name of the physician ordering the blood, and the identification number(s) of RBC

unit(s) taken from the refrigerator. This information is recorded and retained by the blood bank according to statute. The clinical staff is instructed to send a specimen, drawn before blood infusion, to the laboratory as soon as possible so that compatibility testing can begin.

As soon as a patient's blood sample is received, it is tested for ABO/Rh and unexpected antibodies, and crossmatches are begun. RBC units taken from the emergency room refrigerator are crossmatched by testing the patient's serum against samples of the RBC units, which were retained in the blood bank. If a crossmatch is incompatible, the clinical staff is notified immediately so that any adverse reaction can be minimized and therapeutic measures can be instituted promptly.

If more blood is required after ABO and Rh typing is done but before the antibody screen is performed, group-specific uncrossmatched blood is provided. Group-specific uncrossmatched blood is generally made available before all of the group O, uncrossmatched blood can be transfused.

Crossmatched blood is issued as soon as it is available. Cooperation between the blood bank and the blood users is essential to allow this system to provide blood without delay in an emergency while safeguarding the patient as much as possible.

TRANSFUSION POLICIES AT TIMES OF INADEQUATE INVENTORY

An institution must have SOPs to deal with occasional shortages in blood inventory. Such preplanning may minimize the impact of a shortage on an elective surgery schedule or on a specific patient. The inability of a hospital blood bank to meet the transfusion needs of its patients may result either from a shortage of blood within the national/regional system or from a local depletion of blood inventory in spite of an adequate national/regional blood resource. Depletion of a hospital blood inventory may be minimized by the use of an MSBOS because such a schedule promotes effective utilization of a hospital's blood inventory and reduces blood outdating.[23] Frequently, blood crossmatched for a surgical patient is reserved for that patient's use for 48 to 72 hours. However, it may be more efficient to return unused units to inventory, especially if the patient has no alloantibodies or other compatibility problems that require special compatibility test procedures. Units not released might expire within the period in which they are being held, thus wasting an important limited resource.

Use of Blood That Is Not ABO/Rh Identical to the Patient

During times of blood shortage, the surgeon should not feel constrained to only transfuse blood that is ABO/Rh identical to that of the patient. The use of RBC that are not ABO identical but are compatible ("minor incompatibility") is an effective means of increasing the number of available units during a shortage situation.[4] Principles to be followed when switching blood groups and types due to shortages are outlined in Table 22-5.

When nonidentical ABO groups are used, the transfused blood should always be in the form of RBCs rather than whole blood to avoid the transfusion of incompatible ABO alloantibodies.

Table 22-5. Principles to be Followed When Switching Blood Groups and Types Because of Shortages

Patient's Group and Type	Principles to Follow
O-negative	Use only O, Rh-negative if patient is sensitized to D
	Use group O, D-negative, C- and/or E-positive in preference to Rh(D)-positive blood
	Avoid transfusing anything but O, Rh-negative blood to patients (especially female patients) younger than age 45
	Restrict the use of O, Rh-positive blood for O, Rh-negative patients to acute emergency situations, and then use only if the patient either has a negative antibody screen or definitely lacks Rh antibodies
	If massive volumes of blood are required and switching to Rh-positive blood is inevitable, conserve O, Rh-negative blood for other patients, by switching as early as possible
A-negative or B-negative	Use only Rh-negative blood if patient is sensitized to D (i.e., group-specific Rh-negative or O, Rh-negative blood as packed cells if possible)
	Use D-negative, C- and/or E-positive in preference to Rh(D)-positive blood
	Avoid transfusing anything but Rh-negative blood to patients (especially female patients) younger than age 45
	Restrict use of Rh-positive blood to acute emergency situations; then use only if the patient has a negative antibody screen or definitely lacks Rh antibodies
	If massive volumes of blood are required and switching to Rh-positive blood is inevitable, conserve Rh-negative blood for other patients by switching as early as possible
	Conserve group O blood. Only group O can be given to a group O recipient
AB-negative	Use only Rh-negative blood if patient is sensitized to D
	Use D-negative, C- and/or E-positive in preference to Rh(D)-positive blood
	Group A blood may be used (as packed cells if possible) unless the patient has anti-A_1. The patient initially should be switched to group A, then secondarily, may be switched to O. Always do this before switching Rh types (see text)
	Avoid transfusing anything but Rh-negative blood to patients (especially female patients) younger than age 45
	Restrict the use of Rh-positive blood to acute emergency situations and then use only if the patient has a negative antibody screen result or definitely lacks Rh antibodies
	If massive volumes of blood are required and switching to Rh-positive blood is inevitable, conserve Rh-negative blood by switching as early as possible
	Conserve group O blood. Only group O can be given to a group O recipient
O-positive	Group O patients may receive only group O blood
	Rh-negative blood may be used, but this should be avoided due to supply problems
A-positive or B-positive	Group O blood may be given (as packed cells if possible)
	Rh-negative blood may be used, but this should be avoided due to supply problems
AB-positive	Group A blood may be used (as packed cells, if possible) unless the patient has anti-A_1. The patient initially should be switched to group A, then secondarily to group O
	Conserve group O blood. Only group O can be given to a group O recipient
	Rh-negative blood may be used, but this should be avoided due to supply problems

Conversely for plasma, patients with group O blood can receive non-O fresh frozen plasma. In cases of very extreme plasma use, it may be necessary to use ABO-incompatible plasma transfusions. For example, if a patient with group AB blood needed quantities of AB plasma that were so large that the supply was threatened, the patient could be switched first to A RBCs and then, after two or three blood volumes, to group A fresh frozen plasma (even though it contains anti-B antibody). At the end of surgery, the patient could be switched back in the reverse order, with AB fresh frozen plasma first and then to AB RBCs once crossmatches showed compatibility as a result of a sufficient decline in titer of the passive anti-B antibody level.

Use of Rh-Positive Blood for Rh-Negative Patients

When Rh-negative blood is in short supply, it may be necessary to transfuse Rh-positive blood into some Rh-negative patients. Transfusion of Rh-positive blood should be avoided for women with childbearing potential and for female children because of the risk of Rh alloimmunization and subsequent hemolytic disease of the fetus/newborn.[24] Transfusion of Rh-positive blood should also be avoided for patients who have anti-D antibodies (regardless of gender), except for life-threatening situations. On the other hand, group O Rh-positive RBCs may be administered to Rh-negative male patients with very little risk of a reaction. Rh-negative male patients will not have anti-D antibodies unless they have been alloimmunized by a prior transfusion of Rh-positive blood and thus are unlikely to have an acute hemolytic transfusion reaction develop with the transfusion of Rh-positive blood. Rh-negative female patients of childbearing age or older may have been immunized during pregnancy (although this is unusual with modern use of Rh immune globulin to prevent alloimmunization) but will not experience an acute hemolytic transfusion reaction to Rh-positive RBCs if their antibody screening test result is negative.

During life-threatening emergency situations, a surgeon should not feel constrained to transfuse only Rh-negative RBCs to a patient whose Rh type is unknown. In fact, SOPs for the selection of blood for patients whose Rh type is unknown vary widely between institutions. A survey by the College of American Pathologists showed that, of 3,659 surveyed institutions, most routinely provided group O Rh-negative RBCs for emergency uncrossmatched transfusions until the patient's true Rh type was known.[15] However, some institutions routinely provided group O Rh-negative RBC for female patients and group O Rh-positive RBCs for male patients. About 1 percent of institutions provided only group O Rh-positive RBC for all emergency uncrossmatched transfusions before Rh typing regardless of the patient's gender, a policy that we do not recommend.

PATIENTS WITH MULTIPLE ALLOANTIBODIES OR ALLOANTIBODIES TO HIGH-INCIDENCE ANTIGENS OR AUTOANTIBODIES

There are patients for whom an immunohematologic problem will preclude an adequate supply of compatible RBCs in spite of an adequate overall supply of donor blood. These individuals either have RBC autoantibodies, multiple alloantibodies, and/or an alloantibody to a high-incidence antigen. The serologic evaluation of such patients may be complex and time consuming; workups may take hours to days, and it may therefore be necessary to administer a transfusion before the workup is completed. Even after a workup is completed, it may not be possible to find enough compatible units in time for the surgery. Indeed, in some instances, it is impossible to provide compatible RBCs.

In the event a patient's serologic problem cannot be resolved in time or in case a sufficient number of compatible units cannot be found, it becomes the responsibility of the blood bank/transfusion service medical director to apprise the surgeon of the clinical relevance of the particular incompatibility the patient is facing. Because the clinical relevance of an RBC antibody depends in part on the antibody specificity and in vitro reactivity, it should be possible for the blood bank physician to guide the surgeon and blood bank staff on the safest selection of incompatible blood. For example, if multiple antibodies are present and incompatible RBC must be transfused, the donor RBCs should be selected so that they are incompatible with the antibody expected to be the least clinically significant.

The clinical significance of various alloantibodies

and appropriate transfusion policies for patients with multiple alloantibodies or alloantibodies to high-incidence antigens are discussed in Chapter 9, and the transfusion of patients with autoantibodies is considered in detail in Chapter 20.

In Vivo Compatibility Testing

In vivo compatibility testing sometimes provides additional useful information regarding selection of appropriate blood for transfusion. This technique is discussed in Chapter 9, and additional comments about its use in patients with autoantibodies may be found in Chapter 20.

Temporary Use of Incompatible Blood During Massive Transfusion

In certain circumstances, if only a limited number of compatible units can be located, it might be prudent to divide up the compatible units that are available, and use a portion of them for the patient's initial RBC transfusions. Once the patient's blood loss and fluid replacement therapy has diluted the serum alloantibodies, it may be safe to switch to incompatible RBC units under close observation. As soon as the patient's blood loss is under control and the supply of remaining compatible units is sufficient to meet the transfusion needs of the patient, the patient should be switched back to receive compatible RBC units. Such an approach could limit the volume of incompatible RBCs in the patient's circulation. Although this strategy may be complicated by a delayed hemolytic transfusion reaction, only rarely will an intraoperative hemolytic reaction be seen. This strategy has been used successfully on a number of occasions in liver transplant surgery (see Ch. 35).

Other Strategies

Other strategies for minimizing allogeneic transfusion needs include the use of intraoperative RBC salvage, intraoperative hemodilution, and/or preoperative autologous blood collection with or without frozen RBC storage. These strategies are discussed in detail in Chapters 11 and 24.

Another consideration is to obtain directed donor blood from siblings (if available), other family members, or unrelated compatible donors. Use of blood from related donors has the potential to cause graft-versus-host disease; however, this risk can be eliminated by irradiating the donor blood before transfusion. Current AABB guidelines allow for the repeated collection of blood from directed donors without the usual 8-week wait between blood collections.[1] Rare donor blood registries are also available through regional blood suppliers.

Potential Transfusion Reactions

In the event that incompatible blood must be transfused, it is advisable to reduce the likelihood of a nonhemolytic reaction, which could complicate the interpretation of a transfusion reaction. The probability of an allergic or febrile nonhemolytic transfusion reaction can be minimized by using washed RBCs or by leukocyte reduction of the RBCs.[7] Leukocytes can be removed in the blood bank with enough advance warning or on the "floor" by transfusing the blood through a modern leukocyte-reduction filter.

Finally, the clinician must be prepared to deal with the potential of a hemolytic transfusion reaction (see Ch. 41). There must be an awareness by the clinical staff that a reaction might occur and, if it does, to contact the blood bank. Because the morbidity and mortality rates are related to the volume of RBCs transfused, the transfusion should be stopped as soon as a reaction is observed. Preparations should be made to deal with the possibility of hypotension, disseminated intravascular coagulation, and so forth. Fortunately, most acute hemolytic transfusion reactions are not fatal, especially when caused by antibodies other than anti-A and anti-B.

FATAL TRANSFUSION REACTIONS IN SURGICAL PATIENTS

All too often a surgical patient expires soon after a transfusion. When this occurs, a clinical suspicion of a cause and effect may be raised. Although most surgical patient deaths are unrelated to a transfusion reaction, if the possibility is raised that a transfusion might have contributed to a patient's death, an investigation should be done to determine the cause of death and the role (if any) the transfusion might have played as a contributing cause. A transfusion reaction investigation could follow the guidance offered by the 16th edition of the *Standards for Blood*

Banks and Transfusion Services (standards K2.000 through K2.3000).[1] Also see Chapter 41.

In the absence of a clerical error leading to administration of ABO-incompatible blood or of a clinically overt reaction attributed to a transfusion (i.e., acute hemolysis, anaphylaxis, acute respiratory distress, or sepsis), it is unlikely that a transfusion would be responsible for death in the acute setting. Furthermore, if the investigations to determine the cause of death (i.e., a review of the medical records or the performance of an autopsy) reveal no link to a transfusion, then a transfusion-related death may be excluded.

On the other hand, if clinical and laboratory investigation does reveal evidence of one of the following: (1) post-transfusion hemolysis (such a finding in a massive trauma victim must be interpreted with caution because hemoglobinemia and hemoglobinuria may result directly or indirectly from a traumatic injury or may be confused with myoglobinuria), (2) an incompatible transfusion, (3) clinical evidence of an anaphylactic or acute pulmonary reaction to transfusion, or (4) a bacterially contaminated blood component, then there may have been a causal link between the patient's death and a transfusion.

In the event that a blood transfusion is proved to be related to a patient's death, one must be aware that Food and Drug Administration regulations (CFR 606.170 [b]) state the following. "When a complication of blood collection or transfusion is confirmed to be fatal, the Director, Office of Compliance, Center for Biologics Evaluation and Research, shall be notified by telephone or telegraph (sic) as soon as possible; a written report of the investigation shall be submitted to the Director, Office of Compliance, Center for Biologics Evaluation and Research, within 7 days after the fatality by the collecting facility in the event of a donor reaction, or by the facility that performed the compatibility tests in the event of a transfusion reaction."

REFERENCES

1. Klein HG: Standards for Blood Banks and Transfusion Services. American Association of Blood Banks, Bethesda, 1994
2. Shulman IA: Safety in transfusion practices. Red cell compatibility testing issues. Clin Lab Med 12:685, 1992
3. Moore SB, Reisner RK, Losasso TJ, Brockman SK: Morning admission to the hospital for surgery the same day. A practical problem for the blood bank. Transfusion 27:359, 1987
4. Jones F: Accreditation Requirement Manual of the American Association of Blood Banks. American Association of Blood Banks, Arlington, 1992
5. Sazama K: Reports of 355 transfusion-associated deaths: 1976 through 1985. Transfusion 30:583, 1990
6. Shulman IA, Morales J, Nelson JM, Saxena S: Emergency transfusion protocols. Lab Med 20:166, 1989
7. Walker R: Technical Manual of the American Association of Blood Banks. American Association of Blood Banks, Arlington, 1993
8. Saxena S, Wong ET: Does the emergency department need a dedicated stat laboratory? Continuous quality improvement as a management tool for the clinical laboratory (see comments). Am J Clin Pathol 100:606, 1993
9. Friedman BA: An analysis of surgical blood use in United States hospitals with application to the maximum surgical blood order schedule. Transfusion 19:268, 1979
10. Mintz PD, Nordine RB, Henry JB, Webb WR: Expected hemotherapy in elective surgery. N Y State J Med 76:532, 1976
11. Boral LI, Dannemiller FJ, Stanford W et al: A guideline for anticipated blood usage during elective surgical procedures. Am J Clin Pathol 71:680, 1979
12. Mead JH, Anthony CD, Sattler M: Hemotherapy in elective surgery: an incidence report, review of the literature, and alternatives for guideline appraisal. Am J Clin Pathol 74:223, 1980
13. Renner S: Q-Probe 89-08A. Short-term studies of the laboratory's role in quality care. Blood Utilization Data Analysis and Critique. College of American Pathologists, 1990
14. Axelrod FB, Pepkowitz SH, Goldfinger D: Establishment of a schedule of optimal preoperative collection of autologous blood. Transfusion 29:677, 1989
15. Simon T: College of American Pathologists Proficiency Testing Program. 1991 J-C. Northfield, 1991
16. Schwab CW, Shayne JP, Turner J: Immediate trauma resuscitation with type O uncrossmatched blood: a two-year prospective experience. J Trauma 26:897, 1986
17. Gervin AS, Fischer RP: Resuscitation of trauma patients with type-specific uncrossmatched blood. J Trauma 24:327, 1984
18. Lefebre J, McLellan BA, Coovadia AS: Seven years experience with group O unmatched packed red blood

cells in a regional trauma unit. Ann Emerg Med 16: 1344, 1987

19. Linden JV, Paul B, Dressler KP: A report of 104 transfusion errors in New York State (see comments). Transfusion 32:601, 1992

20. Mollison PL, Engelfriet CP, Contreras M: Blood Transfusion in Clinical Medicine. Blackwell Scientific Publications, Oxford, 1993

21. Murphy WG, McClelland DB: Deceptively low morbidity from failure to practice safe blood transfusion: an analysis of serious blood transfusion errors. Vox Sang 57:59, 1989

22. Cooper ES: 1993 CAP Surveys. Comprehensive Transfusion Medicine Survey. 1993 Set J-C. Interlaboratory Comparison Program. Northfield, College of American Pathologists, 1993

23. Rouault C, Gruenhagen J: Reorganization of blood ordering practices. Transfusion 18:448, 1978

24. Issitt PD: Applied Blood Group Serology. Montgomery Scientific Publications, Miami, 1985

Chapter 23

Blood Saving Strategies in Surgical Patients

Richard K. Spence

Two basic approaches exist to limiting the use of allogeneic blood transfusion in the surgical patient. Autologous blood can be substituted for allogeneic blood through predonation, acute normovolemic hemodilution, and autotransfusion. The first two require some action in advance of surgery and are limited primarily to elective surgical cases. Autotransfusion may not be acceptable in the face of bowel injury, cancer, or infection. A second approach to blood conservation has, as a goal, limiting the need for transfusion by reducing surgical blood loss. This approach includes the use of surgical techniques and drugs.

SURGICAL APPROACHES TO REDUCING BLOOD LOSS

Basic Principles

The importance of preventing or controlling blood loss has been known to the surgeon for years. Before the midnineteenth century, major surgical procedures were rarely performed, in part because of the fear of blood loss.[1,2] Most surgery was performed for traumatic injuries, usually those that occurred during wartime. Speed was the essential characteristic of the military surgeon, typified by Ambroise Pare, who emphasized rapid control of traumatic bleeding through the use of cautery and ligature of

vessels.[3] Texts that contain hand-colored illustrations depicting approaches to surgical ligation of blood vessels were an essential part of the surgeon's armamentarium (Fig. 23-1).[4] With the advent of anesthesia and a better understanding of infection came the ability to perform complex operations within the thoracic and abdominal cavities. Careful aseptic and hemostatic technique replaced speed as the hallmark of the surgeon.

The most noted proponent and teacher of this system of surgery was William Stewart Halsted. His thorough, scientific approach to surgery emphasized careful diagnosis and planning before surgery, gentle tissue handling, incisions along avascular anatomic planes to avoid vessels, and meticulous hemostasis.[5] His teachings are known today to all practicing surgeons as the "halstedian principles" of general surgery. Although transfusion was both known to and used by Halsted, this science was in its infancy. Halsted appropriately stressed the importance of *preventing* blood loss over *replacing* blood loss, a philosophy that has seen a resurgence of interest in the last 10 years.

The reader will find the expression "bloodless surgery" used throughout this chapter. The term is in common usage in the surgical literature and refers to a variety of approaches aimed at preventing blood loss and minimizing transfusion (Table 23-1). Bloodless surgery should not be misconstrued to mean surgery without the loss or use of any blood because this goal is clearly not attainable. However, by using the principles and approaches embodied in the term, one can significantly reduce the need for allogeneic transfusion in most patients.

Prevention of Blood Loss

Preventing or minimizing surgical blood loss is important not only as a means of limiting allogeneic blood exposure but also because of its impact on postoperative survival. The latter is demonstrated by our analysis of mortality rates, preoperative hemoglobin levels, and blood losses in Jehovah's Witnesses who refuse any transfusion.[6] To date, we have accumulated data on more than 2,000 Jehovah's Wit-

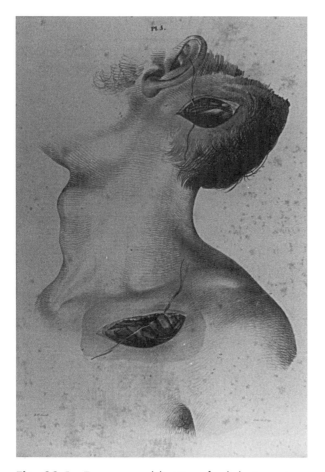

Fig. 23-1. Exposure and ligation of subclavian artery, circa 1812.

Table 23-1. Approach to Bloodless Surgery

Elective surgery
    Determine need for blood based on operation planned
        Schedule autologous predonation where appropriate
    Assess hemoglobin/hematocrit
        Provide medical therapy for anemia where appropriate, e.g., iron therapy for iron deficiency anemia and B_{12} and/or folate for megaloblastic anemia
    Operative procedure
        Choose procedure with least blood loss
        Use careful dissection, cautery, etc. to minimize blood loss
        Use drugs where appropriate, e.g., vasopressin, desmopressin, aprotinin
        Maintain circulating volume with asanguineous fluids
            Crystalloid
            Colloid, e.g., hydroxyethyl starch
        Use hemodilution/autotransfusion where appropriate
Emergency surgery, or if bleeding actively
    Resuscitate with asanguineous fluids
    Stop active bleeding nonoperatively where appropriate with
        Endoscopic sclerosis or coagulation
        Balloon tamponade
        Angiographic embolization
        Drugs
    Perform emergency surgery to stop bleeding if necessary
    Perform staged operation chosen to minimize blood loss

nesses who underwent elective surgery without transfusion. A subgroup of 238 patients who had operations that would have required transfusion based on traditional maximal surgical blood ordering schedules were analyzed to determine the relationship between surgical blood loss, preoperative hemoglobin, and survival (Table 23-2). The preoperative hemoglobin level ranged between 6.0 and 16.4 g/dl, with a mean of 11.4 g/dl. The overall mortality rate was 5 of 238 patients or 2.1 percent. All deaths occurred in those patients with blood losses greater than 500 ml. No deaths occurred with less than 500 ml of blood loss, regardless of the preoperative hemoglobin level. This experience re-emphasizes the importance of careful surgical technique in preventing blood loss.

Table 23-2. Elective Surgery in the Jehovah's Witness

	Number	Deaths (Rate)
Preoperative hemoglobin level		
>10 g/dl	198	3 (1.3%)
<10 g/dl	40	2 (5%)
Estimated blood loss		
>500 ml	93	5 (5.4%)
<500 ml	145	0
Preoperative hemoglobin level/estimated blood loss		
>10 gm/dl >500 ml	72	3 (4.2%)
>10 gm/dl <500 ml	126	0
<10 gm/dl >500 ml (14.3%)	14	2
<10 gm/dl <500 ml	26	0

The sine qua non of minimizing blood loss during surgery is careful, skillful operative technique. Dissection along anatomic, avascular planes is essential and requires a thorough knowledge of anatomy. All potentially vascular structures should be clamped and tied before being cut. Any vessel inadvertently cut or any unexpected bleeding, no matter how minor, must be controlled. Attention to what may seem to be insignificant detail at the time can lead to diminished blood loss. Bleeding from many small vessels can accumulate quickly. In our experience, as much as 100 to 200 ml of blood can be lost from unattended skin and subcutaneous vessels during the course of an operation, especially in the hypertensive patient.

Factors That May Contribute to Bleeding

Bleeding during surgery may also arise from acquired hemostatic defects (see Chs. 8, 18, and 27). Coagulopathy in the trauma patient is generally not dilutional in nature but is related to both the degree and length of hypotension and hypoperfusion.[7] Hypothermia may be a contributing factor.[8] Associated injury to the uterus, lung, or prostate, organs that are rich in plasminogen activators, may result in their release into the circulation and subsequent fibrinolysis.[9] Tissue hypoxia after injury or prolonged cross-clamping of visceral blood supply may also lead to release of plasminogen activators and thromboplastins.

Dilutional Coagulopathy

Coagulation factor and platelet depletion is not as common a cause of intraoperative hemorrhage as many surgeons think. Stored, allogeneic blood maintains sufficient levels to prevent bleeding of all coagulation factors except V and VIII, which decrease over time.[10,11] In the massively transfused patient, dilutional thrombocytopenia begins to appear after 1.5 blood volumes (or 20 units in an adult) have been replaced. In a study of 39 patients who received plasma-depleted blood, either from the blood bank or cell salvage and autotransfusion, Leslie and Toy[12] documented significant platelet decreases in 75 percent of those who received more than 20 units. Prothrombin and partial thromboplastin times were prolonged beyond normal values in 33 percent of patients who received less than 12 units and in all with more than 12 units transfused. Although this study suggests a role for dilution as a cause of coagulopathy in trauma, it is limited by its small numbers and retrospective design.

In general, "cookbook" formulae for "prophylactic" transfusion of fresh frozen plasma (FFP) and platelets according to the number of units transfused should be avoided because they have little value and increase patient risk by multiple donor exposure. Furthermore, they are inadequate to correct consumptive disorders when they occur.[13] Instead, platelets and FFP should be given only to correct proven coagulation abnormalities. Data supporting this approach have been published by Martin et al.,[14] who showed that prophylactic use of FFP did not restore coagulation parameters in dogs subjected to hemorrhagic shock. Similarly, Reed et al.[15] were unable to show any benefit to giving 6 units of platelets or 2 units of FFP prophylactically for every 12 units of red cells transfused in a prospective, randomized study of patients who needed 12 or more units of blood in 12 hours.

Hemolytic Transfusion Reactions

Bleeding can occur as a result of disseminated intravascular cagulation in a patient who has an acute, intravascular hemolytic transfusion reaction, usually a result of ABO incompatibility. Symptoms can take many forms, including hemoglobinuria, fever, chills, coagulopathy, chest pain, and circulatory collapse. In the unconscious, anesthetized patient, acute reactions present either as sudden hypotension in the euvolemic patient and/or unexpected bleeding secondary to disseminated intravascular coagulation.[16] In a study of 104 transfusion errors reported during a 22-month period in New York State, 58 percent were caused solely by personnel outside the blood bank.[17] Forty-three percent resulted from failure to identify correctly either the patient or the unit before transfusion. The message to the surgeon should be clear, that is, as long as human error is a possibility, acute, potentially fatal reactions will occur. Prevention requires constant vigilance, particularly in settings where large volumes of blood are required in a short period of time (e.g., the exsanguinating trauma victim).

Delayed hemolytic transfusion reactions (DHTR) are caused by non-ABO antigen-antibody incompatibility.[16] These occur in patients who have been alloimmunized by pregnancy or prior transfusion but do not have a detectable red blood cell antibody when transfused again. The subsequent transfusion causes an anamnestic response, with the resultant antibody causing hemolysis of the transfused red cells. DHTR may present within 1 to 10 days after transfusion as fever, malaise, hyperbilirubinemia, or a falling hematocrit. The exact incidence of these reactions is unknown, and they are rarely recognized for what they are. Instead, a falling hematocrit in a recently transfused patient is attributed to recurrent or continued bleeding. A real danger exists in continuing to transfuse such patients with incompatible blood. All compatibility tests must be repeated with fresh specimens before additional blood is transfused in a patient with a DTHR.[16] Once the offending antibody has been identified, antigen-negative blood can be transfused (see Ch. 41).

Anesthesia

Both the choice of anesthetic technique and operation can influence the amount of blood lost during surgery. Regional anesthetic techniques have been associated with decreased blood loss in orthopedic surgery. Bridenbaugh[18] showed less blood loss in patients who underwent total hip replacement under continuous epidural anesthesia than in those who received a general anesthetic. Oxygen consumption is reduced 15 to 20 percent under general anesthesia in most patients.[19] Narcotic anesthesia may also re-

duce oxygen consumption by an additional 5 to 10 percent, providing a greater margin of safety. Our anesthesiologists favor narcotic anesthesia, usually with fentanyl, in anemic patients. If inhalational anesthetics are used, isoflurane is usually chosen because it has less inhibitory effect on the heart's conductivity. These anesthetic agents do not directly minimize blood loss, but they provide a somewhat safer environment for the stressed, anemic patient who may need increased cardiac reserves. For example, the use of propofol, an intravenously administered nonbarbiturate hypnotic agent, was associated with a reduction in blood loss compared with standard inhalational agents in a study of endoscopic sinus surgery.[20]

Tools of the Trade

A variety of cutting devices that decrease operative blood loss are available to the surgeon. The use of electrocautery has been shown to reduce blood loss without significant complications in many procedures, including tonsillectomy, gynecologic excisions, laparoscopic cholecystectomy, and abdominal surgery.[21–31] The combination of electrocautery and ultrasonic capability has produced an efficient instrument for dissecting while maintaining a bloodless field.[32] Similarly, both laser and argon beam devices reduce blood loss when used in either open or laparoscopic surgery.[33–35] In an experimental model of splenic injury in swine, Dowling et al.[36] showed that hemostatic control was achieved faster and with less blood loss using argon beam coagulation compared with electrocautery, direct pressure, topical hemostatic agents, or suture ligation. Two reports from China have demonstrated the transfusion-sparing effect of microwave hepatic surgery. Microwave current transmitted through a monopolar needle electrode produced coagulation, reduced blood loss compared with conventional hepatectomy (average = 244 versus 746 ml), and decreased transfusion need.[37] However, this device may produce more septic complications from the coagulum of tissues left behind.[38] In our experience, reduced blood loss is a function more of the surgeon's skill than of the device itself. The individual surgeon should gain experience with these tools to develop optimal surgical technique.

Table 23-3. Hemostatic Agents in Use

Microcrystalline collagen powder
Oxidized cellulose
Positively charged modified collagen
Topical thrombin
Fibrin glue
    Allogeneic
    Autologous

Topical Hemostatic Agents and Fibrin Glue

Collagen hemostat pads, powders, and topical thrombin sprays are helpful in controlling oozing (Table 23-3). These products are applied directly to the wound either in sheet or powder form. The latter can be sprayed onto the cut surface of a solid organ by using a bulb syringe.[39] Fibrin glue, a combination of human fibrinogen, calcium chloride, and aprotinin (Immuno, Vienna, Austria) mixed with bovine thrombin is useful in controlling parenchymal bleeding from the liver and spleen.[40] However, this product is not licensed for use in the United States. The glue is formed by the reaction of fibrinogen and thrombin as they are applied topically or injected just below the cut surface of a solid organ (e.g., liver or spleen) to obtain hemostasis. This product's advantage is that it can obtain good hemostasis in notoriously difficult solid organ bleeding. Comparisons of microcrystalline collagen powder, oxidized cellulose, and positively charged modified collagen with fibrin glue in both experimental and clinical surgery have shown the latter to have more favorable hemostatic properties and greater reliability in terms of preventing postoperative bleeding.[41,42] Fibrin glue also works in the presence of coagulation defects and bacterial contamination commonly seen in trauma patients.[43,44] Caution is advisable if fibrin glue is used in the presence of bacterial contamination or infection because the coagulum produced can be a good culture medium. Antibiotics should be administered systemically or as part of the aerosol glue mixture.[45,46]

Unfortunately, fibrin glue is not without its drawbacks. Bänninger et al.[46] reported on a patient in whom inhibitors to bovine thrombin and human factor V developed after exposure to fibrin glue. Fibrin glue is a blood product and, therefore, may be a source of disease transmission. In answer to this latter problem, autologous fibrinogen can be prepared from either predonated blood or from blood removed during hemodilution at the time of surgery.[47] Gibble and Ness[48] showed that citrate phosphate dextrose (CPD) plasma produces higher yields than acid citrate dextrose (ACD) preparations. Tawes[49] used platelet-rich plasma derived from plasmapheresis of intraoperatively acquired blood to seal vascular grafts. This product has less fibrinogen compared with allogeneic fibrin glue but appears to be effective. It is uncertain whether patients who are Jehovah's Witnesses will accept fibrin glue because it is derived from human blood.

Operative Modifications

A number of operative approaches have been modified from existing techniques or developed anew to minimize blood loss in general, vascular, and orthopaedic surgery. These have been particularly effective in cases that traditionally have had an attendant high blood loss. Some techniques are generic; others are procedure specific. The former group includes preoperative tumor embolization and laparoscopic surgery. Angiographic embolization with either clot, metal coils, or synthetic material can reduce blood loss at the time of surgery.[50,51] Laparoscopic surgical techniques have been shown to reduce blood loss in a wide range of procedures from cholecystectomy to adrenalectomy.[52–57] However, the surgeon must understand that successful bloodless laparoscopic surgery is not inherent in the approach but comes only with practice. The inexperienced surgeon can produce massive bleeding during laparoscopy if correct technique is not used.

Hepatic Surgery

Hepatic surgery frequently leads to bleeding and the need for transfusion. Techniques has been shown to be one of the most important determinants of the need for transfusion in both cancer resection and transplantation.[58,59] Intraoperative ultrasound and/or water-jet dissection, needle localization, and microwave cautery help reduce blood loss.[60–62] Several authors have reported great success using a vascular isolation before parenchymal division or VIP approach to liver resection (Fig. 23-2).[63–69] This includes parenchymal compression, temporary cross-clamping of the portal triad (Pringle maneuver),

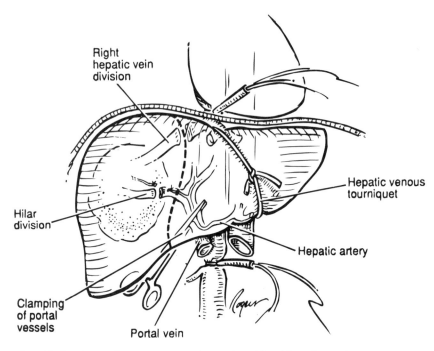

Fig. 23-2. Surgical maneuvers used to reduce blood loss during hepatic surgery.

hepatic venous tourniquet, hilar division, hepatic vein division, and the use of temporary occlusion of the infra- and suprahepatic vena cava (Heaney maneuver). As the name of the approach implies, bleeding is prevented before it occurs. Only two VIP patients in Ryan and Faulkner's[63] series of 34 (6 percent) needed homologous transfusion compared with 18 of 24 patients (75 percent) done without this approach. Makuuchi et al.[65] discharged 87 percent of their hepatectomy patients without the need for whole blood transfusion. Kim et al.[69] reduced blood loss by approximately one-half with this approach. Experienced surgeons working as a team are essential for successful reduction of blood loss during liver surgery.[64,70] Terblanche et al.[64] perform operations with a two-man team of experienced surgeons using 4.5× magnification who complete the resection, with occlusion times averaging 73 minutes.

Vascular Surgery

Modification of operative approaches may minimize blood loss in vascular surgery (Table 23-4). Both the retroperitoneal approach to the abdominal aorta and the exclusion-bypass technique have been re-

ported as superior to traditional surgical approaches and handling of the aorta in terms of blood loss, although some controversy exists. In their study of a standard, transperitoneal approach, Leather et al.[71] estimated blood loss averaged 1,700 ml. By switching to a retroperitoneal approach and excluding the aneurysm, blood loss was decreased to 900 ml, a reduction of almost one-half. Carrel et al.[72] found a similar decrease from 1,300 to 630 ml in 42 retroperitoneal operations compared with 121 transperitoneal cases. In contrast, Cambria et al.[73] found no significant transfusion advantage to using one ap-

Table 23-4. Technical Approaches to Minimizing Blood Loss in Vascular Surgery

Transperitoneal vs. retroperitoneal approach to the abdominal aorta

Exclusion-bypass technique for repair of abdominal aorta

Reversed saphenous vein vs. in situ

Graft choice

    Woven vs. knitted Dacron

    Gelatin/albumin sealed Dacron

    Polytetrafluoroethylene

proach over the other in a series of 69 patients randomized to either a retro- or transperitoneal operation.

Woven Dacron grafts with minimal porosity, gelatin-sealed grafts, and polytetrafluoroethylene (PTFE) essentially eliminate blood loss from extravasation during aortic bypass and replacement, but their effect on reducing transfusion need is questionable. Reid and Pollock[74] reported that gelatin-sealed grafts had "no measurable blood loss at implantation." However, 47 patients still required transfusion for blood loss of greater than 750 ml or on clinical grounds. Fisher et al.[75] performed a comparative analysis of double velour woven Dacron grafts to PTFE using sophisticated blood loss measurement techniques and concluded that neither graft had an advantage over the other in decreasing blood loss or preventing transfusion. Their results may have been skewed by a significantly lower preoperative erythrocyte volume in the Dacron group, which may have accounted for increased transfusion need.

In the lower extremity, Hans et al.[76] noted a greater blood loss with in situ femoral popliteal bypass versus reversed saphenous vein. They attributed this to an increased operative time and more release of blood in testing the vein. By careful attention to detail and limiting bleeding from the anastomosed vein during in situ surgery, we have reduced blood loss in a small number of lower extremity bypass cases to approximately 150 ml, a level below the need for transfusion.[77]

Orthopaedic Surgery

Although blood loss in orthopaedic surgery remains a significant obstacle to avoidance of homologous transfusion, some progress is being made in identifying contributing factors.[78–83] Blood loss during lumbar fusion surgery is greater with a posterior versus an anterior approach, three-level versus two-level fusion, and the use of internal fixation.[80] Two studies of hip surgery have shown that an anterior approach to total hip repair creates less blood loss than a transtrochanteric or posterior approach.[81,84] Blood loss is also greater for exchange arthroplasty compared with internal fixation for hip fractures. Lotke et al.,[82] in a detailed analysis of tourniquet use in total knee replacement, concluded that intraoperative release coupled with immediate, continuous, postoperative

passive motion led to increased blood loss compared with postoperative tourniquet release. Burkart et al.[85] studied this in 100 consecutive knee replacements and demonstrated that tourniquet release had no bearing on overall blood loss. Cemented prostheses and femoral intramedullary plugs offer an advantage in terms of reduced blood loss in knee replacement surgery.[86,87] Delayed hip fracture repair using traction as a temporary measure until red cell mass can be restored may be useful in the severely anemic patient who refuses or cannot be transfused (e.g., the Jehovah's witness).

EMERGENCY SURGERY

Trauma

In elective surgery, the key to success lies in following basic halsteadian principles of careful dissection and attention to detail. The actively bleeding patient or the trauma patient who needs emergency surgery presents a different challenge to the surgeon. Trauma victims and patients with active, visible bleeding from extremities, as a rule, are stabilized quickly and taken from the emergency room to the operating room with only minimal delay. Operative control of bleeding from trauma is essential if blood transfusion is to be minimized. Examples include external fixation to stabilize the fractured pelvis and control venous bleeding and packing of liver fractures followed by a second-look procedure to permit volume restoration and correction of coagulopathy. The need for rapid surgical intervention should not excuse poor technique. The fast, bad surgeon is just as much a liability as the slow, bad surgeon.

Reduction of transfusion need in the trauma patient can be attained primarily through reduction in blood loss. In the bleeding patient, our first priority traditionally has been to correct volume losses and reverse hypotension with infusions of colloid and/or crystalloid solutions. The end point is to stabilize the patient and improve oxygen delivery by increasing cardiac output as quickly as possible. Once the patient is stabilized and is no longer hypovolemic, decisions are made concerning bleeding activity and the need for surgical intervention.

This approach has been questioned recently because of the perception that fluid resuscitation designed to correct hypovolemia may prolong or reinitiate hemorrhage. Several investigators have demonstrated in animal models of uncontrolled hemorrhage that attempts to stabilize the animal with intravenous fluid infusions led to continued blood loss and increased mortality rates.[88,89] This issue was addressed clinically in a prospective study of the effect of fluid resuscitation in hypotensive patients who had sustained penetrating truncal injuries.[90] No significant difference was noted in mortality rates between two groups of patients assigned to either initial or delayed resuscitation, although the trend was toward a higher death rate in the former group. These results can be viewed as supporting the traditional approach to early resuscitation as doing no harm; however, they do not show its benefit. Delaying fluid resuscitation until hemorrhage is controlled appears to be as safe as this traditional approach and may have the added benefit of reducing transfusion need.

Crystalloids and Colloids

Two major resuscitation fluid alternatives to homologous blood transfusion exist—crystalloids and colloids. Both can restore blood pressure—at least temporarily—in the patient in shock after acute blood loss. Colloids have a longer intravascular half-life, but they do not differ significantly from crystalloids in their resuscitative properties (see Ch. 25). A new addition to the family of crystalloids, hypertonic saline (HTS) has been studied extensively in both animals and humans, with mixed results.[91-94] HTS infusions in animal studies have improved hemodynamics after hemorrhage, but they have also increased bleeding, decreased blood pressure, and increased mortality rates.[91,92] Younes et al.[93] randomized 105 patients with hypovolemia treated in the emergency room to either 7.5 percent HTS, a combination of HTS with dextran 70, or saline. Initial mean arterial pressure was higher in HTS groups, and both fluid and blood requirements for overall resuscitation were less. However, there was no effect on mortality rates. A prospective, randomized double-blind trial of a HTS/dextran combination versus lactated Ringer's solution in 166 trauma patients conducted by Vassar et al.[94] showed no significant difference in either bleeding or amount of blood transfused. Outcome was improved only in patients with head injuries. Further studies are needed to assess whether HTS with/without colloid will have a beneficial effect on blood loss and transfusion requirements.

Major Vascular Injuries

Exsanguination remains the critical factor in determining outcome in isolated, major vascular injuries.[95,96] The traditional teaching regarding a retroperitoneal or pelvic hematoma in a blunt trauma patient is to leave it alone for fear of unleashing uncontrollable venous bleeding. In the patient with a suspected large vessel injury, this approach may lead to continued hemorrhage and deterioration. Brathwaite and Rodriguez[97] recommend opening all central and lateral hematomas in blunt trauma victims after proximal and distal aortic control has been established. This approach, based on sound, vascular surgical principles, permits expeditious repair of major injuries while minimizing blood loss.

Angiography remains the standard not only in identifying pelvic vascular injury but also in controlling bleeding by embolization or coil occlusion. Identification of a bleeding vessel with intraoperative ultrasound may avoid the delays and dangers inherent in angiography.[98] Occlusion, either by catheter or direct ligation, is appropriate in smaller vessels and in areas where collateral circulation is sufficient to maintain perfusion of the affected distal tissues or in life-threatening situations. However, occlusion of a proximal iliac vessel can be disastrous, leading to high amputation. Performance of a cross-femoral bypass graft in conjunction with iliac artery ligation can provide limb salvage.[99]

Vascular injuries of the extremities are usually not exsanguinating. Ongoing bleeding can be controlled by direct compression and exploration to attain proximal control followed by either direct repair or bypass.[100] The use of a stent/graft combination to treat a traumatic femoral arteriovenous fistula has been described by Marin et al.[101] These grafts, which can be placed through minimal incisions using angiographic techniques, may lead to dramatic reductions in operative blood loss and patient survival in ruptured aneurysms or similar vascular injuries.

Autotransfusion equipment should be ready so that as much shed blood as possible can be salvaged and returned from the thoracic, abdominal, or thigh compartments. Even though the blood appears to have clotted, such losses can be successfully salvaged, washed, and returned as red cells to the patient. An estimate of blood lost should be made early on so that appropriate replacements can be ordered from the blood bank. One should not be so foolish as to think that emergency surgery can be done without the use of allogeneic or banked blood.

Abdominal Aortic Aneurysms

Early surgery for a leaking or ruptured abdominal aortic aneurysm can lead to a successful outcome in most patients; delay leads to increased mortality rates.[102–104] Insistence on radiologic confirmation of bleeding in a patient with obvious clinical signs of active hemorrhage is to be condemned. Although the use of computed tomography to identify a leaking aneurysm in clinically stable patients has a definite role, one must not make the mistake of assuming that the absence of radiologic evidence of bleeding in those with symptoms supports delaying surgery. Most series promoting the benefits of such scanning contain at least one patient who ruptured a nonleaking aneurysm while hospitalized and awaiting surgery.[105,106] Surgical repair of the symptomatic aneurysm within 24 to 36 hours remains the standard.[102]

Gastrointestinal Bleeding

In contrast to the trauma patient in whom early surgical intervention to stop bleeding is the norm, it is common practice in the patient with gastrointestinal bleeding to determine the need for surgery based on the number of units of blood lost (i.e., transfused) within a 12- to 24-hour period. By using such guidelines, not only do we magnify the risk of allogeneic blood exposure, but we also increase the mortality rate in direct proportion to the number of units transfused.[107,108] Lee et al.[109] studied 101 patients admitted to the intensive care unit with bleeding from varices. Those transfused with more than 10 units in less than 24 hours—30.6 percent of the cohort—had a significantly higher mortality rate compared with others. The use of multiple blood transfusions was a significant independent predictor of death, and both the degree of blood loss and the failure to stop bleeding contributed to the high mor-

Table 23-5. Transfusion and Mortality Rate in Gastrointestinal Bleeding

Mortality rate in upper gastrointestinal bleeding (Data from Sugawa et al.[107])	
More than 5 U PRBC	39/193 (20.2%)
Less than 5 U PRBC	20/369 (5.4%)

Lower gastrointestinal bleeding: effect of age and transfusion (Data from Bender et al.[110])

Age (yr)	0–9 U PRBC	10+ U PRBC
50–69	1/6 (16.7%)	2/9 (22.2%)
70–79	0/1 (0%)	3/7 (42.8%)
80–89	1/13 (7.7%)	4/4 (100%)

Abbreviation: PRBC, packed red blood cells.

tality rate. Bender et al.[110] found that the mortality rate in a group of patients who underwent total abdominal colectomy for massive lower gastrointestinal bleeding was higher in those who were transfused with more than 10 units of blood before surgery (Table 23-5). They recommended immediate surgery in these patients to improve survival. These studies, and those discussed below, suggest that outcomes, defined as both survival and a reduction in the use of allogeneic blood, can be improved significantly by a more aggressive approach to gastrointestinal bleeding.

Early intervention requires early diagnosis. Endoscopy determines the cause of bleeding in the upper gastrointestinal tract and can provide a means of therapy. Failure to stop hemorrhage from an ulcer with electrocoagulation should prompt surgical intervention. Most variceal bleeding can be controlled using a stepwise treatment plan that includes endoscopy, vasopressin infusion, balloon tamponade, and sclerotherapy followed by selective decompression with a shunt for persistent or recurrent bleeding.[111] After confirmation by endoscopy of varices as the bleeding source, vasopressin may be infused at a rate of 0.4 unit/min, increasing to a maximum of 1 unit/min, as needed. Nitroglycerin may be infused concomitantly to minimize coronary vasoconstriction. If bleeding does not stop with this approach, insertion of a Sengstaken-Blakemore tube provides rapid, temporary control. Although the balloon provides only temporary control and rebleeding rates are high after removal, one must remember that the primary goal here is to stop the continued bleeding quickly. Once control is achieved, endoscopic sclerotherapy provides definitive control.

Rebleeding with increased transfusion requirements and mortality rates as high as 45 percent after endoscopic sclerotherapy have led others to evaluate alternative methods of controlling variceal bleeding, including endoscopic ligation, esophageal interruption, and emergency shunting, with the latter being performed either surgically or through an endovascular approach. Stiegmann et al.[112] reduced homologous blood usage and decreased the mortality rate from 44 percent with sclerotherapy to 28 percent using endoscopic ligation in a randomized trial of 129 patients. Burroughs et al.[113] reported decreased rebleeding using staple transection of the esophagus compared with sclerotherapy. However, the morbidity, mortality rate, and blood usage were similar for the two groups compared. Berard[114] states in his report on 108 patients who underwent clip interruption of the esophagus by thoracotomy that this procedure can be done in less than 1 hour without

transfusion and with a mortality rate of 20 percent. Nagasue et al.[115] reduced blood loss from approximately 1,400 to 800 ml using PTFE to construct a modified distal splenorenal shunt. The mortality rate was 11.1 percent using this technique in eight of nine emergency shunts.

Transvenous Intrahepatic Portosystemic Shunts

Use of the transvenous intrahepatic portosystemic shunt, or TIPS, follows catheter-directed vasopressin infusions as the next step in angiographically driven therapy for bleeding varices. This expandable metal shunt can be placed either angiographically between a branch of the hepatic vein and the right or left branch of the hepatic vein and the right or left branch of the portal vein or directly into a small bowel mesenteric vein through a midline laparotomy incision (Fig. 23-3).[116] In Ring et al.'s[117] initial series of 13 patients, creation of a TIPS acutely stopped variceal bleeding by decreasing portal pressure approximately 10 cmH₂O. Four patients had had previous portosystemic shunts; in others, sclero-

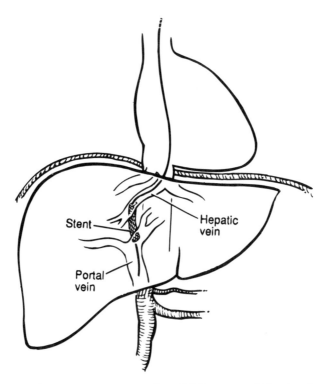

Fig. 23-3. Transvenous intrahepatic portosystemic shunt (TIPS) to control bleeding from portal hypertension.

therapy failed. Bleeding recurred in only one patient after 3 months. Moreover, seven patients derived considerable long-term benefit by going on to successful liver transplantation. This group subsequently reported similar results in more than 100 patients, as have others in smaller series.[118,119]

Jehovah's Witnesses

We prefer definitive therapy (i.e., portocaval shunting) in the Jehovah's Witness after an initial episode of variceal bleeding because rebleeding must be avoided. We have used an end-to-side shunt because of its simplicity and minimal blood loss in four such patients. All survived their initial operation, but one died 8 days postoperatively after the shunt occluded and the patient exsanguinated from his esophageal varices. The other three were discharged from the hospital in good condition. All shunts were done during the hospitalization for the initial bleeding episode. Definitive treatment (i.e., surgery) was not performed until hepatic function had improved. This was facilitated by initial volume replacement, nutritional support, and iron replacement. We believe that this approach, which works well with Jehovah's Witnesses, can be used with other patients to help limit the need for allogeneic transfusion.

PHARMACOLOGIC AGENTS

Several drugs that reduce intraoperative blood loss are available to the surgeon (Table 23-6). Those who perform cardiac or vascular surgery are familiar with the use of protamine to reverse the effect of heparin.

Table 23-6. Pharmacologic Adjuncts to Reduce Blood Loss

Vitamin K
Protamine
Desmopressin
Tranexamic acid
Aminocaproic acid
Aprotinin
Vasopressin
Topical agents
Fibrin glue
Surgicel, Hemopad, etc.

Attention to clotting times and accurate dosing with protamine is necessary. In addition, the surgeon should be aware that heparin may bind temporarily to plasma proteins, preventing complete reversal by protamine. Slow dissociation of this heparin component may produce an anticoagulant effect in the immediate postoperative period, contributing to increased blood loss.[120]

Desmopressin

We use vasopressin intraoperatively during portocaval shunting to constrict dilated vessels in the skin and subcutaneous tissues. A vasopressin analogue, desmopressin (DDAVP) has been used for a number of years in patients with coagulopathies.[83] The drug has no vasopressor activity, but infusions of the hormone lead to increases in the level of circulating factor VIII. DDAVP has a variety of side effects, which range from mild facial flushing and headache through tachycardia and hypertension to tachyphylaxis.

Several trials conducted to evaluate the role of DDAVP in reducing blood loss during cardiac surgical procedures have had mixed results.[121-127] Both Salzman et al.[121] and Czer et al.[122] showed a reduced need for homologous red cell transfusion in a group of cardiac surgical patients treated with the drug. In two separate studies, Dilthey et al.[126] and Sheridan et al.[127] demonstrated a similar reduction in both blood loss and need for transfusion in cardiac surgical patients who had been treated with aspirin before surgery. In contrast, neither Hackman et al.,[123] Rocha et al.,[124] or Reynolds et al.[125] found either a decrease in the need for transfusion or the amount of operative blood loss in similar patients. In their study of DDAVP in lumbar fusion surgery, Johnson and Murphy[80] suggested that the drug was helpful in reducing blood loss, but primarily when losses exceeded 1,000 ml. It is difficult to conclude from these studies anything other than that DDAVP may play a role as an adjunct in reducing operative bleeding. The amounts of blood loss seen in all of these series indicate that the surgeon may need to pay more attention to surgical hemostasis than to drug action.

Aminocaproic Acid and Tranexamic Acid

Hemorrhagic diathesis after cardiopulmonary bypass has been ascribed in part to hyperfibrinolysis caused by increased plasminogen activator. Aminocaproic acid, a synthetic monoamine carboxylic acid, inhibits proteolysis through interference with the conversion of plasminogen to plasmin. Its effect can be measured by monitoring both partial thromboplastin and prothrombin times. Our study of 350 patients undergoing cardiopulmonary bypass, in which patients were randomized either to a treatment or a control group, showed that the aminocaproic acid-treated patients had statistically less bleeding and required less allogeneic blood transfusion than did the control group.[128]

Tranexamic acid, a similar antifibrinolytic agent, has been used successfully to reduce blood loss during cardiac surgery. Nakashima et al.[129] noted significant decreases in postoperative chest tube blood drainage, overall blood loss, and time to hemostasis in a group of 90 patients treated with tranexamic acid compared with a control population. Teasdale et al.[130] found that a similar group of patients treated with tranexamic acid had less blood loss and decreased transfusion need (28 percent transfused versus 49 percent) compared with placebo-treated controls. In this study, aminocaproic acids was also shown to be effective in reducing blood loss.

Aprotinin

Aprotinin, a serine protease inhibitor used in the past to treat pancreatitis and fibrinolysis, has been used successfully to reduce blood loss during cardiac surgery in a number of clinical trials.[131–139] Exactly how the drug accomplishes this is unknown. It may work by interfering with kallikrein and plasmin, by preserving platelet adhesion membrane receptors during cardiopulmonary bypass, or by inhibiting plasmin-mediated fibrinolysis.[133,140,141] Results in more than 200 patients from three controlled, prospective studies have been remarkably similar. Treated patients have all had decreases in postoperative blood loss (up to 45 percent) and the need for allogeneic transfusion.[134–138] Moreover, aprotinin may play an important role in treating patients with aspirin-induced platelet abnormalities. Both Murkin et al.[141] and Wildevuur et al.[134] found significant reductions in both bleeding time and postoperative blood loss in aprotinin-treated patients who had received aspirin before coronary artery bypass. Aprotinin appears to achieve this by maintaining platelet adhesiveness without affecting aspirin-induced inhibition of platelet aggregation. Additional benefit in terms of reducing blood exposure can be achieved by combining aprotinin with autotransfusion.[142] Similar reductions in bleeding and transfusion need have been reported with aprotinin use in both liver transplantation and orthopaedic surgery.[143–145]

Unfortunately, aprotinin therapy is not without toxicity and problems. Anaphylaxis has been reported with its use.[146] To achieve the successes noted, investigators have had to use large doses of the drug intravenously. Administration must be monitored closely to avoid hypotension. Moreover, aprotinin rapidly accumulates in the proximal tubular cells of the kidney and can lead to renal damage. Fraedrich et al.[138] found proteinuria in their patients and suggested that decreasing the dose of aprotinin might be necessary in those with preoperative renal function impairment. Concerns about clotting of coronary artery grafts with aprotinin use have been proved to be unwarranted.[147] It is apparent that aprotinin must undergo further study to document both its safety and efficacy before it is ready for general use. However, the drug holds considerable promise for the surgeon who wishes to reduce intraoperative bleeding, particularly that associated with drug-induced platelet malfunction.

Other Agents

Other pharmacologic agents may be helpful in reducing surgical blood loss. Pentoxifylline, prostacyclin, and bombesin may play a role in controlling bleeding. All three drugs are purported to work on the vascular system: bombesin by counteracting opioid-induced vasodilatation and pentoxifylline and prostacyclin by improving microcirculatory flow and tissue oxygen delivery.[148] The clinical role of these drugs remains unproved, although the latter two may have some benefit in septic or critically ill patients who need to maximize peripheral oxygen consumption. Once bleeding is controlled and the patient is stabilized, attention can be paid to restoring red cell mass, platelets, and clotting factors. Nafamostat mesylate, a protease inhibitor that inactivates coagulation, platelet aggregation, and fibrinolysis, has had initial success in reducing blood loss during cardiac surgery.[149]

This chapter reviewed surgical and pharmacologic approaches to reducing blood loss. Multiple adjuncts, ranging from changes in operative technique to new drugs, are available to the surgeon. These are most helpful when used in conjunction with other modalities such as preoperative autologous donation of blood and autotransfusion.

REFERENCES

1. Bell J: The Principles of Surgery. Philadelphia, 1810
2. Mettler C: History of Medicine. The Classics of Medicine Library, Birmingham, 1986
3. Kaynes G (ed): The Apologie and Treatise of Ambroise Pare. Lacon Educational Books, London, 1951
4. Manec PJ: Traité Théorique et Pratique de la Ligature des Artères. Librairie Médical de Crochard, Paris, 1932
5. Halstead WS: Surgical Papers. Johns Hopkins Press, Baltimore, 1924
6. Spence RK, Carson JA, Poses R et al: Elective surgery without transfusion: influence of preoperative hemoglobin level and blood loss on mortality. Am J Surg 59:320, 1990
7. Stone HH, Strom PR, Mullins RJ: Management of the major coagulopathy with onset during laparotomy. Ann Surg 197:532, 1983
8. Ferrara A, MacArthur JD, Wright HK et al: Hypothermia and acidosis worsen coagulopathy in the patient requiring massive transfusion. Am J Surg 160:515, 1990
9. Ambrus JL, Mittleman A: Hematologic management of the aged and high risk surgical patient. p. 211. In Siegel JH, Chodoff P (eds): The Aged and High Risk Surgical Patient: Medical, Surgical and Anesthetic Management. Grune and Stratton, New York, 1976
10. British Committee for Standardization in Haematology Blood Transfusion Task Force: Guidelines for the transfusion of massive blood. Clin Lab Haematol 10:265, 1988
11. McIntyre AJ: Blood transfusion and hemostatic management in the perioperative period. Can J Anaesth 39:R108, 1992
12. Leslie S, Toy P: Laboratory hemostatic abnormalities in massively transfused patients given red blood cells and crystalloid. Am J Clin Pathol 96:770, 1991
13. Ciavarella D, Reed RL, Counts RB et al: Clotting factor levels and the risk of diffuse microvascular bleeding in the massively transfused patient. Br J Haematol 67$5, 1987
14. Martin DI, Lucas CE, Ledgerwood AM et al: Fresh frozen plasma supplement to massive red blood cell transfusion. Ann Surg 202:505, 1985
15. Reed FL, Ciavarella D, Heimbach DM et al: Prophylactic platelet administration during massive transfusion: a prospective, randomized, double-blind clinical study. Ann Surg 203:40, 1986
16. Aubuchon JP, Busch M, Epstein JS et al: Increasing the safety of blood transfusions. American Red Cross, Washington, DC, 1992
17. Linden JV, Paul B, Dressler KP: A report of 104 transfusion errors in New York State. Transfusion 32:601, 1992
18. Bridenbaugh LD: Regional anesthesia for outpatient surgery—a summary of 12 years' experience. Can J Anaesth 30:548, 1983
19. Bjoraker DG: Blood transfusion. What is a safe hematocrit? Probl Crit Care 5:386, 1991
20. Blackwell KE, Ross DA, Kapur P et al: Propofol for maintenance of general anesthesia: a technique to limit blood loss during endoscopic sinus surgery. Am J Otolaryngol 14:262, 1993
21. Miller E, Paull DE, Morrissey K et al: Scalpel versus electrocautery in modified radical mastectomy. Am Surg 54:284, 1988
22. Pearlman NW, Stiegmann GV, Vance V et al: A prospective study of incisional time, blood loss, pain and healing with carbon dioxide laser, scalpel and electrosurgery. Arch Surg 126:1018, 1991
23. Ward PH, Castro DJ, Ward S: A significant new contribution to radical head and neck surgery. The argon beam coagulator as an effective means of limiting blood loss. Arch Otolaryngol Head Neck Surg 115:921, 1989
24. Trent CS: Electrocautery versus epinephrine-injection tonsillectomy. Ear Nose Throat J 72:520, 1993
25. Tan AK, Rothstein J, Tewfik TL: Ambulatory tonsillectomy and adenoidectomy: complications and associated factors. J Otolaryngol 22:442, 1993
26. Leach J, Manning S, Schaefer S: Comparison of two methods of tonsillectomy. Laryngoscope 103:619, 1993
27. Tchabo JG, Thomure MF, Tomai TP: A comparison of laser and cold knife conization. Int Surg 78:131, 1993
28. Bhatta N, Isaacson K, Flotte T: Injury and adhesion formation following ovarian wedge resection with different thermal surgical modalities. Lasers Surg Med 13:344, 1993
29. Bordelon BM, Hobday KA, Hunter JG: Laser vs electrosurgery in laparoscopic cholecystectomy. A prospective randomized trial. Arch Surg 128:233, 1993

30. Shaha AR: Minimizing the blood loss during flap raising in thyroidectomy. J Surg Oncol 52:153, 1993

31. Andrews BT, Layer GT, Jackson BT: Randomized trial comparing diathermy hemorrhoidectomy with the scissors dissection Milligan-Morgan operation. Dis Colon Rectum 36:580, 1993

32. Muraki J, Addonizio JC, Lastarria E et al: New Cavitron system (CUSA/CEM): its application for kidney surgery. Urology 41:195, 1993

33. Wyman A, Rogers K: Randomized trial of laser scalpel for modified radical mastectomy. Br J Surg 80: 871, 1993

34. Neven P, Shepherd JH, Wilkinson DJ: Radical vulvectomy using the argon enhanced electro-surgical pencil. Br J Obstet Gynaecol 100:789, 1993

35. Helkjaer PE, Eriksen PS, Thomsen CF et al: Outpatient CO_2 laser excisional conization for cervical intraepithelial neoplasia under local anesthesia. Acta Obstet Gynecol Scand 72:302, 1993

36. Dowling RD, Ochoa J, Yousem SA et al: Argon beam coagulation is superior to conventional techniques in repair of experimental splenic injury. J Trauma 31: 717, 1991

37. Zhou XD, Tang ZY, Yu YQ et al: Microwave surgery in the treatment of hepatocellular carcinoma. Semin Surg Oncol 9:318, 1993

38. Lau WY, Arnold M, Guo SK et al: Microwave tissue coagulator in liver resection for cirrhotic patients. Aust N Z J Surg 62:576, 1992

39. Decker CJ: An efficient method for the application of Avitene hemostatic agent. Surg Gynecol Obstet 172: 489, 1991

40. Kram HB, Nathan RC, Stafford FJ et al: Fibrin glue achieves hemostasis in patients with coagulation disorders. Arch Surg 124:385, 1989

41. Kohno H, Nagasue N, Chang YC et al: Comparison of topical hemostatic agents in elective hepatic resection: a clinical prospective randomized trial. World J Surg 16:966, 1992

42. Raccuia JS, Simonian G, Dardik M et al: Comparative efficacy of topical hemostatic agents in a rat kidney model. Am J Surg 163:234, 1992

43. Kuzu A, Aydintug S, Karayalcin K et al: Use of autologous fibrin glue in the treatment of splenic trauma: an experimental study. J R Coll Surg Edinb 37:162, 1992

44. Glimaker H, Bjorck CG, Hallstensson S et al: Avoiding blow-out of the aortic stump by reinforcement with fibrin glue. A report of two cases. Eur J Vasc Surg 7:346, 1993

45. Schwartz RJ, Dubrow TJ, Rival RA et al: The effect of fibrin glue on intraperitoneal contamination in rats treated with systemic antibiotics. J Surg Res 52:123, 1992

46. Bänninger H, Hardegger T, Tobler A et al: Fibrin glue in surgery: frequent development of inhibitors of bovine thrombin and human factor V. Br J Haematol 85:528, 1993

47. Hartman AR, Galanakis DK, Honig MP et al: Autologous whole plasma fibrin gel. Intraoperative procurement. Arch Surg 127:357, 1992

48. Gibble JW, Ness PM: Fibrin glue: the perfect operative sealant? Transfusion 30:741, 1990

49. Tawes RL, Jr: Reducing homologous blood use in vascular surgery. Promotion of hemostasis. In Rutherford R (ed): Seminars in Vascular Surgery 7:82, 1994

50. Siniluoto TM, Luotonen JP, Tikkakoski TA et al: Value of pre-operative embolization in surgery for nasopharyngeal angiofibroma. J Laryngol Otol 107: 514, 1993

51. Wakhloo AK, Juengling FD, Van Velthoven V et al: Extended preoperative polyvinyl alcohol microembolization of intracranial meningiomas: assessment of two embolization techniques. AJNR Am J Neuroradiol 14:571, 1993

52. Go H, Takeda M, Takahashi H et al: Laparoscopic adrenalectomy for primary aldosteronism: a new operative method. J Laparoendosc Surg 3:455, 1993

53. Suzuki K, Kageyama S, Ueda D et al: Laparoscopic adrenalectomy: clinical experience with 12 cases. J Urol 150:1099, 1993

54. Pier A, Gotz F, Bacher C: Laparoscopic appendectomy in 625 cases: from innovation to routine. Surg Laparosc Endosc 1:8, 1991

55. Nowzaraden Y, Westmoreland JC: Laparoscopic cholecystectomy: new indications. Surg Laparosc Endosc 1:71, 1993

56. Corbitt JD, Jr: Laparoscopic cholecystectomy: laser vs electrosurgery. Surg Laparosc Endosc 1:85, 1991

57. Senagore AJ, Lutchefeld MA, Machkeigan JM et al: Open colectomy versus laparoscopic colectomy: are there differences? Am Surg 59:549, 1993

58. Jamieson GG, Corbel L, Campion JP et al: Major liver resection without a blood transfusion: is it a realistic objective? Surgery 112:32, 1992

59. Deakin M, Gunson BK, Dunn JA et al: Factors influencing blood transfusion during adult liver transplantation. Ann R Coll Surg Engl 75:339, 1993

60. Wu CC, Yang MD, Liu TJ: Improvements in hepatocellular carcinoma resection by intraoperative ultrasonography and intermittent hepatic inflow blood occlusion. Jpn J Clin Oncol 22:107, 1992

61. Baer HU, Stain SC, Guastella T et al: Hepatic resection using a water jet dissector. HPB Surg 6:189, 1993
62. Izumi R, Shimizu K, Kiriyama K et al: Hepatic resection guided by needles inserted under ultrasonic guidance. Surgery 114:497, 1993
63. Ryan JA, Jr, Faulkner DJ II: Liver resection without blood transfusion. Am J Surg 157:472, 1989
64. Terblanche J, Krige JEJ, Bornman PC: Simplified hepatic resection with the use of prolonged vascular inflow occlusion. Arch Surg 126:298, 1991
65. Makuuchi M, Kosuge T, Takayama T et al: Surgery for small liver cancers. Semin Surg Oncol 9:298, 1993
66. Hannoun L, Borie D, Delva E et al: Liver resection with normothermic ischaemia exceeding 1 hour. Br J Surg 80:1161, 1993
67. Yamaoka Y, Ozawa K, Kumada K et al: Total vascular occlusion for hepatic resection in cirrhotic patients. Application of venovenous bypass. Arch Surg 127:276, 1992
68. Elias D, Lasser P, Hoang JM et al: Repeat hepatectomy for cancer. Br J Surg 80:1557, 1993
69. Kim YI, Nakashima K, Tada I et al: Prolonged normothermic ischaemia of human cirrhotic liver during hepatectomy: a preliminary report. Br J Surg 80:1566, 1993
70. Nagasue N, Kohno H, Chang YC et al: Liver resection for hepatocellular carcinoma. Results of 229 consecutive patients during 11 years. Ann Surg 217:375, 1993
71. Leather RP, Shah DM, Kaufman JL et al: Comparative analysis of retroperitoneal and transperitoneal aortic replacement for aneurysm. Surg Gynecol Obstet 168:387, 1989
72. Carrel T, Pasic M, Turina M et al: The retroperitoneal approach: an excellent alternative to the transperitoneal route in elective aortic surgery. Int J Angio Winter:1, 1992
73. Cambria RP, Brewster DC, Abbott WM et al: Transperitoneal versus retroperitoneal approach for aortic reconstruction: a randomized prospective study. J Vasc Surg 11:314, 1990
74. Reid DB, Pollock JG: A prospective study of 100 gelatin-sealed aortic grafts. Ann Vasc Surg 5:320, 1991
75. Fisher JB, Dennis RC, Valeri CR et al: Effect of graft material on loss of erythrocytes after aortic operations. Surg Gynecol Obstet 173:130, 1991
76. Hans SS, Masi J, Goyal V et al: Increased blood loss with in situ bypass. Am Surg 56:540, 1990
77. Spence RK: Transfusion practices in vascular surgery. Perspect Vasc Surg 6:14, 1994
78. Toy PTC, Kaplan EB, McVay PA et al: Blood loss and replacement in total hip arthroplasty: a multicenter study. Transfusion 32:63, 1992
79. Surgenor DM, Wallace EL, Churchill WH et al: Red cell transfusions in total knee and total hip replacement surgery. Transfusion 31:531, 1991
80. Johnson RG, Murphy JM: The role of desmopressin in reducing blood loss during lumbar fusions. Surg Gynecol Obstet 171:223, 1990
81. Grzeskiewicz JL, Hall RA, Anderson G et al: Preoperative crossmatch guidelines for total hip arthroplasty. Orthopedics 12:549, 1989
82. Lotke PA, Faralli VJ, Orenatein EM et al: Blood loss after total knee replacement. J Bone Joint Surg [Am] 73:1037, 1991
83. Schulman S: DDAVP—the multipotent drug in patients with coagulopathies. Transfusion Med Rev 5:132, 1991
84. Keene GS, Parker MJ: Hemiarthroplasty of the hip—the anterior or posterior approach? A comparison of surgical approaches. Injury 24:611, 1993
85. Burkart BC, Bourne RB, Rorabeck CH et al: The efficacy of tourniquet release in blood conservation after total knee arthroplasty. Clin Orthop 299:147, 1994
86. Heddle NM, Brox WT, Klama LN et al: A randomized trial on the efficacy of an autologous blood drainage and transfusion device in patients undergoing elective knee arthroplasty. Transfusion 32:742, 1992
87. Raut VV, Stone MH, Wroblewski BM: Reduction of postoperative blood loss after press-fit condylar knee arthroplasty with use of a femoral intramedullary plug. J Bone J Surg [Am] 75:1356, 1993
88. Krausz MM, Meital BZ, Rabinovici R et al: "Scoop and run" or "stabilize" hemorrhagic shock by normal saline or small-volume hypertonic saline. J Trauma 33:6, 1992
89. Bickell WH, Bruttig SP, Millnamoro GA et al: The detrimental effects of intravenous crystalloid after experimental aortotomy in swine. Surgery 110:529, 1991
90. Martin RR, Bickell WH, Pepe PE et al: Prospective evaluation of preoperative fluid resuscitation in hypotensive patients with penetrating truncal injury: a preliminary report. J Trauma 33:354, 1992
91. Lilly MP, Gala GJ, Carlson DE et al: Saline resuscitation after fixed-volume hemorrhage. Role of resuscitation volume and rate of infusion. Ann Surg 216:161, 1992
92. Rabinovici R, Krausz MM, Feuerstein G: Control of bleeding is essential for successful treatment of hemorrhagic shock with 7.5 per cent sodium chloride solution. Surg Gynecol Obstet 173:98, 1991
93. Younes RN, Aun F, Accioly CQ et al: Hypertonic solutions in the treatment of hypovolemic shock: a prospective, randomized study in patients admitted to the emergency room. Surgery 111:380, 1992

94. Vassar MJ, Perry CA, Gannaway WL et al: 7.5% Sodium chloride/dextran for resuscitation of trauma patients undergoing helicopter transport. Arch Surg 126:1065, 1991

95. Jackson MR, Olson DW, Beckett WC, Jr et al: Abdominal vascular trauma: a review of 106 injuries. Am Surg 58:622, 1992

96. Lopez-Viego MA, Snyder WH 3d, Valentine RJ et al: Penetrating abdominal aortic trauma: a report of 129 cases. J Vasc Surg 16:332, 1992

97. Brathwaite CE, Rodriguez A: Injuries of the abdominal aorta from blunt trauma. Am Surg 58:350, 1992

98. Williams DM, Dake MD, Bolling SF et al: The role of intravascular ultrasound in acute traumatic aortic rupture. Semin Ultrasound CT MR 14:85, 1993

99. Samuels LE, Gross CF, DiGiovanni RJ et al: External iliac artery occlusion due to pelvic fracture: management with a cross-femoral bypass graft. South Med J 86:572, 1993

100. van Wijngaarden M, Omert L, Rodriguez A et al: Management of blunt vascular trauma to the extremities. Surg Gynecol Obstet 177:41, 1993

101. Marin ML, Veith FJ, Panetta TF et al: Percutaneous transfemoral insertion of a stented graft to repair a traumatic femoral arteriovenous fistula. J Vasc Surg 18:299, 1993

102. Marston WA, Ahlquist R, Johnson G et al: Misdiagnosis of ruptured abdominal aortic aneurysms. J Vasc Surg 16:17, 1992

103. D'Angelo F, Vaghi M, Mattassi R et al: Changing trends in the outcome of urgent aneurysms surgery. A retrospective study on 170 patients treated in the years 1966–1990. J Cardiovasc Surg (Torino) 34:237, 1993

104. McCready RA, Siderys H, Pittman JN: Ruptured abdominal aortic aneurysms in a private hospital: a decade's experience (1980–1989). Ann Vasc Surg 7:225, 1993

105. Kvilekval KH, Best IM, Mason RA et al: The value of computed tomography in the management of symptomatic abdominal aortic aneurysms. J Vasc Surg 12:28, 1990

106. Seeger JM, Kieffer RW: Preoperative CT in symptomatic abdominal aortic aneurysms: accuracy and efficacy. Am Surg 52:87, 1986

107. Sugawa C, Steffes CP, Nakamura R et al: Upper GI bleeding in an urban hospital. Etiology, recurrence and prognosis. Ann Surg 212:521, 1990

108. Pimpl W, Boeckl O, Heinerman M et al: Emergency endoscopy: a basis for therapeutic decisions in the treatment of severe gastroduodenal bleeding. World J Surg 13:592, 1989

109. Lee H, Hawker FH, Selby W et al: Intensive care treatment of patients with bleeding esophageal varices: results, predictors of mortality, and predictors of the adult respiratory distress syndrome Crit Care Med 20:1555, 1993

110. Bender JS, Weincek RG, Bouwman DL: Morbidity and mortality following total abdominal colectomy for massive lower gastrointestinal bleeding. Am Surg 8:536, 1991

111. Gliedman ML, Langer B, Rikkers LF et al: Management of variceal bleeding. Contemp Surg 41:49, 1992

112. Stiegmann GV, Goff JS, Michaletz-Onody PA et al: Endoscopic sclerotherapy as compared with endoscopic ligation for bleeding esophageal varices. N Engl J Med 326:1527, 1992

113. Burroughs AK, Hamilton G, Phillips A et al: A comparison of sclerotherapy with staple transection of the esophagus for the emergency control of bleeding from esophageal varices. N Engl J Med 321:857, 1989

114. Berard P: Surgical treatment of hemorrhage from ruptured esophageal varices by an orally introduced clip to provoke sclerosis of the lower esophagus and ligation of the peri-esophageal veins through a thoracic approach. Results in 108 cases treated over a period of 5 years. J Chir (Paris) 121:6, 1984

115. Nagasue N, Kohno H, Ogawa Y et al: Appraisal of distal spinal renal shunt in the treatment of esophageal varices: an analysis of prophylactic emergency and elective shunts. World J Surg 13:92, 1989

116. Harville LE, Rivera FJ, Palmaz JC et al: Variceal hemorrhage associated with portal vein thrombosis: treatment with a unique portal venous stent. Surgery 111:585, 1992

117. Ring EJ, Lake JR, Roberts JP et al: Using transjugular intrahepatic portosystemic shunts to control variceal bleeding before liver transplantation. Ann Intern Med 116:304, 1992

118. LaBerge JM, Ring EJ, Gordon RL et al: Creation of transjugular intrahepatic portosystemic shunts with the wall stent endoprosthesis: results in 100 patients. Radiology 187:413, 1993

119. Martin M, Zajko AB, Orons PD et al: Transjugular intrahepatic portosystemic shunt in the management of variceal bleeding: indications and clinical results. Surgery 114:719, 1993

120. Tech KH, Young E, Bradley CA et al: Heparin binding proteins. Contribution to heparin rebound after cardiopulmonary bypass. Circulation to heparin rebound after cardiopulmonary bypass. Circulation 88:II-420, 1993

121. Salzman EW, Weinstein MJ, Wientraub RM et al: Treatment with desmopressin acetate to reduce blood loss after cardiac surgery: a double blind randomized trial. N Engl J Med 314:1402, 1986

122. Czer LSC, Bateman TM, Gray RJ et al: Treatment

of severe platelet dysfunction and hemorrhage after cardiopulmonary bypass: reduction in blood product usage with desmopressin. J Am Coll Cardiol 9:1139, 1987

123. Hackman T, Gascoyne RD, Naiman SC et al: A trial of desmopressin (1-desamino-8-D-arginine vasopressin) to reduce blood loss in uncomplicated cardiac surgery. N Engl J Med 321:1437, 1989

124. Rocha E, Llorens R, Paramo JA et al: Does desmopressin acetate reduce blood loss after surgery in patients on cardiopulmonary bypass? Circulation 77:1319, 1988

125. Reynolds LM, Nicolson SC, Jobes DR et al: Desmopressin does not decrease bleeding during cardiac operation in young children. J Thorac Cardiovasc Surg 106:954, 1993

126. Dilthey G, Dietrich W, Spannagl M et al: Influence of desmopressin acetate on homologous blood requirements in cardiac surgical patients pretreated with aspirin. J Cardiothorac Vasc Anesth 7:425, 1993

127. Sheridan DP, Card RT, Pinilla JC et al: Use of desmopressin acetate to reduce blood transfusion requirements during cardiac surgery in patients with acetylsalicylic acid induced platelet dysfunction. Can J Surg 37:33, 1994

128. DelRossi AJ, Cernaianu AC, Botros S et al: Prophylactic treatment of postperfusion bleeding using EACA. Chest 96:27, 1989

129. Nakashima A, Matsuzaki K, Fukumura F et al: Tranexamic acid reduces blood loss after cardiopulmonary bypass. ASAIO J 39:M185, 1993

130. Teasdale SJ, Norman PH, Carroll JA et al: Prevention of postbypass bleeding with tranexamic acid and epsilon-aminocaproic acid. J Cardiothorac Vasc Anesth 7:431, 1993

131. Feeley TW, Rinsky LA: Use of aprotinin to reduce intraoperative bleeding. West J Med 159:189, 1993

132. Boldt J, Knothe C, Zickman B et al: Aprotinin in pediatric cardiac operations: platelet function, blood loss and use of homologous blood. Ann Thorac Surg 55:1460, 1993

133. D'Ambra MN, Risk SC: Aprotinin, erythropoietin, and blood substitutes. Int Anesthesiol Clin 28:237, 1990

134. Wildevuur RH, Eijsman L, Gu YJ et al: Aprotinin reduces bleeding during cardiopulmonary bypass in aspirin treated patients. J Cardiovasc Surg (Torino) 31:34, 1990

135. vanOeveren W, Jansen NJ, Bidstrup BP et al: Effects of aprotinin on hemostatic mechanism after cardiopulmonary bypass. Ann Thorac Surg 44:640, 1987

136. Royston D, Bidstrup BP, Taylor KM et al: Effect of aprotinin on need for transfusion after repeat open heart surgery. Lancet 2:1289, 1987

137. Bidstrup BP, Royston D, Sapsford RN et al: Reduction in blood loss after cardiopulmonary bypass using high-dose aprotinin (Trasylol): studies in patients undergoing aortocoronary bypass surgery, reoperations and valve replacement for endocarditis. J Thorac Cardiovasc Surg 97:364, 1989

138. Fraedrich G, Eeber GC, Engler H et al: Benefits and risks of aprotinin in open heart surgery. J Cardiovasc Surg (Torino) 31:44, 1990

139. Orchard MA, Goodchild CS, Prentice CR et al: Aprotinin reduces cardiopulmonary bypass-induced blood loss and inhibits fibrinolysis without influencing platelets. Br J Haematol 85:533, 1993

140. Huang H, Ding W, Su Z et al: Mechanism of the preserving effect of aprotinin on platelet function and its use in cardiac surgery. J Thorac Cardiovasc Surg 106:11, 1993

141. Murkin JM, Lux J, Shannon NA et al: Aprotinin significantly decreases bleeding and transfusion requirements in patients receiving aspirin and undergoing cardiac operations. J Thorac Cardiovasc Surg 107:554, 1994

142. Schonberger JP, Bredee J, Speekenbrink RG et al: Autotransfusion of shed blood contributes additionally to blood saving in patients receiving aprotinin (2 million KIU). Eur J Cardiothorac Surg 7:474, 1993

143. Smith O, Hazlehurst G, Brozovic B et al: Impact of aprotinin on blood transfusion requirements in liver transplantation. Transfusion Med 3:97, 1993

144. Grosse H, Lobbes W, Frambach M et al: Influence of high-dose aprotinin on hemostasis and blood requirement in orthotopic liver transplantation. Semin Thromb Hemost 19:302, 1993

145. Janssens M, Joris J, David JL et al: High-dose aprotinin reduces blood loss in patients undergoing total hip replacement surgery. Anesthesiology 80:23, 1994

146. Shulze K, Graeter T, Schaps D et al: Severe anaphylactic shock due to repeated application of aprotinin in patients following intrathoracic aortic replacement. Eur J Cardiovasc Surg 7:495, 1993

147. Lemmer JH, Jr, Stanford W, Bonney SL et al: Aprotinin for coronary artery bypass operations: efficacy, safety, and influence on early saphenous vein graft patency. A multicenter, randomized, double-blind, placebo-controlled study. J Thorac Cardiovasc Surg 107:543, 1994

148. Spence RK: Status of bloodless surgery. Transfusion Med Rev 5:274, 1991

149. Murase M, Usui A, Tomita Y et al: Nafamostat mesylate reduces blood loss during open heart surgery. Circulation 88:II432, 1993

Chapter 24

Alternatives to Allogeneic Transfusion

Linda Stehling, Howard L. Zauder, and Roger Vertrees

There can be no doubt that recognition of the transmission of human immunodeficiency virus by blood has altered transfusion practices in the surgical community. The transfusion trigger has been adjusted downward,[1] surgeons have become more aware of the need for meticulous hemostasis, and pharmacologic alternatives to allogeneic transfusion have been developed.[2] Predonation programs have become more common,[3] as have techniques to conserve blood lost during surgery. It should be noted, however, that the use of two such modalities, acute normovolemic hemodilution[4] and perioperative blood recovery[5] antedated the acquired immunodeficiency syndrome pandemic by more than a decade.

ACUTE NORMOVOLEMIC HEMODILUTION

Acute normovolemic hemodilution (ANH), or acute isovolemic hemodilution, entails the removal of blood from a patient immediately before or shortly after induction of anesthesia, simultaneous replacement with appropriate volumes of acellular fluid, and return of the blood as indicated by intraoperative blood loss.[6] *Limited* ANH is defined as reduction of the hematocrit (Hct) to approximately 28 percent; *extreme* ANH is defined as reduction in Hct to 20 percent or below.[7,8] Although ANH is the purview of the anesthesiologist, transfusion medicine specialists have become involved with the technique as part of comprehensive programs designed to decrease perioperative allogeneic transfusion. Their role may include active assistance in the operating room, approval and monitoring of protocols relating to blood collection and storage, and educating anesthesia and surgical staff regarding locally available autologous blood programs.

Efficacy

ANH has produced decreases in the use of allogeneic blood ranging from 18 to 90 percent in a wide variety of surgical procedures.[9–13] Decreases in allogeneic transfusion and increases in platelet and postoperative hemoglobin values have been reported in cardiac surgical patients.[12] Separate groups have reported a 75 to 85 percent reduction in allogeneic transfusion requirements using either limited or extreme ANH during spine surgery.[14–16] Equally important was the beneficial effect on component therapy. Kafer et al.[14] found that no additional fresh frozen plasma and platelets were required in their ANH group compared with controls who received a mean of 1.8 ± 0.7 units of fresh frozen plasma and 1.2 ± 0.8 units of platelets. Similar decreases have been reported in hemodiluted patients undergoing hepatic resection,[17] colon surgery,[18] and hip arthroplasty.[19,20] A preliminary report of ANH in burn patients treated with tangential excision indicates that allogeneic transfusion may be avoided or at least markedly decreased.[21] The combination of predonation and very modest ANH decreases the need for allogeneic blood in elective abdominal aortic aneurysm surgery.[22]

Unfortunately, historic controls were used for comparison in most of the above series. A recent prospective, controlled comparison of ANH to preoperative autologous blood donation in a group of 50 patients undergoing elective surgery demonstrated that ANH was equally safe and effective in decreasing the need for allogeneic transfusion.[23] All patients underwent standardized anesthetic techniques and modified radical retropubic prostatectomy performed by the same surgeon. The authors concluded, perhaps not unreasonably, that the results of the study could be applied to any elective surgical procedure in which a blood loss of ± 1,000 ml is anticipated.

Advantages

The avoidance of transfusion-transmitted disease and transfusion reactions is an advantage of all autologous transfusion techniques. Acute normovolemic hemodilution, however, also decreases red blood cell (RBC) loss. For example, the patient with a Hct of 45 percent who intraoperatively loses 2,000 ml of blood loses 900 ml of RBCs. If the same patient is hemodiluted to a Hct of 25 percent, the RBC loss is only 500 ml.

Acute normovolemic hemodilution provides the only practical means of obtaining fresh autologous whole blood for transfusion. Unlike preoperatively donated autologous units, blood drawn in the immediate preoperative period does not undergo the biochemical alterations associated with storage. Although some data indicate that ANH does not influence the level of 2,3-diphosphoglycerate (2,3-DPG) and thus the level at which oxygen is "unloaded" at the tissues,[24] recent evidence[25] confirms animal experimentation[26] that indicates that the P_{50} increases from approximately 26.3 to 28.4 mmHg after return of blood drawn during ANH. In contrast, the P_{50} declined from 26.2 to 24.7 mmHg in control patients transfused with stored blood.

Because blood drawn during ANH is kept at room temperature, platelet function is maintained, and the hypothermia associated with administration of refrigerated blood is avoided. The withdrawn blood usually remains in the operating room with the patient, making it readily available and eliminating the ever-present danger of clerical error. Hemolytic and allergic reactions, and the immunomodulatory effect of allogeneic transfusion, are also eliminated.

Logistics

There is no doubt that ANH has a number of logistic advantages over other autologous transfusion modalities. Autotransfusion devices may not be immediately available during emergent or urgent procedures. It is simpler, and probably less expensive, to obtain 2 to 4 units of blood by ANH than to collect a similar volume by preoperative autologous donation. Although the cost differential may not represent a very significant out-of-pocket expense, the cost of a predonated unit per quality-adjusted life year saved, a number scrutinized by administrators and regulators, is astronomical.[27]

The problems of obtaining autologous predonated blood from patients who have limited access to donor facilities is eliminated by ANH. For those patients with cardiac, cerebrovascular, pulmonary, and other significant systemic diseases that may preclude predonation,[28] ANH performed in the operating room under carefully controlled and monitored conditions offers a viable alternative. In urgent or emergent situations when there is no time for the patient to predonate, ANH should certainly be seriously considered. The same may be said of surgery performed in the presence of malignancy or infection where intraperative blood recovery may be contraindicated.

Blood Viscosity and Tissue Perfusion

The potential improvement in tissue perfusion associated with decreased blood viscosity is a further advantage of ANH. Because blood is a non-newtonian fluid, its viscosity varies with flow rate. Oxygen transport is considered optimal at a Hct of 30 percent as long as normovolemia is maintained. An Hct of 40 to 45 percent provides optimal oxygen delivery only at high flow rates. During ANH, reduction in RBC mass and the consequent decrease in viscosity decreases the formation of RBC aggregates. This facilitates flow through microcirculatory beds, increasing oxygen transport to the tissues to approximately normal values at Hct levels between 20 and 25 percent. ANH appears to optimize microvascular vasomotor responses and elevate RBC flux,[29] leading to enhanced oxygen delivery to the periphery and a more homogeneous oxygen supply.[30]

Clinical Applications

Early nonreusable pump oxygenators for cardiopulmonary bypass were primed with fresh, heparinized blood. Demands made on transfusion services were great; disease transmission was common; and the so-called "homologous blood syndrome" characterized by hepatic and pulmonary congestion, portal hypertension, cerebral insufficiency, renal failure, and coagulopathy, was all too common. Although these changes were thought to be due to pooling of blood in the splanchnic circulation,[31] a role for allogeneic blood could not be excluded. Consequently, a "clear" prime for heart-lung machines with normal saline[32] or 5 percent dextrose in water[33] became the standard for most open heart procedures in adult patients. The desire to decrease exposure of patients to allogeneic blood further led to the use of ANH along with the acellular pump prime.[34–36] Theoretically, the decreased viscosity that accompanies ANH should significantly increase tissue blood flow during hypothermic cardiopulmonary bypass; however, conclusive evidence has not been put forth to support this concept. There is some evidence that ANH does minimize bleeding after surgical correction of congenital heart disease.[37]

Although some suggest that ANH be limited to healthy adults, the technique has been successfully used in small children and elderly patients. The technique should be considered in adults with Hct values greater than or equal to 34 percent who are expected to lose more than 1 L of blood. Although it is used most extensively in patients having total joint replacement or spinal surgery, there is experience with ANH for other types of surgery. Patients presenting for vascular,[22,38] gynecologic and general,[18] urologic,[23] and radical cancer surgery[17] are often considered appropriate candidates.

Contraindications

Because the hemoglobin (Hb) level decreases approximately 1 g/dl for each unit of blood removed, anemia represents the major contraindication to ANH. It is inappropriate to use ANH when the Hb is ≤ 11 g/dl. ANH should be avoided when an increase in cardiac output (CO), the major compensatory mechanism, is either impossible or undesirable. ANH may reduce the levels of coagulation factors below those required for hemostasis in patients with low factor concentrations. Inability to excrete large volumes of fluid at the end of the operative procedure precludes ANH in patients with impaired renal function.

Technical Considerations

The volume (V) of blood that can be safely withdrawn during ANH is calculated from a modification of formulae developed for estimating allowable pretransfusion blood loss.[39,40] The calculations are based on the patient's estimated blood volume (EBV), initial Hct (H_0), the desired final Hct (H_f) considered safe for the patient, and the average Hct (H_{av}):

$$V = EBV \times \left(\frac{H_o - H_f}{H_{av}} \right)$$

The EBV is based on age and lean body mass and varies with age and gender, decreasing from 100 ml/kg in the premature infant to 80 ml/kg in the newborn, 70 ml/kg in the adult man, and 65 ml/kg in the adult woman. The EBV approximates 5 L in the 70-kg adult male patient. If the patient has a beginning Hct of 45 percent and the desired final Hct is 30 percent, the amount of blood that may be removed is calculated as follows:

$$5,000 \text{ ml} \times \left(\frac{0.45 - 0.30}{0.38} \right) = 1,973 \text{ ml}$$

Thus, approximately 2,000 ml can be withdrawn. By the same token, 1,000 ml could be withdrawn from a patient with a Hct of 35 percent if a Hct of 25 percent could be tolerated. Obviously, careful monitoring is the final determinant of the volume removed. Many clinicians who use this technique determine the volume of blood to be removed on the basis of a final Hct of approximately 25 percent to provide a margin of safety in the event of sudden, unexpected blood loss.

Hemodilution is initiated immediately before or just after induction of anesthesia but before the beginning of surgery. In patients undergoing open heart surgery for severe coronary artery disease or aortic stenosis who may be unable to compensate for hemodynamic changes secondary to ANH, it is preferable to wait until the patient is heparinized and cannulated. Blood is then removed from the oxygenator tubing before it makes its first pass through the roller pump. Pump flow can be altered to compensate for any hemodynamic alterations associated with blood withdrawal. There is some question as to the quality of blood removed in this manner because some investigators believe heparin has a detrimental effect on platelet function.[41,42]

The circulating blood volume must be maintained at all times by replacement with crystalloid and/or colloid as the blood is withdrawn. In addition to replacing fluid lost by insensible water loss, an adequate volume of crystalloid must also be provided to replace fluid sequestered in damaged tissue, the so-called third space. Crystalloid has a distinct advantage in that excess fluid can be removed readily by administering a diuretic, most commonly furosemide (0.15 to 1.0 mg/kg) 5 to 10 minutes before infusion of the withdrawn blood. Marked, but temporary, peripheral edema resulting from significant fluid shifts may be observed. The presence of peripheral edema must not be equated with pulmonary edema, which does not occur with properly conducted ANH. Colloids, administered in a volume approximately equal to the volume of blood withdrawn, have the advantage of prolonged intravascular retention. Although hemodynamic studies that compare colloid solutions have not demonstrated any difference among diluents,[43] albumin and dextran have rheologic advantages over gelatin and hydroxyethyl starch.[44]

Monitoring requirements depend on the patient's preoperative status, the nature and duration of the surgery, and the anticipated blood loss. Placement of an arterial catheter for blood withdrawal allows direct monitoring of blood pressure and sampling of blood to measure Hct, adequacy of ventilation and oxygenation, and acid-base status. The Hct should be determined serially to follow the progress of ANH and determine whether transfusion is required before completion of surgery. As with all surgery performed under anesthesia, pulse oximetry and capnography are used. A central venous or pulmonary artery catheter is not usually indicated unless extreme ANH is performed. An indwelling urinary catheter should be inserted to serve as both a pathway for egress of copious volumes of urine, provoked by crystalloid administration, and as a means of estimating volume status.

Adequate venous access is essential if volume replacement is to parallel blood withdrawal, thus ensuring isovolemia and hemodynamic stability. Under ideal circumstances, two large-bore (16-gauge) catheters are used. Blood is withdrawn through an arterial catheter, most frequently radial, or a central or large peripheral vein. When an arm vein is used, collection may be expedited by cycling the cuff of a noninvasive blood pressure monitor at 3-minute intervals,[45] a procedure analogous to an awake donor squeezing and releasing a sponge ball during blood donation.

Blood is collected in standard blood bags containing anticoagulant, usually citrate-phosphate-dextrose (CPD). Hemodilution kits containing two blood bags, a Y-type connector set with Luer lock adapter, and a blood recipient identification band are available (autologous blood collection kit 4R5012, Fenwal Division, Baxter Healthcare, Deerfield, IL). The potential for contamination of blood during withdrawal, and for needlestick injury to personnel, is minimized by using the Luer adapter to connect directly to the intravascular catheter or tubing. When blood is collected from the pump oxygenator, a kit with appropriate connectors should be used to access the extracorporeal circuit. A scale should be used to determine the volume of blood removed. Collection bags should be gently agitated to ensure adequate mixing with the anticoagulant solution.

Each unit of blood withdrawn should be labeled with the patient's name, hospital number, time of withdrawal, and sequential number. The blood is kept in the operating room and maintained at room temperature. If transfusion will be delayed more than 8 hours, the bags should be placed on ice in a small cooler. If the blood is not required until after surgery, it should be placed in a monitored blood refrigerator. Refrigerated units must be transfused within 24 hours or discarded.

Physiologic Adaptation to Hemodilution

Acute reduction in Hb level as a result of ANH causes a decrease in arterial oxygen content (CaO_2) and leads to compensatory alterations in physiology that may include rheologic and hemodynamic changes, increased oxygen extraction, and a shift in the oxygen-Hb dissociation curve, favoring the release of oxygen in the periphery. The primary and most intensely studied intrinsic compensatory mechanism activated by ANH is an increase in CO produced by changes in viscosity. CO increases directly as viscosity decreases,[46–48] with the most significant changes occurring when the Hct declines from 45 to 30 percent.[49] Decreases in Hct below 25 percent result in progressive but lesser reductions in viscosity.[50]

Total peripheral vascular resistance (R) is the product of the arterial tone or vascular resistance (Z) and viscosity (n), the inherent resistance to blood flow.

$$R = Z \times n$$

A reduction in RBC mass (and, to a lesser extent, in plasma proteins) decreases viscosity, which lowers aortic input resistance and results in a proportional decrease in R. This decrease in R in turn reduces afterload, shifting the ventricular function curve to the left, which increases the CO.[51] Animal experimentation has demonstrated that a decrease in viscosity results in a proportional increase in venous return. This leads sequentially to increases in the end-diastolic volume (preload) and CO. No changes in cardiovascular reflexes or local changes in vessel caliber were demonstrable.[50]

In 1964, Nunn and Freeman[52] put forth a theoretical concept of oxygen flux, demonstrating a significant reserve in the oxygen transport-oxygen delivery system. This concept was based on the amount of oxygen available per unit time and the amount

of oxygen consumed during that time period. The rate at which oxygen is made available to tissues, oxygen delivery (DO_2), is the product of the CO and CaO_2:

$$DO_2 = CO \times CaO_2$$

Assuming that 1.35 ml of oxygen is bound to 1 g of Hb and that the solubility coefficient of oxygen in human plasma is 0.0003, each liter of blood with a Hb content of 15 g/dl carries 205 ml of oxygen. In normal resting adults, when the CO is 5 L/min, the available oxygen approximates 1,000 ml/min.

$$DO_2 = 5\ L \times 205\ ml/L = 1,025\ ml/min$$

The volume of oxygen consumed (VO_2) is usually 250 ml/min or less in anesthetized patients.[53] The oxygen extraction ratio, or DO_2/VO_2, is 25 percent, which means that only one-quarter of the available oxygen is utilized. This reserve allows the removal of a significant portion of the RBC mass, providing that the total circulating volume remains normal. However, it should be recalled that the venous oxygen content reflects only the content of mixed venous blood collected from the right side of the heart and not that of individual tissues or organs. Tissues with low energy expenditures or high blood flows such as skin and kidney extract only 5 percent of the oxygen delivered; the heart, under basal conditions, removes approximately 55 percent of the oxygen supplied.[54] Although this surfeit of oxygen provides a significant buffer, it is but one part of the equation, with other compensatory mechanisms adding increased safety to ANH.

Manipulations of oxygen content during ANH with methemoglobinemia,[55] hyperbaric oxygenation,[56] oxygen-carrying fluorocarbons[57,58] and high-viscosity dextran[59] have confirmed the importance of viscosity. Murray and Escobar,[55] showed that comparable reductions in CaO_2 produced by either methemoglobinia or ANH led to an increase in cardiac output with the latter but not the former. Dedichen et al.[56] showed that animals hemodiluted during hyperbaric oxygenation had increases in CO similar to those seen at normal atmospheric pressure but showed less of a decrease in CaO_2. Hemodilution with fluorocarbons results in equal increases in CO, but decreases in CaO_2 are markedly reduced because of the contribution of soluble oxygen from the fluorocarbons.[57,58] When high-viscosity diluents such as dextrans are used, Hct and CaO_2 decrease markedly, and CO decreases as viscosity increases.[59]

The role of sympathetic stimulation in increasing CO is less well understood, but certainly of lesser significance than the decrease in viscosity. There is an isolated parallel increase in norepinephrine but not epinephrine levels during ANH.[60] Sympathetic denervation[61] or blockade[62] of the heart results in a blunting of the increase in CO of about one-third.

Influence of Cardiac Disease on Hemodilution

Patients with fixed CO secondary to age or pathologic states may partially compensate for decreased CaO_2 by increasing the amount of oxygen extracted from Hb. Because it is not possible under clinical conditions to examine the oxygen content of the venous effluent from individual tissues or organs, the mixed venous oxygen tension (PvO_2) or the arteriovenous oxygen content difference ($CaO_2 - CvO_2$) is used to reflect the adequacy of oxygenation. A decrease in PvO_2 or an increase in $CaO_2 - CvO_2$ reflects an increase in oxygen utilization and a decrease in the reserve capacity. There is ample evidence that patients who can respond to ANH with an appropriate increase in CO can tolerate Hct levels as low as 20 percent.

Significant changes occur in regional distribution of the augmented CO. Because oxygen extraction by the myocardium is almost complete in normal settings, investigative focus has been shifted to changes in myocardial perfusion.[46,63] Gisselsson et al.[64] demonstrated a 59 percent increase in coronary blood flow in the human coronary sinus at the time CO had increased by 34 percent after ANH had decreased Hct from 37 to 28 percent. Concern that the increase in coronary blood flow may be compromised by coronary artery stenosis has led to the recommendation that patients with coronary artery disease not undergo isovolemic hemodilution.

Although hemodilution is a common occurrence during and after coronary artery bypass surgery, this situation is different from noncardiac surgery. Utiliz-

ing a canine model of coronary artery stenosis, Spahn et al.[65] demonstrated that ANH to a Hct of approximately 22 percent was relatively well tolerated, even in areas of the left ventricle with compromised coronary blood flow. In addition, nonischemic regions of the left ventricle increased their function to compensate for the loss of contractility in the compromised area. Transfusion of small volumes of RBC reversed the effects of ANH and restored regional contractile function. Mean coronary flow was not compromised identically in all dogs, and there was considerable variability in the tolerance of animals to progressive hemodilution when critical coronary stenosis was produced. Utilizing a comparable experimental preparation, other investigators reported myocardial dysfunction with Hct levels as high as 35 percent.[66]

Because of the variability among experimental animals and the discrepancy in findings when similar preparations are used by different investigators, extrapolation to humans is difficult, at best. For example, dogs have significant variations in coronary artery anatomy and a much more highly developed collateral circulation than do humans.[67] In addition, little is known about the tolerance to ANH in the presence of multivessel coronary artery disease. Hemodilution should be undertaken with the greatest caution, if at all, in patients with coronary artery disease undergoing noncardiac surgery.

Indications for Transfusion of Blood Obtained by Hemodilution

It is clear that ANH can help reduce the need for allogeneic blood transfusion in a variety of operations. Its safety has been demonstrated in both pediatric and adult populations, but ANH should be used with caution in the latter if there is any suspicion of coronary artery disease. When reinfusing the withdrawn blood, one must pay attention to the patient's volume status so as not to produce fluid overload. If the anesthesiologist or surgeon routinely finds that blood loss is less than 500 ml in procedures in which ANH has been used, the need for this alternative should be seriously reconsidered.

INTRAOPERATIVE BLOOD RECOVERY

Intraoperative recovery and transfusion of shed blood should be a major component of any blood conservation program. The concept is not new, having been introduced by Blundell[68] in the early part of the nineteenth century. Instrumentation specifically designed for intraoperative blood recovery and reinfusion was first developed in the mid-1960s. Klebanoff, a military surgeon, developed the first commercially available apparatus that utilized disposable components in response to great demands for and a limited supply of blood during the Vietnam conflict.[5] This remarkably simple device combined a DeBakey roller pump, a standard disposable cardiotomy reservoir, and suction and reinfusion tubing. Variable pressure applied to the reservoir determined the rate of blood return to the patient. Systemic anticoagulation was not used, but the reservoir was primed with a heparinized crystalloid solution. Although an air-detecting photoelectric sensor and alarm were added to later versions of the system, it was withdrawn from the market after several cases of air embolism occurred because the sensors could not differentiate liquid from clotted blood in the reservoir. Nevertheless, clinical experience demonstrated the merits of the technique and paved the way for more sophisticated devices.[69]

Blood Recovery Devices

Intraoperative blood recovery devices can be divided into two groups that differ primarily in how the blood is processed before transfusion. Systems either collect blood directly, anticoagulate it, and reinfuse it through filters or collect, wash, and process the blood and provide RBCs for reinfusion. Each of these approaches has its advantages and disadvantages. Some systems without washing capability contain separate chambers for collection and reinfusion; others are constructed with a single collection/reinfusion chamber.[70] These design features offer the advantage of technical simplicity, quick availability, and low per-unit cost compared with cell processing devices. Operating room personnel can use these systems with minimal training, while cell processing units require a dedicated operator.

Collection is similar for both types of devices, with shed blood being aspirated into a collection chamber through a suction wand. The devices either use modifications of double-lumen tubes to add anticoagulant to a mixing chamber distal to the suction tip or the anticoagulant is added to the collection container. In the former, the smaller lumen is connected to a bag of anticoagulant solution. The larger lumen is attached to an appropriate container, usually a cardiotomy reservoir, which is connected to wall suction or an integral vacuum pump. Suction draws both the shed blood and the anticoagulant into the collection chamber.

The vacuum applied to the collection apparatus should approximate 100 mmHg. Although the vacuum can be increased, it should exceed 150 mmHg only when bleeding is excessive, and higher negative pressure is essential for removing blood from the surgical field. Most operating room wall suction is too high to use without a regulator. Excessive pressure, small orifice suction tips, and skimming cause RBC destruction and high free Hb levels in the collected blood.

Heparin (30,000 units/L of saline) or CPD is used as the anticoagulant. Heparin is utilized most often when the patient is or will be fully heparinized; CPD is usually used for other patients. As a general rule, the ratio of citrate solution to blood should range from 1:5 to 1:10 or approximately 70 ml/500 ml recovered blood. With heparin, the flow is regulated so that 15 ml is added to each 100 ml of recovered blood, maintaining a ratio of approximately 1:7. The flow of anticoagulant must be adjusted to compensate for variations in blood loss. More important than the choice of anticoagulant is the meticulous attention to detail by a dedicated operator to ensure that the anticoagulant solution is added in the proper ratio.

Canister Devices

The canister collection system was one of the earliest used for blood recovery.[71] The collected blood is filtered, but not processed. Filters, generally 20 to 80 μ, can remove large debris (e.g., bone chips in orthopaedic cases) and smaller particulate matter (e.g., cellular fragments).

The recovered blood represents "RBCs suspended in plasma," containing platelets, fibrinogen, and clotting factors.[72] Fibrinogen levels can range between 0 and 44 mg/dl. Factors II, V, VII, VIII, IX, and X and antithrombin III have all been detected in clinically significant concentrations, as have complement C3a and C5a.[73,74] Although the presence of coagulation factors is alleged to be one of the primary advantages attributed to shed, unwashed blood, there are no convincing studies that show the superiority of unwashed blood in either preventing coagulopathy or promoting clotting over washed blood.[75,76] In their review of the problem, Dzik and Sherburne[77] point out that all blood collected has undergone partial to complete clotting after contact with tissue and collection apparatus and contains no useful coagulation factors. Platelets in salvaged blood aggregate poorly and systemic heparin and the anticoagulants added in the collection process may interfere with clotting.

Although unwashed blood has been transfused without obvious adverse effect in a variety of settings, there has been an increasing number of disturbing reports of adverse effects attributable to this product in recent years.[78–81] Unwashed blood may contain vasoactive contaminants, activated clotting factors, fibrin degradation products, and free Hb.

Nonwashed, unheparinized blood in particular has measurable amounts of fibrin degradation products, which, if infused in quantity, can produce clinically significant coagulopathies.[72]

Heddle et al. reported a 10 percent incidence of transfusion reactions in those patients who received filtered, unwashed blood postoperatively after knee arthroplasty.[82] These reactions, characterized by increasing blood pressure, chills, fever and rigors, may have been caused by vasoactive contaminants. Woda and Teztlaff[81] reported a case of upper airway edema believed to be secondary to platelet or complement activation after transfusion of unwashed blood. Free Hb has been shown to potentiate ischemic vascular dysfunction in an animal model of reperfusion injury.[83] It can damage renal tubules through the generation of free hydroxyl radicals, especially if circulation to the kidney is compromised, or during acidosis and prolonged hypotension.[77]

These conflicting reports highlight the problem and suggest a solution. Although unwashed blood may contain potentially harmful soluble products, its use appears to be safe if transfusion is limited to small quantities and to appropriate circumstances. Dzik and Sherburne[77] recommend avoiding autotransfusion of unwashed blood in large volumes in the presence of shock, acidosis, or hypoperfusion to avoid renal damage. If the surgeon anticipates small volume losses of 1 to 2 units of blood, the use of an unwashed system appears to be safe. If blood losses are expected to be greater or if they become larger than anticipated, it is safest to rely on a system that washes recovered blood before transfusion. Blood collected in a reservoir not designed for washing can be transferred to a system with such capabilities if blood loss becomes excessive.

Cell Processing Devices

Semicontinuous flow devices collect, filter, wash, concentrate, and return shed blood to the patient.[84] Although commercially available cell processors differ somewhat in their degree of sophistication based on the microprocessor technology used, they share schematic similarities (Fig. 24-1). Recovered blood is usually collected in a 3,000-ml cardiotomy reservoir fitted with a 120-, 40-, or 20-μm filter. Because blood collection is independent of processing, it is frequently cost-effective to set up only the collection portion of the software. If the volume of blood collected is inadequate to process, or is contaminated, the remainder of the apparatus is not opened. If a standard 225-ml centrifuge bowl is used, at least 500 ml of aspirate should be present in the reservoir before manual or automatic initiation of the fill cycle.

Blood is introduced into the centrifuge bowl by a small roller pump (Fig. 24-1). The centrifuge spins at 5,000 rpm and separates blood according to the density of its components. Because of their greater density, RBCs are packed against the outer wall of the bowl as it fills. The level of RBCs in the bowl is sensed by an optical detector or by the operator, and the fill valve is closed, occluding the path from the reservoir to the bowl. Simultaneously, the wash valve is opened, pumping saline into the spinning centrifuge bowl. Washing continues until a predetermined volume of saline, usually 1,000 ml, is pumped through the bowl. The wash valve is then closed, the centrifuge is stopped, the roller pump is reversed, and the empty valve is opened. The washed RBCs are pumped into a holding bag before transfer to a reinfusion bag. The supernatant flows to the collection bag through the outlet port of the centrifuge, taking with it substances less dense than RBCs (e.g., anticoagulant, free Hb, clotting factors, and RBC stroma). A number of cell processing devices are equipped with air and foam detectors that automati-

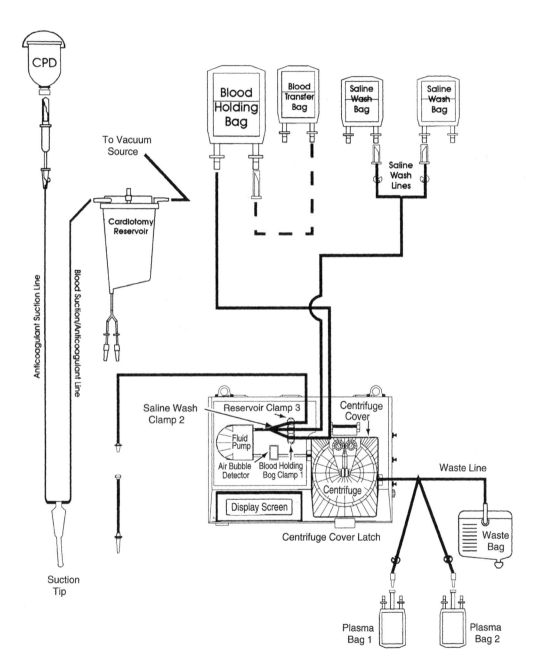

Fig. 24-1. Schematic of cell processing unit configured for collection of PRP. Redirection of the patient collection tubing (solid line lower left) to the cardiotomy reservoir and replacement of the plasma bags with a waste bag prepares the apparatus for cell processing. (Courtesy of Metronic Electromedics.)

cally shut down the roller pump if air is detected, thereby minimizing the danger of air embolism. Depending on the equipment and parameters selected, a processing cycle requires 3 to 10 minutes.

The recovered RBCs are suspended in saline and have an average Hct of 60 percent.[85] The total volume of an average cell pack is 265 ml. Oxygen transport properties and survival of salvaged RBCs are equal or superior to those of stored allogeneic RBCs, and 2,3-DPG levels are higher than those of allogeneic blood.[86,87] Survival of RBCs recovered during spine,[88] aortic,[89,90] and cardiac surgery[91] is comparable to that of allogeneic RBCs. Results are similar whether standard chromium-51 labeling or a dual-isotope technique is used.[85] The final product does not contain anticoagulant, clotting factors, or other blood components such as platelets.[92,93] Therefore, supplemental allogeneic component therapy may be necessary if large volumes of shed blood are replaced with only recovered, washed RBCs.

Levels of plasma Hb in excess of 2,000 mg/dl have been reported in unprocessed blood, but washing removes 50 to 90 percent.[92] Sodium and potassium levels are in the physiologic range. The pH of processed blood is usually alkaline, in contrast to stored blood. Citrate anticoagulant is metabolized by the liver. Although D-dimer levels may be increased up to 85 times in unwashed blood, levels are normal in processed blood.[94] Tumor necrosis factor-β and plasma elastase are present in unprocessed blood but absent after washing.[95,96] Catecholamines are not removed during washing, and significant hypertension has been reported when recovered blood was infused during a pheochromocytoma resection.[97,98]

Clinical Applications

Blood recovery should be considered for any surgical procedure associated with significant blood loss from clean wounds if retrieval is possible without excessive hemolysis. "Significant loss" can be defined variously as blood loss that is expected to exceed 20 percent of the patient's blood volume, an anticipated transfusion need of 1 unit, or a procedure for which 10 percent of patients typically require transfusion. Popovsky et al.[99] consider intraoperative blood recovery cost-effective if 2 or more units are collected and transfused, although Solomon et al.[100] suggest

that greater volumes must be recovered to achieve cost parity with allogeneic blood.

Extensive use has been made of intraoperative blood recovery in cardiac[13,101–108] and vascular surgery[109–117] and during orthopaedic procedures.[118–125] Cosgrove et al.[126] used this technique as early as 1979 in their cardiac surgery patients, reporting that only 6 percent of autotransfused patients required allogeneic blood. Reductions in allogeneic blood use of 50 percent or more are commonplace today in both cardiac and vascular surgical patients.[102–108] Continuous, slow blood loss rather than rapid, high-volume bleeding is the norm in most orthopaedic procedures. Because of this, RBC recovery and transfusion may continue into the early postoperative period (see below). Liver transplant programs commonly use autotransfusion because both the rapidity and volume of blood loss in this procedure call for the expeditious recovery, processing, and return of blood to the patient.[127,128] Because liver transplant recipients are exposed to many donors through blood component usage, the primary goal of autotransfusion is to conserve allogeneic RBC supplies. Experience in gynecology, urology, and neurologic surgery is somewhat limited. Autotransfusion can be used successfully in obstetric patients, but its role is limited (see Ch. 26).

The success or efficacy of autotransfusion usually is reported as either the percentage of patients who avoided allogeneic blood transfusion or the number of units of allogeneic blood not needed in comparison with a control group.[110,121,122,129–132] Unfortunately, most reports are marred by either the use of historical controls or incomplete information on transfusion practices and triggers. These differences in reporting cause some confusion in extrapolating results from one report to another. In general, the percentage of patients relying solely on recovered autologous blood ranges between 20 and 90 percent, depending on the type of procedure. Absolute reductions in the number of allogeneic units transfused range from 2 to 6 units.

Contraindications

Intraoperative blood recovered during or after the use of topical hemostatic agents such as thrombin or microfibrillar collagen hemostat should not be infused.[133,134] Microfibrillar collagen hemostat particles have been shown to pass through 20- to 40-μm filters, embolize to the brain and kidney of animals receiving such blood, and cause extensive perivascular inflammatory reaction.[133,134] Third-generation leukocyte reduction filters such as the Pall RC 100 (Pall Biomedical, East Hills, NY) remove more than 95 percent of the potentially thrombogenic microfibrillar collagen hemostat.[135] Concentrates of the filtrates also do not promote platelet aggregation. Although these filters are effective, they cannot be used when rapid blood loss necessitates transfusion of large volumes of recovered blood in a short time period.

Blood that contains wound irrigants not intended for parenteral use, such as antibiotics or organic iodine preparations, should not be salvaged. Blood should not be aspirated during the application of methylmethacrylate, the cement used to stabilize prosthetic joints. Presumably, the exothermic reaction associated with "curing" of the cement can cause hemolysis. Aspiration should cease before insertion of the acrylic substance into the wound and not recommence until after the area is well irrigated.

Wound Contamination

Bacterial contamination of blood from bowel contents or infected tissues is a relative contraindication to intraoperative blood recovery. Although in vitro studies demonstrate a reduction in the bacterial content of blood after processing, high concentrations of some bacteria, especially anaerobes, persist.[136] However, data from a recent prospective study of autotransfusion in patients who had penetrating abdominal injuries suggest that the technique can be used in potentially contaminated cases.[137] Twenty patients who received salvaged, potentially culture-positive blood (mean, 3.9 L) were compared with 50 patients who received only allogeneic blood (mean, 1.8 L). Broad-spectrum antibiotics were administered to all patients perioperatively. Wound infection rates were identical (25 percent), and no statistically significant increase in site-specific infection rates was identified in the autotransfused group.

The same authors also cultured blood aspirated from the peritoneal cavity of 14 patients with intestinal injuries.[137] No statistical relationship was found between the quantity of bacteria in the aspirated blood and that remaining after processing. Eighty-

four percent of the units were sterile after washing. The investigators cautioned against infusion of potentially contaminated blood in patients with implanted foreign bodies such as heart valves, vascular grafts, or artificial joints or when the use of such materials is anticipated as treatment of concomitant injuries.

Bacteria may also be present in blood retrieved from "clean" wounds. Two studies of patients undergoing cardiac surgery demonstrated that bacteria can be cultured from shed, processed blood in up to 97 percent of patients.[138,139] Positive cultures yielded primarily coagulase-negative staphylococci plus skin or environmental contaminants, which suggests that the most likely sources of contamination were the skin and aspiration of airborne bacteria. Bacteriologic results did not correlate with infectious complications in either study. Whether the addition of an antibiotic to the aspirated blood influenced the results is unknown. Kang et al.[140] report similar results in blood retrieved and processed during orthotopic liver transplantation.

More data are required before retrieval and transfusion of blood from contaminated wounds can be recommended. When there is doubt about the presence of intestinal soilage or infection before an operation, it is reasonable (and economically prudent) to set up the suction apparatus, but not the disposables for the cell processor, until it is determined whether the blood should be processed and transfused. In unusual circumstances in which exsanguination is a potential, intraoperative blood recovery should certainly be considered, even in the presence of contamination.

Cancer Surgery

Recovery of blood shed during cancer surgery is controversial because of theoretical concerns about dissemination of tumor cells. The 1975 case report by Yaw et al.[141] describing malignant cells in shed blood that was collected but not transfused set the stage for future investigations. Two laboratory investigations in which blood was "spiked" with malignant cells have shown that the malignant cells are identifiable in the RBC component after washing.[142,143] Dale et al.[142] labeled two different human tumor cell lines with chromium-51 before processing. After processing, the tumor cells separated with the resuspended RBCs. The tumor cells were presumably viable because only a small amount of isotope had leaked into the effluent or suspension fluid. Miller et al.[143] studied the recovery and viability of four different tumor cell lines added to blood before processing. Cells from all four lines were identified in the RBC concentrate after washing but not in the waste saline wash. Filtration with a 40-μm filter did not eliminate the tumor cells, but none were evident if the RBC concentrate was filtered with a leukocyte reduction filter (Pall RC 100, Pall Biomedical). All but one cell line grew in culture from the unfiltered RBC concentrates.

Filtration may offer some protection against transfusion of malignant cells. Karczewski et al.[144] demonstrated that blood filtered by the Bloodbanker ATS (International Technidyne, Edison, NJ), a gravity-dependent autotransfusion device that contains a 150 μm filter in the blood reservoir and a 170 μm blood tubing screen in the drip chamber, removed an average of 68 percent of human vulvar carcinoma cells that had been seeded into outdated blood. Malignant cells that passed through the device and a 20 μm in-line filter showed morphologic changes, and 62 percent were estimated to have suffered "lethal damage." Clinical studies of blood recovered during resection of primary malignancies showed similar results.

Klimberg's group[145,146] reported on the impact of autotransfusion with recovered, washed blood on genitourinary cancer spread in two series of surgical patients. Twenty-nine of 49 patients who had undergone radical cystectomy were followed a minimum of 1 year postoperatively (mean follow-up = 23.4 months) and were alive at the time of the report. Twenty-five had no evidence of tumor recurrence. Only 5 of 49 similar, consecutively treated patients who underwent radical cystectomy (n = 24), radical prostatectomy (n = 10), radical nephrectomy (n = 13), or similar operations (n = 2) had metastases during a 12- to 23-month follow-up period.[146] The authors concluded that the low incidence of metastases and the pattern of spread did not implicate autotransfusion as a cause of tumor dissemination.

Two studies of hepatic resection for malignancy support the concept that autotransfusion has no adverse effects in cancer surgery. Both Fujimoto et al.[147] and Zulim et al.[148] found that those patients who were autotransfused during hepatic resection for malignancy had neither decreased survival nor increased risk of recurrence compared with patients who received only allogeneic blood. In the former study, cytologic examination of the processed blood revealed no malignancy in any of 100 specimens examined.

All of the published studies are small, the periods of follow-up are relatively short, and data regarding tumor status at the time of operation are incomplete. Considering the presence of malignant cells in processed and unprocessed salvaged blood, further studies are required before routine use of intraoperative blood recovery can be recommended for cancer surgery.

POSTOPERATIVE BLOOD RECOVERY

Collection and transfusion of blood from either the mediastinum or joint spaces has been common practice in many institutions for almost two decades.[75,77,78,107] Transfusion is usually be limited to blood collected during the first 6 postoperative hours, in part because the transfusion of shed blood must begin within 6 hours of initiating the collection. Some authors continue subsequent collections for up to 2 days after surgery when there is continued bleeding.[80] Most collection devices are variations of the Sorensen system that used two bags for collection and transfusion. Newer devices use one bag for collection, anticoagulation, filtration and transfusion. Some units are configured to permit periodic transfusion of the recovered blood.

Controversies relate primarily to efficacy of the technique and whether recovered blood must be processed before infusion. The survival and half-life of recovered and transfused RBCs are normal.[149] Because blood collected is not processed, the same concerns discussed above regarding nonwashed intraoperatively salvaged blood apply. Moreover, the processes of coagulation and fibrinolysis continue in the shed blood, resulting in accumulation of debris that must be filtered before transfusion. The development of clots that make the system unusable is not uncommon. All of the problems inherent in nonwashed blood collection and transfusion are magnified by the slow collection process and extended time in contact with tissue. Blood recovered from the mediastinum has different characteristics from that retrieved after orthopaedic procedures. The potential complications also differ. Therefore, the applications are considered separately.

Cardiac Surgery

Mediastinal blood can be collected in a modified chest drainage system or the cardiotomy reservoir from the cardiopulmonary bypass apparatus for transfusion in aliquots or continuously using an electromechanical pump.[150–152] The Hct depends primarily on the rate of blood loss but is typically 20 to 25 percent.[152–154] Platelet counts in the range of 60 to 70×10^9/L have been reported, but these may vary, depending on measurement technique.[155] More importantly, Kongsgaard et al.[156] showed that recovered platelets are irreversibly activated and would have no hemostatic effects.

Blood within the mediastinum undergoes coagulation and subsequent fibrinolysis. Because the shed blood contains virtually no fibrinogen, the addition of anticoagulant to the collection system is not required.[152] Fibrin degradation products are detected in unwashed mediastinal blood and may be found in patients after its reinfusion.[154] Serum creatine kinase, glutamic oxaloacetic transaminase, and lactate dehydrogenase levels may also be elevated after transfusion of unprocessed mediastinal blood.[157,158] The levels correlate with the volume of drainage infused. However, the presence of fibrin degradation products and these enzymes must not be equated with either disseminated intravascular coagulation or myocardial infarction. The greatest danger posed by their presence is misinterpretation of laboratory tests for DIC and unnecessary blood component administration.

Despite multiple laboratory abnormalities, there do not appear to be adverse effects from transfusion of unwashed mediastinal blood. However, because the potential for coagulation abnormalities exist, it is prudent to either wash the shed blood before reinfusion or to limit the amount of unwashed blood reinfused to 800 to 1,200 ml.

Orthopaedic Surgery

Immediate-return devices are used rather extensively after total hip and knee arthroplasty. The devices were introduced with minimal safety and effi-

cacy data, but clinical studies addressing these issues are finally beginning to appear in the literature. Efficacy is usually defined as a decrease in allogeneic transfusions. Although several investigators report that the percentage of patients receiving allogeneic transfusion is reduced, criteria for transfusion and discharge Hct values are infrequently specified.[159–164] Those studies that reported Hct values for shed blood show a range from 20 to 34 percent.[160,165–167] In the one reported study in which strict transfusion guidelines were used, postoperative autotransfusion resulted in a 42 percent reduction in the number of patients who required allogeneic transfusion.[82]

The average volume of blood recovered and transfused after unilateral knee and hip arthroplasty is approximately 500 ml.[160–165] The RBC volume lost can be calculated using the volume and Hct of the wound drainage. In the study by Umlas et al.[168] of 51 patients, drainage for six hours after total knee and hip arthroplasty was approximately 500 ml and 300 ml, respectively, but the mean RBC losses were only 121 ml and 55 ml. This represented 8.7 and 16.8 percent of overall RBC losses during hospitalization, respectively, and would have supplanted transfusion of less than one-third unit of allogeneic blood after hip surgery and two-thirds of a unit after knee surgery.

Blood collected from a joint space after surgery contains fat, bone chips, and other debris. Particulate matter of 10 to 20 μm can be demonstrated in 20 percent of samples examined with a Coulter counter, but no fat particles greater than 40μm are usually observed.[169] Levels of methylmethacrylate monomer, which were at their highest in the first 5 minutes after initiation of collection, could not be detected by Healy et al.[170] after storage at room temperature for 6 hours, which led the authors to conclude that methylmethacrylate monomer would not be infused under normal clinical conditions.

Like blood shed from the mediastinum, blood collected for 4 hours after total knee arthroplasty contains activated components of the soluble coagulation and fibrinolytic systems.[171,172] Although high levels of D-dimer and C3a desarginine can be measured in the recovered and infused blood, they are no longer present in patients by 12 hours.[166] Bengston et al.[173] detected increased concentrations of anaphylatoxins (C3a and C5a) and terminal complement complexes in shed blood, but infusion of approximately 400 ml of aspirated blood did not cause systemic complement activation. The same group also documented high concentrations of multiple cytokines in shed blood, but only interleukin-6 levels were increased in systemic blood drawn after reinfusion.[174] Febrile reactions have been reported in patients who received unprocessed blood transfused after orthopaedic procedures.[74,175] The incidence appears to increase dramatically with time, from 2 percent for blood collected up to 6 hours[175] to 22 percent when blood collected 6 to 12 hours after surgery was infused.[74] Airway edema, hypotension, and hyperthermia (40.1°C) have been reported after autotransfusion of unwashed blood after total hip or knee arthroplasty.[81,165]

What can be concluded regarding the safety of autotransfusion of blood shed after surgery? Despite laboratory evidence of activation of the coagulation, complement, and fibrinolytic systems and the presence of particulate matter, postoperative autotransfusion appears to be associated with only minimal complications. Transfusion of 1 unit of unprocessed recovered blood appears safe, but there are very limited data regarding administration of larger volumes. Six hours is the maximal recommended collection period before initiation of transfusion. Filtration of shed blood collected after surgery is mandatory. A leukocyte reduction filter (RC 100, Pall Biomedical) during administration is more effective in removing fat particles than a 40-μm screen filter.[162] Some centers provide a further margin of safety by washing all postoperative blood either on site or in the laboratory before infusion.[149,163,164]

Although relatively safe, the actual volume of RBCs transfused may be small.[164] Mechanical problems and insufficient drainage preclude transfusion in about one-third of patients.[176] If only a small amount of blood is collected, administration is probably not worthwhile. Collection is more often efficacious after bilateral total knee arthroplasty than after unilateral knee or hip arthroplasty, but it is difficult to predict blood loss preoperatively. The devices are more expensive than conventional postoperative drainage systems, and processing the blood adds additional expense, particularly if the patient remains in the recovery room while the blood is collected and processed. Umlas et al.[168] estimated the cost of postoperative blood collection devices for the 250,000 arthroplasties performed annually in the United States to be $31 to 35 million.

It seems reasonable to conclude that routine postoperative blood recovery is not justified, but the technique may be useful in selected patients when other sources of autologous blood are limited and blood loss is expected to be excessive.

COLLECTION OF PLATELET-RICH PLASMA

Autologous platelets may be collected in a further attempt to decrease the need for allogeneic blood in cardiovascular surgery patients. Because alterations in platelet function, and decreased platelet counts, are associated with cardiopulmonary bypass, the collection of platelet-rich plasma (PRP) for transfusion after cardiac surgery is an appealing concept. Although platelets can be obtained by apheresis 2 or 3 days before surgery, their short shelf life and the uncertainty that surgery will occur as scheduled make it more desirable to collect PRP in the immediate preoperative period.

One approach is to perform "plasma sequestration" in the immediate preoperative period using a reconfigured cell processing unit (Fig. 24-2). Blood is fractionated by differential centrifugation into a supernatant containing PRP and residual RBCs. The RBCs can be transfused as needed; the PRP is reinfused immediately after cessation of CPB and reversal of heparin. This provides the patient with an infusion of fresh platelets and clotting factors that have not been activated by repeated passage through the heart-lung machine. Design modifications in newer plasma saver devices permit high-yield plateletpheresis in the range of 7.6×10^{11} platelets.[177] This is significantly higher than the standard established by the American Association of Blood Banks which is that plateletpheresis products shall contain a minimum of 3×10^{11} platelets in at least 75 percent of the units tested.[178] A transfusion of 3×10^{11} platelets can be expected to increase the platelet count of a 70-kg person by about 40,000 platelets/μl.

Clinical studies of the efficacy of PRP have yielded conflicting results. Some conducted in a small num-

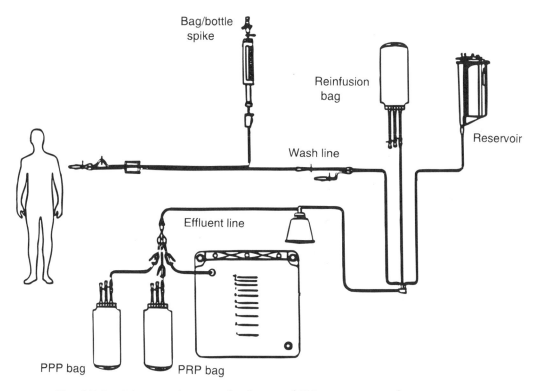

Fig. 24-2. Schematic diagram of collection of PRP using autotransfusion equipment.

ber of patients have demonstrated either no change[179] or a reduction in allogeneic transfusion requirements.[180,181] Jones et al.,[101] using strict criteria for transfusion, limited allogeneic transfusion to 36 percent of patients who received PRP compared with 68 percent of patients in whom PRP was not collected. Two randomized studies, each containing 40 patients, did not demonstrate any advantages in terms of coagulation test findings, postoperative chest tube drainage, or allogeneic transfusions.[182,183]

Blinded, randomized study designs were utilized in two recent investigations. Ereth et al.[184] visually isolated operating room personnel with surgical drapes during collection of PRP in patients having repeat valve surgery. Coagulation parameters did not change, and neither blood loss nor allogeneic transfusion requirements were decreased by PRP administration when results were compared with those in a control group who underwent sham collection.

No criteria for transfusion were specified, and both groups received a median of 10.5 units of allogeneic blood in the first 24 postoperative hours.

Tobe et al.[185] studied 51 patients having primary coronary artery bypass grafting with PRP. Both groups received 8 to 10 ml/kg of PRP, but the control group was transfused immediately after collection; the treatment group was transfused after heparin reversal. Blood components were administered according to predetermined criteria. There were no differences in the surgeon's subjective assessment of coagulation, the number of blood components administered, or postoperative blood loss. The prothrombin time immediately after administration of the PRP was significantly less in the treatment group, but all other laboratory studies were similar at each time period. Both studies have been criticized on the grounds that the number of platelets collected may have been insufficient to produce any clinical effect.[186]

One reason for the difficulty in demonstrating efficacy of PRP in cardiopulmonary surgery is that platelet transfusions are not routinely needed. The National Institutes of Health Consensus Conference on Platelet Transfusion Therapy stated the following: "We believe platelets are overused in some conditions. An example is the prophylactic use of platelets in open-heart surgery, a practice the panel believes is unwarranted."[187] Goodnough et al.[188] also pointed out that platelet transfusions are not routinely needed as prophylaxis against bleeding in cardiac operations. Thus, demonstration of efficacy may be possible only in a small number of patients who stand to benefit from platelet transfusion (e.g., those with exceptionally high volumes of blood loss during surgery). It is difficult to identify this group accurately before surgery. The collection of PRP may have some potential for decreasing exposure to allogeneic blood components during cardiac surgery and deserves further study under more rigorously controlled conditions.

HEMOCONCENTRATION

Blood remaining in the extracorporeal circuit after open heart surgery has an extremely low Hct as a result of dilution with both clear pump prime and the cardioplegia solution. Although cell processing units can be used to concentrate the blood, the advent of hollow-fiber technology made possible the construction of ultrafilters that can be inserted into the extracorporeal bypass circuit to achieve the same goal. Ultrafiltration (i.e., the removal of water and electrolytes from blood by convection transport across a semipermeable membrane) differs from conventional dialysis. With the latter, diffusion occurs because of solute gradient across the membrane. The driving force in ultrafiltration is the pressure gradient across the membrane, which is created by restricting outflow. The fibers are constructed to retain particles with molecular weights greater than 50,000 to 60,000 D.[189]

Infusion of the hemoconcentrate increases the patient's Hct and can decrease allogeneic transfusion requirements. Because heparin is concentrated with the RBCs, additional protamine may be required for heparin reversal.[190] Hct, albumin, total protein content, and colloid osmotic pressure are higher in hemoconcentrated blood than in processed recovered blood.[191] Hemoconcentration is cheaper and easier to perform than cell processing because only a small device is required and no additional personnel are necessary, but total RBC yields may be less.

SUMMARY

The merits of autologous transfusion are unequivocal. However, blood conservation techniques must be utilized appropriately. Withdrawing 1 unit of blood and replacing it with crystalloid or colloid immediately before surgery will do little or nothing to reduce allogeneic transfusion requirements. However, removing 3 to 4 units and inducing normovolemic hemodilution is both efficacious and safe in properly selected and monitored patients. Although unwashed recovered blood contains particulate debris and is associated with multiple biochemical abnormalities, it appears safe for transfusion in limited quantities. The maximal amount that can safely be transfused is unknown. The ultimate role of PRP also remains to be elucidated. Blood recovery after total knee and hip arthroplasty is efficacious in some patients, but routine use does not appear warranted. To achieve the goal of reducing allogeneic transfusions in patients undergoing procedures associated with significant blood loss, a combination of blood conservation techniques is usually indicated.

REFERENCES

1. Zauder HL: Preoperative hemoglobin requirements. Anesthesiol Clin North A 8:471, 1990
2. Royston D: High-dose aprotinin therapy: a review of the first five years' experience. J Cardiothorac Vasc Anesth 6:76, 1992
3. Renner SW, Howanitz PJ, Bachner P: Preoperative autologous blood donation in 612 hospitals. A College of American Pathologists' Q-Probes Study of Quality Issues in Transfusion Practice. Arch Pathol Lab Med 116:613, 1992
4. Beall AC, Yow EM, Bloodwell RD et al: Open heart surgery without blood transfusion. Arch Surg 94:567, 1967
5. Klebanoff G, Watkins D: A disposable autotransfusion unit. Am J Surg 116:475, 1968
6. Stehling L, Zauder HL: Acute normovolemic hemodilution. Transfusion 31:857, 1991

7. Martin E, Hansen E, Peter K: Acute limited normovolemic hemodilution: a method for avoiding homologous transfusion. World J Surg 11:53, 1987

8. Martin E, Ott E: Extreme hemodilution in the Harrington procedure. Bibl Haematol 47:322, 1981

9. Stehling L, Zauder HL: Controversies in transfusion medicine. Perioperative hemodilution: pro. Transfusion 34:265, 1994

10. Weniger J, Shanahn R: Reduction of bank blood requirements in cardiac surgery. Thorac Cardiovasc Surg 30:142, 1982

11. Petry AF, Jost T, Sievers H: Reduction of homologous blood requirements by blood pooling at the onset of cardiopulmonary bypass. J Thorac Cardiovasc Surg 107:1210, 1994

12. Schönberger JPAM, Bredée JJ, Tjian D et al: Intraoperative predonation contributes to blood saving. Ann Thorac Surg 56:893, 1993

13. Scott WJ, Rode R, Castlemain B et al: Efficacy, complications, and cost of a comprehensive blood conservation program for cardiac operations. J Thorac Cardiovasc Surg 103:1001, 1992

14. Kafer ER, Isley MR, Hansen T et al: Automated acute normovolemic hemodilution reduces blood transfusion requirements for spinal fusion. Anesth Analg, suppl. 65:S76, 1986

15. Haberkern M, Dangel P: Normovolaemic haemodilution and intraoperative autotransfusion in children: experience with 30 cases of spinal fusion. Eur J Pediatr Surg 1:30, 1991

16. Olsfanger D, Jedeikin R, Metser U et al: Acute normovolaemic haemodilution and idiopathic scoliosis surgery: effects on homologous blood requirements. Anaesth Intensive Care 21:429, 1993

17. Sejourne P, Poirier A, Meakins JL et al: Effect of haemodilution on transfusion requirements in liver resection. Lancet 2:1380, 1989

18. Rose D, Coutsoftides T: Intraoperative normovolemic hemodilution. J Surg Res 31:375, 1981

19. Rosberg B, Wulff K: Regional lung function following hip arthroplasty and preoperative normovolemic hemodilution. Acta Anaesthesiol Scand 23:242, 1979

20. Barbier-Böhm G, Desmonts JM, Couderc E et al: Comparative effects of induced hypotension and normovolaemic haemodilution on blood loss in total hip arthroplasty. Br J Anaesth 52:1039, 1980

21. Henley M, Tomlinson P, Bailie FB, Obeid EMH: Acute haemodilution in surgery for burns: a preliminary report. Br J Surg 80:1294, 1993

22. Tulloh BR, Brakespear CP, Bates SC et al: Autologous predonation, haemodilution and intraoperative blood salvage in elective abdominal aortic aneurysm repair. Br J Surg 80:313, 1993

23. Ness PM, Bourke DL, Walsh PC: A randomized trial of perioperative hemodilution versus transfusion of preoperatively deposited autologous blood in elective surgery. Transfusion 32:226, 1992

24. Priebe HJ: Hemodilution and oxygenation. Int Anesthesiol Clin 19:237, 1981

25. Parris WCW, Kambam JR, Blanks S, Dean R: The effect of intentional hemodilution on P_{50}. J Cardiovasc Surg (Torino) 29:560, 1988

26. Sunder-Plassmann L, Kessler M, Jesch F et al: Acute normovolemic hemodilution. Changes in tissue oxygen supply and hemoglobin-oxygen affinity. Bibl Haematol 41:44, 1975

27. Birkmeyer JD, Goodnough LT, AuBuchon JP et al: The cost-effectiveness of preoperative autologous blood donation for total hip and knee replacement. Transfusion 33:544, 1993

28. Spiess BD, Sassetti R, McCarthy RJ et al: Autologous blood donation: hemodynamics in a high-risk patient population. Transfusion 32:17, 1992

29. Lipowsky HH, Firrell JC: Microvascular hemodynamics during systemic hemodilution and hemoconcentration. Am J Physiol 250:H908, 1986

30. Messmer K, Sunder-Plassmann L, Jersch F et al: Oxygen supply to the tissues during limited normovolemic hemodilution. Res Exp Med (Berl) 159:152, 1973

31. King RM, White RD: Oxygenators and hemodilution in cardiopulmonary bypass. p. 285. In Tarhan S (ed): Cardiovascular Anesthesia and Postoperative Care. 2nd Ed. Year Book Medical Publishers, Chicago, 1989

32. Panico FG, Neptune WB: A mechanism to eliminate the donor blood prime from the pump-oxygenator. Surg Forum 10:605, 1959

33. Cooley DA, Crawford ES, Howell JF, Beall AC: Open heart surgery in Jehovah's Witnesses. Am J Cardiol 13:779, 1964

34. Hallowell P, Bland JHL, Buckley MJ, Lowenstein E: Transfusion of fresh autologous blood in open-heart surgery. A method for reducing bank blood requirements. J Thorac Cardiovasc Surg 64:941, 1972

35. Zubiate P, Kay JH, Mendez AM et al: Coronary artery surgery. A new technique with use of little blood, if any. J Thorac Cardiovasc Surg 68:263, 1974

36. Cohn LH, Fosberg AM, Anderson WP, Collins JJ, Jr: The effects of phlebotomy, hemodilution and autologous transfusion on systemic oxygenation and whole blood utilization in open heart surgery. Chest 68:283, 1975

37. Milam JD, Austin SF, Nihill MR et al: Use of sufficient hemodilution to prevent coagulopathies following surgical correction of cyanotic congenital heart disease. J Thorac Cardiovasc Surg 89:623, 1985

38. Kramer AH, Hertzer NR, Beven EG: Intraoperative hemodilution during elective vascular reconstruction. Surg Gynecol Obstet 149:831, 1979

39. Gross JB: Estimating allowable blood loss: corrected for dilution. Anesthesiology 58:277, 1983

40. Bourke DL, Smith TC: Estimating allowable hemodilution. Anesthesiology 41:609, 1974

41. Heiden D, Mielke CH, Rodvien R: Impairment by heparin of primary haemostatis and platelet [^{14}C]5-hydroxytryptamine release. Br J Haematol 36:427, 1977

42. Fernandez F, N'guyen P, Van Ryn J et al: Hemorrhagic doses of heparin and other glycosaminoglycans induce a platelet defect. Thromb Res 43:491, 1986

43. Messmer K, Kreimeier U, Intaglietta M: Present state of intentional hemodilution. Eur Surg Res 18:254, 1986

44. Audibert G, Donner M, Lefèvre JC et al: Rheologic effects of plasma substitutes used for preoperative hemodilution. Anesth Analg 78:740, 1994

45. Han D, Rosenblatt M: Collecting blood for autologous transfusion (letter). Anesthesiology 73:1056, 1990

46. Spahn DR, Leone BJ, Reves JG, Pasch T: Cardiovascular and coronary physiology of acute isovolemic hemodilution: a review of nonoxygen-carrying and oxygen-carrying solutions. Anesth Analg 78:1000, 1994

47. Robertie PG, Gravlee GP: Safe limits of isovolemic hemodilution and recommendations for erythrocyte transfusion. Int Anesthesiol Clin 28:197, 1990

48. Lundsgaard-Hansen P: Hemodilution—new clothes for an anemic emperor. Vox Sang 36:321, 1979

49. Laks H, Pilon RN, Klovekorn P et al: Acute hemodilution: its effect on hemodynamics and oxygen transport in anesthetized man. Ann Surg 180:103, 1974

50. Guyton AC, Richardson TQ: Effect of hematocrit on venous return. Circ Res 9:157, 1961

51. Fowler NO, Holmes JC: Blood viscosity and cardiac output in acute experimental anemia. J Appl Physiol 39:453, 1975

52. Nunn JF, Freeman J: Problems of oxygenation and oxygen transport during haemorrhage. Anaesthesia 19:206, 1964

53. Shibutani K, Komatsu T, Kubal K et al: Critical level of oxygen delivery in anesthetized man. Crit Care Med 11:640, 1983

54. Bruns FJ, Fraley DS, Haigh J et al: Control of organ blood flow. p. 87. In Snyder JV (ed): Oxygen Transport in the Critically Ill. Year Book Medical Publishers, Chicago, 1987

55. Murray JF, Escobar E: Circulatory effects on viscosity: comparison of methemoglobinemia and anemia. Am J Physiol 25:594, 1968

56. Dedichen H, Race D, Schenk WG: Hemodilution and concomitant hyperbaric oxygenation. J Thorac Cardiovasc Surg 53:341, 1967

57. Biro GP: Comparison of acute cardiovascular effects and oxygen-supply following haemodilution with dextran, stroma-free haemoglobin solution and fluorocarbon suspension. Cardiovasc Res 16:194, 1982

58. Biro GP: Fluorocarbon and dextran hemodilution in myocardial ischemia. Can J Surg 26:163, 1983

59. Gelin LE, Bergentz SE, Helander CG et al: Hemodynamic consequences from increased viscosity of blood. p. 722. In Copley AL (ed): Hemorheology. Pergamon Press, Oxford, 1968

60. Adams HA, Ratthey K, Rupp D, Hempelmann G: Endokrine Reaktionen bei akuter normovolämischer Hämodilution. Anaesthesist 39:269, 1990

61. Glick G, Plauth WH, Braunwald E: Role of the autonomic nervous system in the circulatory response to acutely induced anemia in unanesthetized dogs. J Clin Invest 43:2112, 1964

62. Clarke TNS, Foex P, Roberts JG et al: Circulatory responses of the dog to acute isovolemic anaemia in the presence of high-grade adrenergic beta-receptor blockade. Br J Anaesth 52:337, 1980

63. Geha AS, Baue AE: Graded coronary stenosis and coronary flow during acute normovolemic anemia. World J Surg 2:645, 1978

64. Gisselsson I, Rosberg B, Ericsson M: Myocardial blood flow, oxygen uptake and carbon dioxide release of the human heart during hemodilution. Acta Anaesthesiol Scand 26:589, 1982

65. Spahn DR, Smith LR, McRae RL, Leone BJ: Effects of acute isovolemic hemodilution and anesthesia on regional function in left ventricular myocardium with compromised coronary blood flow. Acta Anaesthesiol Scand 36:628, 1992

66. Messmer K, Sunder-Plassmann L, Klovekorn WP, Holper K: Circulatory significance of hemodilution: rheological changes and limitations. Adv Microcirc 4:1, 1972

67. Ostadal B, Kolai F: Experimental cardiac hypoxia and ischemia. p. 333. In Deyl Z, Zigha J: Methods in Animal Physiology CRC Press, Boca Raton, FL, 1989

68. Blundell J: Observations on transfusion of blood by

Dr. Blundell with a description of his gravitator. Lancet 2:321, 1828

69. Stehling LC, Zauder HL, Rogers W: Clinical experience with autotransfusion. Anesthesiology 43:334, 1975

70. Vertrees RA: Techniques in autotransfusion. In Cernaiaun AC, DelRossi AJ (eds): Cardiac Surgery '93: Clinical Issues. Plenum Press, 1995

71. Noon GP, Solis RT, Natelson EA: A simple method of intraoperative autotransfusion. Surg Gynecol Obstet 143:65, 1976

72. Harz RS, Smith JA, Green D: Autotransfusion after cardiac operation. Assessment of hemostatic factors. J Thorac Cardiovasc Surg 96:178, 1988

73. Ferrair M, Zia S, Valbonesi M et al: A new technique for hemodilution, preparation of autologous platelet-rich plasma and intraoperative blood salvage in cardiac surgery. Int J Artif Organs 10:47, 1987

74. Faris PM, Ritter MA, Keating EM: Unwashed filtered shed blood collected after knee and hip arthroplasties. J Bone Joint Surg [Am] 73-A:1169, 1991

75. Thurer RL, Hauer JM: Autotransfusion and blood conservation. Curr Probl Surg 19:1, 1982

76. Aubuchon JP: Autologous transfusion and directed donations: current controversies and future directions. Transfusion Med Rev 3:290, 1989

77. Dzik WH, Sherburne B: Intraoperative blood salvage: medical controversies. Transfusion Med Rev 4:208, 1990

78. Glover JL, Broadie TA: Intraoperative autotransfusion. World J Surg 11:60, 1987

79. Claeys L, Horsch S: Autotransfusion of nonwashed shed blood during vascular surgery, abstracted. J Cardiovasc Surg (Torino) 33:89, 1992

80. Tawes RL, Jr, Sydorak GR, DuVall TB: Postoperative salvage: a technological advance in the "washed" versus "unwashed" blood controversy. In Rutherford RB (ed): Blood Transfusion and the Vascular Surgeon. Seminars Vasc Surg. 1994; 7(2):98–103.

81. Woda R, Tetzlaff JE: Upper airway oedema following autologous blood transfusion from a wound drainage system. Can J Anaesth 39:290, 1992

82. Heddle NM, Brox WT, Klama LN et al: A randomized trial on the efficacy of an autologous blood drainage and transfusion device in patients undergoing elective knee arthroplasty. Transfusion 32:742, 1992

83. Ruiz AJ, Chan BBK, Meyerhoefer TA et al: Effects of ischemia and hemoglobin on vascular function in the isolated rabbit aorta. J Vasc Surg 13:487, 1991

84. Stehling L, Zauder HL: Autologous blood salvage procedures. p. 47. In Goldstein J (ed): Biotechnology of Blood. Butterworth-Heinemann, Boston, 1991

85. Thorley PJ, Shaw A, Kent P et al: Dual tracer technique to measure salvaged red cell survival following autotransfusion in aortic surgery. Nucl Med Commun 11:369, 1990

86. O'Hara PJ, Hertzer NR, Santilli PH, Bevan EG: Intraoperative autotransfusion during abdominal aortic reconstruction. Am J Surg 145:215, 1983

87. McShane AJ, Power C, Jackson JF et al: Autotransfusion: quality of blood prepared with a red cell processing device. Br J Anaesth 59:1035, 1987

88. Ray JM, Flynn JC, Bierman AH: Erythrocyte survival following intraoperative autotransfusion in spinal surgery: an in vivo comparative study and 5-year update. Spine 11:879, 1986

89. Kent P, Ashley S, Thorley PJ et al: 24-Hour survival of autotransfused red cells in elective aortic surgery: a comparison of two intraoperative autotransfusion systems. Br J Surg 78:1473, 1991

90. Tawes RL, Jr, Sydorak GR, DuVall TB: Postoperative salvage: the physiological and technological basis for autotransfusion. In Rutherford RB (ed): Blood Transfusion and the Vascular Surgeon, Seminars Vasc Surg 1994; 7(2):91–2

91. Ansell J, Parrilla N, King M et al: Survival of autotransfused red blood cells recovered from the surgical field during cardiovascular operations. J Thorac Cardiovasc Surg 84:387, 1982

92. Yawn DH: Properties of salvaged blood. p. 194. In Taswell HF, Pineda AA (eds): Autologous Transfusion and Hemotherapy. Blackwell Scientific Publications, Boston, 1991

93. Rougej P, Fourquet D, Depoix-Joseph JP et al: Heparin removal in three intraoperative blood savers in cardiac surgery. Appl Cardiopulmonary Pathophysiol 5:5, 1993

94. Lawrence-Brown MMD, Couch C, Halliday M et al: D-dimer levels in blood salvage for autotransfusion. Aust N Z J Surg 59:67, 1989

95. Sieunarine K, Lawrence-Brown MMD, House AK, Goodman MA: Plasma tumour necrosis factor alpha levels in intraoperative salvaged blood. Med Sci Res 19:85, 1991

96. Sieunarine K, Langton S, Lawrence-Brown MMD et al: Elastase levels in salvaged blood and the effect of cell washing. Aust N Z J Surg 60:613, 1990

97. Rice MJ, Violante EV, Kreul JF: The effect of autotransfusion on catecholamine levels during pheochromocytoma. Anesthesiology 67:1017, 1987

98. Sieunarine K, Lawrence-Brown MMD, Brennan D et al: The quality of blood used for transfusion. J Cardiovasc Surg (Torino) 33:98, 1992

99. Popovsky MA, Devine PA, Taswell HF: Intraoperative autologous transfusion. Mayo Clin Proc 60:125, 1985

100. Solomon MD, Rutledge ML, Kane LE, Yawn DH: Cost comparison of intraoperative autologous versus homologous transfusion. Transfusion 28:379, 1988

101. Jones JW, Rawitscher RE, McLean TR et al: Benefit from combining blood conservation measures in cardiac operations. Ann Thorac Surg 51:541, 1991

102. Bell K, Stott K, Sinclair CJ et al: A controlled trial of intra-operative autologous transfusion in cardiothoracic surgery measuring effect on transfusion requirements and clinical outcome. Transfusion Med 2:295, 1992

103. Scott WJ, Kessler R, Wernly JA: Blood conservation in cardiac surgery. Ann Thorac Surg 50:843, 1990

104. Laub GW, Dharan M, Riebman JB et al: The impact of intraoperative autotransfusion on cardiac surgery. A prospective randomized double-blind study. Chest 104:686, 1993

105. McCarthy PM, Popovsky MA, Schaff HV et al: Effect of blood conservation efforts in cardiac operations at the Mayo Clinic. Mayo Clin Proc 63:225, 1988

106. Breyer RH, Engelman RM, Rousou JA, Lemeshow S: Blood conservation for myocardial revascularization. J Thorac Cardiovasc Surg 93:512, 1987

107. Hall RI, Schweiger IM, Finlayson DC: The benefit of the Hemonetics® cell saver apparatus during cardiac surgery. Can J Anaesth 37:618, 1990

108. Tawes RL, Jr: Clinical applications of autotransfusion. In Rutherford RB (ed): Blood Transfusion and the Vascular Surgeon. Seminars Vasc Surg. 1994; 7(2):89–91.

109. Tawes RL, Scribner RG, Duval TB et al: The cell-saver and autologous transfusion: an underutilized resource in vascular surgery. Am J Surg 152:105, 1986

110. Hallett JW, Popovsky M, Ilstrup D: Minimizing blood transfusions during abdominal aortic surgery: recent advances in rapid autotransfusion. J Vasc Surg 5:601, 1987

111. Cali RF, O'Hara PJ, Hertzer NR et al: The influence of autotransfusion on homologous blood requirements during aortic reconstruction. Cleve Clin J Med 51:143, 1984

112. Davies MJ, Cronin KC, Moran P et al: Autologous blood transfusion for major vascular surgery using the Sorenson receptal device. Anaesth Intensive Care 15:282, 1987

113. Stanton PE, Shannon J, Rosenthal D et al: Intraoperative autologous transfusion during major aortic reconstruction procedures. South Med J 80:315, 1987

114. Kalra M, Beech MJ, Al-el-Khaffaf H, Charlesworth D: Autotransfusion in aortic surgery: the Haemocell system 350 cell saver. Br J Surg 80:32, 1993

115. Long GW, Glover JL, Bendick PJ et al: Cell washing versus immediate reinfusion of intraoperatively shed blood during abdominal aortic aneurysm repair. Am J Surg 166:97, 1993

116. Ouriel K, Shortell CK, Green RM, DeWeese JA: Intraoperative autotransfusion in aortic surgery. J Vasc Surg 18:16, 1993

117. Reddy DJ, Ryan CJ, Shepard AD et al: Intraoperative autotransfusion in vascular surgery. Arch Surg 125:1012, 1990

118. Wilson WJ: Intraoperative autologous transfusion in revision total hip arthroplasty. J Bone Joint Surg [Am] 71-A:8, 1989

119. Goulet JA, Bray TJ, Timmerman LA et al: Intraoperative autologous transfusion in orthopaedic patients. J Bone Joint Surg [Am] 71-A:3, 1989

120. Bovill DF, Norris TR: The efficacy of intraoperative autologous transfusion in major shoulder surgery. Clin Orthop 240:137, 1989

121. Behrman MJ, Keim HA: Perioperative red blood cell salvage in spine surgery. Clin Orthop 278:51, 1992

122. Elawad AAR, Öhlin AK, Berntorp E et al: Intraoperative autotransfusion in primary hip arthroplasty. A randomized comparison with homologous blood. Acta Orthop Scand 62:557, 1991

123. Bovill DF, Moulton CW, Jackson WST et al: The efficacy of intraoperative autologous transfusion in major orthopedic surgery: a regression analysis. Orthopedics 9:1403, 1986

124. Lennon RL, Hosking MP, Gray JR et al: The effects of intraoperative blood salvage and induced hypotension on transfusion requirements during spinal surgical procedures. Mayo Clin Proc 62:1090, 1987

125. Cavallieri S, Riou B, Roche S et al: Intraoperative autologous transfusion in emergency surgery for spine trauma. J Trauma 36:639, 1994

126. Cosgrove DM, Thurer RL, Lytle BW et al: Blood conservation during myocardial revascularization. Ann Thorac Surg 28:184, 1979

127. Dzik WH, Jenkins R: Use of intraoperative blood salvage during orthotopic liver transplantation. Arch Surg 120:946, 1985

128. Williamson KR, Taswell HF, Rettke SR, Krom RAF: Intraoperative autologous transfusion: its role in orthotopic liver transplantation. Mayo Clin Proc 64:340, 1989

129. Brown G, Bookallil, Herkes R: Use of the cell saver during elective abdominal aortic aneurysm surgery—influence on transfusion with bank blood. A

retrospective survey. Anaesth Intensive Care 19:546, 1991

130. Giordano GF, Giordano DM, Wallace BA et al: An analysis of 9918 consecutive perioperative autotransfusions. Surg Gynecol Obstet 176:103, 1993

131. Duchateau J, Nevelsteen A, Suy R et al: Autotransfusion during aorto-iliac surgery. Eur J Vasc Surg 4:349, 1990

132. Goodnough LT, Vizmeg K, Marcus RE: Blood lost and transfused in patients undergoing elective orthopedic operation. Surg Gynecol Obstet 176:235, 1993

133. Niebauer GW, Oz MC, Goldschmidt M, Lemole G: Simultaneous use of microfibrillar collagen hemostat and blood saving devices in a canine kidney perfusion model. Ann Thorac Surg 48:523, 1989

134. Robicsek F, Duncan GD, Born GVR et al: Inherent dangers of simultaneous application of microfibrillar collagen hemostat and blood-saving devices. J Thorac Cardiovasc Surg 92:766, 1986

135. Orr MD, Ferdman AG, Maresh JG: Removal of Avitene microfibrillar collagen hemostat by use of suitable transfusion filters. Ann Thorac Surg 57:1007, 1994

136. Timberlake GA, McSwain NE: Autotransfusion of blood contaminated by enteric contents: a potentially life-saving measure in the massively hemorrhaging trauma patient? J Trauma 28:855, 1988

137. Ozmen V, McSwain NE, Nichols RE et al: Autotransfusion of potentially culture-positive blood (CPB) in abdominal trauma: preliminary data from a prospective study. J Trauma 32:36, 1992

138. Ezzedine H, Baele P, Robert A: Bacteriologic quality of intraoperative autotransfusion. Surgery 109:259, 1991

139. Bland LA, Villarino ME, Arduino MJ et al: Bacteriologic and endotoxin analysis of salvaged blood used in autologous transfusions during cardiac operations. J Thorac Cardiovasc Surg 103:582, 1992

140. Kang Y, Aggarwal S, Pasculle AW et al: Bacteriologic study of autotransfusion during liver transplantation. Transplant Proc 21:3538, 1989

141. Yaw PB, Sentany M, Link WJ et al: Tumor cells carried through autotransfusion. Contraindication to intraoperative blood recovery? JAMA 231:490, 1975

142. Dale RF, Kipling RM, Smith MF et al: Separation of malignant cells during autotransfusion. Br J Surg 75:581, 1988

143. Miller GV, Ramsden CW, Primrose JN: Autologous transfusion: an alternative to transfusion with banked blood during surgery for cancer. Br J Surg 78:713, 1991

144. Karczewski DM, Lema MJ, Glaves D: The efficiency of an autotransfusion system for tumor cell removal from blood salvaged during cancer surgery. Anesth Analg 78:1131, 1994

145. Hart OJ, Klimberg IW, Wajsman Z, Baker J: Intraoperative autotransfusion in radical cystectomy for carcinoma of the bladder. Surg Gynecol Obstet 168:302, 1989

146. Klimberg I, Sirois R, Wajsman Z, Baker J: Intraoperative autotransfusion in urologic oncology. Arch Surg 121:1326, 1986

147. Fujimoto J, Okamoto E, Yamanaka N et al: Efficacy of autotransfusion in hepatectomy for hepatocellular carcinoma. Arch Surg 128:1065, 1993

148. Zulim RA, Rocco M, Goodnight JE et al: Intraoperative autotransfusion in hepatic resection for malignancy. Is it safe? Arch Surg 128:206, 1993

149. Umlas J, Jacobson MS, Kevy SV: Survival and half-life of red cells salvaged after hip and knee replacement surgery. Transfusion 33:591, 1993

150. Cosgrove DM, Amiot DM, Meserko JJ: An improved technique for autotransfusion of shed mediastinal blood. Ann Thorac Surg 40:519, 1985

151. Page R, Russell GN, Fox MA et al: Hard-shell cardiotomy reservoir for reinfusion of shed mediastinal blood. Ann Thorac Surg 48:514, 1989

152. Eng J Kay PH, Murday AJ et al: Postoperative autologous transfusion in cardiac surgery: a prospective, randomised study. Eur J Cardiothorac Surg 4:595, 1990

153. Carter RF, McArdle B, Morritt GM: Autologous transfusion of mediastinal drainage blood: a report of its use following open heart surgery. Anaesthesia 36:54, 1981

154. Griffith LD, Billman GF, Daily PO, Lane TA: Apparent coagulopathy caused by infusion of shed mediastinal blood and its prevention by washing of the infusate. Ann Thorac Surg 47:400, 1989

155. Williamson KR, Taswell HF: Intraoperative blood salvage: a review. Transfusion 31:662, 1991

156. Kongsgaard UE, Hovig T, Brosstad F, Geiran O: Platelets in shed mediastinal blood used for postoperative autotransfusion. Acta Anaesthesiol Scand 37:265, 1993

157. Wahl GW, Feins RH, Alfieres G, Bixby K: Reinfusion of shed blood after coronary operation causes elevation of cardiac enzyme levels. Ann Thorac Surg 53:625, 1992

158. Hannes W, Keilich M, Koster W et al: Shed blood autotransfusion influences ischemia-sensitive laboratory parameters after coronary operations. Ann Thorac Surg 57:1289, 1994

159. Flynn JC, Price CT, Zink WP: The third step of total autologous blood transfusion in scoliosis surgery: harvesting blood from the postoperative wound. Spine 16:S328, 1991

160. Majkowski RS, Currie IC: Postoperative collection and reinfusion of autologous blood in total knee arthroplasty. Ann R Coll Surg Engl 73:381, 1991

161. Gannon DM, Lombardi AV, Mallory TH et al: An evaluation of the efficacy of postoperative blood salvage after total joint arthroplasty. J Arthroplasty 1:109, 1991

162. Healy WL, Pfeifer BA, Kurtz SR et al: Evaluation of autologous shed blood for autotransfusion after orthopaedic surgery. Clin Orthop 299:53, 1994

163. Semkiw LB, Schurman DJ, Goodman SB et al: Postoperative blood salvage using the cell saver after total joint arthroplasty. J Bone Joint Surg [Am] 71-A:823, 1989

164. Slagis SV, Benjamin JB, Volz RG, Giordano GF: Postoperative blood salvage in total hip and knee arthroplasty. J Bone Joint Surg [Br] 73-B:591, 1991

165. Clements DH, Sculco TP, Burke SW et al: Salvage and reinfusion of postoperative sanguineous wound drainage. J Bone Joint Surg [Am] 74-A:646, 1992

166. Blevins FT, Shaw B, Valeri CR et al: Reinfusion of shed blood after orthopaedic procedures in children and adolescents. J Bone Joint Surg [Am] 75-A:363, 1993

167. Wixon RL, Kwaan HC, Spies SM et al: Reinfusion of postoperative wound drainage in total hip arthroplasty: red blood cell survival and coagulopathy risk. J Arthroplasty 9:351, 1994

168. Umlas J, Foster RR, Dalal SA et al: Red cell loss following orthopedic surgery: the case against postoperative blood salvage. Transfusion 34:402, 1994

169. Robbins G, Grech H, Howes K: A study of autologous blood collected after joint replacement surgery. Vox Sang 62:152, 1992

170. Healy WL, Wasilewski SA, Pfeifer BA et al: Methylmethacrylate monomer and fat content in shed blood after total joint arthroplasty. Clin Orthop 286:15, 1993

171. Blaylock RC, Carlson KS, Morgan JM et al: In vitro analysis of shed blood from patients undergoing total knee replacement surgery. J Clin Pathol 101:365, 1994

172. Harrap RSJ, Whyte GS, Farrugia A, Jones C: Some characteristics of blood shed into the Solcotrans postoperative orthopaedic drainage/reinfusion system. Med J Aust 157:95, 1992

173. Bengtson JP, Backman L, Stenqvist O et al: Complement activation and reinfusion of wound drainage blood. Anesthesiology 73:376, 1990

174. Arnestad JP, Bengtsson A, Bengtson JP et al: Formation of cytokines by retransfusion of shed whole blood. Br J Anaesth 72:422, 1994

175. Lux PS, Martin JW, Whiteside LA: Reinfusion of whole blood after revision surgery for infected total hip and knee arthroplasties. J Arthroplasty 8:125, 1993

176. Mauerhan DR, Nussman D, Mokris JG, Beaver WB: Effect of postoperative reinfusion systems on hemoglobin levels in primary total hip and total knee arthroplasties. J Arthroplasty 8:523, 1993

177. Klein HG: Standards for Blood Banks and Transfusion Services. 16th Ed. American Association of Blood Banks, Bethesda, 1994

178. Davies GG, Wells DG, Sadler R et al: Plateletpheresis and transfusion practice in heart operations. Ann Thorac Surg 54:1020, 1992

179. Mohr R, Sagi B, Lavee J et al: The hemostatic effect of autologous platelet-rich plasma versus autologous whole blood after cardiac operations: is platelet separation really necessary? J Thorac Cardiovasc Surg 105:371, 1993

180. DelRossi AJ, Cernaianu AC, Vertrees RA et al: Platelet-rich plasma reduces postoperative blood loss after cardiopulmonary bypass. J Thorac Cardiovasc Surg 100:281, 1990

181. Giordano GF, Rivers SL, Chung GKT et al: Autologous platelet-rich plasma in cardiac surgery: effect on intraoperative and postoperative transfusion requirements. Ann Thorac Surg 46:416, 1988

182. Boey SK, Ong BC, Dhara SS: Preoperative plateletpheresis does not reduce blood loss during cardiac surgery. Can J Anaesth 40:844, 1993

183. Wong CA, Franklin ML, Wade LD: Coagulation tests, blood loss, and transfusion requirements in platelet-rich plasmapheresed versus nonpheresed cardiac surgery patients. Anesth Analg 78:29, 1994

184. Ereth MH, Oliver WC, Beynen FMK et al: Autologous platelet-rich plasma does not reduce transfusion of homologous blood products in patients undergoing repeat valvular surgery. Anesthesiology 79:540, 1993

185. Tobe CE, Vocelka C, Sepulvada R et al: Infusion of autologous platelet rich plasma does not reduce blood loss and product use after coronary artery bypass. A prospective, randomized, blinded study. J Thorac Cardiovasc Surg 105:1007, 1993

186. Davies GG, Ruffcorn M, Dooley JB et al: Plateletpheresis before cardiopulmonary bypass: I (letter). Anesthesiology 80:714, 1994

187. National Institutes of Health Consensus Conference:

Platelet transfusion therapy. JAMA 257:1777, 1987

188. Goodnough LT, Johnston MFM, Ramsey G et al: Guidelines for transfusion support in patients undergoing coronary artery bypass grafting. Ann Thorac Surg 50:675, 1990

189. Magilligan DJ, Jr: Indications for ultrafiltration in the cardiac surgical patient. J Thorac Cardiovasc Surg 89:183, 1985

190. Friesen RH, Tornabene MA, Coleman SP: Blood conservation during pediatric cardiac surgery: ultra-filtration of the extracorporeal circuit volume after cardiopulmonary bypass. Anesth Analg 77:702, 1993

191. Boldt J, Kling D, von Bormann B et al: Blood conservation in cardiac operations. Cell separation versus hemofiltration. J Thorac Cardiovasc Surg 97:832, 1989

Emergency Surgery—Trauma and Massive Transfusion

Steven Ross and Elaine Jeter

Trauma is a major health care problem, with an impact on every hospital and blood bank. In the United States, injury is the leading cause of death for individuals in the first four decades of life, and the fourth leading overall cause of death. Approximately 140,000 Americans die from injury every year, and about 9 million sustain disabling injuries as a result of vehicular crashes, falls, suicides, and interpersonal violence. Despite efforts to reduce the severity and incidence of injury, death and disability persist, and trauma continues to exert a major impact on blood resources in the United States.[1]

Although most individuals would associate trauma with blood loss and the need for blood replacement, most trauma patients are managed without blood transfusion. In a 5-year study at Vanderbilt University, only 27 percent of patients admitted to the hospital for trauma required transfusion.[2] In a population of 8,000 trauma patients over a similar period, at one of the author's (S.R.) institution, only 8 percent required emergency transfusion. Despite the low percentage of patients requiring emergency transfusion and the moderate number ultimately requiring transfusion, some of these patients will require "massive transfusion," defined as transfusion of red cells within 24 hours equivalent to the loss of the patient's blood volume. In Wudel's et al.[2] series, 9.6 percent of the blunt trauma patients required 20 or more units of blood. This type of utilization tends to be unscheduled and emergent and traditionally occurs on nights and weekends when blood bank staffing is at its lowest. Institutions caring for trauma patients must be prepared for such occurrences.

The risks associated with exposure to the human immunodeficiency (HIV) and hepatitis viruses in the management of patients with external hemorrhage have led to the institution of universal precautions in handling such patients. Because it is impossible in most states to screen patients routinely for all infectious agents transmissible by blood or to have the results of such screens available before initiating care, such precautions are particularly important in the examination, treatment, and handling of laboratory specimens related to trauma patients. In Charleston, South Carolina, 3.2 percent of trauma patients are HIV positive, a rate that reflects the incidence in the United States in this setting.[3]

It is estimated that, in 1985, there were 2.3 million Americans hospitalized for injury. In addition, 54.4 million individuals suffered injury not requiring hospitalization. The direct cost for the medical care of the hospitalized individuals was $44.8 billion. Data regarding the overall blood consumption of these hospitalized patients and the cost attributable to blood bank charges are not available. It is clear that such costs and efforts are commensurate with the huge burden imposed by trauma as a major public health problem in our society.

SHOCK

The primary indication for administration of intravenous fluids and for the transfusion of blood and blood products in the trauma or emergency surgical patient is shock. Samuel Gross[4] defined shock in 1872 as a "rude unhinging of the machinery of life." Although this definition reflected the late nineteenth century view of the problem, the modern definition and treatment of shock are based on an understanding of its pathophysiology. Most simply stated, shock is the pathophysiologic state of inadequacies in both the delivery of substrate and oxygen and the removal of end products of metabolism from peripheral tissues. Oxygen transport and delivery depends on cardiac output and blood oxygen content. Although a small amount of oxygen can be dissolved in plasma, the primary molecule responsible for oxygen transport is hemoglobin, which is contained in the red blood cell. The justification for blood transfusion instead of nonsanguineous volume resuscitation in trauma patients in shock is based on the ability of hemoglobin to restore oxygen delivery directly. Rapid restoration of oxygen delivery and elimination of the oxygen debt can be a major factor in preventing the development of post-traumatic organ tissue failure.[5]

Classification of Shock

Blalock[6] initially developed a categorization of shock based on cause. Identifying the underlying pathophysiologic cause allows appropriate treatment (Table 25-1). Neurogenic and vasogenic shock in Blalock's classification have been combined into a single classification of shock caused by relaxed vascular tone in the periphery. In this setting, reduction of peripheral vascular resistance and venous compliance creates low blood pressure. In spite of normal or increased cardiac output and oxygen content of the blood, tissue oxygen consumption is decreased, leading to hypoxemia and acidosis. Cardiogenic shock is caused by failure of the pump (i.e., the heart). Although peripheral resistance may be adequate and the oxygen content of the blood may be normal, failure of the pump to provide adequate flow results in decreased tissue perfusion.

Hypovolemic shock is caused by reduction in blood volume after blood loss. This is the most com-

Table 25-1. Classification of Shock

Neurogenic/vasogenic
   Cause: decreased vascular resistance and venous compliance.
   Response: cardiac output normal or increased; oxygen content normal or increased; hypovolemia.
   Result: decreased tissue oxygen consumption, leading to tissue hypoxemia and acidosis.
Cardiogenic shock
   Cause: pump failure.
   Response: cardiac output decreased; peripheral vascular resistance normal or increased; oxygen content normal.
   Result: decreased flow leads to decreased tissue perfusion and decreased oxygen consumption.
Hypovolemic shock
   Cause: reduction in intravascular volume after blood loss, burns, bowel obstruction, etc.
   Response: cardiac output normal or increased; peripheral vascular resistance normal or increased.
   Result: oxygen delivery and consumption decreased because of decreased flow and localized tissue shunting.

mon form of shock seen in the trauma patient and the most likely to require blood transfusion. Hypovolemic shock also occurs commonly in patients with burn injury, bowel obstruction, and other illnesses that cause loss of intravascular volume; with the exception of burns, these problems do not typically lead to transfusion. The basic principles of management of hypovolemic shock are rapid identification of hypovolemia and restitution of lost blood volume. In the trauma patient, loss of volume includes concomitant loss of red cell mass, and restoration of that mass is critical. Given these differences, it is important for the clinician to identify the cause of hypovolemic shock to use transfusion appropriately.

Classification of Blood Loss

Clinicians have used two methods for classifying blood loss. The first relates to the rate of blood loss. Trunkey[7] separated hemorrhage into three classes based on the rate of blood loss. Severe hemorrhage is defined as a rate of blood loss greater than 150 ml/min, which could lead to the loss of one-half of the victim's blood volume within 20 minutes. These patients are relatively easy to recognize because they rapidly show clinical signs of shock such as hypoten-

Table 25-2 Estimated Fluid and Blood Losses[a] Based on Patient's Initial Presentation

	Class I	Class II	Class III	Class IV
Blood loss (ml)	Up to 750	750–1500	1,500–2,000	>2,000
Blood loss (% blood volume)	Up to 15%	15–30%	30–40%	>40%
Pluse rate	<100	>100	>120	>140
Blood pressure	Normal	Normal	Decreased	Decreased
Pulse pressure (mmHg)	Normal or increased	Decreased	Decreased	Decreased
Respiratory rate	14–20	20–30	30–40	>35
Urine output (ml/hr)	>30	20–30	5–15	Negligible
Central nervous system/mental status	Slightly anxious	Mildly anxious	Anxious and confused	Confused and lethargic
Fluid replacement (3:1 rule)[b]	Crystalloid	Crystalloid	Crystalloid and blood	Crystalloid and blood

[a] For a 70-kg male patient.

[b] The guidelines in Table 25-2 are based on the "three-for-one" rule. This rule derives from the empiric observation that most patients in hemorrhagic shock require as much as 300 ml of electrolyte solution for each 100 ml of blood loss. Applied blindly, these guidelines can result in excessive or inadequate fluid administration. For example, a patient with a crush injury to the extremity may have hypotension out of proportion to blood loss and require fluids in excess of the 3:1 guideline. In contrast, a patient whose ongoing blood loss is being replaced requires less than 3:1. The use of bolus therapy with careful monitoring of the patient's response can moderate these extremes.

(From American College of Surgeons Committee on Trauma,[8] with permission.)

sion and tachycardia. Unfortunately, this system is not as helpful in identifying those patients with less severe hemorrhage. For that reason, a classification of hemorrhagic shock based on clinical symptoms is currently in use (Table 25-2).

Class I hemorrhage is considered to be a loss of less then 15 percent of the total blood volume and has the clinical manifestations of a normal pulse rate, blood pressure, and pulse pressure and no changes in signs of tissue perfusion.[8] In class II hemorrhage (15 to 30 percent blood volume loss), the pulse rate is increased, and systolic blood pressure is normal. However, the pulse pressure decreases in response to vasoconstriction and tachycardia, which compensate for decreased perfusion. Capillary refill, which reflects tissue perfusion, is tested easily by pinching and releasing the fingertip while observing how quickly and completely the tissues revert from a blanched to a perfused appearance. Capillary refill may be delayed in class II hemorrhage, and the respiratory rate may be slightly elevated.[9] At this point, patients demonstrate some signs of anxiety as a result of decreased cerebral perfusion. Patients with class III (30 to 40 percent blood loss) present with tachycardia in excess of 120 beats/min, a decrease in systolic blood pressure and pulse pressure, delayed

capillary refill, and a progressively increasing respiratory rate. Urine output may become decreased, and the patient may become confused at this level. In class IV hemorrhage (greater than 40 percent blood loss), clinical signs are those of shock: tachycardia, hypotension, oliguria, and lethargy or coma. Clinical assessment of the patient in severe hemorrhagic shock is usually obvious. It is the patient with class I or II hemorrhagic shock who is difficult to identify.

Clinical assessment should be coupled with laboratory assessment. Initial laboratory studies should be drawn when intravenous lines are placed and should include blood for a both type and crossmatch and hemoglobin and hematocrit levels to assess blood loss. Because an initial low hemoglobin concentration is evidence of ongoing blood loss, these patients should be treated as having massive blood loss.[10]

Consequence of Shock

Shock is associated with loss of thermal regulation and decreased heat production.[11] In addition, the use of a cold environment or cold intravascular fluids can contribute to clinical hypothermia, which lead to coagulopathy in the absence of coagulation factor deficit.[12] Coagulopathy in shock typically follows the activation and/or consumption of coagulation factors. In addition, a fibrinolytic effect occurs after trauma,[13] and both platelets and the intrinsic cascade are activated by trauma and vascular injury.[14] Many patients with ongoing blood loss present with abnormal coagulation study findings. Some specific injuries, most notably cerebral injury, can lead to disseminated intravascular coagulopathy. In the presence of hypothermia, platelet and coagulation function may be normal by laboratory testing but abnormal in the operating room.[12] Care must be taken to warm fluids and to avoid the use of cold banked blood without warming. In addition, active patient warming may be necessary.

Acidosis results from inadequate oxygen delivery and waste product removal. Lactic acid is a product of anaerobic metabolism and accumulates in tissues in the vascular system. Although local acidosis shifts the oxygen dissociation curve to the left and allows better offloading of oxygen, systemic acidosis has a major impact on other metabolic process and on the uptake of oxygen by hemoglobin in the lung. Serum lactate levels or base deficit are frequently used in the identification of early shock in the absence of hypotension.

Ultimately, prolonged shock with delays in resuscitation can lead to multisystem organ failure (MSOF), which with cerebral injury can be attributed to delays or failure to resuscitate patients from shock effectively.[5] Delays in resuscitation have given rise to the popular concept of the "golden hour," during which early, effective treatment of shock can prevent MSOF. Once the golden hour has passed, the patient may be resuscitatable to "normal blood pressure." However, irreversible cellular damage has occurred, and survival is impossible.

MANAGEMENT OF EMERGENCY TRANSFUSION

Transfusion and Trauma Services

Many different factors affect the manner in which a particular institution handles emergency situations and massive transfusions. In many institutions, the physical separation of the transfusion service and the emergency room/trauma center hinder the immediate availability of blood. The turn-around time for immediate (stat) hematology/coagulation testing, staffing of the transfusion service, the availability of

intensive care units and operating room facilities, the level of comfort of the surgical house staff, and the availability of transfusion service/coagulation consultative services are important factors that affect the management of massive transfusions.

Because human error in patient or specimen identification occurs during situations of high emotion in a trauma center and in the operating room, utmost care must be exercised in the identification of the patient for whom blood is ordered or is to be transfused. Patients admitted to a trauma center are frequently unconscious, have no identification among their personal effects, and may not be accompanied by friends or relatives who would be able to provide identification. Another complicating factor occurs when a parent and child with the same name are admitted. A variety of different mechanisms have been used to identify an unknown victim. Unique trauma alphanumeric hospital identification numbers, in lieu of a patient's name on an emergency admission stamp plate, is a popular means of patient identification. Blood samples for laboratory testing, procedural requests, all testing results, and blood issued for this patient are identified with the unique number until the identity of the patient can be determined at which time laboratory and transfusion service results are merged with the patient's identity and any past records on file.

Initial Resuscitation

Intravenous access is critical in shock management. The rate of fluid or blood administration is limited by both the diameter and the length of the tubing through which it flows. A short, large-diameter intravenous catheter is the best possible choice. An 8-French central venous catheter, inserted through the femoral vein or subclavian vein, can reach flow rates of 1,000 ml/min of crystalloid and 500 ml/min of red blood cells when subjected to pressure flow.[15] Because the internal diameter of these intravenous catheters is often larger than the internal diameter of a standard blood administration set, it is frequently necessary to substitute large-diameter, high-flow tubing for standard administration sets to attain such flow rates (Table 25-3).

When blood is administered at high flow rates, it is important to warm the fluids (see above). Several devices have been developed that provide high-flow

Table 25-3. Components of Management of Emergency Transfusion

Use utmost care in the identification of both patient and specimens.
Label using alphanumeric identification numbers.
Red blood cell transfusion
    Large-diameter intravenous catheters and administration sets to attain high flow rates
    Blood warmers
    In-line 170-μm filters
Clinical monitoring to assess response to transfusion

and concurrent warming of blood products.[16] Although some individuals have recommended increasing the temperature of the blood by the addition of saline that has been warmed in a microwave oven, we do not recommend this practice. Without strict quality control, the temperature of the saline may so high as to cause hemolysis. Modern high-flow blood warmers provide a better option. Indeed, the *Standards for Blood Bank and Transfusion Services* of the American Association of Blood Banks states, "When warming of blood is indicated, this should be accomplished during its passage through the transfusion set. The warming system must be equipped with a visible thermometer and, ideally with an audible warning system. Blood must not be warmed above 42°C."[17]

The use of in-line 170-μm filters during the transfusion of blood and packed red blood cells is standard. Similar filters are used with high-flow tubing, which can provide flow rates of blood of 300 ml/min. Although microaggregates smaller than this can pass through the filters, a relationship between these microaggregates and pulmonary dysfunction has not been confirmed.[18] The use of finer filters to remove these particles unnecessarily restricts flow rates and adds no further benefit.

During the course of initial resuscitation, monitoring of pulse, blood pressure, respiratory rate, and urine output is basic. Monitoring of electrocardiographic rhythm is appropriate, particularly with administration of cold blood and blood products, as arrhythmias are not infrequent with hypothermic infusion. Monitoring of core temperature and serial blood pressure is essential to assess the impact of resuscitation. Continued assessment of the neuro-

logic status may give clues to the extent of shock, as a decreasing level of consciousness may be a reflection of shock or progressive neurologic injury. In unstable patients, elderly patients, and those with underlying cardiovascular and pulmonary disease, invasive monitoring of central venous pressure and/or arterial pressures is beneficial. The use of a pulmonary artery flow-directed catheter to monitor cardiac output, oxygen delivery, and consumption is critical to ongoing resuscitation and judgments in fluid management. These catheter-derived measurements foster more appropriate use of transfusion to improve oxygen delivery, rather than merely to treat low blood pressure or a low hemoglobin level.[19]

Fluid Resuscitation

Initial fluid resuscitation is most commonly begun with a crystalloid solution such as normal saline or Ringer's lactate. In most instances, Ringer's lactate is the fluid of choice, as massive fluid resuscitation with normal saline can lead to a hyperchloremic acidosis. For small-volume resuscitation (less than 2 L), both are of equal efficacy. Approximately one-third of administered crystalloid fluids remains in the intravascular space, one-third is excreted, and one-third "leaks" into the interstitial spaces. The initial resuscitation protocol for a patient who presents in shock is to give 2 L of crystalloid by rapid infusion (Table 25-4).[8] If vital signs and perfusion do not improve, then blood transfusion is considered to be appropriate.

When transfusion is initiated, 0.9 percent sodium chloride is the appropriate solution for concomitant intravenous fluids or dilution of packed red cells. Ringer's lactate should not be used because it contains 2.7 mEq/L of calcium, which is sufficient to cause clotting of anticoagulant blood in the bag or intravenous tubing. Red cells in the nutrient/preservative solution Adsol (Baxter Heathcare Corp, Deerfield, IL) may not need additional dilution.

The use of colloids such as 5 percent albumin, plasma protein fraction, and dextran 40 has been advocated in the resuscitation of trauma patients. Polymers of hydroxyethyl starch have been used successfully as a volume expander. Because of expense, coagulopathy initiated by the infused colloid, or difficulties in crossmatching of blood after administration of colloid, these have largely fallen into disfavor

Table 25-4 Responses to Initial Fluid Resuscitation[a]

	Rapid Response	Transient Response	No Response
Vital signs	Return to normal	Transient improvement; recurrence of decreased blood pressure and increased heart rate	Remain abnormal
Estimated blood loss	Minimal (10–20%)	Moderate and ongoing (20–40%)	Severe (>40%)
Need for more crystaloid	Low	High	High
Need for blood	Low	Moderate–high	Immediate
Blood preparation	Type and crossmatch	Type-specific	Emergency blood release
Need for operative intervention	Possibly	Likely	Highly likely
Surgical consultation	Yes	Yes	Yes

[a] 2,000 ml of Ringer's lactate in adults, 20 ml/kg of Ringer's lactate in children, over 10 to 15 minutes.
(From American College of Surgeons Committee on Trauma,[8] with permission.)

in the United States.[19] In addition, colloid resuscitation provides no good clinical advantage over crystalloid resuscitation and may lead to an increase in complication rates related to intravascular fluid retention.[20]

Most recently, small-volume resuscitations with hypertonic saline (3.5 or 7 percent sodium chloride) with and without dextran have been successful in providing intravascular volume expansion beyond administration of the volume of fluid administered.[21] This appears to be particularly useful in patients with severe brain injury, where administration of large volumes of crystalloid solutions can increase cerebral edema (see Ch. 23).

Decision to Transfuse

The decision to transfuse emergently requires a detailed clinical analysis that must include a combination of factors such as the patient's clinical condition; initial hemoglobin concentration; response to fluid resuscitation; coexisting respiratory, cardiac, and vascular conditions; and measurements of tissue oxygenation obtained by cardiac and peripheral monitors (Table 25-5). The primary purpose of emergency transfusion must be to restore perfusion and reverse the effects of shock by ensuring adequate oxygen delivery. A low hemoglobin level in the acutely bleeding patient with signs of shock is evidence of ongoing hemorrhage and should not be misinterpreted as chronic, compensated anemia.[10,22] Moreover, a normal hemoglobin level in an acutely bleeding patient does not mean that the red cell mass is normal but may reflect hemoconcentration from volume loss and a lack of replenishment of plasma volume.

As indicated earlier, clinical assessment of the patient's response to 2 L of crystalloid by rapid infusion provides valuable information regarding volume status and should be a part of the initial resuscitation protocol.[8] Rush[23] showed that a loss of up to 25 percent of a patient's blood volume can be replaced by a balanced salt solution, with volume replacement

Table 25-5. Transfusion Guidelines in Trauma Patients

Purpose: restore oxygen delivery and tissue perfusion; reverse effects of shock
Initial: Observe response to rapid crystalloid/colloid infusion
    Evaluate for ongoing, external bleeding
    Look for injury patterns consistent with high blood loss
        Penetrating injuries to chest, abdomen, neck, proximal extremity
        Pelvic fracture with blunt abdominal trauma
        Severe, multisystem trauma
Intraoperative:
    Monitor clinical signs—heart rate, blood pressure
    Monitor laboratory values—Hct, PT/PTT, fibrinogen
    Joint anesthesia/surgery decision
    Clinical experience and judgment

Abbreviations: Hct, hematocrit; PT, prothrombin time; PTT, partial thromboplastin time.

calculated as approximately three times the amount of the blood loss.

Indications for Early Transfusion

Certain injury patterns prompt the clinician to institute early transfusion. Patients with penetrating injury of the chest, neck, abdomen, or proximal extremities frequently present with hypotension because of injuries to major blood vessels. Although the the evaluation of injury patterns after blunt trauma is more complex, certain injuries are associated with high blood loss, particularly when they are found in a patient presenting with hypotension. Pelvic fracture[24] and severe abdominal injury characteristically have high blood loss and lead to transfusion. Approximately 2 percent of patients with abdominal injury present with "exsanguinating hemorrhage."[25] Ongoing hemorrhage is the cause of death in 41 percent of victims of fatal motor vehicle accidents.[26] Patients with severe multiple system trauma who present in shock should also be considered for early transfusion.

Ongoing blood loss from external sources should be evaluated continuously. Control of external wounds by direct pressure may be valuable. Tourniquet control of extremity bleeding must be viewed as a short-term solution and used with caution as a life saving measure before operative intervention. Scalp wounds are prone to significant ongoing blood loss and should be controlled as soon as possible. In patients who require therapy for other life-threatening injuries, scalp wound may result in significant blood loss, particularly if the patient becomes coagulopathic.

Intraoperative Transfusion

Intraoperatively, the decision to transfuse should be made jointly between the surgeon and the anesthesiologist. Monitoring of vital signs may include invasive techniques to assess arterial blood pressure and central venous pressures (and potentially left heart filling pressures). Monitoring of lactic acid levels or base excess may be considered. Crystalloid and/or colloid solutions are the mainstay of volume replacement. Red blood cell transfusion may become necessary with ongoing blood loss. The need for fresh frozen plasma (FFP) to prevent or correct coagulopathy and the use of platelets may be determined from the clinical presence of capillary or coagulopathic bleeding and laboratory evidence of a deficiency. The need for cryoprecipitate should be based on fibrinogen levels. In the trauma setting, blood losses are often underestimated by both observation and hemoglobin levels. Clinical judgement and experience are important in these cases to avoid the tendency to undertransfuse patients.

Reduction of Blood Loss

Several techniques are available to reduce blood loss during operative intervention. The use of electrocautery in incision has long been identified as a means of decreasing blood loss during abdominal or thoracic exploration. Similarly, the argon beam coagulator has been valuable in incision and in the management of solid organ injury (see Ch. 23).[27] Autotransfusion may be used in exploratory laparotomy or thoracotomy and during emergency management of major orthopaedic injuries.[28] Its use in the presence of bowel injury remains controversial (see Ch. 24).[29] Autotransfusion may reduce the strain on the blood bank for major trauma cases, but it cannot replace the use of allogeneic blood in patients with major ongoing hemorrhage.

Systemic pharmacologic agents are of little value in reducing bleeding in trauma. However, microfibrillar collagen as a topical agent, and other topical coagulants, have long been used in surgery. Fibrin glue has also been reported to be valuable in controlling hemorrhage from solid organ injury (see Ch. 23).[30] When coagulopathic bleeding occurs in the presence of ongoing hemorrhage, packing of the abdominal cavity and wound closure allows return to an intensive care unit where stabilization and correction of coagulopathy can reduce ongoing hemorrhage. This technique has been most useful in hepatic injury but can occasionally be valuable in massive hemorrhage from pelvic, renal, or pancreatic injuries.[31]

Selection of Blood for Transfusion

Whole Blood Versus Component Therapy

Transfusion practice with regard to the use of whole blood versus component therapy varies in different parts of this country and in the world. Since the 1970s, most donated blood in the United States is centrifuged and separated into packed red blood cells, FFP, platelets, and cryoprecipitate. Blood component therapy has provided the optimal means for meeting the specific therapeutic needs of the patient, has minimized the risk of volume overload from whole blood transfusions, and has allowed several patients to benefit from a single blood donation.

In many locations in the United States, whole blood is no longer available for transfusion. Nevertheless, in the setting of massive transfusion, whole blood often is preferred by clinicians because component therapy increases the risk of infectious disease transmission when red cells and FFP are required simultaneously. However, the whole blood lost by the patient and stored whole blood for transfusion are not equivalent. In stored whole blood, platelet function is virtually lost after 48 hours of storage at 4°C. Similarly, there is progressive loss of the labile coagulation factors, namely, factors V and VIII. Factor VIII is most unstable and decreases to 50, 30, and 6 percent of baseline values after 1, 5, and 21 days of storage, respectively. Factor V is also labile and decreases to 50 percent of baseline values after storage for 14 days.[32,33]

Group O Versus Type-Specific Red Blood Cells

In the past, isoagglutination titers were determined on group O whole blood.[34] Units were excluded from use for nongroup O (or type unknown) recipients if the titer exceeded a predetermined value. It is interesting to note that, during a number of previous major wars, the military met its immediate transfusion needs with group O whole blood that had been screened for high-titer anti-A and anti-B antibodies.[35-39] High-titer antibody production results from sensitization by pregnancy, by previous transfusion, and more recently, by immunization of troops with plague vaccine during the war in Vietnam.[40] Passive transmission of these antibodies can occasionally cause hemolysis of recipient A, B, or AB red cells.[41] If patients were then switched to type-specific blood without additional compatibility testing, hemolysis of the type-specific donor cells could also result from the passively acquired antibodies. The probability of these reactions was minimized by using only group O blood with low isoagglutinin titers. However, the use of group O whole blood during initial transfusion resuscitation also necessitates additional testing when switching to type-specific blood and unnecessarily depletes the available group O blood supply. Current American Association of Blood Banks standards states that recipients whose ABO group is not known must receive group O red blood cells.[17]

Because time is of the utmost importance in the exsanguinating patient, it is not always prudent to wait for completion of blood typing tests before initiating red cell transfusions. In these situations, initial blood resuscitation should consist of uncrossmatched group O red cells (Table 25-6).[34,42]

Table 26-6. Blood Availability Time Table for the Operating Room

Time You Can Wait to Transfuse	Type of RBC Product Available	Risks and Comments
5 minutes Immediate transfusion needed	O negative, Uncrossmatched	0.2–0.6% of population has red cell antibody; serious hemolysis rare. Wait for type specific only if a 10–15-min wait does not cause significant risk.
15 minutes After clot arrives in blood bank	Type specific, uncrossmatched	Risk same as O negative uncrossmatched blood. Type-specific blood is no safer. Wait for crossmatched blood if a 45-min wait does not cause significant risk.
45 minutes After clot arrives in blood bank	Type specific, crossmatched (unless red cell antibody present)	No red cell antibody found; blood compatible by crossmatch.
90 minutes to several hours; rarely, even longer	Type specific, crossmatched in a patient with a red cell antibody	Red cell antibody found; antibody identification may take 90 min to several hours. If blood is needed before compatibility testing is completed, hemolysis may occur but transfusion should not be withheld if absolutely necessary; life-threatening morbidity is rare. Communicate with blood bank.

Two to 4 units should be available in a properly monitored blood refrigerator in the trauma room if the transfusion service is at a distant site. During the preparation of red blood cells, the cells are usually centrifuged and resuspended in an additive solution (AS), which extends cell viability and improves flow rates. Only small quantities of residual plasma-containing anti-A and anti-B antibodies (approximately 20 to 30 ml) remain in the red cell concentrates resuspended in AS-1 (Adsol), AS-3 (Nutricel), and AS-5 (Optisol) additive solutions. Consequently, when the patient's blood type is determined, the patient can safely be switched to the specific type needed or a compatible blood type without concern for hemolysis resulting from passive transmission of these naturally occurring antibodies. The use of type-specific blood conserves the frequently limited supply of group O units.

Red cell concentrates prepared in citrate-phosphate-dextrose-adenine (CPDA-1) anticoagulant-preservative solutions may contain as much as 50 to 80 ml of residual plasma. Plasma in this quantity from individuals with high-titer anti-A and/or anti-B antibodies has been known to cause significant hemolysis.[41] Thus, group O CPDA-1 red cells are less desirable than Adsol units for nongroup O recipients and, in addition, have decreased flow rates. After determination of the patients blood type, type-specific CPDA-1 red cells may be used.

Nevertheless, the use of type-specific red cells in the emergency room/trauma center is controversial. The risk of major ABO incompatibility and acute hemolytic transfusion reactions as a result of clerical and technical errors that arise during periods of high emotion are major considerations with regard to the use of type-specific red cells.[35,37,42–45] Errors in patient identification, sample labeling, multiple simultaneous typing procedures, stat testing, and staffing problems increase the risk of clerical errors. Blood administration errors are increased during situations in which multiple trauma patients require urgent transfusion. In some centers, because multiple admissions account for nearly 50 percent of trauma admissions, group O blood is used exclusively in multicasualty situations.[46] When these patients are transferred to the operating room or to an intensive care unit, subsequent transfusions are met with type-specific red cells. Unfortunately, this approach places a heavy demand on the group O blood supply, but it does avoid potential serious errors in ABO incompatibility.

Time delays between recognition of the need for transfusion and the availability of type-specific (uncrossmatched) units have also been cited by opponents to the use of type-specific red cells. Although ABO/Rh typing takes approximately 5 to 10 minutes to perform, 20 minutes to greater than 40 minutes may elapse before the start of blood infusion, depending on specimen collection, transportation, sample handling, and computer processing.

Emergency Compatibility Testing

Twenty to 40 minutes are required for an antibody screen, which is used to detect clinically significant unexpected alloantibodies. (see Ch. 22) For patients with a negative antibody screen finding, crossmatched blood may be available in approximately 10 minutes using an abbreviated immediate-spin crossmatch. The abbreviated crossmatch detects ABO blood group incompatibilities and is greater than 99.9 percent safe when there are no detectable alloantibodies in the patient's serum.[47] In patients with a positive antibody screen result, compatibility cannot be ensured with an immediate-spin crossmatch, and a complete crossmatch (20 to 40 minutes) must be done if time permits (see below). Some institutions with sophisticated computer systems use a computer crossmatch to replace the immediate-spin crossmatch.[48,49] Verification procedures must be in place before initiating the computer crossmatch. Computer crossmatches provide a safe and efficient means of detecting donor-recipient ABO incompatibility without performing a serologic crossmatch and further reduce the turnaround time on stat crossmatches.

Management of Patients With a Positive Antibody Screen Result

Blood group alloantibodies are detected by testing donor serum against two or three different group O reagent cells the phenotypes of which have been identified. These antibodies, if clinically significant, can cause either acute and/or delayed hemolytic transfusion reactions. In vitro agglutination and/or hemolysis is determined at room temperature, at 37°C, and in the antiglobulin phase. Reactions at room temperature usually indicate the presence of cold agglutinins (IgM antibodies) with little or no clinical significance. Reactions at 37°C or in the antiglobulin phase indicate the presence of clinically significant (IgG) antibodies. The risk of significant unexpected antibodies in men with a negative history of transfusion or in women with no history of transfusion or pregnancy is 0.04 percent.[50] The risk of unexpected antibodies increases to 1.0 percent in men and women who are the recipients of previous transfusions or in women who have been pregnant. For women who have been both pregnant and the recipients of transfusions, the risk of unexpected antibodies increases to approximately 3.0 percent. In recent studies, clinically significant antibodies were identified in 1 to 4 percent of patients requiring massive transfusion, none of which were due to anti-D antibody.[51,52]

In patients who have a positive antibody screening test result, life-threatening blood loss may necessitate the transfusion of red cells before antibody identification or screening for antigen-negative units. In these unusual situations, the surgeon/physician and the transfusion medicine physician must decide whether the medical benefits of immediate transfusion justify the risk of a hemolytic transfusion reaction. The class of immunoglobulin (IgG versus IgM), the strength and phase of the reaction, and the extent that complement is likely to be involved are important considerations. Under these circumstances, trauma center and operating room physicians and nursing personnel must be informed of the blood group incompatibility and must be particularly attentive to the signs and symptoms of acute hemolysis (see Ch. 9 and 22).

Group O Rh-Positive Versus Group O Rh-Negative Red Blood Cells

The use of Rh-positive and Rh-negative red cells for transfusion in emergency room/trauma situations varies in different parts of this country. Differing philosophies and practices regarding blood product management contribute to this variation. Most recipients of emergency transfusion fall into two groups: young male patients (nearly 75 percent of patients) with penetrating or blunt trauma without a history of prior transfusion and patients with an acute relapse of some underlying condition that

often has required prior transfusion.[52–54] Because only 6 percent of the blood donor population is group O Rh negative, the universal availability of this product to supply all of the transfusion requirements of emergency room/trauma center patients is generally not attainable. Although the safety and efficacy of group O Rh-positive blood for young healthy males patients was established during the Korean and Vietnam wars[35,39] and in civilian trauma,[42,52,53] many physicians are uncomfortable with the exclusive use of group O Rh-positive blood. Alternatively, many trauma centers have implemented a middle-of-the-road approach regarding this issue. Two to 4 units of group O, Rh-negative red blood cells are used if immediate transfusion is required and, thereafter, if type-specific blood is not available. Group O Rh-negative blood is used for premenopausal female patients who, because of possible future pregnancy, need to be protected from inadvertent sensitization, and for individuals who are already sensitized to the D antigen. If supplies of group O, Rh-negative blood are limited, group O Rh-positive blood is used for male and postmenopausal female patients. Some trauma centers use group O Rh-positive blood for the transfusion requirements of all patients or for all male and postmenopausal female patients, but this policy incurs the risk of a hemolytic transfusion reaction caused by anti-D, which is present in about 0.5 percent of patients.

MASSIVE TRANSFUSION

Definition of Massive Transfusion

Massive transfusion is commonly defined as transfusion approximating or exceeding the patient's blood volume within a 24-hour period (see Ch. 35).[48] However, in many trauma victims, this volume is administered within a shorter time interval. In this setting, blood losses of between 30 to 50 percent of total blood volume may be defined as massive hemorrhage.

Mortality

Although massive hemorrhage may result from gastrointestinal bleeding, ruptured aneurysms, and surgical procedures,[55,56] penetrating and blunt trauma are the leading causes of massive transfusion.[2,14,33,52,57,58] Trauma patients are predominantly young men with an average age in their midthirties.[2,14,51,58,59] Overall survival rates among patients with massive transfusion are 40 to 60 percent and correlate with the number of blood transfusions.[14,51] In one series, survival rates ranged from 38 percent for patients with hepatic failure to 100 percent for obstetric cases.[51] Mobilization of emergency medical personnel, immediate resuscitation and transport, and improved surgical techniques have increased survival rates as high as 70 percent among patients requiring greater than 25 units of blood.[2] Duration and magnitude of shock are critically important factors affecting mortality rates in massively transfused patients.[14,56,58,60,61] Increasing age;[62] severe head injury; abdominal trauma as a source of hemorrhage; pelvic fracture; underlying medical conditions; particularly of hepatic origin; and nontraumatic surgical emergencies are associated with increased mortality rates in relation to blood transfusion.[2,14,58,63]

Injury patterns requiring massive transfusions have been identified after both blunt and penetrating trauma. Most series reviewing the outcome of massive transfusion are based on penetrating trauma.[58] Penetrating injuries of the vessels of the neck, thoracic outlet, aorta, great veins of the chest and abdomen, or major intra-abdominal vascular injuries may require massive transfusion. Penetrating injuries of the liver may also be associated with intrahepatic vascular injury, or parenchymal injury alone may require massive transfusion. Proximal extremity injuries and near amputations may also lead to such requirements. In blunt trauma, injuries of the pelvis, major abdominal and thoracic vessels, liver, spleen, and kidneys can lead to massive hemorrhage requiring massive transfusion. The reported survival rate for massive transfusion in blunt trauma patients is 52 percent.[2]

Dilutional Coagulopathy

Essential to the definition of massive transfusion is an understanding of the principles of exchange transfusion and the concept of a dilutional coagulopathy. The kinetics of exchange transfusion predict that nearly 37 percent of the original blood volume remains after the loss of a single blood volume (10 units in a 70-kg adult).[64] With two or three volume exchanges, the remaining elements drop to levels of approximately 15 and 5 percent, respectively. Not surprisingly, trauma patients who receive massive transfusion are susceptible to having coagulation abnormalities develop. In the past, the loss of coagulation factors and platelets were made up to a limited extent by the replacement of whole blood or by modified whole blood.[33] Modified whole blood is prepared by resuspending red cells in the donor's plasma after platelet concentrates and cryoprecipitates have been removed. It differs from fresh, whole blood in that only 15 percent of platelets, 40 percent of the factor VIII, and about 75 percent of the fibrinogen are retained in the product.[65]

The functional activity of coagulation factors and platelets after a single volume replacement is usually adequate to maintain hemostasis. Dilutional thrombocytopenia is predictable after increasingly larger volumes of blood and fluid replacement[33,66,67] and is clinically manifest by diffuse microvascular bleeding characterized by the onset of oozing from mucosa, raw wounds, and puncture sites. Platelet levels rarely fall below 100,000 until approximately 1.5 times the patient's blood volume has been replaced.[33] Platelet counts above 100,000 usually provide adequate hemostasis unless a qualitative deficit is also present. The exact activity levels needed for hemostasis when multiple factor deficiencies coexist are not well defined. Dilution of coagulation factors during massive transfusion to a level of 30 percent functional activity may be associated with prolongation of the prothrombin (PT) and activated partial thromboplastin (aPTT) times. With diminished factor activity, the prolongation of the PT and aPTT are reagent dependent and, consequently, are not directly correlated with specific functional activity.

Disseminated Intravascular Coagulation

The location and extent of trauma and the duration of shock are important factors in the development of disseminated intravascular coagulation (DIC).[55,60,68,69] In the setting of massive transfusion, DIC is reported to occur in 5 to 30 percent of trauma patients[33,66,70] and is associated with high morbidity and mortality rates of nearly 70 percent.[55,56,71–73] In patients with blunt trauma, tissue injury may cause immediate activation of the clotting system. Tissue and cell fragments enter the bloodstream, which, in the presence of hypoperfusion and circulatory stasis induced by hemorrhage, results in severe DIC. In the patient with severe burns, both hemolysis and tissue necrosis with release of tissue components, cellular enzymes, and lipid-like material into the circulation trigger DIC. Tissue thromboplastins liberated from brain tissue are a common but frequently underrecognized cause of DIC after head trauma.[74] Acidosis-induced endothelial sloughing may also cause activation of the intrinsic clotting cascade.[75]

Regardless of the inciting etiologic mechanism, the development of microvascular thrombosis plays an active role in MSOF, including renal failure, gangrene, hepatic failure, and acute respiratory distress syndrome. Extensive activation of the coagulation system is almost always accompanied by concomitant activation of the fibrinolytic cascade. Consequently, both microthrombi and hemorrhage may be seen.

The development of DIC in the setting of hypothermia is multifactorial. Platelet dysfunction resulting from temperature-dependent diminished thromboxane-B_2 production causes a delay in platelet plug formation.[76] Fibrin clot formation is also delayed because the enzymes of the coagulation cascade are temperature dependent. Finally, large amounts of tissue thromboplastins resulting from tissue damage are released into the systemic circulation and activate the extrinsic clotting cascade.[77] Thus, DIC is frequently seen during cold ischemia and, not surprisingly, has been noted in hypothermic patients after rewarming.[77,78]

Laboratory Testing in Massive Trauma

Laboratory testing and the interpretation of laboratory results in the diagnosis of dilutional coagulopathy and DIC in the massive transfused patient remain controversial. In some trauma patients, the clinical observation of a coagulopathy may not be confirmed by abnormal coagulation (PT and aPTT) test results.[79] Rohrer and Natale[80] showed progressive prolongation of coagulation test results (PT and aPTT) with varying levels of hypothermia. Because coagulation testing is routinely performed at 37°C, rather than at the patient's actual in vivo temperature, it is not surprising that normal coagulation test findings can be obtained. Although these coagulation test results do not reflect in vivo clotting activity, normal findings do indicate that sufficient clotting factors are available for coagulation if normothermia

is restored. On the other hand, coagulation test results may be normal or variably prolonged in the absence of microvascular hemorrhage. In addition, moderate to severe thrombocytopenia may be seen in acute DIC and dilutional coagulopathies.[33]

Fibrin degradation product (FDP) or D-dimer levels are frequently elevated in acute DIC but are not diagnostic of DIC. FDP represent the biodegradation products of the action of plasmin on fibrinogen and fibrin. D-dimers are end products of the action of plasmin on fibrin and may be elevated in the absence of DIC. Platelet factor 4 and β-thromboglobulin are elevated in DIC, but neither of these tests are diagnostic of DIC because the results may be elevated in a variety of intravascular coagulation disorders. The irreversible complexing of some activated clotting factors (thrombin) with antithrombin III (AT III) leads to a significant decrease in functional AT III activity in acute DIC. Assessment of tissue plasminogen activator antigen concentration and activity may also be helpful in the diagnosis of DIC.[81] With the exception of the FDP and D-dimer assays, laboratory turn-around time in the massively bleeding patient is unacceptably long for most of these other assays.

Many investigators believe the laboratory diagnosis of DIC must demonstrate the action of thrombin on the fibrinogen molecule. Thrombin leaves the carboxyl terminals on the α and β fibrinogen chains that produce fibrin monomers and fibrinopeptides A and B. The detection of soluble monomer complexes by hemagglutination technique is a rapid (20 minutes) and specific test to detect activation of thrombin. Although the determination of fibrinopeptide A is sensitive and accurate, the turn-around is unacceptably long (2 hours) in trauma-related microvascular hemorrhage. At the present time, no single laboratory test can be used to confirm or exclude the diagnosis of DIC. However, the combination of a low platelet count, a low fibrinogen level, an elevated D-dimer concentration, and the presence of soluble fibrin monomers in the context of the patient's underlying condition are the most helpful indicators of DIC.

Indications for Replacement of Hemostatic Factors

In the trauma patient, the clinical and laboratory distinction between microvascular hemorrhage caused by a dilutional coagulopathy and DIC may

Table 25-7. Indications for Replacement of Hemostatic Factors in Trauma Patient

Define patient's coagulation status whenever possible with appropriate laboratory tests.
Clinical guidelines
    Extent and location of injury
    Duration of shock
    Response to initial fluid resuscitation
    Risk of complications, e.g., intracranial bleeding
Replace components to correct specific abnormalities.
Guidelines for specific components: replace with
    Platelets if platelet count <80–100 × 10^9/L
    Fresh frozen plasma if PT/PTT >1.5 × normal
    Cryoprecipitate if fibrinogen level <10 g/L

Abbreviations: PT, prothrombin time; PTT, partial thromboplastin time.

be extremely difficult. Nevertheless, every attempt should be made to determine the patient's coagulation status with appropriately selected blood tests and to replace components to correct specific abnormalities.[62,66,82] Practically speaking, because time is of the essence, the decision to administer component therapy to trauma patients with microvascular hemorrhage is often made before the availability of laboratory results (Table 25-7). The location and extent of injury, the duration of shock, the response to resuscitation, and the risk of complicating factors such as intracranial bleeding are important clinical considerations. With prompt management of bleeding, debridement of devitalized tissue, and the skilled use of component therapy, the coagulopathy can usually be controlled.

In the patient with microvascular hemorrhage, general thresholds for component replacement are as follows: transfuse platelets when the count is less than 80 to 100 × 10^9/L, FFP when the PT and/or aPTT are greater than 1.5 times normal, and cryoprecipitate when the fibrinogen level is less than 10 g/L. The prophylactic administration of platelets in the absence of microvascular bleeding is controversial.[33,57,82] Some investigators advocate prophylactic administration of platelets to patients with severe blunt trauma and thrombocytopenia because microvascular bleeding may be occult and precious time and blood may be lost if platelet transfusion is deferred until bleeding has become a problem.[62] Empiric replacement using a standardized regimen of platelet concentrates and FFP that depends on the

amount of blood loss cannot be justified. This results in overtransfusion in many patients, with an accompanying increased risk of disease transmission, and may exhaust available supplies of components. Furthermore, such regimens frequently underestimate transfusion needs in patients who truly need blood products, especially those with a consumptive coagulopathy (see Ch. 18).[82]

COMPLICATIONS OF MASSIVE TRANSFUSION

Blood transfusion has immediate and delayed adverse complications in as many as 10 percent of recipients. In the massively transfused patient, the clinical manifestations of an acute hemolytic reaction may not be recognized because of complications resulting from the injury. Massive transfusion can cause several metabolic problems, including citrate toxicity, hyperkalemia, acidosis, and a shift in the oxygen dissociation curve. The trauma victim that survives the initial injury may succumb to delayed consequences of the resuscitative efforts, for example, transfusion-transmitted disease, and possibly immunosuppression (see Ch. 4). Because the risk of infectious disease transmission is directly related to the number of donor exposures, the indiscriminate or prophylactic use of blood products is not warranted.

Immune Hemolysis

ABO-incompatible hemolytic transfusion reactions are the most common cause of acute fatalities from blood transfusion[45,83] and are frequently the result of human error in patient or specimen identification occurring during situations of high emotion.[36,44] Acute hemolytic reactions are usually caused by naturally occurring isoagglutinins (anti-A or anti-B), which activate complement and result in membrane lysis and liberation of free hemoglobin within the vascular system. The clinical response depends on the quantity of donor red cells, antigen specificity, immunoglobulin type (IgM versus IgG), antibody subclass, antibody thermal amplitude, antibody titer, and the clinical condition of the recipient.[41] The complex interaction of the complement system, the kallikrein-kinin system, the coagulation system, and the neuroendocrine system account for the often catastrophic clinical findings of acute hemolysis caused by ABO incompatibility, namely, acute renal failure, DIC, and death. A hemolytic reaction in a critically injured or massively transfused patient may be overlooked. Clinical findings of hemoglobinuria, hypotension, fever, and microvascular hemorrhage may be attributed to traumatic injury. Prevention of clerical error requires utmost care in patient identification.

Immunosuppression

In the massively transfused patient, infection is common and is one of the leading causes of death (see Ch. 4). However, it is not clear to what extent transfusion is responsible for the susceptibility to infection. Early evidence suggesting an immunosuppressive effect comes from patients with colon and lung cancer.[84–86] Some studies report significantly fewer infections among recipients of autologous transfusion compared with homologous transfusion.[87,88] Other supporters of the immunosuppressive effect of transfusion cite the fact that most infections are nosocomial or distant from the site of injury.[89] The immunosuppressive effects of transfusion and tumor recurrence have been refuted by some investigators.[90–92] The results of experimental studies in animals have been extremely variable, depending on the animal model. Practically speaking, the severity of injury, the amount of bacterial contamination, the pre-existing immunologic state of the trauma victim, and the systemic effects of hemorrhagic shock can impair the immune response to infectious agents. In addition, the mechanism by which immunosuppression might be induced by blood transfusion is unknown.

Citrate Toxicity

To ensure the complete anticoagulation of blood, excess citrate is used to bind calcium and prevent clotting. The citrate load administered during massive transfusion depends on the plasma volume of the blood products administered. CPDA-1 and Adsol red cell concentrates contain 5 and 2 mg/ml of citrate, respectively. However, the plasma from Adsol units contains nearly 30 mg/ml of citrate from the citrate-phosphate-dextrose anticoagulant used in the initial collection.[54] Therefore, during massive transfusion, the plasma-containing blood products (FFP and platelets) are the major source of citrate.

Citrate is excreted in the urine and metabolized rapidly by the liver in normal patients. The end product of its metabolism is bicarbonate. Normal calcium levels are restored by mobilization of skeletal calcium stores. Citrate infusion causes a transient decrease in ionized calcium. However, in patients who have limited ability to metabolize citrate, particularly those with severe hypotension, hypothermia, hepatic injury or pre-existing hepatic disease, citrate toxicity can cause muscle tremors, increased myocardial irritability, and decreased cardiac output.[92] Irreversible ventricular fibrillation may occur at citrate levels of 60 mg/ml. The use of calcium salts should be reserved for selected massively transfused patients with clinical manifestations of citrate toxicity.

Hyperkalemia

Potassium is known to leak from red blood cells during storage. Although the extracellular potassium concentration of AS-1 red cells at 42 days is approximately 60 to 70 mM, the actual potassium content is 7.5 mmol/unit. This metabolic load is transient, as potassium re-enters red cells within a few hours after transfusion. In actual practice, patients may experience a paradoxic hypokalemia resulting from the metabolism of citrate to bicarbonate and increased urinary excretion of potassium.[60] In clinical practice, hyperkalemia may occur during rapid blood transfusion in patients with severe shock or renal dysfunction and in patients with extensive muscle necrosis. In recent years, the ability to infuse large volumes of stored blood rapidly using high-capacity blood warmers has increased the risk of hyperkalemia in these patients.[61] Because hyperkalemia and hypokalemia are associated with cardiac dysfunction, close monitoring of potassium levels is recommended in the massively transfused patient.

2,3-Diphosphoglyceric Acid and Adenosine Triphosphate

The ability of red blood cells to bind and release oxygen is dependent on the ability of 2,3-diphosphoglyceric acid (2,3-DPG) to bind and stabilize deoxyhemoglobin. During red cell storage, normal levels of 2,3-DPG are maintained for approximately 10 days. The subsequent precipitous loss of 2,3-DPG causes the oxygen dissociation curve to shift to the left. Consequently, stored red cells have a greater affinity for oxygen and are less likely to release oxygen. After transfusion, transfused red cells require 3 to 8 hours to regenerate one-half of their 2,3-DPG levels. Complete restoration of 2,3-DPG and normal hemoglobin function occurs within 24 hours.[93] The clinical effect of low 2,3-DPG levels in transfused blood has never been determined but is likely offset by other in vivo variables, including increases in cardiac output, vasodilation, and local acidosis.[94]

The ability of red blood cells to deform during passage through capillaries, which is important in determining resistance of blood to flow, is dependent on cellular adenosine triphosphate (ATP) levels. During storage, the red cell changes shape from a biconcave disc to a sphere as ATP levels decrease. The loss of ATP is anticoagulant dependent. Whole blood in CPDA-1 at 35 days of storage retains only 45 percent of initial ATP levels. Special additive solutions (Adsol) used in the preparation of red cell concentrates have effectively reduced ATP loss (60 to 65 percent of initial levels are retained) and increased red cell storage to 42 days.[95]

REFERENCES

1. Rice DP, MacKenzie EJ, Jones AS et al: Cost of injury in the United States: a report to Congress, 1989. Centers for Disease Control, Atlanta, 1989
2. Wudel JH, Morris JA, Yates K et al: Massive transfusion: outcome in blunt trauma patients. J Trauma 31: 1, 1991
3. Kaplan AJ, Zone-Smith LK, Hannegan C, Norcross ED: The prevalence of hepatitis C in a regional level I trauma center population. J Trauma 33:126, 1992
4. Gross SG: A System of Surgery: Pathological, Diagnostic, Therapeutic and Operative. Lea & Febiger, Philadelphia, 1872
5. Shoemaker WC: Pathophysiology, monitoring, outcome prediction and outcome of shock states. Crit Care Clin 3:307, 1987
6. Blalock A: Shock: further studies with particular reference to effects of hemorrhage. Arch Surg 29:837, 1937
7. Trunkey D: Trauma. Sci Am 249:28, 1983
8. American College of Surgeons Committee on Trauma: Advanced Trauma Life Support Manual. American College of Surgeons, Chicago, 1993
9. Schriger DL, Baraff LS: Capillary refill—is is a useful predictor of hypovolemic states. Ann Emerg Med 20: 601, 1991
10. Knottenbelt JD: Low initial hemoglobin levels in trauma patients: an important indicator of ongoing hemorrhage. J Trauma 31:1396, 1991
11. Jurkovich GJ, Greiser WB, Luterman A, Curreri PW: Hypothermia in trauma victims: ominous predictor of survival. J Trauma 27:1019, 1987
12. Gubler KD, Gentilello LM, Hassantash SA, Maier RV: The impact of hypothermia on dilutional coagulopathy. J Trauma 36:847, 1994
13. Kapash DN, Metzler M, Harrington M et al: Fibrinolytic response to trauma. Surgery 95:473, 1984
14. Kivioja A, Myllynen P, Rokkanen P: Survival after massive transfusions exceeding four blood volumes in patients with blunt injuries. Am Surg 57:398, 1991
15. Millikan JS, Cain TL, Haisbrough J: Rapid volume replacement for hypovolemic shock. J Trauma 24:428, 1984
16. Flauchbaum L, Trooskin S, Pedersen H: Evaluation of blood warming devices with the apparent thermal clearance. Ann Emerg Med 18:355, 1989
17. Klein HG: Standards for Blood Banks and Transfusion Services. 16th Ed. American Association of Blood Banks, Bethesda, 1994
18. Hassy A: When is the microfiltration of whole blood and red cell concentrates essential? When is it superfluous? Vox Sang 50:54, 1986
19. Astiz ME, Rackow EC: Assessing perfusion failure during circulatory shock. Crit Care Clin 9: 299, 1993
20. Weaver DW, Ledgerwood AM, Lucas CE et al: Pulmonary effects of albumin resuscitation for severe hypovolemic shock. Arch Surg 113: 387, 1978
21. Younes RN, Aun F, Accioly CG et al: Hypertonic solutions in the treatment of hypovolemic shock: a prospective randomized study in patients admitted to the emergency room. Surgery 111:380, 1992
22. National Institutes of Health Consensus Conference on Perioperative Red Cell Transfusion: JAMA 260: 2700, 1988
23. Rush G: Volume replacement: why, what, and how much. In Schumer W, Nyhus L (eds): Treatment of Shock. Lea & Febiger, Philadelphia, 1974
24. Mucha P, Welch TJ: Hemorrhage in major pelvic fractures. Surg Clin North Am 68:757, 1988
25. Olsen WR, Redman HC, Hildreth DH: Quantitative peritoneal lavage in blunt abdominal trauma. Arch Surg 104:536, 1972
26. Frey CF, Huelke DF, Gikas PW: Resuscitation and survival in motor vehicle accidents. J Trauma 9:292, 1969
27. Cornwell E, Dunham C, Brathwaite C, Militello P: Use of the argon beam coagulator in critically injured patients. Pan Am J Trauma 1:81, 1989
28. Jacobs LM, Hsich JW: A clinical review of autotransfusion and its role in trauma. JAMA 251:3283, 1984
29. Timberlake GA, McSwain NE: Autotransfusion of

blood contaminated by enteric contents: a potentially life-saving measure in the massively hemorrhaging trauma patient? J Trauma 28:855, 1988

30. Kram HB, del Junco T, Clark SR et al: Techniques of splenic preservation using fibrin glue. J Trauma 30:97, 1990

31. Rotando MF, Schwab CW, McGonigal MD et al: "Damage control": an approach for improved survival in exsanguinating penetrating abdominal injury. J Trauma 35:375, 1993

32. Caggiano V: Red blood cell transfusions. In Silver H (ed): Blood, Blood Components and Derivatives in Transfusion Therapy. American Association of Blood Banks, Arlington, 1980

33. Counts RB, Haisch C, Simon TL et al: Hemostasis in massively transfused trauma patients. Ann Surg 190:91, 1979

34. Barnes A: Transfusion of universal donor and uncrossmatched blood. Bibl Haematol 46:132, 1980

35. Barnes A: Status of the use of universal donor blood transfusion. Clin Lab Sci 4:147, 1973

36. Barnes A, Allen TE: Transfusions subsequent to administration of universal donor blood in Vietnam. JAMA 204:695, 1968

37. Blumberg N, Bove JR: Uncrossmatched blood for emergency transfusion. JAMA 240:2057, 1978

38. Crosby WH, Akeroyd JH: Some immunohematologic results of large transfusions of group O blood in recipients of other blood groups. A study of battle casualties in Korea. Blood 9:102, 1954

39. Crosby WH: The safety of blood transfusion in the treatment of mass casualties. Milit Med 117:354, 1955

40. Camp FR(Jr), Shields CE: Military blood banking identification of the group O universal donors for transfusion of A, B and AB recipients—an enigma of two decades. Mil Med 132:426, 1967

41. Mollison PL, Engelfreit CP, Contreras M (eds): Hemolytic transfusion reactions. In: Blood Transfusion in Clinical Medicine. 9th Ed. Blackwell Scientific Publications, Oxford, 1993

42. Gervin AS, Fischer RP: Resuscitation of trauma patients with type-specific uncrossmatched blood. J Trauma 24:327, 1984

43. Goldfinger D: Uncrossmatched blood for emergency transfusion. JAMA 273:180, 1977

44. Myhre BA: Fatalities from blood transfusion. JAMA 244:1333, 1980

45. Sazama K: Reports of 355 transfusion-associated deaths: 1976 through 1985. Transfusion 30:583, 1990

46. Sohmer PR, Dawson RB: Transfusion therapy in trauma: a review of the principles and techniques used in the MIEMSS program. Am Surg 45:109, 1979

47. Boral LI, Hill SS, Apollon CJ, Folland A: The type and antibody screen, revisited. Am J Clin Pathol 71:578, 1979

48. American Association of Blood Banks: Adverse Effects of Blood Transfusion: In: Technical Manual. 11th Ed. American Association of Blood Banks, Bethesda, 1993

49. Butch SH, Judd WJ, Steiner EA et al: Electronic verification of donor-recipient compatibility: the computer crossmatch. Transfusion 34:105, 1994

50. Giblett ER: Blood group alloantibodies: an assessment of some laboratory practices. Transfusion 17:299, 1977

51. Sawyer PR, Harrison CR: Massive transfusion in adults. Vox Sang 58:199, 1990

52. Schmidt PJ: Use of Rh positive blood in emergency situations. Surg Gynecol Obstet 167:229, 1988

53. Schwab CW, Shayne JP, Turner J: Immediate trauma resuscitation with type O uncrossmatched blood: a two-year prospective experience. J Trauma 26:897, 1986

54. Gervin AS: Transfusion, autotransfusion, and blood substitutes. p. 165. In Moore EE, Mattox KL, Feliciano DV (eds): Trauma. 2nd Ed. Appleton and Lange, Norwalk, 1991

55. Wilson RF, Mammen E, Walt EJ: Eight years of experience with massive blood transfusion. J Trauma 11:275, 1971

56. Rutledge R, Sheldon GF, Collins ML: Massive transfusion. Crit Care Clin 2:791, 1986

57. Harrigan C, Lucas CE, Ledgerwood AM, Mannen EF: Primary hemostasis after massive transfusion for injury. Surgery 98:836, 1985

58. Phillips TF, Soulier G, Wilson RF: Outcome of massive transfusion exceeding two blood volumes in trauma and emergency surgery. J Trauma 27:903, 1897

59. Harrigan C, Lucas CE, Ledgerwood AM: The effect of hemorrhagic shock on the clotting cascade in injured patients. J Trauma 29:1416, 1989

60. Collins JA: Problems associated with the massive transfusion of stored blood. Surgery 75:274, 1974

61. Canizaro PC, Possa ME: Management of massive hemorrhage associated with abdominal trauma. Surg Clin North Am 70:621, 1990

62. Faringer PD, Mullins RH, Johnson RL, Trunkey DD: Blood component supplementation during massive transfusion of AS-1 red cells in trauma patients. J Trauma 34:481, 1993

63. Riska EB, Bostman O, von Donsdorff H et al: Outcome of closed injuries exceeding 20-unit blood transfusion need. Injury 19:273, 1988

64. Marsaglia G, Thomas ED: Mathematical consideration

of cross circulation and exchange transfusion. Transfusion 11:216, 1971

65. Slichter SJ, Counts RB, Henderson R, Harker LA: Preparation of cryoprecipitated factor VIII concentrates. Transfusion 16:616, 1976

66. Mannucci PM, Federici AB, Sirchia G: Hemostasis testing during massive blood replacement. Vox Sang 42: 113, 1982

67. Noe DA, Graham SM, Luff R, Sohmer P: Platelet counts during rapid massive transfusion. Transfusion 22:392, 1982

68. Harke H, Rahman S: Haemostatic disorders in massive transfusion. Bibl Haematol 46:179, 1980

69. Lucas CE, Ledgerwood AM: Clinical significance of altered coagulation test after massive transfusions for trauma. Am Surg 47:125, 1981

70. Braunstein AH, Oberman HA: Transfusion of plasma components. Transfusion 24:281, 1984

71. Wilson RF, Dulchavsky SA, Soullier G, Beckman B: Problems with 20 or more blood transfusions in 24 hours. Am Surg 53:410, 1987

72. Hewson JR, Neame PB, Kumar N et al: Coagulopathy related to dilution and hypotension during massive transfusion. Crit Care Med 13:387, 1985

73. Bodai BI, Smith JP, Blaisell FW: The role of emergency thoracotomy in blunt trauma. J Trauma 22:487, 1982

74. van der Sande JJ, Emeis JJ, Lindeman J: Intravascular coagulation: a common phenomenon in minor experimental head injury. J Neurosurg 54:21, 1981

75. Bick RL: Disseminated intravascular coagulation. CRC Press, Boca Raton, 1983

76. Valeri CR, Cassidy G, Khuri S et al: Hypothermia-induced reversible platelet dysfunction. Ann Surg 205: 175, 1987

77. Mahajan SL, Myers TH, Baldini MG: Disseminated intravascular coagulation during rewarming following hypothermia. JAMA 245:2517, 1981

78. Carden D, Nowak RM: Disseminated intravascular coagulation in hypothermia (letter). JAMA 247:2099, 1982

79. Bick RL: Disseminated intravascular coagulation and related syndromes: a clinical review. Semin Thromb Hemost 14:299, 1988

80. Rohrer MJ, Natale AM: Effect of hypothermia on the coagulation cascade. Crit Care Med 20:1402, 1992

81. Gando S, Tedo I, Kubota M: Post-trauma coagulation and fibrinolysis. Crit Care Med 20:594, 1992

82. Ciavarella D, Reed RL, Counts RB et al: Clotting factor levels and the risk of diffuse microvascular bleeding in the massively transfused patient. Br J Haematol 67: 365, 1987

83. Honig CL, Bove JR: Transfusion-associated fatalities: review of Bureau of Biologics reports 1976–1978. Transfusion 20:653, 1980

84. Blumberg N, Agarwal MM, Chuang C: Relation between recurrence of cancer of the colon and blood transfusion. BMJ 290:1037, 1985

85. Burrows L, Tartter P: Blood transfusions and colorectal cancer recurrence: a possible relationship. Transfusion 23:419, 1983

86. Tartter PI, Burrows L, Kirschner P: Perioperative blood transfusion adversely affects prognosis after resection of stage I (subset NO) non-oat cell lung cancer. J Thorac Cardiovasc Surg 88:659, 1984

87. Mezrow CK, Bergstein I, Tartter PI: Postoperative infection following autologous and homologous blood transfusions. Transfusion 32:27, 1992

88. Murphy P, Heal JM, Blumberg N: Infection or suspected infection after hip replacement surgery with autologous or homologous blood transfusions. Transfusion 31:212, 1991

89. Agarwall N, Murphy JG, Caytenm CG, Stahl WM: Blood transfusion increases the risk of infection after trauma. Arch Surg 128:171, 1993

90. Foster RS, Foster JC, Costanza MC: Blood transfusions and survival after surgery for breast cancer. Arch Surg 119:1138, 1984

91. Ota D, Alverez L, Lichtiger B et al: Perioperative blood transfusion in patients with colon carcinoma. Transfusion 25:392, 1985

92. Bunker JP: Metabolic effects of blood transfusions. Anesthesiology 27:446, 1966

93. Valeri CR, Gray AD, Cassidy GP et al: The 24-hour post-transfusion survival, oxygen transport function, and residual hemolysis of human outdated-rejuvenated red cell concentrate after washing and storage at 4 degrees C for 24 to 72 hours. Transfusion 24:323, 1984

94. Kruskall MS, Mintz PD, Bergin JJ et al: Transfusion therapy in emergency medicine. Ann Emerg Med 17: 327, 1988

95. Wolfe LC: The membrane and lesions of storage in preserved red cells. Transfusion 25:185, 1985

Transfusion Therapy in Obstetrics and Gynecology

Mark E. Boyd

A number of reasons justify the separate consideration of the transfusion needs of women. First, in comparison to men, women are somewhat anemic. They have adapted to that state by improving the efficiency of their red blood cells. This increase in efficiency has been achieved through an elevated level of 2,3-disphosphoglycerate (2,3-DPG) in their erythrocytes. This compound, a by-product of glucose metabolism, decreases the binding of hemoglobin to oxygen and thus increases the ease with which oxygen is released into the tissue. As a result of this change, the need for red blood cell transfusion in women may be less.[1]

Proper therapy requires an understanding of particular problems. The hemorrhagic complications of pregnancy will be unfamiliar to most nonobstetricians. Furthermore, there are practical reasons for the discussion. Obstetric and gynecologic patients make considerable demands on blood transfusion services. These demands do not reflect a high rate of transfusion following either childbirth or gynecologic surgery, since in both instances, the percentage of patients who are transfused is low. The number of units of blood transfused is high simply because the population at risk is enormous; for example, in a single year, nearly 600,000 hysterectomies are performed in the United States[2]; in these operations, approximately 10 percent of patients require transfusions.[3]

Finally, all physicians will have an interest in the history of transfusion therapy as it relates to obstetric practice. Disseminated intravascular coagulation (DIC) was first described in a woman who had an abruptio placentae, incoagulable blood, and a fatal postpartum hemorrhage.[4] The Rh factor was first alluded to in the description of a transfusion reaction in a patient who had a postpartum hemorrhage following delivery of a stillborn hydropic infant.[5] James Blundell's seminal work in blood transfusion was stimulated by his desire to decrease the mortality caused by postpartum hemorrhage.[6]

Because the concerns of physicians who manage obstetric and gynecologic patients are distinct, this chapter is divided into two sections.

OBSTETRICS

There is no need to emphasize that hemorrhage is an important complication of pregnancy. There is, after all, an annual worldwide toll of some 300,000 women who die from postpartum hemorrhage. Fortunately, in the industrialized countries, improved medical care and easier access to blood transfusion have dramatically reduced, but have failed to eliminate, such deaths.[7] Hemorrhage is still the largest single cause of maternal death in the developed world.[8] Although blood transfusion plays a role in treating postpartum hemorrhage, it is a minor one, as discussed later in this chapter. Prevention, plus early recognition and treatment of postpartum hemorrhage are the keys to success in dealing with this problem. The physiologic adaptations that prepare the woman for delivery are discussed and the causes and management of increased blood loss detailed.

Preparation for Delivery

Decisions about transfusion must take into account the dramatic physiologic changes that occur during pregnancy.

Cardiovascular Changes

Within weeks of conception, there is a generalized vasodilation and increase in cardiac output. By the end of the 24th week, cardiac output has increased by 30 percent, at which time it reaches a plateau. For the most part, the increased cardiac output is the result of an increased heart rate.

Plasma volume shows a gradual increase (on the order of 50 percent), from approximately 2,600 to 3,850 ml in a 60-kg woman. The increased flow is divided on a nearly equal basis among the kidneys, the skin, and the uterus. The increased plasma volume will offset some of the blood loss that accompanies delivery.

Since there is a 15 percent increase in red blood cells (1,500 to 1,750 ml), the increase in plasma is disproportionately high, causing the hematocrit to fall to 0.32. The resultant change in blood viscosity reduces the resistance to blood flow and lightens the work for the heart.

Coagulation Factor Changes

The changes in the coagulation factors are more complex. Fetoplacental exchange occurs from pools of blood which are located in the intervillous spaces of the placenta. In these stagnant pools, there is excessive coagulation of the blood, leading to an increase in local fibrinolysis.[9] These actions and reactions may be thought of as a low-grade DIC within the placenta.

Most blood coagulation factors increase during pregnancy. The major change is the increase in circulatory fibrinogen, although there are also substantial increases in factors VII, VIII, and X. An exception to this rule is the decline in platelet numbers.[10] Naturally occurring anticoagulants also increase, in-

cluding antithrombin III (ATIII), which counters factor X, and proteins C and S, which counter factors V and VIII. However, this increase is not proportionate to the increase in blood coagulation factors.

The fibrinolytic system becomes less active. Plasminogen is increased, although its activity is reduced by the placenta-derived plasminogen activator inhibitor type II. These changes produce a hypercoagulable state, which is helpful in the control of bleeding at delivery, in part by facilitating a massive deposit of fibrin onto the open placental site. However, there are negative consequences, as these changes also make pregnant women susceptible to pulmonary emboli and DIC.

Uterine Vasculature Changes

Fibrin infiltrates the smooth muscle in the spiral arteries of the pregnant uterus. As a result, the vessels can both dilate in order to accommodate the increased blood flow that accompanies pregnancy and contract at delivery. A few minutes before birth, some 500 ml/min of blood, one-fourth of the patient's cardiac output, flows through the placenta. The very life of the mother will depend on her ability to arrest this massive blood flow from torn vessels within seconds of delivery. Throughout most of the body, vasospasm and blood clot formation control bleeding. Placental site hemorrhage is controlled by contraction of the uterine musculature, which in turn obliterates the lumen of the intramural spiral vessels. This process would be impossible if they only contained their smooth muscle complement.

Postpartum Hemorrhage

Postpartum hemorrhage is defined as the loss of 500 ml of blood within 24 hours of birth. The definition includes 17 percent of all vaginal deliveries. Within that group, 13 percent lose 500 to 999 ml; the remaining 4 percent lose more than 1,000 ml.[11] Patients who have a hemoglobin level within the normal range withstand the loss of 500 ml of blood without a change in clinical signs.

Etiology of Obstetric Hemorrhage

The leading causes of postpartum hemorrhage are uterine atony, laceration, and DIC. Well over 95 percent of all postpartum hemorrhage occurs because of inadequate contraction of the uterus following delivery of the infant.[12] Anything associated with poor uterine contractions, such as primiparity, induction of labor, prolonged labor, multiple gestation, or amnionitis, is a risk factor for postpartum hemorrhage. In the presence of a well-contracted uterus, bleeding is generally caused by lacerations of the genital tract. In a study of 3,052 women who underwent cesarean delivery, hemorrhage was associated with the use of general anesthesia, preeclampsia, amnionitis, protracted labor and Hispanic ethnicity.[13]

Disseminated Intravascular Coagulation

On occasion, obstetric hemorrhage is caused by failure of the blood to coagulate. In earlier times, the patient was said to have cadaver blood. As this name implies, such a condition could never have been regarded as anything but an ominous sign. Although the poor prognosis is perhaps less true today, at the end stage, most patients who die from postpartum hemorrhage die with DIC.

DIC is the cumulation of a chain of events initiated by the release of excessive amounts of thromboplastin (see below). When factor X is activated, widespread intravascular coagulation results. Coagulation factors are consumed, and a compensatory and excessive fibrinolysis ensues. The fibrinolytic process breaks down the cross-links in fibrin, so that fibrin split products are formed, one of which is the D-dimer fragment. The split products interfere with clot formation and uterine muscle function. The patient bleeds more because the uterus does not contract; the shock worsens because the heart contracts poorly. With ongoing bleeding, oxygen delivery to different organs becomes insufficient, leading to renal tubal necrosis, adult respiratory distress, and/or microangiopathic hemolysis.

It is easier to describe the familiar patterns of coagulation than to decide how to treat the problem. Controlled trials have been impossible for several reasons. DIC in the obstetric patient is uncommon; it has a number of causes and, more often than not, is transient and self-correcting. Treatment should therefore be aimed at its cause, not at its effects, which are always secondary to some pathologic process. DIC will almost always resolve if the uterus is emptied, and the blood volume is maintained. When that is done, the reticuloendothelial system is able to remove activated coagulant factors and to replace the depleted coagulation factors.

Initiating Factors for Disseminated Intravascular Coagulation

DIC may be caused by abruptio placentae, fetal death, ammotic fluid embolism, and pre-eclampsia. In abruptio placentae, a hematoma forms behind the placenta and separates the placenta from the uterus. If the bleeding is extensive (approximately 2,500 ml), the separation will be complete, the mother will go into shock, and the fetus will die. One-third of such cases will be further complicated by DIC.[14] Treatment includes restoration of the depleted blood volume, delivery of the fetus, and correction of any coagulopathy. Cesarean section is performed if blood volume cannot be maintained with transfusion.

Thromboplastin from a dead fetus may initiate the intravascular coagulation. If the circulatory system is intact, this process can be blocked with heparin. Intravascular infusion of amniotic fluid causes pulmonary vascular obstruction and respiratory collapse. Most patients die from the circulatory insult. Of those who survive, nearly one-half will develop DIC. Management in these patients is supportive.

The picture in pre-eclampsia is confusing. These patients have high blood pressure and a low intravascular volume. The DIC that develops is unique. Thrombocytopenia is the most common finding; the liver enzymes are altered, and fibrin split products are often normal.[15] Management depends on delivery of the fetus and on cautious fluid management.

Other Causes of Obstetric Hemorrhage

Placenta Previa

Because the placenta is located on the lower segment of the uterus, the usual mechanisms for control of bleeding are unable to operate. The spiral arteries are not compressed because the muscle in the lower segment is scanty. The placenta is unable to separate cleanly because it has invaded deeply. Finally, the lower segment may be injured during attempts at manual removal of the placenta.

It can be predicted that patients with placenta previa will suffer excessive blood loss and will need a blood transfusion, especially if the patient has had a previous cesarean section.[16] In this circumstance, one-half of the patients will require a hysterectomy in order to control blood loss.[17] It is therefore judicious to ensure that an obstetrician is present who can make an early decision to perform this technically demanding operation.

Chronic Defects of Hemostasis

Chronic defects of hemostasis require specific treatment (see Chs. 8 and 27). Pregnant patients with diseases, such as von Willebrand's disease or idiopathic thrombocytopenic purpura (ITP) or who are obligate carriers of hemophilia are subject to postpartum hemorrhage. For the most part, any postpartum hemorrhage can be managed with oxytocin. Continued bleeding, in particular bleeding from episiotomy or lacerations, will require specific therapy. In addition, patients with ITP may need platelets and intravenous γ-globulin. (see Ch. 45) On occasion, patients who have von Willebrand's disease may have platelet dysfunction as well.[18]

Management of Obstetric Hemorrhage

Obstetric hemorrhage may be massive; most often, it is unpredictable. Well-defined agreed-upon guidelines for the management of severe hemorrhage should be in place, and, at periodic intervals, the plans must be reviewed and rehearsed. Management can be broken down into a number of parts. Patients are usually stabilized by the initial efforts. The early involvement of anesthetists and hematologists is crucial. Definitive surgery should be undertaken before the patient is moribund.

Assessment of the Patient

An apparently simple question presents an unexpectedly difficult problem. There is no easy way to measure obstetric blood loss. The only certainty is that the loss will be underestimated. A good rule of thumb is that the underestimation will be threefold.

Estimating blood loss from changes in a pregnant patients blood pressure or pulse is misleading and potentially dangerous because of the increased intravascular volume.[19] Changes in vital signs come from percentage changes in intravascular volume rather than absolute volume loss. A 60-kg woman has an intravascular blood volume approaching 6,000 ml during pregnancy. She can lose 1,000 ml (15 percent of her intravascular volume) and show no changes in vital signs. After losing 1,500 ml (25 percent of intravascular volume), she may only show a narrowing of pulse pressure and delay in venous filling. With a loss of 2,000 ml (35 percent of intravascular volume), blood pressure will fall, and with loss of 2,500 ml (40 percent of intravascular volume) profound shock occurs. By contrast, the nonpregnant 60-kg woman who has a blood volume of 4,000 ml (2,000 ml less than her pregnant counterpart) will have mild shock with the sudden loss of 750 ml and severe shock with the loss of 1,000 ml.

Assessment is further complicated by the effect of the intravenous fluids. Most patients who are in labor or who are bleeding receive intravenous fluids, which to some extent replace the intravascular volume. In such a circumstance a decline in blood pressure often indicates a blood loss on the order of 2,500 to 3,000 ml, or one-half the patient's blood volume. Another compounding factor is the use of epidural anesthesia with its vasodilation.

A central venous pressure catheter should be inserted if the urine output is inadequate. An insertion site in an arm vein is preferred over the subclavian or jugular veins because DIC may cause hematoma formation at the insertion site. If the patient has cardiac or renal disease, a pulmonary artery catheter is useful.

In most patients, there is no immediate concern for the patient's oxygen-carrying capacity. The first aim is therefore to refill the intravascular compartment so that circulation can be maintained. For every unit of blood that has been lost, 3 units of crystalloid, either isotonic saline or Ringer's lactate, should be infused. If the patient improves, no further treatment is required. The physician should be aware that visual estimates of blood loss typically underestimate actual losses, so replacement formulas must take this into consideration.[19]

Hematologic Studies

Following hemorrhage, periodic blood and platelet counts are conducted. Platelets are not immediately replaced and are a good indication of any ongoing process. The most practical means for monitoring DIC is with the prothrombin time (PT) and partial thromboplastin time (PTT). The specific test for DIC is the thrombin time (TT), which is increased if fibrinogen has been depleted or if fibrin degradation products (FDPs) are increased. Active bleeding can be expected if the fibrinogen is less than 100 mg/dl (normal, 300 to 600 mg/dl). FDPs are measured using a monoclonal antibody (MAb) to the D-dimer fragment. However, management of DIC is not based on the values of fibrinogen or FDPs, since, more often than not, the crisis will be passed by the time they are available.

Nonsurgical Management

Control of bleeding is an important principle that should always be kept in mind. In cases of postpartum hemorrhage, time and nature are not allies, and inaction is always dangerous. The placenta must be removed at an early stage with cord traction, and an oxytocic drug must be given.[20] All patients must be treated, because it is impossible to predict which women will raise their endogenous oxytocin to a satisfactory level.[21] The thrust of management is to cause the postpartum uterus to contract.

The mainstay of treatment is the use of synthetic oxytocin (Syntocinon, Pitocin), which causes a rapid, short-lived contraction of the uterus. An infusion of 20 units of oxytocin in 1,000 ml is used, 10 ml/min, until the uterus is firmly contracted (an initial dose of 1 unit for 5 minutes). Both the dosage and route are arbitrary. A bolus intravenous dosage of 5 units can be used. The results, however, are problematic. It causes a tetanic uterine contraction of the uterus, but it is not recommended because of the risk of transient hypotension. It has also been suggested that the initial dosage in the infusion should be higher than 20 units.[11]

In case of oxytocin failure, the traditional choice is the use of ergometrine, a synthetic alkaloid that exerts a powerful oxytocic effect. This drug is widely used throughout the world. Yet, despite its efficacy and modest price, it has become unpopular in North America because it can cause hypertension and often nausea and vomiting.

A new alternative is the use of the prostaglandin analogue, (15s)-15-methyl prostaglandin $F_{2\alpha}$-tromethamine (HemAbate).[22] It is given as an intramuscular (IM) injection, 0.25 mg, which may be repeated once or twice. In 95 percent of oxytocin failures, it is effective.[12] In the rare instances in which the drug fails, manual examination of the genital tract must be performed. Such an examination usually will reveal other causes, most related to placental disorders or uterine lacerations. Aprotinin (Trasylol), used primarily in cardiac surgery, has been used successfully in one patient with postpartum hemorrhage and coagulopathy after other treatment methods had failed.[23]

Surgery

Hysterectomy may be needed if other treatment approaches fail. If surgery is performed, it should be definitive and undertaken in a timely fashion. A subtotal hysterectomy is often the prudent choice. In former years, peripartum hysterectomy was most often done because of uterine atony. With the availability of HemAbate, this pattern has changed. Placenta accreta occurring in patients with a history of previous cesarean section is the most common reason for emergency peripartum hysterectomy.[24]

Blood loss following cesarean section may be heavy. The method of removal of the placenta can influence the amount of blood loss in these patients. Magann et al.[25] showed in a prospective, randomized study of 100 patients that blood loss was lessened when the placenta was allowed to separate spontaneously compared to manual removal. Cho et al.[26] have described a method of placing circular sutures in the endometrium that helps reduce blood loss following placental separation.

Blood Component Therapy

Packed Red Blood Cells

Physicians in obstetric practice seldom resort to blood transfusion. In recent years, the trend has been noticeable.[28] Overall, the percentage of patients needing blood transfusion after vaginal delivery is 1 percent.[29,30] If cesarean section is performed, this rises to 2 to 6 percent.[13,31] The frequency of blood transfusion at cesarean section is subject to wide variation and has been reported to be as low as 0.1 and as high as 18 percent.[32,33] Nevertheless, in obstetrics, the majority (67 percent) of blood usage follows cesarean section.[34] This is understandable, because the risk factors for cesarean section are risk factors for an atonic uterus. Thus, the patient who undergoes cesarean section will lose blood at surgery and in addition will often be subject to an increased risk of postpartum hemorrhage.

It is best to have agreed-upon indications for red blood cell transfusion rather than relying on ad hoc decisions. The National Institutes of Health (NIH) blood product consensus conferences provide such guidelines.[35] They suggest that patients should not be transfused unless hemoglobin is less than 8 g/dl or packed cell volume (PCV) is less than 24 percent, and the patient is symptomatic or has evidence of ongoing blood loss. Unless these criteria are satisfied, there is no benefit in transfusing a stable patient who has suffered a postpartum hemorrhage because of an atonic uterus.[36] Adoption of the NIH guidelines on obstetric and gynecologic services has resulted in major decreases in the numbers of red blood cell units used and patients transfused.[37,38]

Most patients will have had their blood group determined in the antenatal period; in particularly urgent situations, uncrossmatched ABO and Rh(D) group-specific blood can be used with about a 0.25 percent risk of a transfusion reaction.[39] If the blood group is unknown, group O, Rh(D)-negative uncrossmatched blood can be used with no greater risk than with type-specific uncrossmatched blood. Type-specific blood should be used as soon as possible to conserve supplies of group O blood. A type and screen should be done and, if no unexpected antibodies are found, crossmatched blood, should be available within 20 minutes. By contrast, if unexpected antibodies are found, antibody identification and a full type and crossmatch will be needed (see Chs. 9 and 22).

Fresh Frozen Plasma

The use of fresh frozen plasma (FFP) is poorly defined and has never been scientifically assessed in the obstetric patient. FFP contains all coagulation factors except platelets. It is rich in fibrinogen, factors V and VIII, and antithrombin III (ATIII). The latter is very low in the DIC of obstetrics. FFP is used in order to correct coagulation deficiencies, but it should not be used to restore volume or as part of a replacement formula for patients who have had a massive transfusion (see below).

Cryoprecipitate

In obstetric practice, there is an infrequent need for cryoprecipitate. Since fluid overload is uncommon in obstetrics, the small volume of cryoprecipitate provides no major advantage. Its main use is in the management of DIC (see Ch. 18).

Platelets

Platelets may be low in DIC, or after a massive transfusion, or in patients who have idiopathic thrombocytopenia. They are used if the patient has surgical oozing and a platelet count of less than 50×10^9. Nonetheless, the count may be misleading, because pregnant patients have platelets that are young, large, and more than usually effective. Platelets should be ABO- and Rh specific because they contain some red blood cells. Rh-negative patients who receive platelets from an Rh-positive donor should receive anti-D immunoglobulin (RhoGam) to prevent alloimmunization.

Massive Blood Transfusion

Massive transfusion may be defined as the replacement of the patient's blood volume within 24 hours; in a pregnant woman this would amount to a 10-unit transfusion. Transfusions of this magnitude may lead to a decrease in coagulation factors. In the past, replacement formulas for the transfusion of 1 unit of FFP each with 5 to 6 units of packed cells were used. The formula fell out of favor when it was found that there was little relationship between units of FFP and packed cells and the patient's PT and PTT.[40] Furthermore, when coagulation abnormalities do occur, these formulas do not provide for adequate levels of replacement. Prophylactic component supplementation is both unnecessary and insufficient to correct consumptive disorders[40] (see Chs. 25 and 35).

Autologous Blood Transfusion

In obstetrics, there is little need or justification for autologous blood transfusion. Furthermore, a paucity of literature documents the safety of such donations for the fetus. The chance of needing any blood transfusion is low. Among 16,462 deliveries in Los Angeles, the incidence of at least 2-unit transfusions was 0.16 percent.[41] With the exception of patients who have had an antepartum hemorrhage, it was impossible to predict the need for transfusion.[31,41] Less than one-half of the women who received more than 3 units of blood had any antenatal risk factors.[42] In an analysis of 5,528 deliveries, instrument delivery, Sherman et al.[43] found uterine atony, placenta previa, retained products of conception, abruptio placentae, and coagulopathy to be associated with an increased need for blood products. Since these factors are difficult to predict preoperatively, the use of autologous predonation of blood is inappropriate to meet their needs. Finally, autologous blood transfusion in obstetrics is not cost effective.[41] Its main benefit is in reduction of patient anxiety over possible blood transfusion (see Ch. 11).

GYNECOLOGY

Women are subject to excessive menstrual blood loss (menorrhagia), which can lead to hysterectomy or myomectomy. During both operations, it is common to resort to red blood cell transfusion. This section describes the etiology and diagnosis of, and medical therapy for, menorrhagia. The place of transfusion as it relates to gynecologic surgery, including ectopic pregnancy, is then described.

Menorrhagia

Menorrhagia is defined as the loss of more than 80 ml of blood during the menstrual cycle.[44] Two-thirds of women who suffer such a loss will develop iron deficiency anemia.[45]

Diagnosis

It is distressing to have to acknowledge that much of our treatment is based on notoriously inaccurate data. If menstrual loss is carefully measured, the clinical diagnosis of menorrhagia will be confirmed in only 50 percent of cases.[46] The measurement involves the calorimetric quantification of the amount of blood on soiled napkins.[46] Medical literature dealing with menorrhagia is suspect unless the diagnosis has been confirmed in this way, but in practice we must depend on the less accurate clinical observation and indirect laboratory evaluation.

Menstrual history will correlate with excessive blood loss if the patient uses more than two pads at any one time, if the pads are changed more than once every 2 hours, if super pads are used, or if there is soiling of underclothes and nightclothes.[47]

Iron deficiency anemia can be taken as objective evidence of menorrhagia. In addition, it is useful to determine the ferritin level, which falls before the

hemoglobin does. However, it is unnecessary to measure thyroid function and progesterone levels or to screen for bleeding dyscrasias in every instance.

In selected patients, a pelvic ultrasound is done. If endometrial cancer is suspected, an endometrial biopsy is obtained. The traditional investigation of abnormal uterine bleeding is dilation and curettage (D&C), but this expensive and inefficient procedure has been superseded by hysteroscopy and directed biopsy.[48]

Etiology

In most instances, menorrhagia is the exaggeration of a normal physiologic event, menstruation. The excessive loss of blood is caused by an impairment in hemostasis at the endometrial level. The condition is brought on by a disturbance in prostaglandin balance and an increase in the local fibrinolytic process. For the most part, menorrhagia is seldom caused by a pathologic lesion or by a hormonal disturbance.

Bleeding from any traumatized surface is arrested within minutes by vasospasm and by the deposit of fibrin clot inside and outside the torn blood vessels. Menstruation, which is bleeding from the endometrial surface, is an exception to this rule because the bleeding continues over a number of days. It does so because the fibrinolytic system is activated locally and dissolves the fibrin clot within the uterus.[49] The process is initiated by plasminogen activator which increases in the latter part of the menstrual cycle.[50] Fibrinolytic activity can be confirmed by analysis of menstrual blood: menstrual blood does not contain fibrinogen; it has fibrin split products, and it does not clot. Fibrinolytic activity is especially active in women who have menorrhagia.[51,52]

There is evidence that prostaglandins are involved in the control of menstrual bleeding. Their precursor, arachidonic acid, and, phospholipase, the enzyme that governs its release, are present in high concentrations in the endometrium. The concentration of arachidonic acid follows the rise and fall of progesterone, although the proportions of the different prostaglandins change in patients who have menorrhagia, with the replacement of the vasoconstrictor $PGF_{2\alpha}$ by the vasodilatory PGE_2 and PGD_2.[53] Finally, medication that lowers the prostaglandin level diminishes menstrual bleeding.

Uterine fibroids, especially submucosal fibroids,

are an important cause of excessive menstrual loss. Patients with menorrhagia often have intramural fibroids, endometrial polyps, or minor degrees of adenomyosis, but 25 percent of patients who do not have menorrhagia have the same findings.[54] An occasional patient will have excessive loss as a result of a bleeding disorder.[55] Endometriosis, pelvic inflammatory disease (PID),[56] or thyroid disease[57] are not proven causes of menorrhagia.

Treatment

Medical Treatment

The aim of medical therapy is to control excessive menstrual loss by diminishing prostaglandin formation or fibrinolytic activity. This control can be achieved either directly by using nonsteroidal anti-inflammatory drugs (NSAIDs) or antifibrinolytic agents or indirectly by causing endometrial atrophy. If the endometrium is atrophic, there is little prostaglandin formation or fibrinolytic activity.

NSAIDs, which prevent the breakdown of arachidonic acid to its active component, cyclic endoperoxide, are often used as the first line of treatment because they are inexpensive, have few side effects, and can be used for long periods. Mefenamic acid is prescribed as 500 mg tid. Despite these advantages, the decrease in blood loss that results (20 percent) may be insufficient to return menstrual loss to normal.[58,59]

Antifibrinolytic agents are more effective because they reduce blood loss by 54 percent.[60,61] They do present some practical problems. Prescribed as tranexamic acid, 3 to 6 g/day, these drugs have never been popular in North America because they cause gastrointestinal side effects and may cause thrombotic complications.

At the endometrial level progesterone acts as an antiestrogenic agent. If used for prolonged periods (at least 1 month), it causes endometrial atrophy and thereby reduces blood loss.[62] The use of progesterone in this way is not to be confused with the short-term use of medroxyprogesterone (Provera) in the regulation of anovulatory cycles.[63] Provera will produce regular menses in anovulatory patients, but the total blood loss is unchanged.

There are a number of ways to prescribe progesterone. In the usual circumstances, an oral contraceptive, which contains a potent progestational agent, is used. The result is a 50 percent decrease in blood loss.[63] The same hormone can be released from an intrauterine device (IUD) or subdermal implants. In both instances, there is a marked diminution of blood loss.[64,65]

Danazol, through its effect on gonadotropin secretion, causes endometrial atrophy and a 60 percent decrease in menstrual loss.[61] Side effects from a minimal dose of 200 mg/day will cause one-half of patients to stop therapy within 2 or 3 months.

Complete suppression of ovarian function can be achieved with the use of gonadotropin-releasing hormone (GnRH) analogues. The pituitary is downregulated; menstruation ceases in 1 or 2 months, but the medication's side effects and its expense are such that it is usually reserved for preoperative preparation.

Hysterectomy

Hysterectomy is the definitive treatment for menorrhagia. It is often resorted to because medical therapy was ineffective or had unacceptable side effects. One-half of all hysterectomies are undertaken for menorrhagia or fibroids, and many of the operations for fibroids are performed because of the associated bleeding.[66–68]

There is an advantage to hysterectomy. The vast majority of patients are satisfied with operations that are done because of abnormal bleeding. Hysterectomy has the further benefit that associated symptoms such as dysmenorrhea, uterine prolapse, or urinary stress incontinence can be relieved at the same time.

Nevertheless, its disadvantages are also noteworthy. There is a considerable mortality; abdominal hysterectomy for benign disease is associated with 1 death for every 1,600 operations.[69] The morbidity may be as high as 40 percent.[67] Furthermore, the operation is an expensive one.

Preparation. Blood group and antibody screen testing are sufficient for abdominal and vaginal hysterectomy. A full crossmatch is appropriate if the patient has large pelvic masses or if radical surgery is to be performed. It is also appropriate if the patient has extensive pelvic inflammatory disease or is to undergo vaginal hysterectomy and repair.[70] The community experience with blood transfusion should be considered.

The use of predeposited autologous blood donation (PAD) for uncomplicated hysterectomy is controversial. Etchason et al.[71] showed that PAD in general is not cost effective, since there is a high wastage rate of the autologous units collected. The only support for its use appears to come from those who use autologous transfusion to lower an unusually high (18 percent) rate of allogeneic transfusion of women undergoing hysterectomy.[72] The substitution of autologous blood for allogeneic blood can reduce the risks associated with the latter in the 10 percent of patients who are transfused. Each physician should decide whether PAD will be beneficial, based on a review of his or her practice pattern, type of patient, and transfusion practices (see Ch. 11).

Metoprolol given as part of the patient's preoperative management may be helpful in reducing transfusion need. Jakobsen and Blom[73] have reported success in reducing blood loss associated with hypertensive responses during hysterectomy with this drug. Blood loss was reduced by approximately one-half in a randomized double-blind placebo-controlled study of patients undergoing elective hysterectomy.

Red Blood Cell Transfusion. Preoperative transfusion is infrequently given prior to hysterectomy. The large majority of transfusions that are done in association with hysterectomy are intraoperative. The infrequent use of preoperative transfusion is illustrated by the experience of Samra et al.[74] Of 48 transfused patients, 46 were transfused intraoperatively, and 2 were transfused in the immediate postoperative period.

The need for transfusion can generally be foreseen. Patients who have pelvic abscesses, severe endometriosis, large fibroids, or ovarian cancer or who undergo radical pelvic surgery are likely to have increased intraoperative blood loss. Intraoperative transfusion is initiated by intraoperative blood loss and resultant changes in the patient's vital signs that do not abate with crystalloid infusion. Patients who are anemic as a result of menorrhagia may require

early use of transfusion. Blood transfusion is performed in approximately 10 to 15 percent of patients undergoing a hysterectomy. The experience of Williamson and Greaves[75] is typical. Among 149 abdominal hysterectomies, 13 patients (9 percent) were transfused. The transfused patients received a mean of 2.92 units, but two patients received 8 or more units. In earlier times, transfusion rates were higher and averaged 15 percent.[67,76] The numbers of units transfused usually will approximate the number of units that are lost. In the series of Samra et al.,[74] all patients with blood loss of more than 1,000 ml were transfused.

Surgical Technique. Refinement of surgical techniques will result in a substantial decrease in operative blood loss and need for transfusion. Control of blood loss in the pelvis is especially dependent on proper exposure. The transverse muscle-cutting Maylard incision gives good access to the pararectal and paravesical spaces. Dissection of these spaces will allow for early ligature of the ovarian and uterine blood vessels. Pelvic surgeons should bear this in mind and make it the aim of their operation.

There are two areas that may be the site of particularly dangerous intraoperative bleeding. Trauma to the great veins of the pelvis may be the cause of frightening hemorrhage. Any pelvic vein can be ligated to control hemorrhage, but the prudent choice may be to ask the assistance of a vascular surgeon to repair major vessels. Bleeding from the presacral vessels often fails to respond to any of the usual maneuvers. Strangely enough, household thumbtacks have sometimes proved a lifesaving means of controlling venous bleeding from the sacral lacuna.[77]

Internal iliac ligation is sometimes done for uncontrollable pelvic hemorrhage. It may be useful for dealing with bleeding that originates from the vaginal wall, although the operation often fails because the internal iliac has numerous vertical and horizontal anastomoses. It anastomoses on the same side through the lumbar, middle sacral, and superior hemorrhoidal vessels and, to a lesser extent, to the opposite side. The ligation will reduce the pulse pressure in the uterine artery by 85 percent and the uterine blood flow by 48 percent.[78,79] In a stable postoperative patient, arterial embolization may be helpful.[80]

Endometrial Ablation

Menorrhagia can be managed by resecting or destroying the endometrium. The operation carries the immediate risks of excessive fluid absorption and uterine trauma, but the major concern with the operation is its inconsistent results. Furthermore, there is an ongoing chance that the patient will become pregnant and a long-term concern about the detection of endometrial cancer. The operation cannot, therefore, be recommended until controlled trials confirm both its safety and its efficacy.

Myomectomy

Following myomectomy, the transfusion rate is 20 percent.[81] Good surgical technique, which involves the use of a red rubber catheter as a tourniquet and Stansky vascular clamps, will reduce operative blood loss.[82] Further, but less important reductions come from the use of a dilute vasopressin (Pitressin; Parke-Davis, Morris Plains, NJ) solution, 20 units in 20 ml of normal saline, which is injected along the uterine incision line.

Ectopic Pregnancy

Over the past decade, with the improvement of medical care and blood transfusion services, the likelihood that a patient will die from ectopic pregnancy has decreased. Yet in spite of this improvement, ectopic pregnancy accounts for 12 percent of maternal deaths.[83] It is worrisome that one-half of the deaths occur among teenagers and nonwhite women who have not sought medical care. Other studies have also confirmed that substandard medical care contributes to a large proportion of these deaths.[8]

Some deaths occurred as a result of undue delay in diagnosis; that is, the attending physician had failed to consider the diagnosis in a woman of reproductive age who complained of abdominal pain. Other occasions involved the failure to do a laparoscopy on patients with a positive pregnancy test and an empty uterus on ultrasound examination. Still other deaths were caused by delayed or inadequate transfusions. Some patients succumbed while waiting for a transfusion that had been delayed for a full crossmatch. The opposite error also occurred, and patients died because of overtransfusion of solutes and blood.

REFERENCES

1. Friedman BA, Burns TL, Schork MA: An analysis of blood transfusion of surgical patients by sex: a quest for the transfusion trigger. Transfusion 20:179, 1980
2. Graves EJ: National Hospital Discharge Survey: Annual Summary, 1990. DHHS Publication no. PHS 92-1773. Vital and Health Statistics, series 13, no. 112. National Center for Health Statistics, Washington, DC, 1992
3. Friedman AJ, Haas ST: Should uterine size be an indication for surgical intervention in women with myomas? Am J Obstet Gynecol 168:751, 1993
4. DeLee JB: A case of fatal hemorrhagic diathesis, with premature detachment of the placenta. Am J Obstet Dis Wom Child 44:785, 1901
5. Levine P, Stetson R: An unusual case of intra-group agglutination. JAMA 113:126, 1939
6. Blundell J: Experiments on the transfusion of blood by the syringe. Medicochir Trans 9:56, 1818
7. Sachs BP, Brown DAJ, Driscoll SG et al: Maternal mortality in Massachusetts: trends and prevention. N Engl J Med 316:667, 1987
8. Great Britain Department of Health: Report on Confidential Enquires into Maternal Deaths in the United Kingdom 1988–1990. HMSO, London, 1994
9. Gerbasi FR, Bottoms S, Farag A, Mammen E: Increased intravascular coagulation associated with pregnancy. Obstet Gynecol 75:385, 1990
10. Burrows RF, Kelton JG: Thrombocytopenia at delivery: a prospective survey of 6715 deliveries. Am J Obstet Gynecol 162:731, 1990
11. McDonald SJ, Prendiville WJ, Blair E: Randomized controlled trial of oxytocin alone versus oxytocin and ergometrine in active management of third stage of labour. BMJ 307:1167, 1993
12. Oleen MA, Mariano JP: Controlling refractory atonic postpartum hemorrhage with Hemabate sterile solution. Am J Obstet Gynecol 162:205, 1990
13. Combs CA, Murphy EL, Laros RK Jr: Factors associated with hemorrhage in cesaerean deliveries. Obstet Gynecol 77:77, 1991
14. Pritchard JA, Brekken AL: Clinical and laboratory studies on severe abruptio placentae. Am J Obstet Gynecol 97:681, 1967
15. Leduc L, Wheeler JM, Kirshon B et al: Coagulation profile in severe preeclampsia. Obstet Gynecol 79:14, 1992
16. Kruskall MS, Leonard S, Klapholz H: Autologous blood donation during pregnancy: analysis of safety and blood use. Obstet Gynecol 70:938, 1987
17. Clark SL, Yeh Sy, Phelan JP et al: Emergency hysterec-

tomy for obstetric hemorrhage. Obstet Gynecol 64: 376, 1984

18. Greer IA, Lowe GD, Walker JJ, Forbes CD: Haemorrhagic problems in obstetrics and gynaecology in patients with congenital coagulopathies. Br J Obstet Gynaecol 98:909, 1991

19. Duthie SJ, Ven D, Yung GL et al: Discrepancy between laboratory determination and visual estimation of blood loss during normal delivery. Eur J Obstet Gynecol Reprod Biol 38:119, 1991

20. Prendiville WJ, Harding JE, Elbourne DR, Stirrat GM: The Bristol third stage trial: active versus physiological management of third stage of labour. BMJ 297:1295, 1988

21. Thornton S, Davison JM, Baylis PH: Plasma oxytocin during third stage of labour: comparison of natural and active management. BMJ 297:167, 1988

22. Hayashi RH, Castillo MS, Noah ML: Management of severe postpartum hemorrhage with a prostaglandin F_{2alpha} analogue. Obstet Gynecol 63:806, 1984

23. Valentine S, Williamson P, Sutton D: Reduction of haemorrhage with aprotinin. Anaesthesia 48:405, 1993

24. Sturdee DW, Rushton DI: Caesarean and post-partum hysterectomy 1968–1983. Br J Obstet Gynaecol 93: 270, 1986

25. Magann EF, Dodson MK, Albert JR et al: Blood loss at time of cesaerean section by method of placental removal and exteriorization versus in situ repair of the uterine incision. Surg Gynecol Obstet 177:389, 1993

26. Cho JY, Kim SJ, Cha KY et al: Interrupted circular suture: bleeding control during cesarean delivery in placenta praevia accreta. Obstet Gynecol 78:876, 1991

27. Naif RW, Chauhim SP, Chevalier SP et al: Prediction of hemorrhage at Cesarean delivery. Obstet Gynecol 77:77, 1991

28. Klapholz H: Blood transfusion in contemporary obstetrical practice. Obstet Gynecol 75:940, 1990

29. Gilbert L, Porter W, Brown VA: Postpartum haemorrhage. A continuing problem. Br J Obstet Gynaecol 94:67, 1987

30. Combs CA, Murphy EL, Laros RK: Factors associated with hemorrhage with vaginal birth. Obstet Gynecol 77:69, 1991

31. Dickason LA, Dinsmoor MJ: Red blood cell transfusion and cesarean section. Am J Obstet Gynecol 167: 327, 1992

32. Reisner LS: Type and screen for cesarean section: a prudent alternative. Anesthesiology 58:476, 1983

33. Gilstrap LC, Hauth JC, Hankins GDV et al: Effect of type of anesthesia on blood loss at cesarean section. Obstet Gynecol 69:328, 1987

34. Kamani AA, McMorland GH, Wadsworth LD: Utilization of red blood cell transfusion in an obstetric setting. Am J Obstet Gynecol 159:1177, 1988

35. National Blood Resource Education Program (US): Indications for the Use of Red Blood Cells, Platelets and Fresh Frozen Plasma. NIH Publication No. 89-2974A. US Department of Health and Human Services, Washington, DC, 1989

36. Morrison JC, Floyd RC, Martin RW et al: Blood transfusions after postpartum hemorrhage due to uterine atony. J Matern Fetal Invest 1:209, 1991

37. Morrison JC, Sumrall DD, Chevalier SP et al: The effect of provider education on blood utilization practices. Am J Obstet Gynecol 169:1240, 1993

38. Rosen NR, Bates LH, Herod G: Transfusion therapy: improved patient care and resource utilization. Transfusion 33:341, 1993

39. Blood Transfusion in Clinical Medicine: Mollison PL, Engelfriet CP, Contreras M (eds): Blackwell Scientific, 9th Ed., London, 1993, p. 111

40. Ciavarella D, Reed RL, Counts RB et al: Clotting factor levels and the risk of diffuse microvascular bleeding in the massively transfused patient. Br J Haematol 67: 365, 1987

41. Combs CA, Murphy EL, Laros RK: Cost-benefit analysis of autologous blood donation in obstetrics. Obstet Gynecol 80:621, 1992

42. Sherman SJ, Greenspoon JS, Nelson JM, Paul RH: Identifying the obstetric patient at high risk of multiple-unit blood transfusions. J Reprod Med 37:649, 1992

43. Sherman SJ, Greenspoon JS, Nelson JM et al: Obstetric hemorrhage and blood utilization. J Reprod Med 38:929, 1993

44. Hallberg L, Hogdahl AM, Nilsson L, Rybo G: Menstrual blood loss—a population study. Acta Obstet Gynecol Scand 45:320, 1966

45. Fairhurst E, Pale TL, Fidge BD: A comparison of anaemia and storage iron deficiency in working women. Proc Nutr Soc 36:98A, 1977

46. Fraser IS, McCarron G, Markham R: A preliminary study of factors influencing perception of menstrual blood loss volume. Am J Obstet Gynecol 149:788, 1984

47. Fraser IS: Treatment of menorrhagia. Bailliere's Clin Obstet Gynaecol 3:391, 1989

48. Gimpelson RJ, Rappold HD: A comparative study between panoramic hysteroscopy with directed biopsies and dilatation and curettage. Am J Obstet Gynecol 158:489, 1988

49. Christiaens GC, Sixma JJ, Haspels AA: Morphology of hemostasis in menstrual endometrium. Br J Obstet Gynaecol 87:425, 1980

50. Gleeson N, Devitt M, Sheppard BL, Bonnar J: Endometrial fibrinolytic enzymes in women with normal menstruation and dysfunctional uterine bleeding. Br J Obstet Gynaecol 100:768, 1993

51. Bonnar J, Sheppard BL, Dockerey CJ: The haemostatic system and dysfunctional uterine bleeding. Res Clin Forums 5:27, 1983

52. Hourihan HM, Sheppard BL, Brosens IA: Endometrial hemostasis. In D'Arcangues C, Fraser IS, Newton JR, Odlind V (eds): Contraception and Mechanisms of Endometrial Bleeding. Cambridge University Press, Cambridge, 1990

53. Smith SK, Abel MH, Kelly RW, Baird DT: Prostaglandin synthesis in the endometrium of woman with ovular dysfunctional uterine bleeding. Br J Obstet Gynaecol 88:434, 1981

54. Fraser IS: Hysteroscopy and laparoscopy in women with menorrhagia. Am J Obstet Gynecol 162:1264, 1990

55. van Eijkeren MA, Christiaens GC, Haspels AA, Sixma JJ: Measured menstrual blood loss in women with a bleeding disorder or using oral anticoagulant therapy. Am J Obstet Gynecol 162:1261, 1990

56. Fraser IS, McCarron G, Markham R et al: Measured menstrual blood loss in women with menorrhagia associated with pelvic disease or coagulation disorder. Obstet Gynecol 68:630, 1986

57. Scott JC, Mussey E: Menstrual patterns of myxedema. Am J Obstet Gynecol 90:161, 1964

58. Dockeray CJ, Sheppard BL, Bonnar J: Comparison between mefenamic acid and danazol in the treatment of established menorrhagia. Br J Obstet Gynaecol 96:840, 1989

59. Fraser IS, McCarron G: Randomized trial of 2 hormonal and 2 prostaglandin-inhibiting agents in women with a complaint of menorrhagia. Aust NZ Obstet Gynaecol 31:66, 1991

60. Andersch B, Milsom I, Rybo G: An objective evaluation of flurbiprofen and tranexamic acid in the treatment of idiopathic menorrhagia. Acta Obstet Gynecol Scand 67:645, 1988

61. Nilsson L, Rybo G: Treatment of menorrhagia. Am J Obstet Gynecol 110:713, 1971

62. Cameron IT, Haining RH, Lumsden MA et al: The effects of mefenamic acid and norethisterone on measured menstrual blood loss. Obstet Gynecol 76:85, 1990

63. Fraser IS: Treatment of ovulatory and anovulatory dysfunctional uterine bleeding with oral progestogens. Aust NZ J Obstet Gynaecol 30:353, 1990

64. Andersson JK, Rybo G: Levonorgestrel-releasing intrauterine device in the treatment of menorrhagia. Br J Obstet Gynaecol 97:690, 1990

65. Milsom I, Andersson JK, Andersch B, Rybo G: A comparison of flurbiprofen, tranexamic acid, and a levonorgestrel-releasing intrauterine contraceptive device in the treatment of idiopathic menorrhagia. Am J Obstet Gynecol 164:879, 1991

66. Easterday CL, Grimes DA, Riggs JA: Hysterectomy in the United States. Obstet Gynecol 62:203, 1983

67. Dicker RC, Greenspan JR, Strauss LT et al: Complications of abdominal and vaginal hysterectomy among women of reproductive age in the United States. Am J Obstet Gynecol 144:841, 1982

68. Lee NC, Dicker RC, Rubin GL, Ory HW: Confirmation of the preoperative diagnoses for hysterectomy. Am J Obstet Gynecol 150:283, 1984

69. Boyd ME, Groome PA: The morbidity of abdominal hysterectomy. Can J Surg 36:155, 1993

70. Mintz PD, Sullivan MF: Preoperative crossmatch ordering and blood use in elective hysterectomy. Obstet Gynecol 65:389, 1985

71. Etchason J, Calhoun L, Petz LD et al: Cost effectiveness analysis of a predeposited autologous donation (PAD) program. Blood, suppl 1. 82:394a, 1993

72. Chambers LA, Kruskall MS: Preoperative autologous blood donation. Transfus Med Rev 4:35, 1990

73. Jakobsen CJ, Blom L: Effect of preoperative metoprolol on cardiovascular and catecholamine response and bleeding during hysterectomy. Eur J Anaesthesiol 9:209, 1992

74. Samra SK, Friedman BA, Beitler PJ: A study of blood utilization in association with hysterectomy. Transfusion 23:490, 1983

75. Williamson LM, Greaves M: Blood usage for elective surgery. A reappraisal of the need for autologous transfusion. Clin Lab Haematol 11:233, 1989

76. Amirikia H, Evans TN: Ten-year review of hysterectomies: trends, indications, and risks. Am J Obstet Gynecol 134:431, 1979

77. Timmons MC, Kohler MF, Addison WA: Thumbtack use for control of presacral bleeding, with description of an instrument for thumbtack application. Obstet Gynecol 78:313, 1991

78. Burchell RC: Internal iliac artery ligation: hemodynamics. Obstet Gynecol 24:737, 1964

79. Clark SL, Phelan JP, Yeh SY et al: Hypogastric artery ligation for obstetrical hemorrhage. Obstet Gynecol 66:353, 1985

80. O'Hanlan KA, Trambert J, Rodriguez-Rodriguez L et

al: Arterial embolization in the management of abdominal and retroperitoneal hemorrhage. Gynecol Oncol 34:131, 1989

81. LaMorte AI, Lalwani S, Diamond MP: Morbidity associated with abdominal myomectomy. Obstet Gynecol 82:897, 1993

82. Boyd ME: Practical Gynecologic Surgery: Principles in Practice. Urban & Schwarzenberg, Baltimore, 1989

83. Cartwright PS: Incidence, epidemiology, risk factors, and etiology. p. 32. In Stovall TG, Ling FW (eds): Extrauterine Pregnancy: Clinical Diagnosis and Management. McGraw-Hill, New York, 1993

Chapter 27

Management of Surgical Patients with Special Problems

Richard K. Spence

Operating on a patient with congenital bleeding disorder may be one of the most challenging and frightening tasks confronting the surgeon—challenging because of the need to control bleeding with unfamiliar methods, frightening because of the unpredictable nature of the patient's response to conventional therapy. Fortunately, significant therapeutic advances aided by a clearer understanding of the major disorders—the hemophilias and von Willebrand's disease—offer some help with these problems.

Successful management of patients with hemophilia or von Willebrand's disease requires a basic knowledge of the diseases as a first step. Both disorders are also discussed in Chapter 8; this chapter emphasizes treatment guidelines for the surgeon.

CONGENITAL COAGULATION FACTOR DEFICIENCIES

Hemophilia A and B

Hemophilia A is defined as an inherited deficiency of the procoagulant factor VIII, also known as antihemophilic factor (AHF). Hemophilia B is an inherited deficiency of functional procoagulant factor IX, also known as plasma thromboplastin component (PTC), or Christmas factor. Both protein cofactors are essential for normal blood coagulation. Since both are X chromosome linked, they appear as a clinical deficiency in hemizygous males, with the disorder transmitted through carrier females.[1]

Factors VIII and IX are synthesized in a variety of tissues, with exact sites still not completely known.[2] The liver appears to be the predominant production site, as evidenced by the reversal of hemophilia, following successful orthotopic liver transplantation.[3] Both factors circulate in an inactive form as procoagulants. Factor VIII forms a noncovalent complex with von Willebrand factor (vWF), which protects it from proteolysis and allows it to concentrate at bleeding sites. It is cleaved by thrombin to initiate activity, a process requiring calcium and phospholipid. Factor IX can be activated through either the intrinsic pathway via tissue factor and/or activated factors VII and IX or the extrinsic pathway via tissue factor and activated factor IX.[4] Both processes require calcium.

The incidence of the hemophilias is probably in the range of 20 per 100,000 males.[1] Hemophilia A makes up 80 percent of this number. Clinical manifestations are similar for both and, because the disorders are heterogeneous, clinical severity correlates well with extent of the factor deficiency.[5] Normal plasma concentrations for factors VIII and IX are usually defined in comparison to a reference standard presumed to have 100 percent levels. Normal ranges for both factors are 50 to 200 percent of the standard, or 0.5 to 2.0 U/ml.[1]

Severe deficiencies are defined as those in which less than 1 percent of normal plasma levels are detectable. These patients have a history of easy bruising, spontaneous hemarthroses, and muscle bleeding. Gingival bleeding and epistaxis are common; bleeding from minor cuts may be minimal in amount but persistent. Spontaneous hematoma formation in the psoas muscle or in muscles of the retroperitoneum may mimic appendicitis. Closed-space hemorrhage into muscles of the forearm may lead to Volkmann's ischemic contracture.[6]

Similar hemorrhage into the confined spaces of the neck may cause airway obstruction or nerve entrapment. Surgeons should be alerted to the possible existence of hemophilia in the male patient who presents with one of these problems anew.[7] Hematuria may develop, leading to renal colic.[8] Intracranial bleeding following minor trauma is a serious problem, causing death in 25 percent of affected patients.[1,9] Gastrointestinal bleeding is unusual.

Moderately severe hemophiliacs are those with 1 to 5 percent of normal factor levels. These patients tend to have fewer episodes of spontaneous bleeding. Hemorrhage is seen most often with identifiable trauma. Post-traumatic bleeding is usually delayed because platelets produce initial hemostasis.[1] Mild hemophiliacs, with 6 to 25 percent of normal factor concentrations, typically bleed only following surgery or after severe injury. Because these patients may escape diagnosis until adult life, they represent the potential problem of prolonged and potentially fatal postoperative bleeding for the surgeon.

Management

The treatment of hemophilia has undergone steady evolution over the past 30 years. Successful treatment using whole blood transfusion was first described by Lane[10] in 1840. Factor VIII-rich cryoprecipitates, first produced during the 1960s, became the mainstay of therapy for the next 20 years.[11] Subsequent improvement through purification of factor concentrates lead to the production of lyophilized virus-inactivated products (reviewed in Ch. 8). These concentrates have greatly reduced the risk of transmission of the hepatitis and eliminated human immunodeficiency virus (HIV), with only anecdotal cases still being reported.[12,13] Virus-free recombinant DNA-derived factor VIII, available since the late 1980s, has proved both safe and effective.[14] An added benefit of recombinant factor VIII is its acceptability by the rare Jehovah's Witness with hemophilia. A surgical cure of hemophilia is available in the form of orthotopic liver transplantation.[3]

The surgeon should be familiar with some general principles of therapy in the hemophilic patient. The activity of replacement factors is calculated in units, 1 unit being the activity of the factor found in 1 ml of pooled citrated fresh frozen plasma (the reference standard noted above). Sufficient factor must be given to allow for the distribution, metabolism, and clearance of the product, all of which are reflected in the factor half-life.[15] Factor VIII has a half-life of 8 to 12 hours; factor IX survives considerably longer, with a half-life of 24 hours. Therapeutic effectiveness must be determined by both clinical response and by repeated assays of factor VIII or IX, as patients will vary in response and may have inhibitor antibodies. Measurements of bleeding time or prothrombin time/activated partial thromboplastin time (PT/aPTT) should not be used, as these are misleading.[15]

In patients with hemophilia A, factor VIII levels 80 to 100 percent of normal should be attained prior to surgery by infusion of factor concentrates. Mild hemophiliacs who have some normal factor VIII may respond to DDAVP (desmopressin), given in doses of 0.3 g/kg IV, by elevating circulating factor VIII levels two- to four-fold.[16] Surgery has been performed successfully in patients with factor VIII levels as low as 5 percent, using only DDAVP therapy.[16–18] DDAVP works by releasing vWF from storage sites; vWF then binds to factor VIII, stabilizes it, and carries it in the circulation. Since DDAVP does not directly increase factor VIII, it is ineffective in patients with severe hemophilia.[19] Factor VIII levels should be kept within the 30 to 50 percent range by reinfusing concentrate at 8- to 12-hour intervals during the postoperative period. An alternative approach is to use a dose-adjusted continuous infusion of factor VIII.[20] Therapy typically continues for 7 to 10 days or longer, depending on the extent and type of surgery performed.

Dosage

The dose of factor VIII needed can be calculated on the assumption that each unit of factor VIII infused per kilogram body weight raises plasma VIII levels 2 percent.[21] For example, a 70-kg patient who is to undergo surgery will need an 80 to 100 percent plasma factor VIII level preoperatively. Assuming that the patient has no circulating factor VIII, an initial infusion to attain a 100 percent level will require 3,500 units (100 percent × 70 kg = 7000/2), followed by repeat infusions of 2,800 to 3,000 units (80 to 85 percent × 70 kg = 5,600 − 6,000/2) every 8 to 12 hours, to compensate for the short half-life of factor VIII over the next 7 to 10 days. It must be remembered that the calculated dose is only an estimate. It is critical to measure postinfusion factor VIII levels for at least 1 to 2 days postoperatively and correct as needed.

Levels of factor IX for surgery in hemophilia B patients should be raised initially to at least 80 to 100 percent of normal, and maintained at 40 percent for 2 to 3 days, then 20 percent for 7 to 10 days.[1] Infusion doses can be calculated in a fashion similar to that used for factor VIII, with two important differences: (1) the half-life of factor IX is approximately 24 hours, and (2) each unit of factor IX replacement given per kilogram body weight will increase plasma IX levels by only 1 percent. If we assume complete absence of factor IX in our 70-kg male with hemophilia B, we must give 5,600 units initially (80 percent × 70 kg = 5,600 units), followed by 2,800 units every 24 hours (longer half-life) for 2 to 3 days, then 1,400 U/day for 7 to 10 days.

In hemophilia B, fresh frozen plasma can be used if the amount needed is small and bleeding is expected to be minimal. Otherwise, factor IX concentrates should be used. Unfortunately, when administered as prothrombin complex concentrates these products frequently contain other procoagulants, such as factors II, VII, and X. Administration of large doses has been associated with thrombotic complications, including deep vein thrombosis and pulmonary embolism.[22] The simultaneous administration of subcutaneous heparin (5,000 units every 8 hours) with factor IX concentrate may minimize this problem.[1] Recently, purified factor IX concentrates have become available and should be considered, taking into account costs and availability.

Inhibitors of Factor VIII

Unfortunately, otherwise straightforward therapy in the hemophiliac is complicated by the presence of IgG inhibitor antibodies specific for factor VIII. Their incidence ranges from 5 percent to 10 percent of all patients with hemophilia A, and up to 15 per-

cent in those with the severe form of the disease.[23] Most antibodies are detectable 2 to 3 days after exposure to factor VIII. Inhibitor activity is determined in Bethesda units, relying on a 2-hour incubation of dilutions of a patient's plasma with normal plasma. A sample that demonstrates residual factor VIII activity of 50 percent of normal is considered to contain 1 Bethesda unit of inhibitor/ml of plasma. Patients are separated into low (less than 5 units), moderate (5 to 30 units), and high (greater than 30 units) responders. Those with low titers make up 20 to 25 percent of affected patients; "high-responders" represent 65 to 75 percent.[1] The presence of inhibitors should be suspected if transfused factor VIII does not have the expected effect or has a shorter than usual half-life.

Surgery in Patients With Inhibitors to Factor VIII

Because of the high incidence and serious effect of inhibitors, all hemophiliacs who are surgical candidates should be evaluated for the presence of inhibitors; titers should be measured to determine their responder category. Three therapeutic choices are available to the surgeon if inhibitors are present: (1) to raise factor VIII levels by infusing more product, either human or porcine, (2) if the titer is high, to perform maneuvers to lower it, or (3) to use hemostatic material that bypasses the need for factor VIII, that is, recombinant factor VII or IX concentrates. These approaches may be used in combination with beneficial effect. Patients with inhibitors are best managed in consultation with a hematologist or specialist in bleeding disorders.

Moderately high inhibitor levels can be lowered by plasmapheresis or extracorporeal immunoadsorption with staphylococcal protein A columns, followed by either replacement with porcine factor VIII or the use of factor IX to attain hemostasis.[24,25] If human factor VIII concentrate is used in the presence of inhibitors, Kasper[26] recommends an initial bolus of 70 to 140 U/kg, followed by either a continuous infusion of 4 to 14 U/kg or replacement with 40 U/kg plus 20 U/kg for every Bethesda unit each hour. In all cases, factor VIII levels must be assayed frequently and doses adjusted accordingly.

Alternatives to human factor VIII concentrates are available. Porcine concentrates may be used successfully, although approximately 25 percent of patients have cross-reacting inhibitors. A multicenter trial in 38 patients with severe bleeding, inhibitors and treatment failure showed an 84 percent response rate following infusion of porcine factor VIII.[27,28]

Both recombinant factor VIIa and factor IX act as bypassing agents.[23,29] The mechanism of action is uncertain, but these factors complex with tissue factor at the site of injury, leading to direct activation of the final common coagulation pathway through factor X, producing local hemostasis. Hedner et al and others[29,30] reported a small clinical experience in patients undergoing major surgery using recombinant factor VIIa with mixed results. Direct monitoring of factor VII levels is needed to guide therapy, with trough levels of greater than 5 U/ml required for hemostasis. The addition of tranexamic acid or ε-amino-caproic acid to prevent fibrinolysis of the hemostatic plug formed may be beneficial. The thrombotic side effects seen with factor IX must be taken into consideration if this product is to be used.[24]

Induction of immunotolerance to inhibitors has been accomplished by a variety of regimens, which have included the infusion of very large doses of factor VIII, alone or in conjunction with activated factor IX concentrates, corticosteroids, or cyclophosphamide.[31]

von Willebrand's Disease

von Willebrand's disease was first described in 1924 by Erich von Willebrand in Finland.[32] It is defined as the congenital presence of abnormal or reduced amounts of vWF.[33] Unlike the hemophilias, von Willebrand's disease follows an autosomal inheritance pattern and has numerous variations. Estimates of incidence vary from 3 to 4/100,000 to as high as 5 to 10/1,000, or roughly 1 percent of the population.[34]

The disorder can be classified by major type I, II, or III, each of which has subtypes. Type I, or classic von Willebrand's disease, is characterized a partial deficiency of vWF (IA) or dysfunctional vWF (IB).[35] Type I, the most common form, is found in 70 to 80 percent of affected patients.[33] Type II disease has three subgroups, all of which are characterized by reductions in factor VIII/vWF complex activities and the presence of abnormal multimers.[19,33] Type III von Willebrand's disease is defined as a severe quantitative deficiency of vWF. Spontaneous bleeding in von Willebrand's disease usually appears as mucocutaneous hemorrhage (e.g., epistaxis, menorrhagia,

and postpartum hemorrhage). Gastrointestinal hemorrhage has been reported as a manifestation of acquired disease but is uncommon in the congenital form.[36] Bruising in excess of that expected following minor trauma or bleeding at surgery (e.g., dental extraction or tonsillectomy) is a typical presentation.[37]

Diagnosis

Standard tests of coagulation function are of only limited use in the diagnosis of von Willebrand's disease. Bleeding time is almost always prolonged in severe von Willebrand's disease but may be normal in milder forms.[38] In severe cases, factor VIII, which depends on binding to vWF to circulate in the plasma, may be reduced, leading to prolongation of the activated partial thromboplastin time (aPTT).[33] However, aPTT is not reliable, as it may be normal in clinically significant disease. Factor VIII levels should be determined separately. Laboratory diagnosis of the disorder relies on detection of vWF:Ag by quantitative immunoelectrophoresis or enzyme-linked immunosorbent assay (ELISA). However, levels may be misleading because vWF is an acute-phase reactant that may be elevated immediately after surgery, trauma, stress, or pregnancy.[39]

Multiple assays for the different types of von Willebrand's disease must be performed to make an accurate diagnosis.[40] Determination of vWF multimers is a standard part of every evaluation, as treatment may vary, depending on the subgroup and plasma multimer concentration.[33] Assays for standard or complex multimers can be performed using immunoelectrophoresis. It is of note that 65 percent of patients with von Willebrand's disease are blood type O.[41]

Management

Treatment for von Willebrand's disease is usually unnecessary, except at surgery.[42] Three goals should be kept in mind: (1) elevate vWF plasma levels, (2) replace abnormal vWF with normal vWF, and (3) restore levels of factor VIII. vWF levels should be increased preoperatively to 80 to 100 U/dl and maintained above 40 U/dl for 2 to 3 days postoperatively. Factor VIII levels should be monitored to ensure they are maintained above 40 U/dl for 4 to 5 days or longer, depending on the extent of the surgery.

DDAVP, which releases vWF and factor VIII from storage, increasing plasma levels three- to four-fold, should be the first line of therapy, especially in patients with type IA disease.[19] However, DDAVP is contraindicated in patients with type 2B or type 3 von Willebrand's disease because of the potential for the development of a hypercoagulable state in the former and a lack of response in the latter. This drug is usually given intravenously in a dose of 0.3 g/kg body weight in 25 to 30 ml of saline over 30 minutes. The dose is repeated every 12 to 24 hours, depending on response, determined by checking vWF ristocetin cofactor activity (vWF:R:Co).[43] This assay is used to determine the efficacy of treatment, because the bleeding time is not reliable. Side effects of DDAVP can be considerable; they include facial flushing, headache, tachycardia, and hypotension.[19] Because these are caused by vasodilation, they can be minimized by slowing the infusion rate.

Abnormal vWF can be replaced with normal vWF using either cryoprecipitate or those commercial factor VIII concentrates that contain vWF. Dosages are calculated on the assumption that each unit of factor VIII contains 1 unit of vWF and that the half-life of vWF is similar to factor VIII, although it is longer in reality. A 1-U/kg dose of vWF will increase plasma levels by 2 U/dl. Factor VIII levels are restored as though the patient had hemophilia. It is important to remember that patient response will vary depending on the type of von Willebrand's disease.

Other Congenital Coagulation Factor Deficiencies

Deficiencies of factors VII, II, X, V, and XII all have been reported.[1,44] All are rare and appear as a result of autosomal defects. Bleeding is usually not spontaneous, occurring only at surgery or during the postoperative period. Treatment is with fresh frozen plasma or specific factor replacement.[1]

Summary

Tables 27-1 and 27-2 summarize treatment of the hemophilias and von Willebrand's disease in the surgical patient. It is essential that the surgeon learn

Table 27-1. Perioperative Treatment of Bleeding Disorders

Disorder	Preoperative	Postoperative
Hemophilia A (Factor VIII)	*Goal:* Raise FVIII to 80–100% *Approach:* FVIII concentrate; no. of units = % × kg BW)/2 If inhibitors present: 70–150 U/kg bolus, then 5–15 U/kg qh or 40 U/kg plus 20 U/kg for each Bethesda unit qh human FVIII Plasmapheresis to remove inhibitor; replace FVIII with porcine or recombinant FVIII Recombinant FIX or VII	*Goal:* Maintain FVIII at 80–100% for 10–14 days *Approach:* Same as for preop; reinfuse every 8–12h (or longer if surgery extensive) Monitor FVIII levels as guide to therapy
Hemophilia B (factor IX)	*Goal:* Factor IX levels to 80–100% *Approach:* FIX concentrate; no. at of units = % × kg BW Use FFP if deficit and surgery minimal *Note:* FIX concentrate may cause thrombosis, consider adding heparin 5,000 units SC q8h	*Goal:* Maintain FIX levels at 40% for 2–3 days; then at 20% for 7–10 days or longer, depending on response. *Approach:* Same as preop; monitor FIX levels as guide to therapy
von Willebrand's disease (vWF)	*Goals:* Raise vWF to 80–100 U/dl Replace abnormal vWF Raise FVIII as needed *Approach:* (except in types 2B and 3): DDAVP: 0.3 g/kg IV in 20-ml saline over 30 minutes; repeat q12–24h if DDAVP not effective or not indicated, use FVIII concentrate Replace FVIII as needed	*Goals:* Maintain vWF at 40 U/dl for 2–3 days or longer as needed Maintain FVIII at 80–100% levels for 4–5 days or longer; monitor vWF:R:Co and FVIII as guide to therapy

Abbreviations: FVII, FVIII, FIX, factors VII, VIII, IX; vWF, von Willebrand factor.

Table 27-2. Plan for Surgical Patients With Inherited Bleeding Disorder

1. Preoperative consultation with experienced hematologist.
2. Explain risks of surgery and factor therapy in advance.
3. Look for inhibitor antibodies and measure titers.
4. If surgery is for a lesion that occurred because of suboptimal management of the underlying disease, especially hemophilia, maximize preoperative treatment to normalize as much as possible.
5. Avoid any and all aspirin or nonsteroidal anti-inflammatory drugs (NSAIDs) or platelet inhibiting medications.
6. Schedule surgery for a time when full laboratory facilities are available on ongoing basis to measure levels (e.g., early in week).
7. Ensure availability of enough replacement factor for at least 2 weeks at blood bank.
8. Consider combining major and minor operations (e.g., abdominal and dental surgery).
9. Avoid intramuscular injections during the perioperative period.

the basics of management of the most common coagulopathies. However, one should not rely on these guidelines alone to treat patients with these disorders, because of their heterogeneous and somewhat unpredictable nature. Perioperative consultation and close cooperation with the transfusion medicine specialist (hematologist or blood banker, or both) is essential to ensure a favorable outcome.

THE JEHOVAH'S WITNESS PATIENT

From time to time, the surgeon may be called to treat a member of the Jehovah's Witness faith. This can be a positive or a negative experience for both, depending on how much the surgeon understands about the beliefs of the Jehovah's Witness and the constraints they may place on medical care. In our experience, many physicians have an incorrect understanding of the Witnesses' position and covertly consider them to be medical nihilists. If the surgeon is to make intelligent, informed choices in dealing with Jehovah's Witness patients, it is essential to have a clear understanding of their position on medical care, specifically transfusion.

The Jehovah's Witness religion began as a Bible study group founded in the early 1800s. Known as Milleniasts, this group believed in the imminent second coming of Christ and His rule over the earth for the ensuing 1,000 years. Reorganized during the 1870s by Charles Taze Russell, the religion expanded the role of Bible study and began promoting its beliefs through the publication of religious tracts and books. In 1884, the group became known as the Zion's Watch Tower Tract Society. Joseph Franklin Russell assumed the religious group's leadership in 1916, using his talents as an attorney and organizer to restructure the followers into a centrally run religion, which became known as the Jehovah's Witnesses in 1931. Under his tutelage, the Jehovah's Witnesses further developed their goals of Bible study and community missionary work. The religion is currently run by a governing body based in Brooklyn, New York.

Of primary concern to surgeons is the Jehovah's Witness refusal to accept blood transfusion. This belief is based on a strict interpretation of passages from the Bible:

Every moving thing that liveth shall be meat for you; even as the green herb have I given you all things. But the flesh of the life thereof, ye shall not eat (Genesis 9:3–4).
For it [blood] is the life of all flesh; the blood of it is for the life thereof: therefore I say unto the children of Israel, ye shall eat the blood of no manner of flesh: for the life of all flesh is the blood thereof. Whosoever eateth it shall be cut off (Leviticus 17:14).

One can argue interminably that these passages should not be interpreted to include blood transfusion. However, the true Jehovah's Witness cannot be dissuaded and frequently counters any philosophic or religious arguments with sound scientific reasons as to why blood transfusion is inherently dangerous.[45]

Physicians tend to underestimate the importance of this prohibition against blood transfusion. To the Jehovah's Witness, acceptance of transfusion is not a minor infraction, punishable by a slap on the wrist. The consequences of transfusion for the Jehovah's Witness include excommunication from the church, forfeiture of a chance for eternal life, and severance of the individual's relationship with God. To die while upholding one's religious beliefs, in this case, refusing transfusion, is an ancient and accepted practice in the world's religions. Although the physician may not agree with this position, especially regarding transfusion, one must understand that the potential for life everlasting is an enormous incentive, especially when the alternative is so negative. Each surgeon must make a personal decision as to whether this prohibition against transfusion is acceptable. If not, Jehovah's Witness patients should be referred or transferred to physicians who are willing to accept them. Time should not be wasted in misguided attempts to convince the Witness by argument and logic or in waiting for the situation to worsen, in hopes that the patient will convert at the operating room door. Unfortunately, we have seen just such actions rob actively bleeding patients of a chance for survival.

Alternatives to Transfusion

Although Jehovah's Witnesses do not accept blood transfusion, this restriction is confined primarily to the use of allogeneic blood products or autologous blood that is separated from the body for a period of time (i.e., autologous predonation). These prohibitions do not prevent most Witness patients from accepting the use of cardiopulmonary bypass, hemodilution, dialysis, and intraoperative blood salvage and reinfusion.[46] Hemodilution can be performed by collecting blood into bags previously connected at the infusion port to an intravenous line and to the patient via a three-way stopcock for reinfusion. In this setup, the circuit from the patient back to the patient is never broken. Autotransfusion devices can be revised in a similar fashion by dedicating an intravenous line from the collection device to the patient to maintain a closed circuit[47] (Fig. 27-1).

From time to time, the Watchtower will publish

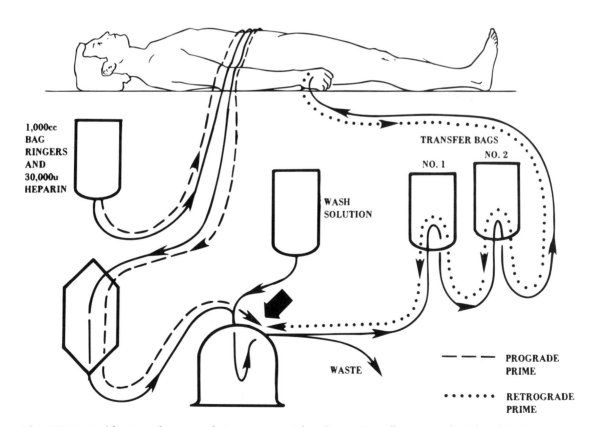

Fig. 27-1 Modification of autotransfusion setup as "closed circuit" to allow use in the Jehovah's Witness.

guidelines concerning transfusion issues, with the instruction to the Jehovah's Witness that the decision to use an alternative is a matter of individual conscience. Such is the case with recombinant human erythropoietin (rHuEPO) (Ortho Biotech, Raritan, NJ) (see also Ch. 47), which contains a small amount of human albumin. Albumin, when used as a volume expander, is considered an unacceptable blood product. Because the amount contained in rHuEPO is so small and it is not intended to be used as a blood product, the albumin is generally acceptable. In our experience, only a very small percentage of Jehovah's Witnesses have refused rHuEPO use. Although perhaps best given preoperatively, rHuEPO can be effective if used postoperatively or after a bleeding episode.[48-50]

Contrary to popular belief, Jehovah's Witnesses do not refuse all medical care but tend to seek the best in medical treatment. As a group, they are among the most educated consumers the surgeon will ever encounter and are very knowledgeable, especially in areas of alternatives to transfusion. Their church has established local liasion committees, consisting of church members whose goals are to act as a liasion between the physician and the patient and to provide the physician with a clear understanding of the Witnesses' position, the use of alternatives, and other considerations. Recently, these committees have established relationships with regional hospitals, known as Centers for Bloodless Surgery, where Witness patients can be referred. Such centers have physicians trained in blood alternative strategies who will honor the Witness patient's wishes regarding transfusion.[47]

THE RISK OF SEVERE ANEMIA IN JEHOVAH'S WITNESSES

Is major surgery possible in the Jehovah's Witness without undue risk? Both our experience and that of many others in performing surgery that carries with it a risk of blood loss has shown clearly that it is.[47,51-55] Nevertheless, as with any patient, severe anemia does pose risk (see Ch. 7).

Viele and Weiskopf[56] reviewed the medical literature from 1970 to early 1993 and found reports of 134 Jehovah's Witness patients who had a hemoglobin level of up to 8 g/dl or a hematocrit of 24 percent

or less who were treated without transfusions. There were 50 reported deaths (overall mortality, 37 percent); Viele and Weiskopf concluded that 23 of the deaths resulted exclusively or primarily from anemia. It is important to note that, with the exception of three patients with cardiac disease who died after cardiac surgery and two patients for whom no individual laboratory data were available, all patients whose deaths were attributed primarily or exclusively to anemia died with hemoglobin concentrations <5 g/dl or an equivalent hematocrit.

Medicolegal Considerations

Legal actions regarding Jehovah's Witnesses have helped define treatment approaches for the surgeon. Controversial areas include transfusion of the minor, the use of emergency transfusion, and determinations of competency.[57] Traditionally, the courts have ruled in favor of the physician in a decision to transfuse a minor child of Jehovah's Witness parents, based on the doctrine of parens patriae, or the power of the state to preserve the lives of minors.[58,59] However, courts are beginning to distinguish between life-threatening and non-life-threatening situations in regard to transfusion.[58] Physicians may be required to document the life-threatening nature of an illness and to justify the benefits of transfusion, that is, to prove to the court that a transfusion will indeed be needed to save a child's life. In our experience, judges have required the physician to limit transfusion to the circumstances presented at a court hearing and to report back to the court the success or failure of the transfusion. In other words, blanket orders "to transfuse as needed" are becoming rare. Similarly, if a surgical procedure is not needed to save a child's life and can safely be postponed until the child reaches adulthood, such a procedure may be denied by the court if it involves transfusion.

The teenage patient, or mature minor, is viewed differently by the courts. If a child has married or joined the armed forces or has been legally emancipated, he or she is considered a competent adult with all rights and privileges. Some courts have upheld the teenage Jehovah's Witness' refusal to accept blood after being convinced of the individual's understanding of the nature and consequences of his or her actions. The Illinois Supreme Court recently found in favor of a 17-year-old girl with leukemia who opposed a transfusion because of her religious beliefs.[58]

Early and open discussion with both parents of the Jehovah's Witness minor patient and the child are desirable.[59] The surgeon should consider how essential transfusion is to the patient's outcome and whether or not alternatives are available. A wide variety of surgical procedures, including those with unavoidable attendant blood loss, have been performed safely in Jehovah's Witness children using combinations of hemodilution, hypothermic anesthesia, and intraoperative salvage.[59]

The question frequently arises as to the legality of transfusing the unconscious Jehovah's Witness in an emergency. The traditional approach to this problem is to stabilize the patient first, using blood transfusion as needed, seeking consent later. Most states will permit transfusion in this setting, provided there is no advance directive known to the physician prohibiting transfusion and the transfusion is needed to save the patient's life. One may need to be able to prove the latter after the fact. Most Jehovah's Witnesses carry a card proclaiming them as such and describing their refusal of blood and blood products. One must consider this card to be valid and binding, since it carries the weight of an advance directive. Some states have recognized the card's validity by law.[60] In *Malette v. Shulman*, the Court of Ontario established this precedent by awarding damages to a Jehovah's Witness who was transfused despite the fact that she had such a card.[61]

Informed consent with the Jehovah's Witness or, for that matter, with any other patient should include a discussion of the potential of life-threatening hemorrhage and its consequences.[62,63] This need to include such discussions has been made clear in two recent decisions regarding Jehovah's Witnesses. In a case similar to *Malette v. Shulman* discussed above, the Michigan Court of Appeals ruled in favor of a surgeon who transfused his patient during a routine dilation and curettage (D & C) when bleeding became life-threatening.[64] The decision to uphold the surgeon's actions was based in large part on the fact that the patient did not fully comprehend that she might die during the operation if a transfusion became necessary and was not given. In a similar case in New Jersey, in which a patient bled during a hysterectomy, the surgeon sought a court order to transfuse on the basis of the inability to inform the unconscious patient contemporaneously of the change in circumstances (i.e., bleeding) that now threatened her life. Given the life-threatening circumstances, the court allowed the husband to act as a surrogate and to grant permission to transfuse, even though the patient was a known Jehovah's Witness. However, in their decision the court recognized that by failing to discuss the potential for life-threatening hemorrhage with the patient, the surgeon had not fulfilled his obligation to provide adequate informed consent. The appellate court subsequently upheld the decision while reaffirming the right of a Jehovah's Witness to refuse a blood transfusion while he or she is competent—or when incompetent—through an advance directive or Living Will. It is prudent, therefore, that the surgeon discuss the possibility of life-threatening hemorrhage and the possible need for transfusion with all patients before surgery. It is important to remember that the patient's refusal to accept such a transfusion does not protect the surgeon from liability for any negligent actions that may necessitate transfusion.

We have listed in Table 27-3 our recommenda-

Table 27-3. Guidelines for Dealing With the Jehovah's Witness

1. Discuss issues with patient, including the possibility of life-threatening hemorrhage and possible death, if not transfused.
2. Document discussions in the record or as part of a refusal of treatment form.
3. If unable or unwilling to treat, stabilize, and transfer to a sympathetic institution such as a Center for Bloodless Surgery.
4. Accept the limitation—don't harrass an already traumatized patient or family.
5. Contact the local JW liasion committee for information and help.
6. Seek legal assistance for minor or unconscious/incompetent adult.
7. In an emergency or with a unconscious patient, look for an advance directive (e.g., cardiac), and discuss with third party.
8. Stop the bleeding!!! You cannot replace any blood that has been lost.
9. Monitor blood pressure, and don't resuscitate to excessive levels with an actively bleeding patient. This only increases the blood loss.
10. Learn about and use alternatives.

tions for dealing with the Jehovah's Witness patient. This includes both the issues described above and actions to be taken if the surgeon feels uncomfortable or ill-equipped to deal with the Witness. One should take a careful look at the standard refusal of blood transfusion forms in use in most hospitals to ensure that it is comprehensive enough to cover all possible complications of surgery. If not, the surgeon should specifically document these in the record. In its 1988 report, the Presidential Commission on HIV recommended that all hospitals adopt reasonable strategies to avoid homologous transfusion, including the use of alternatives such as those discussed earlier.[65] The surgeon should check into what is available at his or her hospital and should analyze his or her practice to see where improvements can be made. If a patient is to be transferred to a Center for Bloodless Surgery or a sympathetic institution, arrangements should be made expeditiously to prevent unfavorable outcomes caused by ongoing bleeding.

REFERENCES

1. Brettler DB, Levine PH: Clinical manifestations and therapy of inherited coagulation factor deficiencies. p. 169. In Colma RW, Hirsh J, Marder VJ, Salzman EW (eds): Hemostasis and Thrombosis: Basic Principles and Clinical Practice. 3rd Ed. JB Lippincott, Philadelphia, 1994
2. Hoyer LW, Wyshock EG, Colman RW: Coagulation cofactors: factors V and VIII. p. 109. In Colma RW, Hirsh J, Marder VJ, Salzman EW (eds): Hemostasis and Thrombosis: Basic Principles and Clinical Practice. 3rd Ed. JB Lippincott, Philadelphia, 1994
3. Fischbach P, Scharrer I: Therapeutic impact of orthotopic liver transplantation on disorders of hemostasis. Semin Thromb Hemost 19:250, 1993
4. Limentani SA, Furie BC, Furie B: The biochemistry of factor IX. p. 94. In Colma RW, Hirsh J, Marder VJ, Salzman EW (eds): Hemostasis and Thrombosis: Basic Principles and Clinical Practice. 3rd Ed. Colma RW, Hirsh J, Marder VJ, Salzman EW (eds) JB Lippincott, Philadelphia, 1994
5. Hoyer LW: Factor VIII: new perspectives. Transfus Med Rev 1:113, 1987
6. Tountas CP, Ferris FO, Cobb SW: Exertional compartment syndrome in covert mild hemophilia. A case report. Acta Haematol 88:194, 1992
7. Hoskinson J, Duthrie RB: Management of musculo-skeletal problems in hemophiliacs. Orthop Clin North Am 9:455, 1978
8. Rizza CR, Matthews JM: Management of the hemophilic child. Arch Dis Child 47:451, 1972
9. Eyster ME, Gill FM, Blatt PM et al: Central nervous system bleeding in hemophiliacs. Blood 51:1179, 1978
10. Lane S: Haemorrhagic diathesis: successful transfusion of blood. Lancet 1:1, 1840
11. Pool JG, Hershgold EJ, Pappenhagen AR: High potency anti-haemophilic factor concentrate prepared from cryoglobulin precipitate. Nature 203:312, 1964
12. Goedert JJ, Kessler CK, Aledort LM et al: A prospective study of HIV-1 infection and the development of AIDS in patients with hemophilia. N Engl J Med 32:1141, 1989
13. Kasper CK, Lusher JM, and the Transfusion Practices Committee: Recent evolution of clotting factor concentrates for hemophilia A and B. Transfusion 33:422, 1993
14. Lusher JM, Arkin S, Abilsgaard CF et al: Recombinant factor VIII for the treatment of previously untreated patients with hemophilia A. Safety, efficacy and development of inhibitors. N Engl J Med 328:453, 1993
15. Shulman NR: Surgical care of patients with hereditary disorders of blood coagulation. Mod Treat 5:61, 1968
16. Mannucci PM: Desmopressin: a nontransfusional form of treatment for congenital and acquired bleeding disorders Blood 72:1449, 1988
17. Mariana G, Caivarella N, Mazzucconi MG et al: Evaluation of the effectiveness of DDAVP in surgery or in bleeding episodes in hemophilia and von Willebrand's disease. A study on 43 patients. Clin Lab Haematol 6:229, 1984
18. Rudowski WJ, Scharf R, Ziemski JM: Is major surgery in hemophiliac patients safe? World J Surg 11:378, 1987
19. Schulman S: DDAVP—The multipotent drug in patients with coagulopathies. Transfus Med Rev 5:132, 1991
20. Martinowitz U, Schulman S, Gitel S et al: Adjusted dose continuous infusion of Factor VIII in patients with hemophilia A. Br J Haematol 82:729, 1992
21. Brettler DB, Levine PH: Clinical manifestations and therapy of inherited coagulation disorders. p. 169. In Coleman RW, Hirsh J, Marder VJ, Salzman EW (eds): Hemostasis and Thrombosis. Basic Principles and Clinical Practice. JB Lippincott, Philadelphia, 1994.
22. Kasper CK: Clinical use of Factor IX concentrates: report on thromboembolic complications. Thromb Haemost 33:642, 1975
23. Feinstein DI: Immune coagulation disorders p. 169. In Colma RW, Hirsh J, Marder VJ, Salzman EW (eds):

Hemostasis and Thrombosis: Basic Principles and Clinical Practice. 3rd Ed. JB Lippincott, Philadelphia, 1994

24. Francesconi M, Korniger C, Thaler E et al: Plasmapheresis: its value in the management of patients with antibodies to Factor VIII. Hemostasis 11:79, 1982

25. Nilsson IM, Jonsson S, Sundquist SB et al: A procedure for removing high titer antibodies by extracorporeal protein A-Sepharose adsorption in hemophilia. Blood 58:38, 9181

26. Kasper CK: The management of hemophiliacs with inhibitors. p. 71. In Westphal RG, Smith DM (eds): Treatment of Hemophilia and von Willebrand's disease: new developments. American Association of Blood Banks, Arlington, VA, 1989

27. Brettler DB, Forsberg AD, Levine PH et al: The use of porcine factor VIII concentrate (hyate:C) in the treatment of patients with inhibitor antibodies to factor VIII. Arch Intern Med 149:1381, 1989

28. Hay CRM, Bolton-Maggs P: Porcine Factor VIIIc in the Management of Patients with Factor VIII Inhibitors. Transfus Med Rev 5:145, 1991

29. Hedner U, Glazer, Falcj J: Recombinant activated factor VII in the treatment of bleeding episodes in patients with inherited and acquired bleeding disorders. Transfus Med Rev 7:78, 1993

30. Gringeri A, Santagostino E, Mannucci PM: Failure of recombinant activated factor VII during surgery in a hemophiliac with high-titer factor VIII antibody. Haemostasis 21:1, 1991

31. Nilsson IM: The management of hemophilia patients with inhibitors. Transfus Med Rev 6:285, 1992

32. Jorpes EJ: EA von Willebrand och von Willebrand's sjukdom. Nord Med 67:729, 1962

33. Montgomery RH, Coller BS: Von Willebrand disease. p. 134. In Colma RW, Hirsh J, Marder VJ, Salzman EW (eds): Hemostasis and Thrombosis: Basic Principles and Clinical Practice. 3rd Ed. JB Lippincott, Philadelphia, 1994

34. Rodeghiero F, Castaman G, Dini E: Epidemiologic investigation of the prevalence of vWd. Blood 69:454, 1987

35. Mannucci PM, Lombardi R, Bader R et al: Heterogeneity of type I von Willebrand's disease: evidence for a subgroup with an abnormal von Willebrand factor. Blood 66:796, 1985

36. White LA, Chisholm M: Gastro-intestinal bleeding in acquired von Willebrand's disease: efficacy of high-dose immuno-globulin where substitution treatments failed. Br J Haematol 84:332, 1993

37. Wahlberg TH, Blomback M, Hall P et al: Application of indicators, predictors and diagnostic indices in coagulation disorders. I. Evaluation of a self-administered questionnaire with binary questions. Methods Infect Med 19:194, 1980

38. Rodgers RP, Levin J: A critical reappraisal of the bleeding time. Semin Thromb Hemost 16:1, 1990

39. Kuitenen A, Hyuygen M, Salmenper AM et al: Anaesthesia affects plasma concentrations of vasopressin, von Willebrand's factor and coagulation Factor VIII in cardiac surgical patients. Br J Anaesth 70:173, 1993

40. Lombardi R, Mannucci PM, Seghatchian MJ et al: Alterations of Factor VIII:vWF in clinical conditions associated with an increase in its plasma concentration. Br J Haematol 49:61, 1981

41. Gill JC, Endres Brooks J, Bauer PJ et al: The effect of ABO blood group on the diagnosis of vWd. Blood 69:1691, 1987

42. Slaughter TF, Mody EA, Oldham HN Jr et al: Management of a patient with type IIC von Willebrand's disease during coronary artery bypass graft surgery. Anesthesiology 78:195, 1993

43. Scott JP, Montgomery RR: Therapy of vWd. Semin Thromb Hemost 19:37, 1993

44. Aznar J, Villa P, Vay A et al: Functional anomaly of Factor XII, letter. Haemostasis 22:345, 1992

45. Jehovah's Witnesses and the Question of Blood. Watchtower Bible and Tract Society, New York, 1977, pp. 38–49

46. Ridley DT: Accommodating Jehovah's Witnesses Choice of Nonblood Management. Perspect Healthcare Risk Mgmt 10:17, 1990

47. Spence RK, Alexander JB, DelRossi AJ et al: Transfusion guidelines for cardiovascular surgery: lessons learned from operations in Jehovah's Witnesses. J Vasc Surg 16:835, 1992

48. Madura JA: Use of erythropoietin and parenteral iron dextran in a severely anemic Jehovah's Witness with colon cancer. Arch Surg 128:1168, 1993

49. Schiff SJ, Weinstein SL: Use of recombinant human erythropoietin to avoid blood transfusion in a Jehovah's Witness requiring hemispherectomy. J Neurosurg 79:600, 1993

50. Atabek U, Alvarez R, Pello MJ et al: Erythropoietin accelerates hematocrit recovery in severe post-surgical anemia. Am Surg 61:74, 1995

51. Spence RK, Carson JA, Poses R et al: Elective surgery without transfusion: influence of preoperative hemoglobin level and blood loss on mortality. Am J Surg 59:320, 1990

52. Carson JL, Spence RK, Poses RM et al: Severity of anemia and operative mortality and morbidity. Lancet 2:727, 1988

53. Jehovah's Witness cases raise critical issues for RMs, editorial. Hosp Risk Management 12:101, 1990

54. Spence RK, Cernaiainu AC, Carson J et al: Transfusion and Surgery. 30:1101, 1993

55. Kitchen CS: Are transfusions overrated? Surgical outcome of Jehovah's Witnesses, editorial. Am J Med 94: 117, 1993

56. Viele MK, Weiskopf RB: What can we learn about the needs for transfusion from patients who refuse blood? The experience with Jehovah's Witnesses. Transfusion 34:396, 1994

57. Finfer S, Howell S, Miller J et al: Managing patients who refuse blood transfusions: an ethical dilemma. Major trauma in two patients refusing blood transfusion. BMJ 308:1423, 1994

58. Goldman EB, Oberman HA: Legal aspects of transfusion of Jehovah's Witnesses. Transfus Med Rev 5:263, 1991

59. Luban NC, Leikin SL: Jehovah's Witnesses and transfusion: the pediatric perspective. Trans Med Rev V:4; 253, 1991

60. In re *Green,* 292 A 2d 387 (1971)

61. In re *EG,* No. 66089 Illinois Supreme Court, November 13, 1989

62. Jehovah's Witness cases raise critical issues for RMs, editorial. Hosp Risk Management 12:101, 1990

63. Fontanarosa PB, Giorgio GT: Managing Jehovah's Witnesses: medical, legal and ethical challenges, editorial. Ann Emerg Med 20:1148, 1991

64. Battery Claim of Jehovah's Witness Rejected by Michigan Court, editorial. Hosp Law Newsl 9:4, 1992

65. Report of the Presidential Commission on the Human Immunodeficiency Virus Epidemic. US Government Printing Office, Washington, DC, 1988, p. 78

Chapter 28

Fetal and Perinatal Transfusion Therapy

Daniel W. Skupski, Carl F.W. Wolf, and James B. Bussel

The development of fetal blood sampling and fetal blood transfusions for the management of Rh disease pioneered and established fetal transfusion therapy. Subsequently, fetal transfusion therapy has been expanded not only to other anemias but to other cytopenias as well. Large series of fetuses undergoing blood sampling, including one of more than 5,000 samplings, have described normal fetal hematologic values at varying gestational ages, clearly a prerequisite for fetal assessment and transfusion therapy.[1,2]

Despite the effectiveness of anti-D prophylaxis for Rh alloimmunization, the great majority of fetal transfusions are still performed for this indication. Severely affected fetuses have only transfusion as a lifesaving therapy, requiring as many as four to six transfusions. Studies of fetal alloimmune thrombocytopenia are providing methodology and indications for fetal platelet transfusions, as well as investigation of therapy administered to the mother designed to increase the fetal platelet count and avoid fetal platelet transfusions. Management schemes including transfusion are continually being developed and amended to reduce mortality in these disorders. Table 28-1 presents the indications for intrauterine fetal transfusion (IUT) therapy.

Where will ongoing studies lead in the future? Sophisticated diagnostic techniques are required to diagnose otherwise unsuspected severe fetal cytopenias. Early diagnosis until now has relied on ultrasound, amniocentesis, and fetal blood sampling. Ultrasonography needs to be further refined or new technology developed, so that fetal anemia less severe than that associated with hydrops fetalis can be detected. DNA-based diagnosis from fetal cells in the amniotic fluid, chorionic villus samplings, or the maternal circulation has become available. These methods of diagnosis are less invasive than fetal blood sampling and can therefore be more routinely used as they are further developed.

This chapter reviews (1) Rh alloimmunization and erythroblastosis fetalis, (2) other fetal cytopenias, and (3) immunohematologic and blood-processing techniques pertinent to perinatal transfusion therapy.

ANEMIA: IMMUNE DISEASE

Serologic History

Hydrops fetalis was first described by Plater[3] in 1641 and defined by Ballantyne[4] in 1892, who delineated the criteria for diagnosis. The association of hydrops fetalis with anemia and circulating erythroblasts in the fetus was first reported by Diamond et al.[5] in 1932. A major advance occurred in 1940 with the discovery of the rhesus (Rh) factor by Landsteiner and Weiner.[6] This resulted directly in the understanding that anti-red cell antibodies mediate severe

Table 28-1. Indications for Intrauterine Fetal
Transfusion Therapy: Present and Future

1. Anemia
   A. Fetal red blood cell alloimmunization
   B. Nonimmune fetal hydrops secondary to parvovirus B-19 infection[a]
   C. Homozygous α-thalassemia[b]
   D. Congenital dyserythropoietic anemia[b]
2. Thrombocytopenia
   A. Fetal alloimmune thrombocytopenia
   B. Maternal autoimmune chronic ITP causing fetal thrombocytopenia
   C. TAR (thrombocytopenia with absent radii)[b]
   D. Infections (i.e., CMV)[b]

[a] Most nonimmune hydrops is cardiac in origin and does not involve anemia.
[b] No reported cases managed by intrauterine transfusion therapy.

fetal hemolytic anemia.[7] Pickles[8] gives an excellent review of these early historical developments.

Technologic History

Several subsequent technological developments have resulted in the current approach to the management of hemolytic disease of the fetus and newborn (HDFN). Amniocentesis was the first technique to allow direct access to the intrauterine environment. In 1961, Liley[9] first reported the correlation of elevated amniotic fluid delta OD450 (indicative of the bilirubin level) with the severity of fetal anemia in those pregnancies affected by Rh alloimmunization. Liley[10] also introduced the technique of intraperitoneal transfusion (IPT) to the severely affected fetus in 1963.

The next breakthrough was ultrasound technology, permitting better and safer visualization than was available with fluoroscopy. In 1981, the first intravascular fetal transfusion was performed, using a fetoscope.[11] Subsequently, percutaneous cordocentesis was developed.[12] This procedure involved the placement of a needle through the maternal abdominal wall into the umbilical cord under ultrasound guidance, allowing direct access to the fetal circulation. With this technique, it was possible to obtain fetal blood for a blood count more safely and easily than with fetoscopy, and it was possible to transfuse the fetus if necessary.

Different approaches to fetal blood sampling have recently been used at certain centers, including fetal

ductus venosus puncture and even fetal cardiac puncture. The role of these newer modalities remains to be established.

Prevention of Rh Immunization

Transplacental Hemorrhage

Detectable transplacental hemorrhage (TPH) occurs at delivery in 75 percent of all pregnancies,[13] frequently during the third trimester of pregnancy, during any intrauterine invasive procedure (Table 28-2), and during any pregnancy-related bleeding complication (Table 28-2). The amount of blood required to result in primary sensitization is unclear, but anamnestic stimulation may occur with a TPH of as little as 0.1 ml of fetal blood, explaining the almost uniform occurrence of erythroblastosis in subsequent Rh(D)-positive fetuses, once primary maternal sensitization has occurred.

Table 28-2. Current Recommendations for the Use of Rh Immunoglobulin[a]

For all Rh-negative nonimmunized women:

1. A single intramuscular dose of 300 micrograms of Rh immunoglobulin at 28 to 32 weeks gestation.
2. Another dose of 300 μg of Rh immunoglobulin within 72 hours of the birth of a D-positive infant.
3. A 300-μg intramuscular dose of Rh immunoglobulin during the first half of pregnancy for women undergoing threatened abortion, spontaneous abortion, ectopic pregnancy, or any vaginal bleeding thought to be of uterine origin.[b]
4. Immune prophylaxis (300 μg) for any procedures that increase the risk of transplacental hemorrhage, such as chorionic villus sampling, amniocentesis, cordocentesis, placental biopsy, percutaneous or open fetal surgery, or external cephalic version.[b]
5. A maternal Kleihauer-Bettke test for all cases in which transplacental hemorrhage is suspected during pregnancy or at delivery (e.g., bleeding from placenta previa or abruptio placenta). A corresponding increase in the dose of Rh immunoglobulin if the Kleihauer-Bettke test reveals more than 30 ml fetal whole blood (15 ml fetal red cells) in the maternal circulation.

[a] Blood group, Rh type, and antibody screen are recommended for all pregnant women at their first prenatal visit, and again before the administration of Rh immunoglobulin at any time during pregnancy or postpartum.
[b] During the first trimester (i.e., before 13 weeks gestation), a dose of 50 μg of Rh immunoglobulin is also acceptable.
(Adapted from the American College of Obstetricians and Gynecologists,[100] with permission.)

Rh Immunoglobulin

The development of Rh immunoglobulin (RhIg) in the 1960s was a major advance in the prevention of HDFN.[14,15] RhIg is a preparation of hyperimmune γ-globulin using pooled donor plasma obtained from Rh-negative sensitized donors with high titers of anti-D antibody. Initially, it was made from the plasma of women who had previously had fetuses affected by Rh alloimmunization. Subsequently, as the incidence of the disease declined, donors are used whose titers are maintained by periodic vaccination.[16]

With the institution of immune prophylaxis, the incidence of Rh(D) alloimmunization in Rh-incompatible pregnancies decreased from 1 percent to 0.2 percent when RhIg was given in doses of 100 to 300 μg within 72 hours of delivery.[17] This further decreased to 0.07 percent (7 in 10,000) with the introduction of a second dose of RhIg early in the third trimester.[18] The current recommendations for the prevention of RBC alloimmunization, including when to consider additional or increased doses of RhIg, are presented in Table 28-2.[19,20]

Red Blood Cell Alloimmunization and Hemolytic Disease of the Fetus and Newborn

Subsequent Rh-positive pregnancies in a woman with Rh alloimmunization typically lead to worsening severity of fetal disease. Antibodies to the Rh(D) antigen usually only cause fetal hemolytic disease at a titer of greater than 1:16.[21] In general, the greater the titer, the greater the risk of severe hemolytic disease in the fetus. However, the titer is an unreliable guide to the severity of fetal anemia, as is an increase in titer, which may be seen even with an Rh-negative fetus.

Atypical blood group antibodies represent an increasing fraction of cases of HDFN as a result of the effectiveness of anti-D prophylaxis. They may cause severe hemolytic disease in the fetus, even at titer(s) of less than 1:8 (i.e., anti-Kell).[22] Many antibody specificities have been claimed to have caused HDFN, including nearly every one that can occur as IgG able to cross the placenta, but only a few have been reported to cause moderate or severe hemolytic disease. The atypical antibodies that are able to cause moderate or severe hemolytic disease in the fetus are -c, -C, -C^W, -C^X, -e, -E, -E^W, -ce, -Ce^S, -Rh32, -Go^a, Be^a, -Evans, -Riv, -K or Kell, -Jk^a or Kidd, -Js^a, -Js^b, -Ku, -Fy^a, -M, -N, -s, -U, -PP$_1$P^k, -Di^b, -Lan, -LW, -Far, -Good, -Wr^a, and -Zd.[23,24] Maternal antibodies against immunodominant sugar antigens, such as Lewis, P, and I, are not causes of HDFN because the corresponding antigens are weak and almost lacking on fetal red cells and are fully expressed only after birth. Also, antibodies to these antigens are frequently IgM isotype and, accordingly, do not cross the placenta. The A, B, and H antigens are also weaker than those on cells from adults.[25] Because of the possibility of severe fetal anemia despite low antibody titer, the good but imperfect ability to predict fetal anemia by amniotic fluid bilirubin studies, and the inability to diagnose fetal anemia definitively by ultrasound until hydrops fetalis appears, fetal blood sampling is usually the management option of choice if antibodies known to cause moderate or severe hemolytic disease in the fetus appear (see below).

The natural history of HDFN, in cases in which the fetus is severely affected, is one of hemolysis, resulting in an anemia as the bone marrow fails to increase production sufficiently to keep up with the red cell destruction. In Rh disease, this may be due in part to the presence of the Rh(D) antigen on erythroid precursors. Marked erythroid hyperplasia extends outside the bone marrow, resulting in extramedullary hematopoiesis (EMH). As a result of EMH, hepatosplenomegaly develops, and hypoproteinemia occurs secondary to decreased hepatic production of plasma proteins. In HDFN, fetal hydrops (total body edema or anasarca) is attributed to the combination of severe anemia and marked hypoproteinemia, resulting in high-output cardiac failure in the setting of reduced intravascular volume. Total body edema is an end-stage process of third-space fluid accumulation, which has causes other than RBC alloimmunization. Hydrops fetalis is classically divided between anemic and nonanemic hydrops (Table 28-3). Anemic hydrops is divided into two categories: immune and nonimmune.

Ultrasound has been instrumental in detecting fetal hydrops, permitting intervention prior to fetal death. The fluid accumulations recognizable in the fetus by ultrasound are ascites, pericardial effusions, pleural effusions, skin and scalp edema, a thickened placenta due to edema, and hydramnios (excess am-

Table 28-3. Causes of Hydrops Fetalis

Anemic	Nonanemic
1. Immune hemolysis from RBC alloimmunization	1. Cardiovascular (arrhythmia, supraventricular tachycardia)
2. Fetal infection with parvovirus B9 (nonimmune)	2. Chromosomal (Turner syndrome)
3. Hematologic (homozygous α- or β-thalassemia) (nonimmune)	3. Infectious (enterovirus, adenovirus)
	4. Structural—mass effect (e.g., chest mass, sacrococcygeal teratoma, diaphragmatic hernia, cystic hygroma, other large fetal masses)
	5. Metabolic diseases (e.g., glycogen storage diseases)

niotic fluid accumulation). Two or more of these conditions must be present for the diagnosis of hydrops fetalis, which would be an immediate indication for fetal blood sampling and, if anemia is confirmed, transfusion; fetal echocardiography for the detection of arrhythmias would be the other primary test (Table 28-3).

Typically, the earliest occurrence of hydrops fetalis secondary to HDFN is at 18 to 20 weeks gestation in very severely affected cases, a time when fetal blood sampling and transfusion can first be instituted. Although still controversial, it is possible that the use of doppler waveform measurements to describe fetal blood flow will provide additional diagnostic information indicative of impending fetal hydrops. Early intervention, before progression to unmistakable hydrops fetalis, may thus be possible.

The consequence of untreated RBC alloimmunization, in Rh-incompatible pregnancies where the fetus is severely affected, is often that of fetal death or very premature delivery. In moderately affected cases, the fetus does not develop significant anemia during the pregnancy but, upon delivery, especially if premature, the newborn's liver is unable to conjugate the excess bilirubin that is released by ongoing RBC destruction, and unconjugated bilirubin levels rise dramatically during the first hours or days of life, resulting in kernicterus. Bilirubin deposition in cells of the central nervous system (CNS) produces widespread brain damage. The result is mental impairment, spasticity, choreoathetosis, and severe neurologic deficits—all permanent. Neonatal management combining phototherapy, exchange transfusion, hydration, and other supportive care is required in these cases. In milder cases of RBC

alloimmunization, there can be a marked rise in unconjugated bilirubin in the serum of the neonate, which does not reach levels known to place the neonate at risk of kernicterus.[26] Late anemia is not an uncommon finding in neonates with positive Coombs tests, even when the hemolytic disease is mild or moderate and requires no fetal or immediate neonatal blood transfusion.[27] For these infants, hemoglobin or hematocrit testing should be done during the second or third week of life, to detect impending severe late anemia, which tends to present most commonly during the fourth week of life.

Management of RBC Alloimmunization

Noninvasive Measures

Non-stress testing (NST) to detect fetal heart rate (FHR) changes due to severe anemia, ultrasound to detect impending fetal hydrops, and serial maternal antibody titer(s) are all helpful as initial noninvasive measures in the management of the alloimmunized pregnancy. NST uses a continuous doppler technique for the monitoring of the FHR and has been useful in detecting FHR changes that are secondary to anemia, most notably the sinusoidal FHR pattern seen after 24 to 26 weeks and classically associated with RBC alloimmunization[28,29] (Figure 28-1). NST begins at 26 to 28 weeks gestation and should be performed weekly. Ultrasound monitoring can begin in the second trimester (or before the gestational age of onset of disease of any previously affected child); it is also performed on a weekly basis. Maternal antibody titers are usually performed once per month but are the least helpful parameter. Since the severity of disease is difficult to predict, and un-

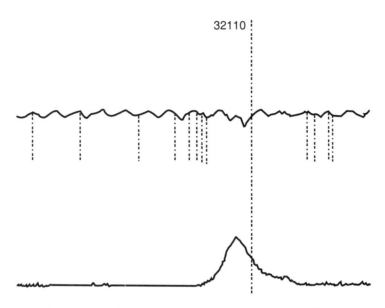

Fig. 28-1. Sinusoidal fetal heart rate pattern. (From Sibai et al.,[98] with permission.)

recognized small TPH can result in rapid increase in antibody titer and worsening of disease, these noninvasive methods of monitoring the alloimmunized pregnancy are of paramount importance.

Amniocentesis

Amniocentesis allows indirect assessment of the degree of fetal hemolysis by determination of the level of bilirubin in the amniotic fluid (delta OD450). The normal levels have been designated by Liley[9] as zone I. An increase in delta OD450 indicates fetal hemolysis (i.e., zones II and III on the curve developed by Liley). Delta OD450 normally decreases as gestation progresses and the trend of an increasing delta OD450 is characteristic of worsening hemolytic disease.[9] A level in zone III indicates the need for intervention, that is, assessment of the fetal hematocrit by cordocentesis, possible intrauterine fetal transfusion, or immediate early delivery. If delta OD450 measurements remain in zone I of the Liley curve, serial amniocenteses may be continued.

Classically, serial amniocenteses were the mainstay of management of RBC alloimmunization. They began at 28 weeks gestation, were performed every 3 to 4 weeks if the delta OD450 remained in zone I or low zone II, and were performed every 1 to 2

weeks if the delta OD450 was elevated to mid to high zone II, with the option of intraperitoneal transfusion if the delta OD450 levels reached zone III. Delta OD450 measurements are less reliable prior to 28 weeks gestation.

The current practice at almost all referral centers that actively treat RBC alloimmunization is to proceed promptly to cordocentesis when the delta OD450 levels reach high zone II or III. If amniocentesis, performed for an anti-D titer of greater than 1:16, demonstrates an elevation of the delta OD450 into zone III, 99 percent of these fetuses will be shown by cordocentesis to have severe hemolytic disease,[30] with hematocrits at least 2 SD below the mean for gestational age,[17] indicating the need for IUT.

A recently developed advantage of amniocentesis (or chorionic villus sampling) is the ability to determine the fetal Rh(D) type by the use of the polymerase chain reaction (PCR) for DNA amplification in the first or early second trimester.[31] This is important if the father is heterozygous for the D locus, as there is no "d" antigen allowing confirmation of zygosity status. Second-trimester amniocentesis has a pregnancy loss rate of only 0.5 percent[32-34] compared with 1 to 2 percent for cordocentesis.[35,36] If the fetus is determined to be Rh negative by PCR, no cordocentesis and no further amniocenteses are required.

Cordocentesis

Percutaneous cordocentesis permits direct assessment of fetal anemia by obtaining a sample of fetal blood and rapidly determining the fetal hematocrit or the complete blood count (CBC)[37] (Fig. 28-2). Cordocentesis has been available for more than 8 years and has been shown to have a procedure-related loss rate of 1 to 2 percent.[35,36] Most referral centers prefer cordocentesis over amniocentesis as the method for evaluating RBC alloimmunization, especially when there has been a previously affected child, because cordocentesis directly specifies the severity of fetal disease[17] (Fig. 28-3). This direct measurement is important in attempting to avoid the higher mortality from cordocentesis or IUT that occurs in the hydropic fetus as compared to the nonhydropic fetus.

The development of high-resolution ultrasound with color doppler enhancement of blood flow has facilitated visualization of the umbilical vein at the level of the cord insertion into the placenta (Fig. 28-4). Venous turbulence upon saline injection visualized by ultrasound initially demonstrates placement of the needle within the umbilical vessels.[38] The confirmation that the specimen is fetal is obtained by the use of the RBC mean corpuscular volume (MCV). Fetal blood can be distinguished from maternal blood, since the adult MCV is significantly lower than that of the fetus; even intermixing can be detected (Fig. 28-5). It is important to note that the distinction between fetal and maternal MCV becomes obscured after the first intrauterine transfusion (IUT) and late in gestation; in these cases, greater reliance is placed on the visualization of turbulence within the umbilical vessels. Other ways of distinguishing between fetal and maternal blood exist, including the Kleihauer-Betke test, but none can be performed rapidly

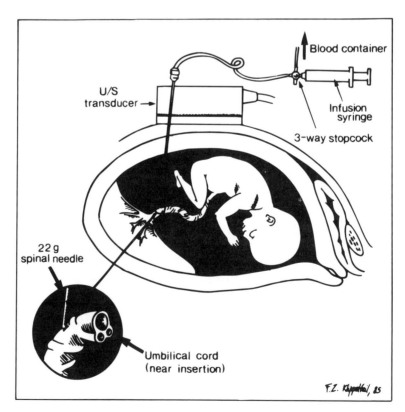

Fig. 28-2. In utero direct intravascular transfusion. U/S = ultrasound. (From Grannum et al.,[99] with permission.)

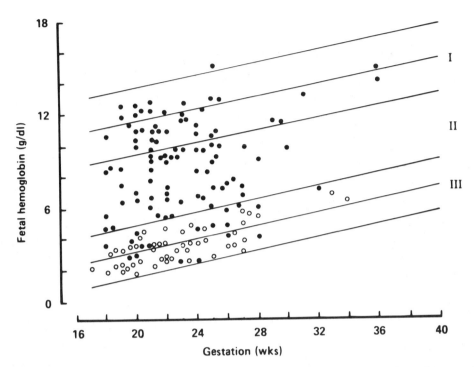

Fig. 28-3. Pretransfusion fetal hemoglobin concentrations in 48 hydropic (open symbols) and 106 nonhydropic fetuses (closed symbols) from red cell isoimmunized pregnancies at the first fetal blood sampling. Values are plotted on the reference range of fetal hemoglobin for gestation. The individual 95 percent confidence intervals of the hemoglobin for gestation of the normal fetuses define zone I and the individual 95 percent confidence intervals of the hemoglobin for gestation of the hydropic fetuses define zone III. Zone II indicates moderate anemia. (From Nicolaides et al.,[50] with permission.)

enough to be clinically useful other than for retrospective confirmation.

Cordocentesis through an anterior placenta is technically simpler but is known to cause TPH. An anamnestic maternal response is thought to be produced in these cases, and subsequent worsening of fetal and/or neonatal hemolysis is possible. Worsening disease cannot be ascribed with certainty to the intervention of cordocentesis, because the natural progression of disease in RBC alloimmunization is one of increasing maternal antibody titer and worsening fetal hemolysis as gestation progresses. TPH, and thus presumed iatrogenic worsening of RBC alloimmunization, is much less likely to occur when the placenta is not traversed at amniocentesis or cordocentesis (i.e., with a posterior umbilical cord insertion). Some centers have chosen to perform cordocentesis without traversing an anterior placenta; the

clinical consequences to the fetus of this practice are not established.

Fetal Hematology

The large number of cordocenteses performed has allowed the description of normal fetal blood parameters. These values can be derived from a very small volume of blood. Most CBC machines require 0.2 ml or less of whole blood to provide a complete CBC and histogram. The fetal blood type and direct antiglobulin ("Coombs") test can be obtained on 0.05 ml. A reticulocyte count can be obtained manually from 1 drop of blood for a smear.

Normal fetal hematologic indices have been derived largely from fetuses at risk for genetic or infectious diseases who were sampled and found not to be affected and therefore are "completely normal." Figure 28-6 summarizes these values, which have

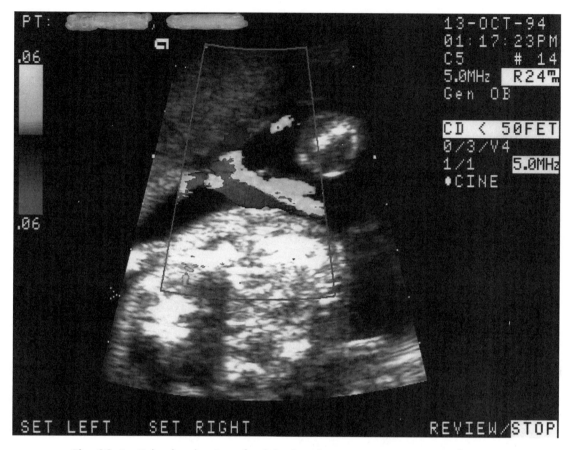

Fig. 28-4. Color doppler view of umbilical cord insertion into an anterior placenta.

been reported from several centers.[39-41] Normal fetal blood chemistries,[42] coagulation factor levels,[39] and 2,3-diphosphoglycerate (DPG) levels[43] have also been reported for different gestational ages.

Intrauterine Transfusion

Intraperitoneal Transfusion

Intraperitoneal (IPT) was the first treatment available for the severely anemic fetus affected by immune hemolytic disease. IPT is still used, albeit infrequently. The indications for IPT include situations in which intravascular access is difficult: a morbidly obese patient (especially when the umbilical cord insertion into the placenta is posterior within the uterus); late in gestation, when the enlarging fetus may obscure access to a posterior cord insertion; massive hydramnios obscuring access to a posterior

cord insertion; and frequently in twin gestations when one or both umbilical cord insertions are not accessible. In some of these cases, intrahepatic vein or direct cardiac puncture (rather than IPT) may be chosen as a more efficacious method of fetal transfusion. The complication rate of IPT is higher than that of intravascular transfusion, and IPT is ineffective in already hydropic fetuses, presumably because the peritoneal lymphatics will no longer carry the transfused red cells into the systemic circulation. Finally, IPT does not permit determination of the fetal hematocrit.

Intravascular Transfusion

Intravascular transfusion (IVT) is performed by cordocentesis, and donor RBCs are transfused directly into the umbilical circulation of the fetus. Based on

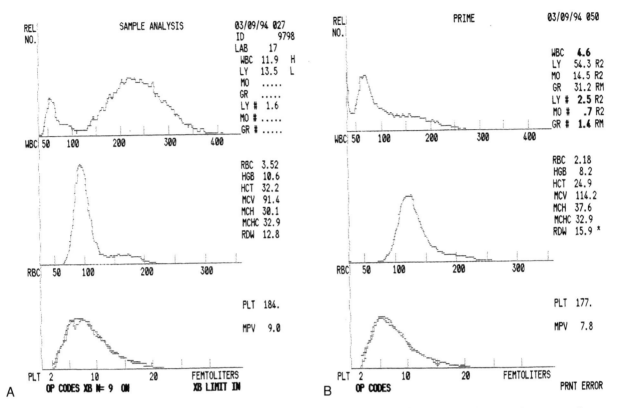

Fig. 28-5. Maternal **(A)** and fetal **(B)** hemograms showing marked difference in red corpuscle mean cell volume (MCV).

the normal fetal blood counts described in the previous section, any degree of fetal anemia is considered sufficient to transfuse the fetus because of the inability to resample frequently and the possibility that the anemia will progress rapidly once it has occurred. In practice, a hematocrit of less than 30 percent is generally the threshold for transfusion. Only in exceptional circumstances will transfusion not be rapidly instituted, such as (1) a stable serial fetal hematocrit of 25 to 30 (by cordocentesis), (2) other indication for cordocentesis (e.g., alloimmune thrombocytopenia) in a mother known not to have RBC alloimmunization, or (3) a very mature fetus.

Generally, donor blood that is group O, Rh negative, and lacking the antigens to which the mother is sensitized is used for transfusion to the fetus. In the case of sensitization to atypical blood group antigens, it is acceptable to use Rh-positive blood for

transfusion if the fetus is found to be Rh positive, provided the mother is Rh positive as well.

A substantial experience has now been accrued at several centers using washed maternal red cells for the treatment of severe hemolytic disease of the fetus.[44] We believe that all pregnant women who have RBC alloimmunization and whose fetuses must undergo IUT should be informed of the option of using maternal autologous blood (if compatible). Maternal blood negative for disease markers may be donated and used for the first transfusion, prior to knowledge of the fetal blood type. The theoretical, albeit small, risk of ABO incompatibility must be reviewed with each patient in this setting, if the maternal blood to be used is other than type O blood.[45] Repeated use of maternal blood, where possible, will avoid exposure of both mother and fetus to multiple donors. We use frozen deglycerolized red cells, al-

Test	Study	16	17	18	19	20	21	22	23	24	25	26	27	28	29	30	31	32	33	34
RBC (x 10 12/L)	1				2.66 ± 0.29		2.96 ± 0.26		3.06 ± 0.26					3.52 ± 0.32						
	2		2.5 ± 0.1							2.9 ± 0.2										
	3				2.8 ± 0.3		2.8 ± 0.35		3.0 ± 0.3		3.1 ± 0.3		3.1 ± 0.3		3.2 ± 0.35		3.3 ± 0.3		3.4 ± 0.3	
Hemoglobin (g/dl)	1					11.47 ± 0.78	12.28 ± 0.89			12.40 ± 0.77					13.35 ± 1.17					
	2		11.0 ± 0.7						12.1 ± 0.8											
	3																			
Hematocrit (%)	1				35.86 ± 3.29		38.53 ± 3.21			38.59 ± 2.41			41.54 ± 3.31							
	2		33.0 ± 2.0						36.0 ± 2.0											
	3																			
MCV (fl)	1				133.92 ± 8.83		138.06 ± 6.17			126.19 ± 6.23			118.17 ± 5.75							
	2		134.0 ± 11.0						121.0 ± 8.0											
	3																			
WBC (x 10 9/L)	1				4.20 ± 0.83		4.19 ± 0.84			3.95 ± 0.69				4.44 ± 0.85						
	2		4.7 ± 0.8						4.3 ± 0.9											
	3				2.3 ± 1.0		2.4 ± 1.0		2.5 ± 1.1		2.7 ± 1.1		2.9 ± 1.0		4.0 ± 1.0		4.2 ± 1.0		4.5 ± 1.2	
Platelets (10 9/L)	1				242.1 ± 34.48		258.2 ± 53.65			259.4 ± 42.45				253.5 ± 36.6						
	2		185.0 ± 31.0						218.0 ± 21.0											
	3																			

Fig. 28-6. Normal fetal hematologic indices (mean ±SD) for fetuses undergoing cordocentesis for diagnosis of genetic abnormalities or infectious diseases who were found to be unaffected. (Data from Forrestier, et al.,[39] DeWaele et al.,[40] and Weiner et al.[41])

lowing us to ignore the donor cytomegalovirus (CMV) serostatus. Also there is evidence that filtration leukoreduction also may be effective in minimizing viral transmission[46] (see Ch. 39).

Fetal blood from the first cordocentesis in each patient with HDFN must be sent for blood typing, since after transfusion of donor blood there will be great difficulty in typing the fetal blood. Depending on gestational age and fetal weight, 1 to 4 ml of fetal blood may be readily obtained during each cordocentesis. At the first cordocentesis, generally 0.5 to 1.0 ml is collected in a microhematocrit tube for the determination of hemoglobin, hematocrit, and MCV; an additional 0.5 to 1.0 ml is provided to the blood bank for typing of fetal blood and performance of the direct antiglobulin test (DAT).

Selection and Preparation of Red Blood Cells for Intrauterine Fetal Transfusion

The red cells selected for IUT must be compatible with a current sample of the mother's serum in crossmatch. At each opportunity, the mother's antibody titer(s) should be determined for comparison with previous measurements, and a panel of reagent red cells, selected to lack the antigens known to be involved, should be tested with maternal serum to ensure that no additional antibody specificities have appeared since the last examination. Red cells intended for IUT must then be shown to lack all antigens to which the mother is sensitized. It is desirable to report the details of immunohematologic studies of the mother's, father's, and fetal blood samples, so that the laboratory findings, and therefore the precise condition being treated, are clear to all members of the treatment team as the pregnancy proceeds. Two sample reports prepared on the occasion of percutaneous umbilical blood sampling (PUBS) are reproduced in Table 28-4 and 28-5. Such comprehensive reports are especially useful when multiple antibody specificities are involved and not all of them are affecting the fetus, as in the second example.

Blood products are prepared for IUT in similar ways to blood prepared for any transfusion, but with several additional measures taken. Donor red cells are tested to be negative for sickle hemoglobin. To prevent graft-versus-host disease (GVHD), the cells should be irradiated. Our practice is to irradiate with 3,000 rad (30 Gy) of γ-radiation, usually 2 to 3 hours and no more than 6 hours before use to minimize loss of intracellular potassium,[47] although such a policy may be more stringent than necessary because only small volumes of plasma are transfused.[48]

Table 28-4. Blood Bank Consultation Report for Pregnancy Affected by RBC Alloimmunization With Anti-C and Anti-D Antibodies

CONSULTANT REPORT: DATE: _____

    Date of specimen: 08 March 1994
    Mother's Blood: O Rh: NEG
        Probable Rh genotype: rr (cde/cde)
        Antibody detected: anti-C (1:512) and anti-D (1:128)
    Father's blood: A Rh: Pos
        Probable Rh genotype: R_1r (CDe/cde)
    Fetal blood type: O Rh: POS
        Probable Rh genotype: R_1r (CDe/cde)
        Direct Coombs result: Positive
        Red cell elution result: anti-C and anti-D

Testing of the mother's serum for anti-red cell antibodies reveals anti-C with a titer of 1:512 and anti-D with a titer of 1:128. The maternal red cells are negative for the C and D antigens. The direct Coombs test on fetal RBC is positive with broad-spectrum and monospecific anti-IgG anti-human globulin and negative with anticomplement antiserum. Anti-C and anti-D were demonstrated in elution studies from fetal red cells.

Interpretation: The positive direct Coombs test on the fetal RBCs indicates that maternal anti-C and anti-D antibodies have crossed the placenta and are reacting with the fetal C and D antigens. The mother was probably sensitized to C and D during this or previous pregnancies with fetuses that had inherited C and D antigens from the father, or previous transfusions. These results suggest that anti-C and anti-D are potentially clinically significant in this case.

Conclusion: Maternal anti-C and anti-D antibodies are responsible for the fetus's positive direct Coombs. Current titer of anti-C is 1:512 and anti-D is 1:128.

Table 28-5. Blood Bank Consultation Report for Pregnancy Affected by RBC Alloimmunization With Anti-c

REPORT:	Additional Antigens
Date of specimen: 04 February 1994	
Mother's blood: A Rh: Positive	
Probable Rh genotype: R_1R_1 (DCe/DCe)	Fy^a (−) Fy^b (+)
Antibody detected: Anti-c (1:32)	
Antibody detected: Anti-E (1:8)	
Antibody detected: Anti-Fy^a (1:4)	
Father's blood: A Rh: Negative	
Probable Rh genotype: rr (dce/dce)	Fy^a (+) Fy^b (+)
Fetal blood type: A Rh: Positive	
Probable Rh genotype: R_1r (DCe/dce)	Fy^a (−) Fy^b (+)
Direct Coombs result: Positive	
Red cell elution result: Positive, anti-c	

Testing of the maternal serum for anti-red cell antibodies reveals (1) anti-c (previously detected) with a titer of 1:32, (2) anti-E (previously detected) with a titer of 1:8; and (3) a newly detected anti-Fy^a with a titer of 1:4. The maternal red cells are c, E and Fy^a negative. The fetal red cells are *c positive* and E and Fy^a negative. The direct Coombs test on fetal RBC is positive with broad spectrum and monospecific anti-IgG antiserum and negative with anti-complement antiserum. An elution was performed on the fetal red cells and only *anti-c antibody* was recovered.

Interpretation: The mother has multiple red cell antibodies, suggesting sensitization during this and/or previous pregnancies. For the current pregnancy, the fetal-red cells are positive for the c antigen. The positive direct Coombs test and positive elution demonstrating anti-c on the fetal red cells suggests that the maternal anti-c antibody is crossing the placenta and reacting with the fetal c red cell antigen. (Of note, initial testing done on fetal blood samples from 2/3/94 revealed a negative direct Coombs test and a negative elution. More recent testing on fetal blood samples from 2/14/94 revealed a weakly positive direct Coombs test with IgG antisera, as well as the positive elution demonstrating anti-c. The reason for the initial negative DAT and eluate is unclear, particularly in light of the clinical picture. Additional special studies were performed, demonstrating the maternal anti-c antibody to be IgG subclass IgG3.

Conclusion: Maternal anti-c antibodies titer 1:32 are responsible for the positive direct Coombs in the fetus. Anti-c alone is detected as the cause of the positive direct Coombs test in the fetus. Maternal anti-E and Fy^a antibodies should not present a problem for the current pregnancy.

The red cells should also be rendered as free of extraneous plasma and other cells as practicable. We process them as frozen thawed and deglycerolized cells resuspended in 0.2 percent dextrose in saline. If maternal red cells are used, the donation is divided in half before freezing, to permit use on two occasions. The final automated cell deglycerolization washing step is lengthened to ensure a high final hematocrit of approximately 85 percent to minimize the volume to be transfused. The higher red cell concentration is crucial to the success of IUT. During gestation, the small total fetal blood volume mandates use of a highly concentrated suspension to avoid overloading the fetoplacental intravascular volume. There is a suggestion that the extremely high viscosity of a too highly concentrated blood product may be detrimental to the transfused cells and to the fetus,[49] especially at the high rates of

transfusion undertaken when fetal transfusion is performed: 1 to 5 ml/min (greater than 1 to 5 ml/kg/min). Thus, donor hematocrits of more than 90 percent are currently not recommended.

Because we use frozen deglycerolized red cells, the product is not leukoreduced by filtration. If frozen deglycerolized cells are not used, other precautions should be taken to avoid transmission of CMV, such as the use of seronegative donors and possibly leukoreduction by filtration. When prepared for transfusion, the net weight of the cells is measured, and a microhematocrit is done to confirm the desired concentration. In our most recent 26 cases, the mean hematocrit was 83 percent (SD ± 6 percent), and net weight provided (not all transfused) averaged 222 g. In addition, in order to minimize the nonfunctional hemoglobin/bilirubin load in the fetus, the degree of hemolysis in the final red cell preparation is measured by visual comparison of the microhematocrit supernatant color with a calibrated color standard. The average free hemoglobin was 145 mg/dl (SD ± 109; range 25 to 450), and values of more than 600 mg/dl are cause for rejecting the unit.

Calculation of Volume of Transfused Red Cells Needed

A substantial experience has accumulated to guide the calculation of the volume of blood needed to correct various degrees of fetal anemia.[50] This is based on calculations of the fetoplacental blood volume at any given gestational age.[51–53] Figure 28-7 is adapted from Nicolaides et al.[50] and shows how the fetal hematocrit, the concentration of transfused red cells, the estimated fetal weight and the desired post-transfusion hematocrit are used to calculate the amount of red cells to transfuse. The total volume for any one IUT is usually within the range of 20 to 120 ml.

Most IUT procedures take between 20 and 60 minutes, during which time the fetus is transfused at a rate of approximately 5 ml/kg/min. This extraordinary rate, 300 ml/kg/h, is only used in major trauma in the setting of rapid exsanguination. Many centers administer a paralytic agent such as pancuronium to the fetus, to prevent the fetus from dislodging the needle during the procedure.[54,55] Generally, the fetus tolerates the volume load very well, probably due to capacitance within the placental vasculature. Fetal intolerance to this large rapid intravascular volume load is generally manifested in FHR abnormalities, especially bradycardia. If any abnormalities are seen, the transfusion is interrupted. If the abnormality is mild and the FHR rapidly returns to baseline with cessation of the transfusion, the transfusion may be reinstituted (within minutes).

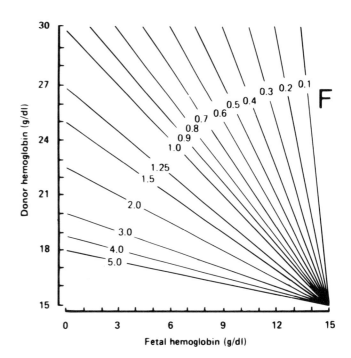

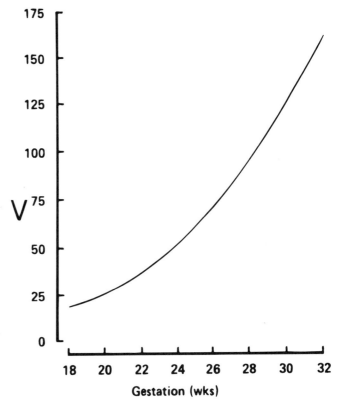

Fig. 28-7. Nomogram for calculating volume of donor blood (ml) necessary to correct fetal anemia. The value F is multiplied by the value V. For example, for a fetus at 24 weeks gestation, the V value is 50. If the pretransfusion fetal hemoglobin is 5 g/dl and the donor blood hemoglobin is 26 g/dl (value F = 0.9), 45 ml of donor blood will have to be transfused to achieve a post-transfusion fetal hemoglobin of 12.5 g/dl (normal mean for gestation). (From Nicolaides et al.[50] with permission.)

Timing of Intrauterine Transfusion

Cordocentesis is the procedure of choice in patients with a history of a child severely affected by HDFN, in anti-D Rh disease with a very high titer (greater than 1:128), in any other atypical blood group antibody disease known to be clinically significant, and when fetal hydrops is present. Delta OD450 determinations have been shown to be unreliable indicators of fetal hemolysis in patients with atypical antibodies.[30] In a patient who is found to be sensitized for the first time during a pregnancy, cordocentesis is chosen in most cases at 26 weeks gestation, the beginning of the third trimester, to determine fetal blood type and hematocrit. There are two reasons for choosing this gestational age. The first is that the third trimester is the time of greatest risk of worsening disease due to fetal hemolysis. The second is that 26 weeks is the point at which a fetus may be able to survive outside the uterus in the event of a procedure-related complication requiring delivery of the fetus (discussed below). If a previous fetus had been affected by immune hydrops or if hydrops is detected early in the current gestation, cordocentesis may be instituted as early as 18 weeks. Cordocentesis may not be necessary if amniocentesis for PCR determination of the fetal Rh(D) locus has shown a negative fetal blood type.

If the risk of severe disease and significant fetal hemolysis is high (based on the factors listed previously), the first cordocentesis may be performed with packed and concentrated red cells prepared and available in the room. When blood is prepared for an IUT, the blood must be drawn up in the syringes and blood tubing prior to the procedure; thus, the unit cannot be reused. This is because the success of an IUT depends on having a procedure of short duration. If allogeneic donor blood is being used, care is taken to control the position of the blood–saline interface, so that donor exposure can be avoided if the procedure must be aborted for any reason. At the New York Hospital-Cornell Medical Center, the pregnancy (or fetal) loss rate from 1991 to 1994 has been 5 losses out of 161 procedures (3.1 percent). Four of these five losses occurred in patients who underwent a procedure of greater than 60 minutes (i.e., needle in the uterus for more than 60 minutes). Because of this experience, we always strive for as short a duration for the procedure time as is safely possible.

In many cases, however, cordocentesis is performed at 26 weeks gestation without preparing for immediate blood transfusion to the fetus. This is usually chosen if the pregnancy is the first in which the patient is alloimmunized, or if the anti-D antibody titer is relatively low (i.e., 1:16 to 1:64). Under these circumstances, there is a significant chance that there will not be a fetal anemia. If a significant fetal anemia is revealed, the patient will be brought back for a repeat procedure, with blood available for transfusion. The timing of the repeat procedure depends on the level of fetal anemia. All attempts are made to avoid fetal hydrops, which is rarely evident at fetal hematocrit levels of greater than or equal to 20 percent (5 SD below the mean for gestational age), but almost always present when the hematocrit falls to 10 percent or less.[17] The timing of repeat procedures is based on the observation that the fetal hematocrit in cases of RBC alloimmunization severely affecting the fetus generally falls at a rate of one hematocrit point per day[56] and can therefore be predicted once the post-transfusion hematocrit is known. However, this figure is more reliable after one or two IVTs have been completed, and the fall-off is due to the stable decay of transfused cells. For example, if the fetal hematocrit is 25 percent at an initial cordocentesis, a repeat procedure would be indicated within 5 days for performance of an IUT. Pre-IUT fetal hematocrits have been seen as low as 5 percent in the hydropic fetus but often range between 15 to 30 percent for those fetuses who are severely affected but not hydropic. Attempts are made to achieve post-IUT fetal hematocrits within the range of 35 to 50 percent. This is achieved by a combination of the calculation of volume needed (see above) and a mid-transfusion sampling of the fetal hematocrit after a majority of the calculated volume needed has been transfused.

Generally, the frequency of IUT is about every 2 to 4 weeks, although occasionally IUT is required every 7 to 10 days, depending on the rate of fall in hematocrit in the individual patient. A pilot study at our institution suggested that the number and frequency of IUTs could be decreased by the use of larger volume transfusions without any apparent increase in fetal mortality or morbidity, or any increase in the pregnancy loss rate (i.e., preterm delivery). A minor increase in fetal bradycardia was noted with the larger volume transfusions, although all were completed without other complications.

Once serial IUTs have been initiated, the last procedure is timed to be at approximately 34 to 36 weeks gestation. This allows for a time period of 2 to 3 weeks after the procedure for maturation of the fetal lungs, so that delivery can be performed as close to term as possible.

Complications of Intrauterine Transfusion

The complications of IUT are numerous, but fortunately uncommon in experienced hands. Table 28-6 lists the complications and their management.

Neonatal Management

After the delivery of a fetus suffering from severe intrauterine alloimmune hemolysis, there are abrupt changes in the biochemical environment and physiology of the neonate. In addition to anemia, increas-

ing bilirubin levels may result in brain damage if left untreated. Initially, phototherapy is tried; if this fails, the next step is exchange transfusion. The level of bilirubin at which phototherapy or an exchange transfusion is initiated depends on the degree of prematurity of the neonate, the degree of illness of the infant, and the rate of rise of the bilirubin. In general, even a very sick premature newborn would rarely have an exchange transfusion at a bilirubin of less than 10 mg/dl and a term well newborn would almost always start phototherapy at a bilirubin of greater than 15 mg/dl. Comprehensive reviews of this topic are widely available.[55] A double volume exchange with antigen-negative, whole blood, or reconstituted whole blood (RBC plus plasma) is usually used. The blood volume also depends on the degree of prematurity but is high even in a term newborn, approximately 100 ml/kg.

In the severely affected fetus, IUT is not only lifesaving for the fetus but has a positive effect on the neonatal course. Babies are typically born less jaun-

Table 28-6. Complications of Intrauterine Transfusions and Their Management

Complications	Management	Frequency
1. Fetal heart rate abnormalities (bradycardia, tachycardia, severe variable decelerations)	Stop transfusion until resolution of FHR abnormality: if unremitting, delivery	Common
2. Preterm labor	Tocolysis (depending on circumstances and only if transfusion is successful)	Uncommon
3. Preterm premature rupture of membranes	No vaginal examinations, NSTs; observation	Uncommon
4. Abruptio placenta	For mild abruption, observation; for significant abruption, delivery	Rare
5. Inability to access umbilical circulation	Fetal cardiac puncture, fetal hepatic vein puncture, IPT	Uncommon
6. Umbilical cord hematoma	Emergent delivery (always associated with FHR abnormalities)	Rare
7. Direct fetal exsanguination	Emergent delivery	Rare
8. Fetal death	Delivery of stillborn	Rare
9. Chorioamnionitis	Delivery with antibiotic treatment in labor	Rare
10. Maternal blood transfusion reaction	Expectant, symptomatic	Rare
11. Maternal abdominal wall/rectus hematoma	Expectant, surgery if patient is unstable from hemorrhage.	Rare
12. Worsening of hemolytic disease due to increased transplacental hemorrhage or other unknown factors	More frequent IUTs	Unknown
13. Puncture of umbilical artery	Remove needle and replace in umbilical vein	Uncommon

Abbreviations: FHR, fetal heart rate; IPT, intraperitoneal transfusion; IUT, intrauterine transfusion.

diced, only mildly anemic for gestational age (if transfused effectively), without hydrops or significant hepatosplenomegaly. Transfusions are not invariably needed, and exchange transfusion is distinctly uncommon. Occasionally, these babies are even sent to the well-baby nursery.

Recent studies have documented the apparent suppression of erythropoiesis by IVT.[58,59] Neonatal erythropoietin levels were shown to be inappropriately low, and hemoglobin fell to levels of less than 6 g/dl without compensatory reticulocytosis by 3 to 6 weeks postnatal age.[58] Subsequently, selective marrow erythroid hypoplasia was seen in three of three neonates; a pilot study of erythropoietin administration suggested that failure of red cell production was a second major cause of the anemia. Currently, we are conducting a double-blind, randomized, placebo-controlled trial of the use of erythropoietin in the late anemia of newborns with Rh alloimmune hemolysis who received at least two IVTs. Our guidelines for postnatal transfusion of RBC are to give 15 ml/kg for a hemoglobin of 7 g/dl or less without reticulocytosis. Clearly, as in any patient, the development of symptoms of anemia (i.e., tachycardia and/or tachypnea) can be an indication to modify these guidelines. This "late" anemia can persist for up to 4 months.

Other Causes of Immune Fetal Anemia

Maternal Autoimmune Hemolytic Anemia

The estimated incidence of autoimmune hemolytic anemia (AIHA) is about 1:100,000, much more rare than autoimmune thrombocytopenia. However, AIHA does occur during pregnancy, and severe immune hemolysis may pose a risk to the mother and fetus. However, only a small percentage of affected women deliver infants who have hemolytic disease of the newborn and exchange transfusion has only rarely been necessary.[60] It is impossible to define indications for cordocentesis precisely, but amniocentesis to measure the delta OD450 may be indicated if the mother's AIHA causes severe anemia and does not respond to therapy.[60,61] Weekly monitoring of the FHR with both NST and ultrasound may be indicated when significant degrees of anemia are present.

ANEMIA: NONIMMUNE DISEASE

Parvovirus B19 infection

Parvovirus B19 is the etiologic agent responsible for so-called fifth (exanthematous) disease or "slapped cheeks" in children. Parvovirus can infect the adult, usually producing very mild flu-like symptoms and/or a rash, and has been documented to cause anemia and hydrops in the fetus of patients who develop an infection while pregnant. If a pregnant woman is known to be exposed, primary parvovirus infection can be determined by maternal serologic IgM positivity; these fetuses are at risk of in utero infection. If it is determined that the infant has an intrauterine infection, the pregnancy should be monitored by weekly ultrasound examinations to detect fetal hydrops. Cordocentesis may be performed: precise clinical indications have not been defined.

Hematopoietic cells are believed to be infected by the virus, causing severe anemia. The sequelae are fetal hydrops (nonimmune) and, if the anemia remains untreated, fetal death in a substantial proportion of cases.[62–64] IUT has been shown to alleviate the anemia and hydrops and to allow subsequent resolution of the infection (i.e., no further anemia or hydrops recurs and no further IUTs are necessary). Anecdotal data suggest that these fetuses do not have lasting sequelae. Transfusion is handled similarly to transfusion of fetuses affected by RBC alloimmunization.

Homozygous α-Thalassemia

Three long-term survivors affected with homozygous α-thalassemia have been reported; none received IUT.[65–67] Postnatal management of these infants is similar to that used for homozygous β-thalassemia: transfusions and chelation therapy to minimize tissue iron accumulation. All three survivors have suffered severe neurologic sequelae for reasons that remain uncertain.

The lack of a replacement for the α chain in α-thalassemia, as compared to the γ chain replacing the β chain in β-thalassemia, results in severe fetal anemia and fetal demise in α- but not β-thalassemia. Prenatal diagnosis is possible for both α- and β-thalassemia. Successful institution of a prenatal screening program for α-thalassemia could result in the development of a fetal transfusion program in cases in which the parents are unwilling or it is too late for elective termination of the pregnancy. Currently, however, there are no reports of fetal transfusion therapy for this disease.

Congenital Dyserythropoietic Anemias

Three recent cases have been described in which hydrops fetalis developed in cases later diagnosed as congenital dyserythropoietic anemia.[68–70] These cases emphasize the need for the study of unexplained anemias after birth, including a bone marrow aspirate, since marrow dyserythropoiesis is the diagnostic feature of these dyserythropoietic anemias. The use of the sucrose hemolysis and the Ham acid hemolysis (HAM) tests are helpful, as are more specialized testing of the red blood cell, available only on a research basis. However, because any marrow recovering from a severe insult and/or anemia may demonstrate dyserythropoiesis,[71] careful consideration of the findings, and possibly a repeat bone marrow following attainment of a stable hemoglobin, are required to confirm the diagnosis. Suspecting these cases other than by detection of fetal hydrops by ultrasound or by family history is not yet possible.

IMMUNE DISEASE: THROMBOCYTOPENIA

Alloimmune Thrombocytopenia

Fetal and neonatal alloimmune thrombocytopenia (AIT) develops as a result of maternal sensitization to fetal platelet antigens. AIT is the platelet equivalent of hemolytic disease of the fetus and newborn. IgG antiplatelet antibodies produced by the mother are directed against the platelet antigens that the mother lacks and that the fetus inherits from the father.

The most commonly involved platelet antigen (polymorphism), Pl^{A1} (HPA-1a), is expressed on platelet glycoprotein GPIIIa, but other platelet specific antigens on GPIIIa as well as other platelet glycoproteins can be involved. The Pl$^{A1/2}$ (HPA-1a/1b) polymorphism is the most clinically important in Caucasians but virtually never occurs in Orientals. By contrast, the Yuk/Pen (HPA-4) polymorphism is an important cause of AIT in Orientals but is not found in Caucasians. Bak (HPA-3) incompatibility

appears to be rare but can be severe when it occurs. In contrast, Br (HPA-5) incompatibility seems to be clinically milder than Pl^{A1} incompatibility.[72] Other antigens have not yet had sufficient cases reported for the spectrum of clinical disease to be well defined. An important factor in this disorder is that, although platelet count is often severely low, platelet function appears to be only mildly impaired.

Sensitization is presumed to occur by the same mechanism as in RBC alloimmunization, that is, maternal immune stimulation by the foreign fetal antigen. Genetic restrictions on immune response limit the number of Pl^{A1}-negative women who actually become sensitized in the setting of parental incompatibility, such that only approximately 1 in 20 Pl^{A1}-negative women with a Pl^{A1} positive fetus will develop AIT.[73] These antiplatelet IgG antibodies are transported across the placenta, where they mediate fetal immune thrombocytopenia. Unfortunately, no routine prenatal screening test has been designed to prevent AIT since, unlike RBC alloimmunization, 40 percent of cases involve the first sibling in the family.

As in RBC alloimmunization, a woman who has had one child with AIT is at high risk of having another affected child, depending on the specific antigen incompatibility and paternal zygosity. The natural course of disease in AIT is one of progressive thrombocytopenia in the fetus as pregnancy continues and often with worsening of the thrombocytopenia from one pregnancy to the next, similar to RBC alloimmunization.[74,75]

The most serious complication of AIT, in either the fetus or neonate, is intracranial hemorrhage (ICH). ICH is known to occur in a proportion of cases when the fetal or neonatal platelet count is below 20,000/μl and is identified in approximately 20 percent of cases overall, as many as one-half of which occur before birth. ICH in AIT is typically intraparenchymal, unlike ICH due to prematurity, wherein the neonates mainly have intraventricular hemorrhages. ICH may lead to permanent neurologic sequelae, such as seizures, learning disabilities, and mental retardation, or to death.

Management

The severity of thrombocytopenia early in gestation and the relatively high risk of antenatal ICH combined with developments of fetal blood sampling

(FBS) and fetal platelet transfusion have resulted in a number of centers attempting the management of fetal thrombocytopenia. The challenge is to increase the fetal platelet count and prevent ICH in utero, since management of neonatal AIT during the postnatal period is relatively straightforward.

We believe that maternally administered intravenous γ-globulin (IVIg) is the treatment of choice for the pregnancy at risk for AIT (documented by a previously affected child). Low-dose prednisone treatment was attempted and then essentially abandoned as insufficiently effective; the results have not yet been published in peer-reviewed form.[76] We have now treated 72 pregnant women with IVIg, both with and without concomitant glucocorticoids. The initial results of the pilot study of that experience were published in 1988[74] and 1992.[77]

More recently, we completed a study of 54 pregnancies in which thrombocytopenic fetuses (based on fetal blood samples required prior to entry) affected by AIT received 1 g/kg/week of IVIg administered to the mother and were randomized for the addition of 1.5 mg/day of dexamethasone. Response was monitored at a second FBS 4 to 6 weeks later. The nonresponders (according to a protocol definition) were either delivered (n = 3) or entered on a salvage arm of the protocol (n = 9) consisting of continued IVIg and the addition of 60 mg/day of prednisone.

The addition of low-dose dexamethasone had no effect on the platelet increase in response to therapy. Combining the data from the two groups treated with IVIg (with and without dexamethasone), the mean platelet increase from the first FBS to the second FBS and to birth was substantial (greater than 30,000/μl) despite the tendency of AIT to worsen as gestation progresses. Comparison of the birth platelet count of the treated fetus to that of the previous sibling showed a mean increase of well over 50,000/μl, with 40 of 51 patients having greater counts than the previous sibling despite the tendency in AIT to worsen in subsequent gestations. The addition of prednisone was effective in 5 out of 10 of the unresponsive cases treated.

Unfortunately, it became clear, during the course of this study, that there was an increased tendency to fatal exsanguination at FBS when the fetal platelet count was less than 20,000/μl. We now recommend immediately obtaining (1 to 2 minute) the fetal platelet count at FBS with the needle left in position. To be safe, if the fetal platelet count is less than 50,000/μl, we recommend transfusion of platelets (see below). Using this policy, we have experienced no further fetal losses.

Early cesarean section is an option, but cannot be the sole therapy when many cases are documented to have severe fetal thrombocytopenia prior to 30 weeks of gestation, one as early as 16 weeks of gestation.[78] Furthermore, early ICH (prior to 30 weeks gestation) has been documented in well over 10 cases. We use early cesarean section adjunctively depending upon the fetal platelet count. If the count is low (with or without treatment), we would deliver, except under extreme circumstances, at or after 34 weeks following proof of fetal lung maturity.

Other investigators have suggested that serial fetal platelet transfusions are the preferred therapy for severely affected fetuses with marked thrombocytopenia (fetal platelet count less than 20,000/μl) and severe hemorrhagic complications (ICH) in a previous infant. Our unpublished data clearly demonstrates that the majority of fetuses with platelet counts less than 20,000/μl respond to IVIG. Fortunately fetuses in whom the previous sibling has suffered an early ICH (prior to 30 weeks gestation) are rare; unfortunately, treatment information in these fetuses is correspondingly limited. The optimal form of management for this most severely affected group is therefore uncertain at this time.

The general use of fetal platelet transfusions for the more typical case (previous sibling with low platelet count and with or without "late" ICH) has much less to favor it. Unlike RBC alloimmunization, where IUT is the treatment of choice in severe cases, the effectiveness of treatment of AIT by platelet transfusions is limited by the shorter lifespan of platelets. Platelet transfusions have to be given weekly to maintain the fetal platelet count, for which there is ample evidence of clinical effectiveness with post-transfusion platelet counts well over 100,000/μl. However, weekly cordocentesis and fetal platelet transfusions are relatively invasive and fetal mortality has been reported.[79] Accordingly, we feel that weekly fetal platelet transfusions should be reserved for those patients who are IVIg nonresponders, since none of the 73 maternal-fetal pairs in two trials reported by our center suffered any fetal or neonatal ICH despite more than 15 previous siblings having suffered ICH. There is, however, one reported case of ICH at 31 weeks gestation in a fetus suffering from alloimmune thrombocytopenia who had received 11 weeks of IVIg therapy (at a dosage of 1 g/kg maternal body weight/week).[80]

In summary, the optimal management of fetal thrombocytopenia secondary to alloimmune thrombocytopenia remains to be completely defined. Nonetheless, we believe that medical management with IVIg with or without steroids is effective therapy for most cases with platelet transfusion reserved optimally for cases failing medical management or possibly for the most severe cases. At this time, it would also seem appropriate to monitor the efficacy of therapy with fetal blood sampling, covered by platelet transfusion, in order to be able to alter therapy (including early delivery, combined IVIg and prednisone, or weekly fetal platelet transfusions) for cases not responding to initial management. The optimal antenatal management of the pregnancy at risk of AIT is therefore not yet resolved.[78]

Selection and Preparation of Platelets for Intrauterine Fetal Transfusion

Platelet transfusions to the fetus with alloimmune thrombocytopenia (AIT) are done with platelets that are known to be negative for the antigen responsible for the incompatibility in question; most commonly this is Pl^{A1} (HPA-1a, Zwa). Allogeneic antigen-negative platelets have proved efficacious.[81] However, owing to availability and situations in which the antigen in question is still unknown, the preferred platelet donor in most instances is the mother. Thus, we prefer to use maternal concentrated, irradiated, filtration-leukoreduced platelets, collected from a unit of whole blood or by platelet apheresis, for transfusion to the fetus.[82] The mother should meet the usual requirements for directed donation and for autologous donation in pregnancy, but exceptions to the criteria can be considered by the obstetricians and transfusion medicine physicians in individual cases. Red cells are returned to the mother after the platelets have been separated. There are several advantages to the use of maternal platelets, in addition to their ready availability. The risk that the transfusion will transmit disease to the mother is elimi-

nated, as is the risk of sensitizing the mother to additional red or white cell antigens. Also, preliminary evidence suggests that HLA incompatibility may affect the fetal response to platelet transfusion if multiple transfusions are contemplated.[82] Thus, using maternal platelets to provide a partial HLA match may allow the fetus to respond to multiple platelet transfusions with a higher fetal platelet count and with longer survival of the donor platelets. It has also been suggested that platelet crossmatching may be of use (Thomas S. Kickler, personal communication, 1994).

If the mother is seropositive for hepatitis C virus (HCV), human T-cell leukemia virus (HTLV), human immunodeficiency virus (HIV), or hepatitis B virus (HBsAg or anti-HBc) or has an elevated alanine aminotransferase (ALT) level, the use of maternal platelets should be avoided. However, in some cases, as when the mother is seropositive for CMV, their use may be considered if allogeneic platelets are not available or are unacceptable to the mother. In the latter instance, leukoreduction filtration of the maternal platelet preparation would reduce the CMV content, and data are accumulating that such filtration may effectively prevent CMV transmission.[83] The role of maternal anti-CMV in protecting the fetus from intrauterine transfusion of CMV-infected leukocytes is unclear, but the potential for harm to the fetus by CMV is present.[84]

Platelet transfusions to the fetus are generally of smaller volumes than RBC transfusions. Thus, deliberate packing of platelets beyond the usual concentration achieved for ordinary platelet concentrates is not mandatory. The classic approach is to centrifuge the platelets to remove the supernatant plasma in order to remove anti-Pl^{A1} antibody. The platelets are then resuspended in an appropriate solution[85] and irradiated in much the same manner as are red cells destined for transfusion. Platelet concentrates are technically more difficult to prepare than red blood cells, requiring careful attention to centrifugation speeds and controlled time for resting and agitation after processing and before use to dissociate aggregates. These difficulties and the possible loss of function of transfused platelets handled in this manner has led to the obtaining of platelets in as concentrated a fashion as possible (to minimize the quantity of antiplatelet antibody) and their transfusion to the fetus without additional handling other than for irradiation. The optimal approach remains to be clarified.

We calculate the volume of platelet concentrate needed by an empiric method. We transfuse 1 to 5 ml of platelet concentrate for a fetus of less than 30 weeks gestation and 5 to 10 ml for a fetus over 30 weeks. This assumes that platelet concentrates contain 55 billion platelets in about 40 ml average volume, thus providing 1 billion platelets per ml and that the average fetoplacental blood volume for a fetus prior to 30 weeks is approximately 150 ml. Since a platelet count of 100,000 per microliter (μl) is 100,000,000 per ml, then 10 ml of platelet concentrate would provide an increase of 100,000/μl to the fetus who has a blood volume of 100 ml. In practice, while waiting for a pretransfusion fetal platelet count, we begin to transfuse platelets slowly, to prevent the disastrous occurrence (in a severely affected fetus) of needle dislodgement and exsanguination.

Different methods of harvesting platelets (apheresis machine versus manual harvesting from whole blood with subsequent replacement of red cells to the mother) may result in widely differing concentrations of platelets in the concentrate to be transfused to the fetus. Thus, a platelet count post-transfusion is needed in each instance to ensure adequacy of the fetal platelet count before the cordocentesis needle is removed. Using this empiric method for platelet transfusions, we know of no cases of overtransfusion of platelets, and no cases of fetal exsanguination.

A different method for the calculation of the volume of donor platelets necessary has been elucidated by Kaplan et al.[75] and Murphy et al.[81] The formula is as follows:

Volume of concentrate to be infused =
(desired increment of platelet count ×
fetoplacental blood volume)/
platelet count of concentrate

Charts are available for the derivation of fetoplacental blood volume that are dependent on gestational age.[51–53] This calculation requires that a platelet count be performed on the concentrate to be transfused, and still requires that a platelet count be performed on fetal blood post-transfusion before the removal of the needle. Ensuring the correct volume of platelet concentrate to be transfused is important, as fetal cardiac arrest has happened in association with overtransfusion of platelets.[86]

Autoimmune Thrombocytopenia

Idiopathic (autoimmune) thrombocytopenia (ITP) is the term used to describe an autoimmune disease in which autoantibodies develop to the patient's own platelet antigens. The result is the accelerated destruction of platelets with the clinical consequence of thrombocytopenia and an increased risk of bleeding episodes. There is an extensive review on the pathophysiology of this disease.[87]

Maternal ITP may itself worsen during pregnancy but management of the mother is not the subject of this discussion. One of the major concerns of the obstetrician dealing with a pregnant woman with ITP, however, is the potential occurrence of neonatal thrombocytopenia. In cases of ITP, unlike in AIT, the risk of significant thrombocytopenia in the neonate is not high. The mechanism for fetal thrombocytopenia is presumed to be transplacental passage of the IgG anti-platelet autoantibodies responsible for the maternal thrombocytopenia, the details of which are a matter of continued speculation and ongoing research. Clinically significant neonatal thrombocytopenia occurs in the setting of maternal ITP in less than 15 percent of cases and ICH occurs in 1 to 2 percent overall.[88,89]

Management

Maternal treatment consists of steroid medications and IVIg. Both medications have been shown to increase the maternal platelet count when disease appears to be active. Limited data have shown that the effect of maternal treatment on the fetal platelet count is at best uncertain.[90] Samuels et al.[91] were unable to show a relationship of maternal treatment with neonatal platelet count, but the patient groups were not controlled. Christiaens et al.[92] demonstrated that low-dose β-methasone, equivalent to 15 mg of prednisone per day, administered to the mother during the last 2 to 3 weeks of pregnancy had no effect on the fetal platelet count in a randomized study. However, more recent data exploring the comparison of serial neonatal platelet counts of mothers who have two or more children suggests that aggressive maternal treatment may increase the fetal platelet count, but this area requires formal study.[93] The lack of proven antenatal ICH and the rarity of any ICH in the neonate has failed to demonstrate a need for this form of treatment.

Cordocentesis

There is no consensus regarding the use of cordocentesis in cases of ITP. The risk of thrombocytopenia in the fetus whose mother has ITP is approximately 10 to 15 percent.[88,89] The risk of ICH in these thrombocytopenic infants is itself approximately 10 percent or an estimated risk of neonatal ICH, or only 1 percent of all pregnancies in women with ITP.[91] Indeed, one recent review was only able to report on four cases of ICH in infants born to mothers with ITP.[94] It is not known whether elective cesarean delivery decreases ICH in thrombocytopenic infants, but this supposition has been used as a justification for cordocentesis in cases of ITP.

If cordocentesis is performed at 37 or 38 weeks gestation (prior to the onset of labor), the presence of fetal thrombocytopenia has been used as an indication for cesarean delivery. The procedure related risk of cordocentesis is at least 1 percent, even at this gestational age; some investigators have therefore questioned the use of cordocentesis for this indication, because the incidence of ICH in these infants is low.[95,96] If one believes that cesarean section would substantially reduce the risk of ICH in fetuses with severe thrombocytopenia and that cesarean section should be avoided in the great majority of cases (80 to 90 percent) in which the fetal platelet count will be normal, the procedure is justified. It is important, however, to perform cordocentesis in near proximity to facilities where an emergent cesarean delivery could be performed if either unremitting fetal bradycardia or persistent bleeding from the puncture site in the umbilical cord occur. The need for "prophylactic" platelet transfusion to prevent hemorrhage at cordocentesis as described above for AIT is not defined.

Systemic Lupus Erythematosus

In general, the fetal thrombocytopenia and neonatal thrombocytopenia in systemic lupus erythematosus (SLE) are thought to be similar to that seen in ITP. Insufficient cases have been studied prospectively, to be sure that the situation is comparable to that

of maternal ITP. Maternal placental insufficiency, a common complication of SLE, may have detrimental effects on fetal well-being unrelated to the fetal platelet count.

Thrombocytopenia Absent Radii

Increasingly, the use of routine prenatal ultrasound may lead to the diagnosis of TAR syndrome (thrombocytopenia with absent radii) by virtue of the lack of radii. The severe thrombocytopenia and high rate of ICH in the neonatal period raise the question of intrauterine platelet transfusion therapy, at least to safeguard the delivery. This remains unresolved. The gene responsible for TAR has been recently identified so that the use of recombinant DNA techniques for prenatal diagnosis may be possible in the future.

INTRAUTERINE BONE MARROW TRANSPLANT

Intrauterine bone marrow transplantation (BMT) has been performed for prenatally diagnosed congenital conditions in which there is inadequate hematopoiesis of the cellular blood components or increased destruction of these cells. The advantage is thought to be that engraftment of donor tissues can be given to a fetus who is immunoincompetent, thus avoiding the problem of graft rejection and graft-versus-host disease (GVHD). Two types of donor tissues have been used: donor human bone marrow, or fetal liver and thymus. Both of these latter tissues are thought to contain the desired component—the totipotential stem cell. Conditions in which intrauterine BMT has been attempted (on a research basis only) are listed in Table 28-7. A recent review

Table 28-7. Fetal Conditions in Which Intrauterine Hematopoietic Stem Cell Transplantation Has Been Attempted

Rh alloimmunization
α-Thalassemia
β-Thallassemia
Metachromatic leukodystrophy
Bare lymphocyte syndrome
Severe combined immunodeficiency syndrome
Chediak-Higashi syndrome
Hurler syndrome

listed 13 cases at 6 centers.[97] Engraftment is thought to have occurred in only 4 of the cases. GVHD and bacterial contamination of the fetal tissues used are thought to have resulted in the death of several of the fetuses.

CONCLUSION

Major advances in the diagnosis and treatment of the fetus affected by anemia or thrombocytopenia have been made with the advent of ultrasound combined with invasive access to the fetus. Refinements in the management of these fetal cytopenias continue as the knowledge of the pathophysiology and biochemical environment of the fetus affected by them expands. The transfusion guidelines described in this chapter—including indications for IUT, techniques of preparation of blood products, and modes of transfusion—will therefore be subject to change in the near future.

REFERENCES

1. Hohlfeld P, Forestier F, Kaplan C et al: Fetal thrombocytopenia: a retrospective survey of 5194 fetal blood samplings. Blood 84:1851, 1994
2. Nicolini U, Nicolaides P, Fisk NM et al: Fetal blood sampling from the intrahepatic vein: analysis of safety and clinical experience with 214 procedures. Obstet Gynecol 76:47, 1990
3. Plater F: Observationum Basle, 1641, p. 748
4. Ballantyne JW: The Diseases and Deformities of the Foetus. Oliver & Boyd, 1892–1895
5. Diamond LK, Blackfan KP, Baty JM: Erythroblastosis fetalis and its association with universal edema of the fetus, icterus gravis neonatorum and anemia of the newborn. J Pediatr 1:269, 1932
6. Landsteiner K, Weiner AS: An agglutinable factor in human blood recognized by immune sera for Rhesus blood. Proc Soc Exp Biol Med 43:223, 1940
7. Levine P: Isoimmunization in pregnancy and the pathogenesis of erythroblastosis fetalis. p. 505. In Karsner HT, Hooker SB (eds): 1941 Yearbook of Pathology and Immunology. Yearbook, Chicago, 1941
8. Pickles MM: Haemolytic Disease of the Newborn. Blackwell Scientific, Oxford, 1949
9. Liley AW: Liquor amnii analysis in the management of pregnancy complicated by rhesus immunization. Am J Obstet Gynecol 82:1359, 1961
10. Liley AW: Intrauterine transfusion of foetus in haemolytic disease. BMJ 2:1107, 1963
11. Rodeck CH, Holman CA, Karicki J et al: Direct intravascular fetal blood transfusion by fetoscopy in severe rhesus isoimmunization. Lancet 1:625, 1981
12. Rodeck CH, Nicolaides KH, Warsof SL et al: The management of severe rhesus isoimmunization by fetoscopic intravascular transfusions. Am J Obstet Gynecol 150:769, 1984
13. Bowman JM, Pollock JM, Penston LE: Fetomaternal transplacental hemorrhage during pregnancy and after delivery. Vox Sang 51:117, 1986
14. Freda VJ, Gorman JG, Pollack W: Successful prevention of sensitization to Rh with an experimental anti-Rh gamma$_2$ globulin antibody preparation. Fed Proc 22:374, 1963
15. Freda VJ, Gorman JG, Pollack W, Bowe E: Prevention of Rh hemolytic disease: ten years' clinical experience with Rh immune globulin. N Engl J Med 292:1014, 1975
16. Bowman JM, Friesen AD, Pollack JM, Taylor WE: WinRho: Rh immune globulin prepared by ion exchange for intravenous use. Can Med Assoc J 123:1121, 1980
17. Nicolaides KH: Management of red blood cell isoimmunized pregnancies. In Chervenak FA, Isaacson GC, Campbell S (eds): Ultrasound in Obstetrics and Gynecology. Little, Brown, Boston, 1993
18. Bowman JM, Pollock JM: Antenatal Rh prophylaxis: 28 week gestation service program. Can Med Assoc J 118:627, 1978
19. Prevention of D Isoimmunization. American College of Obstetricians and Gynecologists Technical Bulletin 147. Washington, DC, 1990
20. de Almeida V, Bowman JM: Massive fetomaternal hemorrhage: Manitoba experience. Obstet Gynecol 83:323, 1994
21. Bowell PJ, Wainscoat JS, Peto TEA et al: Maternal anti-D concentrations and outcome in rhesus haemolytic disease of the newborn. BMJ 285:327, 1982
22. Leggat HM, Gibson JM, Barron SL, Reid MM: Anti-Kell in pregnancy. Br J Obstet Gynaecol 98:162, 1991
23. Mollison PL, Engelfriet CP, Contreras M: Haemolytic disease of the fetus and newborn. p. 545. In Mollison PL (ed): Blood Transfusion in Clinical Medicine. 9th Ed. Blackwell Scientific, Oxford, 1993
24. Bowman JM: Hemolytic disease (erythroblastosis fetalis). p. 739. In Creasy RK, Resnik R (eds): Maternal–fetal Medicine: Principles and Practice. 3rd Ed. WB Saunders, Philadelphia, 1994
25. Marsh WL, Reid ME, Kuriyan M, Marsh NJ (eds): A Handbook of Clinical and Laboratory Practices in the

Transfusion of Red Blood Cells. Monita Press, Monita, VA, 1993

26. Tarczy-Hornoch P, Hodson WA: Neonatology, editorial. JAMA 271:1682, 1994

27. Mollison PL: Haemolytic disease of the newborn. p. 675. In Mollison PL (ed): Blood Transfusion in Clinical Medicine. 6th Ed. Blackwell Scientific, Oxford, 1979

28. Rocard F, Schifrin BS, Goupil F et al: Non-stressed fetal heart rate monitoring in the antepartum period. Am J Obstet Gynecol 126:699, 1976

29. Visser GHA: Antepartum sinusoidal and decelerative heart rate patterns in Rh disease. Am J Obstet Gynecol 143:538, 1982

30. Nicolaides KH, Rodeck CH, Mibashan MD et al: Have Liley charts outlived their usefulness? Am J Obstet Gynecol 155:90, 1986

31. Bennett PR, Le Van Kim C, Colin Y et al: Prenatal determination of fetal RhD type by DNA amplification. N Engl J Med 329:607, 1993

32. Medical Research Council: Diagnosis of genetic disease by amniocentesis during the second trimester of pregnancy. Report No. 5. Medical Research Council, 1977

33. Lowe CU, Alexander D, Bryla D, Seigel D: The NICHD Amniocentesis Registry: The Safety and Accuracy of Midtrimester Amniocentesis. DHEW Publications No. NIH 78-190. U.S. Department of Health, Education and Welfare. Washington, DC, 1978

34. Medical Research Council: An assessment of the hazards of amniocentesis. Br J Obstet Gynaecol 85:1, 1978

35. Ghidini A, Sepulveda W, Lockwood CJ, Romero R: Complications of fetal blood sampling. Am J Obstet Gynecol 168:1339, 1993

36. Duchatel F, Aury JF, Mennesson B, Muray JM: Complications of ultrasound-guided percutaneous umbilical blood sampling: analysis of a series of 341 cases and review of the literature. Eur J Obstet Gynecol Reprod Biol 52:95, 1993

37. Laifer SA, Kuller JA, Hill LM: Rapid assessment of fetal hemoglobin concentration with the HemoCue system. Obstet Gynecol 76:723, 1990

38. Seeds JW, Bowes WA, Chescheir NC: Echogenic venous turbulence is a critical feature of successful intravascular intrauterine transfusion. Obstet Gynecol 73:488, 1989

39. Forestier F, Daffos F, Galacteros F et al: Hematologic values of 163 normal fetuses between 18 and 30 weeks of gestation. Pediatr Res 20:342, 1986

40. de Waele M, Foulon W, Renmans W et al: Hematologic values and lymphocyte subsets in fetal blood. Am J Clin Pathol 89:742, 1988

41. Weiner CP, Sipes SL, Wenstrom K: The effect of fetal age upon normal fetal laboratory values and venous pressure. Obstet Gynecol 79:713, 1992

42. Forestier F, Daffos F, Rainaut M et al: Blood chemistry of normal human fetuses at midtrimester of pregnancy. Pediatr Res 21:579, 1987

43. Soothill PW, Lestas AN, Nicolaides KH et al: 2,3-Diphosphoglycerate in normal, anaemic and transfused human fetuses. Clin Sci 74:527, 1988

44. Gonsoulin WJ, Moise KJ, Milam JD et al: Serial maternal blood donations for intrauterine transfusion. Obstet Gynecol 75:158, 1990

45. DePalma L, Criss VR, Roseff SD, Luban NLC: Formation of alloanti-E in an 11 week old infant. Transfusion, suppl. 31:52S, 1991

46. Eisenfeld L, Silver H, McLaughlin J et al: Prevention of transfusion-associated cytomegalovirus infection in neonatal patients by the removal of white cells from blood. Transfusion 32:205, 1992

47. Hall TL, Barnes A, Miller JR et al: Neonatal mortality following transfusion of red cells with high plasma potassium levels. Transfusion 33:606, 1993

48. Strauss RG: Routinely washing irradiated red cells before transfusion seems unwarranted. Transfusion 30P:675, 1990

49. Moise KJ, Mari G, Fisher DJ et al: Acute fetal hemodynamic alterations after intrauterine transfusion for treatment of severe red blood cell alloimmunization. Am J Obstet Gynecol 163:776, 1990

50. Nicolaides KH, Clewell WH, Mibashan RS et al: Fetal haemoglobin measurement in the assessment of red cell isoimmunization. Lancet i:1073, 1988

51. MacGregor SN, Socol ML, Pielet BW et al: Prediction of fetoplacental blood volume in isoimmunized pregnancy. Am J Obstet Gynecol 159:1493, 1988

52. Queenan JT: Amniotic fluid analysis. p. 73. In Queenan JT (ed): Modern Management of the Rh Problem. 2nd Ed. Harper & Row, Hagerstown, MD, 1977

53. Nicolaides KH, Clewell WH, Rodeck CH: Measurement of human fetoplacental blood volume in erythroblastosis fetalis. Am J Obstet Gynecol 157:50, 1987

54. Copel JA, Grannum PA, Harrison D, Hobbins JC: The use of pancuronium bromide to produce fetal paralysis during intravascular transfusion. Am J Obstet Gynecol 158:170, 1988

55. Bernstein HH, Chitkara U, Plosker H et al: Use of atracurium besylate to arrest fetal activity during intrauterine transfusions. Obstet Gynecol 72:813, 1988

56. MacGregor SN, Socol ML, Pielet BW et al: Prediction of hematocrit decline after intravascular fetal transfusion. Am J Obstet Gynecol 161:1491, 1989

57. Avery ME, First LR (eds): Pediatric Medicine. 2nd Ed. Williams & Wilkins, Baltimore, 1994, p. 224

58. Millard DD, Gidding SS, Socol ML et al: Effects of intravascular, intrauterine transfusion on prenatal and postnatal hemolysis and erythropoiesis in severe fetal isoimmunization. J Pediatr 117:447, 1990

59. Scaradavou A, Inglis S, Peterson P et al: Suppression of erythropoiesis by intrauterine transfusions in hemolytic disease of the newborn: use of erythropoietin to treat the late anemia. J Pediatr 123:279, 1993

60. Petz LD, Garratty G: Acquired Immune Hemolytic Anemias. Churchill Livingstone, New York, 1980 p. 321

61. Chaplin H, Cohen R, Bloomberg G et al: Pregnancy and idiopathic autoimmune haemolytic anaemia: a prospective study during 6 months gestation and 3 months post-partum. Br J Haematol 24:219, 1973

62. Carrington D, Gilmore DH, Whittle MJ et al: Maternal serum alphafetoprotein; a marker of fetal aplastic crises during intrauterine human parvovirus infection. Lancet 1:433, 1987

63. Schwarz TF, Roggendorf M, Hottentrager B et al: Human parvovirus B19 infection in pregnancy. Lancet 2:566, 1988

64. Anand A, Gray ES, Brown T et al: Human parvovirus infection in pregnancy and hydrops fetalis. N Engl J Med 316:183, 1987

65. Bianchi DW, Beyer EC, Stark AR et al: Normal long-term survival with alpha-thalassemia. J Pediatr 108:716, 1986

66. Lam TK, Chan V, Fok TF et al: Long-term survival of a baby with homozygous alpha-thalassemia-1. Acta Haematol 88:198, 1992

67. Beaudry MA, Ferguson DJ, Pearse K et al: Survival of a hydropic infant with homozygous alpha-thalassemia-1. J Pediatr 108:713, 1986

68. Carter C, Darbyshire PJ, Wickramasinghe SN: A congenital dyserythropoietic anaemia variant presenting as hydrops fetalis. Br J Haematol 72:289, 1989

69. Williams G, Lorimer S, Merry CC et al: A variant congenital dyserythropoietic anaemia presenting as hydrops foetalis. Br J Haematol 76:438, 1990

70. Roberts DJ, Nadel A, Lage J, Rutherford CJ: An unusual variant of congenital dyserythropoietic anaemia with mild maternal and lethal fetal disease. Br J Haematol 84:549, 1993

71. Nathan DG, Oski FA (eds): Hematology of Infancy and Childhood. 3rd Ed. WB Saunders, Philadelphia, 1987, p. 207

72. Kaplan C, Morel-Kopp MC, Kroll H et al: HPA-5b [Br(a)] neonatal alloimmune thrombocytopenia: clinical and immunological analysis of 39 cases. Br J Haematol 78:425, 1991

73. Shulman NR, Marder VJ, Heller MC, Collier EM: Platelet and leukocyte isoantigens and their antibodies: serologic, physiologic and clinical studies. Prog Hematol 4:222, 1964

74. Bussel JB, Berkowitz RL, McFarland JG et al: Antenatal treatment of neonatal alloimmune thrombocytopenia. N Engl J Med 319:1374, 1988

75. Kaplan C, Daffos F, Forestier F et al: Management of alloimmune thrombocytopenia: antenatal diagnosis and in utero transfusion of maternal platelets. Blood 72:340, 1988

76. Giovangrandi Y, Daffos F, Kaplan C et al: Very early intracranial haemorrhage in alloimmune fetal thrombocytopenia, letter. Lancet 336:310, 1990

77. Lynch L, Bussel JB, McFarland JG et al: Antenatal treatment of alloimmune thrombocytopenia. Obstet Gynecol 80:67, 1992

78. Waters A, Murphy M, Hambley H, Nicolaides K: Management of alloimmune thrombocytopenia in the fetus and neonate. p. 155. In Nance SJ (ed): Clinical and Basic Science Aspects of Immunohematology. American Association of Blood Banks, Arlington, VA, 1991

79. Murphy MF, Waters AH, Doughty A et al: Antenatal management of fetomaternal alloimmune thrombocytopenia—report of 15 affected pregnancies. Transfus Med 4:281, 1994

80. Kroll H, Kiefel V, Giers G et al: Maternal intravenous immunoglobulin treatment does not prevent intracranial haemorrhage in fetal alloimmune thrombocytopenia. Transfus Med 4:293, 1994

81. Murphy MF, Pullon HWH, Metcalfe P et al: Management of fetal alloimmune thrombocytopenia by weekly in utero platelet transfusions. Vox Sang 58:45, 1990

82. Murphy MF, Metcalfe P, Waters AH et al: Antenatal management of severe feto-maternal alloimmune thrombocytopenia: HLA incompatibility may affect responses to fetal platelet transfusions. Blood 81:2174, 1993

83. Hillyer CD, Emmens RK, Zago-Novaretti M, Berkman EM: Methods for the reduction of transfusion-transmitted cytomegalovirus infection: filtration versus the use of seronegative donor units. Transfusion 34:929, 1994

84. Fowler KB, Stagno S, Pass RF et al: The outcome of congenital cytomegalovirus infection in relation to maternal antibody status. N Engl J Med 326:663, 1992

85. Pineda AA, Zylstra VW, Clare DE et al: Viability and

functional integrity of washed platelets. Transfusion 29:524, 1989

86. Rodeck CH, Roberts LJ: Successful treatment of fetal cardiac arrest by left ventricular exchange transfusion. Fetal Diagn Ther 9:213, 1994

87. McMillan R: Chronic idiopathic thrombocytopenic purpura. N Engl J Med 304:1135, 1981

88. Burrows RF, Kelton JG: Low fetal risks in pregnancies associated with idiopathic thrombocytopenic purpura. Am J Obstet Gynecol 163:1147, 1990

89. Bussel JB, Druzin ML, Cines DB, Samuels P: Thrombocytopenia in pregnancy, letter. Lancet 337:251, 1991

90. Kaplan C, Daffos F, Forestier F et al: Fetal platelet counts in thrombocytopenic pregnancy. Lancet 336:979, 1990

91. Samuels P, Bussel JB, Braitman LE et al: Estimate of the risk of thrombocytopenia in the offspring of pregnant women with presumed immune thrombocytopenic purpura. N Engl J Med 323:229, 1990

92. Christiaens GC, Nieuwenhuis HK, von dem Borne AE et al: Idiopathic thrombocytopenic purpura in pregnancy: a randomized trial on the effect of antenatal low dose corticosteroids on neonatal platelet count. Br J Obstet Gynaecol 97:893, 1990

93. Bussel JB, Christiaens G: Birth platelet counts in sequential newborns of mothers with ITP: Do the platelet counts change with subsequent babies? abstracted. Blood, suppl. 82:202a, 1993

94. Cook RL, Miller RC, Katz VL, Cefalo RC: Immune thrombocytopenic purpura in pregnancy: a reappraisal of management. Obstet Gynecol 78:578, 1991

95. Weiner CP: Thrombocytopenia and cordocentesis, letter. Am J Obstet Gynecol 161:1091, 1989

96. Weiner CP: Cordocentesis and immune cytopenia, letter. Am J Obstet Gynecol 163:1371, 1990

97. Cowan MJ, Golbus M: In utero stem cell transplants for inherited diseases. Am J Pediatr Hematol Oncol 16:35, 1994

98. Sibai BM, Lipshitz J, Schneider JM et al: Sinusoidal fetal heart rate pattern. Obstet Gynecol 55:637, 1980

99. Grannum PAT, Copel JA, Plaxe SC et al: In utero exchange transfusion by direct intravascular transfusion severe erythroblastosis fetalis. N Engl J Med 314:1431, 1986

100. The American College of Obstetricians and Gynecologists: Technical Bulletin 147. ACOG, Washington, D.C., Oct. 1990

Chapter 29

Neonatal Erythropoiesis and Red Blood Cell Transfusions

Ronald G. Strauss

Newborn infants, particularly prematures with birthweight of less than 1.3 kg, are given multiple red blood cell (RBC) transfusions during the first weeks of life. The mechanisms responsible vary at different periods of time during early infancy. During the first 2 to 3 weeks of life, severe respiratory disease may predispose to repeated blood sampling for laboratory studies and, consequently, to replacement transfusions. During later weeks, the inability to mount an effective erythropoietin (EPO) response to falling RBC values (hematocrit or hemoglobin concentration) may lead to additional transfusions to treat the "anemia of prematurity."

Remarkable advances in diminishing the severity of acute respiratory disease (e.g., maternal corticosteroid administration, surfactant therapy for premature infants, and use of less damaging mechanical ventilators) have reduced the need, in some neonates, for early RBC transfusions. Another key factor is the adoption of more conservative transfusion practices by neonatologists. To illustrate, the pattern of RBC transfusions given to small premature neonates at the University of Iowa is shown in Table 29-1. The number of RBC transfusions given to infants from birth until either discharge or 60 days of age has fallen dramatically, with nearly all transfusions in 1993 given to infants with birthweight of less than 1.0 kg. Although not shown in Table 29-1, when the 31 infants studied during 1993 were subdivided, 94

percent of these with birth weight of less than 1.0 kg received RBC transfusions, as compared with only 27 percent of those weighing 1.0 to 1.3 kg. It is important to note that this reduction in RBC transfusions occurred without the use of recombinant EPO—a finding that also emphasizes the need to evaluate concurrent control subjects when studying therapeutic interventions such as EPO.

Anemia remains a major problem for many premature infants. The current pathophysiology of this disorder, considerations for EPO therapy, and principles of RBC transfusion practice are analyzed in this chapter.

PATHOPHYSIOLOGY OF NEONATAL ANEMIA

During the first weeks of life, all infants experience a decline in circulating RBC volume (mass), generally expressed as hematocrit or blood hemoglobin concentration. This decline results both from physiological factors and, in sick premature infants, from phlebotomy blood losses. In healthy term infants, the nadir hemoglobin value rarely falls below 9 g/dl at approximately 10 to 12 weeks of age.[1] This decline occurs earlier and is more pronounced in premature infants, even in those without complicating illnesses, in whom the mean hemoglobin concentration falls to approximately 8 g/dl in infants of 1.0 to 1.5-kg birthweight and to 7 g/dl in infants weighing less

Table 29-1. Patterns of Neonatal RBC Transfusions at the University of Iowa

	Year of Study		
	1989	1991	1993
Infants less than 1.5 kg	49	52	31[b]
% given RBCs	78	67	61
RBC transfusions[a]			
Mean	10.0	8.2	3.8
Range	1–40	2–46	1–12
≥4 Tx	82%	41%	37%
≥15 TX	26%	14%	0%

Abbreviations: RBC, red blood cell; Tx, transfusion.
[a] Only transfused infants considered.
[b] Infants with birthweight of less than 1.3 kg studied in 1993.

than 1.0 kg.[2,3] Because this postnatal drop in hemoglobin level is universal and is well tolerated in term infants, it is commonly referred to as the "physiologic" anemia of infancy. In premature infants, however, this decline in hemoglobin may be associated with clinical signs abnormal enough to prompt transfusions. Accordingly, the acceptance of this anemia as a normal benign event has been questioned.[4,5]

A key reason for the lower nadir hemoglobin values of premature infants than those of term infants is the former group's relatively diminished EPO output in response to anemia.[2,3,6–9] Although anemia provokes EPO production in premature infants, the levels achieved are lower than those observed in older persons with comparable degrees of anemia.[8] When related quantitatively, rising EPO levels and falling blood hemoglobin concentrations correlate weakly in premature infants.[9] Low EPO output, accepted as a mechanism for physiologic anemia, may also limit compensation for anemia in the newborn due to "nonphysiological" mechanisms (e.g., RBC loss due to bleeding, hemolysis). Erythroid progenitor cells in the blood[10] and bone marrow[11] of premature infants are quite responsive to EPO in vitro. Although erythroid colonies derived from fetal and adult subjects display different growth patterns in culture,[12] the bulk of information available supports the hypothesis that the inadequate production of EPO, rather than an abnormal response of erythroid progenitors to this growth factor, is the major cause of physiologic anemia.

The mechanisms responsible for the diminished EPO output by premature neonates are undefined. One mechanism of apparent importance in premature infants is the reliance, during the first weeks of life, on the liver as the primary site of EPO production, rather than on kidney.[13] As established by animal studies, the sequence of EPO production in normal fetuses is liver, followed by kidney. In lambs, EPO production by fetal liver begins to decrease after 120 to 130 days of gestation (term: 145 to 150 days), at which time renal EPO production increases.[14] However, at term, 70 to 75 percent of EPO produced in response to anemia continues to be generated by the liver. This dependency on hepatic production of EPO is important because liver is less sensitive to anemia and tissue hypoxia than is kidney,[14] hence the relatively dampened EPO response in the fetus and neonate to the falling RBC mass. The switch to renal EPO production in lambs is related to the time of conception, not birth, and it is complete by about 40 days after birth. Viewed from a teleologic perspective, decreased EPO production under conditions of tissue hypoxemia in utero may offer an advantage to the fetus. If this were not the case, normal levels of fetal hypoxemia could stimulate high EPO output, with resulting polycythemia and hyperviscosity in utero. Following birth, however, diminished EPO responsiveness to tissue hypoxemia results in ineffective erythropoietic compensation—like that routinely observed in the physiologic anemia of infancy. Production of EPO by human neonatal liver or kidney tissue has not been measured directly. However, macrophages from human cord blood generated normal quantities of EPO mRNA and protein, suggesting satisfactory synthetic capability.[15]

As another mechanism possibly contributing to low EPO levels, plasma levels of EPO are undoubtedly influenced by metabolism (clearance), as well as production. Thus, pharmacokinetic studies of EPO during the perinatal period are likely to be important both in understanding the physiology involved and in designing successful therapeutic trials for use of recombinant EPO (i.e., optimal dose, schedule, and route of administration). Data in human infants[16,17] suggest that low plasma EPO levels may result from increased clearance or volume of distribution of this hormone, or both, in neonates relative to adults. Thus, low EPO plasma levels may be due to a combination of low production, coupled with high turnover. In addition, pharmacokinetics of subcutaneous doses are variable, suggesting erratic absorption, a fact that must be considered when evaluating EPO therapy studies.

Physiologic factors influencing EPO biology are critical in the pathogenesis of neonatal anemia, as is rapid growth early in life that leads to a commensurate need for greatly increased RBC mass. A contributing practical factor is the need for repeated blood sampling to monitor critically ill neonates. Small premature infants—the most critically ill—require the most frequent blood sampling and suffer the greatest proportional loss of RBCs because their circulating RBC volumes are small. Although attempts have been made to minimize sampling, to employ percutaneous monitoring devices, and to miniaturize testing assays, the mean volume of blood removed for sampling has been reported to range from 0.8 to 3.1 ml/kg/day during the first few weeks of life. When the volumes removed are expressed in terms of total RBCs lost, the quantities during an entire hospitalization range from 30 percent to more than 300 percent of the total circulating RBC volume of neonates at birth. Because of the diminished erythropoietic response to anemia, such losses could lead to severe anemia within a short time, unless the RBCs are replaced by transfusions.

RECOMBINANT EPO TO TREAT NEONATAL ANEMIA

Because infants mount an ineffective EPO response to anemia, the administration of recombinant EPO has been touted as promising therapy.[18-20] Initial studies revealed mixed results; several reasonable criticisms can be made. Most early studies enrolled fairly small numbers of subjects, and only a few were of a randomized, placebo-controlled design. In addition, EPO and iron administration (dose, schedule, and route) were quite variable. Key factors leading to failure in these early studies were probably related to less than optimal EPO administration (dose and schedule), to pharmacokinetic differences between newborns and adults, and/or

to inadequate availability of iron to sustain erythropoiesis stimulated to high rates by EPO therapy. With respect to the last, some anemic adults with kidney disease respond to EPO only if treated with parenteral iron.[21] Except for one relatively recent study,[22] in which intravenous iron was given, all other studies of infants have employed oral iron. In support of using larger therapeutic doses of EPO, high "pharmacologic" doses of EPO have been effective in patients with disease processes associated with anemia, when they have failed EPO given in the lower more "physiologic" doses, patterned after those used to treat anemic renal patients.[23] In addition, high doses of EPO have proved effective in increasing hemoglobin levels in newborn rats.[24]

Although failing to establish the efficacy of EPO as treatment for neonatal anemia, early reports of EPO therapy in neonates provided important information for later studies. For example, studies conducted by Halperin and co-workers[25-27] employed historical controls and noted only marginal effects when small numbers of infants were given EPO subcutaneously three times per week for 1 month at doses of 75 to 600 U/kg/dose plus oral iron (2 to 8 mg/kg/day) and vitamin E (5 to 20 mg/day). A dose-dependent reticulocytosis occurred, and only 3 of the 18 infants, those with low baseline hematocrits of 21 to 23 percent, were given transfusions.[27] Although 3 of 18 infants exhibited absolute neutrophil counts of less than 0.5 $\times 10^9$/L, no infections were noted. In another early study, Beck et al.[28] conducted an uncontrolled trial in which stable, older premature infants were given weekly doses of EPO intravenously at 10 to 200 U/kg/ week. Reticulocyte counts increased, but not in relation to EPO dose. Likewise, hemoglobin levels rose, but without an EPO dose-dependent effect. All but one infant had transiently lowered neutrophil counts, with several patients exhibiting values lower than 1.0 $\times 10^9$/L. No infections occurred. Overall, definitive conclusions cannot be drawn from these studies[25-28] because of the lack of controls, the small number of subjects, the use of varying EPO doses, and the inconsistent responses observed.

Studies in which control infants were evaluated concurrently to assess the role of recombinant EPO in the management of neonatal anemia are summa-

Table 29-2. Studies of Recombinant Erythropoietin to Treat Neonatal Anemia Involving Concurrent Control Infants

Investigators	Infants Age/Wt[a]	Controls	EPO Dose	EPO Effects
Shannon et al.[29]	Age 21 days, 896 g	Randomized 10S, 10C	100 U/kg, 2×/wk (IV)	Early reticulocytes None on transfusions
Shannon et al.[31]	Age 20 days, 819 g	Randomized 4S, 4C	100–200 U/kg, 5×/wk (SC)	Higher reticulocytes Higher hematocrits Fewer (?) transfusions
Shannon et al.[32]	Age 24 days, 981 g	Randomized 77S, 80C	100 U/kg, 5×/wk (SC)	Higher reticulocytes Higher hematocrits Fewer transfusions
Ohls and Christensen[33]	Age 41 days, 1,426 g	Randomized 10S, 9C	200 U/kg, 3×/wk (SC)	Higher reticulocytes Higher erythropoiesis Fewer transfusions
Carnielli et al.[22]	Age 2 days, 1,328 g	Randomized 11S, 11C	400 U/kg, 3×/wk (IV)	Higher reticulocytes Higher hematocrits Fewer transfusions
Soubasi et al.[34]	Age ≤7 days, 1,197 g	Randomized 25S, 19C	150 U/kg, 2×/wk (SC)	Higher reticulocytes Fewer transfusions
Bechensteen et al.[35]	Age 21 days, 1,423	Randomized 14S, 15C	100 U/kg, 3×/wk (SC)	Higher reticulocytes Higher hematocrits Fewer (?) transfusions
Messer et al.[36]	Age 10 days, 1,265 g	Nonrandomized 31S, 20C	100–300 U/kg, 3×/wk (SC)	Higher reticulocytes Higher hematocrits Fewer (?) transfusions
Emmerson et al.[37]	Age 7 days, 1,363 g	Randomized 16S, 8C	50–150 U/kg, 2×/wk (SC)	Higher reticulocytes Fewer (?) transfusions
Maier et al.[38]	Age 3 days, 1,150 g	Randomized 120S, 121C	250 U/kg, 3×/wk (SC)	Fewer transfusions

Abbreviations: S, study; C, control (e.g., 10 study, 10 control infants).
[a] Mean or median age and weight at enrollment.

rized in Table 29-2. The first randomized placebo-controlled trial conducted by Shannon et al.[29] found no improvement with respect to hematocrit, transfusion requirements, overall reticulocyte count, calculated erythrocyte mass, or rate of growth. Infants with low phlebotomy losses (of less than 20 ml during the study) may have benefited, as none of four infants treated with EPO needed transfusions, compared to three of five controls. Another possible EPO effect was the more rapid rise of reticulocytes in EPO versus control infants. Serum EPO levels and blood platelet, leukocyte, and neutrophil counts did not differ in EPO-treated infants as compared with those given placebo. The lack of clinically important benefits likely was due to the low dose of EPO given and to the probable occurrence of iron deficiency. Although all 20 in-

fants were prescribed oral iron (3 mg/kg/day), six did not receive complete therapy. Additional information was provided about these 20 infants in another report.[30]

The findings in this initial study led to a small randomized pilot study in which eight infants were given either EPO, 100 to 200 U/kg/day SC, or placebo, 5 days per week for 6 weeks.[31] All infants were given iron, 6 mg/kg/day PO. Although the number of subjects was quite small, EPO infants exhibited higher reticulocyte counts and hematocrits than those of controls. A benefit with transfusion requirements possibly occurred, but the number of subjects was too small for meaningful statistical analysis. This pilot study[31] led to a multicenter, randomized, placebo-controlled trial.[32] Although the data support the efficacy of EPO in treating the anemia present in very small—but older, stable infants—the findings are surprisingly modest.[32] At least one RBC transfusion was given during the study period to 57 percent of EPO-treated infants versus 69 percent of controls. The mean number of RBC transfusions given per infant was 1.1 for EPO versus 1.6 for control infants, and the mean volume of RBCs given per infant was 16.4 ml for EPO versus 23.9 ml for controls. Importantly, on average, infants received more than three RBC transfusions before entering the EPO versus placebo phase of the study. Thus, EPO had limited impact on the overall RBC needs throughout both the prestudy and study periods (4.4 versus 5.3 transfusions). Clearly, EPO did not eliminate the need for RBC transfusions—even in older, stable infants, in whom phlebotomy blood losses were minimal.

Ohls and Christensen[33] randomized stable premature infants with anemia, who were relatively large and advanced in age, to receive either EPO or RBC transfusions—the latter given to raise the hematocrit initially to 40 percent or greater. The transfused infants, in a sense, served as controls; they were transfused again if the hematocrit fell to 30 percent or lower and if signs of anemia were present. Recipients of EPO received oral iron (2 mg/kg/day) and 25 units of vitamin E. It was not stated whether transfused infants received these nutrients as well. Infants receiving EPO showed increased serum erythropoietin, hematocrit, reticulocyte count, and bone marrow erythroid activity, compared to transfused infants. These findings were not unexpected, since the RBC transfusions as given were likely to suppress erythropoiesis.[1,3,8] EPO-treated infants did not require transfusions during the study. Mean blood neutrophil counts were significantly lower in EPO infants than controls (1.8 versus 3.9×10^9/L), but only one infant in each group fell below 1.0×10^9/L. EPO increased colony forming units-erythroid (CFU-E) in the marrow, but burst forming units-erythroid (BFU-E), colony forming units-granulocyte, macrophage (CFU-GM), and colony forming units-mixed lineage (CFU-MIX) were no different in EPO-treated versus transfused infants. Although EPO seemed to exert effects on marrow erythropoiesis, the findings are difficult to apply to clinical practice because control subjects were transfused to fairly high hematocrit levels—a situation that lowered reticulocyte counts

and rendered them somewhat transfusion dependent due to marrow suppression. It would have been interesting to document the transfusion requirements and erythropoietic response of a group of control infants given placebo plus iron and vitamin E and permitted to experience modest degrees of symptomatic anemia without being given RBC transfusions.

The randomized trial of conducted by Carnielli et al.[22] provides promising results in neonates studied shortly after birth. Study infants were given EPO and iron (20 mg/kg/week) intravenously from day 2 of life until discharge. Control prematures were given neither EPO nor, unfortunately, iron. Thus, two variables (EPO and iron) that might affect response were present rather than only one (EPO). Infants were fairly large in size, with a mean birthweight slightly greater than 1.3 kg. Importantly, the criteria for transfusion were quite liberal, and the sustained high hematocrit suppressed reticulocyte counts in control infants. Thus, the applicability of the findings to neonatal transfusion practice in the United States might be debated. Nonetheless, the need for RBC transfusions was significantly decreased by EPO. In EPO-treated versus control infants, the number of RBC transfusions was 0.8 versus 3.1, and the volume of RBCs transfused was 14 ml/kg versus 48 ml/kg. Blood neutrophil and platelet counts were normal and were similar in both groups.

In the study by Soubasi et al.,[34] attempts were made to identify factors in neonates that might predict a successful response to EPO. Although infants were randomized to either an EPO or a control group, there was no mention of a placebo, and the possibility of bias due to lack of blinding must be considered. As another source of potential variability, prescribed oral iron (3 mg/kg/day, beginning on day 15 of life), could be discontinued at the discretion of the attending physician. For analysis, infants were divided into two groups—"uncomplicated" or "complicated"—the latter defined as requiring mechanical ventilation for at least 3 days. Reticulocyte counts were increased by EPO, but hematocrits did not differ between groups because they were maintained by RBC transfusions. The need for transfusions was significantly less in "uncomplicated" EPO-treated infants than controls (three of nine EPO-treated infants transfused versus six of seven controls). By contrast, EPO did not benefit "complicated" infants because a high incidence of transfusions was required for both EPO-treated and control infants. No differences in platelet or leukocyte units were found between groups, and neutropenia (less than 1×10^9/L) was not observed.

Bechensteen et al.[35] evaluated EPO in stable premature infants, in whom unusual efforts were made to ensure optimal protein and iron balance. A randomized, but not placebo-controlled, study was conducted at four centers. Breast milk feedings were supplemented with 9 g/L of human breast milk protein, and ferrous fumarate (18 mg of elemental iron) was given daily. The dose of oral iron was doubled if the serum iron fell to less than 90 μg/dl (16 μmol/L)—a situation that occurred in 26 of the 29 infants. After 1 week of therapy, reticulocyte and blood hemoglobin concentrations were significantly higher in the EPO-treated group. None of the 14 EPO infants was transfused with RBCs versus 4 of the 15 controls. In the absence of placebo and blinding to diminish bias, differences in transfusion practice are difficult to interpret—particularly with few study subjects. However, modest doses of EPO seemed to benefit stable premature infants who were well nourished with protein and iron.

Messer et al.[36] studied increasing doses of EPO given to premature infants until approximately 7 weeks of age. The study was not randomized; controls were infants whose parents refused EPO therapy. Moreover, the need for RBC transfusions was judged by attending physicians, who were not blinded to therapy. The decline in hematocrit values with advancing age was slower in EPO-treated infants, but hematocrits were influenced by frequent RBC transfusions—19 percent of EPO-treated infants versus 45 percent of controls were transfused. Transient neutropenia (less than 1.5×10^9/L) occurred in 61 percent of EPO-treated infants and in 50 percent of controls (not significantly different). Iron utilization increased with higher doses of EPO; Messer and colleagues postulated that EPO would be most effective for older, stable premature infants able to take large doses of oral iron (15 mg/kg/day).

Emmerson et al.[37] randomized infants to receive either EPO or placebo until discharge. Randomization was deliberately set at 2:1, favoring EPO, and 36 infants were planned to be recruited. However, two EPO-treated infants died suddenly of sudden infant

death syndrome (SIDS) 1 month after discharge. Although SIDS could not be ascribed to EPO, the study was terminated early, making it impossible to establish statistical significance for some of the trends observed. Reticulocyte counts were higher in EPO-treated infants than controls and fewer transfusions (not statistically different) were given. Forty-seven percent of EPO-treated infants received transfusions (10 ml/kg) versus 88 percent of infants who received placebo (19.6 ml/kg). Physicians were blinded and ordered transfusions per predetermined criteria, which included prophylactic transfusions at a hemoglobin level of 8 g/dL. EPO-treated infants exhibited (not statistically significant) increased blood platelets, decreased neutrophils, and increased weight gain. Serum ferritin fell, and both RBC folate and hemoglobin F increased in EPO-treated infants, suggesting stimulation of erythropoiesis.

Maier et al.[38] report results of a multicenter European trial in which premature infants were randomized either to receive EPO until day 42 or to serve as controls. Controls were not given placebo, but extensive measures were taken in an attempt to blind physicians involved in their nursery care. All infants were given iron, 2 mg/kg PO, beginning on day 14. Results reported were obtained from a somewhat selected group of infants. Of 598 infants entered, only 241 (40 percent) were evaluated, and 177 (30 percent) actually completed the study per protocol. Most infants were relatively large, with only 25 percent of the 241 evaluated infants weighing less than 1.0 kg and being most likely to need transfusions (51 percent weighed less than 1.25 kg and 49 percent greater than 1.25 kg). RBC transfusions were given uniformly per predetermined guidelines, with indications that were quite liberal (e.g., infants without signs of anemia and an hematocrit of less than 27 percent were transfused prophylactically). During the first 2 weeks of life, EPO had no apparent effect, as transfusion rates were similar in EPO-treated and control infants. However, EPO was successful overall in diminishing RBC transfusions. EPO-treated infants were given a mean of 0.87 transfusions (median of 0.09 ml/kg) versus controls, each given a mean of 1.25 transfusions (median of 0.41 ml/kg). Of interest, 28 percent of EPO-treated infants maintained an hematocrit of 32 percent or greater throughout the study without transfusions versus only 4 percent of controls—raising the possibility that the ability to sustain a higher hematocrit in untransfused infants might serve as a secondary goal for EPO, in addition to the primary goal of decreasing the overall need for transfusions. Although toxicity was not a major problem, infections were slightly increased (not significantly), and growth rate was decreased in EPO-treated infants. Infections could not be related to neutropenia.

In conclusion, EPO deficiency is a major mechanism responsible for neonatal anemia, and therapy for this disorder with recombinant EPO is promising—particularly for stable, older premature neonates. However, since relatively few transfusions are given to these infants, especially those weighing more than 1.0 kg, the genuine need for EPO to diminish transfusions can be questioned. Unfortunately, efficacy has not been established for EPO in infants who receive the most transfusions (less than 1.0 kg early in life, when they are sick), and its value awaits further study. Although enticing, a great deal must be learned about the efficacy and potential toxicity of EPO before it is widely prescribed as standard therapy for the anemia of prematurity. Additional studies are warranted with careful consideration of EPO dose, schedule, route of administration, interactions with iron, and use in combination with other hematopoietic growth factors. Of note, EPO levels in premature infants receiving theophylline therapy were unexpectedly higher than those in infants not receiving theophylline.[39] Thus, the potential for drug interactions must also be considered.

The full spectrum of potential toxicity must be defined before EPO is widely prescribed. In particular, the clinical and biological effects of iron utilization are worrisome. Insufficient quantity and/or bioavailability of iron have limited success of several therapeutic trials to date. Recombinant EPO therapy seems able to shunt iron into erythropoiesis pathways, as evidenced by decreased serum ferritin and increased serum transferrin receptor levels in premature infants.[40] It remains to be shown whether iron commitment to erythropoiesis that has been greatly accelerated by EPO might lead to iron deficiency in other tissues, such as muscle and brain.

Another potentially adverse factor is cost.[41] Data are insufficient to permit an accurate cost analysis of EPO therapy for neonatal anemia. Moreover, re-

sults of the analysis will vary among institutions. However, an estimate of costs can be made using assumptions that apply to the University of Iowa Hospitals and Clinics (UIHC). The major assumption is that the value of EPO is determined primarily by the number of RBC transfusions avoided in EPO-treated infants. One vial of EPO (2,000 units) costs $18.20 at UIHC. In the United States multicenter trial,[26] EPO was given as 100 U/kg, Monday to Friday, for 6 weeks (i.e., 30 doses). The vials are not manufactured as multidose vials, but it is possible to dispense more than 1 dose/vial, if desired, using a laminar-flow hood and devising a means for sterile storage between doses. Thus, the number of vials needed per infant will vary among institutions. If a new vial is used for each of the 30 doses, the cost to supply EPO for each infant is $546—if one vial is used for all 5 doses/week, the cost per infant is $109. Obviously, if several infants are being treated concurrently, costs can be reduced by dispensing EPO for all of them from the same vial. The cost at UIHC to prepare and transfuse one aliquot (15 ml/kg) of CMV-seronegative and irradiated RBCs is $90. If three aliquots are taken from the same unit, the total cost is $130 versus $270, if three aliquots are taken from three separate units. Thus, transfusion costs will vary, depending on institutional transfusion practices.

Using UIHC costs as noted above, data from the United States multicenter trial[32] can be analyzed. The total RBC transfusion need of each EPO infant was a mean of 4.4 transfusions (3.3 transfusions before entry plus 1.1 transfusion during the study). The total RBC transfusion need of each control infant was 5.3 transfusions (3.7 before entry plus 1.6 during study). Thus, approximately one RBC transfusion per infant was avoided by EPO (4.4 versus 5.3), so that the "break-even" point for EPO costs at UIHC would be $90—the cost of one transfusion. As was found for the European multicenter study,[38] the United States multicenter trial likely will not find EPO to be cost effective—the major problem being that not enough RBC transfusions are avoided by EPO therapy, as currently prescribed. Possible ways to improve EPO cost effectiveness are to minimize EPO wastage (e.g., smaller quantities of EPO per vial or multidose vials), avoid more RBC transfusions, and give EPO selectively (i.e., treat only those infants predicted to need transfusions and withhold EPO from those who will not).

Some of these issues will be addressed by future studies. Pending these results, it might be anticipated that EPO will be recommended for infants with birthweight 800 to 1,300 g, who are in stable condition and able to take oral iron at a dose of 4 to 8 mg/kg/day. A reasonable EPO dose would be 300 to 500 U/kg/week given as 2 to 3 subcutaneous doses. For other groups of infants (e.g., very small with severe illness or relatively large with little need for transfusion), EPO probably should be given only in study settings.

RED BLOOD CELL TRANSFUSIONS TO TREAT NEONATAL ANEMIA

Transfusion practices for neonates are controversial, variable, and based on limited scientific information. This lack of a rational approach stems from incomplete knowledge of the cellular and molecular biology of hematopoiesis during the perinatal period and of the physiologic effects of neonatal anemia, as well as a lack of complete understanding of the infant's response to RBC transfusions. Data from clinical studies of infants are sparse and difficult to interpret because of the precarious and heterogeneous medical condition of these tiny patients. Even the deceptively simple task of obtaining sufficient blood to conduct definitive studies is a major impediment because of small total blood volumes and difficult vascular access. Although, in some instances, the value of RBC transfusions is clear (e.g., to treat anemia that has caused congestive heart failure), in others it is not.

Generally, RBC transfusions are given in modest volumes (15 ml/kg per dose) to maintain a level of hematocrit believed to be most desirable for each neonate's clinical status (Table 29-3). It is widely recognized that this clinical approach is imprecise, and more physiologic indications for RBC transfusions, such as circulating RBC mass, available oxygen, and measurements of oxygen delivery and tissue extraction, have been suggested.[42] However, the means by which these techniques can best be applied to everyday practice remain to be defined. Clearly established indications for neo-

Table 29-3. Guidelines for Small-Volume Red Blood Cell Transfusions Given to Neonates

Maintain >40 percent hematocrit (hct) for severe[a] cardiopulmonary disease
Maintain >30 percent hct for moderate[a] cardiopulmonary disease
Maintain >30 percent hct for major surgery
Maintain >25 percent hct for symptomatic anemia
Unexplained breathing disorders
Unexplained poor growth

[a] Must be defined locally (e.g., "severe" pulmonary disease might be defined as requiring mechanical ventilation with >0.35 FiO₂ and "moderate" as anything less).

natal RBC transfusions, based on controlled scientific studies, do not exist. In many clinical situations, the need for RBCs seems logical, but an understanding of the efficacy and risks is incomplete. Because of the limited data available, it is important that pediatricians critically evaluate the guidelines suggested in Table 29-3 and apply them in light of neonatal practice at their respective institutions. The rationale for each of the guidelines listed in Table 28-3 is discussed in the following paragraphs.

Maintain hematocrit of greater than 40 percent during severe cardiopulmonary disease. In neonatal patients with severe respiratory disease, defined as those requiring relatively large quantities of oxygen and ventilator support, it is customary to maintain the hematocrit above 40 percent (blood hemoglobin greater than 13 g/dl). Proponents believe that transfused RBCs containing adult hemoglobin, with its superior interaction with 2,3-diphosphoglycerate (2,3-DPG) and better oxygen off-loading than that of fetal hemoglobin, are likely to provide optimal oxygen delivery throughout the period of diminished pulmonary function. Although this practice is widely recommended, little evidence is available to establish its efficacy, to define its optimal use (i.e., the best level of hematocrit for each degree of pulmonary dysfunction), or to document its risks.[43] In a study of 10 infants with severe (oxygen-dependent) bronchopulmonary dysplasia,[42] physiologic end points (increased systemic oxygen transport and decreased oxygen use) improved after small-volume RBC transfusions. However, blood hemoglobin levels alone failed to predict which infants would benefit from transfusion.[42] Although more information is needed to define the precise indication for and benefits of RBC transfusions, as based either on hematocrit levels or measurements of tissue oxygenation, it is logical to presume that infants with less severe cardiopulmonary disease require less vigorous support, hence the lower hematocrit level suggested for those with only moderate disease (Table 28-3).

Consistent with the rationale for optimal oxygen delivery in neonates with severe respiratory disease, it seems logical to maintain the hematocrit at greater than 40 percent in neonates with severe cardiac disease leading either to cyanosis or to congestive heart failure. Regarding the latter, isovolemic exchange transfusions were used to treat nine infants with ventricular septal defects and large left-to-right shunts.[44] The postpartum decline in hematocrit had produced a fall in blood viscosity that resulted in decreased pulmonary vascular resistance and increased left-to-right shunting. Exchange transfusion increased the mean blood hemoglobin level from 9.9 to 14.6 g/dl, a change that increased pulmonary vascular resistance and decreased both left-to-right shunting and pulmonary blood flow. Heart rate and left ventricular stroke volume fell without compromising oxygen transport to the tissues. Extending these observations to neonatal patients with patent ductus arteriosus, Rosenthal[45] suggested that RBC transfusions might increase pulmonary vascular resistance, enhance ductal closure, and alleviate high-output cardiac failure. The efficacy of RBC transfusions in the treatment of severe patent ductus arteriosus and other forms of neonatal cardiac disease requires more study.

Maintain hematocrit at greater than 30 percent for major surgery. The need to achieve a specific hematocrit preoperatively and to maintain a desired value during surgery has been a controversial issue, even in adult patients. For many years, a minimum value of 30 percent hematocrit or 10 g/dl/hemoglobin was preferred. Recently, acceptance of much lower values has been encouraged, particularly for patients able to compensate for anemia. Definitive studies are not available to establish the optimal hematocrit value for neonates facing major surgery. However, it seems reasonable to maintain an hematocrit of greater than 30 percent because of limited ability of the neonate's heart, lungs, and vasculature to compensate for anemia, the inferior off-loading of oxygen due to the diminished interaction between fetal hemoglobin and 2,3-DPG, and the developmental impairments of neonatal renal, hepatic, and neurologic function. This transfusion guideline is simply a recommendation. It should be applied with flexibility to individual infants facing different kinds of surgery, in concert with local transfusion practices.

Maintain hematocrit of greater than 25 percent for symptomatic anemia. Stable neonates do not require RBC transfusions unless they exhibit clinical problems presumed to be related to the degree of anemia present. Proponents of RBC transfusion therapy for symptomatic anemia believe that the low RBC mass contributes to tachypnea, dyspnea, apnea, tachycardia, bradycardia, feeding difficulties, and lethargy and that these problems can be alleviated by RBC transfusions. Conceivably, tachypnea, dyspnea, and apnea could be exacerbated by anemia as a consequence of decreased oxygen delivery to the respiratory center of the brain.[46] In sick premature infants, when anemia and severe apnea occur together, it is tempting to believe that transfusion of RBCs might increase oxygen delivery and decrease the number of apneic spells. In support, RBC transfusions were shown to diminish irregular breathing patterns and episodes of bradycardia in anemic preterm infants when the mean hematocrit was increased from 27 percent to 36 percent.[47] However, others found no benefit of RBC transfusions on breathing patterns.[48]

Some neonatologists consider poor weight gain an indication for RBC transfusions, particularly if the hemoglobin concentration is below 10 g/dl (hematocrit lower than 30 percent) and if other signs of distress (e.g., tachycardia, respiratory difficulty, weak suck, less vigorous cry, and diminished activity) are evident. Support for this practice was suggested by studies of infants with bronchopulmonary dysplasia in whom growth failure was ascribed to increased metabolic expenditure to support the work of labored breathing.[49] Stockman and Clark[50] investigated the effects of RBC transfusion on weight gain in relatively stable premature infants. Thirteen infants with birthweight of less than 1.5 kg were studied for 1 week before and after transfusion. The mean hemoglobin concentration was raised from 8.5 to 11.4 g/dl, and the rate of weight gain increased from 20.8 to 28.0 g/day. Increased weight gain after transfusion was associated with a low pretransfusion hematocrit and a post-transfusion fall in metabolic rate (measured by oxygen consumption). These investigators considered anemia as only one of several possible causes for growth failure; they recommended RBC transfusions to treat unexplained growth failure only in infants with subnormal hemoglobin levels and clinical manifestations of anemia.

In support, Blank et al.[51] found no advantage for the prophylactic use of small-volume RBC transfusions in otherwise well, growing, premature infants. Fifty-six premature infants were randomly assigned to either a prophylactic transfusion group (hemoglobin maintained at greater than 10 g/dl) or an elective transfusion group in which RBCs were transfused only to treat marked clinical manifestations of anemia. Only 4 of 30 infants in this latter group were transfused electively, once each for apnea. Characteristics at birth were similar with a mean gestational age about 30 weeks and birthweight about 1.2 kg for prophylactic and elective transfusion groups, respectively. At discharge, the elective transfusion infants exhibited significantly (P <0.01) greater anemia and reticulocyte counts than those receiving prophylactic transfusions (hemoglobin 9.10 ± 1.67 versus 11.75 ± 1.72 g/dl, and reticulocytes = 6 ± 3 versus 3 ± 2 percent). Despite these differences, both groups were comparable in the number of days required to regain birthweight, in discharge weight, in the length and cost of hospitalization, and in the frequency and severity of clinical problems. Thus, no value was demonstrated for prophylactic RBC transfusions to maintain a hematocrit of greater than 30 percent in stable, growing premature infants who were otherwise healthy.[51]

In a similar study, Ross et al.[52] randomly assigned 16 preterm infants, over 1 month of age and clinically stable, either to receive a RBC transfusion or to be observed (nontransfusion group). Infants with hematocrits of 29 percent or less were studied for 3 days before and after receiving 10 ml/kg of packed RBCs. Factors that identified infants most likely to benefit from RBC transfusions included a pretransfusion heart rate of greater than 152/min, presence of apnea/bradycardia requiring intervention, and an elevated blood lactate level. Additional studies are needed to identify infants for whom RBC transfu-

sions are likely to provide a clinical benefit (i.e., the symptoms, signs, and laboratory values that predict success).

Red blood cell product for transfusion. The RBC product chosen by most for small-volume neonatal transfusions is a packed RBC concentrate (hematocrit of 70 to 90 percent). Most RBC transfusions are infused slowly (2 to 4 hours) at a dose of about 15 ml/kg body weight. Because of the small quantity of extracellular fluid (RBC storage media) given at these high hematocrit values and the slow rate of transfusion, the type of anticoagulant/preservative medium selected is believed not to pose risks for the majority of premature infants.[53] Similarly, the traditional use of relatively fresh RBCs (less than 7 days of storage) is being challenged in hopes that donor exposure can be diminished by using a single unit of RBCs for each infant, regardless of the duration of RBC storage.[54] Neonatologists who object to this practice and insist on transfusing fresh RBCs generally raise two objections: the rise in plasma potassium (K^+) and the drop in RBC 2,3-DPG that occurs during extended storage. After 42 days of storage, plasma K^+ levels are ≤ 50 mEq/L (0.05 mEq/ml), a value that, at first glance, seems alarmingly high. By simple calculations, however, the dose of bioavailable K^+ transfused (i.e., ions in the extracellular fluid) is quite small. An infant weighing 1 kg, given a 15-ml/kg transfusion of packed RBCs (hematocrit 80 percent), will receive 3 ml of extracellular fluid, or only 0.15 mEq of K^+, and it will be transfused slowly. This dose is quite small compared to the usual daily K^+ requirement of 2 to 3 mEq/kg. However, it must be remembered that this rationale may not apply to large-volume transfusions in which larger doses of K^+ may be harmful, especially if infused rapidly.

As for the second objection, 2,3-DPG is totally depleted from RBCs by 21 days of storage, and this is reflected by a P50 value that falls from about 27 torr in fresh blood to 18 torr at outdate. The last value corresponds to the P50 expressed by RBCs obtained from the blood of many normal premature infants at birth. Thus, the P50 of older transfused RBCs is comparable to that of RBCs produced endogenously by the infant's own bone marrow. Moreover, these older adult RBCs provide an advantage over infant RBCs because the P50 of transfused RBCs (but not endogenous RBCs) increases rapidly after transfusion, as 2,3-DPG regenerates within hours. Although the regeneration of 2,3-DPG in transfused RBCs has not been studied in infants, there is no reason to think it would differ from that in adults, provided marked hypoglycemia or hypophosphatemia were not present. Thus, small-volume transfusions with older RBCs appear to pose no substantive risks to relatively stable, premature infants, and their acceptance as a suitable blood component likely will diminish donor exposure.

Regardless of the RBC product selected for transfusion, it will present the risk of transmitting donor infections such as CMV, and it will contain viable lymphocytes and pose the risk of transfusion-associated GVHD. The need to provide special blood components for neonates to prevent these problems is controversial.[43,55,56] Regardless, the vast majority of institutions provide either CMV-seronegative or filtered blood products to neonates, and approximately one-half γ-irradiate cellular components.[55] Thus, standards of practice have been established. Accordingly, RBC transfusions should be given per the same local practices as are platelet and granulocyte transfusions, regarding CMV seronegativity, leukocyte filtration, and γ-irradiation.[55,56]

OVERALL APPROACH TO NEONATAL ANEMIA

Currently, the mechanisms responsible for, and the management of, neonatal anemia are undergoing continuous change. Although all premature infants sustain a fall in red blood cell mass during the first weeks of life, anemia of a severity to require RBC transfusions occurs almost exclusively in infants with birthweight of less than 1.0 kg. During the first 3 weeks of life, RBC transfusions are given primarily to infants with severe respiratory disease that has necessitated phlebotomy blood losses, with the goal of maintaining hematocrit levels indicated in Table 29–3. During this period, efforts should be made in at least two areas: (1) measures to diminish respiratory disease that include corticosteroid administration to women with threatened delivery of premature infants, surfactant therapy for high-risk neonates and optimal ventilator therapy; and (2) consideration for delayed clamping of the umbilical cord as a means to provide an increased RBC mass at birth.[57] The latter requires further study because

of the potential risks of erythrocytosis with hyperviscosity and delayed resuscitation of extremely premature neonates.

Transfusions following the first 3 weeks of life are given primarily for the anemia of prematurity. The role of EPO therapy to treat this condition is undefined. However, it seems reasonable to treat stable infants weighing 0.8 to 1.3 kg with EPO, 300 to 500 U/kg/week SC, as 2 to 3 divided doses plus oral iron, 4 to 8 mg/kg/day. The efficacy and potential toxicity of EPO in sick, very small infants (less than 1.0 kg) or in stable, large infants (more than 1.3 kg) needs further definition, before EPO can be prescribed routinely. Despite success in minimizing respiratory disease and in using EPO optimally, many premature infants will require RBC transfusions. When these transfusions are unavoidable, efforts should be made to limit donor exposure. This is most likely to be accomplished by supplying all RBC needs from a single unit of blood, without regard to the length of storage.[58,59] Attempts to minimize donor exposure by collecting and storing placental blood (i.e., autologous transfusion) is a technique that warrants further study[60] but poses too many potential problems for use at present.[61]

ACKNOWLEDGMENTS

This work was supported in part by Research Career Development Award K04 HD00255, Transfusion Medicine Academic Award K07 HL01426, and Program Project Grant P01HL46925-01A1 from the National Institutes of Health.

REFERENCES

1. Strauss RG: Current issues in neonatal transfusions. Vox Sang 51:1, 1986
2. Dallman PR: Anemia of prematurity. Annu Rev Med 32:143, 1981
3. Stockman JA: Anemia of prematurity. Current concepts in the issue of when to transfuse. Pediatr Clin North Am 33:111, 1986
4. Wardrop CAJ, Holland BM, Beale KEA et al: Nonphysical anemia of prematurity. Arch Dis Child 53:855, 1978
5. Holland BM, Jones JG, Wardrop CAJ: Lessons from the anemia of prematurity. Hematol Oncol Clin North Am 1:355, 1987

6. Stockman JA III, Garcia JF, Oski FA: The anemia of prematurity. Factors governing the erythropoientin response. N Engl J Med 296:647, 1977

7. Brown MS, Phibbs RH, Garcia JF, Dallman PR: Postnatal changes in erythropoietin levels in untransfused premature infants. J Pediatr 103:612, 1983

8. Stockman JA III, Graeber JE, Clark DA et al: Anemia of prematurity: determinants of the erythropoietin response. J Pediatr 105:786, 1984

9. Brown MS, Garcia JF, Phibbs RH, Dallman PR: Decreased response of plasma immunoreactive erythropoietin to "available oxygen" in anemia of prematurity. J Pediatr 105:793, 1984

10. Shannon KM, Naylor GS, Tordildson JC et al: Circulating erythroid progenitors in the anemia of prematurity. N Engl J Med 317:728, 1987

11. Rhondeau SM, Christensen RD, Ross MP et al: Responsiveness to recombinant human erythropoietin of marrow erythroid progenitors from infants with "anemia of prematurity." J Pediatr 112:935, 1988

12. Holbrook ST, Christensen RD, Rothstein G: Erythroid colonies derived from fetal blood display different growth patterns from those derived from adult marrow. Pediatr Res 24:605, 1988

13. Brown MS, Garcia JF, Phibbs RH, Dallman PR: Decreased response of plasma immunoreactive erythropoietin to "available oxygen" in anemia of prematurity. J Pediatr 105:793, 1984

14. Zanjani ED, Ascensao JL, McGlave PB et al: Studies in the liver to kidney switch of erythropoietin production. J Clin Invest 67:1183, 1981

15. Ohls RK, Yan LI, Trautman MS, Christensen RD: Erythropoietin production by macrophages from preterm infants: implications regarding the cause of the anemia in prematurity. Pediatr Res 35:169, 1994

16. Ruth V, Widness JA, Raivio KO: Postnatal changes in serum Ep in relation to hypoxia before and after birth. J Pediatr 116:950, 1990

17. Brown MS, Jones MA, Ohls RK, Christensen RD: Single-dose pharmacokinetics of recombinant human erythropoietin preterm infants after intravenous and subcutaneous administration. J Pediatr 122:655, 1993

18. Christensen RD: Recombinant erythropoietic growth factors as an alternative to erythrocyte transfusion for patients with "anemia of prematurity." Pediatrics 83:793, 1989

19. Stockman JA III: Erythropoietin: off again on again. J Pediatr 112:906, 1988

20. Phibbs RH, Shannon K, Mentzer WC: Rationale for using recombinant human erythropoietin to treat the anemia of prematurity. p. 324. In Baldamus CA, Scigalla P, Wieczorek L, Koch KM (eds): Erythropoietin:

From Molecular Structure to Clinical Application. Vol. 76. Skarger, Basel, 1989

21. Eschbach JW, Egrie JC, Downing MR et al: Correction of the anemia of end-stage renal disease with recombinant human erythropoietin. J Engl J Med 316:73, 1987

22. Carnielli V, Montini G, DaRiol R et al: Effect of high doses of human erythropoietin on the need for blood transfusions in preterm infants. J Pediatr 121:98, 1992

23. Ludwig H, Fritz E, Kotzmann H et al: Erythropoietin treatment of anemia associated with multiple myeloma. N Engl J Med 322:1693, 1990

24. Koenig JM, Christensen RD: Effect of erythropoietin on granulocytopoiesis: in vitro and in vivo studies in weaningly rats. Pediatr Res 27:583, 1990

25. Halperin DS, Wacher P, Lacourt G et al: Effects of recombinant human erythropoietin in infants with the anemia of prematurity: a pilot study. J Pediatr 116:779, 1990

26. Halperin DS: Use of recombinant erythropoietin in treatment of the anemia of prematurity. Am J Pediatr Hematol Oncol 13:351, 1991

27. Halperin DS, Felix M, Wacker P et al: Recombinant human erythropoietin in the treatment of infants with anemia of prematurity. Eur J Pediatr 151:661, 1992

28. Beck D, Masserey E, Meyer M, Calame A: Weekly intravenous administration of recombinant human erythropoietin in infants with the anemia of prematurity. Eur J Pediatr 150:767, 1991

29. Shannon KE, Mentzer WC, Abels RI et al: Recombinant human erythropoietin in the anemia of prematurity: results of a placebo-controlled pilot study. J Pediatr 118:949, 1991

30. Phibbs RH, Shannon KM, Mentzer WC: Potential for treatment of anaemia of prematurity with recombinant human erythropoietin: preliminary results. Acta Haematol, (suppl 1). 87:28,1992

31. Shannon KM, Mentzer WC, Abels RI et al: Enhancement of erythropoiesis by recombinant human erythropoietin in low birth weight infants: a pilot study. J Pediatr 120:586, 1992

32. Shannon KM, Keith JP, Mentzer WC et al: Recombinant human erythropoietin stimulates erythropoiesis and reduces erythrocyte transfusions in very low birth weight preterm infants. Pediatrics 95:1, 1995

33. Ohls RK, Christensen RD: Recombinant erythropoietin compared with erythrocyte transfusion in the treatment of anemia of prematurity. J Pediatr 119:781, 1991

34. Soubasi V, Kremenopoulos G, Diamandi E et al: In which neonates does early recombinant human erythropoietin treatment prevent anemia of prematurity?

Results of a randomized controlled study. Pediatr Res 34:675, 1993

35. Bechensteen AG, Haga P, Halvorsen S et al: Erythropoietin, protein, and iron supplementation and the prevention of anemia of prematurity. Arch Dis Child 69:19,1993

36. Messer J, Haddad J, Donato L et al: Early treatment of premature infants with recombinant human erythropoietin. Pediatrics 92:519, 1993

37. Emmerson AJB, Coles HJ, Stern CMM, Pearson TC: Double blind trial of recombinant human erythropoietin in preterm infants. Arch Dis Child 68:291, 1993

38. Maier RF, Obladen M, Scigalla P et al: The effect of recombinant human erythropoietin on the need for transfusion in very low birth weight infants. N Engl J Med 330:1173, 1994

39. Gonzales MT, Sherwood JB, Brion LP, Schulman M: Erythropoietin levels during theophylline treatment in premature infants. J Pediatr 124:128, 1994

40. Kivivuori SM, Heikinheimo M, Teppo AM, Siimes MA: Early rise in serum concentration of transferrin receptor induced by recombinant human erythropoietin in very-low-birth-weight infants. Pediatr Res 36:85, 1994

41. Shireman TI, Hilsenrath PE, Strauss RG et al: Recombinant human erythropoietin vs. transfusions in the treatment of anemia and prematurity, a cost-benefit analysis. Arch Pediatr Adolesc Med 148:582, 1994

42. Alverson DC, Isken VH, Cohen RS: Effect of booster blood transfusions on oxygen utilization in infants with bronchopulmonary dysplasia. J Pediatr 113:722, 1988

43. Strauss RG: Transfusion therapy in neonates. Am J Dis Child 145:904, 1991

44. Lister G, Hellenbranc WE, Kleinman CS, Talner NS: Physiologic effects of increasing hemoglobin concentration in left-to-right shunting in infants with ventricular septal defects. N Engl J Med 306:502, 1982

45. Rosenthal A: Hemodynamics in physiologic anemia of infancy. N Engl J Med 306:538, 1982

46. Kattwinkel J: Neonatal apnea: pathogenesis and therapy. J Pediatr 90:342, 1977

47. Joshi A, Gerhardt T, Shandloff P, Bankalari E: Blood transfusion effect on the respiratory pattern of preterm infants. Pediatrics 80:79, 1987

48. Keyes WG, Donohur PK, Spivak JL et al: Assessing the need for transfusion of premature infants and role of

hematocrit, clinical signs and erythropoietin level. Pediatrics 84:412, 1989

49. Kurzner SI, Garg M, Bautista DB et al: Growth failure in infants with bronchopulmonary dysplasia: nutrition and elevated resting metabolic expenditure. Pediatrics 81:379, 1988

50. Stockman JA, Clark DA: Weight gain: a response to transfusion in selected preterm infants. Am J Dis Child 138:828, 1984

51. Blank JP, Sheagren TG, Vajaria J et al: The role of RBC transfusion in the premature infant. Am J Dis Child 138:831, 1984

52. Ross MP, Christensen RD, Rothstein G et al: A randomized trial to develop criteria for administering erythrocyte transfusions to anemic preterm infants 1 to 3 months of age. J Perinatol 9:246, 1989

53. Luban NLC, Strauss RG, Hume HA: Commentary on the safety of red blood cells preserved in extended storage media for neonatal transfusions. Transfusion 31:229, 1990

54. Strauss RG, Sacher RA, Blazina JF et al: Commentary on small-volume red cell transfusions for neonatal patients. Transfusion 30:565, 1990

55. Strauss RG, Levy GJ, Sotelo-Avila et al: A national survey of transfusion practices. II. Blood component therapy. Pediatrics 91:520, 1993

56. Strauss RG: Selection of white cell-reduced blood components for transfusions during early infancy. Transfusion 33:352, 1993

57. Holland BM, Wardrop CAJ: Anaemias of the premature infant. p. 121. In Turner TL (ed): Perinatal Haematological Problems. John Wiley & Sons, New York, 1991

58. Lill EA, Mannino FL, Lane TA: Prospective, randomized trial of the safety and efficacy of a limited donor exposure transfusion program for premature neonates. J Pediatr 125:92, 1994

59. Lee DA, Slagle TA, Jackson TM, Evans CS: Reducing blood donor exposures in low birth weight infants by the use of older, unwashed packed red blood cells. J Pediatr 126:280, 1995

60. Bifano EM, Dracker RA, Lorah K, Palit A: Collection and 28-day storage of human placental blood. Pediatr Res 36:90, 1994

61. Strauss RG: Autologous transfusions for neonates using placental blood, a cautionary note. Am J Dis Child 146:21, 1992

Hemorrhagic Complications in Newborns

Maureen Andrew and Lu Ann Brooker

The diagnosis and management of acquired and congenital bleeding disorders in newborns differs from older children and adults, reflecting unique aspects of blood coagulation at birth. This chapter briefly reviews developmental hemostasis, bleeding disorders in newborns, and treatment using a variety of blood component therapies.

The preparation and availability of blood component therapy began in the 1950s. Cryoprecipitate was first prepared from human plasma by Judith Pool in 1964. The purification of individual coagulation factors in the form of concentrates quickly followed. Implementation of plasma component therapy in newborns has been facilitated by the development of modern neonatal intensive care units (ICUs) beginning in the late 1960s. Plasma products are used for the treatment of acquired hemostatic disorders and, less frequently, for the treatment of specific congenital deficiencies of coagulation proteins.

The identification of publications providing information on specific disease states was initiated by a computerized search of the medical literature employing the MEDLINE database from 1966 to February 1994, using combinations of key words appropriate for each disorder. The bibliographies of the retrieved articles were checked for any additional studies, and recent journal publications were searched independently.

DEVELOPMENTAL HEMOSTASIS

Both the diagnosis and treatment for newborns with hemorrhagic or thrombotic complications are distinctly different from older patients, reflecting the relative immaturity of the hemostatic system at birth.[1-7] The following discussion briefly summarizes our current understanding of developmental hemostasis and its relevance to specific pathologic states. A detailed summary of hemostasis in general is provided in Chapter 8.

The Procoagulants

Coagulation proteins do not cross the placenta from mother to fetus.[8-10] Rather, the factors are synthesized by the fetus beginning in the first trimester of pregnancy.[11-18] At birth, the levels of the vitamin K-dependent coagulant factors (FII, FVII, FIX, FX) and the contact factors (FXII, FXI, prekallikrein, PK; and high-molecular-weight kininogen [HMWK]) are approximately 50 percent of adult values.[2-7] Plasma concentrations of other coagulant proteins (fibrinogen, FXIII, FVIII, FV) are present in concentrations similar to adults.[2-7] von Willebrand factor (vWF) levels are increased, with a disproportional increase in high-molecular-weight multimers.[19,20] The net effect of these differences at birth is a decreased capacity to generate thrombin (50 percent) compared to adult plasma.[21-25] The plasma concentration of prothrombin is the critical determinant of the amount of thrombin generated in newborn plasma.[21,25,26] During the first weeks of life, plasma levels of the vitamin K-dependent and contact factors rapidly increase and are within the adult range by 6 months of age.[5-7]

At birth, some proteins are present in "fetal" forms. Fetal fibrinogen is characterized by increased sialic acid content compared to adult fibrinogen.[27-29] However, the physiologic significance of "fetal" fibrinogen is unknown. The amino acid concentrations, the rate of release of FPA by thrombin and cross-linking are similar to adult fibrinogen.[27-29]

Inhibitors of Coagulation

Inhibitors of coagulation proteins are also synthesized by the fetus and do not cross the placenta. Plasma concentrations of protein C and protein S (vitamin K-dependent inhibitors) are approximately 35 percent of adult values, with lower limits of normal at 10 percent of adult values.[1,15,30-40] Protein C is present in a "fetal," form characterized by a two-fold increase in single-chain protein C but similar anticoagulant activities to protein C in adult plasma.[41] Protein S circulates in adult plasma in both a free form (active) and complexed with C_4B binding protein.[42,43] Although total protein S levels are very low at birth, the available protein S is completely in the free or active form, thereby compensating for the absence of C_4B binding protein.[43] The overall activity of the protein C/protein S inhibitory system is dependent on the presence and function of thrombomodulin (TM), an endothelial cell receptor for thrombin. Although the effect of age on endothelial expression of TM is unknown, plasma concentrations of TM are increased at birth and during the first years of life.[44] This observation raises the possibility that endothelial expression of TM may compensate for low levels of protein C at birth.[44]

Plasma concentrations of the direct thrombin inhibitors, antithrombin III (ATIII) and heparin cofactor II (HCII), are approximately 50 percent of adult values at birth.[1-4,15,30-39,45,46] By contrast, plasma concentrations of α_2M are increased at birth and are approximately twice adult values by 6 months of age.[47,48] The net effect of this unique balance of direct thrombin inhibitors in newborn plasmas is a slower rate of thrombin inhibition, but a similar overall capacity to inhibit thrombin, compared to adult plasma.[49,50]

The Fibrinolytic System

Components of the fibrinolytic system are also synthesized by the fetus and present at birth.[5-7,30,51-57] Plasma concentrations of the key enzyme, plasminogen, and its major inhibitor, α_2-antiplasmin (α_2AP), are reduced to 50 percent and 80 percent of adult values, respectively.[5-7,30,51-57] By contrast, plasma concentrations of the major activator of fibrinolysis, tissue plasminogen activator (tPA), and the major inhibitor of tPA, plasminogen activator inhibitor 1 (PAI1) are increased compared to adult values. The increased levels of tPA and PAI1 in newborns likely reflect release from the endothelium in the early postnatal period because cord values of for both proteins are considerably lower than values from newborns.[52] Although it has not been measured in newborn plasma, cord plasma concentrations of urokinase plasminogen activator (uPA) are reduced.[58] The PAI2 level in women in the third trimester of pregnancy is 240 ± 27 ng/ml[59] and cord plasma likely reflects that value.

The capacity of the neonatal fibrinolytic system to generate plasmin and to lyse fibrin clots is significantly decreased compared to adult plasmas. Supplementation of newborn plasmas with plasminogen increases the capacity of newborn plasmas to lyse fibrin clots. Although plasminogen is present in a "fetal" form at birth,[60,61] there is no evidence that this impairs its capacity to lyse fibrin clots.

Summary

In order to diagnose and treat newborns with hemostatic problems correctly, it is critically important to interpret laboratory screening tests and specific coagulation protein assays in the context of normal physiology. Although cord values have been helpful in understanding the ontogeny of hemostasis, they do not always reflect values during the early postnatal period. Table 30-1 provides values for screening tests and plasma concentrations of coagulation proteins during the first month of life compared to the adult. Reference ranges for older infants and children are also available but are not discussed in this review.[47]

Table 30-1. Reference Values for Coagulation Tests in Healthy Full-Term Infants During the First 6 Months of Life[a]

Test	Day 1		Day 5		Day 30		Adult	
	M	B	M	B	M	B	M	B
Coagulation tests								
PT (sec)	13.0	(10.1–15.9)[b]	12.4	(10.0–15.3)[b]	11.8	(10.0–14.3)[b]	12.4	(10.8–13.9)
INR	1.00	(0.53–1.62)	0.89	(0.53–1.48)	0.79	(0.53–1.26)	0.89	(0.64–1.17)
APTT (sec)	42.9	(31.3–54.5)	42.6	(25.4–59.8)	40.4	(32.0–55.2)	33.5	(26.6–40.3)
TCT (sec)	23.5	(19.0–28.3)[b]	23.1	(18.0–29.2)	24.3	(19.4–29.2)[b]	25.0	(19.7–30.3)
Fibrinogen (gl)	2.83	(1.67–3.99)[b]	3.12	(1.62–4.62)[b]	2.70	(1.62–3.78)[b]	2.78	(1.56–4.00)
II (U/ml)	0.48	(0.26–0.70)	0.63	(0.33–0.93)	0.68	(0.34–1.02)	1.08	(0.70–1.46)
V (U/ml)	0.72	(0.34–1.08)	0.95	(0.45–1.45)	0.98	(0.62–1.34)	1.06	(0.62–1.50)
VII (U/ml)	0.66	(0.28–1.04)	0.89	(0.35–1.43)	0.90	(0.42–1.38)	1.06	(0.67–1.43)
VIII (U/ml)	1.00	(0.50–1.78)[b]	0.88	(0.50–1.54)[b]	0.91	(0.50–1.57)[b]	0.99	(0.50–1.49)
vWF (U/ml)	1.53	(0.50–2.87)	1.40	(0.50–2.54)	1.28	(0.50–2.46)	0.92	(0.50–1.58)
IX (U/ml)	0.53	(0.15–0.91)	0.53	(0.15–0.91)	0.51	(0.21–0.81)	1.09	(0.55–1.63)
X (U/ml)	0.40	(0.12–0.68)	0.49	(0.19–0.79)	0.59	(0.31–0.87)	1.06	(0.70–1.52)
XI (U/ml)	0.38	(0.10–0.66)	0.55	(0.23–0.87)	0.53	(0.27–0.79)	0.97	(0.67–1.27)
XII (U/ml)	0.53	(0.13–0.93)	0.47	(0.11–0.83)	0.49	(0.17–0.81)	1.08	(0.52–1.64)
PK (U/ml)	0.37	(0.18–0.69)	0.48	(0.20–0.76)	0.57	(0.23–0.91)	1.12	(0.62–1.62)
HK (U/ml)	0.54	(0.06–1.02)	0.74	(0.16–1.32)	0.77	(0.33–1.21)	0.92	(0.50–1.36)
XIII$_a$ (U/ml)	0.79	(0.27–1.31)	0.94	(0.44–1.44)[b]	0.93	(0.39–1.47)[b]	1.05	(0.55–1.55)
XIII[b] (U/ml)	0.76	(0.30–1.22)	1.06	(0.32–1.80)	1.11	(0.39–1.73)[b]	0.97	(0.57–1.37)
Inhibitor levels								
ATIII (U/ml)	0.63	(0.39–0.87)	0.67	(0.41–0.93)	0.78	(0.48–1.08)	1.05	(0.79–1.31)
α_2M (U/ml)	1.39	(0.95–1.83)	1.48	(0.98–1.98)	1.50	(1.06–1.94)	0.86	(0.52–1.20)
C_1E-INH (U/ml)	0.72	(0.36–1.08)	0.90	(0.60–1.20)[b]	0.89	(0.47–1.31)	1.01	(0.71–1.31)
α_1AT (U/ml)	0.93	(0.49–1.37)	0.89	(0.49–1.29)[b]	0.62	(0.36–0.88)	0.93	(0.55–1.31)
HCII (U/ml)	0.43	(0.10–0.93)	0.48	(0.00–0.96)	0.47	(0.10–0.87)	0.96	(0.66–1.26)
Protein C (U/ml)	0.35	(0.17–0.53)	0.42	(0.20–0.64)	0.43	(0.21–0.65)	0.96	(0.64–1.28)
Protein S (U/ml)	0.36	(0.12–0.60)	0.50	(0.22–0.78)	0.63	(0.33–0.93)	0.92	(0.60–1.24)
Fibrinolytic system								
Plasminogen (U/ml)	1.95	(1.25–2.65)	2.17	(1.41–2.93)	1.98	(1.26–2.70)	3.36	(2.48–4.24)
TPA (ng/ml)	9.6	(5.0–18.9)	5.6	(4.0–10.0)[b]	4.1	(1.0–6.0)[b]	4.9	(1.4–8.4)
α_2AP (U/ml)	0.85	(0.55–1.15)	1.00	(0.70–1.30)[b]	1.00	(0.76–1.24)[b]	1.02	(0.68–1.36)
PAI-1 (U/ml)	6.4	(2.0–15.1)	2.3	(0.0–8.1)[b]	3.4	(0.0–8.8)[b]	3.6	(0.0–11.0)
PAI-2 (ng/ml)	240	(213–267)[59]	—		—		<10[59]	
uPA (ng/ml)	0.18	(0.08–0.28)[57]	—		—		0.32	(0.18–0.46)[57]

Abbreviations: PT prothrombin time; APTT, activated partial thromboplastin time; TCT, thrombin clotting time; VIII, factor VIII procoagulant; vWF, von Willebrand factor; PK, prekallikrein; HK, high-molecular-weight kininogen; INR, international normalized ratio.

[a] All factors except fibrinogen are expressed as units per milliliter (U/ml), where pooled plasma contains 1.0 U/ml. All values are expressed as mean (M), followed by the lower and upper boundary encompassing 95 percent of the population (B). Between 40 to 77 samples were assayed for each value for the newborn. Some measurements were skewed due to a disproportionate number of high values. The lower limit, which excludes the lower 2.5 percent of the population, has been given.

[b] Values indistinguishable from those of the adult.

(From Andrew et al.[7] with permission.)

BLEEDING DISORDERS

Newborns presenting with bleeding complications may have an acquired or congenital hemostatic defect. Although acquired problems are more common, congenital deficiencies often first present in early infancy and need to be considered in otherwise healthy infants who are bleeding excessively from minor trauma.[62–64] The most frequent causes of bleeding in healthy full-term infants are an immune thrombocytopenia, vitamin K deficiency, or a congenital factor deficiency. By contrast, sick newborns who bleed are more likely to have disseminated intravascular coagulation (DIC) or liver disease.

The sites and consequences of bleeding differ in newborns compared to children or adults. An underlying hemostatic impairment may be manifested by oozing from the umbilicus, bleeding into the scalp with large cephalohematomas, bleeding following circumcision, and bleeding from peripheral blood sampling sites. Unfortunately, the first sign of impaired hemostasis in a healthy infant may be an intracranial hemorrhage (ICH). Because newborns have very small total blood volumes (approximately 200 to 400 ml), what would be minor bleeding for an adult can rapidly result in shock for newborns.

The correct diagnosis of underlying hemostatic defects in newborns depends on the clinical presentation, as well as initial laboratory screening tests, which include a prothrombin time (PT) expressed as an international normalized ratio (INR), activated partial thromboplastin time (APTT), thrombin clotting time (TCTs), fibrinogen level, platelet count, a peripheral blood smear and, in some cases, bleeding time. Additional assays such as specific factor assays or markers of activation of the coagulation, or fibrinolytic systems, may be indicated. Once the hemostatic disorder is identified, coagulation factor replacement provides an important part of therapy. Abnormal laboratory values in the absence of clinical symptoms, especially if there is anticipated resolution of the primary problem, do not necessarily require treatment.

Acquired Bleeding Disorders

Disseminated Intravascular Coagulation

The term DIC was first used in the 1960s to describe diffuse fibrin deposition in the microvasculature at autopsy. The advent of sensitive markers of in vivo activation of coagulation and fibrinolysis have extended the definition of DIC. The term DIC is broadly used currently to describe patients in whom both the coagulation and fibrinolytic systems are activated, with or without significant fibrin deposition, consumption of coagulation proteins, or hemorrhagic complications. A Medline search using the words DIC and newborn identified 42 publications, of which 19 were case reports, 4 were review articles, 12 were case series, and 7 were controlled trials. The following discussion reflects these studies.

The most common causes of DIC in newborns are shock, sepsis, asphyxia, and respiratory distress syndrome (RDS).[65-78] Improving perinatal care has significantly reduced the number of infants with serious clinical manifestations of DIC and led to the identification of a large group of infants with mild or no clinical consequences of DIC.[78-82]

The laboratory diagnosis of severe DIC remains unchanged and consists of prolongation of screening tests (PT, APTT), depletion of selected coagulation proteins (fibrinogen, FV, FVIII), increased fibrinogen/fibrin-split products, thrombocytopenia, and a microangiopathic hemolytic anemia.[65-77] However, the availability of sensitive markers of in vivo thrombin and plasmin generation has broadened the diagnosis of DIC without necessarily changing the criteria for treatment of the hemostatic problem.

The cornerstone of treatment for DIC remains effective control of the underlying problem(s). If the underlying problem(s) cannot be corrected, intervention with plasma products may, at best, be temporarily helpful. However, in the presence of significant bleeding or thrombotic consequences of DIC, and anticipated resolution of the primary problems, intervention therapy with plasma products is indicated. Therapeutic options for improving hemostasis in infants with DIC include fresh frozen plasma (FFP), cryoprecipitate, and factor concentrates (i.e., ATIII concentrates, prothrombin complex concentrates) and exchange transfusions.

Only one recent randomized controlled trial specifically addressed the issue of coagulation protein replacement in newborns with DIC.[83] In this study, mortality from DIC was evaluated in 33 infants who were randomized to a control group (n = 11), or treatment by exchange transfusion (n = 11) or treatment with FFP (n = 11). It was concluded that intervention did not affect survival: however, the sample size was too small, and the severity of the illness (75 percent survival rate) too minimal to test the hypothesis adequately. The remaining five controlled studies do not necessarily reflect current neonatal intensive care treatment because they were conducted between 1968 and 1983.[84-88] These five trials evaluated the effect of coagulation protein replacement on abnormal coagulation profiles, ICH, and death (Table 30-2). Of the five trials, three focused on large groups of sick low-birthweight infants and full-term infants following asphyxia episodes.[85-87] One group reported a beneficial effect of FFP on the thrombotest, as well as the decrease in mortality.[88] Another noted that the use of FFP in addition to cryoprecipitate and factor IX concentrates corrected the coagulation tests in 80 percent of infants.[84] The variable

Table 30-2. Clinical Trials Assessing the Potential Benefits of Plasma Products in Newborns With Coagulopathies

Investigators	No.	Outcome		Comment
Gross et al.[83] (1982)		Death		No effect on the PT, APTT, or
Treatment (ET)	11	4 (35%)		fibrinogen level
Treatment (FFP)	11	5 (45%)		
Control	11	3 (27%)		
Turner et al.[155] (1981)		Death		
Treatment (FFP, Cryo, factor IXC)	39	23 (59%)		PT, APTT, and fibrinogen level
Control	39	22 (56%)		improved in the treatment group
Waltt et al.[85] (1973)		Death	ICH	
Treatment (factor IXC)	40	19 (47%)	12 (30%)	TT lower in the control group
Control	40	16 (40%)	4* (10%)	on day 1
De Lemos et al.[86] (1973)		Death		
Treatment (ET)	20	5 (25%)		Prolonged APTT associated
Treatment (FEP)	20	16 (80%)		with a poorer outcome
Hambleton and Appleyard[87] (1973)		Death		
Treatment (FFP)	33	9 (27%)	2 (6%)	Minor improvements in the PT
Control	33	10 (30%)	3 (<9%)	and APTT
Gray et al.[88] (1968)		Death		
Treatment (FFP)	26	1 (4%)		TT lower in infants who died
Control	48	9 (19%)		

Abbreviations: FFP, fresh frozen plasma; ET, exchange transfusion; C, concentrate; PT, prothrombin time; APTT, activated partial thromboplastin time; TT, thrombotest; IVH, intraventricular hemorrhage; Cryo, cryoprecipitate; ICH, intracranial hemorrhage; FIXC, factor IX concentrate.

ª A significant difference between groups of at least *P* < 0.05.

response to FFP reported in the various series and case reports probably reflects the different disease states and the amounts of FFP used. In addition, one small study assessed the potential benefits of ATIII concentrates in addition to heparin.[89] In this study, 21 preterm infants were treated with ATIII concentrates and coagulation parameters returned to normal by 48 hours of age.

Liver Disease

The coagulopathies of liver disease in newborns are similar to adults and reflect failure of hepatic synthetic functions superimposed on a physiologic immaturity, activation of the coagulation and fibrinolytic systems, poor clearance of activated coagulation factors, and the loss of hemostatic proteins into ascitic fluid.[90] Secondary effects of liver disease affect platelet number and function.[91–93] Thrombocytopenia reflects impaired platelet production due to direct viral invasion of megakaryocytes, splenic sequestration, and accelerated clearance.[94–97] A Med-

line search was conducted using the key words of blood coagulation disorders, liver disease, and newborn. Ten publications were identified, five of which were case reports and five review articles.[98–107] The following discussion reflects these studies.

The laboratory abnormalities induced by acute liver disease include a prolonged PT and low plasma concentrations of several coagulation proteins, including fibrinogen.[108,109] Chronic liver failure with cirrhosis is also characterized by a coagulopathy[110–113] and mild thrombocytopenia due to splenic sequestration.[114,115] Secondary vitamin K deficiency due impaired absorption from the small intestine may occur, particularly from intra- and extrahepatic biliary atresia.[116]

The common pathologic causes of hepatic dysfunction in newborns are viral hepatitis, hypoxia, total parenteral nutrition (TPN), shock, fetal hydrops, and other disorders. Patients with clinical bleeding may benefit temporarily from replacement of coagulation proteins with FFP, cryoprecipitate, and/or exchange transfusion. However, without recovery of hepatic function, replacement therapy is futile. Vitamin K should be administered to infants suspected of having cholestatic liver disease. Prothrombin complex concentrates containing FII, FVII, FIX, FX should, in general, be avoided in newborns due to the high risk of transmitting hepatitis.

Periventricular-Intraventricular Hemorrhage

The most frequent form of ICH in premature infants is periventricular-intraventricular hemorrhage (PIVH).[117] The hemorrhage, which usually begins within the first 6 hours of life, begins in the fragile microvasculature of the subependymal germinal matrix.[117-123] The latter rupture into the adjacent ventricle in approximately 80 percent of newborns and may initiate an arachnoiditis obstructing cerebrospinal fluid (CSF) flow. The secondary consequences of PIVH include destruction of the germinal matrix with cyst formation, progressive ventricular dilation, and periventricular infarction. Hemorrhagic infarction usually occurs by day 4 of life, in 15 to 20 percent of infants with PICH.[124,125] The hemorrhagic infarction is frequently asymmetric and is located in the periventricular white matter.[120,121,124-130] Bedside ultrasound through the anterior fontanelle and computed tomography (CT) have permitted accurate detection of PIVH, determination of the natural history, and assessment of the effects of specific therapeutic interventions.[118,131-139] The incidence of PIVH in premature infants is decreasing, probably reflecting improving neonatal care.

Etiology of PIVH

The etiology of PIVH in premature infants is multifactorial and incompletely understood. The mechanism of primary importance is fluctuation of cerebral blood flow.[140-147] Other contributing mechanisms include increased fragility of the germinal matrix capillaries, oxidative damage to endothelium, and impairment of hemostasis.[148-151]

Therapeutic Intervention

The numerous clinical trials completed with the objective of decreasing the incidence and severity of PIVH have been recently reviewed.[152] The therapeutic interventions have included agents that affect cerebral blood flow (prenatal phenobarbital, postnatal

phenobarbital, indomethacin, pancuronium bromide), drugs that affect cell membranes (ethamsylate, vitamin E), and products that enhance hemostasis (ethamsylate, vitamin K, FFP, tranexamic acid, platelet concentrates). Only the studies testing interventions directed at altering hemostasis are discussed in the following section.

Trials of Coagulation Factor Replacement Prior to the 1980s

The immature physiologic state of hemostasis in premature infants and the association of pathologic alterations of hemostasis with PIVH form the rationale for intervention studies directed at enhancing hemostasis.[83,85,88,148,150,153-157] Six clinical trials with coagulation factor replacement were conducted between 1968 and 1981.[87,88,155,158-160] The results of these early trials cannot be extrapolated to current practice because of the significant improvements in neonatal intensive care management and the availability of ultrasound for diagnosing PIVH. Since 1980, trials testing drugs or blood products that enhance specific aspects of hemostasis have been tested in infants at risk of PIVH (Table 30-3).

Antenatal Administration of Vitamin K

Beginning antenatally, vitamin K was administered to mothers to increase the plasma activity of vitamin K-dependent coagulation proteins in premature infants. Of the three clinical trials conducted to test this hypothesis, two reported a benefit and one did not.[161-163] A placebo control group was not present in any study. Despite randomization, imbalances in the two positive studies between treatment and control groups may have conferred a positive bias for vitamin K. Both positive studies reported an effect on coagulation tests that might reflect the administration of vitamin K. The negative study did not identify a positive effect on the infants' coagulation system. For all these reasons, antenatal vitamin K administration for the prevention of PIVH cannot be recommended. This statement is not to be confused with the well-substantiated need for postnatal vitamin K supplementation.

Blood Products

Three blood products have been tested in randomized controlled trials (RCTs) in PIVH (Table 30-3). FFP was tested in one such conducted in 1985.

Table 30-3. PIVH Prevention Studies

Study	Number of Patients	Weight (kg)	Dose-1 (mg/kg)	Dose-2 (mg/kg)	PIVH
Transexamic Acid					
Hensey[165]	105	1.25	25 (IV)	25 × 20	↔
Blood Products					
Beverley[148] (FFP)	73	1.5	10 ml	10 ml × 1	↓
Shirata[164] (FFP)	21	—	100 units	None	↓
Andrew[156,157] (Platelet-C)	154	1.5	10 ml	10 ml × 1–3	↔
Indomethacin					
Kreuger[401]	32	1.5	0.2	none	—
Hanigan[179]	111	1.3	0.1	0.1 × 3	↓
Ment[180]	36	1.25	0.1	0.1 × 2	↓
Bandstra[402]	199	1.3	0.2	0.1 × 2	↓
Bada[403]	141	1.5	0.2	0.1 × 2	↓
Mahoney	104	1.3	0.2	0.1 × 2	—
Ment[178]	48	1.25	0.6	0.1 × 8	↓
Rennie[181]	50	1.75	0.2	0.2 × 2	↔
Vincer	30	1.5	0.2	0.2 × 2	—
Ethamsylate					
Morgan[174]	73	1.5	12.5	12.5 × 16	↓
Benson[176]	330	1.5	12.5	12.5 × 16	↓
Vitamin K					
Pomerance[162]	53	1.5	10	10 × 2	↓
Morales[161]	100	1.5	10	10 E 5d	↓
Kazzi[163]	98	2.5	10	20 Ed	↔

Treated newborns received 10 ml/kg of FFP on admission and at 24 hours of age.[148] Of the treated newborns, 5 of 36 developed ICH, compared to 15 of 37 newborns, a significant difference. However, without a placebo control, it is possible that the beneficial effect observed was the result of "stabilizing the circulation," rather than improving hemostasis. In a second study of a blood product, factor XIII concentrates were given to premature infants to prevent ICH by enhancing fibrin cross-linking.[164] Although this study reported a significant effect, the analysis was performed on a small subset of infants who were not balanced. Furthermore, there is no strong biologic rationale to support the likely benefit of factor XIII concentrates, as plasma concentrations of factor XIII are well within the adult range at birth (Table 30-3). In a third study of a blood product, platelet concentrates were administered to thrombocytopenic infants because of the close association of PIVH and thrombocytopenia[156,157] (Table 30-3). One hundred fifty-four premature infants, thrombocytopenic during the first 72 hours of life, were randomized to a control or treated group. Treated infants received platelet concentrates to maintain platelet counts above 150×10^9/L. No beneficial effect on ICH was shown in this study, which was designed to detect 25 percent effect or greater.

Inhibition of Fibrinolysis

An inhibitor of fibrinolysis, tranexamic acid, was tested in PIVH because of increased fibrinolytic activity at birth.[151,165] Tranexamic acid has been shown to reduce the incidence of recurrent subarachnoid hemorrhage in adults[166,167] and to prevent bleeding after oral surgery in high-risk patients.[168,169] In this study, 105 infants were randomized to receive tranexamic acid or placebo on day 1 of life and for 4 subsequent days. No significant effect was demonstrated (Table 30-3).

Stabilization of Capillary Membranes

The microvasculature of the germinal matrix is fragile and thereby susceptible to rupture. Ethamsylate is a drug that may stabilizes capillary membranes and increases platelet adhesiveness. In addition, ethamsylate is an inhibitor of prostaglandin synthesis with potential effects on the cerebral vasculature. Ethamsylate reduces capillary bleeding during selected surgical interventions in humans (ear, nose, and throat surgery)[170-172] and reduces the incidence of PIVH in the Beagle puppy model.[173] Two randomized controlled trials and one controlled trial have reported a reduction in PIVH with ethamsylate (Table 30-3).[174-176] However, before ethamsylate can be generally recommended, neurodevelopmental follow-up is needed because of the remaining possibility that treatment could cause brain ischemia.[152]

Regulation of Cerebral Blood Flow

Cerebral blood flow is regulated in part by prostaglandins, such as prostacyclin (PGI_2) and thromboxane A_2 (TXA_2). PGI_2 is a potent vasodilator that inhibits platelet aggregation, and TXA_2 is a potent vasoconstrictor that promotes platelet aggregation. In the Beagle puppy model, indomethacin, a drug that blocks the enzyme cyclooxygenase, significantly decreased the incidence of ICH. Indomethacin reduced plasma concentrations of 6-keto-$PGF_{1\alpha}$ and TXB_2, the stable metabolites of PGI_2 and TXA_2.[177] A recently conducted metanalysis of 9 randomized controlled trials shows idomethaacin treatment reduces the risk for PIVH[152] (Table 30-3).

Recommendations

Several confounding variables may have contributed to differing results in the trials discussed. Of particular importance is the declining incidence of PIVH during the 1980s probably reflecting improving perinatal care. Ongoing clinical studies are necessary to test potentially beneficial therapeutic agents within the context of improving clinical care. No firm recommendations can be made for any of the intervention modalities discussed because of a lack of consistent results and neurodevelopmental follow-up.[173]

Respiratory Distress Syndrome

RDS, an acute lung disorder that primarily affects premature infants, is characterized by diffuse atelectasis, hyaline membrane formation, permeability edema, and right-to-left shunting of pulmonary blood flow.[178-180] Increased pulmonary surface tension secondary to surfactant deficiency is an important mechanism that contributes to RDS.[181]

Potential Role of Coagulation

One of the pathologic characteristics of RDS is fibrin deposition at both intra-alveolar and intravascular sites.[178-180] This observation has led several investigators to look for evidence of activation of coagulation in infants with RDS. Early studies reported decreased plasma concentrations of some coagulation proteins and inhibitors. However, these tests were neither sensitive nor specific for sensitive paracoagulation tests, F1.2, TAT, and D-dimer, have been measured in newborns with a spectrum of mild to severe RDS.[78] There was a direct correlation between increasing thrombin generation, decreased ATIII levels, and severity of RDS.[78] Furthermore, there is evidence that fibrin deposition within the lung likely contributes to the severity of lung disease.[182-185] In a piglet model of neonatal acute lung injury, increasing plasma concentrations of ATIII by the infusion of ATIII concentrates decreased the severity of the lung disease.[186]

Intervention Trials Influencing Hemostasis

The possible role of coagulation in acute neonatal lung disease has provided the rationale for four intervention studies directed at decreasing fibrin deposition by the use of anticoagulants and thrombolytic therapy (Table 30-4).

Anticoagulation Therapy

Two anticoagulants, heparin and ATIII concentrates, have been tested in RDS.[187,188] In the first trial conducted in 1971, high-risk low-birthweight infants were randomized to receive heparin or placebo (saline), with nurses blinded to treatment. Eighty-one infants were entered; 39 to heparin and 42 to placebo. In the primary analyses, there was no difference in the number of deaths, incidence of RDS, or bleeding. However, on a subanalysis in which seven moribund infants treated with heparin and three moribund infants treated with saline were excluded, the authors suggested that there was a positive effect on mortality.[187] The second trial was a randomized controlled trial in which 45 newborns received ATIII concentrates and 53 received standard care alone.[188] There was no difference in duration of ventilation, ICH, or mortality.[188] ATIII concentrates are commercially available (Table 30-5) but cannot be recommended for use alone or as adjunc-

Table 30-4. Clinical Trials Assessing the Potential Benefits of Anticoagulant or Thrombolytic Therapy in Newborns With RDS

		Outcome		
Investigators	N	Deaths (%)	RDS (%)	ICH (%)
Markarian[187] et al.				
Heparin	39	17 (44%)	26 (68.8%)	40% mild 10% severe
Saline	42	16 (38%)	22 (53.3%)	0% mild 61% severe
Muntean and Rosseger[188]				
ATIIIC	45	9 (20%)	23 (51%)	—
	53	8 (15%)	28 (53%)	—
Ambrus et al.[189]				
UK-plasmin	32	9 (28%)	32 (100%)	7 (22%)
Placebo	28	17 (61%)	28 (100%)	6 (21%)
Ambrus et al.[190]				
Plasminogen C	251	6 (2%)	35 (14%) mild 19 (7%) severe	1 (0.4%)
Placebo	249	20 (8%)	22 (9%) mild 31 (12%) severe	1 (0.4%)

Abbreviations: Number (No.), respiratory distress syndrome (RDS), intracranial hemorrhage (ICH), urokinase (UK), antithrombin III concentrate (ATIIIC), plasminogen concentrate (plasminogen C).

Table 30-5. Clinical Inhibitor Concentrates

Concentrate	Manufacturer	Source	Viral Inactivation Method	Purity (Units FIX/mg)	Dose Guidelines
ATIII	Immuno	Human plasma	Aqueous heat-treated 60°C for 10 hr	1.0–2.5 U/mg	IU req'd = kg × desired increase × 1.0
Thrombate III	Miles	cold ethanol method of Cohn lyophilized modification			IU req'd = kg × [desired increase − baseline ATIII] ÷ 4
ATIII	Cutter	From Cohn fraction IV-I-affinity chromatography— ultra + difiltration	Heat-treated in solution at 60°C for 10 hr	>6.4 U/mg	IU req'd = kg × desired increase × 0.7
Protein C	Immuno	MAb chromatography from FIX complex	Vapor-treated	14 U/mg	IU req'd = kg × desired increase × 0.45

Abbreviations: IU, international units; kg, kilograms, ATIII antithrombin III; MAb, monoclonal antibody; req'd, required; FIX, factor IX.

tive for heparin in neonatal RDS, unless further trials demonstrate their benefit.

Fibrinolytic Therapy

In 1966, the value of urokinase-activated human plasmin was tested in a randomized, placebo-controlled double-blind study of 60 infants with severe RDS. Results indicated a substantially increase in survival rate without toxicity.[189] In a second double-blind randomized study, 500 premature infants were treated with plasminogen or placebo intravenously within 60 minutes of birth. There was a substantial decrease in severe clinical respiratory distress, death caused by hyaline membrane disease, and total mortality in the plasminogen-treated infants, as compared to the controls.[190] Although these two trials support the role of fibrinolytic therapy in RDS, they were both conducted prior to 1970. Plasminogen concentrates are commercially available and cannot be recommended for use in neonatal RDS unless further trials demonstrate their benefit in the context of modern neonatal intensive care management. Future clinical trials are needed to assess the benefits of antithrombotic or thrombolytic therapy in RDS.

Vitamin K Deficiency

Vitamin K deficiency was one of the first acquired bleeding disorders in pediatrics for which both an etiology and successful therapy were identified.[191] The earliest description of hemorrhagic disease of the newborn (HDN) was bleeding on days 1 to 5 of life in otherwise healthy breast-fed infants.[191] The importance of vitamin K in blood coagulation was discovered serendipitously in 1929, when spontaneous hemorrhaging was observed by Dam et al.[192] in chicks fed a fat-free diet. Vitamin K deficiency was rapidly implicated in HDN[30,193–195] and treatment of affected infants with vitamin K followed.[30,196–198] The following discussion focuses on the diagnosis and treatment of the infant with bleeding secondary to vitamin K deficiency. The issue of prophylactic vitamin K deficiency in newborns is not discussed, and the reader is referred to recent reviews.[199–201]

Function of Vitamin K in Coagulation

Vitamin K is required for the production of the active forms for FII, FVII, FIX, and FX, as well as the inhibitors protein C and S. Vitamin K-dependent proteins contain a series of 10 to 13 des-carboxyglutamic acid residues within their N-terminal region. Vitamin K is an essential cofactor for the post-translational carboxylation of these glutamic acid residues to δ-carboxyglutamic acid residues.[202–204] δ-carboxyglutamic acid residues serve as calcium binding sites required for participation in coagulation by binding to negatively charged phospholipid surfaces.[204–206]

Clinical Presentation of Vitamin K Deficiency

Although vitamin K deficiency may occur at any age, infants are particularly at risk of hemorrhagic complications. Physiologically, plasma concentrations of the vitamin K-dependent proteins at birth are only 50 percent of adult values. The additive insult of vitamin K deficiency rapidly results in significant impairment of the capacity to generate thrombin with resultant bleeding complications.[5–7,30,207–209]

The classic form of vitamin K deficiency, or HDN, presents on days 2 to 5 of life in otherwise healthy full-term infants, who are usually breast fed.[30,191,207–210] The spectrum of bleeding manifestations includes gastrointestinal bleeding, widespread ecchymosis, bleeding from puncture sites for postnatal screening tests, and sometimes intracranial hemorrhage. The reasons for this clinical presentation are that the stores of vitamin K are low in newborns due to low placental transfer of vitamin K,[211,212] breast milk has very low concentrations of vitamin K,[213,214] there is a low intake of milk in the first days of life, and the gut is sterile.[215,216] Infants fed formulas rarely develop vitamin K deficiency because formulas are supplemented with high concentrations of vitamin K. The classic form of vitamin K deficiency is rarely seen in countries in which newborn infants receive supplemental vitamin K at birth.[217] In the absence of vitamin K prophylaxis, the frequency of HDN is variable, depending on the population studied, the frequency of breast milk feeding, and supplementation with vitamin K-fortified formula.[217] In the United States, the frequency of HDN, in the absence of prophylaxis, may be as high as 1.7 percent for some areas of the country.[218]

An earlier, often more serious, form of vitamin K deficiency can occur shortly following birth in infants whose mothers have been taking drugs that interfere with the already marginal placental transport of vitamin K.[217] Drugs that have been implicated include warfarin, anticonvulsants, rifampin, and isoniazid. Unfortunately, these infants may present with significant bleeding, such as ICH. Occasionally, no underlying predisposing factor is identified.

A late form of vitamin K deficiency can occur beyond the first week of life. The delayed presentation is often associated with a variety of diseases that can compromise the supply of vitamin K. These disorders include chronic diarrhea, diarrhea in breast-fed infants, infants with cystic fibrosis, α_1-antitrypsin deficiency, hepatitis, celiac disease, and other rare causes.[219-226] In one report, an epidemic of HDN was caused by warfarin-contaminated talcs.[227] As for the early presentation of vitamin K deficiency, these infants often present with serious bleeding problems.

Laboratory Diagnosis of Vitamin K Deficiency

In the presence of vitamin K deficiency, the screening tests, including PT (INR), APTT, and thrombotest, will be prolonged. These tests are not specific and confirmatory tests for vitamin K deficiency are often helpful. However, treatment of an infant with suspected vitamin K deficiency should not be delayed for confirmatory tests. One diagnostic approach is to measure one or more vitamin K-dependent factor and a non-vitamin K-dependent factor. The limitation of this approach is that it is not specific, and infants have physiologically low levels of the vitamin K-dependent factors. A second approach is to measure the des-δ-carboxyglutamic acid forms of vitamin K-dependent factors, also known as PIVKA (protein induced by vitamin K absence). PIVKA can be measured directly[222,228-233] or as discrepancies between coagulant activity and immunologic concentrations of vitamin K-dependent proteins.[234] One rapid method is to use the snake venom, *Echis carinatum*, which cleaves thrombin from both decarboxylated and carboxylated forms of prothrombin in the absence of Ca^{2+}.[235] Discrepancies between prothrombin functional activity and prothrombin concentration measured by the *Echis* assay provides a clinically useful confirmation of vitamin K deficiency.

Treatment of Vitamin K Deficiency

The treatment of vitamin K deficiency depends upon the clinical status of the patient and the cause of the deficiency. The clinical spectrum of vitamin K deficiency ranges from patients with no symptoms, with mild bleeding, and with life-threatening bleeding.

Vitamin K Replacement

All vitamin K-deficient infants should receive treatment with vitamin K, either subcutaneously or intravenously, depending on the clinical circumstances; one should not wait for confirmatory tests from the laboratory before treatment. For therapeutic purposes, neither oral vitamin K nor intramuscular vitamin K is advisable. Severe anaphylactoid reactions with hypotension that can be fatal have complicated intravenous vitamin K administered to older patients.[217] Although the latter has not been described in newborns, it seems prudent to give intravenous vitamin K slowly to newborns as well. Following parenteral administration, approximately 50 percent of the vitamin K will be in the liver within 1 hour, and the coagulation abnormality will be corrected within 2 to 6 hours. If the same dose is given orally, only 20 percent of the amount will be in the liver within 2 hours, and the coagulation defect does not correct for 6 to 8 hours.

Plasma Products

Depending on the severity of the bleeding, patients may benefit from replacement of the vitamin K-dependent proteins with plasma products. The therapeutic options are plasma (stored or fresh frozen), and prothrombin complex concentrates (PCC). Administering 10 to 20 ml/kg of plasma should increase plasma concentrations of FII, FVII, FIX, and FX by approximately 0.1 to 0.2 U/ml. FFP is particularly useful when the precise nature of the coagulation factor deficiency is unknown or if there is secondary DIC. Patients with life-threatening or significant hemorrhage into the central nervous system (CNS) may benefit from increasing plasma concentrations of vitamin K-dependent factors to more than 50 percent of normal, immediately. Unfortunately, this cannot be achieved with plasma because of the volume requirements. PCCs at a minimum dose of 50 U/kg, in addition to systemic vitamin K, are indicated (Table 30-6). PCCs entail a number of potential risks to patients, including the transmission of hepatitis. Patients should also receive hepatitis B immunoglobulin intramuscularly and hepatitis vacci-

Table 30-6. Prothrombin Complex Concentrates and Factor IX Concentrates

| Concentrate | Manufacturer | Source | Viral Inactivation Method | Purity (Units FIX/mg) | Ratio of Other Factors | | | Dose Guidelines (IU required = kg multiplied by) |
					II	VII	X	
PCC								
Konyne 80	Miles	Human plasma	80°C dry, 74 hr	2.0	0.70	0.07	0.85	Desired increase × 1.0
Bebulin VH	Immuno	Human plasma	2-step vapor-heated	1.9	1.00	0.01	0.14	Desired increase × 1.2
FEIBA	Immuno	Human plasma	2-step vapor-heated	1.6	1.23	0.76	0.43	50 U/kg, q12h
Factor IX								
Alphanine SD	Alpha	Human plasma	SD (polysorbate 80)	69 ± 16	<0.01	<0.01	<0.05	Desired increase × 1.0

Abbreviations: SD, solvent detergent (solvent is 0.3% tri-*n*-butyl phosphate [TNBP] with 1 percent of the detergent indicated, usually incubated 6 hours at ambient temperature prior to purification step; IU, international units; PCCs, prothrombin complex concentrates; FIX, Factor IX; DEAE, diethylaminoethyl.

nation as soon as the coagulopathy is corrected and within 24 hours of receiving the factor IX concentrate.

Nonimmune Thrombocytopenia

Definition of Thrombocytopenia in Newborns

Healthy infants and fetuses have platelet counts in the same range as adults. Therefore, a platelet count of less than 150×10^9/L is the currently accepted definition of thrombocytopenia for all infants.[18,35,236] On average, premature infants have slightly lower platelet counts but still within the normal adult range (150 to 450×10^9/L).[18,30] Studies of fetuses at 18 to 30 weeks gestation show a stable mean platelet count of approximately 250×10^9/L without any change over the 12-week period.[18] The mean platelet volume of newborn platelets is similar to that of adults, with values usually less than 10 fL, averaging 7 to 9 fL.[237–240] Postnatally, the mean platelet volume may increase slightly over the first 1 to 2 weeks of life, concomitant with an increase in platelet count.

Epidemiology

Thrombocytopenia is probably the most common hemostatic abnormality in sick newborn infants.[241–243] The definition of thrombocytopenia in newborns is the same as in adults: a platelet count of less than 150×10^9/L. Consequently, platelet counts of less than 150×10^9/L are abnormal and require investigation and sometimes treatment. Like

many other aspects of neonatal hemostasis, the pathophysiologic causes and consequences of thrombocytopenia in newborns are an active area of study. A single prospective cohort study[153,240] and several retrospective reviews[154,239,244–246] provide the most reliable information available on the frequency, natural history, mechanisms, and clinical impact of thrombocytopenia in newborns. There is general agreement that thrombocytopenia is indicative of an underlying pathologic process; however, the clinical relevance of mild thrombocytopenia remains to be proved. Because of difficulties collecting and processing blood samples from a neonate, it is important to ensure that the infant is truly thrombocytopenic, by examining a stained blood film.

Approximately 22 percent of infants develop thrombocytopenia in a tertiary care neonatal ICU.[240] For some infants, the thrombocytopenia appears trivial (the platelet count is 100 to 150×10^9/L); however, for more than one-half of affected infants, the platelet count falls to below 100×10^9/L. Twenty percent of thrombocytopenic infants have platelet counts of less than 50×10^9/L. The natural history of thrombocytopenia in sick infants is remarkably consistent: the thrombocytopenia is present by day 2 of life in 75 percent of infants, reaching a nadir by day 4 in 75 percent of infants, and recovering to greater than 150×10^9/L by day 10 of life in approximately 90 percent of infants. This remarkably consistent natural history suggests that common mechanisms and precipitating events are responsible for neonatal thrombocytopenia.

Pathogenesis

Thrombocytopenia can be caused by increased platelet destruction, decreased platelet production, platelet pooling in an enlarged spleen, or a combination of these mechanisms. Characterization of mechanisms responsible for thrombocytopenia is important because it has practical implications in assessing the risk of bleeding and management of affected infants. For example, transfusion of platelets into infants with consumptive thrombocytopenia may be of limited benefit, since the same processes destroying the infant's platelets will also consume the transfused platelets. Clinical and laboratory findings that help define each group are summarized in Table 30-7.

Table 30-7. Neonatal Nonimmune Thrombocytopenia

Decreased production
    Amegakaryocytic thrombocytopenia
        TAR syndrome
        Chromosomal abnormalities
        Amegakaryocytic thrombocytopenia with microcephaly
        Wiskott-Aldrich syndrome
    Constitutional aplastic anemia
        Thrombocytopenia absent radii
        Fanconi's anemia
        Amegakaryocytic thrombocytopenia
    Infiltrative disorders
        Congenital leukemia
        Congenital neuroblastoma
        Contenital leukemoid reactions
        Osteoporosis
Consumptive Thrombocytopenia
    DIC
    Giant hemangioma
    Thrombosis (associated with CVLs, renal and umbilical veins, aorta, and IVC)
    Thrombotic thrombocytopenic purpura (TTP)
    Necrotizing enterocolitis
    Hemolytic anemia
    Exchange transfusion
    Hyperbilirubinemia
    Phototherapy
    Intrauterine growth retardation (IUGR)
    Polycythemia
    Infection induced
    Hypothermia
    Asphyxia
    Perinatal aspiration
    Respiration distress syndrome (RDS)
    Total parenteral nutrition (TPN)
    Inborn errors of metabolism

Based on measurements of mean platelet volume, the presence of megakaryocytes, and platelet survival, increased platelet destruction is the mechanism responsible for thrombocytopenia in most infants.[240,247,248] Splenic sequestration contributes to thrombocytopenia in some infants.[247] The mean platelet volume, although similar to that of adults at birth, increases significantly by day 7 of life in thrombocytopenic infants.[240] Sick nonthrombocytopenic infants also increase mean platelet volume by day 7 and show a fall in platelet count, suggesting that increased consumption of platelets occurs in many sick infants, although they do not develop thrombocytopenia. Newborn marrow samples are not always adequate, and quantitation of megakaryocytes may not be reliable. However, at autopsy, thrombocytopenic infants have similar numbers of megakaryocytes compared to nonthrombocytopenic infants in bone marrow biopsies.[240] The strongest evidence of platelet consumption comes from uniformly short radiolabeled platelet survival in thrombocytopenic infants.[240,247,248] The lowest platelet counts, longest duration of thrombocytopenia, and highest mean platelet volume all correlate with the shortest platelet survival.[247] Evidence of hypersplenism is documented by a reduced percentage recovery of labeled platelets in some infants[247] and enhanced splenic sequestration. Although platelet survival has not been measured in healthy full-term infants, platelet survival is similar in newborn and adult rabbits.[249]

Thrombocytopenia due to increased platelet destruction can be divided into those mediated by immune or by nonimmune events. Immune thrombocytopenia is defined as an increased rate of platelet clearance, caused by platelet-associated IgG (PAIgG) or complement. Elevated PAIgG levels are not diagnostic of idiopathic thrombocytopenic purpura (ITP) but are associated with a variety of thrombocytopenic disorders. Approximately 50 percent of infants with a platelet count of less than 100×10^9/L, have increased amounts of PAIgG on their platelets (Fig. 30-1). The cause of the elevated PAIgG levels in most of these infants has not been identified. Other investigators also report elevated PAIgG levels in thrombocytopenic neonates with sepsis[250] and in babies born to mothers with pre-eclampsia.[245] Neither sepsis nor pre-eclampsia occurs frequently enough

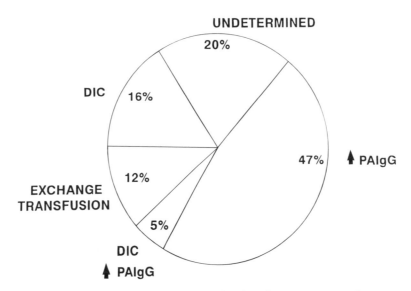

Fig. 30-1. Mechanisms responsible for thrombocytopenia in infants.

to provide a complete explanation for the large number of infants with elevated PAIgG.

Nonimmune causes of thrombocytopenia include DIC and thrombocytopenia secondary to exchange transfusion (Table 30-7). Exchange transfusions and intrauterine transfusions cause thrombocytopenia by a dilutional effect, depending on the amount of blood transfused.[251] Following an exchange transfusion, the platelet count begins to rise within days and rapidly reaches pre-exchange levels. Finally, for some infants, a likely mechanism cannot be identified, except that the thrombocytopenia is secondary to increased destruction.

Indications for Platelet Transfusions in Nonimmune Thrombocytopenia

The indication for administering platelet transfusions in most thrombocytopenic infants is a contentious issue and poses a therapeutic dilemma to clinicians. Specifically, do the benefits of raising platelet counts outweigh the risks associated with administration of an additional blood product? While there is extensive clinical information, including therapeutic intervention trials, linking thrombocytopenia with significant bleeding in older patients,[252–255] there is a paucity of information for newborns. Physiologic aspects of hemostasis (see previous sections) may place newborns at risk of bleeding at somewhat

higher platelet counts than for children and adults.[5,6,21,50,256–258]

Full-term Infants

The available information suggests that healthy full-term infants with platelet counts of more than approximately 50×10^9/L are at low risk of serious, spontaneous bleeding. However, platelet counts below approximately 50×10^9/L place some otherwise healthy full-term neonates at significant risk of ICH,[259–262] at least in infants with immune-mediated thrombocytopenia[259,260] or with thrombocytopenia/absent radius (TAR) syndrome.[261,262] Depending on the etiology, anticipated duration, and other risk factors for bleeding in infants with nonimmune thrombocytopenia, consideration should be given to the use of platelet concentrates when platelet counts are less than 50×10^9/L.

Premature Infants

In contrast to full-term infants, platelet counts of 50 to 100×10^9/L in premature infants have been linked to increased clinical bleeding, prolonged bleeding times, and increased frequency of ICH.[149,153,240,263] In one study, premature infants with platelet counts of less than 100×10^9/L had an 80 percent incidence of ICH, compared to a 40 percent incidence in those with platelet counts greater than $100 \times 10^9/L$.[153] Other studies have not found an association between thrombocytopenia and ICH.[154] A recent randomized controlled trial evaluated the potential benefits of early intervention with platelet concentrates in premature infants with platelet counts of less than $150 \times 10^9/L$.[240] Both the platelet counts and bleeding times improved significantly, indicating that the infusion of platelets positively affected platelet vessel wall interaction. The main clinical outcome was ICH, which was discussed in a previous section. A subanalysis of control infants with platelet counts of less than $60 \times 10^9/L$ showed that these infants received more blood products than the treated group and control infants with platelet counts greater than $60 \times 10^9/L$, perhaps reflecting increased bleeding in this subpopulation of infants. A reasonable recommendation, based on this study, is that nonbleeding premature infants with platelet counts greater than approximately $60 \times 10^9/L$ do not require prophylactic platelet transfusions.

Inherited Bleeding Disorders

Historically, exsanguination from ritual circumcision of Jewish male babies performed on the eighth day of life may be the first descriptions of bleeding in newborns with hemophilia, the most common congenital factor deficiency to present in newborns. Over the past century, congenital deficiencies have

been reported for all known coagulation proteins. The following discussion provides a general overview of the inheritance, clinical presentation, diagnosis, and treatment of congenital coagulation factor deficiencies in the neonatal period.

Inheritance

Deficiencies in factors II, VII, V, XI, and XII, PK, and HMWK are autosomally inherited, and rare, with consanguinity present in many families. Deficiencies of FXII, PK, and HMWK do not result in hemorrhagic complications and are not considered further. Deficiencies in factors VIII and IX are sex-linked and the most common congenital bleeding disorders to present in newborns. Rarely, combined deficiencies of FII, FVII, FIX, and FX or of FV and FVIII present in the neonatal period.[264,265]

Clinical Presentation

Most newborns with congenital coagulation factor deficiencies do not present with bleeding in the perinatal period, unless there is a hemostatic challenge. By contrast, unexplained bleeding in an otherwise healthy newborn should be carefully investigated because it may reflect the presentation of a congenital coagulation factor deficiency. With few exceptions, only severe forms of congenital coagulation factor deficiencies present with bleeding in newborns. Table 30-8 summarizes the number of newborns in

Table 30-8. Cases of Congenital Factor Deficiencies Presenting With Bleeding in Newborns[a]

Factor	No. of Patients	ICH	Circumcision	Umbilicus	Hematoma	Puncture Site	Cephalohematoma	Subgaleal	GI
Fibrinogen	7	0	2	5	1	—	—	—	—
II	1	0	—	—	—	—	—	—	1
V	4	2	—	1	1	—	—	—	—
VII	12	11	1	2	—	2	1	—	2
VIII	144	23	75	3	4	17	9	10	2
IX	27	3	16	2	3	3	1	1	—
vWF	4	1	—	1	2	1	—	—	—
X	5	4	—	—	—	1	1	—	2
XI	1	0	1	—	—	—	—	—	—
XIII	25	4	—	24	4	13	—	—	—
II,V,IX,X	1	0	—	—	—	—	—	—	—
V + VIII	1	0	—	—	—	—	—	—	—

Abbreviations: ICH, intracranial hemorrhage; GI, gastrointestinal; vWF, von Willebrand factor.
[a] All sites of bleeding are included for each patient.

the literature who bled at birth due to a congenital coagulation protein deficiency. The most common sites of bleeding include circumcision, umbilical, ICH, scalp, and peripheral heelsticks. The frequency of ICH may reflect a reporting bias as less clinically important sites of hemorrhage may not be reported as frequently. Although less common than ICH, subgaleal bleeding with concurrent shock and DIC may be the initial presentation of a congenital factor deficiency.[266]

Intracranial Hemorrhage

ICH is rare in full-term infants[267] and usually secondary to significant primary problems. When ICH occurs for unexplained reasons in full-term infants, the newborn should be carefully evaluated for congenital or acquired hemostatic defects.[62,268–276] Unfortunately, the diagnosis of ICH may be delayed due to the nonspecific nature of the early clinical presentation, which includes lethargy, apnea, vomiting, and irritability. Further delays can occur when secondary coagulopathies such as DIC occur[277–280] and when the plasma concentration of the coagulation protein in question is physiologically low in newborns. The more extreme clinical presentation of ICH is usually recognized early, characterized by seizures, meningismus, and a tense fontanelle.

Severe congenital deficiencies of fibrinogen, FII, FV, FVII, FVIII, FIX, FX, FXI, and FXIII are all capable of causing ICH at birth. Deficiency of FVIII is the most common cause of ICH from coagulation factor deficiencies.[64] The incidence of ICH in newborns is unknown and is probably changing, reflecting improved perinatal care and improved techniques for making the diagnosis. The widespread use of ultrasound during pregnancy has resulted in detection of ICH in utero and provided a safe modality for monitoring fetuses at risk. In utero factor replacement has also been accomplished in a few infants.[260]

Diagnosis

The diagnosis of a previously unexpected inherited coagulation protein deficiency is usually made by abnormal coagulation screening tests and subsequent specific coagulation protein assays. Studies of the parents are invaluable when physiologic levels overlap with pathologic levels. Subsequently, or in identified families, molecular techniques are now available for prenatal and postnatal diagnoses of most coagulation protein deficiencies.

Plasma concentrations of any coagulation protein must be interpreted within the context of age-specific physiologic values. Homozygous deficiencies of FV, FVII, and FXIII result in levels less than 0.01, 0.03, and 0.01 U/ml, respectively, which is easily distinguishable from physiologic values. Similarly, severe forms of both FVIII and FIX deficiency are defined by levels of less than 0.01 U/ml and are easily distinguished from physiologic values. By contrast, homozygous deficiencies of FII, FX, and FXI are defined by levels of less than 0.20, 0.10, and 0.15 U/ml, respectively, all of which overlap with physiologic levels. One might expect that patients would have values less than the physiologic range, but this has not been demonstrated.

Treatment

The fundamental principle of treatment is to increase the plasma concentration of the deficient coagulation protein to a minimal hemostatic level. A minimal hemostatic level of a particular coagulation protein varies and is dependent on the protein and the nature of the hemostatic challenge. The plasma products available for treatment include plasma, cryoprecipitate, and factor concentrates. Currently, factor concentrates are available for fibrinogen, FII, FVII, FVIII, FIX, and FXIII, and a combination of FII, FVII, FIX, and FX. Factor concentrates are not available for FV, FX, and FXI. Although there are several potential indications for specific factor replacement in newborns, the recommendations are limited to the treatment of congenital factor deficiencies.

Pharmacokinetics

The recovery of coagulation proteins is likely decreased in newborns compared to adults, reflecting a larger volume of distribution per body weight and altered pharmacokinetics.[248,281–283] For example, clearance of both fibrinogen and ATIII is faster in healthy newborns than in adults.[248,281–283] No pharmacokinetic studies of either FVIII or FIX in newborns with hemophilia were identified in the literature. However, clearance of FVIII is faster in boys compared to men.[284] The reason for the increased clearance of coagulation proteins in healthy newborns is unknown but could, in part, reflect an increased basal metabolic rate.[285]

In addition to physiologic differences, pathologic states such as DIC or RDS accelerate the consumption of coagulation proteins. For example, premature newborns with RDS have a shortened fibrinogen survival compared to that of healthy infants.[248] Despite the widespread use of FFP, there are no studies of coagulation protein recovery following the administration of FFP in neonates.

Laboratory Monitoring of Replacement Therapy

Replacement therapy must be accompanied by laboratory monitoring. However, monitoring poses additional problems for newborns because venous access is difficult, only small samples can be obtained, and the laboratory frequently must use microtechniques.[286] Despite these difficulties, determining the effectiveness of coagulation factor replacement therapy is recommended.

Doses

The dose and frequency of coagulation factor replacement are directly determined by the clinical situation and target plasma concentration. Some general guidelines can be provided. For serious bleeding, such as in an infant with ICH, plasma concentrations of the deficient protein should be maintained well within the normal range for several days. For minor bleeding, such as umbilical or into soft tissues, lower doses may be used for shorter periods. Prophylactic therapy should be used for infants undergoing circumcision or other hemostatic challenges.

Complications of Replacement Therapy

Potential complications of replacement therapy include allergic reactions; inhibitor formation, volume overload, and transmission of infection. The MEDLINE search did not identify any reports of allergic reactions or inhibitor formation in the neonatal period. The earliest age at which inhibitors to FVIII were reported was at 3 months of age,[287] and the risk of inhibitor formation appears to be similar for rFVIII and plasma-derived products.[287] In neonatal ICUs, volume overload is rarely a problem due to general awareness of the problem, and the use of

more concentrated products. By contrast, the risk of transmission of viral infection remains the complication of greatest concern for newborns. A review of this problem is beyond the scope of this chapter; readers are referred to recent reviews.[288–291]

SPECIFIC CONGENITAL COAGULATION PROTEIN DEFICIENCIES

A MEDLINE search was conducted using the key words of coagulation factor deficiency, specific factors, bleeding, and newborn; bibliographies of identified publications were searched as well. Sixty-two publications describing 226 infants who bled from a congenital factor deficiency at birth were identified (Table 30-8). These reports form the basis for the current guidelines provided for each coagulation factor deficiency in newborns.

Fibrinogen Deficiency

Literature Review

Four publications identified seven newborns with bleeding due to afibrinogenemia[292–295] (Table 30-8). The sites of bleeding were umbilical, soft tissue, and following circumcision. Plasma products used for replacement therapy were whole blood, cryoprecipitate, FFP, and fibrinogen concentrates. Two of the seven infants died from bleeding complications.

Current Treatment Guidelines

The options for fibrinogen replacement include FFP, cryoprecipitate, and fibrinogen concentrates (Table 30-9). A fibrinogen concentrate has been produced but is not available or approved for use in Canada. Of these products, cryoprecipitate is usually the therapy of choice because it is widely available, has a higher concentration of fibrinogen than FFP, and fibrinogen concentrates are not available in many countries. Replacement therapy can be given every 3 to 4 days due to the long half-life of fibrinogen. A reasonable minimum hemostatic level is approximately 1.0 g/L. Prophylactic therapy should be considered on an individual basis.

Factor II Deficiency

Literature Review

Only one publication reporting one newborn with a mild gastrointestinal bleed due to severe FII deficiency was identified[296] (Table 30-8). No replace-

Table 30-9. Coagulation Factor Proteins

Factor	Plasma Concn	Half-life	Minimum Hemostatic Value	Replacement Therapy
Fibrinogen	1.56–4.00 g/L[406]	3–5 days[406]	0.5–1.0 g/L[406]	Plasma Cryo[406]
II	0.10 mg/ml[407]	72 hr[407]	0.40 U/ml[407]	Plasma PCC FIIC[407]
V	4–14 μg/ml[409]	12–36 hr[409]	0.25 U/ml[409]	FFP Cryo[409]
VII	300–500 ng/ml	3–7 hr[410]	0.15 U/ml[410]	Plasma PCC FVIIC[410]
VIII	0.2 μg/ml[411]	8–12 hr[411]	0.30 U/ml[411]	FVIIIC[411]
IX	4 μg/ml[412]	24 hr[412]	0.10 U/ml[412]	PCC FIXC[412]
vWF	3–12 μg/ml[358]	1–4 hr[358]	0.25–0.50 U/ml[358]	Cryo FVIIIC[358]
X	4–10 μg/ml	24–56 hr[414]	0.10 U/ml[414]	Plasma PCC[414]
XI	2–7 μg/ml[415]	40–80 hr[415]	0.20 U/ml[415]	Plasma
XIII	A: 15 μg/ml[418] B: 21 μg/ml[418]	4–14 days[418]	0.10 U/ml[418]	Plasma Cryo FXIIIC[418]
ATIII	0.30 mg/ml[419]	17–26 hr[419]	0.38–0.49[419]	Plasma ATIIIC[419]
Protein C	0.004 mg/ml[420]	10 hr[420]	0.38–0.49[420]	FFP PCC
Protein S	25 μ/ml[420]	24 hr	0.40–0.55	FFP[420]

Abbreviations: Cryo, cryoprecipitate; FFP, fresh frozen plasma; PCC, prothrombin complex concentrate; C, concentrate.

ment therapy was given. Reviews of adult patients with FII deficiency have reported bleeding to occur following invasive events such as circumcision and venipunctures or as soft tissue hematomas, but not as umbilical cord bleeding or hemarthroses.[297]

Current Treatment Guidelines

The options for FII replacement include FFP, PPC, and FII concentrates (Table 30-9). Currently, PCC is the usual therapy of choice because it is widely available, has a higher concentration of FII than FFP, and FII concentrates are not available in most countries. However, FII concentrates are being manufactured and may be available if specifically requested.

Factor V Deficiency

Literature Review

Three publications identified four newborns bleeding due to severe FV deficiency[260,298,299] (Table 30-8). Two infants presented with ICH[260,299]—one with umbilical bleeding,[298] and one with a soft tissue bleed.[298] Replacement therapy consisted of whole blood, FFP, and local measures. One infant with ICH died at 6 days of age.[260] Although thrombotic complications occur in some patients with FV deficiency, this has not been reported in newborns.[300]

Current Treatment Guidelines

Currently, only FFP is available as a replacement source for FV (Table 30-9).

Factor VII Deficiency

Literature Review

Eight publications identified 12 newborns bleeding due to severe FVII deficiency[260,301-307] (Table 30-8). The sites of bleeding were multiple; however, 11 of the 12 newborns had ICH, and all died due to the ICH.[260,301-306] Infants in the first year of life are also at an increased risk of ICH.[306] Replacement therapy consisted of exchange transfusion, whole blood, FFP, serum, prothrombin complex concentrates (PCC), and FVII concentrates (FVIIC). In general, patients with FVII levels of less than 1 percent have severe hemorrhages equivalent to those in severe hemophilia. Patients with FVII levels of greater than 5 percent generally have mild hemorrhagic episodes. Congenital FVII deficiency may occur in infants with the Dubin-Johnson syndrome[308] or Gilbert syndrome.[309]

In Utero Diagnosis

In 1988, Daffos et al.[260] used fetal blood sampling to diagnose FVII deficiency at 24 weeks of age, and the fetus was transfused in utero at 37 weeks with 200 units of FVII concentrate. Subsequently, the baby was born without hemorrhagic complications and did not bleed as a newborn.

Current Treatment Guidelines

The options for FVII replacement include FFP, PCC, plasma-derived FVII concentrate, and recombinant FVIIa (Table 30-9). Of these products, FVII concentrates are the agent of choice because they are available, are highly concentrated, and are more specific than PCC. A plasma-derived FVII concentrate is manufactured by Immuno (Austria). This manufacturer suggests that for initial therapy in adults, 1 unit of FVII per kilogram of body weight will result in a plasma increase of 2 percent. For maintenance therapy, 1 unit FVII per kilogram of body weight will result in a 2.5 percent increase in plasma levels. In the literature, two newborns[307,310] were treated with 200 IU of FVII concentrate. Although FVII concentrates have a potentially important role in the treatment of haemophiliacs who developed inhibitors, their use in newborns is confined to the FVII-deficient patient.[311] The short half-life of FVII necessitates treatment every 8 to 12 hours, depending on the bleeding complication. A reasonable minimum hemostatic level is approximately 0.15 U/ml. Prophylactic therapy should be considered on an individual basis.

Factor VIII Deficiency

Severe FVIII deficiency is the most common congenital disorder to present in the neonatal period (Table 30-8). The severity of FVIII deficiency is determined by the plasma concentration of FVIII, with less than 1 percent severe, 1 to 5 percent moderate, and 5 to 50 percent mild.[312] Newborns who bleed due to FVIII deficiency usually have the severe form. However, a small number of moderate and mild hemophiliacs have presented following a hemostatic challenge, usually circumcision.[277,313-319] Large cohort studies have reported that approximately 10 percent of children with hemophilia are clinically symptomatic in the neonatal period,[64] a further 40 percent present by 1 year of age, and by 1.5 years more than 70 percent have had a major bleeding event.[64] By contrast, in less severe FVIII deficiency, a major hemorrhage occur in only 2.5 percent of patients by the end of the neonatal period.[64]

Literature Review

Twenty publications identified 144 male infants, with bleeding due to FVIII deficiency in the neonatal period.[266,277,278,313-329] Seventy-five infants (53 percent) presented with bleeding following circumcision, and 23 (16 percent) presented with ICH.[277,313,316,317,319,320,322,324,326,327,329] Eight infants died in the newborn period due to bleeding.[277,278,319,326] In contrast to older infants and children, bleeding into joints is extremely rare in the neonatal period.[330] Severe FVIII deficiency can, on rare occasion, occur in females with clinical presentation in the neonatal period. The Medline search also identified three female infants with a history of bleeding at birth from puncture sites and into the skin. The FVIII levels were less than 0.01 U/ml in two infants and 0.04 U/ml in the third.[331,332] All three girls were diagnosed later in life and did not receive any form of replacement therapy at birth.

Past Therapy

Treatments were not reported for 97 of the 144 male infants. For the reported 47 infants, treatment reflected the decade in which they were born. During the 1960s, 10 cases were treated with exchange transfusion (n = 5), whole blood (n = 1), and a combination of FFP and whole blood (n = 4).[313–316] During the 1970s, 11 cases were treated with exchange transfusion (n = 2), whole blood (n = 3), a combination of FFP and whole blood (n = 3), and FVIIIc (n = 3).[317,318,320–323] In the 1980s, 26 cases were treated with FVIIIC (n = 8)[266,277,278,319,324–326,328,329] a combination of FFP and cryoprecipitate (n = 17), and one had no therapy. Alternative therapy to FVIII replacement has been used in newborns undergoing circumcision. In one study of 10 severe patients, local fibrin glue was used instead of infusion of FVIII.[333] Only two of three patients who bled postoperatively required FVIII concentrate.

Current Treatment Guidelines

Options for FVIII replacement include FFP, cryoprecipitate, and FVIII concentrates (Table 30-9). Of these products, FVIII concentrates are the therapy of choice because they are widely available, have a higher concentration of FVIII, and, due to the purification procedures, are safer than FFP or cryoprecipitate. The FVIII concentrates available from the Red Cross and other sources are listed in Table 30-10. Based on data from older children and adults, 1 unit of FVIII per kilogram of body weight will raise the plasma concentration of FVIII by 2 percent. However, the pharmacokinetics for FVIII have not been reported in newborns, and the recovery of FVII should by measured for any concentrates listed in Table 30-10.

FVIII concentrates can be considered as plasma-derived or as recombinant FVIII (rFVIII). In general, there are three types of FVIII concentrate: intermediate, high, and recombinant DNA-derived products.[334] Intermediate products are purified from the cryoprecipitates of large pools of human donor plasma by various modifications of the original method.[335] They are virally inactivated by either vapor heating (i.e., heating in suspension at 60°C for 20 hours), by pasteurization (i.e., heating in aqueous solution at 60°C for 10 hours), or by a solvent-detergent method consisting of tri-*n*-butly-phosphate (TNBP) and detergents such as sodium cholate, Triton X-100, or polysorbate 80.[291] Intermediate-purity concentrates have specific activities of 1.5 units FVIII/mg of protein. High-purity concentrates have specific activities of approximately 200 units FVIII/mg of protein and have been further purified by an additional step consisting of an immunoaffinity column coated with monoclonal antibodies (mAb). The choice of FVIIIc is determined to some extent by the products available. In general, a rFVIIIC is the preferred product with high-purity plasma products being a second choice. Based on data from older children and adults, 1 unit of FVIII/kg will raise the plasma concentration of FVIII by 2 percent. However, the pharmacokinetics for FVIII have not been reported in newborns, and the recovery of FVIII should be measured for any newborn receiving FVIIC. Dosing guidelines are provided in Table 30-10.

There is complete agreement that affected newborns should receive factor VIII concentrates for

Table 30-10. Clinical Factor VIII Concentrates

Concentrate	Manufacturer	Source	Viral Inactivation Method	Dose Guidelines (IU required = kg multiplied by)
Haemate P	Hoechst-Roussel	Human plasma	Pasteurized 60°C for 10 hr wet	Desired increase ×0.5
AHF VIII-HP	Miles	Human plasma	SD (polysorbate 80)	Desired increase ×0.4
Hyate: C porcine	Porton	Porcine plasma	—	Desired increase ×0.68
High Purity Hemofil-M	Baxter	MAb	SD (Triton X-100)	Desired increase ×0.5
Kogenate	Baxter	Recombinant	—	Desired increase ×0.5

Abbreviations: IU international units; kg, kilograms; MAb, monoclonal antibody; SD, solvent-detergent.

bleeding episodes and planned hemostatic challenges.[336] Whether infants should be placed on prophylactic regimens is not clear but is being seriously considered.

Factor IX Deficiency

Literature Review

Ten publications identified 27 newborns with bleeding secondary to severe FIX deficiency[313,316,319,326, 327,329,337–340] (Table 30-8). Twelve infants bled following circumcision, and three presented with ICH.[313,316,319,327,329,337,340] The severity of FIX deficiency is identical to FVIII. Diagnosis of the milder forms of FIX deficiency is complicated by physiologic levels of FIX that can be as low as 0.15 U/ml and, in the rare infant, the potential for concurrent vitamin K deficiency. The 27 newborns bled from diverse sites at presentation (Table 30-8). Replacement therapy was in the form of FFP (n = 4), PCC (n = 1), and FIXC (n = 1).

Current Treatment Guidelines

Options for FIX replacement include FFP, PCC, and FIX concentrates (Table 30-9). Of these products, FIX concentrates are the therapy of choice. Currently available FIX concentrates are listed in Table 30-6. Based on adults, approximately 1 unit of FIX concentrate per kilogram of body weight will increase the plasma concentration by 1 percent. This risk of DIC, thrombotic complications, and viral transmission with PCCs prepared in the 1970s and 1980s has led to the development of purified FIX concentrates. Highly purified FIX concentrates may be safer because they are isolated by mAb-conjugated immunoaffinity chromatography and virally inactivated by solvent-detergent methods.[341] At this time, FIX concentrates are the treatment of choice for newborns with congenital FIX deficiency.

Prothrombin Complex Concentrates

PCCs contain the vitamin K-dependent proteins, FII, FVII, FIX, and FX. The currently available PCCs are listed in Table 30-6. The disorders in newborns in which PCCs should be considered are severe vitamin K deficiency with an ICH; combined congenital deficiency of FII, FVII, FIX, and FX; congenital FX deficiency; and when individual products are not available. A dose of 1 unit of FIX/kg should raise the

plasma concentration of FIX by 1 percent. Although not precise, similar calculations can be used for initial dosing of the other coagulation proteins present in the PCC (Table 30-6).

Factor X Deficiency

Literature Review

Five publications identified five newborns with bleeding due to severe FX deficiency[342–346] (Table 30-8). Four of the five infants had ICH, two subsequently died, and one remained in a coma.[342] One of the four ICH was diagnosed in utero and, despite prophylactic PCC in the first months of life, the infant died from an ICH.[344] Other sites of bleeding were umbilical, gastrointestinal, and intra-abdominal.[342,343,345] Replacement therapy included whole blood, FFP, and PCC.

Treatment Guidelines

If PCCs are unavailable, FFP can be used. When PCC are available, this is the product of choice (Table 30-9).

Factor XI Deficiency

FXI deficiency occurs sporadically in all populations but has a particularly high frequency in individuals of Ashkenazi Jewish descent. FXI deficiency is different from other coagulation protein deficiencies in that bleeding symptoms do not correlate with the FXI level, nor do all patients with FXI deficiency bleed. Bleeding often occurs following trauma or surgery which in newborns is frequently circumcision.[347]

Literature Review

Only one publication was identified reporting one newborn with severe FXI deficiency (Table 30-8). The infant was a 3-day-old who bled from the circumcision site with a FXI level of 0.07 U/ml.[347] He was successfully treated with small amounts of FFP.

Treatment Guidelines

Either FFP or cryoprecipitate can be used for the treatment of FXI-deficient patients (Table 30-9).

Factor XIII Deficiency

Literature Review

Ten publications identified 25 newborns with bleeding due to homozygous FXIII deficiency[320,348–356] (Table 30-8). Delayed bleeding from the umbilicus is the classic presentation for FXIII deficiency. Twenty-four of the 25 infants had delayed bleeding from the umbilicus. Two infants had an ICH within 2 months of birth.[355,356] One infant died during the neonatal period.[354] In later life, ICH occurs in 25 percent of reported cases.[354] Replacement therapy was administered with whole blood, FFP, cryoprecipitate, and FXIIIC.

Treatment Guidelines

Either cryoprecipitate or FXIII concentrates can be used for the treatment of FXIII-deficient patients (Table 30-9). Newborns with FXIII deficiency should be placed on a prophylactic regimen of FXIII replacement because of the high incidence of ICH, plasma concentrations of FXIII of more than 1 percent are effective and the very long half-life of FXIII permits once monthly therapy.[340] The currently available FXIII concentrate is Fibrogammin (Hoechst-Roussel, Canada). In adults, the manufacturer suggests 7 to 10 U/kg of body weight (500 to 750 units) at intervals of 4 weeks. The one neonate treated with FXIII concentrate was given monthly doses of 250 units. At this time, FXIII concentrates provide one option for newborns with severe congenital FXIII deficiency. Consideration should be given to lifelong prophylactic therapy.

Familial Multiple Factor Deficiencies

Congenital deficiencies of two or more coagulation proteins have been reported for 16 different combinations of coagulation factors.[357]

Literature Review

Bleeding in the neonatal period has only be reported for two infants with combined factor deficiencies. One infant was FII, FVII, FIX, and FX deficient and presented with spontaneous bruising and umbilical stump bleeding, which continued until 3 months of age, when the infant was treated with FFP.[265] A second infant, who was FV and FVIII deficient, presented with serious bleeding (undescribed) during the first week of life.[264] FFP was administered without improvement.

Treatment Guidelines

The product of choice will vary, depending on the specific factors affected. However, FFP is the only plasma product that contains all coagulation proteins and may provide initial therapy.

von Willebrand's Disease

von Willebrand's disease (vWD) is a complex disease reviewed in detail elsewhere.[350,358,359] Although vWD is the most common congenital bleeding disorder, patients rarely present in the neonatal period. vWF is an acute-phase reactant, and the plasma concentration of vWF in newborns with vWD is increased as is the proportion of high-molecular-weight multimers.[19,20] In the classic form of vWD, (type I), the inheritance is dominant, with mild bleeding and decreased plasma concentration of vWF. In type II vWD, the vWF protein is structurally altered; several subtypes are known. Type III vWD, or severe vWD, is characterized by very low plasma concentrations of FVIII and vWF.

Literature Review

In the medline search, three publications identified four newborns with bleeding secondary to vWD[360–362] (Table 30-8). One infant was identified at birth with type I vWD by use of the polymerase chain reaction.[361] The infant was asymptomatic and had a vWF:AG level of 2.03 U/L, and vWF:RCo of 0.56 U/L. One infant, with type IIA vWD presented with umbilical bleeding and later with epistaxis which was life-threatening.[363] Two infants with type IIB vWD presented with bleeding as newborns (blood sampling sites, soft tissue) and repeated platelet counts of less than $50 \times 10^9/L$.[360] In addition, the bleeding time and APTT were prolonged, the vWF multimeric structure was characterized by the absence of the high-molecular-weight forms, and the patient's platelets aggregated at much lower ristocetin concentrations than did controls.[360] Details on therapy for the infants with type II vWD were not provided. One infant presented on day 7 of life with an intracerebral and subdural hemorrhage.[362] The FVIII level was 0.03 U/ml, and the vWF:AG and vWF:RCO were undetectable. This infant was treated with an intermediate-purity FVIII concentrate at a dose of 60 U/kg twice a day for 10 days, followed by once daily dosing for 10 days. The bleeding stopped, and the infant's neurologic status was normal.[362] Another infant, with a defect in the ability of vWF to bind FVIII, presented with several intramuscular haematomas and a post-traumatic haemorrhage of the scale.[364] vWF concentrate was used effectively to treat.

Concentrates for von Willebrand Disease

Therapeutic choices consist of cryoprecipitate,[365-367] vWF concentrates,[364] and some FVIII concentrates[368,369] (Table 30-9). Some FVIII concentrates fail to correct the bleeding time or control hemorrhage in vWD,[370] whereas others contain vWF multimers with structures of similar to normal plasma vWF multimers,[359,363, 371, 372] for example, Haemate P (Table 30-10).

PLASMA PRODUCTS

Fresh Frozen Plasma

The Pediatric Hemotherapy Committee of the American Association of Blood Banks has developed guidelines for auditing transfusion in pediatric patients.[336] (Table 30-11). The indications for FFP in

Table 30-11. Criteria for Transfusion of Plasma Products[a]

Fresh frozen plasma
    Bleeding, or an invasive procedure, in a patient with a coagulation factor deficiency or a markedly prolonged prothrombin, and/or partial thromboplastin times
    Replacement therapy in antithrombin III or protein C or S deficiencies
    Replacement therapy during therapeutic plasma exchange for disorders in which fresh-frozen plasma is beneficial
Cryoprecipitate
    Bleeding, or an invasive procedure in von Willebrand's disease
    Bleeding, or an invasive procedure, in hypofibrogenemia or dysfibrinogememia
    Replacement therapy in factor XIII deficiency
Clotting factor concentrates
    Bleeding, active or anticipated, in patients with documented coagulation factor deficiencies, such as hemophilia A or B
    Severe or variant forms of von Willebrand's disease
Albumin
    Acute correction of hypoalbuminemia *when clinically* indicated
    Correction of hypovolemia when colloid infusion is indicated
    Replacement therapy in therapeutic plasma-exchange procedures

[a] Italicized statements require additional definition by each local transfusion committee. (From American Association of Blood Banks,[422] with permission.)

newborns are adapted from the guidelines for older children and provided in Table 30-11. In general, FFP is used to replace coagulation proteins in infants with acquired and some congenital deficiencies. However, infants with these disorders who are not bleeding, may not require coagulation factor replacement, particularly if the underlying problem is resolving. Information about the benefits of FFP in sick newborns comes from two randomized controlled studies,[83,148] four controlled trials,[84,86-88] and several case series. These studies used FFP for the prevention of ICH, and the management of DIC (see previous sections).

Indications

The indications for FFP in neonates include (1) reconstitution of red blood cell concentrates in the setting of massive transfusions (e.g., exchange transfusion or cardiovascular surgery), (2) hemorrhage secondary to vitamin K deficiency, (3) DIC, and (4) bleeding in patients with congenital coagulation factor deficiencies when more specific treatment is either unavailable or inappropriate. FFP is preferable to stored liquid plasma because FV and FVIII are labile. A common dosing regimen is 10 to 20 ml/kg every 12 to 24 hours, depending on the clinical situation.

Nonindications

The use of prophylactic FFP transfusions to prevent ICH in premature infants is controversial,[148,150,373] and a firm recommendation about this practice cannot be made. Although still being used to adjust the hematocrit values for small-volume RBC transfusions to neonates, this practice is not recommended because FFP offers no apparent medical benefit and exposes infants to an additional donor.[374,375] In addition, FFP use in partial exchange transfusion for the treatment of neonatal hyperviscosity syndrome is unnecessary, as safer colloid solutions are available.[374,375] FFP is not indicated for correction of hypovolemia or as immunoglobulin replacement therapy, because safer alternatives exist.[374,375]

Guidelines

The approach used by the Canadian Red Cross is to supply group AB FFP, split into three bags, using a closed system, for all infants under 3 months of age.

Plasma used to wash donor blood for exchange transfusion should be the same as for the infant's blood group.

Cryoprecipitate

Cryoprecipitate, prepared by thawing FFP at 4°C, provides a concentrated form of fibrinogen, FXIII, vWF, and FVIII compared to FFP (approximately a fivefold increase). FXI is present, but not in increased concentrations compared to FFP. The benefits of cryoprecipitate as a single agent have not been evaluated in sick newborns. A commonly used dose of cryoprecipitate is 20 ml/kg.

Indications

Cryoprecipitate is an important source of coagulation factor replacement in newborns with congenital FXIII deficiency and congenital hypofibrinogenemia. Although FXIII concentrates are preferable to cryoprecipitate for FXIII replacement, they are not uniformly or rapidly available. Cryoprecipitate is also a useful adjunct to therapy for acquired hypofibrinogenemia such as DIC and extracorporeal membrane oxygenation.

Nonindications

Historically, cryoprecipitate was an important source of FVIII for newborns with hemophilia A and the rarer infant with severe vWD. Cryoprecipitate is no longer recommended as the first choice for treatment of these two disorders because of the availability of safer products.

Conclusions

The use of coagulation factor replacement in newborns is a rapidly changing area of medicine. New products are rapidly coming into clinical practice. It continues to be very important to test these products in appropriate clinical trials before giving firm recommendations for their use in newborns.

OTHER USES OF PLASMA PRODUCTS IN NEWBORNS

Hypovolumia and Shock

Infants are very susceptible to hypovolemic shock because of their small blood volume and exposure to predisposing events at the time of birth.[376] Also, the high risk of serious bacterial infections in the postnatal period can lead to the development of septic shock. Plasma products are important therapeutic modalities for supporting neonates in shock. FFP and albumin are the two most commonly used products, although packed red blood cells and stored plasma may also be used, depending on the underlying events.[376] Although FFP is frequently used inappropriately in the child or adult for volume expansion, it is frequently an agent of choice in the newborn[377] because sick newborn infants in shock often develop DIC.

Hypoalbuminemia

Albumin

Serum albumin levels are physiologically low in the newborn; the level of albumin correlates with gestational age.[378-381] Most infants at less than 36 weeks gestation have a serum albumin concentration of less than 30 g/L. Combined disorders can lower the level of albumin even further. Hypoalbuminemia in the newborn has been associated with peripheral and pulmonary edema.[382] Numerous investigators have reported case series describing an improvement in peripheral edema or RDS following infusion of albumin, which enhances urine output. The optimal role, if any, for albumin infusions in the sick infant remains to be clarified.[382-385]

Hyperbilirubinemia

Serum bilirubin binds to albumin, producing a drop in the circulating level of bilirubin.[386] Unbound bilirubin can cross the blood-brain barrier in the newborn and cause kernicterus. Albumin infusions in conjunction with exchange transfusions have been used to decrease the concentration of unbound bilirubin.[387]

Neonatal Hyperviscosity

Polycythemia with secondary hyperviscosity is a relatively frequent event in the newborn.[388-393] These infants can be symptomatic at birth. Clinical signs of hyperviscosity include impaired cardiorespiratory, gastrointestinal, renal, and CNS functions. The benefits of therapeutic intervention are debated, but some investigators have described benefit from a partial plasma-exchange transfusion.[389,394-396]

ACKNOWLEDGMENTS

Dr. M. Andrew is a Career Investigator of the Heart and Stroke Foundation of Canada. This work was supported by a grant-in-aid from the Medical Research Council of Canada.

REFERENCES

1. Hathaway WE, Bonnar J: Bleeding disorders in the newborn infant. p. 115. In Oliver TK Jr (ed): Perinatal Coagulation. Monographs in Neonatology. Grune & Stratton, Orlando, FL, 1978
2. Hathaway W, Corrigan J: Report of scientific and standardization subcommittee on neonatal hemostasis. Thromb Haemost 65:323, 1991
3. Hathaway WE, Bonnar J: Hemostatic Disorders of the Pregnant Woman and Newborn Infant. Elsevier Science, New York, 1987
4. Corrigan JJ: Normal hemostasis in fetus and newborn. Coagulation. p. 1368. In Polin RA, Fox WW (eds): Neonatal and Fetal Medicine. Physiology and Pathophysiology. Grune & Stratton, Orlando, FL, 1991
5. Andrew M, Paes B, Milner R et al: Development of the human coagulation system in the full-term infant. Blood 70:165, 1987
6. Andrew M, Paes B, Milner R et al: Development of the human coagulation system in the healthy premature infant. Blood 72:1651, 1988
7. Andrew M, Paes B, Johnston M: Development of the hemostatic system in the neonate and young infant. Am J Pediatr Hematol Oncol 12:95, 1990
8. Cade JF, Hirsh J, Martin M: Placental barrier to coagulation factors: its relevance to the coagulation defect at birth and to haemorrhage in the newborn. BMJ 2:281, 1969
9. Andrew M, O'Brodovich H, Mitchell L: The fetal lamb coagulation system during normal birth. Am J Hematol 28:116, 1988
10. Kisker CT, Robillard JE, Clarke WR: Development of blood coagulation—a fetal lamb model. Pediatr Res 15:1045, 1981
11. Heikenheimo R: Coagulation studies with fetal blood. Biol Neonate 7:319, 1964
12. Holmberg L, Henriksson P, Ekelund H, Astedt B: Coagulation in the human fetus, comparison with term newborn infants. J Pediatr 85:860, 1974
13. Jensen AH, Josso S, Zamet P et al: Evolution of blood clotting factors in premature infants during the first ten days of life: a study of 96 cases with comparison between clinical status and blood clotting factor levels. Pediatr Res 7:638, 1973
14. Mibashan RS, Rodeck CH, Thumpson JK et al: Plasma assay of fetal factors VIIIc and IX for prenatal diagnosis of haemophilia. Lancet 1:1309, 1979
15. Bleyer WA, Hakami N, Shepard TH: The development of hemostasis in the human fetus and newborn infant. J Pediatr 79:838, 1971
16. Forestier F, Daffos F, Rainaut M et al: Vitamin K dependent proteins in fetal hemostasis at mid trimester pregnancy. Thromb Haemost 53:401, 1985
17. Barnard DR, Simmons MA, Hathaway WE: Coagulation studies in extremely premature infants. Pediatr Res 13:1330, 1979
18. Forestier F, Daffos F, Galacteros F et al: Hematological values of 163 normal fetuses between 18 and 30 weeks of gestation. Pediatr Res 20:342, 1986
19. Katz JA, Moake JL, McPherson PD et al: Relationship between human development and disappearance of unusually large von Willebrand factor multimers from plasma. Blood 73:1851, 1989
20. Weinstein MJ, Blanchard R, Moake JL et al: Fetal and neonatal von Willebrand factor (vWF) is unusually large and similar to the vWF in patients with thrombotic thrombocytopenia purpura. Br J Haematol 72:68, 1989
21. Xi M, Beguin S, Hemker HC: The relative importance of the factors II, VII, IX and X for the prothrombinase activity in plasma of orally anticoagulated patients. Thromb Haemost 62:788, 1989
22. Vieira A, Ofosu F, Andrew M: Heparin sensitivity and resistance in the neonate: an explanation. Thromb Res 63:85, 1991
23. Schmidt B, Ofosu FA, Mitchell L et al: Anticoagulant effects of heparin in neonatal plasma. Pediatr Res 25:405, 1989
24. Bussel JP, Berkowitz RL, McFarland JG et al: Antenatal treatment of neonatal alloimmune thrombocytopenia. N Engl J Med 319:1374, 1988
25. Andrew M, Schmidt B, Mitchell L et al: Thrombin generation in newborn plasma is critically dependent on the concentration of prothrombin. Thromb Haemost 63:27, 1990
26. Andrew M, Mitchell L, Vegh P, Ofosu F: Thrombin regulation in children differs from adults in the absence and presence of heparin. Thromb Haemost 72:836, 1994
27. Witt I, Muller H, Kunter LJ: Evidence for the existence of fetal fibrinogen. Thromb Haemost 22:101, 1969
28. Hamulyak K, Nieuwenhuizen W, Devillee PP, Hemker HC: Re-evaluation of some properties of fibrinogen purified from cord blood of normal newborns. Thromb Res 32:301, 1983

29. Galanakis DK, Mosesson MW: Evaluation of the role of in vivo proteolysis (fibrinogenolysis) in prolonging the thrombin time of human umbilical cord fibrinogen. Blood 48:109, 1976

30. Aballi AJ, de Lamerens S: Coagulation changes in the neonatal period and in early infancy. Pediatr Clin North Am 9:785, 1962

31. Gross SJ, Stuart MJ: Hemostasis in the premature infant. Clin Perinatol 4:259, 1977

32. Buchanan GR: Neonatal coagulation: normal physiology and pathophysiology. Clin Haematol 1:85, 1978

33. Montgomery RR, Marlar RA, Gill JC: Newborn Haemostasis. Clin Hematol 14:443, 1985

34. Gibson B: Neonatal haemostasis. Arch Dis Child 64:503, 1989

35. Gobel U, Voss HC, Petrich C et al: Etiopathology and classification of acquired coagulation disorders in the newborn infant. Klin Wochenschr 57:81, 1979

36. Buchanan GR: Coagulation disorders in the neonate. Pediatr Clin North Am 33:203, 1986

37. McDonald MM, Hathaway WE: Neonatal haemorrhage and thrombosis. Semin Perinatol 7:213, 1983

38. Strothers J, Boulton F, Wild R et al: Neonatal coagulation, letter. Lancet 1:408, 1975

39. Bahakim H, Gader A, Galil A et al: Coagulation parameters in maternal and cord blood at delivery. Ann Saudi Med 10:149, 1990

40. Karpatkin M, Manucci PM, Mannuccio Manniuci P et al: Low protein C in the neonatal period. Br J Haematol 62:137, 1986

41. Greffe BS, Marlar RA, Manco-Johnson M: Neonatal protein C: molecular composition and distribution in normal term infants. Thromb Res 56:91, 1989

42. Moalic P, Gruel Y, Body G et al: Levels and plasma distribution of free and C_4b-BP-bound protein S in human fetuses and fullterm newborns. Thromb Res 49:471, 1988

43. Schwarz HP, Muntean W, Watzke H et al: Low total protein S antigen but high protein S activity due to decreased C_4b-binding protein in neonates. Blood 71:562, 1988

44. Aurousseau MH, Amiral J, Boffa MC: Level of plasma thrombomodulin in neonates and children, abstracted. Thromb Haemost 65:1232, 1991

45. Peters M, Jansen E, ten Cate JW et al: Neonatal antithrombin III. Br J Haematol 58:579, 1984

46. Manco-Johnson M: Neonatal antithrombin III deficiency. Am J Med, suppl 3B. 87:1989

47. Andrew M, Vegh P, Johnston M et al: Maturation of the hemostatic system during childhood. Blood 80:1998, 1992

48. Ganrot PO, Schersten B: Serum α_2-macroglobulin concentration and its variation with age and sex. Clin Chim Acta 15:113, 1967

49. Schmidt B, Mitchell L, Ofosu F, Andrew M: Alpha-2-macroglobulin is an important progressive inhibitor of thrombin in neonatal and infant plasma. Thromb Haemost 62:1074, 1989

50. Shah JK, Mitchell LG, Paes B et al: Thrombin inhibition is impaired in plasma of sick neonates. Pediatr Res 31:391, 1992

51. Corrigan J: Neonatal thrombosis and the thrombolytic system. Pathophysiology and therapy. Am J Pediatr Hematol Oncol 10:83, 1988

52. Corrigan J, Sluth JJ, Jeter M, Lox CD: Newborn's fibrinolytic mechanism: components and plasmin generation. Am J Hematol 32:273, 1989

53. Kolindewala JK, Das BK, Dube B, Bhargava B: Blood fibrinolytic activity in neonates: effect of period of gestation, birth weight, anoxia and sepsis. Ind Pediatr 24:1029, 1987

54. Runnebaum IB, Maurer SM, Daly L, Bonnar J: Inhibitors and activators of fibrinolysis during and after childbirth in maternal and cord blood. J Perinat Med 17:113, 1989

55. Ambrus CM, Jung O, Ambrus JL et al: The fibrinolysin system and its relationship to disease in the newborn. Am J Pediatr Hematol Oncol 1:251, 1979

56. Ginsberg JS, Hirsh J, Rainbow AJ, Coates G: Risks to the fetus of radiologic procedures used in the diagnosis of maternal venous thromboembolic disease. Thromb Haemost 61:189, 1989

57. Reverdiau-Moalie P, Gruel Y, Delahousse B et al: Comparative study of the fibrinolytic system in human fetuses and in pregnant women. Thromb Res 61:489, 1991

58. Ekelund H, Hedner U, Nilsson I: Fibrinolysis in the newborn. Acta Paediatr Scand 59:33, 1970

59. Kruithof EKO, Tran-Thang C, Gudinchet A et al: Fibrinolysis in pregnancy: a study of plasminogen activator inhibitors. Blood 69:460, 1987

60. Edelberg JM, Enghild JJ, Pizzo SV, Gonzalez-Gronow M: Neonatal plasminogen displays altered cell surface binding and activation kinetics. Correlation with increased glycosylation of the protein. J Clin Invest 86:107, 1990

61. Summaria L: Comparison of human normal, fullterm, fetal and adult plasminogen by physical and chemical analyses. Haemostasis 19:266, 1989

62. Girolami A, De Marco L, Dal Bo Zanon R et al: Rarer quantitative and qualitative abnormalities of coagulation. Clin Hematol 14:385, 1985

63. Kunzer W: Die blugerinnung bei neugeborenen und ihre storungen. Wien Klin Wochenschr 80:159, 1968

64. Smith PS: Congenital coagulation protein deficiencies in the perinatal period. Semin Perinatol 14:384, 1990

65. Hathaway WE, Mull MM, Pechet GS: Disseminated intravascular coagulation in the newborn. Pediatrics 43:233, 1969

66. Abildgaard CF: Recognition and treatment of intravascular coagulation. J Pediatr 74:163, 1969

67. Watkins MN, Swan S, Caprini JA et al: Coagulation changes in the newborn with respiratory failure. Thromb Res 17:153, 1980

68. Markarian M, Lindley A, Jackson JJ, Bannon A: Coagulation factors in pregnant women and premature infants with and without the respiratory distress syndrome. Thromb Haemost 17:585, 1967

69. Appleyard WJ, Cottom DG: Effect of asphyxia on thrombotest values in low birthweight infants. Arch Dis Child 45:705, 1970

70. Anderson JM, Brown JK, Cockburn F: On the role of disseminated intravascular coagulation on the pathology of birth asphyxia. Dev Med Child Neurol 16:581, 1974

71. Zipursky A, Jaber HM: The hematology of bacterial infection in newborn infants. Clin Hematol 7:175, 1978

72. Chessells JM, Wigglesworth JS: Coagulation studies in severe birth asphyxia. Arch Dis Child 46:253, 1971

73. Chessells JM, Wigglesworth JS: Haemostatic failure in babies with rhesus isoimmunization. Arch Dis Child 46:38, 1971

74. Chessells JM, Wigglesworth JS: Coagulation studies in preterm infants with respiratory distress and intracranial hemorrhage. Arch Dis Child 47:564, 1972

75. Altstaff LB, Dennis LH, Sundell H et al: Disseminated intravascular coagulation and hyaline membrane disease. Biol Neonate 19:227, 1971

76. Edson JR, Blaese RM, White JG, Krivit W: Defibrination syndrome in an infant born after abruptio placentae. J Pediatr 72:342, 1968

77. Corrigan JJ: Activation of coagulation and disseminated intravascular coagulation in the newborn. Am J Pediatr Hematol Oncol 1:245, 1979

78. Schmidt BK, Vegh P, Weitz J et al: Thrombin/antithrombin III complex formation in the neonatal respiratory distress syndrome. Am Rev Respir Dis 145:767, 1992

79. Boyd JF: Disseminated fibrin thromboembolism among neonates dying more than 48 hours after birth. J Clin Pathol 22:663, 1969

80. Boyd JF: Disseminated fibrin thromboembolism among neonates dying within 48 hours of birth. Arch Dis Child 42:401, 1967

81. Boyd JF: Disseminated fibrin thromboembolism in stillbirths; a histological picture similar to one form of maternal hypofibrinogenemia. J Obstet Gynaecol Br 73:629, 1966

82. Schmidt B, Vegh P, Andrew M, Johnston M: Coagulation screening tests in high risk neonates: a prospective cohort study. Arch Dis Child 67:1196, 1992

83. Gross S, Filston HC, Anderson JC: Controlled study of treatment for disseminated intravascular coagulation in the neonate. J Pediatr 100:445, 1982

84. Turner T: Randomized sequential control trial to evaluate effect of purified factor II, VII, IX, and X concentrate, cryoprecipitate and platelet concentrate in management of preterm low birthweight and mature asphyxiated infants with coagulation defects. Arch Dis Child 51:810, 1981

85. Waltt H, Kurz R, Mitterstieler G et al: Intracranial haemorrhage in low birth weight infants and prophylactic administration of coagulation factor concentrates. Lancet 1:1284, 1973

86. De Lemos RA, McLaughlin GW, Koch HF, Diserens HW: Abnormal partial thromboplastin time and survival in respiratory distress syndrome. Effect of exchange transfusion, abstracted. Pediatr Res 7:396, 1973

87. Hambleton G, Appleyard WJ: Controlled trial of fresh frozen plasma in asphyxiated low birthweight infants. Arch Dis Child 48:31, 1973

88. Gray OP, Ackerman A, Fraser AJ: Intracranial hemorrhage and clotting defects in low birth weight infants. Lancet 1:545, 1968

89. Nowak-Gottl U, Groll A, Kreuz WD et al: Treatment of disseminated intravascular coagulation with antithrombin III concentrate in children with verified infection. Klin Padiatr 204:134, 1992

90. Kelly DA, Summerfield JA: Hemostasis in liver disease. Semin Liver Dis 7:182, 1987

91. von Breedin K: Hamorrhagische diathesen bei lebererkrankungen unter besonderer berucksichtigung der thrombocytenfunction. Acta Haematol 27:1, 1962

92. Rubin MH, Weston MJ, Bullock G: Abnormal platelet function and ultrastructure in fulminant hepatic failure. Q J Med 46:339, 1977

93. Weston MJ, Langley PG, Rubin MH: Platelet function in fulminant hepatic failure and effect of charcoal haemoperfusion. Gut 18:897, 1977

94. Osborn JE, Shahidi NT: Thrombocytopenia in murine cytomegalovirus infections. J Lab Clin Med 81:53, 1973

95. Chesney PJ, Taher A, Gilbert EM: Intranuclear inclusions in megakaryocytes in congenital cytomegalovirus infection. J Pediatr 92:957, 1978

96. Zinkham WH et al: Blood and bone marrow findings in congenital rubella. J Pediatr 71:512, 1967

97. Lafer CZ, Morrison AN: Thrombocytopenic purpura progressing to transient hypoplastic anemia in a newborn with rubella syndrome. Pediatrics 38:499, 1966

98. Bortolotti F, Vajro P, Barbera C et al: Hepatitis C in childhood: epidemiological and clinical aspects. Bone Marrow Transplant, suppl 1. 12:21, 1993

99. Kulhanjian J: Fever, hepatitis and coagulopathy in a newborn infant. Pediatr Infect Dis 11:1069, 1992

100. Telfer MC: Clinical spectrum of viral infections in hemophilic patients. Hematol Oncol Clin North Am 6:1047, 1992

101. van Saene HKF, Stoutenbeek CP, Faber-Nijholt R, van Saene JJM: Selective decontamination of the digestive tract contributes to the control of disseminated intravascular coagulation in severe liver impairment. J Pediatr Gastroenterol Nutr 14:436, 1992

102. Kuhn W, Rath W, Loos W, Graeff H: The Hellp syndrome. Clinical and laboratory test results. Rev Fr Gynecol Obstet 87:323, 1992

103. Meili EO: Treatment of hemophilia. Schweiz Med Wochenschr 43:82, 1991

104. Dresse MF, David M, Hume H et al: Successful treatment of Kasabach-Merritt syndrome with prednisone and epsilon-aminocaproic acid. Pediatr Hematol Oncol 8:329, 1991

105. Noseda G, Roy C, Phan P et al: Acute hepatic insufficiency disclosing congenital syphilis. Arch Fr Pediatr 47:445, 1990

106. Rathgeber J, Rath W, Wieding JU: Anesthesiologic and intensive care aspects of severe pre-eclampsia with HELLP syndrome. Anaesth Intensive Care 25:206, 1990

107. Kurzel RB: Can acetaminophen excess result in maternal and fetal toxicity? South Med J 83:953, 1990

108. Dupuy JM, Frommel D, Alagille D: Severe viral hepatitis B in infants. Lancet 1:191, 1975

109. Mindrum G, Glueck HI: Plasma prothrombin time in liver disease: its clinical and prognostic significance. Ann Intern Med 50:1370, 1959

110. Hope PL, Hall MA, Millward-Sadler GH, Normand IC: Alpha-1-antitripsin deficiency presenting as a bleeding diathesis in the newborn. Arch Dis Child 57:68, 1982

111. Olivera JE, Elearte R, Erice B: Galactosemia of early diagnosis with psychomotor retardation. An Esp Pediatr 4:267, 1986

112. Mercier JC, Bourillon A, Beaufils F: Hereditary fructose intolerance with early onset. Arch Fr Pediatr 10:945, 1976

113. di-Battista C, Rossi L, Marcelli P: Hereditary tyrosinemia in acute form. Pediatr Med Chir 3:101, 1981

114. Aster RH: Pooling of platelets in the spleen: role in the pathogenesis of "hypersplenic" thrombocytopenia. J Clin Invest 45:645, 1966

115. Stein SF, Harker LA: Kinetic and functional studies of platelets, fibrinogen, and plasminogen in patients with hepatic cirrhosis. J Lab Clin Med 99:217, 1982

116. Blanchard RA et al: Acquired vitamin K-dependent carboxylation deficiency in liver disease. N Engl J Med 305:242, 1981

117. Volpe JJ: Intraventricular hemorrhage in the premature infant—current concepts. Part I. Ann Neurol 25:3, 1989

118. Dolfin T, Skidmore MB, Fong KW et al: Incidence, severity and timing of subependymal and intraventricular hemorrhages in preterm infants born in a perinatal unit as detected by serial real-time ultrasound. Pediatrics 71:541, 1983

119. Ment LR, Duncan CC, Ehrenkranz RA: Intraventricular hemorrhage of the preterm neonate. Semin Perinat 11:132, 1987

120. Papile L-A, Burstein J, Burstein R: Incidence and evolution of subependymal and intraventricular hemorrhage: a study of infants with birth weights less than 1,500 gm. J Pediatr 92:529, 1978

121. Tsiantos A, Victorin L, Relier JP: Intracranial hemorrhage in the prematurely born infant: timing of clots and evaluation of clinical signs and symptoms. J Pediatr 85:854, 1974

122. Hambleton G, Wigglesworth JS: Origin of intraventricular hemorrhage in the preterm infant. Arch Dis Child 51:651, 1976

123. Szymonowicz W, Yu VYH: Timing and evolution of periventricular haemorrhage in infants weighing 1250 g or less at birth. Arch Dis Child 59:7, 1984

124. Guzzetta F, Shackelford GD, Volpe S et al: Periventricular intraparenchymal echodensities in the premature newborn: critical determinant of neurological outcome. Pediatrics 78:995, 1986

125. Gould SJ, Howard S, Hope PL, Reynolds EOR: Periventricular intraparenchymal cerebral haemorrhage in preterm infants: the role of venous infarction. J Pathol 151:197, 1987

126. Shinnar S, Molteni A, Gammon K et al: Intraventricular hemorrhage in the premature infant: a changing outlook. N Engl J Med 306:1464, 1982

127. Ahmann Pa, Lazzara A, Dykes FD et al: Intraventricular hemorrhage in the high-risk preterm infant: incidence and outcome. Ann Neurol 7:118, 1980

128. Levene MI, de Vries L: Extension of neonatal intraventricular hemorrhage. Arch Dis Child 59:631, 1984

129. Rushton DI, Preston PR, Durbin GM: Structure and evolution of echo dense lesions in the neonatal brain. Arch Dis Child 60:798, 1985

130. Takashima S, Mito T, Ando Y: Pathogenesis of periventricular white matter hemorrhages in preterm infants. Brain Dev 8:25, 1986

131. Volpe JJ: Neonatal intraventricular hemorrhage. N Engl J Med 304:886, 1981

132. White LW: CT brain scanning in neonates: indications and practices. Appl Radiol 8:58, 1979

133. Bejar R, Curbelo V, Coen RW et al: Diagnosis and follow-up of intraventricular and intracerebral hemorrhages by ultrasound studies of infant's brain through the fontanelles and sutures. Pediatrics 66: 661, 1980

134. Mack LA, Wright K, Hirsch JH: Intracranial hemorrhage in premature infants: accuracy of sonographic evaluation. AJR 137:245, 1981

135. Pape KE, Bennett-Britton S, Szywonowicz W et al: Diagnostic accuracy of neonatal brain imaging: A postmortem correlation of computed tomography and ultrasound scans. J Pediatr 102:275, 1983

136. Graziani LJ, Pasto M, Stanley C et al: Cranial ultrasound and clinical studies in preterm infants. J Pediatr 106:269, 1985

137. Sinha SK, Davies JM, Sims DG, Chiswick ML: Relation between periventricular haemorrhage and ischaemic brain lesions diagnosed by ultrasound in very preterm infants. Lancet 2:1154, 1985

138. Perlman JM, Nelson JS, McAlister WH, Volpe JJ: Intracerebellar haemorrhage in a premature newborn: diagnosis by real-time ultrasound and correlation with autopsy findings. Pediatrics 71:159, 1983

139. Trounce JQ, Fagan D, Levene MI: Intraventricular haemorrhage and periventricular leucomalacia: ultrasound and autopsy correlation. Arch Dis Child 61: 1203, 1986

140. Perlman JM, McMenamin JB, Volpe JJ: Fluctuating cerebral blood-flow velocity in respiratory distress syndrome. N Engl J Med 309:204, 1983

141. Perlman JM, Hill A, Volpe JJ: The effect of patent ductus arteriosus on flow velocity in the anterior cerebral arteries: ductal steal in the premature newborn infant. J Pediatr 99:767, 1981

142. Lou HC: Perinatal hypoxic-ischaemic brain damage and intraventricular haemorrhage: a pathogenic model. Arch Neurol 37:585, 1980

143. Sonesson S-V, Winberg P, Lundell BPW: Early postnatal changes in intracranial arterial blood flow velocities in term infants. Pediatr Res 22:461, 1987

144. Tweed A, Cote J, Lou H et al: Impairment of cerebral blood flow autoregulation in the newborn lamb by hypoxia. Pediatr Res 20:516, 1986

145. Greisen G, Johansen K, Ellison PH et al: Cerebral blood flow in the newborn infant: comparison of Doppler ultrasound and ^{133}xenon clearance. J Pediatr 104:411, 1984

146. Ment LR, Duncan CC, Ehrenkranz RA et al: Intraventricular hemorrhage in the preterm neonate: timing and cerebral blood flow changes. J Pediatr 104:419, 1984

147. Goddard J, Lewis RM, Armstrong DL, Zeller RS: Moderate, rapidly induced hypertension as a cause of intraventricular hemorrhage in the newborn beagle model. J Pediatr 96:1057, 1980

148. Beverley DW, Pitts-Tucker TJ, Congdon J et al: Prevention of intraventricular haemorrhage by fresh frozen plasma. Arch Dis Child 60:710, 1985

149. McDonald MM, Johnson ML, Rumack CM et al: Role of coagulopathy in newborn intracranial haemorrhage. Pediatrics 74:26, 1984

150. Beverley DW, Chance GW, Inwood MJ et al: Intraventricular haemorrhage and haemostasis defects. Arch Dis Child 59:444, 1984

151. Gilles FH, Price RA, Kevy SV, Berenberg W: Fibrinolytic activity in the ganglionic eminence of the premature human brain. Biol Neonate 18:426, 1971

152. Horbar JD: Prevention of periventricular-intraventricular hemorrhage. p. 562. In Sinclair JC, Bracken MB (eds): Effective Care of the Newborn Infant. Oxford University Press, Oxford, 1992

153. Andrew M, Castle V, Saigal S et al: Clinical impact of neonatal thrombocytopenia. J Pediatr 110:457, 1987

154. Lupton BA, Hill A, Whitfield MF et al: Reduced platelet count as a risk factor for intraventricular haemorrhage. Am J Dis Child 142:1222, 1988

155. Turner T, Prouse CV, Prescott RJ, Cash JD: A clinical trial on the early detection and correction of hemostatic defects in selected high-risk neonates. Br J Haematol 47:65, 1981

156. Andrew M, Caco C, Vegh P et al: Benefits of platelet transfusions in premature infants: a randomized controlled trial, abstracted. Thromb Haemost 65:721, 1991

157. Andrew M, Caco C, Vegh P et al: A randomized controlled trial of platelet transfusions in thrombocytopenic premature infants. J Pediatr 123:285, 1993

158. Thomas DB, Burnard ED: Prevention of intraventricular haemorrhage in babies receiving artificial ventilation. Med J Aust 1:933, 1973

159. Watl H, Fodisch NJ, Kurz R et al: Intracranial haemorrhage in low-birth weight infants and prophylactic administration of coagulation-factor concentrate. Lancet 1:1284, 1973

160. Gupta JM, Starr H, Fincher P, Lam-Po-Tang PRLC: Intraventricular haemorrhage in the newborn. Med J Aust 2:338, 1976

161. Morales WJ, Angel JL, O'Brien WF et al: The use of antenatal vitamin K in the prevention of early neonatal intraventricular hemorrhage. Am J Obstet Gynecol 159:774, 1988

162. Pomerance JJ, Teal JG, Gogdok JF et al: Maternally administered antenatal vitamin K_1: effect on neonatal prothrombin activity, partial thromboplastin time, and intraventricular hemorrhage. Obstet Gynecol 70:235, 1987

163. Kazzi NJ, Ilagen MB, Liang KC: Maternal administration of vitamin K does not improve the coagulation profile of preterm infants. Pediatrics 84:1045, 1989

164. Shirahata A, Nakamura T, Shimono M et al: Blood coagulation findings and the efficacy of factor XIII concentrate in premature infants with intracranial hemorrhages. Thromb Res 57:755, 1990

165. Hensey OJ, Morgan MEI, Cooke RWI: Tranexamic acid in the prevention of periventricular hemorrhage. Arch Dis Child 59:719, 1984

166. Fodstad H, Forssell A, Liliequist B, Schaunong M: Antifibrinolysis with tranexamic acid in aneurysmal subarachnoid haemorrhage: a consecutive controlled clinical trial. Neurosurgery 8:158, 1981

167. Bartlett JR: Subarachnoid haemorrhage. BMJ 283:1347, 1981

168. Sindet-Pederson S, Stenbjerb S: Effect of local antifibrinolytic treatment with tranexamic acid in hemophiliacs undergoing oral surgery. J Oral Maxillofac Surg 44:703, 1986

169. Sindet-Pederson S, Ramstrom G, Bernvil S, Blomback M: Hemostatic effect of tranexamic acid mouthwash in anticoagulant-treated patients undergoing oral surgery. N Engl J Med 320:840, 1989

170. Papatheodossiou N: A double blind clinical trial on dicynone in tonsillectomy. Med Hyg 31:1818, 1973

171. Symes JM, Offen DN, Lyttle JA et al: The effect of dicynene on blood loss during and after transurethral resection of the prostate. Br J Urol 47:203, 1975

172. Harrison RF, Campbell S: A double blind trial of ethamsylate in the treatment of primary intrauterine-device menorrhagia. Lancet 2:283, 1976

173. Ment LR, Ehrenkranz RA, Duncan CC: Intraventricular hemorrhage of the preterm neonate: prevention studies. Semin Perinatol 12:359, 1988

174. Morgan MEI, Ben JWT, Cooke RWI: Ethamsylate reduces the incidence of periventricular haemorrhage in very low birth weight babies. Lancet 1981; 2:830–831.

175. Cooke RWI, Morgan MEI: Prophylactic ethamsylate for periventricular haemorrhage. Arch Dis Child 59:82, 1984

176. Benson JWT, Drayton MR, Hayward C et al: Multicentre trial of ethamsylate for prevention of periventricular haemorrhage in very low birthweight infants. Lancet 2:1297, 1986

177. Ment L, Stewart W, Scott D, Duncan C: Beagle puppy model of intraventricular hemorrhage: randomized indomethacin prevention trial. Neurology 33:179, 1983

178. Bachofen M, Weibel ER: Structural alterations of lung parenchyma in the adult respiratory distress syndrome. Clin Chest Med 3:35, 1982

179. Gajl-Peczalska K: Plasma protein composition of hyaline membrane in the newborn as studies by immunofluorescence. Arch Dis Child 39:226, 1964

180. Gitlin D, Kumate J, Urrusti J, Morales C: The selectivity of the human placenta in the transfer of plasma proteins from mother to fetus. J Clin Invest 43:1938, 1964

181. Avery ME, Mead J: Surface properties in relation to atelectasis and hyaline membrane disease. Am J Dis Child 97:517, 1959

182. Seeger W, Stohr G, Wolf HRD: Alteration of surfactant function due to protein leakage: special interaction with fibrin monomer. J Appl Physiol 58:326, 1985

183. Saldeen T: Fibrin-derived peptides and pulmonary injury. Ann NY Acad Sci 384:319, 1982

184. Fukuda Y, Ishizaki M, Masuda Y et al: The role of intraalveolar fibrosis in the process of pulmonary structural remodelling in patients with diffuse alveolar damage. Am J Pathol 126:171, 1987

185. Damiano VV, Cherian PV, Frankel FR et al: Intraluminal fibrosis induced unilaterally by lobar instillation of $CdCl_{22}$ into the rat lung. Am J Pathol 137:883, 1990

186. Schmidt B, Davis P, LaPointe H et al: Efficacy of thrombin inhibition in a piglet model of neonatal acute lung injury, abstracted. Thromb Haemost 69:1020, 1993

187. Markarian M, Luchenco LO, Rosenblut E: Hypercoagulability in premature infants with special reference to the respiratory distress syndrome and hemorrhage. II. The effect of heparin. Biol Neonate 17:98, 1971

188. Muntean W, Rosseger H: Antithrombin III concen-

trate in preterm infants with IRDS: an open, controlled, randomized clinical trial, abstracted. Thromb Haemost 62:288, 1989

189. Ambrus CM, Weintraub DH, Ambrus JL: Studies on hyaline membrane disease. III. Therapeutic trial of urokinase-activated human plasmin. Pediatrics 38: 231, 1966

190. Ambrus CM, Choi TS, Cunnanan E et al: Prevention of hyaline membrane disease with plasminogen. A cooperative study. JAMA 237:1837, 1977

191. Townsend CW: The haemorrhagic disease of the newborn. Arch Pediatr 11:559, 1894

192. Dam CPH: Cholesterinstoffwechsel in Huhnereierin und Huhnchen. Biochem Z 215:475, 1929

193. Bruchsaler FS: Vitamin K and the prenatal and postnatal prevention of hemorrhagic disease in newborn infants. J Pediatr 18:317, 1941

194. Dam H, Tage-Hansen E, Plum P: K-avitaminose hos spaede born som aarag til hemorrhagisk diathese. Ugesk Laeger 101:896, 1939

195. Brinkhous KM, Smith HP, Warner ED: Plasma prothrombin level in normal infancy and in hemorrhagic disease of the newborn, abstracted. Am J Med Sci 193:475, 1937

196. Quick AJ, Grossman: Concentration of prothrombin in blood of babies (3 to 7 days old). Proc Soc Exp Biol Med 40:647, 1939

197. Nygaard KK: Prophylactic and curative effect of vitamin K in hemorrhagic disease of the newborn (hypothrombinemia hemorrhagica neonatorum). A preliminary report. Acta Obstet Gynecol Scand 19:361, 1939

198. Waddell WW, Guerry D: The role of vitamin K in the etiology, prevention, and treatment of hemorrhage in the newborn infant. Part II. J Pediatr 15:802, 1939

199. Loughnan PM, McDougall PN: The efficacy of oral vitamin K1: implications for future prophylaxis to prevent haemorrhagic disease of the newborn. J Pediatr Child Health 29:171, 1993

200. Bussel JB, Grabowski EF: Coagulation disorders in children. Curr Opin Pediatr 5:88, 1993

201. Von Kries R, Greer FR, Suttie JW: Assessment of vitamin K status of the newborn infant. J Pediatr Gastroenterol Nutr 16:231, 1993

202. Furie B, Furie BC: Molecular basis of vitamin K-dependent γ-carboxylation. Blood 75:1753, 1990

203. Stenflo J, Fernlund P, Egan W, Roepstorff P: Vitamin K-dependent modifications of glutamic acid residues in prothrombin. Proc Natl Acad Sci USA 71:2730, 1974

204. Nelsestuen GL, Zytkovicz TH, Howard JB: The mode of action of vitamin K. Identification of γ-carboxyglu-

tamic acid as a component of prothrombin. J Biol Chem 249:6347, 1974

205. Nelsestuen GL: Role of gamma-carboxyglutamic acid: an unusual protein transition required for calcium-dependent binding of prothrombin to phospholipid. J Biol Chem 251:5648, 1976

206. Borowski M, Furie BC, Bauminger S, Furie B: Prothrombin requires two sequential metal-dependent conformational transitions to bind phospholipid. J Biol Chem 261:14969, 1986

207. Lane PA, Hathaway WE: Medical progress: vitamin K in infancy. J Pediatr 106:351, 1985

208. Kries RV, Shearer MJ, Gobel U: Vitamin K in infancy. Eur J Pediatr 147:106, 1988

209. Rose SJ: Neonatal hemorrhage and vitamin K. Acta Haematol 74:121, 1985

210. Shapiro AD, Jacobson LJ, Aramon ME et al: Vitamin K deficiency in the newborn infant: prevalence and perinatal risk factors. J Pediatr 109:675, 1986

211. Mandelbrot L, Guillaumont M, Forestier F et al: Placental transfer of vitamin K1 and its implications in fetal haemostasis. Thromb Haemost 60:39, 1988

212. Hamulyak K, de Boer-van den Berg MAG: The placental transport of [3H] vitamin K1 in rats. Br J Haematol 65:335, 1987

213. Haroon Y, Shearer MJ, Rahim S et al: The content of phylloquinone (vitamin K1) in human milk, cow's milk and infant formula foods determined by high-performance liquid chromatography. J Nutr 112: 1105, 1982

214. Von Kries R, Shearer MJ, McCarthy PT et al: Vitamin K1 content of maternal milk: influence of the stage of lactation, lipid composition, and vitamin K1 supplements given to the mother. Pediatr Res 22:513, 1987

215. Gellis SS, Lyon RA: The influence of the diet of the newborn infant on the prothrombin index. J Pediatr 19:495, 1941

216. Widdershoven J, Motohara K, Endo F et al: Influence of the type of feeding on the presence of PIVKA-II in infants. Helv Paediatr Acta 41:25, 1986

217. Andrew M, Schmidt B: Hemorrhagic and thrombotic complications in children. p. 989. In Colman RW, Hirsh J, Marder VJ, Salzman EW (eds): Hemostasis and Thrombosis: Basic Principles and Clinical Practice. JB Lippincott, Philadelphia, 1994

218. Sutherland JM, Glueck HI: Hemorrhagic disease of the newborn; breast feeding as a necessary factor in the pathogenesis. Am J Dis Child 113:524, 1967

219. Editorial: Late onset of hemorrhagic disease of the newborn. Nutr Rev 43:303, 1985

220. Matsuda I, Nishiyama S, Motohara K et al: Late neonatal vitamin K deficiency associated with subclinical liver dysfunction in human milk fed infants. J Pediatr 114:602, 1989

221. Goldschmidt B, Bors S, Szabo A: Vitamin K-dependent clotting factors during longterm parenteral nutrition in fullterm and preterm infants. J Pediatr 112:108, 1988

222. Motohara K, Endo F, Matsuda I: Screening for late neonatal vitamin K deficiency by acarboxyprothrombin in dried blood spots. Arch Dis Child 62:370, 1987

223. Forbes D: Delayed presentation of haemorrhagic disease of the newborn. Med J Aust 2:136, 1983

224. Payne NR, Hasegawa DK: Vitamin K deficiency in newborns: a case report in α-1-antitrypsin deficiency and a review of factors predisposing to hemorrhage. Pediatrics 73:712, 1984

225. Chaou W-T, Chou M-L, Eitzman DV: Intracranial hemorrhage and vitamin K deficiency in early infancy. J Pediatr 105:880, 1984

226. Motohara K, Endo F, Matsuda I: Vitamin K deficiency in breast-fed infants at one month of age. J Pediatr Gastroenterol Nutr 5:931, 1986

227. Martin-Bouyer G, Linh PD, Tuan LC: Epidemic of haemorrhagic disease in Vietmanese infants caused by warfarin-contaminated talcs. Lancet 1:230, 1983

228. Motohara K, Kuroki Y, Kan H et al: Detection of vitamin K deficiency by use of an enzyme-linked immunosorbent assay for circulating abnormal prothrombin. Pediatr Res 19:354, 1985

229. Widdershoven J, Kollee L, van Munster P et al: Biochemical vitamin K deficiency in early infancy: diagnostic limitation of conventional coagulation tests. Helv Paediatr Acta 41:195, 1986

230. Bloch CA, Rothberg AD, Bradlow BA: Mother-infant prothrombin precursor status at birth. J Pediatr Gastroenterol Nutr 3:101, 1984

231. Widdershoven J, Lambert W, Motohara K et al: Plasma concentrations of vitamin K_1 and PIVKA-II in bottle-fed and breast-fed infants with and without vitamin K prophylaxis at birth. Eur J Pediatr 148:139, 1988

232. Fujimura Y, Okubo Y, Sakai T et al: Studies on precursor proteins PIVKA-II, -IX, and -X in the plasma of patients with "hemorrhagic disease of the newborn." Haemostasis 14:211, 1984

233. Motohara K, Endo F, Matsuda I: Effect of vitamin K administration on acarboxy prothrombin (PIVKA-II) levels in newborns. Lancet 2:242, 1985

234. Fujimura Y, Mimura Y, Kinoshita S et al: Studies on vitamin K-dependent factor deficiency during early childhood with special reference to prothrombin activity and antigen level. Haemostasis 11:90, 1982

235. Corrigan JJ, Earnst D: Factor II antigen in liver disease and warfarin induced vitamin K deficiency: correlation with coagulation activity using *Echis* venom. Am J Hematol 8:249, 1980

236. Beverley DW, Inwood MJ, Chance GW et al: "Normal" haemostasis parameters: a study in a well-defined inborn population of preterm infants. Early Hum Dev 9:249, 1984

237. Kipper S, Sieger L: Whole blood platelet volumes in newborn infants. J Pediatr 101:763, 1982

238. Arad ID, Alpan G, Sznajderman SD, Eldor A: The mean platelet volume (MVP) in the neonatal period. Am J Perinatol 3:1, 1986

239. Mehta P, Vasa R, Newman L, Karpatkin M: Thrombocytopenia in the high-risk infant. J Pediatr 97:791, 1980

240. Castle V, Andrew M, Kelton JG et al: Frequency and mechanism of neonatal thrombocytopenia. J Pediatr 108:749, 1986

241. Pearson HA, McIntosh S: Neonatal thrombocytopenia. Clin Haematol 7:111, 1978

242. Gill FM: Thrombocytopenia in the newborn. Semin Perinatol 7:201, 1983

243. Andrew M, Kelton JG: Neonatal thrombocytopenia. Clin Perinatol 11:359, 1984

244. Austin N, Darlow BA: Transfusion-associated fall in platelet count in very low birthweight infants. Aust Paediatr J 24:354, 1988

245. Samuels P, Main EK, Tomaski A et al: Abnormalities in platelet antiglobulin tests in preeclamptic mothers and their neonates. Am J Obstet Gynecol 157:109, 1987

246. Ballin A, Koren G, Kohelet D, Burger R et al: Reduction of platelet counts induced by mechanical ventilation in newborn infants. J Pediatr 111:445, 1987

247. Castle V, Coates G, Kelton J, Andrew M: [111]Indium oxine platelet survivals in the thrombocytopenic infant. Blood 70:652, 1987

248. Feusner JH, Slichter SJ, Harker LA: Acquired haemostatic defects in the ill newborn. Br J Haematol 53:73, 1983

249. Castle V, Coates G, Mitchell L et al: The effect of hypoxia on platelet survival and site of sequestration in the newborn rabbit. Thromb Haemost 59:45, 1988

250. Tate DY, Carlton GT, Johnson D et al: Immune thrombocytopenia in severe neonatal infections. J Pediatr 98:449, 1981

251. Podolsak B: Thrombopoiesis in newborn infants after exchange blood transfusion. Z Kinderheilkd 114:13, 1973

252. Slichter SJ: Platelet transfusion therapy. Hematol Oncol Clin North Am 4:291, 1990

253. Gaydos LA, Freireich EJ, Mantel N: The quantitative relation between platelet count and hemorrhage in patients with acute leukemia. N Engl J Med 266:905, 1962

254. Roy AJ, Jaffe N, Djerassi I: Prophylactic platelet transfusions in children with acute leukemia: a dose response study. Transfusion 13:283, 1973

255. Aderka D, Praff G, Santo M, Weinberger A: Bleeding due to thrombocytopenia in acute leukemias and re-evaluation of the prophylactic platelet transfusion policy. Am J Med Sci 291:147, 1986

256. Andrew M, Mitchell L, Paes B et al: An anticoagulant dermatan sulphate proteoglycan circulates in the pregnant women and her fetus. J Clin Invest 89:321, 1992

257. Matzch T, Bergqvist D, Bergqvist A et al: No transplacental passage of standard heparin or an enzymatically depolymerized low molecular weight heparin. Blood Coagul Fibrinolysis 2:273, 1991

258. Stuart J, Breeze EG, Picken AM, Wood BS: Capillary-blood coagulation profile in the newborn. Lancet 2:1467, 1973

259. Bussel JB, Tanli S, Peterson HdC: Favorable neurological outcome in 7 cases of perinatal intracranial hemorrhage due to immune thrombocytopenia. Am J Pediatr Hematol Oncol 13:156, 1991

260. Daffos F, Forestier F, Kaplan C, Cox W: Prenatal diagnosis and management of bleeding disorders with fetal blood sampling. Am J Obstet Gynecol 158:939, 1988

261. Hall JG, Levin J, Kuhn JP et al: Thrombocytopenia with absent radius. Medicine (Baltimore) 48:411, 1969

262. Hedberg VA, Lipton JM: Thrombocytopenia with absent radii. A review of 100 cases. Am J Pediatr Hematol Oncol 10:51, 1988

263. Setzer ES, Webb IB, Wassenaar JW et al: Platelet dysfunction and coagulopathy in intraventricular hemorrhage in the premature infant. J Pediatr 100:599, 1982

264. Mazzone D, Fichera A, Pratico G, Sciacca F: Combined congenital deficiency of factor V and factor VIII. Acta Haematol 68:337, 1982

265. McMillan CW, Roberts HR: Congenital combined deficiency of coagulation factors II, VII, IX and X. N Engl J Med 274:1313, 1966

266. Rohyans JA, Miser AW, Miser JS: Subgaleal hemorrhage in infants with hemophilia: report of two cases and review of the literature. Pediatrics 70:306, 1982

267. Hayden CK, Shattuck KE, Richardson CJ et al: Subependymal germinal matrix hemorrhage in fulterm neonates. Pediatrics 75:714, 1985

268. Scher MS, Wright FS, Lockman LA, Thompson TR: Intraventricular hemorrhage in the fulterm neonate. Arch Neurol 39:769, 1982

269. Jackson JC, Blumhagen JD: Congenital hydrocephalus due to prenatal hemorrhage. Pediatrics 72:344, 1983

270. Serfontein GL, Rom S, Stein S: Posterior fossa subdural hemorrhage in the newborn. Pediatrics 65:40, 1980

271. Gunn TR, Mok PM, Becroft DMO: Subdural hemorrhage in utero. Pediatrics 76:605, 1985

272. Cartwright GW, Culbertson K, Schreiner RL, Garg BP: Changes in clinical presentation of term infants with intracranial hemorrhage. Dev Med Child Neurol 21:730, 1979

273. Palma PA, Miner ME, Morriss FH, Jr: Intraventricular hemorrhage in the neonate at term. Am J Dis Child 133:941, 1979

274. Chaplin ER Jr, Goldstein GW, Norman D: Neonatal seizures, intracerebral hematoma, and subarachnoid hemorrhage in fulterm infants. Pediatrics 63:812, 1979

275. Guckos-Thoeni U, Boltshauser E, Willi UV: Intraventricular hemorrhage in fulterm neonates. Dev Med Child Neurol 24:704, 1982

276. Mackay RJ, Crespigny L, Laurence J et al: Intraventricular hemorrhage in term neonates: diagnosis by ultrasound. Aus Paediatr J 18:205, 1984

277. Bray GL, Luhan NL: Hemophilia presenting with intracranial hemorrhage. Am J Dis Child 141:1215, 1987

278. Schmidt B, Zipursky A: Disseminated intravascular coagulation masking neonatal hemophilia. J Pediatr 109:886, 1986

279. Baugh RF, Deemar KA, Zimmerman JJ: Heparinase in the activated clotting time assay: monitoring heparin-independent alterations in coagulation function. Anesth Analg 74:201, 1992

280. Karpatkin S, Strick N, Karpatkin M, Siskind AW: Cumulative experience in the detection of antiplatelet antibody in 234 patients with idiopathic thrombocytopenic purpura, systemic lupus erythematosus and other clinical disorders. Am J Med 52:776, 1972

281. Andrew M, Mitchell L, Berry L et al: Fibrinogen has a rapid turnover in the healthy newborn lamb. Pediatr Res 23:249, 1988

282. Karitzky D, Kleine N, Pringsheim W, Kunzer W: Fibrinogen turnover in the premature infant with and without idiopathic respiratory distress syndrome. Acta Paediatr Scand 60:465, 1971

283. Schmidt B, Wais U, Pringsheim W, Kunzer W: Plasma

elimination of antithrombin III is accelerated in term newborn infants. Eur J Pediatr 141:225, 1984

284. Manno CS, Butler RB, Cohen AR: Low recovery in vivo of highly purified factor VIII in patients with hemophilia. J Pediatr 121(5 pt 1):814, 1992

285. Pencharz PB, Steffee WP, Cochran W et al: Protein metabolism in human neonates: Nitrogen-balance studies, estimated obligatory losses of nitrogen and whole-body turnover of nitrogen. Clin Sci Mol Med 52:485, 1977

286. Johnston M, Zipursky A: Microtechnology for the study of the blood coagulation system in newborn infants. Can J Med Technol 42:159, 1980

287. Addiego J, Kasper C, Abildgaard C et al: Frequency of inhibitor development in haemophiliacs treated with low-purity factor VIII. Lancet 342:462, 1993

288. Lusher JM, Warrier I: Hamophilia A. Hematol Oncol Clin North Am 6:1021, 1992

289. Mannucci PM, Columbo M: Virucidal treatment of clotting factor concentrates. Lancet 2:782, 1988

290. Pierce GF, Lusher JM, Brownstein AP et al: The use of purified clotting factor concentrates in hemophilia. Influence of viral safety, cost, and supply on therapy. JAMA 261:3434, 1989

291. Brettler DB, Levine PH: Factor concentrates for treatment of hemophilia: which one to choose? Blood 73:2067, 1989

292. Manios SG, Schenck W, Kunzer W: Congenital fibrinogen deficiency. Acta Pediatr Scand 57:145, 1968

293. Gilchrist GS, Piepgras DG, Roskos RR: Neurological complications in hemophilia. p. 45. In Hilgartner M, Pochedly C (eds): Hemophilia in the Child and Adult. Raven Press, New York, 1989

294. Zenny JC, Chevrot A, Sultan Y et al: Lesions hemorragiques intra-osseuses des afibrinemies congénitales. A propos d'un nouveau cas. J Radiol 62:263, 1981

295. Fried K, Kaufman S: Congenital afibrinogenemia in 10 offspring of uncle-niece marriages. Clin Genet 17:223, 1980

296. Gill FM, Shapiro SS, Schwartz E: Severe congenital hypoprothrombinemia. J Pediatr 93:264, 1978

297. Lewis JH, Spero JA, Ragni MV, Bontempo FA: Transfusion support for congenital clotting deficiencies other than haemophilia. Clin Hematol 13:119, 1984

298. Seeler RA: Parahemophilia. Factor V deficiency. Med Clin North Am 56:119, 1972

299. Whitelaw A, Haines ME, Bolsover W et al: Factor V deficiency and antenatal ventricular hemorrhage. Arch Dis Child 59:997, 1984

300. Roberts HR, Lefkowitz JB: Inherited disorders of prothrombin conversion. p. 200. In Colman RW,

Hirsh J, Marder VJ, Salzman EW (eds): Hemostasis and Thrombosis. Basic Principles and Clinical Practice. JB Lippincott, Philadelphia, 1994

301. Rabiner SF, Winick M, Smith CH: Congenital deficiency of factor VII associated with hemorrhagic disease of the newborn. Pediatrics 25:101, 1960

302. Matthay KK, Koerper MA, Ablin AR: Intracranial hemorrhage in congenital factor VII deficiency. J Pediatr 94:413, 1979

303. van Creveld S, Veder HA, Blans MM: Congenital hypoproconvertinemia. Ann Pediatr 187:373, 1956

304. Girolami A, Cattorozi Y, Mengarda G, Lazzarin M: Congenital factor VII deficiency: a case report. Blut 27:236, 1973

305. van Creveld S, Veder HA, Kleinherenbrink W: Congenital hypoproconvertinemia II. Ann Pediatr 190:316, 1958

306. Ragni MV, Lewis JH, Spero JA et al: Factor VII deficiency. Am J Hematol 10:79, 1981

307. Schubert B, Schindera F: Congenital factor VII deficiency in a newborn, abstracted. Hamophilie Symposion 1988

308. Seligsohn U, Shani M, Ramot B: Dubin-Johnson syndrome in Israel II. Association with factor VII deficiency. Q J Med 39:569, 1970

309. Seligsohn U, Shani M, Ramot B: Gilbert syndrome and factor VII deficiency. Lancet 1:1398, 1970

310. Cox AC, Rao GHR, Gerrard JM, White JG: The influence of vitamin E quinone on platelet structure, function and biochemistry. Blood 55:907, 1980

311. Schmidt ML, Smith HE, Gamerman S et al: Prolonged recombinant activated factor VII (rFVIIa) treatment for severe bleeding in a factor-IX-deficient patient with an inhibitor. Br J Haematol 78:460, 1991

312. Adcock DM, Brozna J, Marlar RA: Proposed classification and pathologic mechanisms of purpura fulminans and skin necrosis. Semin Thromb Haemost 16:333, 1990

313. Schulman I: Pediatric aspects of the mild hemophilias. Med Clin North Am 46:93, 1962

314. Kozinn PJ, Ritz ND, Moss AH, Kaufman A: Massive hemorrhage—scalps of newborn infants. Am J Dis Child 108:413, 1964

315. Kozinn PJ, Ritz ND, Horowitz AW: Scalp hemorrhage as an emergency in the newborn. JAMA 194:179, 1965

316. Baehner RL, Strauss HS: Hemophilia in the first year of life. N Engl J Med 275:524, 1966

317. McCarthy JW, Coble LL: Intracranial hemorrhage and subsequent communicating hydrocephalus in a neonate with classical hemophilia. J Pediatr 51:122, 1973

318. Umetsu M, Chiba Y, Horino K et al: Cytomegalovirus-mononucleosis in a newborn infant. Arch Dis Child 50:396, 1975

319. Yoffe G, Buchanan GR: Intracranial haemorrhage in newborn and young infants with hemophilia. J Pediatr 113:333, 1988

320. Volpe JJ, Manica JP, Land VJ, Coxe WS: Neonatal subdural hematoma associated with severe hemophilia A. J Pediatr 88:1023, 1976

321. Cohen DL: Neonatal subgaleal hemorrhage in hemophilia. J Pediatr 93:1022, 1978

322. Eyster ME, Gill FM, Blatt PM et al: Hemophilia Study Group: Central nervous system bleeding in hemophiliacs. Blood 51:1179, 1978

323. Koch JA: Haemophilia in the newborn. A case report and literature review. S Afr Med J 53:721, 1978

324. Pettersson H, McClure P, Fitz C: Intracranial hemorrhage in hemophilic children. Acta Radiol 25:161, 1984

325. Bisset RAL, Gupta SC, Zammit-Maempel I: Case report: radiographic and ultrasound appearances of an intra-mural haematoma of the pylorus. Clin Radiol 39:316, 1988

326. Kletzel M, Miller CH, Becton DL et al: Postdelivery head bleeding in hemophilic neonates. Am J Dis Child 143:1107, 1989

327. Ljung R, Petrini P, Nilsson IM: Diagnostic symptoms of severe and moderate haemophilia A and B. Acta Paediatr Scand 79:196, 1990

328. Oski FA: Blood coagulation and its disorders in the newborn. p. 137. In Oski FA, Naiman JL (eds): Hematologic problems in the newborn. WB Saunders, Philadelphia, 1982

329. Hartmann JR, Diamond LK: Hemophilia and related hemorrhagic disorders. Practitioner 178:179, 1957

330. Rosendaal FR, Smit C, Briet E: Hemophilia treatment in historical perspective: a review of medical and social developments. Ann Hematol 62:5, 1991

331. Stormorken H, Hessel B, Lunde J, Holmsen IB: Severe factor VIII deficiency in a chromosomally normal female. Thromb Res 44:113, 1986

332. Mannucci PM, Coppola R, Lombardi R et al: Direct proof of extreme lyonization as a cause of low factor VIII levels in females. Thromb Haemost 39:544, 1978

333. Martinowitz U, Varon D, Jonas P et al: Circumcision in hemophilia: the use of fibrin glue for local hemostasis. J Urol 148:855, 1992

334. Seremetis SV, Aledort LM: Congenital bleeding disorders. Rational treatment options. Drugs 45:541, 1993

335. Hershgold EJ, Pool JG, Pappenhagen AR: The potent antihemophilic globulin concentrate derived from a cold insoluble fraction of human plasma characterization and further data on preparation and clinical trial. J Lab Clin Med 67:23, 1966

336. Blanchette VS, Hume HA, Levy GJ et al: Guidelines for auditing pediatric blood transfusion practices. Am J Dis Child 145:787, 1991

337. Wiltgen Trotter C, Hasegawa DK: Hemophilia B. Case study and intervention plan. JOGN Nurs 12:82, 1983

338. Schwartz ID, Root AW: Hypercalcemia associated with normal I^{125}-dihydroxyvitamin D concentrations in a neonate with factor IX deficiency. J Pediatr 114:509, 1989

339. Pegelow CH, Borromeo Antigua MC, Daghastani D, Setzer Bandstra E: Plasma support for surgery in a premature infant with factor IX deficiency, letter. Am J Dis Child 143:638, 1989

340. Stowell KM, Figueiredo MS, Brownlee GG et al: Haemophilia B Liverpool: a new British family with mild haemophilia B associated with a-6 G to A mutation in the factor IX promoter. Br J Haematol 85:188, 1993

341. Kim HC, McMillan CW, White GC et al: Clinical experience of a new monoclonal antibody purified factor IX: Half-life, recovery, and safety in patients with hemophilia B. Semin Hematol, suppl 2. 27:30, 1990

342. Girolami A, Molaro G, Calligaris A, De Luca G: Severe congenital factor X deficiency in 5-month-old child. Thromb Haemost 24:175, 1970

343. Machin SJ, Winter MR, Davies SC, Mackie IJ: Factor X deficiency in the neonatal period. Arch Dis Child 55:406, 1980

344. De Sousa C, Clark T, Bradshaw A: Antenatally diagnosed subdural haemorrhage in congenital factor X deficiency. Arch Dis Child 63:1168, 1988

345. Sandler E, Gross S: Prevention of recurrent intracranial hemorrhage in a factor X deficient infant. Am J Pediatr Hematol Oncol 14:163, 1992

346. Ruane BJ, McCord FB: Factor X deficiency—a rare cause of scrotal haemorrhage, letter. Irish Med J 83:163, 1990

347. Kitchens CS: Factor XI: a review of its biochemistry and deficiency. Semin Thromb Haemost 17:55, 1991

348. Duckert F, Jung E, Shmerling DH: Hitherto undescribed congenital haemorrhagic diathesis probably due to fibrin stabilizing factor deficiency. Thromb Haemost 5:179, 1960

349. Barry A, Delage M: Congenital deficiency of fibrin stabilizing factor: observation of a new case. N Engl J Med 272:943, 1965

350. Vosburgh E: Rational intervention in von Willebrands disease. Hosp Pract 28:31, 1993

351. Fisher S, Rikover M, Naor S: Factor 13 deficiency with severe hemorrhage diathesis. Blood 28:34, 1966

352. Britten AFH: Congenital deficiency of factor XIII (fibrin-stabilizing factor). Am J Med 43:751, 1967

353. Ozsoylu S, Altay C, Hisconmez G: Congenital factor XIII deficiency: observation of two cases in the newborn period. Am J Dis Child 122:541, 1971

354. Francis J, Todd P: Congenital factor XIII deficiency in a neonate. BMJ 2:1532, 1978

355. Abbondanzo SL, Gootenberg JE, Lofts RS, McPherson RA: Intracranial hemorrhage in congenital deficiency of factor XIII. Am J Pediatr Hematol Oncol 10:65, 1988

356. Merchant RH, Agarwal BR, Currimbhoy Z et al: Congenital factor XIII deficiency. Ind Pediatr 29:831, 1992

357. Mammen EF, Murano G, Bick RL: Combined congenital clotting factor abnormalities. Semin Thromb Haemost 9:55, 1983

358. Lethagen S: Von Willebrand's disease. Pathogenesis and clinical aspects. Crit Rev Oncol Hematol 15:1, 1993

359. Scott JP, Montgomery RR: Therapy of von Willebrand disease. Semin Thromb Haemost 19:37, 1993

360. Donner M, Holmberg L, Nilsson IM: Type IIB von Willebrand's disease with probable autosomal recessive inheritance and presenting as thrombocytopenia in infancy. Br J Haematol 66:349, 1987

361. Bignall P, Standen GR, Bowen DJ et al: Rapid neonatal diagnosis of von Willebrand's disease by use of the polymerase chain reaction, letter. Lancet 336:638, 1990

362. Gazengel C, Fischer AM, Schlegel N et al: Treatment of type III von Willebrand's disease with solven/detergent-treated factor VIII concentrates. Nouv Rev Fr Hematol 30:225, 1988

363. Pasi KJ, Williams MD, Enayat MS, Hill FG: Clinical and laboratory evaluation of the treatment of von Willebrand's disease patients with heat-treated factor VIII concentrate (BPL 8Y). Br J Haematol 75:228, 1990

364. Mazurier C, Gaucher C, Jorieux S et al: Evidence for a von Willebrand factor defect in factor VIII binding in three members of a family previously misdiagnosed mild hemophilia A and hemophilia carriers: consequences for therapy and genetic counselling. Br J Haematol 76:372, 1990

365. Perkins HA: Correction of the hemostatic defects in von Willebrand's disease. Blood 30:375, 1967

366. Green D, Potter EV: Failure of AHF concentrate to control bleeding in von Willebrand's disease. Am J Med 60:357, 1976

367. Nilsson IM, Hedner U: Characteristics of various factor VIII concentrates used in the treatment of haemophilia A. Br J Haematol 37:543, 1977

368. Kohler M, Hellstern P, Wenzel E: The use of heat-treated factor VIII concentrates in von Willebrand's disease. Blut 50:25, 1985

369. Fukui H, Nishino M, Terada S et al: Haemostatic effect of a heat-treated factor VIII concentrate (Haemate P) in von Willebrand's disease. Blut 56:171, 1988

370. Blatt PM, Brinkhous KM, Culp HR et al: Antihemophilic factor concentrate therapy in von Willebrand disease. JAMA 236:2770, 1976

371. Pasi KJ, Hill FG: In vitro and in vivo inhibition of monocyte phagocytic function by factor VIII concentrates: correlation with concentrate purity. Br J Haematol 76:88, 1990

372. Skidmore SJ, Pasi KJ, Mawson SJ et al: Serological evidence that dry heating of clotting factor concentrates prevents transmission of non-A, non-B hepatitis. J Med Virol 30:50, 1990

373. Van De Bor M, Briet E, Van Bel F et al: Hemostasis and periventricular-intraventricular hemorrhage of the newborn. Am J Dis Child 140:1131, 1986

374. Sacher RA, Strauss RG, Luban NLC et al: Blood component therapy during the neonatal period: a national survey of red cell transfusion practice. Transfusion 30:271, 1985

375. Hume H: Pediatric transfusions: quality assessment and assurance. p. 55. In Sacher RA, Strauss R (eds): Contemporary Issues in Pediatric Transfusion Medicine. American Association of Blood Banks, Arlington, VA, 1989

376. Benitz WE: The pharmacology of neonatal resuscitation and cardiopulmonary intensive care. Part 1—Immediate resuscitation. West J Med 144:704, 1986

377. Oberman HA: Inappropriate use of fresh-frozen plasma. JAMA 253:556, 1985

378. Cartlidge PHT, Rutter N: Serum albumin concentrations and oedema in the newborn. Arch Dis Child 61:657, 1986

379. Zlotkin SH, Casselman CW: Percentile estimates of reference values for total protein and albumin in sera of premature infants (<37 weeks of gestation). Clin Chem 33:411, 1987

380. Thom H, McKay E, Gray DWG: Protein concentrations in the umbilical cord plasma of premature and mature infants. Clin Sci 33:433, 1967

381. Hyvannen M, Zeltzer P, Oh W, Stiehm ER: Influence of gestational age on serum levels of alpha-1-fetoprot-

ein, IgG globulin, and albumin in newborn infants. J Pediatr 82:430, 1973

382. Greenough A, Greenall F, Gamsu HR: Immediate effects of albumin infusion in ill premature neonates. Arch Dis Child 63:307, 1988

383. Bignall S, Bailey PC, Bass CA et al: The cardiovascular and oncotic effects of albumin infusion in premature infants. Early Hum Dev 20:191, 1989

384. Cochran EB, Hogue SL: Prediction of serum albumin concentration after albumin supplementation in pediatric patients receiving parenteral nutrition. Clin Pharm 10:704, 1991

385. Kanarek KS, Williams PR, Blair C: Concurrent administration of albumin with total parenteral nutrition in sick newborn infants. JPEN J Parent Ent Nutr 16:49, 1992

386. Ivarsen PR, Brodersen R: Displacement of bilirubin from adult and newborn serum albumin by a drug and fatty acid. Dev Pharmacol Ther 12:19, 1989

387. Grossman MF, Backal MP: Use of albumin in neonatal exchange transfusions. J Am Osteopath Assoc 66:656, 1967

388. Buchanan GR: Transfusion Therapy: Coagulation factors. p. 1606. In Nathan DG, Oski FA (eds): Hematology of Infancy and Childhood. WB Saunders, Philadelphia, 1991

389. Urbaniak S, Cash JD: Blood replacement therapy. Br Med Bull 33:273, 1977

390. Honig GR, Abildgaard CF, Forman EF et al: Some properties of the anticoagulant factor of aged pooled plasma. Thromb Haemost 22:151, 1969

391. Canadian Red Cross Society Blood Services: Clinical Guide to Transfusion. 1987, pp. 1–84

392. Glassman AB: Pediatric transfusion: considerations by age and blood component. South Med J 75:22, 1982

393. William OH: Neonatal polycythemia and hyperviscocity. Pediatr Clin North Am 33:523, 1986

394. Black VD, Lubchenco LO, Koops BL et al: Neonatal hyperviscosity. Randomized study of effect of partial plasma exchange transfusion on long term outcome. Pediatrics 75:1048, 1985

395. Maertzdorf WJ, Tangelder G, Slaaf DW, Blanco CE: Effects of partial plasma exchange transfusion on cerebral blood flow velocity in poly cythaemic preterm, term and small for date newborn infants. Eur J Pediatr 148:774, 1989

396. Bada HS, Korones SB, Kolni HW et al: Partial plasma exchange transfusion improves cerebral hemodynamics in symptomatic neonatal polycytemia. Am J Med Sci 291:11, 1986

397. Krueger RC Jr, Schwartz NB: An improved method of sequential alcian blue and ammoniacal silver staining of chrondoitin sulfate proteoglycan in polyacrylamide gels. Anal Biochem 167:295, 1987

398. Hanigan WC, Kennedy G, Roemisch F et al: Administration of indomethacin for the prevention of periventricular-intraventricular hemorrhage in high-risk neonates. J Pediatr 112:941, 1988

399. Ment LR, Duncan CC, Ehrenkranz RA: Randomized low dose indomethacin trial for prevention of intraventricular hemorrhage in very low birth weight neonates. J Pediatr 112:948, 1988

400. Bandstra ES, Montalvo BM, Goldberg RN et al: Prophylactic indomethacin for prevention of intraventricular hemorrhage in premature infants. Pediatrics 82:533, 1988

401. Bada HS, Green RS, Pourcyrous M et al: Indomethacin reduces the risks of severe intraventricular hemorrhage. J Pediatr 115:631, 1989

402. Mahony L, Caldwell RL, Girod DA et al: Indomethacin therapy on the first day of life in infants with very low birthweight. J Pediatr 106:801, 1985

403. Ment LR, Duncan CC, Ehrenkranz RA: Randomized indomethacin trial for prevention of intraventricular hemorrhage in very low birth weight infants. J Pediatr 107:937, 1985

404. Rennie JM, Doyle J, Cooke RWI: Early administration of indomethacin to preterm infants. Arch Dis Child 61:233, 1986

405. Vincer M, Allen A, Evans J et al: Early intravenous indomethacin prolongs respiratory support in very low birth weight infants. Acta Paediatr Scand 76:894, 1987

406. Mammen EF. Fibrinogen abnormalities. Semin Thromb Haemost 9:1, 1983

407. Mammen EF: Factor II abnormalities. Semin Thromb Haemost 9:13, 1983

408. Hoyer LW, Wyshock EG, Colman RW: Coagulation cofactors: Factors V and VIII. p. 109. In Colman RW, Hirsh J, Marder VJ, Salzman EW (eds): Hemostasis and Thrombosis. Basic Principles and Clinical Practice. JB Lippincott, Philadelphia, 1994

409. Mammen EF: Factor V deficiency. Semin Thromb Haemost 9:17, 1983

410. Mammen EF, Murano G, Bick RL: Factor VII abnormalities. Semin Thromb Haemost 9:19, 1983

411. Mammen EF, Murano G, Bick RL: Factor VIII abnormalities. Semin Thromb Haemost 9:22, 1983

412. Mammen EF, Murano G, Bick RL: Factor IX abnormalities. Semin Thromb Haemost 9:28, 1983

413. Edmunds LH, Salzman EW: Hemostatic problems, transfusion therapy, and cardiopulmonary bypass in surgical patients. p. 956. In Colman RW, Hirsh J,

Marder VJ, Salzman EW (eds): Hemostasis and Thrombosis: Basic Principles and Clinical Practice. JB Lippincott, Philadelphia, 1994

414. Mammen EF: Factor X abnormalities. Semin Thromb Haemost 9:31, 1983

415. Mammen EF, Murano G, Bick RL: Factor XI deficiency. Semin Thromb Haemost 9:34, 1983

416. DeLa Cadena RA, Wachtfogel Y, Colman RW: Contact activation pathway: inflammation and coagulation. p. 219. In Coleman RW, Hirsh J, Marder VJ, Salzman EW (eds): Hemostasis and Thrombosis. Basic Principles and Clinical Practice. JB Lippincott, Philadelphia, 1994

417. Ichinose A, Davie EW: The blood coagulation factors: their cDNAs, genes, and expression. p. 19. In Colman RW, Hirsh J, Marder VJ, Salzman EW (eds): Hemostasis and Thrombosis. Basic Principles and Clinical Practice. JB Lippincott, Philadelphia, 1994

418. Mammen EF, Murano G, Bick R: Factor XIII deficiency. Semin Thromb Haemost 9:10, 1983

419. Mammen EF, Murano G, Bick RL: Inhibitor abnormalities. Semin Thromb Haemost 9:42, 1983

420. Broze GJ Jr, Miletich JP: Biochemistry and physiology of protein C, protein S, and thrombomodulin. p. 259. In Colman RW, Hirsh J, Marder VJ, Salzman EW (eds): Hemostasis and Thrombosis. Basic Principles and Clinical Practice. JB Lippincott, Philadelphia, 1994

421. Hirsh J, Prins MH, Samama M: Approach to the thrombophilic patient for hemostasis and thrombosis: Basic principles and Clinical practice. p. 1543. In Colman RW, Hirsh J, Marder VJ, Salzman EW (eds): Hemostasis and Thrombosis. Basic Principles and Clinical Practice. JB Lippincott, Philadelphia, 1994

422. American Association of Blood Banks: Guidelines for Conducting Pediatric Transfusion Audits. AABB, Bethesda, MD, 1992

Chapter 31

Neonatal Myelopoiesis and Immunomodulation of Host Defenses

Joseph Rosenthal and Mitchell S. Cairo

Neonatal sepsis is a major cause of morbidity and mortality in newborns, particularly preterm infants. The high incidence of neonatal sepsis is attributed to, among other factors, the immaturity of the neonatal host defense systems. Defects in all components of the immune system have been demonstrated. The risk of developing neonatal sepsis depends on the degree of prematurity, predisposing maternal conditions, and extent of life-support procedures required postnatally.[1,2] The overall incidence is estimated to be in the range of 1 to 10 patients per 1,000 live births. However, a seven- to eleven-fold increase in the risk of infection has been observed among premature and low-for-gestational-age newborns.[1–3] The mortality rate from neonatal bacterial sepsis ranges from 15 to 75 percent, and is dependent on the maturity of host defense mechanisms, the causative organism, associated complications at the time of diagnosis, and time of initiation of appropriate antibiotic and supportive therapy.

The processes of neutrophil proliferation and differentiation, storage and release, and normal functions of neutrophils are essential for successful anti-bacterial activity. Although defects in antibody-mediated immunity and the complement system in the newborn have been described,[4–6] the defects that may play the most important role in susceptibility to infection are the quantitative and qualitative alterations that have been documented in neutrophils and other phagocytic cells.

GRANULOPOIESIS

Stem Cells and Progenitor Cells

In 1961, Till and McCulloch[7] were the first to demonstrate that when bone marrow cells are transfused into lethally irradiated mice, separate colonies of hematopoietic cells can be identified in the spleen of the recipient. Each colony, containing neutrophils, monocytes, erythrocytes, megakaryocytes, eosinophils, and basophils, is derived from an individual cell, and many of the colonies contain cells that are capable of such colony formation when transplanted into a second irradiated animal. Such cells, which are capable of unlimited self-renewal, have been refered to as pluripotent stem cells. The hematopoietic stem cell is therefore a cell that is not committed to any particular hematopoietic lineage and has the capacity for proliferation as well as for differentiation into mature blood cells. The earliest form of the committed myeloid progenitor cell is termed a

Supported by grants from the Pediatric Cancer Research Foundation, the Walden W. and Jean Young Shaw Foundation, the CHOC-PSF Research and Education Foundation and the Sandoz Pharmaceuticals Bone Marrow Transplant Fellowship Grant.

colony-forming-unit granulocyte, erythrocyte, macrophage, and megakaryocyte (CFU-GEMM). CFU-GEMM are not true pluripotent cells since they have a limited self-renewal capacity. CFU-GEMM differentiate into more committed progenitors, such as the granulocyte-macrophage colony-forming unit (CFU-GM) and the erythroid burst-forming unit. These are further differentiated to form committed and unilineage colony-forming units such as the granulocyte CFU, macrophage CFU, eosinophil CFU, basophil CFU, and the erythroid burst-forming unit. The differentiation and maturation of bone marrow progenitor cells into peripheral blood effector cells involve complex interactions between the bone marrow microenvironment, progenitor cells, and hematopoietic growth factors.

Neonatal Neutrophil Proliferative Pool

In a series of studies, Christensen et al. have documented significant differences in myeloid progenitor pools and cell kinetics in fetal and neonatal rats when compared to adult rats. Differences have been identified in CFU-GM pool size per gram of body weight, anatomic location of CFU-GM, and cell cycle. In the newborn rat, the myeloid progenitor pool, which is the number of CFU-GM, is only 25 percent of that of adult rats and requires 4 weeks of maturation to reach adult levels.[8] Additionally, in spite of a lower number, the CFU-GM of the newborn rat is in a state of near-maximal proliferative capacity—the maximal rate of proliferation being 75 to 80 percent—whereas that of adult CFU-GM is only 25 percent.[8] Similar high proliferative rates have been documented in peripheral blood of neonates approaching maximal levels in premature subjects.[9] The latter observation might be significant in understanding the mechanisms behind the increased susceptibility of premature neonates to infection, because the CFU-GM proliferative rate is so high in many normal, noninfected fetuses that production of additional neutrophils does not appear possible, even during a bacterial infection.[10]

Neonatal Neutrophil Storage Pool

Concomitantly with reduced numbers of myeloid progenitor cells, the neonatal rat possesses reduced numbers (25 percent) of neutrophil storage pool (NSP) cells, defined as the percentage of metamyelocytes, bands, and polymorphonuclear neutrophil (PMN) forms in nucleated cells in the bone marrow, compared to normal adult values attained by 4 weeks of age.[11] The neutrophil storage pool increases in rats by fourfold per gram of body weight between birth and 6 weeks of age.[11]

Microenvironment

The processes of intramedullar migration, adhesion, proliferation, and differentiation of hematopoietic cells are normally regulated by stromal cells, fibroblasts, endothelial cells, macrophages, and adventitial reticulum cells.[12] The cell-to-cell information required for these functions is transmitted by diffusable growth factors via cell junctions of the hematopoietic progenitor cells and the stromal cells.

Colony-Stimulating Factors

The regulation of hematopoiesis is a complex biologic process involving multifactorial mechanisms. A relatively small and common set of pluripotent stem cells gives rise to large numbers of functionally diverse mature cells. Cell proliferation and differentiation is regulated and controlled by highly specified protein factors, affecting single- and multiple-lineage hematopoiesis. These growth-promoting factors are named colony-stimulating-factors (CSFs) (also refered to as cytokines or hematopoietic growth factors). CSFs are a group of glycoproteins with a molecular weight of 18 to 90 kd, defined by their abilities to support proliferation and differentiation of hematopoietic cells of various lineages (Fig. 31-1).

Although most CSFs possess similar and sometimes overlapping activities, no sequence homology or common secondary structure exists between any of the CSFs except interleukin 6 (IL-6) and granulo-

Fig. 31-1. Role of colony-stimulating factors (CSF) in the evolution from the pluripotent stem cell to mature effector myeloid cell. SCF, stem cell factor; CFU, colony-forming unit; IL, interleukin; GEMM, granulocyte, erythroid, macrophage, megakaryocyte; ?, putative factor; G, granulocyte; GM, granulocyte macrophage; EO, eosinophil; M, macrophage; Baso, basophil.

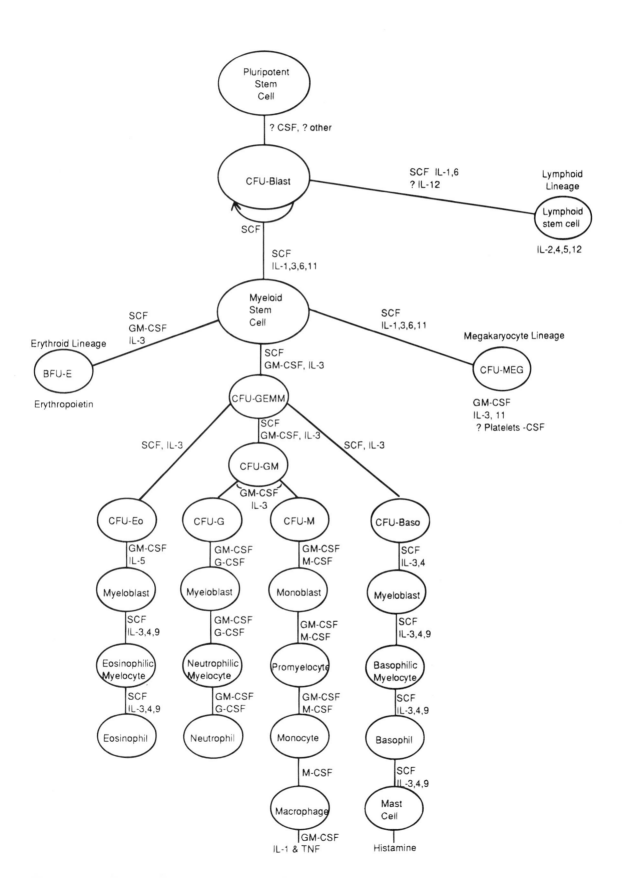

cyte colony-stimulating factor (G-CSF). Most factors are synthesized with a hydrophobic leader peptide that is proteolytically cleaved from the active molecule. The carbohydrate component is variable according to the tissue source, is not required for receptor binding or activation, and may play a role in protecting these proteins from degradation. Attempts to derive or synthesize small segments of the CSFs have failed to generate the biologic effects of the whole molecule, suggesting that a complex three-dimension configuration of the molecule is essential for biologic activity.

Each growth factor is coded for by a single unique gene and a cluster of genes. GM-CSF, IL-3, IL-4, IL-5, G-CSF, and M-CSF (macrophage colony-stimulating factor) receptors are located on the long arm of chromosome 5 in humans. The full implication of this clustering remains to be determined.

The rate of hematopoiesis and specific lineage proliferation and differentiation is controlled by up-regulation of receptors induced by growth factors and by down-regulation by inhibitors such as interferons, macrophage-inhibiting protein 1α, transforming growth factor-β, and tumor necrosis factor (TNF).[13] There are at least two classes of CSFs that influence hematopoiesis and effector cell differentiation. Class I includes IL-1, IL-3, IL-6, IL-11, stem cell factor (SCF, Steel factor), and the recently identified IL-12. These factors affect the production of multilineage blood cell formation and regulate the proliferation of early committed progenitor cells. The class II factors act on committed cell progenitors and have effects on the activation and function of mature effector cells. These are GM-CSF, G-CSF, M-CSF, and erythropoietin.

CSFs appear to be the major regulators of increased peripheral blood cell production during states of sepsis or increased demand.[14-16] Of these factors, only GM-CSF and G-CSF are available for clinical use at this time. Both are recombinant products, similar in activity to the naturally occurring proteins. Numerous studies in adults have documented that both factors are capable of stimulating the proliferation of myeloid progenitor cells in the bone marrow, inducing the release of the bone marrow NSP, and enhancing mature neutrophil effector function.[17,18]

NEONATAL LEUKOCYTE COUNT IN HEALTH AND DISEASE

Hematopoietic progenitor cells are first observed in the yolk sac at 3 weeks' gestational age. Progenitor cells from the vascular system of the yolk sac migrate into the liver to form the fetal liver extramedullary hematopoiesis. Neutrophils are the last of the fetal blood cells to appear, possibly because the fetus exists in a sterile environment and is unlikely to acquire an infection. The total granulocyte number is lower at 18 to 21 weeks' gestational age than at the end of pregnancy (2.8×10^8/L and 1.77×10^9/L, respectively).[19] This late maturation of the neutrophil system might be responsible, at least in part, for the high incidence of bacterial infections and sepsis in the premature newborn.

The total white blood cell count and differential provides a useful clinical tool for evaluation of a variety of medical situations. Increased numbers of mature neutrophils are released to the peripheral blood from the bone marrow in response to different stimuli generated by infection, providing the cells necessary for host resistance to bacterial infection. Relating the total white blood cell count to adult values has been of little clinical use in the evaluation of neonatal sepsis because of the variation in values and the overlap in values between normal and sick infants.[20-22] The number of circulating neutrophils increases immediately following birth. The peak values occur between 12 and 14 hours of age, with a minimum of 7,800 cells/μl and a maximum of 14,500 cells/μl. Following this peak, the cell count starts to decline. The minimum value of 1,750 total neutrophils/μl is established by 72 hours of age, and the maximum level of 5,400 neutrophils/μl is not reached until 120 hours (Fig. 31-2). According to the criteria set by Manroe et al.,[14] neutropenia in the presence of respiratory distress in the first 72 hours had an 84 percent likelihood of signifying bacterial infection. A "shift to the left," meaning the release of younger, immature nonsegmented cells to the peripheral blood in response to infection, has also been of value for early diagnosis of bacterial infection.[4,5,8,23,24] A variety of methods has been used for evaluation of the shift to the left, such as the absolute band count, the band/segment ratio, the band/total neutrophil ratio, and the immature/total neutrophil ratio.[4,5,8,23-26]

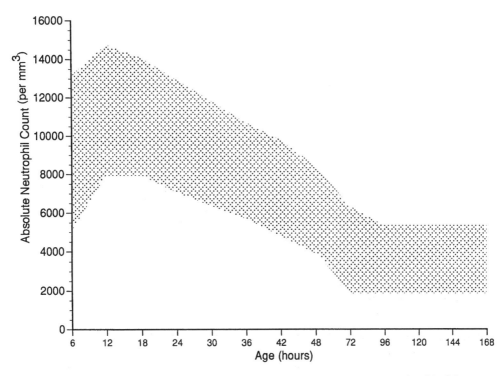

Fig. 31-2. The shaded area represents the range of total absolute neutrophil counts in healthy full-term neonates during the first week of life.

Peripheral neutropenia is a common finding in neonatal sepsis and is associated with a poor prognosis.[2] Neutropenia may be caused by any one or a combination of several disturbances in production, maturation, or release. The pathophysiologic mechanisms responsible for neonatal neutropenia may be either exhaustion of myeloid precursor cells or inadequate responses to proliferative or maturation signals.

The mechanisms of neutropenia and depletion of the bone marrow neutrophil storage pool, which occur in neonatal sepsis, have been studied in the neonate rat. Following infection with group B *Streptococcus*, adult rats respond with a transient decrease in circulating neutrophil counts followed by a significant increase associated with a two- to threefold increase of the progenitor pool (CFU-GM) and an increase in the CFU-GM proliferative rate to 75 percent of maximal capacity.[10,27] In contrast, neonate animals under the same conditions decrease CFU-GM by almost 50 percent and fail to increase

their myeloid proliferative rate above 70 to 80 percent of maximal capacity. Most importantly, during experimental sepsis, neonate rats further deplete their already-reduced NSP reserves by almost 80 percent, compared to a decline of 33 percent in adult rats.[10,27,28]

Similar incidences of neutropenia during neonatal sepsis have been documented in human neonates.[9,29] It has been hypothesized that the septic newborn is also unable to replenish neutrophil reserves because the myeloid storage pool and the NSP are small and the myeloid proliferative rate is already maximal and cannot be increased.

An additional explanation for neutropenia in the septic newborn is a defect in the regulation of bone marrow neutrophil release. A release of 10 percent of bone marrow reserves has been documented in adult rats treated with a subcutaneous inflammatory stimulus, compared to greater than 80 percent release in neonate rats treated under the same experimental conditions.[30]

In summary, neutropenia in the neonate is likely to be a result of several factors: (1) both the myeloid progenitor pool and the NSP contain relatively small reserves; (2) the myeloid proliferative rate is near maximum and cannot meet the increasing demands in a septic state; and (3) there is a defect in regulation of release and mobilization of the neutrophil from the bone marrow reserves to the peripheral blood.

Neonatal Colony-Stimulating Factor Levels

The biology of endogenous CSFs in fetal and neonatal life is yet unknown and data regarding their levels are conflicting. Laver et al.[31] have studied the plasma levels of G-CSF and GM-CSF and the frequency of GM-CFUs in the umbilical cord blood of normal full-term neonates. Plasma levels of G-CSF and GM-CSF at birth were significantly higher than adult levels. Meister et al.[32] have compared IL-3, IL-6, GM-CSF, and erythropoietin cord blood levels of 19 preterm and 20 full-term neonates. While no statistical differences between the two groups were found in levels of IL-6, IL-3, and GM-CSF, levels of erythropoietin were significantly higher in cord blood of term infants. Cairo et al.[33] compared circulating serum levels of stem cell factor (SCF) and G-CSF in preterm and term neonates with adults. There were no significant differences in SCF serum levels between preterm and term neonates and adults. In addition, there were no differences in G-CSF levels between third-trimester maternal levels and matched full-term newborns. However, G-CSF levels were higher in preterm neonates compared with full-term infants and adults. Russell et al.[34] have studied G-CSF levels at birth and their relationship with neutrophil count and various perinatal conditions. High G-CSF levels at birth were associated with infection and maternal pregnancy-induced hypertension, but not with gestational age. Gessler et al.[35] reported G-CSF serum levels at birth with respect to neutrophil count, infection, and gestational age. Serum concentrations of G-CSF in full-term and preterm neonates without infection reached peak levels within the first 7 hours of life (mean values: 261 pg/ml and 126 pg/ml in full-term and preterm neonates, respectively). Levels fell to normal adult range (< 50 pg/ml) between 4 and 7 days of age, and were unchanged at at 2 to 3 weeks of age. Peak G-CSF levels preceded peak neutrophil levels between 7

and 12 hours of life, which was similar to the interval noted between exogenous administration of recombinant G-CSF and neutrophilia seen in other clinical settings.[36-38] Mean serum concentrations of G-CSF at birth were higher in neonates older than 37 weeks' gestation compared with neonates of 32 to 37 weeks' gestation. These differences resulted in higher neutrophil counts in full-term neonates. Full-term and preterm neonates with signs of bacterial infection soon after birth had significantly higher levels of G-CSF compared with noninfected neonates. Neonates born to mothers with maternal pregnancy-induced hypertension tended to have lower but not significantly different G-CSF levels and neutrophil counts compared with healthy neonates. The lower G-CSF levels in offsprings of mothers with maternal pregnancy-induced hypertension could explain, in part, the neutropenia reported in these infants.[39]

In summary, although the data are conflicting, it seems that higher levels of G-CSF and possibly GM-CSF are correlated with gestational age, presence of infection, and maternal pregnancy-induced hypertension.

Neonatal Neutrophil Function

Numerous reports have documented functional defects in vitro in neutrophils obtained in neonates with sepsis. Effective neutrophil activity depends on normal propagation of three phases of neutrophil function: chemotaxis, phagocytosis, and intracellular killing. Chemotaxis is the first step in the inflammatory response, consisting of a series of processes that starts with stimuli from the invading microorganism and continuing with the directed migration of the PMN to the site of invasion, while changes in biochemical activity and shape are taking place. Defects in chemotaxis of the neonatal neutrophil include abnormal motility of neutrophils derived from cord blood, decreased deformability, decreased generation of filamentous actin, defective adherence, decreased migration, and irreversible aggregation when exposed to chemotactic factors.[19-25]

Phagocytosis is the second phase of neutrophil activity. The phagocytic activity of neonatal neutrophils has been reported to be similar to that of neutrophils obtained from adults when assayed in the presence of normal adult serum or plasma.[21,26] However, when assayed under conditions of "stress," neonatal neutrophils appear to have deficient phagocytosis.[21]

The ultimate phase of neutrophil activity after it has successfully recognized and phagocyted the microorganism is the intracellular killing of the invader. The major bactericidal function of the neutrophil is carried out by an oxygen-dependent chain of reactions that are called the respiratory burst, in which toxic oxygen metabolites, such as hydrogen peroxide, superoxide anion, and hydroxyl radicals, are produced. Superoxide anion production in PMNs obtained from neonates is comparable to that in adults cells; however, hydroxyl radical production is decreased.[26,40] Direct bacterial killing tests measuring the actual killing capacity of PMNs have shown decreased activity by neonatal PMNs during overwhelming stress or infection.[41,42]

In summary, although the data is not conclusive, the large body of information available provides indirect evidence that neonatal neutrophil functions are decreased either by humural or cellular defects. These defects in chemotaxis, phagocytosis, and intracellular killing appear to play a significant role in the increased susceptibility to infection in the neonate.

GRANULOCYTE TRANSFUSION

The quantitative and qualitative abnormalities in myelopoiesis and circulating neutrophils found in the newborn have suggested a possible role for granulocyte (neutrophil) transfusions in addition to antimicrobial therapy in the treatment of overwhelming sepsis. The results of clinical trials in adults seem to be inconclusive. While a significant overall benefit for granulocyte transfusion was found in some studies,[43,44] such an effect could not be demonstrated in others.[45,46] Possible explanations for this inconsistency include the low number of harvested neutrophils obtained with early apheresis technology, the defective neutrophil functions occurring with some of these techniques, and the extremely short ex vivo and in vivo life span of neutrophils compared to red blood cells and platelets. A meta-analysis of results of the controlled studies of PMN transfusions in adults has demonstrated that granulocyte transfusions are likely to offer benefit to infected neutro-

penic patients only when an adequate number of compatible granulocytes is given.[47]

The efficacy of granulocyte transfusion in neonatal sepsis was first evaluated in animal models. The administration of human or dog granulocytes during experimental group B streptococcal sepsis (GBS) has resulted in a significant improvement of survival in newborn rats and dogs, respectively.[27,48] Several controlled clinical studies evaluating granulocyte transfusion for neonatal sepsis were done. Laurenti et al.[49] demonstrated that a group of 20 premature newborn infants with sepsis who received between 2 and 15 daily granulocyte transfusions in addition to antibiotics had a significantly lower mortality rate compared to a control group of 18 newborns who were treated with antibiotics alone (10 percent versus 72 percent, respectively; $P < .001$). In a controlled randomized study, Christensen et al.[50] reported the effect of leukocyte transfusions in patients with severe depletion of their neutrophil storage marrow pool (consisting of leukocytes, bands, and metamyelocytes). The survival rate was 100 percent in a group of 7 patients who received a single PMN transfusion obtained by continous-flow centrifugation leukapheresis (0.7×10^9), compared to 11 percent (1 of 9 patients) in the control group.

Cairo et al. conducted two prospective and randomized trials to evaluate the potential role of granulocyte transfusion in treating human neonatal sepsis.[51,52] Infants were eligible for each study if they met the following criteria: weighing more than 1,000 g, age over 28 days, and admittance to the neonatal intensive care unit with signs and symptoms of overwhelming neonatal sepsis. These criteria allow for inclusion of patients presenting clinically with neonatal sepsis, an emergency situation calling for immediate decisions without the luxury of waiting for a definitive diagnosis. In the first study,[51] 35 newborns with at least one criterion of neonatal sepsis were randomized to receive either granulocyte transfusion or no other adjuvant therapy in addition to standard antimicrobial therapy. Twenty-one septic infants received leukapheresed granulocytes obtained by continous-flow centrifugation leukapheresis (0.5 to 1×10^9), and 14 infants were randomized to the control group. Survival rate was 20 of 21 (95 percent) and 9 of 14 (64 percent) in the treatment and control groups, respectively ($P < .05$). Twenty of 35 patients had age-corrected neutropenia, and only 3 of 35 (9 percent) were found to have a depleted NSP. In the second study,[52] 35 patients were randomized to receive either granulocyte transfusion or intravenous immunoglobulin (IVIG) as adjuvant therapy to antibiotics. There was a significantly different survival rate in the group receiving granulocyte transfusion (100 percent; 21/21) compared with the group receiving IVIG (64 percent; 9/14; $P < .03$).

In contrast to the studies using leukapheresed granulocytes, two controlled studies using granulocyte concentrates in buffy coat showed no advantage in the treatment of neonatal sepsis. Baley et al.[53] reported in a randomized prospective study the role of buffy coat transfusion in neutropenic neonates with presumed sepsis (14) or necrotizing enterocolitis (11). All patients had age-corrected peripheral neutropenia; however, marrow depleted NSP (< 7 percent) was present in only 9 of 25 patients (36 percent). The buffy coats were obtained and stored for a maximum of 24 hours before use. The mean total number of PMNs obtained by this method (0.35×10^9) was significantly lower than the number usually obtained by leukapheresis. The survival rates in the 14 patients with sepsis were 50 percent and 63 percent in the treatment and control groups, respectively. Survival of the 11 patients with necrotizing enterocolitis was 83 percent for the patients given PMN transfusions and 80 percent for the controls. This study evaluated three separate neonatal populations: those under 1,500 g with presumed sepsis, those over 1,500 g with presumed sepsis, and those with necrotizing enterocolitis. Results were reported

as a single group, whereas in reality these were three different groups, each with a different clinical course and outcome, requiring separate randomization. Wheeler et al.[54] looked at the role of stored buffy coat transfusions in the treatment of neonatal sepsis with marrow NSP depletion. The dose of PMNs was similar to that reported by Baley (0.4×10^9). Only 4 neonates with NSP depleted marrow received PMN transfusions. The mortality was equal in both groups. In contrast to studies reporting successful use of PMN transfusions using leukopheresed PMNs, Baley and Wheeler used buffy coat from units of whole blood–harvested PMNs. Buffy coat preparations have a significant advantage of immediate availability and are somewhat less expensive. However, buffy coat preparations have not been proven to be efficacious in sepsis with neutropenia in other settings. Differences in in vivo neutrophil function, a shortened lifespan of PMNs in stored blood, and the lower number of granulocytes in buffy coat preparations may account for the different results in these studies. Table 31-1 summarizes the results of studies investigating the use of granulocyte transfusions in neonatal sepsis.

Granulocyte transfusion seems to be more effective in sepsis in neonates than it in adults. One possible explanation is that the average of cells per harvest is 1 to 2×10^{10}, only about 10 percent of the daily adult granulocyte production, but about twice the average daily production of a neonate. In addition, differences in the distribution of transfused granulocytes in organs of newborn and adult experimentally septic rats have been documented by Baley

Table 31-1. Use of Granulocyte Transfusion in the Treatment of Neonatal Sepsis

Author	Observation	Granulocyte Transfusion (%)	Control (%)	Dose of PMN	Number Transfusions	Method	Statistical Analysis
Laurenti et al.[49]	Mortality[b]	2/20 (10)	13/18 (72)	0.75×10^9	2–15	CFL	$P < .01$
	Mortality[a]	1/10 (10)	10/11 (91)				$P < .001$
Christiansen et al.[50]	Survival	7/7 (100)	1/9 (11)	0.7×10^9	1	CFL	NA
Baley et al.[53]	Survival	3/6 (50)	5/8 (63)	0.35×10^9	1–3	BC	NS
Wheeler et al.[54]	Survival	2/4 (50)	2/5 (40)	0.5×10^9	1	BC	NS
Cairo et al.[51,52]	Survival	41/42 (98)	18/28 (64)	$0.75–1 \times 10^9$	5	CFL	$P < .05$

[a] Overall survival
[b] Survival for very low birth weight ($<$1,500 g) infants.
Abbreviations: NA, not available; CFL, continuous-flow leukapheresis filtration; BC, buffy coat; NS, not significantly different; PMN, polymorphonuclear neutrophils.

et al.[53] The investigators transfused Cr-labeled human granulocytes in animals several hours after inoculation of either group B *Streptococcus* or placebo, and demonstrated that granulocyte transfusion had different effects on newborn rats compared to adult rats. Both granulocytes and bacteria could penetrate the brain and lungs more readily in neonates than in adults.

Several questions still remain to be answered regarding the future use of granulocyte transfusion in the treatment of neonatal sepsis. Issues awaiting further study include selection criteria to define the groups of patients who require early granulocyte transfusion, the optimal number of harvested granulocytes, optimal doses, and the role of plasma factors, such as intravenous gammaglobulins and cytokines, which influence the opsonization and phagocytosis of PMNs. The benefits of PMN transfusion must be weighed against reported side effects, such as fluid overload and congestive heart failure, the potential for graft-versus-host disease if the product is not irradiated, pulmonary failure, cytomegalovirus, human immunodeficiency virus, hepatitis infections, and alloimmunization. Until further information is gathered, granulocyte transfusion should be considered as an adjuvant therapy to antibiotics only for situations highly suspicious for bacterial sepsis. The diagnosis of neonatal sepsis is most likely to be based on the clinical presentation and immediately available laboratory findings, such as age-corrected neutropenia, Gram stains, and serologic evidence of infection. The use of colony-stimulating factors capable of inducing both progenitor cell proliferation and differentiation may potentially limit the use of granulocyte transfusions to patients with significantly depleted NSP and peripheral neutropenia.

A definitive conclusion regarding the use of granulocyte transfusion awaits further investigation in larger randomized, prospective, and multicenter trials. The benefit demonstrated in patients receiving granulocyte transfusion may in fact be secondary to other factors found in the apheresis material, such as fibronectin, complement, and cytokines.[52] Granulocyte transfusions are associated with morbidity, are difficult to obtain and expensive, and their benefits must be carefully contrasted with their possible side effects.[52] Granulocyte transfusions should be considered as an additional treatment to antibiotic therapy limited to neonates with very strong evidence of bacterial septicemia with age-corrected neutropenia.[14]

The granulocyte product should be obtained by leukapheresis from a donor who has been tested seronegative for human immunodeficiency virus, cytomegalovirus, syphilis, and hepatitis viruses. Preferably, there should be erythrocyte compatability between the donor and neonate. The volume for a single transfusion should be 15 ml/kg, containing 1 to 2×10^9 granulocytes/kg. If the neonate is premature or if there is other evidence suggesting immune deficiency, the product should be 25 Gy (see Ch. 42). Such doses do not damage mature neutrophils or platelets, although they may have some effect on the red cells.[55] A course of treatment should consist of five transfusions over the first five days of life. Additional courses might be necessary if neutropenia and sepsis persist.

INTRAVENOUS IMMUNOGLOBULIN

Rationale for Use in Neonates

In addition to the quantitative and qualitative neutrophil defects, reduced activity of other arms of immunity may further compromise the antimicrobial defenses of neonates. IgG is acquired transplacentally by the fetus. Since most of the IgG is transferred in the late phases of gestation, premature neonates have decreased levels of IgG.[56] Transplacentally transferred immunoglobulins are limited to those acquired by the mother through previous exposures. Newborns—especially preterm infants—may have both a low concentration and an inadequate spectrum of opsonic IgG. IVIG preparations have been shown to contain opsonic antibodies against bacteria with polysacharide capsules.[57–60] Therefore, IVIG may theoretically enhance the immune systems efforts against bacterial infection. Several animal studies have suggested that immunoglobulin may be of value in correcting some of the immunologic defects of premature and full-term newborns. Under controlled experimental conditions, investigators were able to demonstrate that prophylactic or therapeutic administration of IVIG to neonatal animals resulted in improved survival and a decrease in incidence of infection.[48,58,61–63] These preliminarily promising data prompted the investigation of IVIG administration as a strategy for the prevention and treatment of life-threatening infections in newborns.

Effects of Administration in Neonates

Infusion of IVIG results in an increase in serum IgG levels. It has been shown to enhance the capacity of serum from human neonates to deposit IgG antibodies onto bacteria.[64] In addition, IVIG increased the opsonization of various types of group B *Streptococci* toward ingestion and killing by neutrophils from adults.[65]

Use of IVIG in human newborns is safe; no unwanted effects were observed when IVIG was administered to healthy premature newborns.[66,67] Premature neonates who received 750 to 1,000 mg/kg IVIG weekly during their hospitalization maintained higher IgG levels compared to babies who did not receive IVIG.[66,67] von Muralt et al.[68] tried a different approach by transfusing IVIG to pregnant women with signs of infection who were at risk of preterm delivery. Mothers were randomized to receive low doses of IVIG (12 g, 1 day) or high (24 g, 5 days) or received no treatment as a control group. None of the mothers or newborn infants experienced adverse side effects from IVIG. Levels of IVIG in maternal serum and cord blood were the same in the low-dose and control groups. Levels in the high-dose group were higher; however, an increase in cord blood IgG level occured only when treatment was given after 32 weeks' gestation. Therefore, this approach cannot be used for IVIG therapy in premature infants since IVIG seems to be of greater importance in this age group.

Prevention of Sepsis

Several studies have evaluated the role of IVIG in preventing sepsis in neonates and especially in preterm babies. Whereas some studies suggest that IVIG may provide protection against overwhelming neonatal sepsis when given early after birth,[69–73] other studies have shown no difference between IVIG and placebo in preventing infection.[74–76] Haque et al.[69] gave 50 normal newborn infants weighing less than 1,500 g 125 mg/kg IVIG on day 1; another 50 infants received IVIG on days 1 and 8, and 50 control newborn infants did not receive IVIG. Eight of the 50 control patients developed sepsis, compared to 4 of

100 patients receiving IVIG, suggesting a beneficial effect for IVIG prophylactic therapy. Chirico et al.[70,77] reported 83 preterm neonates and high-risk full-term babies who received either 500 mg/kg IVIG every week for 4 weeks or no IVIG therapy. IVIG was given within 24 hours of birth. The differences between the IVIG-treated and control groups in this study were statistically significant: 31 of 40 (77 percent of control babies developed infection and 13 (32 percent) died, whereas 22 of 43 (51 percent) of IVIG-treated patients developed infection and 7 (16 percent) died. Among the high-risk infants, IVIG had no significant benefit compared to standard therapy.

Clapp et al.[71] have evaluated the efficacy of maintaining therapeutic immunoglobulin levels of over 700 mg/dl in 115 preterm babies who were randomized to receive prophylactic IVIG or placebo; an additional group of patients was not randomized and received no therapy. Sepsis was documented in 0 of 56 (0 percent), 7 of 59 (12 percent), and 9 of 85 (11 percent) in IVIG-treated, placebo-treated, and nonrandomized patients, respectively. The incidence of infection differed significantly between the treated and nontreated patients in this study ($P <$ .01). Serum levels of IgG were maintained around the "target level" of 700 mg/dl in patients who received IVIG, and none of these infants acquired nosocomial sepsis, whereas all patients in the placebo group in whom sepsis developed had serum IgG levels of less than 400 mg/dl. These data indicate that administration of IVIG to maintain sufficient levels of IgG may protect newborn infants and decrease the incidence of neonatal sepsis from nosocomial infection.

Conway et al.[78] reported results in 63 preterm newborn infants randomized either to receive prophylactic IVIG 200 mg/kg within 48 hours of life, then every 3 weeks during hospitalization, or to a no-therapy control group. Of the 55 evaluable patients, significantly fewer babies in the treatment group had infection (8 of 29 versus 17 of 26; $P <$ .01). However, the difference was not significant when only culture-proven sepsis was considered (8 versus 14; $P <$ .09) in the IVIG-treated group and controls, respectively.

Stabile et al.[74] compared the efficacy of IVIG in preventing neonatal sepsis. Ninety-four patients were randomized to receive 500 mg/kg IVIG given daily for the first 4 days of life and then weekly until 4 weeks of age or no therapy. Proven sepsis was documented in 5 of 46 (13 percent) and 3 of 48 (8 percent) of IVIG and control infants, respectively (P = .48). Mortality rates were 4 of 5 (80 percent) and 1 of 3 (33 percent) in the IVIG and control groups. Magny et al.[75] reported 235 preterm neonates at very high risk (with an endotracheal tube or umbilical catheter on admission) who were treated either with 500 mg/kg IVIG for the first 4 days of life and biweekly thereafter or with albumin. Infections occurred in 45 of 120 (38 percent) and 36 of 115 (31 percent) of IVIG-treated and albumin-treated patients and were not significantly different.

Results of three large prospective multicenter controlled studies with contradictive conclusions have been recently reported. Baker et al.[73] reported results of 588 very low birth weight (VLBW) newborns (< 1,500 g) who were randomized to receive either 500 mg/kg body weight IVIG on days 1 and 7 and every two weeks thereafter or albumin as placebo. Results of treatment were assessed at 56 days in both groups. The risk of first infection was lower and the duration until first infection occurred was longer in the IVIG-treated group. The overall duration of hospitalization for infection was 80 versus 100 days (P < .05) in the IVIG and control groups, respectively. During the 56 days, 10 of 287 (3 percent) patients given IVIG and 14 of 297 (5 percent) newborns given placebo died.

Bussel[72] reported a study of VLBW neonates (< 1,300 g) in which each newborn received a total of 5 days of IVIG at 1 g/day, four doses between days 1 and 5, and one on day 15, or an albumin placebo. Preliminary analysis showed that in the first 30 days, sepsis developed in 9 of 61 patients given IVIG and in 16 of 65 given placebo (P = .065). At 70 days, the number of patients who developed sepsis was similar in the two groups—20 and 23 in the IVIG and placebo groups, respectively. The level of serum IgG was significantly higher in the IVIG than in the placebo group for days 7 through 42. The data from both studies (Baker et al. and Bussel et al.) suggest that infusion of IVIG may be effective in decreasing the incidence of sepsis during the first month of life, but were at least nondecisive regarding the effect of IVIG on the overall rate of infection in newborn infants of VLBW.

The most conclusive results have been reported by Fanaroff et al.[76] This study of 2,416 VLBW newborn infants who were assigned to receive IVIG or placebo in phase I of the study, or IVIG and no therapy in phase II, has shown no significant differences between the IVIG and control groups. Infants weighing less than 1,000 g received 900 mg/kg IVIG and infants weighing 1,000 to 1,500 g were given 700 mg/kg. Nosocomial infection of the blood, meningitis, or urinary tract infections occurred in 208 of 1,204 patients (17.3 percent) given IVIG and 231 of 1,212 (19.1 percent) in the control group. Septicemia occurred in 15.5 percent and 17.2 percent of IVIG and control patients, respectively. The duration of hospitalization, complication of prematurity, and mortality were unaffected by IVIG therapy. The conclusion of this study was that prophylactic use of IVIG failed to reduce the incidence of nosocomial infections in VLBW infants.

Cairo et al. have prospectively studied newborns who were randomly selected to receive—in addition to standard supportive care—either granulocyte transfusion or IVIG.[52] There was a significantly different survival rate in the group receiving granulocyte transfusion (21 of 21; 100 percent) compared with the IVIG group (9 of 14; 64 percent; P < .03). This pilot study suggested a possible advantage for the use of granulocyte transfusion over IVIG in the adjuvant treatment of neonatal neutropenia and overwhelming bacterial sepsis. Table 31-2 summarizes studies investigating the efficacy of prophylactic IVIG.

Treatment of Sepsis

Four studies have shown that using IVIG with antibiotics for treatment of neonatal sepsis had no clear benefit over treatment with antibiotics alone. Sidiropoulos et al.[79] reported 82 neonates treated for presumed sepsis with antibiotics alone or antibiotics plus daily IVIG for 6 days. The total IVIG dose was 1.6 to 2.4 g/kg and 3.9 g/kg in preterm and full-term babies, respectively. There were no significant differences between the two groups with respect to morbidity and mortality in this study; the mortality rate in the preterm group was slightly lower in the antibiotics plus IVIG group. In a long-term follow-up, there were no differences between treatment groups in development, somatic growth, and immu-

Table 31-2. Use of IVIG in Prevention of Neonatal Sepsis

Author	Observation	IVIG (%)	Control (%)	IVIG Treatment	Statistical Significance
Haque et al.[69]	Infection[a]	2/50 (4)	8/50 (16)	120 mg/kg on day 1	$P < .005^c$
	Infection [b]	2/50 (4)	8/50 (16)	120 mg/kg on days 1, 8	
Chirico et al.[70]	Infection	2/43 (5)	8/40 (20)	500 mg/kg/week	$P = .044$
Clapp et al.[71]	Sepsis	0/56 (0)	16/144 (11)[d]	IVIG given to maintain IgG level >700 mg/dl	$P < .05$
Conway et al.[78]	Infection	8/29 (28)	17/26 (65)	200 mg/kg within 48 hr, then q3 weeks	$P < .01$
Stabile et al.[74]	Infection	5/46 (13)	3/48 (8)	500 mg/kg/day, days 1, 2, 3; then once a week	$P = .48$
Magny et al.[75]	Infection	45/120 (38)	36/115 (31)	500 mg/kg/day, days 0, 1, 2, 3, 17, 31	NS
Bussel[72]	Sepsis[e]	9/60 (15)	16/65 (25)	1 g/day × 4 days; then 1 g on day 15	$P = 0.065$
	Sepsis[f]	20/60 (33)	23/61 (38)		NS
Baker et al.[73]	Infection (first)	70/287	104/297 (35)	500 mg/kg/day, days 1, 7; then q2 weeks	rr = 0.7
	Sepsis (% infection)	50/81 (62)	75/118 (64)		NS
Fanaroff et al.[76]	Infection[d]	208/1204 (17)	231/1,212 (19)	700 or 900 mg/kg q14 days	NS
	Sepsis[d]	186/1204 (15)	209/1,212 (17)		NS

[a] First infection
[b] Overall infections.
[c] Both IVIG treatment groups combined versus control.
[d] Placebo and no therapy groups combined.
[e] Sepsis within the first 30 days of life.
[b] Sepsis within the first 70 days of life.
Abbreviations: relative risk, 95% confidence; IVIG, intravenous immunoglobulin.

nologic functions.[79] Haque et al.[80] reported on 150 preterm neonates who, in addition to receiving antibiotics, were randomized to one of three treatment groups—120 mg/kg of IVIG at birth, the same dose at birth and on day 8 after birth, or untreated controls. The IVIG product in this study was IgM-enriched: each 250 mg of the product contained 190 mg IgG and 30 mg each IgM and IgA. Sepsis was documented in 21 of 30 (70 percent) and 23 of 30 (77 percent) of immunoglobulin-treated and placebo-treated groups, respectively. Mortality rates were 1/21 (5 percent) of immunoglobulin-treated patients and 4/23 (23 percent) of placebo-treated patients. The results were not significantly different when an appropriate analysis was used (Fisher's exact test).[81] The addition of IgM to the product in this study seems to be physiologically insignificant. Friedman et al.[82] reported results of treatment with IVIG and antibiotics in 12 neonates with neutropenia and high titers of GBS antigens. The patients were compared with 12 historical controls with neutropenia and high GBS antigen titers treated with antibiotics alone. Mortality in the IVIG treated group was 2 of 12 (17 percent) compared with 7 of 12 (58 percent) in the historical control group. There was no significant difference between the groups ($P < .01$). However, this study, as well as others, suggested that IVIG may enhance recovery from neutropenia: PMN count at 24 hours after initiation of therapy was 8,000/mm^3 in the IVIG group versus 2,000/mm^3 in the antibiotics-alone group.

Weisman and Lorenzetti[83] reported the results of a large multicenter, double-blind, placebo-controlled study. In this study, 753 preterm neonates were treated 12 hours or less after birth with antibiotics and IVIG (500 mg/kg) or albumin (5 mg/kg). Total serum IgG was higher for 7 days in the IVIG group. During these first 7 days, the mortality rate was significantly higher in the albumin group. Whereas it seems that death was delayed by treat-

Table 31-3. Use of IVIG for Treatment of Neonatal Sepsis

Author	Observation	IVIG (%)	Control (%)	Comment	Statistical Significance
Sidiropolous et al.[79]	Sepsis[a]	20/41 (49)	15/41 (37)	Efficacy shown in preterm babies; long-term follow-up showed no unwanted effect of use of IVIG	NS
	Mortality	2/21 (10)	4/15 (27)		$P = .16$
	Preterm mortality	1/31 (8)	4/9 (44)		$P = .04$
Haque et al.[80]	Sepsis[a]	21/30 (70)	23/30 (77)	Efficacy of IgM-enriched preparation not proven	$P < .001$
	Mortality	1/21 (5)	4/23 (17)		
Friedman et al.[82]	Mortality	2/12 (17)	7/12 (58)	Demonstrated effect on recovery from neutropenia	$P < .01$
Weisman and Lorenzetti[83]	Mortality	1/14 (7)	5/17 (29)	Improved survival in IVIG group for first 7 days; no difference on day 56	
Total	Sepsis	41/71 (58)	38/71 (54)		
	Mortality[b]	5/60 (8)	20/61 (33)		
	Mortality[c]	6/67 (9)	20/66 (30)		

[a] Proven sepsis.
[b] All treated newborns.
[c] Preterm low birth weight newborns.
Abbreviations: not significantly different; IVIG, intravenous immunoglobulin.

ment with IVIG, there was no difference in survival at 56 days. Table 31-3 summarizes studies of use of IVIG in treatment of established sepsis.

Current studies do not establish the efficacy of IVIG for either treating or preventing neonatal bacterial infections. Although the use of IVIG in preterm neonates with low levels of IgG is sound, given the current available data the prophylactic use of IVIG cannot be considered the standard of medical care in full-term or preterm neonates. Since the use of IVIG, especially in high doses, is associated with necrotizing enterocolitis, its use for prophylaxis therapy should be limited to the investigational setting only.

Infected neonates with overwhelming sepsis may benefit from IVIG as adjunctive therapy to antibiotics. Current data suggest that 500 to 1,000 mg/kg/dose would be appropriate for therapy. Repeat doses may need to be given every 2 weeks. Studies investigating the use of hyperimmune IVIG or monoclonal antibodies in treatment of neonatal sepsis are warranted.

COLONY-STIMULATING FACTORS

Effects on Neonatal Neutrophil Kinetics

Cairo et al.[84] have previously demonstrated that rhG-CSF, given to neonatal rats, induces neutrophilia similar to that seen in adult animals. Administration of rhG-CSF to newborn rats over a period of 7 days postnatally resulted in a profound peripheral neutrophilia within 24 hours and a sustained and increased response for the following 7 days. At the end of 7 days, an increase in bone marrow NSP without the depletion of early bone marrow progenitor cells has been documented.[84] The effect of single-pulse rhG-CSF in the treatment and prophylaxis of experimental GBS was recently evaluated in neonatal rats. Administration of a single intraperitoneal dose of rhG-CSF at the time of experimental GBS resulted in a synergistic effect on survival compared to animals treated with antibiotics alone (91 percent versus 28 percent, respectively; $P < .001$).[85] Additionally, Cairo et al. demonstrated the efficacy of rhG-CSF prophylaxis in newborn rats over control animals who received no adjuvant prophylactic CSF therapy.[84] In this study, newborn rats were treated with placebo or rhG-CSF for 7 days and were then inoculated with experimental GBS and then treated with or without antibiotics. Seventy-two hours after experimental GBS inoculation, there was still 100 percent survival in the rhG-CSF and antibiotic-treated group, as compared with survival of only 50 percent in the placebo and antibiotic group ($P <$ .001).

A similar effect has been demonstrated for rhGM-CSF. Newborn rats infected intraperitoneally with GBS were treated with rhGM-CSF 7 to 19 hours later. The mortality was 67 percent and 37 percent ($P =$ .003) and peritoneal cultures were positive in 86 percent and 44 percent ($P =$ .017) in the control and rhGM-CSF groups, respectively.[86] Several studies have addressed the effect of simultaneous administration of cytokines. Cairo et al. recently demonstrated that recombinant rat stem cell factor (rrSCF), an early-acting hematopoietic growth factor on neonatal rat hematopoiesis, does not induce a significant increase in the peripheral neutrophil or platelet count when administered alone.[87] However, when administered simultaneously with rhG-CSF, there was a significant increase in the peripheral neutrophil count, an increase in bone marrow NPS, and an increase in bone marrow as well as extramedullary myeloid proliferative rate compared with rhG-CSF alone. These effects were associated with a decreased mortality rate during experimental GBS compared to the effect of rhG-CSF alone.

Cairo et al. have also demonstrated that 14-day administration of rhIL-11, a new hematopoietic cytokine isolated from primate stromal cells, results in an increase in platelet count in neonatal rats, with little effect on the circulating neutrophil count.[88] The combination of rhIL-11 administered either sequentially or simultaneously with rhG-CSF induces an increase in peripheral neutrophil count, bone marrow NSP, bone marrow CFU-GM, and CFU-GM proliferative rate over similar administration of rrSCF with rhG-CSF.[87] Although the combination of rhIL-11 and rhG-CSF induced an increase in circulating neutrophils, it failed to reduce the mortality rate during experimental GBS infection in newborn rats. Other mechanisms besides augmentation of myelopoiesis may play a role in the difference in the prophylactic capacity between the combinations of rhIL-11 with rhG-CSF[88] and rrSCF with rhG-CSF.[87] An increase in bone marrow mast cell pool seen by treatment with rrCSF but not with IL-11 may play a role in enhancing neonatal rat host defense. These studies suggest that a combination of two or more cytokines may be needed for an optimal and comprehensive moduation of host defense.

Effects on Neutrophil Function

CSFs have been reported to enhance multiple functions in granulocytes obtained from adults, including enhanced phagocytosis,[89,90] superoxide production,[91] lysosomal secretion,[89] membrane depolarization responses,[92] and adhesion.[93] GM-CSF was also reported to act as a chemoattractant on one hand and as an inhibitor of migration on the other.[94,95] In contrast to the vast data collected on granulocytes obtained from adults, little is known of the effects of rhGM-CSF on functions of neutrophils derived from neonates. Cairo et al. demonstrated that chemotaxis, superoxide anion generation, and bacterial killing were enhanced by rhGM-CSF.[96] In vitro studies have documented enhanced neutrophil C3bi expression and increased adhesion and aggregation of neutrophils from cord blood incubated with rhGM-CSF.[97]

Production, Expression, and Membrane Receptors in Neonates

Recent studies have evaluated the affinity and number of CSF receptors on effector neutrophils and CSF production and mRNA expression in stimulated mononuclear cells obtained from neonatal and adult specimens. Cairo et al. investigated the affinity and quantity of rhGM-CSF receptors in neutrophils and GM-CSF production and GM-CSF mRNA expression from activated neonatal and adult T cells.[98] While the affinity and number of GM-CSF receptors were similar in neonatal and adult neutrophils, the GM-CSF production and GM-CSF mRNA expression were reduced in activated T cells derived from neonates compared to those from adults. Another set of investigations has shown that G-CSF and IL-3 production from stimulated adult mononuclear cells was higher than that from cord blood ($P <$ .007 and $<$ .02, respectively).[99] Additionally, there were significantly more G-CSF and IL-3 mRNA transcripts from adult than from cord mononuclear cells. No differences were found in affinity, binding, and number of G-CSF receptors on cord and adult peripheral effector cells. These studies suggest that (1) reduced endogenous production and decreased mRNA expression of CSFs and other cytokines may predispose the newborn to immature myeloproliferative response and to functional defects of the effector neutrophils and (2) an exogenous supply of CSFs will be met by a normal number of membrane receptors with normal affinity, which theoretically will allow propagation of the quantitative and qualitative effects of these cytokines.

Pilot Clinical Studies

A recent study investigated the safety, pharmacokinetics, and biologic efficacy of administration of rhG-CSF to newborn infants with sepsis.[100] Forty-two newborn infants (26 to 40 weeks' gestation) with presumed sepsis within the first 3 days of life were randomized to receive either placebo or varying doses of rhG-CSF. The growth factor was given for 3 days at doses of 1, 5, or 10 μg/kg every day or 5 or 10 μg/kg divided twice a day. The half-life of rhG-CSF was 4.4 ± 0.4 hours. Intravenous rhG-CSF was well tolerated at all gestational ages treated and was not associated with any recognized acute toxicity. RhG-CSF induced a significant increase in the absolute neutrophil count within 24 hours after doses of 5 and 10 μg/kg given either every 24 or divided every 12 hours. The increased neutrophil count was maintained for 96 hours, 48 hours after the last rhG-CSF dose. Bone marrow aspirates demonstrated a dose-dependent increase in the NSP after treatment with rhG-CSF. In addition, C3bi expression was significantly increased at 24 hours after 10 μg/kg of rhG-CSF given every 24 hours. The enhancement of neonatal neutrophil C3bi expression indicates that rhG-CSF may induce functional maturation in neonatal neutrophils.

Several other clinical investigations using CSFs in the treatment of neonatal sepsis are under way. These studies focus on investigating the use of rhG-CSF in large multicenter phase III studies as well as the use of other cytokines in the treatment of neonatal sepsis. Future clinical research should look at the long-term effects, if any, of treating newborn infants with CSFs.

In summary, the neonate's increased susceptibility has been attributed to neutropenia and decreased bone marrow NSP reserves and immature or defective neonatal neutrophil functions. The recombinant CSFs have been proven in animal models and in clinical experience in humans to stimulate the proliferation of myeloid progenitors and mature neutrophils and to enhance functional activation of mature effector neutrophils. Neonates at high risk of developing neonatal sepsis may ultimately benefit from treatment with combinations of rhGM-CSF, rhG-CSF, and other cytokines for both proliferative and functional enhancing therapy for the granulocyte.

REFERENCES

1. Siegel J, McCracken G: Sepsis neonatorum. N Engl J Med 304:642, 1981
2. Polin R, St. Geme J: Neonatal Sepsis. Adv Pediatr Infect Dis 7:25, 1992
3. Boyer K, Gadzala C, Burd L et al: Selective intrapartum chemoprophylaxis of neonatal group B streptococcal early-onset disease. I. Epidemiologic rationale. J Infect Dis 148:795, 1983
4. Mills E, Bjorksten B, Quie P: Deficient alternative complement pathway activity in newborn sera. Pediatr Res 13:1341, 1979
5. Edwards M, Buffone G, Fuselier P et al: Deficient classical complement pathway activity in newborn sera. Pediatr Res 17:685, 1983
6. Hill H: Host defenses in the neonate: prospects for enhancement. Semin Perinatol 9:2, 1985
7. Till J, McCulloch E: A direct measurement of the radiation sensitivity of normal mouse bone marrow cells. Radiat Res 14:213, 1961
8. Christensen R, Rothstein G: Pre- and post-natal development of granulocyte stem cells (CFUc) in the rat. Pediatr Res 18:599, 1984
9. Christensen R, Harper T, Rothstein G: Granulocyte-macrophage progenitor cells in term and preterm neonates. J Pediatr 109:1047, 1986
10. Christensen R, Hill H, Rothstein G: Granulocytic stem cell (CFU-C) proliferation in experimental group B streptococcal sepsis. Pediatr Res 17:278, 1983
11. Erdman S, Christensen R, Bradley P, Rothstein G: Supply and release of storage neutrophils: A developmental study. Biol Neonate 41:132, 1982
12. Torok-Storb B: Cellular interactions. Blood 72:373, 1988
13. Robinson N, Quesenberry P: Hematopoietic growth

factors: overview and clinical applications, part I. Am J Med Sci 300:163, 1990

14. Manroe B, Weinberg A, Rosenfeld C, Browne R: The neonatal blood count in health and disease. J Pediatr 95:89, 1979

15. Philip A, Hewitt J: Early diagnosis of neonatal sepsis. Pediatr 65:1036, 1980

16. Zipursky A, Palko J, Milner R, Akenzua G: The hematology of bacterial infections in premature infants. Pediatr 57:839, 1976

17. Clark S, Kamen R: The human hematopoietic colony-stimulating factors. Science 236:1229, 1987

18. Sieff C: Hematopoietic growth factors. J Clin Invest 79:1549, 1987

19. Anderson D, Hughes B, Smith C: Abnormal mobility of neonatal polymorphonuclear leukocytes: Relationship to impaired redistribution of surface adhesion sites by chemotactic factor or colchicine. J Clin Invest 68:863, 1981

20. Miller M: Chemotactic function in the human neonate: humoral and cellular aspects. Pediatr Res 5:487, 1971

21. Miller M: Phagocyte function in the neonate: selected aspects. Pediatr 64:709, 1979

22. Anderson D, Pickering L, Feigin R: Leukocyte function in normal and infected neonates. J Pediatr 85:420, 1974

23. Mease A, Burgess D, Thomas P: Irreversible neutrophil aggregation: a mechanism of decreased newborn neutrophil chemotactic response. Am J Pathol 104:98, 1981

24. Krause P, Herson V, Boutin-Lebowitz J et al: Polymorphonuclear leukocyte adherence and chemotaxis in stressed and healthy neonates. Pediatr Res 20:296, 1986

25. Klein R, Fischer T, Gard S et al: Decreased mononuclear and polymorphonuclear chemotaxis in human newborns. Pediatr 60:467, 1977

26. Ambruso D, Bentwood B, Henson P: Oxidative metabolism of cord blood neutrophils: Relationship to content and degranulation of cytoplasmic granules. Pediatr Res 18:1148, 1984

27. Christensen R, Macfarlane J et al: Blood and marrow neutrophils during experimental group B streptococcal infection: quantification of the stem cell, proliferative, storage and circulating pools. Pediatr Res 16:549, 1982

28. Christensen R, Shigeoka A, Hill H, Rothstein G: Circulating and storage neutrophil changes in experimental type II group B streptococcal sepsis. Pediatr Res 14:806, 1980

29. Christensen R, Rothstein G: Exhaustion of mature marrow neutrophils in neonates with sepsis. J Pediatr 96:316, 1980

30. Christensen R, Rothstein G: Efficiency of neutrophil migration in the neonate. Pediatr Res 14:1147, 1980

31. Laver J, Duncan E, Abboud M: High levels of granulocyte and granulocyte-macrophage colony-stimulating factors in cord blood of normal full-term neonates. J Pediatr 116:627, 1990

32. Meister B, Herold M, Mayr A et al: Interleukin-3, interleukin-6, granulocyte-macrophage colony-stimulating factor and erythropoietin cord blood levels of preterm and term neonates. Eur J Pediatr 152:569, 1993

33. Cairo M, Gillan E, Buzby J et al: Circulating Steel factor (SLF) and G-CSF levels in preterm and term newborn and adult peripheral blood. Am J Pediatr Hematol Oncol 15:311, 1993

34. Russell A, Davies E, McGuigan S et al: Plasma granulocyte-colony stimulating factor concentrations ([G-CSF]) in the early neonatal period. Br J Haematol 86:642, 1994

35. Gessler P, Kirchmann N, Kientsch-Engel R et al: Serum concentrations of granulocyte colony-stimulating factor in healthy term and preterm neonates and in those with various diseases including bacterial infections. Blood 82:3177, 1993

36. Gabrilove J: Clinical applications of granulocyte colony stimulating factor (G-CSF). Growth Factors 6:187, 1992

37. Lieschke G, Burgess A: Granulocyte colony-stimulating factor and granulocyte-macrophage colony-stimulating factor. N Engl J Med 327:28, 1992

38. Stute N, Santana V, Rodman J et al: Pharmacokinetics of subcutaneous recombinant human granulocyte colony-stimulating factor in children. Blood 79:2849, 1992

39. Koenig J, Christensen R: Incidence, neutrophil kinetics, and natural history of neonatal neutropenia associated with maternal hypertension. New Engl J Med 321:557, 1989

40. Shigeoka A, Charette R, Wyman M, Hill H: Defective oxidative metabolic responses of neutrophils from stressed neonates. J Pediatr 98:392, 1981

41. Quie P, Mills E: Bactericidal and metabolic function of polymorphonuclear leukocytes. Pediatr 64:719, 1979

42. Wright W, Ank B, Stiehm E: Decreased bacterial capacity of leukocytes of stressed newborns. Pediatr 56:579, 1975

43. Vogler W, Winton E: A controlled study of the efficacy of granulocyte transfusions in patients with neutropenia. Am J Med 63:548, 1977

44. Herzig R, Herzig G, Graw R et al: Successful granulocyte transfusion therapy for gram-negative septicemia. A prospectively randomized controlled study. N Engl J Med 296:701, 1977
45. Fortuny I, Bloomfield C, Hadlock D et al: Granulocyte transfusion: a controlled study in patients with acute nonlymphocytic leukemia. Transfusion 15:548, 1975
46. Winston D, Ho W, Gale R: Therapeutic granulocyte transfusions for documented infections. A controlled trial in ninety-five infectious granulocytopenic episodes. Ann Intern Med 97:509, 1982
47. Strauss R: Therapeutic granulocyte transfusion in 1993. Blood 81:1675, 1993
48. Santos J, Shigeoka A, Hill H: Functional leukocyte administration in protection against experimental neonatal infection. Pediatr Res 114:1408, 1980
49. Laurenti F, Ferro R, Isacchi G et al: Polymorphonuclear leukocyte transfusion for the treatment of sepsis in the newborn infant. J Pediatr 98:118, 1981
50. Christensen R, Rothstein G, Anstall H, Bybee B: Granulocyte transfusions in neonates with bacterial infection, neutropenia, and depletion of mature neutrophils. Pediatr 70:1, 1982
51. Cairo M: Granulocyte transfusions in neonates with presumed sepsis. Pediatr 80:738, 1987
52. Cairo M, Worcester C, Rucker R et al: Randomized trial of granulocyte transfusions versus intravenous immune globulin therapy for neonatal neutropenia and sepsis. J Pediatr 120:281, 1992
53. Baley J, Stork E, Warkentin P, Shurin S: Buffy coat transfusions in neutropenic neonates with presumed sepsis: a prospective randomized trial. Pediatrics 80:712, 1987
54. Wheeler J, Chauvenet A, Johnson C et al: Buffy coat transfusions in neonates with sepsis and neutrophil storage pool depletion. Pediatrics 79:422, 1987
55. Huestis DW, Glasser L: The neutrophil in transfusion medicine. Transfusion 34:630, 1994
56. Ballow M, Cates KL, Rose JC et al: Development of the immune system in very low birth weight (less than 1500 g) premature infants: concentrations of plasma immunoglobulins and patterns of infections. Pediatr Res 20:899, 1986
57. Bortolussi R, Issekutz T, Burbridge S, Schellekens H: Neonatal host defense mechanisms against listeria monocytogenes infection: the role of lipopolysaccharides and interferons. Pediatr Res 25:311, 1989
58. Fischer G, Wilson S, Hunter K: Functional characteristics of a modified immunoglobulin preparation for intravenous administration: summary of studies of opsonic and protective activity against group B streptococci. J Clin Immunol 2:31, 1982
59. Fischer G, Hemming V, Hunter K: Intravenous immunoglobulin in the treatment of neonatal sepsis: therapeutic strategies and laboratory studies. Pediatr Infect Dis 5:171, 1986
60. Hill H, Augustine N, Shigeoka A: Comparative opsonic activity of intravenous gamma globulin preparations for common bacterial pathogens. Am J Med 76:61, 1984
61. Harper T, Christensen R, Rothstein G: Effect of intravenous immunoglobulin G on neutrophil kinetics during experimental group B streptococcal infection in neonatal rats. Rev Infect Dis 8 (suppl.):S401, 1986
62. Harper T, Christensen R, Rothstein G: The effect of administration of IgG to newborn rats with E coli sepsis and meningitis. Pediatr Res 22:455, 1987
63. Redd H, Christensen R, Fisher G: Circulating and storage neutrophils in septic neonatal rats treated with immune globulin. J Infect Dis 157:705, 1988
64. Lassiter H, Speranza M, Hall R, Meade V, Christensen R, Packer C: Complement C3 deposition onto bacteria by neonatal serum is not enhanced after the infusion of intravenous immunoglobulin. J Perinatol 10:27, 1990
65. Diamond E, Puruggganan H, Choi H: Effect of prophylactic gamma globulin administration on infection morbidity in premature infants. Ill Med J 139:668, 1966
66. Homan S, Kurth C, Meade V, Hall R: Prophylactic intravenous immunoglobulin (IVIG) in the low birth weight (LBW) infant: infusion effects (abstract). Pediatr Res 23:464, 1988
67. Christensen R, Hardman T, Thornton J, Hill H: A randomized, double-blind, placebo-controlled investigation of the safety of intravenous immune globulin administration to preterm neonates. J Perinatol 9:126, 1989
68. von Muralt G, Sidiropoulos D: Experience with intravenous immunoglobulin treatment in neonates and pregnant women. Vox Sang 51:22, 1986
69. Haque K, Zaidi M, Haque S et al: Intravenous immunoglobulin for prevention of sepsis in preterm and low birth weight infants. Pediatr Infect Dis J 5:622, 1986
70. Chirico G, Rondini G, Plebani A et al: Intravenous gamma globulin therapy for prophylaxis of infection in high-risk neonates. J Pediatr 110:437, 1987
71. Clapp D, Kliegman R, Baley J et al: Use of intravenously administered immune globulin to prevent nosocomial sepsis in low birth weight infants: report of a pilot study. J Pediatr 115:973, 1989

72. Bussel J: Intravenous gammaglobulin in the prophylaxis of late sepsis in very-low-birth-weight infants: preliminary results of a randomized, double-blind, placebo-controlled trial. Rev Infect Dis 12 (suppl. 4): S457, 1990

73. Baker C, Melish M, Hall R et al: Intravenous immune globulin for the prevention of nosocomial infection in low-birth-weight neonates. The Multicenter Group for the Study of Immune Globulin in Neonates. N Engl J Med 327:213, 1992

74. Stabile A, Miceli Sopo S, Romanelli V et al: Intravenous immunoglobulin for prophylaxis of neonatal sepsis in premature infants. Arch Dis Child 63:441, 1988

75. Magny J-F, Bremard-Oury C, Brault D et al: Intravenous immunoglobulin therapy for prevention of infection in high-risk premature infants: report of a multicenter, double-blind study. Pediatr 88:437, 1991

76. Fanaroff A, Korones S, Wright L et al: A controlled trial of intravenous immune globulin to reduce nosocomial infections in very-low-birth-weight infants. N Engl J Med 330:1107, 1994

77. Chirico G, Rondini G, Regazzi M, Ugazio A: Pharmacokinetics and effectiveness of intravenous immunoglobulin in neonates (letter). J Pediatr 112:326, 1988

78. Conway S, Ng P, Howel D et al: Prophylactic intravenous immunoglobulin in preterm infants: a controlled trial. Vox Sang 59:6, 1990

79. Sidiropoulos D, Boehme U, von Muralt G et al: Immunoglobulin supplementation in prevention or treatment of neonatal sepsis. Pediatr Infect Dis J 5: S193, 1986

80. Haque K, Zaidi M, Bahakim H: IgM-enriched intravenous immunoglobulin therapy in neonatal sepsis. Am J Dis Child 142:1293, 1988

81. Weisman L, Cruess D, Fischer G: Standard versus hyperimmune intravenous immunoglobulin in preventing or treating neonatal bacterial infections. Clin Perinatol 20:211, 1993

82. Friedman C, Wender D, Temple D, Rawson J: Intravenous gamma globulin as adjunct therapy for severe group B streptococcal disease in the newborn. Am J Perinatol 7:1, 1990

83. Weisman L, Lorenzetti P: High intravenous doses of human immune globulin suppress neonatal group B streptococcal immunity in rats. J Pediatr 115:445, 1989

84. Cairo M, Plunkett J, Mauss D, van de Ven C: Seven-day administration of recombinant human granulocyte colony-stimulating factor to newborn rats: modulation of neonatal neutrophilia, myelopoiesis, and group B streptococcus sepsis. Blood 76:1788, 1990

85. Cairo M, Mauss D, Kommareddy S et al: Prophylactic or simultaneous administration of recombinant human granulocyte colony stimulating factor in the treatment of group B streptococcal sepsis in neonatal rats. Pediatr Res 27:612, 1990

86. Wheeler J, Givner L: Therapeutic use of recombinant human granulocyte-macrophage colony-stimulating factor in neonatal rats with type III group B streptococcal sepsis. J Infect Dis 165:938, 1992

87. Cairo M, Plunkett J, Nguyen A, van de Ven C: Effect of stem cell factor with and without granulocyte colony-stimulating factor on neonatal hematopiesis: in vivo induction of newborn myelopoiesis and reduction of mortality during experimental group B streptococcal sepsis. Blood 80:96, 1992

88. Cairo M, Plunkett J, Nguyen A et al: Effect of interleukin-11 with and without granulocyte colony-stimulating factor on in vivo neonatal rat hematopoiesis: induction of neonatal thrombocytosis by interleukin-11 and synergistic enhancement of neutrophilia by interleukin-11 + granulocyte colony-stimulating factor. Pediatr Res 34:56, 1993

89. Burgess A, Begley C, Johnson G et al: Purification and properties of bacterially synthesized human granulocyte-macrophage colony stimulating factor. Blood 69:43, 1987

90. Fleischmann J, Golde D, Weisbart R, Gasson J: Granulocyte-macrophage colony-stimulating factor enhances phagocytosis of bacteria by human neutrophils. Blood 68:708, 1986

91. Weisbart R, Kwan L, Golde D, Gasson J: Human GM-CSF primes neutrophils for enhanced oxidative metabolism in response to the major physiological chemoattractants. Blood 69:18, 1987

92. Sullivan R, Griffin J, Simons E et al: Effects of recombinant human granulocyte and macrophage colony-stimulating factors on signal transduction pathways in human granulocytes. J Immunol 139:3422, 1987

93. Arnaout M, Wang E, Clark S, Sieff C: Human recombinant granulocyte-macrophage colony-stimulating factor increases cell-to-cell adhesion and surface expression of adhesion-promoting surface glycoproteins on mature granulocytes. J Clin Invest 78:597, 1986

94. Gasson J, Weisbart R, Kaufman S et al: Purified human granulocyte-macrophage colony stimulating factor: Direct action on neutrophils. Science 226: 1339, 1984

95. Wang J, Colella S, Allavena P, Mantovani A: Chemo-

tactic activity of human recombinant granulocyte-macrophage colony-stimulating factor. Immunol 60: 439, 1987

96. Cairo M, van de Ven C, Toy C et al: Recombinant human granulocyte-macrophage colony stimulating factor primes neonatal granulocytes for enhanced oxidative metabolism and chemotaxis. Pediatr Res 26: 395, 1989

97. Cairo M, van de ven C, Toy C et al: GM-CSF primes and modulates neonatal PMN motility: upregulation of C3bi (Mo1) expression with alteration in PMN adherence and aggregation. Am J Pediatr Hematol Oncol 13:249, 1991

98. Cairo M, Suen Y, Knoppel E et al: Decreased stimu-

lated GM-CSF production and GM-CSF gene expression but normal numbers of GM-CSF receptors in human term newborns compared to adults. Pediatr Res 30:362, 1991

99. Cairo M, Suen Y, Knoppel E et al: Decreased G-CSF and IL-3 production and gene expression from mononuclear cells of newborn infants. Pediatr Res 31:574, 1992

100. Gillan E, Christensen R, Suen Y et al: A randomized, placebo-controlled trial of recombinant human granulocyte-colony stimulating factor administration in newborn infants with presumed sepsis: significant induction of peripheral and bone marrow neutrophilia. Blood 84:1427, 1994

Transfusion Support of Children with Hematologic and Oncologic Disorders

Heather Hume

This chapter focuses on the transfusion support of children with malignancies, congenital or acquired bone marrow failure syndromes, thalassemia and sickle cell disease (SCD), and other congenital hemolytic anemias. The transfusion support of patients with bleeding disorders is addressed elsewhere in this book.

The long-term survival of patients in all these categories is continually improving. Event-free survival for childhood acute lymphoblastic leukemia (ALL) exceeds 70 percent; more than 50 percent of children with cancer will be long-term survivors.[1,2] Children with severe acquired aplastic anemia who undergo bone marrow transplantation from an human leukocyte antigen (HLA)-compatible related donor have long-term survival and event-free survival rates of 96 percent and 71 percent, respectively.[3] Thalassemia patients are now surviving into the third decade of life; 50 percent of people with sickle cell anemia survive beyond the fifth decade.[4,5] Modern blood transfusion therapy is an integral part of the treatment of all these disorders and can contribute to the improved outlook for many of these patients. We must therefore continue to strive to provide optimal transfusion support, including, where appropriate, the use of specialized blood components, while minimizing as much as possible both the short- and long-term risks associated with transfusion therapy. Ideally, a transfusion medicine ex-

pert should be part of the team treating every child with a hematologic or oncologic disorder requiring multiple transfusions.

MALIGNANCIES

The majority of the studies addressing the transfusion support of patients with malignancies have involved children or adults undergoing treatment for acute leukemia. Because more intensive chemotherapeutic regimes are being used in the treatment of solid tumors in childhood, many of these patients now also require transfusion support. The issues involved in the transfusion support of these two groups of pediatric patients (i.e., patients with leukemia or solid tumors) are very similar and are therefore discussed together in the following sections. The same principles of blood transfusion support are also applicable to children undergoing autologous or allogeneic bone marrow transplantation. Special problems unique to the bone marrow transplantation setting are discussed in Chapter 34.

Red Blood Cell Transfusions

Anemia in children with malignances is usually due to bone marrow hypoplasia secondary to chemotherapy and/or to bone marrow infiltration with malignant cells. In some cases, in particular in the presence of nonhematologic malignancies, it may also be a reflection of the anemia of chronic disease (i.e., a defect in iron use combined with relatively low levels of endogenous erythropoietin).[6,7] Occasionally, anemia may be due to bleeding in association with thrombocytopenia and/or disseminated intravascular coagulation. In very small children, blood removed for laboratory testing may also be a contributing factor in the development of anemia. Finally, in a few cases, anemia in this group of patients may be due to other factors. For example, severe anemia due to B19 parvovirus infection and responsive to intravenous immunoglobin therapy has been reported in children with leukemia.[8,9] Immune hemolytic anemia, known to occur with penicillin use, has more recently been described with cephalosporins[10] (a class of antibiotics frequently used in this population), and hemolytic anemia, caused by a number of mechanisms (microangiopathic hemolytic anemia, immune hemolytic anemia, and oxidative hemolysis), has been associated with the use of some chemotherapeutic agents.[11]

In considering the indications for red blood cell (RBC) transfusions in this or any other pediatric population, it is important to remember that normal hemoglobin and hematocrit values are lower in children than adults. Normal ranges of hemoglobin values for children are shown in Table 32-1. These lower normal values may be explained at least partially by the finding that young children have slightly higher erythrocyte 2,3-diphosphoglycerate (2,3-DPG) levels than do adults, resulting in slightly higher P_{50} levels and a slightly lower hemoglobin oxygen affinity.[13]

While pediatric patients with malignancies may occasionally require RBC transfusions for acute anemia secondary to bleeding, the majority of RBC transfusions are given for a more slowly developing hypoproliferative anemia. The approach to the transfusion of patients with chronic anemia, as previously recommended by Petz and Tomasulo, can therefore be applied.[14] In summary, they propose the following cardinal principles: (1) do not transfuse simply on the basis of a given hemoglobin or hematocrit level; (2) try to establish which symptoms and signs are caused by anemia; (3) determine if the symptoms and signs that were attributed to anemia are alleviated by transfusion; and (4) determine that temporary relief of symptoms warrants the risks of continued transfusion.

Determining which symptoms are due to anemia may be difficult in this setting. For example, in a patient undergoing intensive therapy for a malignancy, fatigue may be caused or influenced by a variety of physical and/or psychological factors other than anemia. Children with other hypoproliferative disorders, such as iron deficiency anemia or Diamond-Blackfan anemia (DBA), often tolerate hemoglobin levels below 7.0 g/dl surprisingly well. In patients with chronic anemia, the eyrthrocyte 2,3-DPG levels are usually increased, resulting in an increased level of tissue oxygenation at any given hemoglobin level. It has been calculated that 2,3-DPG–induced changes may compensate for up to one half the expected oxygen deficit in association with anemia.[15,16] RBC 2,3-DPG levels have been shown to be increased in iron-deficiency anemia and a variety of other anemias.[17,18] Whether similar increases occur in children with malignancies has not been well studied. One older study in a small number of children with anemia and acute leukemia or solid tumors did show that the 2,3-DPG levels were appropriately elevated at diagnosis and in children receiving chemotherapy only. However, children with anemia and acute leukemia who had received both RBC transfusions and intensive chemotherapy did not have elevated 2,3-DPG levels.[19] Unfortunately, this study is too small to allow any generalizations concerning the RBC transfusion support of patients with malignancies.

It has been claimed that in patients with anemia and thrombocytopenia, maintaining hemoglobin levels in the near-normal range may decrease bleeding at a given platelet level.[20] However, there are no

Table 32-1. Normal Hemoglobin and Hematocrit Values in Children

Age	Hemoglobin (g/dl)		Hematocrit	
	Mean	− 2 SD	Mean	− 2 SD
2 months	11.5	9.0	0.35	0.28
0.5–2.0 years	12.0	10.5	0.36	0.33
2–6 years	12.5	11.5	0.37	0.34
6–12 years	13.5	11.5	0.40	0.35

(Adapted from Nathan and Oski,[12] with permission.)

studies in humans to substantiate this claim. Studies in humans with normal platelet counts have shown an inverse relationship between the bleeding time and the hematocrit level, as have studies in thrombocytopenic and nonthrombocytopenic animals.[21,22] Nevertheless, it is not known whether the prolongation of the bleeding time attributable to anemia actually increases the risk of bleeding.

There is evidence to suggest that maintaining a high hemoglobin level may shorten periods of neutropenia in children with malignant disease. In a prospective, randomized controlled study, published in 1976, of 30 children with various malignant diseases, children transfused to maintain a hemoglobin of 13.0 to 16.0 g/dl had a significantly more rapid rise in granulocyte count, lower incidence of infection, and lower incidence of interruption of chemotherapy than did children transfused to maintain a hemoglobin level of 8.5 to 12.0 g/dl.[23] The same group of investigators subsequently confirmed these results in a second prospective, controlled trial of 26 anemic, neutropenic children, all of whom had newly diagnosed ALL.[24] They hypothesized that suppression of erythropoiesis by hypertransfusion could lead to a greater influx of cells from the pluripotential stem-cell compartment into the granulocytic pathway. However, given the risks associated with transfusion therapy and the potential hypercoaguable state associated with malignant disease, it is unlikely that physicians today would be willing to maintain hemoglobin levels of 13 to 16 g/dl.

Recommendations have also been made that a near-normal hemoglobin level should be maintained in children undergoing radiotherapy.[25] Some cancer treatment protocols recommend this even when radiotherapy is being administered for microscopic disease only. Presumably, the justification for this recommendation is that the tumor tissue of anemic patients may be poorly oxygenated, and this in turn may lead to a suboptimal response to radiotherapy. However, the only tumor in which possible support for this hypothesis has been documented is carcinoma of the cervix.[14,26] Therefore, it appears unwarranted to administer RBC transfusions in order to maintain hemoglobin levels in the normal range in pediatric patients undergoing radiotherapy until such time as studies specific to childhood malig-

nancies are performed and the actual benefits can be assessed.

In summary, whereas many claims and recommendations have been made regarding the RBC transfusion support of children undergoing treatment for malignancies, very few scientific studies are available to assess the validity of these recommendations. Therefore, further study is merited. In light of the currently available data, it would appear reasonable to administer RBC transfusions to most patients with a hemoglobin level of less than 7.0 g/dl. Alternatively, if the hemoglobin level is above 7.0 g/dl and the patient is asymptomatic, there should be additional justification (other than the hemoglobin level per se) for administering a RBC transfusion. Possible situations in which a transfusion might be warranted include a falling hemoglobin level that is likely to decrease below 7.0 g/dl or the need to continue administering intensive chemotherapy in the immediate future, such as during remission induction therapy.

With the availability of human recombinant erythropoietin (rHuEPO), the possibility of increasing hematocrit levels and/or decreasing RBC transfusion requirements in oncology patients has begun to be investigated. Adult patients with anemia and malignant tumors have decreased endogenous erythropoietin levels when compared with patients with similar degrees of anemia due to iron deficiency, and they do not have the expected inverse linear relationship between serum erythropoietin levels and hemoglobin concentration.[7] The erythropoietin response is further blunted following the administration of chemotherapy. It is less clear whether such a relationship also exists in children. In a study performed in 12 children receiving chemotherapy, including cisplatin for malignant tumors, there was an inverse relationship between serum erythropoietin levels and hemoglobin concentrations in all patients (10/12) retaining at least 40 percent of their pretreatment renal function.[27]

The observations in adults have led to several studies of the use of rHuEPO in the treatment of anemia associated with cancer and cancer chemotherapy.[28–33] The data available to date suggest that the administration of rHuEPO in these patients does result in enhanced reticulocytosis and/or increased hematocrit levels as compared to those found in placebo-treated or historical controls. Reduced RBC transfusion requirements were observed in some, but not all, of these studies. Further studies, particularly in children, are required to determine the eventual role of rHuEPO in the supportive care of children with malignancies.

In general, the approach to the management of the acutely bleeding pediatric oncology patient should be the same as that for any child with hemorrhagic shock. The first steps, then, include the establishment of an adequate airway and assisted ventilation if necessary, attempts to control the bleeding (which in this population may more often include the use of antifibrinolytic agents, platelet transfusions, and/or fresh frozen plasma transfusions), and rapid volume expansion with Ringer's lactate. In acutely bleeding children without underlying hematologic disease, RBC transfusion is generally required after blood losses of more than 20 to 30 percent of the total blood volume in children 2 years of age or older; in infants younger than 6 months of age, RBC transfusion is required after losses of 15 percent of the total blood volume.[34] In children with malignancies, RBC transfusion may be required after smaller blood losses if the child was anemic prior to the onset of hemorrhage.

Platelet Transfusions

Before the availability of platelets for transfusion, hemorrhage in patients with severe thrombocytopenia was frequently fatal. In a report from the National Cancer Institute, hemorrhage was considered to have been the major cause of death in 52 percent of 414 acute leukemic patients studied from 1954 to 1963.[35] With the introduction of plastic blood collection systems in the late 1960s, platelets became available for the treatment of patients with thrombocytopenic bleeding. Since that time, deaths caused by hemorrhage have gradually decreased to the point that only 3 percent of adults with acute nonlymphoblastic leukemia now have lethal hemorrhagic complications.[36]

In the 1970s and 1980s, several studies addressed the issue of prophylactic versus therapeutic platelet transfusions for thrombocytopenic patients with acute leukemia.[37–42] These studies were carefully reviewed by Feusner in 1984.[43] In summary, it can be concluded from these studies that platelets given prophylactically do decrease the incidence of significant bleeding episodes in patients with leukemia, but these studies did not demonstrate a longer survival in patients transfused prophylactically versus those transfused only in the presence of active bleeding. Despite this, several experts began in the late 1970s to recommend the use of prophylactic platelet transfusions.[44–48] There are likely several reasons for this, among them the easy availability of platelets, the relative lack of discussion of viral disease transmission when considering the transfusion support of patients with malignant diseases, the lack of clear evidence in adults, at least, that platelet refractoriness is related to the amount of exposure (discussed further below), and the desire to avoid death or permanent sequelae caused by a potentially preventable event (i.e., hemorrhage) even if such an outcome is rare.

Nevertheless, the debate of prophylactic versus therapeutic platelet transfusion therapy continues.[36,49,50] In a survey conducted recently by the Transfusion Practices Committee of the American Association of Blood Banks, 70 percent of 126 institutions treating pediatric hematology/oncology patients reported that platelet transfusions were given primarily prophylactically whereas 20 percent transfused platelets primarily therapeutically and 10 percent followed a policy combining both approaches.[50a]

For those physicians and institutions that choose to use prophylactic platelet transfusions, the current debate centers around the choice of a platelet count at which to routinely administer platelet concentrates. In the reviews cited above—published in the late 1970s—advocating the use of prophylactic platelet transfusion for leukemic patients, it was often suggested that the platelet count be maintained above 20×10^9/L. A few studies suggest that in practice, in some centers at least, prophylactic transfusions are sometimes given at even higher platelet levels.[51,52] In particular, 21 percent of pediatric institutions responding to the survey mentioned above stated that they administered prophylactic platelet transfusions at a platelet count higher than 20×10^9/L.

The figure of 20×10^9/L appears to have been derived from a much-quoted study by Gaydos et al., published in 1962.[53] In this study, the authors tried to determine if there was a threshold platelet level above which bleeding rarely occurred and below which it commonly occurred. They conducted a retrospective review of 92 patients (40 patients $\geq$ 21 years old and 52 patients < 21 years old) with acute leukemia. They determined the percent of days with bleeding manifestations at various platelet levels. Grossly visible hemorrhage was visible on less than 1 percent of days at all platelet levels higher than 20×10^9/L, on 4 percent of days where platelet counts were 10 to 20×10^9/L, on 6 percent of days with platelet counts of 5 to 10×10^9/L, and then gradually increasing to a maximum of 31 percent of days at platelet counts lower than 1×10^9/L. Sixteen of the 92 patients suffered fatal intracranial hemorrhage: 8 were in "blastic crisis" (not further defined by the authors) and had a median platelet count of 10×10^9/L; the remaining 8 were not in blastic crisis—7 had a platelet count lower than 5×10^9/L, and 1 had a platelet count of 5 to 10×10^9/L. It must also be remembered that when this study was performed, the platelet inhibitory effects of aspirin were not yet appreciated and so many of these patients were likely receiving aspirin. Although the authors concluded that no clear "threshold" platelet count could be identified, this study has often been cited in the choice of a platelet count of 20×10^9/L for prophylactic transfusion.

The necessity of maintaining a minimum platelet count of 20×10^9/L in all patients with malignancies has since been questioned. In a consensus development conference addressing platelet transfusion therapy sponsored by the National Institutes of Health in 1986, the panel concluded that patients with severe thrombocytopenia may benefit from prophylactic transfusions but that the commonly used threshold value of 20×10^9/L may sometimes be safely lowered.[54] Even more conservative recommendations have recently been published. Slichter, in a review published in 1991, recommended that only patients with platelet counts lower than 5×10^9/L should routinely be given prophylactic platelet transfusions, and that for those with platelet counts higher than 5×10^9/L, clinical judgment should used to assess the need for platelet therapy.[55] Beutler likewise suggested abandoning the practice of routinely transfusing patients whenever the platelet count decreases below 20×10^9/L; he too suggests that if any level

is to be chosen for prophylactic transfusions in a stable patient, it should be 5×10^9/L, with prophylactic transfusions at higher platelet counts being reserved for patients in whom additional risk factors exist.[56]

The rationale for these more conservative recommendations is based on results of older studies as well as more recent ones addressing the safety of lowering threshold levels for prophylactic platelet transfusions. Among the studies cited above addressing the issue of prophylactic versus therapeutic platelet transfusions, one was a retrospective review of 70 children with ALL studied during induction and first remission.[42] Platelets were given only for significant bleeding associated with a platelet count below 20×10^9/L. In this study there were no deaths due to hemorrhage, and 84 percent of patients achieved complete remission without a single platelet transfusion, in spite of the fact that 49 percent had a platelet count below 20×10^9/L at some time during the induction phase. Unfortunately, the actual platelet nadirs were not specified.

More recently, Aderka et al. published a retrospective study reviewing the safety of their policy of using prophylactic platelet transfusion only for platelet counts below 10×10^9/L and comparing the bleeding tendency at platelet counts above and below 10×10^9/L in patients with ALL and acute non-lymphoblastic leukemia (ANLL).[57] In all, 117 episodes of thrombocytopenia (platelet count lower than 20×10^9/L) were studied. There were 67 episodes of bleeding, of which 85 percent were minor and 15 percent were major (severe hematuria, hematemesis, melena). There were no intracranial hemorrhages and there was only 1 death due to hemorrhage, this occurring in a patient with a platelet count of 5×10^9/L. All the severe bleeding episodes occurred in patients with decreasing platelet counts and concomitant fever. At platelet counts of 10 to 20×10^9/L versus platelet counts lower than 10×10^9/L, patients with ALL had more bleeding episodes than patients with ANLL. In both groups, there were more episodes of bleeding with platelet counts of 10 to 20×10^9/L in leukemia-related thrombocytopenia versus chemotherapy-related thrombocytopenia.

In a study published by Gmür et al. in 1991, the

authors reported the results of routinely using prophylactic platelet transfusions in 104 patients with newly diagnosed acute leukemia only if the platelet count was 5×10^9/L.[58] Prophylactic platelet transfusions were administered to patients with platelet counts of 6 to 10×10^9/L in the presence of fresh minor hemorrhagic manifestations or fever and to patients with platelet counts of 11 to 20 $\times 10^9$/L in the presence of coagulation disorders and/or heparin therapy. Using this protocol, a platelet transfusion was withheld on 69 percent of days when a morning platelet count was 6 to 20×10^9/L. Thirty-one major bleeding episodes occurred in the 104 patients; 3 patients died of complications related to bleeding—1 because of unavailability of platelets due to platelet refractoriness, 1 nonthrombocytopenic patient with disseminated intravascular coagulation (DIC) and heparin therapy, and 1 thrombocytopenic patient with acute promyelocytic leukemia and unrecognized spinal cord hematoma.

The German BFM study group reported the causes of early death in 294 children with ANLL.[59] Thirty (10 percent) patients died prior to or in the first 12 days of therapy, and of these 30 deaths, 12 were due to hemorrhage alone. Of these 12 patients, 8 had white blood cell (WBC) counts higher than 100×10^9/L, 2 had platelet counts lower than 20 $\times 10^9$/L, and 2 had platelet counts between 50 and 100 $\times 10^9$/L. The authors noted that several of the hemorrhagic deaths occurred during the period of rapid blast reduction. Thus, it appears that children with ANLL and hyperleucocytosis are at high risk of early hemorrhagic death and that such hemorrhages often occur in spite of platelet levels higher than 50 $\times 10^9$/L.

Patients with acute promyelocytic leukemia (ANLL, FAB M3) are also at high risk of hemorrhage during induction therapy: rates of early fatal hemorrhage of 9 to 26 percent have been reported in these patients.[60–62] This bleeding tendency is associated with the presence of disseminated intravascular coagulation and fibrinolysis thought to be related to the release of procoagulant substances from the promyelocytic granules.

The incidence of hemorrhage in patients with solid tumors and thrombocytopenia has been addressed in at least two reports, although neither specifically studied children.[63,64] Based on these stud-

ies, the risk factors for hemorrhage in patients with solid tumors are similar to those in leukemic patients, although one additional consideration is the predisposition to hemorrhage associated with local tumor invasion.

In summary, given the presently available data, the use of either therapeutic or prophylactic platelet transfusions for children with thrombocytopenia associated with malignancies can be justified. However, the exclusive use of therapeutic transfusions should be considered only in settings where frequent evaluations by an experienced team of physicians can be carried out and where platelet concentrates, if necessary, can be quickly obtained and administered. Alternatively, for physicians or institutions electing to transfuse platelets prophylactically, consideration should be given to using a threshold platelet count at which platelets are routinely administered that is below 20×10^9/L. Just as the indication for a RBC transfusion should not be determined solely on the basis of a hemoglobin level, the decision to administer a platelet transfusion should also be individualized, taking into account the clinical situation as well as the platelet level.

Prophylactic platelet transfusions are indicated for thrombocytopenic patients undergoing invasive procedures. At least one study suggests that major surgical procedures can be safely performed in leukemic patients at platelet counts of 50×10^9/L.[65] However, there are relatively few published guidelines concerning two of the most common invasive procedures that patients with hematologic or other malignancies undergo, namely lumbar puncture and the insertion of permanent indwelling central venous catheters. Tomasulo and Petz reported an informal survey of 40 physicians that suggested that the risk of lumbar puncture in thrombocytopenic patients is not great at platelet counts over 20×10^9/L, although there was insufficient information from which to draw a definite conclusion.[66] Regarding the insertion of central lines, it has been suggested that a platelet count of 20×10^9/L may be sufficient in children, although many physicians would likely prefer to have a higher platelet count before performing this procedure; again, definite recommendations are difficult to propose.[25] Bone marrow aspiration and biopsy can be safely performed (with respect to local bleeding) at any platelet level. Suggested guide-

Table 32-2. Suggested Guidelines for Prophylactic Platelet Transfusions in Children with Hypoproliferative Thrombocytopenia Associated with Malignant Disease

Platelet count $<10 \times 10^9/L$

Platelet count $<20 \times 10^9/L$ and bone marrow infiltration, fever, mucositis, DIC, anticoagulation therapy, a platelet count likely to fall below $10 \times 10^9/L$ prior to next possible evaluation, or risk of bleeding due to local tumor invasion

Platelet count $<30–40 \times 10^9/L$ and severe DIC (e.g., during induction therapy for promyelocytic leukemia), extreme hyperleukocytosis, or prior to lumbar puncture or central venous line insertion

Platelet count $<50–60 \times 10^9/L$ and major surgical intervention

Abbreviations: DIC, disseminated intravascular coagulation.

lines for prophylactic platelet transfusions for children with hypoproliferative thrombocytopenia associated with malignant disease are summarized in Table 32-2.

Finally, it is important to remember that mechanisms other than hypoproliferation may occasionally cause thrombocytopenia in patients with malignancies. Patients with sepsis or acute promyelocytic anemia may have DIC, patients with Hodgkin's disease may have an immunologic-mediated thrombocytopenia, and occasionally a patient may develop drug-dependent platelet antibodies, as, for example, has been recently described with vancomycin.[67]

Granulocyte Transfusions

Between 1977 and 1982, the role of therapeutic granulocyte transfusions was the subject of several papers, including reports of seven controlled studies. These studies have been fully reviewed[68] and suggest a benefit for selected neutropenic patients with bacterial infections, providing adequate numbers of granulocytes are given. Despite this, granulocytes are not frequently used and at least two investigators suggest that if an "abuse" of granulocyte transfusions exists today, it lies in underuse rather than inappropriate or overuse of this blood component.[68–70] Reasons for the decreased use of granulocytes in the late 1980s, as discussed in these reviews, probably included concerns about adverse transfu-

sion reactions combined with a lack of conviction of potential efficacy.

In 1981, Wright et al. reported lethal pulmonary reactions associated with the combined use of amphotericin B and granulocyte transfusions.[71] However, since then, other investigators have not observed lethal reactions with combined therapy and have reported significant pulmonary reactions in patients receiving either modality alone as well as those receiving both amphotericin B and granulocytes.[72–74] Thus, the use of amphotericin B is not currently considered a contraindication to use of granulocyte transfusions or vice versa, although most authors would suggest separating each treatment by a period of 4 to 6 hours.[68,75] However, the efficacy granulocyte transfusions in treating fungal infections remains undetermined.[76]

Lack of efficacy may occur if inadequate doses (less than 1×10^9 granulocytes/kg/transfusion in smaller patients or less than 2 to 3×10^{10} granulocytes/kg/transfusion in larger patients) are used or if the possibility of HLA alloimmunization is not taken into consideration.[68] Patients with evidence of HLA alloimmunization should receive HLA-matched or leukocyte-crossmatched granulocytes.[68,70]

More recently, the availability of hematopoietic growth factors, in particular granulocyte-macrophage colony-stimulating factor (GM-CSF) and granulocyte colony-stimulating factor (G-CSF), which can decrease the duration of periods of severe neutropenia and the incidence of severe infections in patients undergoing cancer chemotherapy, has likely decreased the need for granulocyte transfusions.[77–79] However, granulocyte transfusions should still be considered for those patients with documented or strongly suspected bacterial (and possibly fungal) infections unresponsive to antibiotics and who remain severely neutropenic (absolute neutrophil count $< 0.2 \times 10^9/L$) in spite of treatment with GM-CSF or G-CSF or for whom this treatment in unavailable or contraindicated.

The indications for granulocyte transfusions should be determined locally. On a practical level, most children with acute leukemia (or other malignancies) have little need for granulocyte transfusions, since their periods of severe bone marrow depression are fairly short and response to antibiotics is good. However, bone marrow transplant recipients or patients undergoing second or subsequent remission inductions may have prolonged periods of profound neutropenia. Ongoing analyses of infectious deaths in these patients should be conducted locally. If potentially curable patients are dying of bacterial and/or fungal infections during periods of severe but temporary neutropenia, consideration should be given to the increased use of granulocyte transfusions.

For further discussion of the theoretic and practical aspects of granulocyte transfusion, see Chapters 17 and 31.

INHERITED BONE MARROW FAILURE SYNDROMES

The inherited bone marrow failure syndromes are rare hematologic disorders characterized by reduced bone marrow production of blood cells resulting in single or multiple peripheral blood cytopenias. These syndromes include DBA, severe congenital neutropenia, Shwachman-Diamond syndrome, amegakaryocytic thrombocytopenia, thrombocytopenia with absent radii, Fanconi's anemia, and dyskeratosis congenita. Blood transfusion therapy plays an important role in the supportive therapy of many of these patients. The principles of transfusion support are the same for a given cytopenia, regardless of the specific syndrome. To illustrate these principles, the transfusion support of patients with DBA, severe congenital neutropenia, and Fanconi's anemia (FA) are discussed in this section.

Congenital Red Cell Aplasia: Diamond-Blackfan Anemia

DBA is the most common name given to a syndrome of RBC aplasia presenting in childhood. The current diagnostic criteria, as outlined by Alter and Young, are (1) normochromic, macrocytic or normocytic anemia developing early in childhood, (2) reticulocytopenia, (3) normocellular bone marrow with selective deficiency of RBC precursors, (4) normal or slightly decreased leukocyte counts, and (5) normal or increased platelet counts.[80]

The majority of patients with DBA have significant anemia: in approximately 60 infants diagnosed with DBA in the first 2 months of life, the median hemoglobin level was 4.0 g/dl, with a range of 1.5 to 10

g/dl.[80] All patients with DBA and significant anemia should receive an initial course of prednisone therapy, since approximately 50 percent can be expected to have an satisfactory response.[80] In patients who are unresponsive to corticosteroids, or in whom the side effects of corticosteroid therapy (particularly delayed growth) are considered unacceptably high, a program of chronic RBC transfusion therapy is usually undertaken. For patients with severe anemia (hemoglobin levels lower than 6.0 g/dl), the benefits of regular RBC transfusion, in particular increased energy level and improved growth, clearly justify its use. RBC transfusions of 10 to 15 ml/kg (see also the section on RBC transfusions below) are administered at 3- to 6-week intervals as required to maintain a minimum pretransfusion hemoglobin level of 6.0 to 7.0 g/dl.

For patients with moderate degrees of anemia (e.g., 6.0 to 7.0 g/dL), the long-term complications, in particular secondary iron overload and the eventual necessity for chelation therapy (see the section on thalassemia syndromes below), must be carefully weighed against the anticipated benefits before deciding to embark on such a course of treatment. Patients whose hemoglobin levels remain above 7.0 to 8.0 g/dl (with or without corticosteroid therapy) do not require regular RBC transfusions. Approximately 15 to 20 percent of DBA patients will have a spontaneous remission.

Several studies investigating the efficacy of hematopoietic growth factors, in particular, erythropoietin and interleukin 3 (IL-3), in the treatment of DBA have been performed.[81–84] Erythropoietin, even in doses as high as 2,000 U/kg/day administered subcutaneously, does not result in increased reticulocyte counts or increased hemoglobin levels.[81] In one study, the administration of Il-3 did result in a sustained response in two patients in whom bone marrow precursors and peripheral blood reticulocytes were present prior to IL-3 therapy. However, in another study, IL-3 was not found to induce erythropoiesis in any of 13 DBA patients with markedly reduced to absent recognizable bone marrow erythroid elements.[84] The variability in responses to IL-3 treatment may be another manifestation of the heterogeneity of this syndrome.

DBA can be cured with allogeneic bone marrow transplantation.[85,86] This therapy should be considered for all DBA patients who are transfusion dependent and who have a related HLA-compatible donor.

Severe Congenital Neutropenia: Kostmann Syndrome

Kostmann syndrome is a rare bone marrow failure syndrome consisting of extreme neutropenia (absolute neutrophil counts usually lower than $0.2 \times 10^9/$ L) and severe pyogenic infections presenting in early infancy and is often associated with early death. Patients do not have anemia nor thrombocytopenia (unless associated with a superimposed infection). Bone marrow examination reveals normal cellularity with absent or markedly decreased myeloid precursors, often with a maturation arrest at the myelocyte or promyelocyte stage.

Most patients with Kostmann syndrome will receive prophylactic antibiotics. Established infections are treated with appropriate antibiotics. Recent studies have shown that treatment with the hematopoietic growth factor G-CSF (although not GM-CSF) may be beneficial in this disorder.[83,87] Granulocyte transfusions should be considered for patients with documented or strongly suspected severe bacterial or fungal infections unresponsive to antibiotics and G-CSF.

Congenital Aplastic Anemia: Fanconi's Anemia

Until recently, the diagnosis of FA was made in patients with familial aplastic anemia associated with specific congenital anomalies (most commonly cutaneous hyperpigmentation, short stature, skeletal anomalies involving the arms, and renal or cardiac abnormalities). Currently, FA is defined as the presence, upon cytogenetic testing, of characteristic chromosomal breaks after clastogenic stress, with or without aplastic anemia or congenital abnormalities.[80] While the majority of patients diagnosed clinically have been between 3 and 14 years of age, FA has been diagnosed in very young infants as well as adults. Patients often present with isolated thrombocytopenia or neutropenia prior to the onset of pancytopenia. However, most patients do eventually develop severe aplastic anemia. Approximately 10 percent of FA patients will develop leukemia; in some patients, this is the initial mode of presentation.

Based on reports of cases published between 1927

and 1990, the predicted mean survival is 16 years of age.[80] When the only treatment used was supportive blood transfusion therapy, almost all patients died within 3 to 4 years of the onset of aplastic anemia. Survival following the onset of aplastic anemia was slightly prolonged to approximately 5 to 7 years in patients treated with androgens.[80]

Patients with FA can be cured by bone marrow transplantation (BMT) from a related HLA-compatible donor.[88,89] However, it must be ascertained that the donor does not have FA and the preparative cytotoxic regimen for BMT must take into consideration the FA patient's chromosomal fragility. Owing to these difficulties in the preparative regime, BMT using unrelated donors or less than completely matched family donors is not currently recommended.[80] There have been recent reports of successful BMT of FA patients using umbilical cord blood from non-FA, HLA-compatible siblings.[90,91]

The anemia associated with FA is a slowly developing hypoproliferative anemia, and in that sense the consideration of when to administer an RBC transfusion is similar to that discussed above for patients with malignancies or DBA. However, unlike the anemia in patients with malignancies, the anemia of FA is permanent, and unlike DBA patients, patients with FA and no appropriate BMT donor are likely to die of FA before they are at risk of significant morbidity or mortality from secondary hemochromatosis. Taking into consideration these two factors, the physician may decide, depending on the clinical condition of the patient, to maintain a slightly higher minimum hemoglobin level in the FA patient than in the other two groups of patients. Alternatively, if BMT is a possibility, data from thalassemia patients suggest that the prevention of iron overload may lead to an increased chance of successful BMT (see the section on thalassemia syndromes below).

Studies specifically addressing the question of prophylactic versus therapeutic platelet transfusions are not available for either congenital or acquired thrombocytopenia caused by bone marrow failure. Although, as discussed previously, several authors have suggested maintaining platelet counts at $20 \times 10^9/L$ in patients with malignancies, many authors do not advocate the same approach for patients with aplastic anemia. (This fact may constitute another argument in favor of the individualization of platelet transfusion therapy in all patients with hypoproliferative thrombocytopenias). One rationale for the more conservative approach in this group of patients may be the fact that they are less likely to have additional risk factors for spontaneous hemorrhage such as mucositis, DIC, septicemia, bone marrow infiltration, and so forth. A reasonable approach to the platelet transfusion support of patients with FA is that suggested by Slichter for all patients with hypoproliferative thrombocytopenia, namely prophylactic platelet transfusion at platelet counts lower than 5×10^9/L, platelet transfusions as judged necessary in the presence of additional risk factors for bleeding at platelet counts of 5 to 20×10^9/L, and a search for other etiologies if significant bleeding occurs at platelet counts above 20×10^9/L.[55]

SEVERE ACQUIRED APLASTIC ANEMIA

The definition of severe acquired aplastic anemia (SAAA) is the same in children as in adults—namely, a hypocellular bone marrow biopsy and of two of the three following criteria: an absolute neutrophil count lower than 0.5×10^9/L, a platelet count lower than 20×10^9/L, and a corrected reticulocyte count below 1 percent (approximately equal to an absolute reticulocyte count lower than 25×10^{12}/L).[80]

Allogeneic BMT from a related HLA-compatible donor is the treatment of choice for SAAA. Patients without such a donor are treated with an immunotherapy regime that usually includes corticosteroids, antithymocyte globulin (ATG), and cyclosporine.[80] Some patients who do not respond to a first course of ATG will respond to a second course. Patients without an HLA-compatible related BMT donor and who are unresponsive to immunotherapy may be candidates for an allogeneic BMT from an phenotypically HLA-compatible unrelated donor. Alternatively, these patients may be treated with supportive therapy only, which currently includes blood transfusion therapy and possibly treatment with hematopoietic growth factors, in particular G-CSF.[92]

The prognosis for patients with SAAA who do not undergo BMT or respond to immunotherapy is very difficult to predict. Prior to the availability of modern transfusion and antibiotic therapy, there were almost no long-term survivors. The improvement in

these supportive modalities has increased survival, although precise survival figures are not available.

The indications for RBC and platelet transfusions in children with SAAA are similar to those discussed above for children with inherited bone marrow failure syndromes. However, if BMT is to be performed rapidly, there may be advantages to withholding transfusions where possible.[1] Patients with SAAA are at high risk of developing HLA alloimmunization and should receive only leukodepleted RBC and platelet concentrates (see the section on platelet alloimmunization and leukocyte-depletion filters). Granulocyte transfusions should be considered only for life-threatening infections unresponsive to antibiotics and hematopoietic growth factors.

Traditionally, RBC transfusion-dependent patients with SAAA have not been treated with iron chelators. However, as some SAAA patients are now surviving long enough to develop significant secondary hemochromatosis, consideration may need to be given to the introduction of chelation therapy in selected patients with SAAA.

THALASSEMIA SYNDROMES

The thalassemia syndromes are a heterogeneous group of genetic disorders that have in common deficient synthesis of the α, β, and/or δ polypeptide chains of normal hemoglobins. The distribution of thalassemia is similar to that of malaria, extending from the Mediterranean basin through the Middle East and India to Southeast Asia. Clinically, the thalassemia syndromes are divided into thalassemia minor, which is characterized by a mild, clinically asymptomatic microcytic anemia; thalassemia major, in which blood transfusions are necessary for survival beyond infancy; and thalassemia intermedia, in which a moderate degree of anemia, sometimes leading to transfusion support, is present. Genetically, thalassemia minor is usually found in a heterozygous carrier of an abnormal globin gene, whereas patients with thalassemia major or intermedia are homozygous or doubly heterozygous for globin gene defects. A full description of the genetic and clinical aspects of the thalassemia syndromes is beyond the scope of this chapter; interested readers are referred to McDonagh and Nienhuis[93] and Lukens.[94]

RBC Transfusions in β-Thalassemia Syndromes

Prior to the introduction of RBC transfusion therapy for β-thalassemia major in the 1950s, β-thalassemia major was an uniformly fatal disease. Initially, children were transfused only to hemoglobin levels of 5.0 to 6.0 g/dl, a level sufficient to ensure survival but insufficient to suppress the exuberant erythroid bone marrow hyperplasia characteristic of this disorder. Consequently, patients survived into their second decade but developed severe skeletal deformities, osteoporosis, and splenomegaly. So-called hypertransfusion regimens, in which endogenous erythroid production is suppressed by maintaining a minimum pretransfusion hemoglobin level of 9 to 10 g/dl, were therefore gradually introduced in the 1960s, and 1970s and remain the most common approach today.[4] During the 1980s, investigators evaluated the possibility of further improving the quality of life of thalassemic patients by introducing a "supertransfusion" regimen in which the minimum pretransfusion hemoglobin level was kept entirely within the normal range.[95] However this regimen led, not surprisingly, to a significant increase in transfusion requirements and has since been abandoned by most physicians caring for thalassemia patients.[4]

Another approach investigated during the 1980s was the possibility of decreasing transfusion exposure and increasing transfusion intervals through the use of young RBCs, so-called neocytes. Neocytes, with an average age of 12 to 21 days, can be collected by erythrocytapheresis or by fractionation of standard whole blood units using a cell processor. The studies performed in the 1980s reported only modest decreases of 12 to 16 percent in transfusion requirements; the use of neocyte transfusions was therefore abandoned.[96,97] More recently, the use of a newly developed neocyte-separation set (Neocel System, Cutter Biological, Berkeley, CA) has been reported.[98] Using this system, the average transfusion interval was increased by 6 days, leading to an estimated 15 percent reduction in transfused iron load. Nevertheless, the costs of this system were significantly higher and donor exposure per transfusion episode was doubled. It is thus also unlikely that the use of neocyte transfusions for thalassemic patients will now increase despite the availability of this new system.

One of the most difficult determinations facing physicians treating thalassemia patients is the necessity of instituting a chronic RBC transfusion program for patients with thalassemia intermedia and hemoglobin levels of 6.0 to 7.0 g/dl. In addition to the considerations discussed above for patients with DBA with this degree of anemia, the physician must take into account the fact that untransfused thalassemia intermedia patients may development bone deformities due to bone marrow erythroid hyperplasia, and even without RBC transfusions, these patients may develop clinically significant hemochromatosis secondary to the increased intestinal iron absorption induced by their inefficient erythropoiesis.[4] If a transfusion program is embarked upon, the goals of transfusion therapy components are the same as those outlined above for thalassemia major patients. The transfusion intervals can usually be longer, although it is often more difficult to completely suppress endogenous erythropoiesis in thalassemia intermedia patients than in thalassemia major patients.

Treatment of Iron Overload

To maintain pretransfusion hemoglobin levels of 9 to 10 g/dl, patients with β-thalassemia major require RBC transfusions approximately every 3 weeks. Since the body has no mechanism for iron excretion, such a transfusion program inevitably results in iron overload that, if not prevented, causes death from lethal cardiac toxicity in the second or third decade of life.[4] The prevention of iron overload is achieved by the use of the iron-chelating agent deferoxamine. This agent is effective only if administered slowly by an intravenous or subcutaneous infusion. Deferoxamine can be administered by patients at home using a small portable infusion pump that permits continuous slow delivery through a butterfly needle placed subcutaneously in the abdomen. Most patients choose to install the pump at bedtime, thus allowing the deferoxamine to infuse during sleeping hours. Deferoxamine treatment is usually started when serum ferritin is greater than 1,500 mg/ml and/or the unsaturated iron binding capacity exceeds 80 percent and the child is at least 3 years old.[4,93,94] Deferoxamine treatment in younger children may lead to growth failure and, with minimal iron load, is not efficacious and is potentially toxic.[4,99,100] Obviously, deferoxamine is a very cumbersome therapy; it is also very expensive. Because of these problems, there has been an effort to develop oral iron chelators. At present, a number of oral iron chelators are under investigation in the hope that one such treatment will eventually be able to replace deferoxamine therapy.[4]

Practical Aspects of RBC Transfusion Support

Before the administration of the first RBC transfusion, an extended RBC phenotype should be performed. RBC alloimmunization has been reported to occur in up to 20 to 30 percent of thalassemia patients, although it may occur less frequently in patients beginning RBC transfusions prior to 3 years of age.[101–104] The use of RBC units phenotyped for rhesus and K antigens has been reported to decrease the incidence of alloimmunization.[103] The use of leukodepleted and/or washed units is discussed below. Patients with thalassemia may be candidates for a limited donor exposure program (see the section below on strategies to decrease allogeneic donor exposure).

Patients with β-thalassemia major can be cured by bone marrow transplantation from a related HLA-compatible donor.[105,106] The donor may be a heterozygous carrier for a thalassemic gene. BMT in low-risk patients (i.e., those without hepatomegaly or liver fibrosis and in whom iron-chelation therapy was started at an early age and was adequately maintained) results in 98 percent long-term survival and 94 percent event-free survival rates.[105] Even in older high-risk patients, the actuarial probabilities of long-term survival and event-free survival after BMT are 85 percent and 80 percent, respectively.[107] Thus, any patient with β-thalassemia major and a related HLA-compatible donor should be considered a potential BMT candidate, and appropriate measures should be taken to prevent HLA alloimmunization and, if cytomegolovirus (CMV)-seronegative, the transmission of CMV (see below).

SICKLE CELL DISEASE

The term *sickle cell disease* includes persons with homozygous HbSS (also referred to as sickle cell anemia) as well as those who are doubly heterozygous for HbSC or HbS/β-thalassemia. Worldwide, SCD is one of the most common genetic disorders. In equa-

torial Africa, the frequency of HbS heterozygotes reaches 35 percent; among African-Americans, approximately 8 percent are heterozygous for HbS and 1 in 200 to 500 newborns have SCD.[108–111] HbS and HbC are abnormal hemoglobins, each resulting from a point mutation at the codon for the sixth amino acid of the β-globin chain (HbS: glutamine → valine; HbC: glutamine → lysine). Those homozygous for HbS have a moderately severe hemolytic anemia (mean hemoglobin levels for HbSS adults is 7.5 g/dl, with a range of 5.5 to 9.5 g/dl), although those with HbSC disease have no or only mild anemia.[109] In addition to hemolysis, the presence of HbS (either alone or in the presence of HbC) induces, through a complex series of interactions, changes in microrheology, which in turn result in the well-known episodes of severe pain and other acute complications, as well as chronic and irreversible organ damage. For a full discussion of the pathophysiology of SCD, see Platt and Dover[108] and Lukens.[109]

Indications for RBC Transfusions

The administration of RBC transfusions in the management and/or prevention of the complications of SCD is so frequent that almost all adult HbSS patients and many HbSC or HbS/β-thalassemia patients have been transfused at least once and often multiple times.[112] RBC transfusions are administered to SCD patients for two reasons—to increase oxygen-carrying capacity in the anemic patient and/or to replace the abnormal HbS by normal HbA. Depending on the complication and the goal of transfusion, RBC transfusions may be administered as simple transfusions or exchange transfusions, with either being used acutely or in a chronic transfusion program.

Simple RBC transfusions (approximately 10 ml/kg) are used acutely to treat acute major splenic sequestration and aplastic or hyperhemolytic crises, as well as other selected complications.[112] In acute splenic sequestration, the spleen rapidly increases in size, leading to sequestration of blood in the spleen. In young children, the splenic sequestration may be sufficiently severe to lead to life-threatening hypovolemic shock. B19 parvovirus infections in patients with SCD results in temporary aplasia, which may be severe, with hemoglobin levels of 3.0 g/dl or less, thus requiring simple RBC transfusions. Transfusions are not indicated for uncomplicated painful episodes. However, occasionally an exaggerated hemolysis, associated with an episode of pain, may herald the onset of multiorgan failure syndrome, which appears to respond to RBC transfusion.[112]

The necessity of RBC transfusion prior to surgery in the SCD patient—either simple transfusion to attain a certain total hemoglobin level or exchange transfusion to reduce the HbS level—has been debated in the literature. A large, multicenter study addressing this issue has recently been completed and should provide definitive guidelines for transfusion in this setting (E. Vichinsky, personal communication, 1994).

A study addressing the role for RBC transfusion therapy in the pregnant SCD patient demonstrated that prophylactic RBC transfusions did not decrease the incidence of obstetric complications.[113] Prophylactic RBC transfusions are therefore not recommended during pregnancy, although transfusion therapy is recommended for such complications as toxemia, septicemia, severe anemia, acute chest syndrome, or anticipated surgery.[114]

In children with cerebral vascular accidents (CVA) associated with SCD, the administration of regular RBC transfusions to maintain a HbS level below 30 percent in the first 2 years after the CVA and below 50 percent thereafter has been shown to prevent recurrent CVAs.[115–118] Unfortunately, it appears that there is no time at which RBC transfusions can be stopped in these children without running the risk of recurrent CVA.

RBC transfusions are currently used by most physicians, either acutely or chronically, for a variety of other complications, including acute pulmonary disease (acute chest syndrome), priapism, and leg ulcers. However, their role and the best type (i.e., simple versus exchange transfusion, acute versus chronic transfusions) for these and other complications require further investigation before definitive recommendations can be made. For a fuller discussion of the indications for RBC transfusion in SCD, see Wayne et al.[112]

Complications and Practical Aspects of RBC Transfusion

In addition to the potential complications of RBC transfusions common to all recipients, there are complications that are either unique or more common in SCD patients.

A major problem in the transfusion support of SCD patients is RBC alloimmunization. The Cooperative Study for SCD reported an overall alloimmunization rate of 18.6 percent in 1,814 transfused SCD patients, with 3.2 percent having four or more RBC alloantibodies.[119] In a smaller study of 102 transfused SCD patients, 30 percent developed RBC alloantibodies and 14 percent experienced delayed hemolytic transfusion reactions.[120] Delayed transfusion reactions in SCD patients may present as an acute pain episode in a recently transfused patient.[121] In addition there are reports of delayed transfusion reactions in SCD that have been accompanied by a severe autoimmune hemolysis.[122–124] The high rate of sensitization to RBC antigens is likely due, at least in part, to racial differences between the blood-donor and SCD recipient population. The development of multiple RBC antibodies in SCD patients who are at risk of future complications requiring RBC transfusion may place some of these patients in life-threatening situations, owing to lack of availability of compatible blood. These observations have led to discussions in the literature as to whether all chronically transfused SCD patients should receive antigen-matched blood. Certainly an extended RBC phenotype should therefore be performed on all SCD patients prior to first transfusion. As a minimum, many centers treating large numbers of SCD patients will attempt to provide RBC units that are K-negative and matched for rhesus antigens (D, C, E, c, e). A number of experts have further suggested providing more extended RBC phenotyping of units for transfusion to SCD patients or meeting their transfusion requirements with blood selected from random black blood donors.[125,126] A recent retrospective review of one center's policy of using units matched for the K, C, E, S, and Fy^a or Fy^b antigens showed that none of the 40 patients who received antigen-matched transfusions showed any evidence of alloimmunization, whereas 16 (34.8 percent) of the 46 patients who received both antigen-matched and non–antigen-matched transfusions developed clinically significant alloantibodies.[127] However, since at least 60 to 70 percent of SCD patients do not develop clinically significant alloantibodies, not all experts are convinced that prophylactic extended antigen matching is the best management approach for chronically transfused

SCD patients. A reasonable alternative approach would be the provision of blood selected to match the patient's phenotype only after an initial antibody becomes detectable.[128]

RBC units for transfusion to SCD patients should be screened for the presence of HbS and found to be negative. This will avoid confusion when the goal of transfusion is to decrease the HbS level to a predetermined level and will prevent the use of blood from a donor with undiagnosed HbSC disease.

In vitro, the viscosity of HbS has been shown to increase to potentially clinically significant levels if the hematocrit exceeds 35 percent.[129] Therefore, when transfusing SCD patients, especially in the presence of high HbS levels, the hematocrit should not be allowed to increase above 35 percent. Neurologic events, including headache, seizures, and CVA, have been described after exchange transfusion in SCD.[130] It has been postulated that some of these events may have been caused by hyperviscosity, although other factors may also have been important in at least some of the patients.

As with any group of repeatedly transfused patients, febrile and allergic reactions may occur in SCD patients. The use of specialized components to prevent these reactions is discussed below.

BMT can cure SCD; its role in the treatment of SCD is currently under investigation.[131,132] For patients who are candidates for BMT, appropriate measures should be taken to prevent HLA alloimmunization and, where indicated, the transmission of CMV (see below).

SCD patients in chronic transfusion programs will develop secondary iron overload. The net amount of iron infused can be decreased by using partial exchange transfusion. An algorithm for planning partial manual exchange transfusions in children has been published.[133] Recently, it has been reported that the development of hemachromatosis can be further delayed or even prevented by the use of automated erythrocytopheresis.[134] However, patients who develop significant secondary hemochromatosis should be placed on deferoxamine chelation therapy similar to that described above for transfusion-dependent thalassemia patients.

CONGENITAL HEMOLYTIC ANEMIAS OTHER THAN SICKLE CELL DISEASE

Occasionally, children with congenital hemolytic anemias other than SCD will require regular or intermittent RBC transfusion support. Although these disorders are rare, the most common among them include hemolytic anemias due to pyruvate kinase deficiency, an unstable hemoglobin, or a severe (uncommon) form of hereditary spherocytosis. Unlike SCD or thalassemia syndromes, in which RBC transfusions are given both to suppress endogenous erythropoiesis and to increase oxygen carrying capacity, RBC transfusions in other congenital hemolytic anemias are given only to improve tissue oxygen delivery. The decision to administer RBC transfusions to children with these disorders, either chronically or intermittently, should be made using the same principles outlined above for children with malignancies or DBA. In addition, factors unique to each particular etiology should be considered. For example, in children with pyruvate kinase deficiency, the enzyme blockage is such that there is an increase in the red cell 2,3-DPG level, which significantly increases oxygen off-loading.[135]

The transfusion requirements in several of these disorders, including pyruvate kinase deficiency and severe hereditary spherocytosis, are usually decreased after splenectomy. The indication for and the timing of splenectomy must take into account the risks of splenectomy versus the risks of continuing RBC transfusion support.

PRATICAL ASPECTS OF PROVIDING TRANSFUSION SUPPORT

RBC Transfusions

During the first 4 months of life, the choice of ABO blood group for RBC transfusions must be based upon consideration the possible presence of maternal anti-A/B antibodies. All children who are likely to receive multiple RBC transfusions should have an extended RBC phenotype performed prior to the first RBC transfusion. This group includes patients with congenital or acquired aplastic anemia, SCD, thalassemia major or intermedia, or other transfusion-dependent congenital anemias. It is not necessary for patients with leukemia or other malignancies unless the patient is a candidate for bone marrow transplantation. Knowing a patient's extended RBC phenotype will assist in the identification of irregular RBC antibodies should they develop. However, except as previously discussed for patients with thalassemia syndromes or SCD, extended phenotyping of RBC units is not necessary in the absence of irregular RBC alloantibodies.

The quantity of blood to administer in simple RBC transfusions depends on the storage medium, the pretransfusion hemoglobin level, and the patient's weight. If the hemoglobin level is 5.0 g/dl or more and if blood stored in CPDA-1 (hematocrit, 0.70 to 0.75) is used, a transfusion of 10 ml/kg is usually administered. This can be expected to raise the hemoglobin level by approximately 3.0 g/dl. To obtain the same result using blood stored in an extended storage medium (hematocrit, 0.50 to 0.60) 14 ml/kg should be administered. For patients who weigh less than 20 kg, the volume of an entire RBC unit is too large to be administered during one transfusion. To minimize donor exposure, attempts should be made to use the whole unit, either by giving two or three small transfusions over a 24-hour period if the unit is opened nonsterilely or by entering the unit using a sterile docking device and transfusing appropriately sized aliquots before the unit's original expiration date. Additional strategies to limit donor exposure are discussed below.

If the anemia has developed slowly and the hemoglobin level is less than 5.0 g/dl, it may be necessary to administer RBC transfusions more slowly to avoid precipitating cardiac failure from circulatory overload. A transfusion regimen for the treatment of children with severe anemia of gradual onset without clinical signs of cardiac decompensation has recently been described.[136] The authors successfully treated 22 such children using RBCs with a hematocrit of 0.7 to 0.8 at a continuous infusion rate of 2 ml/kg/hr until the desired hemoglobin level was achieved.

If a severely anemic child has signs of cardiac decompensation, a partial exchange transfusion should be performed. Guidelines for performing partial manual exchange transfusions have been published.[133,137] Alternatively, where available, automated RBC exchanges can be performed even in critically ill pediatric patients.[138]

Several authors recommend using RBC units that have been stored for fewer than 7 to 10 days for patients on chronic transfusion programs. Two factors are given for these recommendations: the higher concentrations of 2,3-DPG and the increased 24-hour post-transfusion survival in units stored for fewer than 10 days as opposed to units stored for 35 to 42 days. In adults, it has been shown that intraerythrocyte 2,3-DPG levels are restored in transfused RBCs within 24 hours; thus, the first factor is not valid.[139] With respect to the second factor, there are no published data available to determine whether such an approach would actually decrease transfusion requirements. However, as discussed above for thalassemia patients, the use of neocyte-enriched RBC units resulted in only a small decrease in transfusion requirements that was much lower than predicted and not considered sufficient to justify the expense or the increased donor exposure of such a program.[96–98] This suggests that relatively short storage periods for RBC units would also not significantly affect RBC transfusion requirements.

Patients on chronic transfusion programs do frequently develop allergic and/or febrile nonhemolytic transfusion reactions. Therefore, prior to the availability of leukodepletion filters, many authors recommended the use of frozen, deglycerolized RBCs for these patients; currently, some authors recommend using leukodepletion filters beginning with the first RBC transfusion. However, not all patients develop reactions; an alternate strategy is to provide leukodepleted and/or washed RBCs as necessary, depending on the nature of the reactions should they occur. Leukodepleted units may first be provided using the centrifuge-cool-spin technique[140]; if reactions persist, leukodepletion with third-generation filters may be used. Occasionally, in multiply transfused patients, reactions persist despite the use of washed RBC units administered with leukodepletion filters; these may respond to premedication with high-dose corticosteroids.

Platelet Transfusions

Platelets possess intrinsic ABH antigens and extrinsically absorbed A and B antigens.[141,142] Nevertheless, ABO-incompatible platelets (i.e., platelets with A and/or B antigens given to a donor with a corresponding antibody) are usually clinically effective. However, in some patients, particularly those receiving multiple platelet transfusions, there may be a poorer post-transfusion response than that obtained with ABO-compatible platelets, and some studies have suggested that the transfusion of ABO-incompatible platelets is associated with the development of platelet refractoriness.[143–145] Also, there are reports of acute intravascular hemolysis after the transfusion of platelet concentrates containing ABO antibodies incompatible with the recipient's RBCs.[146–148] Therefore, it would seem prudent, particularly in small children, in whom the volume of plasma may be relatively large with respect to the patient's total blood volume, to try to use ABO-matched platelets. If ABO-matched platelets are not available, units with plasma compatible with the recipients RBCs should be chosen. If this is also not possible, units with low titers of anti-A or -B should be selected.

Platelets do not carry Rh antigens.[149] However the quantity of RBCs in platelet concentrates is sufficient to induce Rh sensitization even in immunosuppressed cancer patients.[150–152] Rh sensitization caused by platelet transfusions in Rh-negative patients with malignancy can be prevented by the administration of Rh immunoprophylaxis.[153,154] Thus if platelets from an Rh-positive donor or a donor of unknown Rh phenotype are given to an Rh-negative recipient, administration of Rh immunoprophylaxis should be considered, especially for female patients. The amount of anti-D immunoglobulin necessary to prevent sensitization depends on the number of contaminating RBCs in the platelet concentrates. A dose of 25 μg (125 IU) of anti-D immunoglobulin will protect against 1 ml RBCs.[155] It is preferable to use a preparation of anti-D that can be administered intravenously, if available.

A suitable starting platelet dosage that can be expected to raise the platelet level by 50×10^9/L is 1 random donor unit/10 kg body weight. An equivalent dose for platelets obtained by apheresis is approximately 5 ml/kg. Patients with increased platelet consumption (e.g., with septicemia or DIC) or patients with splenomegaly may require larger amounts of platelets.

Platelet Alloimmunization and Leukodepletion Filters

The mechanisms and management as well as the prevention of platelet refractoriness are of considerable current interest. Several excellent reviews have recently been published.[156–160] Therefore, the subject will be discussed only briefly here, with emphasis on some aspects relevant to the transfusion support of children.

Studies performed in the 1970s and early 1980s documenting the frequency of platelet refractoriness and/or HLA alloimmunization in adult patients with leukemia indicated that this problem occurred in approximately 50 percent of patients.[157] More recent studies suggest that the incidence may now be somewhat lower, around 25 to 30 percent.[161,162] Very few studies documenting the frequency of platelet refractoriness and/or HLA alloimmunization have been reported specifically in children, and in particular, there is almost no literature available on the current incidence of this problem. The only study specifically addressing HLA alloimmunization in children was published in 1981; hence, it reported on children treated prior to that time.[163] It was a retrospective study of 100 children with leukemia or solid tumors and 8 children with aplastic anemia, all of whom had been heavily transfused: each patient had received at least 10 units of platelets, the mean number of platelet units administered was 72, and 24 of the leukemia patients had received granulocyte transfusions. Among the acute leukemia patients, 20 of 45 developed HLA antibodies, although in 10, the antibodies subsequently became undetectable; 7 of 28 and 7 of 8 patients with solid tumors and aplastic anemia, respectively, developed HLA antibodies.

Saarinen and colleagues, in reporting on the use of leukocyte-free blood components to prevent platelet refractoriness, compared their study group to a historical reference group of patients who had not received leukocyte-free components.[164] The latter group consisted of 21 patients treated between 1978 and 1984; 3 had aplastic anemia, 13 had acute leukemia, and 10 were patients with solid tumors. Overall, 11 of 21 patients developed platelet refractoriness (alloimmunization was not studied); the details for each subgroup were not reported. The same group, in a second study evaluating the role of leukodepletion, again described a reference group of 10 pediatric patients who had been exposed to nonleukodepleted components.[165] Of the 10 patients, 5 had acute leukemia, 2 had solid tumors, and 1 had aplastic anemia. Three of the 10 (2 with leukemia, 1 with neuroblastoma) developed HLA antibodies.

Although these studies indicate that platelet refractoriness and/or HLA alloimmunization do occur in children, it is impossible to estimate, with such small numbers, the true significance of this problem in pediatric hematology/oncology patients. In addition, these studies have included only a few patients with the most common pediatric malignancy—namely, ALL. The incidence of platelet refractoriness may be lower in this group of patients for two reasons: first, they are almost always treated with corticosteroids, and second, in the absence of relapse they receive relatively small numbers of RBC and platelet transfusions. As shown in Table 32-3, in patients with ALL diagnosed in our hospital over a 1-year period, a median of four RBC and four platelet transfusions per patient were administered over a follow-up period of 2 to 3 years from diagnosis. Patients with acute nonlymphoblastic leukemia received a much larger number of transfusions.

The question of whether the incidence of platelet alloimmunization can be reduced by limiting the number of transfusions and/or limiting the number of different donors may have practical importance for children, who can be supported with relatively small numbers of donors. For adult patients, such an approach is generally considered of little use.[158] Dutcher et al., in a study of 106 adult patients with ANLL, found no relationship between the number of platelet transfusions given and the rate of alloimmunization.[166] The overall rate of alloimmunization was 38 percent; 52 percent of patients receiving four or fewer platelet transfusions became immunized, compared with 34 percent of patients receiving more than four transfusions. These results differ from those reported by Saarinen, who observed that no patient receiving fewer than 10 platelet transfusions (or about 50 units of platelet concentrates) developed platelet refractoriness.[164] In another European study, the incidence of platelet refractoriness in recipients of single random-donor apheresis platelets as compared with patients receiving platelet transfusions from pooled random donors was evaluated.[167] There was a clear difference between the number of patients who became refractory to multiple-donor platelet transfusions (14/27; 52 percent) versus single-donor platelets (4/27; 15 percent). There was also a difference in the number who developed lymphocytotoxic antibodies—15/27 (56 percent) versus 4/27 (15 percent), respectively. The mean number of platelet transfusions in the two groups was 5.5 and 6 (versus 9.3 in the study by Dutcher et al.[166]). These observations suggest that it may be possible to prevent alloimmunization in selected pediatric patients who are unlikely to require prolonged platelet transfusion support (e.g., patients with ALL) by decreasing the number of donor exposures through the use of single-donor apheresis platelets.

The prevention of platelet alloimmunization by the use of leukoreduced blood components has been reported by several investigators.[164,165,168–172] The majority of these studies, including the two performed by Saarinen exclusively in pediatric patients, do suggest that leukodepletion can effectively prevent HLA alloimmunization and its related platelet refractoriness. Nevertheless, opinions remain varied regarding recommendations for the routine use of leukodepletion filters.[158,173,174] The recently completed TRAP study (Trial to Reduce Alloimmunization to Platelets) may permit the development of guidelines. However, this study addresses only adult patients with acute nonlymphoblastic leukemia; therefore, definitive guidelines for children cannot yet be made. Nevertheless, some tentative recom-

Table 32-3. Blood Transfusion Support of Children with ALL or ANLL[a]

	Median No. Transfusions (Range)	Median No. Units (Range)
ALL (*n* = 33)		
RBC	4 (1–17)	4 (1–19)
Platelets	4 (0–45)	10 (0–60)
Total donor exposure		12 (1–77)
ANLL (*n* = 8)		
RBC	15 (4–51)	15 (4–52)
Platelets	25 (4–99)	79 (9–661)
Total donor exposure		98 (15–738)

Abbreviations: ALL, acute lymphoblastic leukemia; ANLL, acute nonlymphoblastic leukemia; RBC, red blood cells.

[a] Diagnosed at Hôpital Ste-Justine, Montreal, Quebec, Canada, June 1989–May 1990; follow-up through March 1992.

mendations can be proposed. Patients with severe acquired aplastic anemia appear to be at high risk of developing platelet refractoriness. In addition, they are potential candidates for long-term platelet transfusion therapy and/or bone marrow transplantation. They should therefore receive leukodepleted components. The use of leukodepletion should also be considered for other pediatric hematology/oncology patients who will require long-term platelet transfusion support or who may undergo BMT. Clinical situations in which children might undergo BMT are somewhat debatable and may depend partly on local protocols; a suggested list is given in Table 32-4. The use of leukodepletion filters for potential BMT patients may serve the dual purpose of preventing CMV transmission (see below and Chapter 39). Finally, as discussed previously, patients requiring

Table 32-4. Potential Pediatric BMT Candidates for Whom Prevention of HLA Alloimmunization and Transfusion-Transmitted CMV[a] Should be Considered

Patients with ANLL, relapsed ALL, or advanced or relapsed solid malignant tumors treated with protocols, including autologous BMT

Patients with the following diagnoses who have a related HLA-compatible BMT donor:
    CML
    SAAA
    ANLL
    Selected very high risk patients with ALL in first remission (e.g., age <12 months, presence of a Philadelphia chromosome)
    Relapsed ALL
    Thalassemia major
    Transfusion-dependent or life-threatening congenital bone marrow failure syndrome
    Other selected hematologic diseases (e.g., familial hemophagocytic lymphohistiocytosis, osteopetrosis)

Patients with the following diagnoses who have an unrelated HLA-compatible BMT donor:
    CML
    SAAA
    Selected patients with relapsed ANLL or ALL
    Other selected hematologic disorders (e.g., osteopetrosis, congenital amegakaryocytic thrombocytopenia)

Abbreviations: CMV, cytomegalovirus; ANLL, acute nonlymphoblastic leukemia; ALL, acute lymphoblastic leukemia; BMT, bone marrow transplantation; CML, chronic myelogenous leukemia; SAAA, severe acquired aplastic anemia.

chronic RBC transfusions may develop febrile, non-hemolytic transfusion reactions that persist in spite of the use of centrifuge-cool-spin units and may therefore benefit from the use of leukodepletion filters.

Among the potential problems associated with the use of leukodepletion filters—one that may be relatively more important for pediatric than for adult patients—is the fact that there is a 5 to 10 percent RBC loss and a 10 to 20 percent platelet loss after filtration, potentially increasing the number of RBC and/or platelet units that must be transfused.[175,176] Some of the filters must be rinsed with relatively large quantities of saline and this, too, may cause practical difficulties in very small patients.

Prevention of Cytomegalovirus Transmission

CMV exists in a latent state in the leukocytes (probably T lymphocytes and monocytes) of CMV-seropositive people and can be transmitted via the transfusion of blood components containing viable leukocytes,—namely, RBC, platelet, and granulocyte concentrates and liquid plasma. Depending on geographic location, approximately 30 to 50 percent of blood donors are CMV-seropositive, although not all CMV-seropositive donors are infectious. The consequences of transfusion-transmitted CMV appear to depend mainly on recipient factors. Immunocompetent CMV-seronegative recipients may seroconvert and occasionally may have a mononucleosis-like syndrome but do not develop permanent or severe CMV disease. Severely immunodeficient recipients, on the other hand, may develop severe pneumonitis, hepatitis, and disseminated and often fatal disease.[177–179]

The transmission of CMV by transfusion can be prevented by the exclusive use of cellular blood components from CMV-seronegative donors.[177–179] As discussed further in Chapter 39, it is also likely that CMV transmission can be prevented by the use of third-generation leukodepletion filters.

The only CMV-seronegative pediatric patients discussed in this chapter for whom blood components at low risk of CMV transmission are currently recommended are those undergoing or highly likely to undergo autologous or allogeneic bone marrow transplantation (Table 32-4). CMV-seronegative patients who require chronic transfusion support but for whom BMT is not an option (e.g., thalassemia patients without a related HLA-compatible donor) or for whom the chances of eventually undergoing a BMT are small (e.g., the majority of children with acute lymphoblastic leukemia) are not considered candidates for blood components at low risk of CMV transmission. Whereas a small number of these patients may eventually undergo BMT, the time between the initiation of transfusion support and eventual BMT may be quite long. Although it is true that the risks of serious morbidity and mortality of BMT are decreased in patients who are CMV-seronegative at the time of transplantation, it is not clear that providing components at low risk for CMV transmission will significantly decrease the frequency of CMV seroconversion over a prolonged period. In a brief report on the prevalence of CMV antibody in pediatric oncology patients and cystic fibrosis patients in the same community, the overall seroprevalence was significantly higher in the oncology group.[180] However, the incidence of seropositivity did not correlate with the number of cellular blood products received. This study demonstrates that more needs to be learned about the sources of CMV infection in pediatric patients and the impact that the use of blood components at low risk of CMV transmission would have on CMV seroconversion rates before the use of such products in all CMV seronegative pediatric oncology patients can be recommended.

γ-Irradiation to Prevent Transfusion-Associated Graft-Versus-Host Disease

Because the topic of γ-irradiation for prevention of transfusion-associated graft-versus-host disease is also covered fully in Chapter 42, only a few aspects particularly pertinent to pediatric hematology/oncology patients are outlined here.

The necessity of irradiating cellular blood components to prevent transfusion-associated graft-versus-host disease (TA-GVHD) in pediatric patients remains controversial in many situations. Patients who should definitely receive γ-irradiated cellular blood components include those with severe congenital immunodeficiency syndromes, those undergoing autologous or allogeneic BMT, and those receiving blood components donated by family members. As well, most experts would recommend irradiating blood components for patients with Hodgkin's dis-

ease.[181–185] There have been several reports of fatal TA-GVHD in children receiving chemotherapy for acute leukemia or solid malignant tumors other than Hodgkin's disease (including non-Hodgkin's lymphoma, neuroblastoma, and rhabdomyosarcoma).[180–185] Some of these children were in remission from their underlying disease. Therefore, consideration should be given, where possible, to irradiating cellular blood components for all children undergoing chemotherapy and/or radiotherapy for the treatment of malignant disease. Recently, there have been reports of TA-GVHD in patients receiving HLA-matched platelets from HLA-homozygous donors.[186,187] Considering these reports, as well as calculations as to the frequency of HLA-homozygous donors, it has been recommended that all HLA-matched cellular blood components should be irradiated.[186–188] Although reports of TA-GVHD in patients with SAAA are rare, these patients now receive more aggressive immunosuppressive therapy than in the past and consideration may be given to irradiating cellular blood components for these patients. Alternatively, γ-irradiation is not indicated for patients with the other disorders discussed in this chapter, including those receiving transfusions for thalassemia syndromes, SCD, or congenital bone marrow failure syndromes (unless, of course, they are undergoing BMT). Suggested guidelines for the irradiation of cellular blood products for pediatric patients (excluding the neonatal period) are summarized in Table 32-5.

Table 32-5. Guidelines for γ-Irradiation of Cellular Blood Components for Pediatric Patients Other Than Neonates

Well-established indications:
    Severe congenital immunodeficiency
    Autologous or allogeneic bone marrow transplantation
    Blood from first- or second-degree relatives
    Hodgkin's disease
    HLA-matched cellular blood components from unrelated donors
Other possible indications:
    Any patient undergoing chemo- and/or radiotherapy for malignant disease
    Patients with aplastic anemia receiving immunosuppressive therapy
    Solid organ transplant recipients

Potassium levels in the extracellular fluid of RBCs stored after irradiation increase more rapidly than those of nonirradiated units.[189,190] Concern has thus been expressed about the safety of these units for transfusion, particularly to very small recipients. However, careful calculations suggest that the increased potassium levels should not pose a problem for most recipients.[190] Thus, routine washing of irradiated units seems unwarranted. Problems might arise if large volumes were used and/or if the recipient had significantly compromised renal function. Until more data are available on the quality of units stored following irradiation, it would seem prudent to irradiate blood components as close to the time of transfusion as possible.

Strategies to Decrease the Number of Allogeneic Donor Exposures

As discussed in the preceding sections, many pediatric hematology and oncology patients require multiple blood transfusions. However, because the volumes required in each transfusion episode are often small, attempts to limit allogeneic donor exposures in this population may often be possible. Although there is little available data correlating the risk of transfusion-transmitted viral disease with the number of allogeneic donor exposures, it seems logical to assume that such a relationship does exist. Simple calculations support this assumption.[191] The possibility of decreasing HLA-alloimmunization through the use of single-donor apheresis platelets versus pooled random donor platelets is discussed above. Finally, in certain patients undergoing BMT, particularly those with aplastic anemia or those with donors other than HLA-compatible family members, successful outcome is inversely related to the number blood transfusions administered prior to transplantation.[1,192–194]

The first and possibly the most important strategy in limiting donor exposure is to administer blood transfusions only if absolutely necessary. A second and equally simple strategy is to ensure the optimum utilization of each blood unit. As discussed above, when transfusing RBC units to very small patients, attempts should be made to use the whole unit. This can usually be accomplished by giving the patient 2 or 3 aliquots over the 24-hour period after the unit has been opened or by using a sterile docking device.

Likewise, a standard unit of fresh frozen plasma can be divided into smaller aliquots, although the disappearance of the labile coagulation factors with storage at 4°C must be taken into consideration. Where available, the use of single-donor apheresis platelets rather than pooled random-donor platelets can significantly decrease the number of donor exposures in selected children. In addition, attention should be paid to ensure that the number of random-donor units requested is not more than that actually required for the child's weight and the desired platelet increment.

The use of autologous blood to limit allogeneic donor exposure is obviously not often possible in this population. However, there are a few situations where it might be considered. Patients from whom autologous bone marrow is being collected and cryopreserved for future potential use can donate their own blood prior to the intervention. Second, in certain selected cases, intraoperative blood salvage and autotransfusion might be considered. The question of whether intraoperative blood salvage and autotransfusion result in the reinfusion of malignant cells and the development of metastatic disease has been fully reviewed.[195] At least some investigators have not found this to occur. However, in most children it is likely that even a very small risk of metastatic spread would be considered more harmful than the risk currently associated with allogeneic blood transfusion. Autologous transfusions have also been used in selected patients with sickle cell anemia, particularly for those patients who have developed multiple erythrocyte antibodies.[196,197] However, the administration of autologous blood is not appropriate for those situations in which a goal of transfusion is to decrease the percentage and/or absolute amount of HbS in circulation.

Another approach to decreasing allogeneic blood exposure in children is the use of "limited-exposure" blood donor programs (i.e., the use of one or a very small number of dedicated donors to provide the patient's total blood needs).[198,199] There has been a report of the successful use of such a program to meet the blood transfusion requirements of children undergoing elective surgery who are unable to donate autologous blood.[200] This approach could also be used to provide the RBC transfusion requirements of selected children on chronic transfusion programs, particularly if the transfusion requirements are relatively modest as, for example, may be the case for certain infants and young children with DBA or congenital hemolytic anemia due to pyruvate kinase deficiency. The use of limited-exposure blood donor programs for the transfusion support of young children with leukemia or other malignancies can be considered in selected cases, although it may be difficult to organize because the need for blood components, especially platelets, is not always predictable. However, there has been at least one report of its successful application to minimize the number of donor exposures in an newborn undergoing BMT.[201] While attention must be paid so that the quality of blood components prepared and/or the safety for the donor of participating in limited donor exposure programs is not compromised, preliminary reports suggest that donors can safely donate blood more often than every 56 days, the interval usually required between donations of allogeneic blood.[202]

Finally, as discussed in several sections above, the role of hematopoietic growth factors to decrease the blood transfusion requirements of children with hematologic and neoplastic diseases is currently a very active area of research. A full discussion of the findings to date is beyond the scope of this chapter; the interested reader is referred to several excellent recent articles and reviews; see references 77 through 79, 83, 92, and 203 through 206, as well as Chapter 47.

REFERENCES

1. Rivera GK, Pinkel D, Simone JV et al: Treatment of acute lymphoblastic leukemia. 30 years' experience at St. Jude Childrens' Research Hospital. N Engl J Med 329:1289, 1993
2. Suton WW, Fernbach DJ, Vietti TJ: Clinical Pediatric Oncology, 3rd ed. CV Mosby, St. Louis, 1984
3. Sanders JE, Storb R, Anasetti C et al: Marrow transplant experience for children with severe aplastic anemia. Am J Pediatr Hematol Oncol 16:43, 1994
4. Piomelli S: Management of Cooley's anemia. Baillieres Clin Haematol 6:287, 1993
5. Platt OS, Brambilla DJ, Rosse WF et al: Mortality in sickle cell disease. Life expectancy and risk factors for early death. N Engl J Med 330:1639, 1994
6. Means RT, Krantz SB: Progress in understanding the pathogenesis of the anemia of chronic disease. Blood 80:1639, 1992
7. Miller CB, Jones RJ, Piantadosi S et al: Decreased erythropoietin response in patients with the anemia of cancer. N Engl J Med 322:1689, 1990
8. Rao SP, Miller ST, Cohen BJ: Severe anemia due to B19 parvovirus infection in children with acute leukemia in remission. Am J Pediatr Hematol Oncol 12:194, 1990
9. Kurtzman G, Young N: Clinical spectrum of bone marrow failure due to chronic B19 parvovirus infection and the immunologic mechanism responsible for persistence. Blood 72:45A, 1988
10. Garratty G: Immune cytopenia associated with antibiotics. Transf Med Rev 7:255, 1993
11. Doll DC, Weiss RB: Hemolytic anemia associated with antineoplastic agents. Cancer Treatment Reports 69:777, 1985
12. Nathan DG, Oski FA: Hematology of Infancy and Childhood, 4th ed. WB Saunders, Philadelphia, 1993
13. Card RT, Brain MC: The "anemia" of childhood: evidence for a physiologic response to hyperphosphatemia. N Engl J Med 228:388, 1973
14. Petz LD, Tomasulo PA: Red cell transfusion. p. 1. In Kolins J, McCarthy LJ (eds): Contemporary Transfusion Practice. American Association of Blood Banks, Arlington, VA, 1987
15. Oski FA: Red cell 2,3-diphosphoglycerate levels in subjects with chronic hypoxemia. N Engl J Med 280:1165, 1969
16. Oski FA, Marshall BE, Cohen PJ et al: The role of the left-shifted or right-shifted oxygen-hemoglobin equilibrium curve. Ann Intern Med 74:44, 1971
17. Hjelm M: The content of 2,3-diphosphoglycerate and some other phospho compounds in human erythrocytes from healthy adults and subjects with different types of anemia. Forsvarsmedicin 5:219, 1969
18. Torrance JD, Jacobs P, Restrepo A et al: Intraerythrocytic adaptation to anemia. N Engl J Med 283:165, 1970
19. Festa RS, Asakura T: Oxygen dissociation curves in children with anemia and malignant disease. Amer J Hematol 7:233, 1979
20. Greenhaum BH, Herman JH: Transfusion therapy in pediatric oncology. Pediatr Ann 17:687, 1988
21. Hellem AJ, Borchgrevink CF, Ames SB: The role of red cells in haemostasis: The relation between haematocrit, bleeding time and platelet adhesiveness. Brit J Haemat 7:42, 1961
22. Blajchman MA, Bordin JO, Bardossy L, Heddle NH: The contribution of the haematocrit to thrombocyto-

penic bleeding in experimental animals. Br J Haematol 86:347, 1994

23. Smith PJ, Ekert H: Evidence of stem-cell competition in children with malignant disease. Lancet 1:776, 1976

24. Toogood IRG, Ekert H, Smith PJ: Controlled study of hypertransfusion during remission induction in childhood acute lymphoblastic leukemia. Lancet 2:862, 1978

25. Buchanan GR: Hematologic supportive care of the pediatric cancer patient. p 973. In Pizzo PA, Poplack DG (eds): Principles and Practice of Pediatric Oncology. 2nd Ed. JB Lippincott, Philadelphia, 1993

26. Bush RS: The significance of anemia in clinical radiation therapy. Int J Radiat Oncol Biol Phys 12:2047, 1986

27. Bray GL, Reaman GH: Erythropoietin deficiency: A complication of cisplatin therapy and its treatment with recombinant human erythropoietin. Am J Pediatr Hematol Oncol 13:426, 1991

28. Miller CB, Platanias LC, Mills SR et al: Phase I–II trial of erythropoietin in the treatment of cisplatin-associated anemia. J Natl Cancer Inst 84:98, 1992

29. Henry DH, Abels RI: Recombinant human erythropoietin in the treatment of cancer and chemotherapy-induced anemia: results of double-blind and open-label follow-up studies. Semin Oncol 21:21, 1994

30. Cascinu S, Fedeli A, Fedeli SL, Catalano G: Cisplatin-associated anaemia treated with subcutaneous erythropoietin. A pilot study. Br J Cancer 67:156, 1993

31. Cascinu S, Fedeli A, Del Ferro E et al: Recombinant human erythropoietin treatment in cisplatin-associated anemia: a randomized, double-blind trial with placebo. J Clin Oncol 12:1058, 1994

32. Ayash LJ, Elias A, Hunt M et al: Recombinant human erythropoietin for the treatment of the anaemia associated with autologous bone marrow transplantation. Br J Haematol 87:153, 1994

33. Locatelli F, Zecca M, Beguin Y et al: Accelerated erythroid repopulation with no stem-cell competition effect in children treated with recombinant human erythropoietin after allogeneic bone marrow transplantation. Br J Haematol 84:752, 1993

34. Guay J, Hume H, Gauthier M, Tremblay P: Choc hémorragique. p. 173. In Lacroix J, Gauthier M, Beaufils F (eds): Urgences et Soins Intensif Pédiatriques. Les Presses de l'Université de Montréal, Montreal, 1994

35. Hersh EM, Bodey GP, Nies BA, Freireich EJ: Causes of death in acute leukemia. JAMA 193:105, 1965

36. Schiffer CA: Prophylactic platelet transfusion. Transfusion 32:295, 1992

37. Higby DJ, Cohen E, Holland JF, Sinks L: The prophylactic treatment of thrombocytopenic leukemic patients with platelets. A double blind study. Transfusion 14:440, 1974

38. Roy AJ, Jaffe N, Djerassi I: Prophylactic platelet transfusions in children with acute leukemia. A dose response study. Transfusion 13:283, 1973

39. Murphy S, Litwin S, Herring LM et al: Indications for platelet transfusion in children with acute leukemia. Am J Hematol 12:347, 1982

40. Gockerman JP, Davis J: Platelet transfusion in acute leukemic patients. Blood 54:122A, 1979

41. Solomon J, Bofenkamp T, Fahey JL et al: Platelet prophylaxis in acute nonlymphoblastic leukemia. Lancet 1:267, 1978

42. Ilett SJ, Lilleyman JS: Platelet transfusions requirements of children with newly diagnosed lymphoblastic leukemia. Acta Hematol 62:86, 1979

43. Feusner J: The use of platelet transfusions. Am J Pediatr Hematol Oncol 6:255, 1984

44. Schiffer CA: Some aspects of recent advances in the use of blood cell components. Br J Haematol 39:289, 1978

45. Hoak JC, Koepeke JA: Platelet transfusions. Clin Haematol 5:69, 1976

46. Aisner J: Clinical use of platelet transfusion for patients with cancer. p. 39. In: Platelet Physiology and Transfusion. American Association of Blood Banks, Arlington, VA, 1980

47. Kelton JG, Blajchman MA: Platelet transfusions. Can Med Assoc J 121:1353, 1979

48. Tomasulo PA, Lenes BA: Platelet transfusion therapy. p. 63. In Menitove JE, McCarthy LJ (eds): Hemostatic Disorders and the Blood Bank. American Association of Blood Banks, Arlington, VA, 1984

49. Baer MR, Bloomfield CD: Controversies in transfusion medicine. Prophylactic platelet transfusion therapy: pro. Transfusion 32:377, 1992

50. Patten E: Controversies in transfusion medicine. Prophylactic platelet transfusion revisited after 25 years: con. Transfusion 32:381, 1992

51a. Pisciotto PT, Benson K, Hume H et al: Transfusion, June 1995 (in press)

51. Hume HA, Ali A, Decary F, Blajchman MA: Evaluation of pediatric transfusion practice using criteria maps. Transfusion 31:52, 1991

52. McCullough J, Steeper TA, Connelly DP et al: Platelet utilization in a university hospital. JAMA 259:2414, 1988

53. Gaydos LA, Freireich EJ, Mantel N: The quantitative relation between platelet count and hemorrhage in

patients with acute leukemia. N Engl J Med 266:905, 1962

54. National Institutes of Health, Consensus Development Conference: Platelet transfusion therapy. JAMA 257:1777, 1987

55. Slichter SJ: Platelet transfusions a constantly evolving therapy. Thromb Haemost 66:178, 1991

56. Beutler E: Platelet transfusions: The 20,000/μL trigger. Blood 81:1411, 1993

57. Aderka D, Praff G, Santo M et al: Bleeding due to thrombocytopenia in acute leukemias and reevaluation of the prophylactic platelet transfusion policy. Am J Med Sci 291:147, 1986

58. Gmür J, Burger J, Schanz U et al: Safety of stringent prophylactic platelet transfusion policy for patients with acute leukaemia. Lancet 338:1223, 1991

59. Creutzig U, Ritter J, Budde M et al: Early deaths due to hemorrhage and leukostasis in childhood acute myelogenous leukemia. Cancer 60:3071, 1987

60. Cunningham I, Gee TS, Reich LM et al: Acute promyelocytic leukemia: treatment results during a decade at Memorial Hospital. Blood 73:1116, 1989

61. Kantarjian HM, Keating MJ, Walters RS et al: Acute promyelocytic leukemia. Am J Med 80:789, 1986

62. Rodeghiero F, Avvisati G, Castaman G et al: Early deaths and anti-hemorrhagic treatment in acute promyelocytic leukemia. A GIMEMA retrospective study in 268 consecutive patients. Blood 75:2112, 1990

63. Belt RJ, Leite C, Haas CD, Stephens RL: Incidence of hemorragic complications in patients with cancer. JAMA 239:2571, 1978

64. Dutcher JP, Schiffer CA, Aisner J et al: Incidence of thrombocytopenia and serious hemorrhage among patients with solid tumors. Cancer :557, 1984

65. Bishop JF, Schiffer CA, Aisner J et al: Surgery in leukemia: a review of 167 operations on thrombocytopenic patients. Am J Hematol 26:147, 1987

66. Tomasulo PA, Petz LD: Platelet transfusions. p. 427. In Petz LD, Swisher SN (eds): Clinical Practice of Transfusion Medicine, 2nd ed. Churchill Livingstone, New York, 1989

67. Christie DJ, Van Buren N, Lennon SS, Putnam JL. Vancomycin-dependant antibodies associated with thrombocytopenia and refractoriness to platelet transfusions in patients with leukemia. Blood 75:518, 1990

68. Strauss RG: Granulocyte transfusions: uses, abuses and indications. p. 65. In Kolins J, McCarthy LJ (eds): Contemporary Transfusions Practice. American Association of Blood Banks, Arlington, VA, 1987

69. Strauss RG: Therapeutic granulocyte transfusions in 1993. Blood 81:1675, 1993

70. Schiffer CA: Granulocyte transfusions: an overlooked therapeutic modality. Transfusion Med Rev 4:2, 1990

71. Wright DG, Robichaud KJ, Pizzo PA et al: Lethal pulmonary reactions associated with the combined use of amphotericin B and leukocyte transfusions. N Engl J Med 304:1185, 1981

72. Dana BW, Durie BGM, White RF et al: Concomitant administration of granulocyte transfusions and amphotericin B in neutropenic patients: absence of significant pulmonary toxicity. Blood 57:90, 1981

73. Haber RH, Oddone EZ, Gurbel PA, Stead WW: Acute pulmonary decompensation due to amphotericin B in the absence of granulocyte transfusions (letter). N Engl J Med 315:836, 1986

74. Dutcher JP, Kendall J, Norris D et al: Granulocyte transfusion therapy and amphotericin B: adverse reactions? Am J Hematol 31:102, 1989

75. Slichter SJ: Transfusion and bone marrow transplantation. Transf Med Rev 2:1, 1988

76. Bhatia S, McCullough J, Perry EH et al: Granulocyte tranfusions: efficacy in treating fungal infections in neutropenic patients following bone marrow transplantation. Transfusion 34:226, 1994

77. Morstyn G: The impact of colony stimulating factors on cancer chemotherapy. Br J Haematol 75:303, 1990

78. Asano S: Human granulocyte colony-stimulating factor: its basic aspects and clinical applications. Am J Pediatr Hematol Oncol 13:400, 1991

79. Furman WL, Crist WM: Potential uses of recombinant human granulocyte-macrophage colony-stimulating factor in children. Am J Pediatr Hematol Oncol 13:388, 1991

80. Alter BP, Young NS: The bone marrow failure syndromes. p. 216. In Nathan DG, Oski FA (eds): Hematology of Infancy and Childhood. 4th Ed. WB Saunders, Philadelphia, 1993

81. Niemeyer CM, Baumgarten E, Holldack et al: Treatment trial of recombinant human erythropoietin in children with congenital hypoplastic anemia. Contrib Nephrol 88:276, 1991

82. Dunbar CE, Smith DA, Kimball J et al: Treatment of Diamond-Blackfan anemia with hematopoiesis growth factors, granulocyte-macrophage colony-stimulating factor and interleukin-3: sustained remission following IL-3. Br J Haematol 79:316, 1991

83. Gillio AP, Gabrilove JL: Cytokine treatment of inherited bone marrow failure syndromes. Blood 81:1669, 1993

84. Olivieri NF, Feig SA, Valentino L et al: Failure of recombinant human interleukin-3 therapy to induce

erythropoiesis in patients with refractory Diamond-Blackfan anemia. Blood 83:2444, 1994

85. Lenarsky C, Weinberg K, Guinan E et al: Bone marrow transplantation for constitutional pure red cell aplasia. Blood 71:226, 1988

86. Greinix HT, Storb R, Sanders JE et al: Long-term survival and cure after marrow transplantation for congenital hypoplastic anaemia (Diamond-Blackfan syndrome). Br J Haematol 84:515, 1993

87. Bonilla MA, Gillio AP, Ruggiero M et al: Effects of recombinant human granulocyte colony-stimulating factor on neutropenia in patients with congenital agranulocytosis. N Engl J Med 320:1574, 1989

88. Gluckman E, Berger R, Dutreix J: Bone marrow transplantation for Fanconi anemia. Semin Hematol 21:20, 1984

89. Alter BP: Fanconi's anemia: Current concepts. Am J Pediatr Hematol Oncol 14:170, 1992

90. Gluckman E, Broxmeyer HE, Auerbach AD et al: Hematopoietic reconstitution in a patient with Fanconi's anemia by means of umbilical-cord blood from an HLA-identical sibling. N Engl J Med 321:1174, 1989

91. Broxmeyer HE, Hangoc G, Cooper S et al: Growth characteristics and expansion of human umbilical cord blood and estimation of its potential for transplantation in adults. Proc Natl Acad Sci USA 89:4109, 1992

92. Kojima S, Matsuyama T: Stimulation of granulopoiesis by high-dose recombinant human granulocyte colony-stimulating factor in children with aplastic anemia and very severe neutropenia. Blood 83:1474, 1994

93. McDonagh KT, Nienhuis AW: The thalassemias. p. 783. In Nathan DG, Oski FA (eds): Hematology of Infancy and Childhood. 4th Ed. WB Saunders, Philadelphia, 1993

94. Lukens JN: The thalassemias and related disorders. p. 1102. In Lee GR, Bitheu TC, Forester J et al (eds): Wintrobe's Clinical Hematology. 9th Ed. Lea & Febiger, Philadelphia, 1993

95. Propper RD, Button LN, Nathan DG: New approaches to the transfusion management of thalassemia. Blood 55:55, 1980

96. Cohen AR, Schmidt JM, Martin MB et al: Clinical trial of young red cell transfusions. J Pediatr 104:865, 1984

97. Marcus RE, Wonke B, Bantock HM et al: A prospective trial of young red cells in 48 patients with transfusion-dependent thalassaemia. Br J Haematol 60:153, 1985

98. Collins AF, Gonçalves-Dias C, Haddad S et al: Comparison of a transfusion preparation of newly formed red cells and standard washed red cell transfusions in patients with homozygous β-thalassemia. Transfusion 34:517, 1994

99. De Virgiliis S, Congia M, Frau F et al: Deferoxamine-induced growth retardation in patients with thalassemia major. J Pediatr 113:661, 1988

100. Olivieri NF, Buncic JR, Chew E et al: Visual and auditory neurotoxicity in patients receiving subcutaneous deferoxamine infusions. N Engl J Med 314:869, 1986

101. Coles SM, Klein HG et al: Alloimmunization in two multitransfused patient populations. Transfusion 21:462, 1981

102. Blumberg N, Ross K et al: Should chronic transfusion be matched for antigens other than ABO and Rh(o)D? Vox Sang 47:205, 1984

103. Michail-Merianou V, Pamphili-Panousopoulou L et al: Alloimmunization to red cell antigens in thalassemia: comparative study of usual versus better-match transfusion programmes. Vox Sang 52:95, 1987

104. Spanos T, Karageeorga M et al: Red cell alloantibodies in patients with thalassemia. Vox Sang 58:50, 1990

105. Lucarelli G, Galimberti M, Polchi P et al: Marrow transplantation in patients with thalassemia responsive to iron chelation therapy. N Engl J Med 329:840, 1993

106. Giardini C, Angelucci E, Lucarelli G et al: Bone marrow transplantation for thalassemia. Am J Pediatr Hematol Oncol 16:6, 1994

107. Lucarelli G, Galrmberti M, Polchi P et al: Bone marrow transplantation in adult thalassemia. Blood 80:1603, 1992

108. Platt OS, Dover GJ: Sickle cell disease. p. 732. In Nathan DG, Oski FA (eds): Hematology of Infancy and Childhood. 4th Ed. WB Saunders, Philadelphia, 1993

109. Lukens JN: Hemoglobinopathies S, C, D, E and O and associated diseases. p. 1061. In Lee GR, Bitheu TC, Forester J et al (eds): Wintrobe's Clinical Hematology. 9th Ed. Lea & Febiger, Philadelphia, 1993

110. Wethers D, Pearson H, Gaston M: Newborn screening for sickle cell disease and other hemoglobinopathies. Pediatrics 83:813, 1989

111. Motulsky AG: Frequency of sickling disorders in U.S. blacks. N Engl J Med 288:31, 1973

112. Wayne AS, Kevy SV, Nathan DG: Transfusion management of sickle cell disease. Blood 81:1109, 1993

113. Koshy M, Burd L, Wallace D et al: Prophylactic red cell transfusion in pregnant patients with sickle cell disease. N Engl J Med 319:1447, 1988

114. Koshy M, Burd L: Management of pregnancy in

sickle cell syndromes. Hematol Oncol Clin North Am 5:585, 1991

115. Ohene-Frempong K: Stroke in sickle cell disease: demographic, clinical, and therapeutic considerations. Semin Hematol 28:213, 1991

116. Wang WC, Kovnar EH, Tonkin IL et al: High risk of recurrent stroke after discontinuance of five to twelve years of transfusion therapy in patients with sickle cell disease. J Pediatr 118:377, 1991

117. Miller ST, Jensen D, Rao SP: Less intensive long-term transfusion therapy for sickle cell anemia and cerebrovascular accident. J Pediatr 120:54, 1992

118. Cohen AR, Martin MB, Silber JH et al: A modified transfusion program for prevention of stroke in sickle cell disease. Blood 79:1657, 1992

119. Rosse WF, Gallagher D, Kinney TR et al: Transfusion and alloimmunization in sickle cell disease. Blood 76: 1431, 1990

120. Vichinsky EP, Earles A, Johnson RA et al: Alloimmunization in sickle cell anemia and transfusion of racially unmatched blood. N Engl J Med 322:1617, 1990

121. Diamond WJ, Brown FL, Bitterman P et al: Delayed hemolytic transfusion reaction presenting as sickle-cell crisis. Ann Intern Med 93:231, 1980

122. Friedman DF, Kim HC, Manno CS: Hyperhemolysis associated with red cell transfusion in sickle cell disease. Transfusion 33:6S, 1993

123. Cummins D, Webb G, Shah N, Davies SC: Delayed haemolytic transfusion reactions in patients with sickle cell disease. Postgrad Med J 67:689, 1991

124. Lankiewicz MW, Shirez RS, Ness PM, Charache S: Delayed hemolytic transfusion reactions DHTR) in sickle cell disease (SCD): evidence for autologous RBC destruction (abstract). Transfusion 33:22S, 1993

125. Ambruso DR, Githens JH, Alcorn R et al: Experience with donors matched for minor blood group antigens in patients with sickle cell anemia who are receiving chronic transfusion therapy. Transfusion 27:94, 1987

126. Sosler SD, Jilly BJ, Saporito C, Koshy M: A simple, practical model for reducing alloimmunization in patients with sickle cell disease. Am J Hematol 43:103, 1993

127. Tahhan HR, Holbrook CT, Braddy LR et al: Antigen-matched donor blood in the transfusion management of patients with sickle cell disease. Transfusion 34: 562, 1994

128. Ness PM: To match or not to match: the question for chronically transfused patients with sickle cell anemia. Transfusion 34:558, 1994

129. Jan K, Usami S, Smith JA: Effects of transfusion on the rheological properties of blood in sickle cell anemia. Transfusion 22:17, 1982

130. Rackoff WR, Ohene-Frempong K, Month S et al: Neurologic events after partial exchange transfusion for priapism in sickle cell disease. J Pediatr 120:882, 1992

131. Vermylen C, Cornu G: Bone marrow transplantation for sickle cell disease. The European experience. Am J Pediatr Hematol Oncol 16:18, 1994

132. Walters MC, Thomas ED: Bone marrow transplantation for sickle cell disease. The United States experience. Am J Pediatr Hematol Oncol 16:22, 1994

133. Piomelli S, Seaman C, Ackerman K et al: Planning an exchange transfusion in patients with sickle cell syndromes. Am J Pediatr Hematol Oncol 12:268, 1990

134. Kim HC, Dugan NP, Silber JH et al: Erythrocytapheresis therapy to reduce iron overload in chronically transfused patients with sickle cell disease. Blood 83: 1136, 1994

135. Mentzer WC: Pyruvate kinase deficiency and disorders of glycolysis. p. 634. In Nathan DG, Oski FA (eds): Hematology of Infancy and Childhood. 4th Ed. WB Saunders, Philadelphia, 1993

136. Jayabose S, Tugal O, Ruddy R et al: Transfusion therapy for severe anemia. Am J Pediatr Hematol Oncol 15:324, 1993

137. Berman B. Krieger A, Naiman JL: A new method for calculating volumes of blood required for partial exchange transfusion. J Pediatr 94:86, 1979

138. Fosburg M, Dolan M, Propper R et al: Intensive plasma exchange in small and critically ill pediatric patients: techniques and clinical outcome. J Clin Apheresis 1:215, 1983

139. Heaton A, Keegan T, Holme S: In vivo regeneration of red cell, 2,3-diphosphoglycerate following transfusion of DPG-depleted AS-1, AS-3, and CPDA-1 red cells. Br J Haematol 71:131, 1989

140. Meryman HT, Hornblower M: The preparation of red cells depleted of leukocytes. Review and evaluation. Transfusion 26:101, 1986

141. Dunstan RA: The origin of ABH antigens on human platelets. Blood 65:615, 1985

142. Kelton JG et al: The amount of blood group A substance on platelets is proportional to the amount in the plasma. Blood 59:980, 1982

143. Brand A, Sintnicolaas K, Claas FHJ, Eernisse JG: ABH antibodies causing platelet transfusion refractoriness. Transfusion 26:463, 1986

144. Lee EJ, Schiffer CA: ABO incompatibility can influence the results of platelet transfusion. Results of a randomized trial. Transfusion 29:384, 1989

145. Carr R, Hutton JL, Jenkins JA et al: Transfusion of ABO mismatched platelets leads to early platelet refractoriness. Br J Haematol 75:408, 1990

146. Pierce RN, Reich LM, Mayer K: Hemolysis following platelet transfusions from ABO-incompatible donors. Transfusion 25:60, 1985

147. Ferguson DJ: Acute intravascular hemolysis after a platelet transfusion. Can Med Assoc J 138:523, 1988

148. Reis MD, Coovadia AS: Transfusion of ABO-incompatible platelets causing severe hemolytic reaction. Clin Lab Haematol 11:237, 1989

149. Dunstan RA, Simpson MB, Rosse WF: Erythrocyte antigens on human platelets. Absence of the Rhesus, Duffy, Kell, Kidd, and Lutheran antigens. Transfusion 24:243, 1984

150. Goldfinger D, McGinnis MH: Rh incompatible platelet transfusion—risks and consequences of sensitizing immunosuppressed patients. N Engl J Med 284:942, 1971

151. McLeod BC, Piehl MR, Sassetti RJ: Alloimmunization to RhD by platelet transfusions in autologous bone marrow transplant recipients. Vox Sang 59:185, 1990

152. Baldwin ML, Ness PM, Scott D et al: Alloimmunization to D antigen and HLA in D-negative immunosuppressed oncology patients. Transfusion 28:330, 1988

153. Heim MU, Bock M, Kold HJ et al: Intravenous anti-D gammaglobulin for the prevention of rhesus isoimmunization caused by platelet transfusions in patients with malignant diseases. Vox Sang 62:165, 1992

154. Zeiler T, Wittmann G, Zingsem J et al: A dose of 100 IU intravenous anti-D gammaglobulin is effective for the prevention of RhD immunisation after RhD-incompatible single donor platelet transfusion. Vox Sang 66:243, 1994

155. National Blood Transfusion Service Immunoglobulin Working Party: Recommendations for the use of anti-D immunoglobulin. Prescribers J 31:137, 1991

156. Slichter SJ: Prevention of platelet alloimmunization. p. 83. In Murawski K (ed): Transfusion Medicine: Recent Technological Advances. Alan R. Liss, New York, 1986

157. Slichter SJ: Mechanisms and management of platelet refractoriness. p. 95. In Nance ST (ed): Transfusion Medicine in the 1990's. American Association of Blood Banks, Arlington, 1990

158. Schiffer CA: Prevention of alloimmunization against platelets. Blood 77:1, 1991

159. Lane TA, Anderson KC, Goodnough LT et al: Leukocyte reduction in blood component therapy. Ann Intern Med 117:151, 1992

160. Freedman JJ, Blajchman MA, McCombie N: Canadian Red Cross Society Symposium on leukodepletion: report of proceedings. Transfus Med Rev 8:1, 1994

161. Lee EJ, Schiffer CA: Serial measurement of lymphocytoxic antibody and response to non-matched platelet transfusions in alloimmunized patients. Blood 70:1727, 1987

162. Schiffer CA, Dutcher JP, Aisner J et al: Randomized trial of leukocyte-depleted platelet transfusion to modify alloimmunization in patients with leukemia. Blood 62:815, 1983

163. Holohan TV, Terasaki PI, Deisseroth AB: Suppression of transfusion-related alloimmunization in intensively treated cancer patients. Blood 58:122, 1981

164. Saarinen UM, Kekomaki R, Siimes MA et al: Effective prophylaxis against platelet refractoriness in multitransfused patients: use of leukocyte-free blood components. Blood 75:512, 1990

165. Saarinen UM, Koskimies S, Myllyla G: Systematic use of leukocyte-free blood components to prevent alloimmunization and platelet refractoriness in multitransfused children with cancer. Vox Sang 65:286, 1993

166. Dutcher JP, Schiffer CA, Aisner J, Wiernik PH: Alloimmunization following platelet transfusion: the absence of a dose-response relationship. Blood 57:395, 1981

167. Gmur J, vonFelten A, Osterwaldei B et al: Delayed alloimmunization using random single donor platelet transfusions: a prospective study in thrombocytopenic patients with leukemia. Blood 62:473, 1983

168. Murphy MF, Metcalfe P, Thomas H et al: Use of leucocyte-poor blood components and HLA-matched-platelet donors to prevent HLA alloimmunization. Br J Haematol 62:529, 1986

169. Andreu G, DeWilly J, Leberre C et al: Prevention of HLA immunization with leukocyte-poor packed red cells and platelet concentrates obtained by filtration. Blood 72:964, 1988

170. Sniecinski I, O'Donnell MR, Nowicki B et al: Prevention of refractoriness and HLA-alloimmunization using filtered blood products. Blood 71:1402, 1988

171. vanMarwijk Kooy M, vanProoijen HC, Moes M et al: The use of leukocyte-depleted platelet concentrates for the prevention of refractoriness and primary HLA alloimmunization; a prospective, randomized trial. Blood 77:201, 1990

172. Oksanen K, Kekomaki R, Ruutu R et al: Prevention of alloimmunization in patients with acute leukemia by use of white cell-reduced blood components—a randomized trial. Transfusion 31:588, 1991

173. Heddle NM: The efficacy of leukodepletion to improve platelet transfusion response: a critical appraisal of clinical studies. Transfus Med Rev 8:15, 1994

174. Reesink HW, Nydegger WE, Brand A et al: Should all platelet concentrates issued be leukocyte-poor? Vox Sang 52:57, 1992

175. Pietersz RNI, Steneker I, Reesink HW et al: Comparison of five different filters for the removal of leukocytes from red cell concentrates. Vox Sang 62:76, 1992

176. Meryman HT: Transfusion-induced alloimmunization and immunosuppression and the effects of leukocyte depletion. Transfus Med Rev 3:180, 1989

177. Adler SP: Transfusion-associated cytomegalovirus infection. Rev Infect Dis 5:977, 1983

178. Adler SP: Cytomegalovirus and transfusions. Transfus Med Rev 2:235, 1988

179. Preiksaitis JK: Indications for the use of cytomegalovirus seronegative blood products. Transfus Med Rev 5:1, 1991

180. Preiksaitis JK, Roberts S, Desai S, Vaudry WL: Increased prevalence of CMV seropositivity in pediatric oncology patients (letter). Transfusion 30:573, 1990

181. Leitman SF, Holland PV: Irradiation of blood products: indications and guidelines. Transfusion 25:293, 1985

182. Anderson KC, Weinstein HJ. Transfusion-associated graft-versus-host disease. N Engl J Med 323:315, 1990

183. Anderson KC, Goodnough LT, Sayers M et al: Variation in blood component irradiation practice: Implications for prevention of transfusion-associated graft-versus-host disease. Blood 77:2096, 1991

184. Greenbaum BH: Transfusion-associated graft-versus-host disease: historical perspectives, incidence, and current use of irradiated blood products. J Clin Oncol 9:1889, 1991

185. Linden JV, Pisciotti PT: Transfusion-associated graft-versus-host disease and blood irradiation. Transfus Med Rev 6:116, 1992

186. Shivdasani RA, Haluska FG, Dock NL et al: Brief report: graft-versus-host disease associated with transfusion of blood from unrelated HLA-homozygous donors. N Engl J Med 328:766, 1993

187. Benson K, Marks AR, Marshall MJ, Goldstein JD: Fatal graft-versus-host disease associated with transfusions of HLA-matched, HLA-homozygous platelets from unrelated donors. Transfusion 34:432, 1994

188. Grishaber JE, Birney SM, Strauss RG: Potential for transfusion-associated graft-versus-host disease due to apheresis platelets matched for HLA class I antigens. Transfusion 33:910, 1993

189. Ramirez AM, Woodfield DG, Scott R, McLachlan J: High potassium levels in stored irradiated blood. Transfusion 27:444, 1987

190. Strauss RG: Routinely washing irradiated red cells before transfusion seems unwarranted. Transfusion 30:675, 1990

191. Hume H: The transfusion support of pediatric patients with acquired or congenital bone marrow hypoplasia. In Wilson SM, Levitt JS, Strauss RG (eds): Improving Transfusion Practice for Pediatric Patients. American Association of Blood Banks, Arlington, VA, 1991

192. Storb R, Weiden PL: Transfusion problems associated with transplantation. Semin Hematol 18:163, 1981

193. Kerman NA, Flomenberg N, Dupont B, O'Reilly RJ: Graft rejection in recipients of T-cell depleted HLA-nonidentical marrow transplants for leukemia. Transplantation 43:842, 1987

194. Rowe JM, Ciobanu N, Ascensao J: Recommended guidelines for the management of autologous and allogeneic bone marrow transplantation. Ann Intern Med 120:143, 1994

195. Dzik WH, Sherburne B: Intraoperative blood salvage: medical controversies. Transfus Med Rev 3:208, 1990

196. Castro OL: Long-term cryopreservation of red cells from patients with sickle cell disease. Transfusion 25:70, 1985

197. Castro O: Autotransfusion: a management option for alloimmunized sickle cell patients? p. 117. In Scott RB (ed): Advances in the Pathophysiology, Diagnosis, and Treatment of Sickle Cell Disease. 2nd Ed. Alan R. Liss, New York, 1982

198. Strauss RG: Directed and limited-exposure donor programs for children. p. 1. In Sacher RA, Strauss RG (eds): Contemporary Issues in Pediatric Transfusion Medicine. American Association of Blood Banks, Arlington, VA, 1989

199. Strauss RG, Barnes A, Blanchette VS et al: Directed and limited-exposure blood donations for infants and children. Transfusion 30:68, 1990

200. Strauss RG, Wieland MR, Randels MJ, Koerner TAW: Feasibility and success of a single-donor red cell program for pediatric elective surgery patients. Transfusion 32:747, 1992

201. Karandish S, DePalma L, Quinones RR, Luban NLC: Minimal allogeneic donor exposure with the use of dedicated donors and a sterile connecting device in

a newborn undergoing bone marrow transplantation. Am J Pediatr Hematol Oncol 16:90, 1994

202. Becker LM, Weitekamp LA, Kleis DG et al: Minimal donor exposure: low risk/high benefit. Transfusion 33:80S, 1993

203. Ascensao JL, Bilgrami S, Zanjani ED: Erythropoietin biology and clinical applications. Am J Pediatr Hematol Oncol 13:376, 1991

204. Guinan EC, Sieff CA, Oette DH, Nathan DG: A phase I/II trial of recombinant granulocyte-macrophage colony-stimulating factor for children with aplastic anemia. Blood 76:1077, 1990

205. Goodnough LT, Anderson KC, Kurtz S et al: Indications and guidelines for the use of hematopoietic growth factors. Transfusion 33:944, 1993

206. Gordon MS, Hoffman R: Growth factors affecting human thrombocytopoiesis: potential agents for the treatment of thrombocytopenia. Blood 80:302, 1992

Chapter 33

Extracorporeal Therapy for Infants and Children

Sherwin V. Kevy

The modern era of apheresis was inaugurated by the development of a single-arm instrument capable of separating plasma from cells and a continuous flow instrument for collection of granulocytes from donors.[1,2] Current automated instrumentation utilizes microprocessor technology to separate the desired component and recombine the remaining components to the donor or patient. This chapter discusses the therapeutic applications of plasma exchange (PE) and removal of cellular components (cytopheresis), which include red blood cells (red cell exchange and erythrocytopheresis), white cells (leukocytopheresis), and extracorporeal membrane oxygenation support. Emphasis is given to those modifications necessary for the treatment of the pediatric patient.

TYPES OF SEPARATORS

The instrumentation may be either continuous or discontinuous and achieve separation by centrifugation or filtration. In centrifugal instruments, separation of the components is achieved according to density by altering the centrifugal force and blood flow rate. Continuous-flow centrifugal instrumentation utilizes optical sensors and computerization to detect the desired interface, which allows a specific component to be removed continuously and the remainder to be returned to the patient combined with

the replacement fluid. These instruments require two venapunctures or a double-lumen catheter. They also have the option to be run in the manual mode, which allows the operator to adjust to a change in the clinical condition of the patient. Intermittent-flow centrifugal cell separators essentially batch process. Once the desired component is collected, the centrifuge stops, and the residual components are returned along with the replacement fluid. Discontinuous procedures require a single venipuncture but can utilize a double-lumen catheter. More important, the patient is intermittently hypovolemic or hypervolemic. This may not be an important consideration in adults or adolescents, it can, however, create a serious problem in a small or unstable child.[3]

In filtration instruments, blood is passed through hollow fibers or between flat membranes with pore sizes small enough to prevent passage of cellular elements. Separation efficiency is a function of pore size, membrane composition, and transmembrane pressure. These machines have a small extracorporeal volume and can separate plasma from whole blood but cannot isolate cellular components. They are ideal for PE in pediatric patients, but unfortunately one manufacturer (Cobe BCT, Lakewood, CO) has phased out their instrument because of a lack of versatility.

The ideal treatment for disorders mediated by an abnormal component is selective removal, thus eliminating the need for replacement fluid and avoiding the loss of essential plasma constituents. The newer continuous-flow centrifugal instruments can incorporate cryoprecipitation, charcoal columns, dextran sulfate precipitation, and immunoadsorbent columns.[4-7] These techniques, although more applicable to adults, have been utilized in pediatric patients.

VASCULAR ACCESS

The difficulties associated with vascular access in children were initially considered to be a major obstacle to the use of apheresis in this group.[3] Older children and adolescents frequently have peripheral veins that can accommodate a 17-gauge needle for the draw line and a 18- or 19-gauge needle for the return to sustain the required minimal blood flow rates ($\pm$ 20 ml/min). A limiting factor can be the frequency with which the procedure has to be performed. In such instances, we routinely apply Emla (Astra Pharmaceutical Co., Westboro, MA) to the insertion site, a mixture of lidocaine and prilocaine, 1 to 2 hours before the treatment. This markedly reduces discomfort and has enabled us to perform twice-weekly procedures.

Infants and children require the placement of alternative access. Central venous lines (CVLs) are the most common. The catheters must be relatively rigid so that patency is maintained in the presence of the increased negative pressure during the draw phase. A 7-French catheter can be placed in infants weighing as little as 4 kg; in larger children and adolescents, a 9-, 10-, or 11-French catheter is used. There are a number of different types available; we prefer to use double-lumen side-by-side temporary and permanent catheters.

Catheters placed in the femoral vein or centrally through the subclavian or internal jugular vein are suitable for the brief periods usually used in PE in childhood. The femoral site presents a greater risk of infection in infants and toddlers and limits mobility. The femoral site is ideal for a planned single procedure such as a red cell exchange for a complication of sickle cell anemia. Centrally placed lines require general anesthesia, whereas femoral lines can usually be placed under conscious sedation. The lines must be evaluated for adequacy of flow before and after being sutured in place. A test that we have found to be useful is to attach an empty 10-ml syringe

to the line and draw back steadily. If the syringe can be filled without excessive pressure and without "catching," the line will allow the necessary flow rates. If there is any catching during aspiration, despite how easily blood draws in between the catching, the line is not adequate. Positional change of the patient or an adjustment of the line frequently improves the flow.

Patency of the catheter between procedures can be maintained by several methods. In most instances, we flush the catheter with 2 or 3 ml of a heparin solution (10 units/ml) every 12 hours. Another option is to instill a heparin solution, 1,000 units/ml and aspirate before the next treatment. Several centers have had success instilling normal saline into central lines.

BLOOD VOLUME HEMATOCRIT

Maintenance of a constant blood volume and red cell mass is the technical modification necessary to treat children using instruments essentially designed for adults. The extracorporeal circuit volume of separators, including a blood warmer, varies between 275 and 350 ml, which can represent a significant fraction of the child's blood volume. Because the circuits are primed with saline, the patient's hematocrit falls because of dilution during the initial phase of the procedure.[3,8]

We routinely prime the cell separator with leukodepleted red cells when the extracorporeal circuit is 12 percent or greater of the child's blood volume, in most children who weigh less than 20 kg, or when the patient is anemic or unstable. The hematocrit of the prime should be at least 50 percent or 15 to 35 percentage points greater than the patient's to maintain or raise the child's hematocrit. The red cells initially are diluted with saline; therefore the prime should be bled into the waste bag until the desired hematocrit is reached. On completion of the procedure, blood is left in the separator to maintain isovolemia. Details of the procedure for red cell priming of the various instruments can be found in the operator's manual.

If the infant or child is volume overloaded before the start of the procedure, excess fluid can be removed. This is accomplished by gradually decreasing the replacement rate from the collection rate.

The most common situation in which this is necessary occurs when the patient has received a large volume of fresh frozen plasma in an attempt to correct a coagulopathy. In such situations, the replacement rate is decreased from 1 to 5 ml less than the removal rate. The volume that can be removed depends on both the patient's size and blood pressure change during the procedure.

ANTICOAGULATION

The general principle is to utilize the minimal amount of anticoagulant to prevent clotting. Depending on the type of separator, this can be accomplished with heparin, acid-citrate-dextrose (ACD), or both. For adolescents with normal coagulation, any regimen recommended by the manufacturer of the separator is acceptable. Infants and young children, especially those being treated in intensive care units or with liver failure, require modification in agent and dose. Before initiation of the procedure, baseline studies should include prothrombin time (PT), activated partial thromboplastin time (PTT), fibrinogen level, platelet count, and activated clotting time (ACT). The latter is particularly useful in critically ill children because the degree of anticoagulation can be monitored instantaneously and adjusted as necessary.

Heparin has been used in dialysis for decades and can be adapted for pediatric apheresis. As detailed below, children, especially those receiving fresh frozen plasma as replacement, are particularly prone to hypocalcemia. Our standard heparin regimen for adolescents is an initial bolus of 2,000 units followed by an infusion of 40 units/min into the draw line. In patients at high risk for bleeding, the heparin dose is titrated utilizing the ACT. Our initial bolus varies from 0 to 40 units/kg, depending on the pretreatment ACT, to attain an ACT of 150 to 300 seconds (our normal is 90 to 120 seconds). Concomitantly, a minimal heparin infusion, 1 to 5 units/min, is started. ACTs are repeated every 20 to 30 minutes during the procedure; additional heparin is given as needed to maintain the ACT in the desired range. In the patient with a severe coagulopathy, the procedure is often started without anticoagulation. Small boluses of heparin are administered to maintain the ACT in the desired range. Patients with hypercoagu-

lability (e.g., sickle cell disease), who have pretreatment ACTs less than 75 seconds require an initial heparin bolus of 50 to 100 units/kg and a corresponding increase in the heparin infusion.

Citrate, administered as ACD as an infusion into the draw line, prevents clotting by reducing levels of ionized calcium. The ratio utilized ranges from 1:8 to 1:12 when ACD is used alone and from 1:20 to 1:30 when used in combination with heparin. The side effects of citrate are due to hypocalcemia. Infusion ratios of 1:8 to 1:12 achieve a citrate dose 0.6 to 1 mg/kg/min, which can lower the calcium level by 20 to 30 percent.[9,10] This produces mild symptoms in about one-quarter of adults and adolescents undergoing therapeutic apheresis.[11]

Pediatric patients at high risk are those in renal and/or hepatic failure, those receiving fresh frozen plasma as replacement solution, and small children. Citrate intoxication in children is characterized by agitation, pallor, sweating, and abdominal pain without emesis, which can progress to tachycardia and hypotension. In infants and obtunded children, hypotension is often the only indication of hypocalcemia.[3] If any of these signs or symptoms appear, the procedure should be stopped, an ionized calcium level should be obtained from a peripheral site (normal 1.14 to 1.29 mmol/L), and calcium should be administered as indicated. Our preference is to administer calcium chloride in such situations because of the higher content of ionized calcium. Because citrate has not been shown to be safer than heparin and because of its frequent side effects, we utilize heparin in virtually all apheresis procedures.

REPLACEMENT SOLUTIONS

It is essential that the replacement solution have a protein oncotic pressure and an electrolyte content similar to that of the plasma being removed. Solutions most commonly used are 5 percent albumin, fresh frozen plasma, and plasma protein fraction. Several centers utilize saline in situations when less than 10 percent of the blood volume is being replaced.[12]

Five percent albumin is the standard replacement solution for PE because it is largely free of side effects. If multiple PEs are performed within a brief period, we usually add additional potassium and calcium to maintain electrolyte balance. Plasma protein fraction has similar properties but has been associated with hypotensive reactions.[13]

Fresh frozen plasma should be utilized only for situations in which its use is absolutely necessary. These are characterized by a need for clotting factors, such as hepatic failure, or specific disease entities, such as thrombotic thrombocytopenic purpura (TTP).[14,15] Cryoprecipitate-poor frozen plasma is considered the replacement fluid of choice for TTP in many centers.[16]

Routine replacement of coagulation factors removed by PE is rarely if ever indicated. A single 1.5 volume plasma exchange produces a 50 to 70 percent reduction in coagulation factors and other proteins.[17] This is not sufficient to induce bleeding in children with normal pretreatment coagulation status.[18] All clotting factors except for fibrinogen return to normal levels within 12 to 24 hours after PE.[19] The latter may be depressed for 48 hours or longer.

Plasma may be needed in instances in which greater than 2 plasma volumes are removed or when daily therapy is required. In such situations, we supplement the albumin solution with 15 ml/kg of fresh frozen plasma toward the end of the PE. Fibrinogen levels of less than 100 mg/dl should be corrected with cryoprecipitate. An option that we have utilized is to prepare autologous cryoprecipitate from the first 200 to 500 ml of plasma removed, depending on the anticipated volume of the PE. Leukodepleted red cells and platelets can be used as part of the replacement solution to correct anemia or thrombocytopenia. Intravenous gamma globulin (IVIG), if indicated because of repeated exchanges or clinical condition, is administered after completion of the IPE. Our practice is to administer 400 mg/kg, with the exception being our recent modification of our Guillain-Barré protocol (see subsequent section).

DOSE AND FREQUENCY

Optimal therapy is the minimal frequency and dose necessary to halt progression of the disease and therefore must be individualized. The effect of PE on levels of known mediators and clinical symptoms must be determined and the results used to determine further therapy. However, in many conditions, there is often little or no correlation between mediator level and clinical symptoms.

In acute life- or organ-threatening diseases 1.5 to 2 plasma volumes are exchanged daily until there is evidence of clinical effect. This is generally accomplished with three to five treatments. Children who require inotropic support must be monitored closely because much of the drug(s) effect is removed during plasma exchange. Active disease states are treated with 1.3 to 1.5 plasma volumes on alternate days. The interval is extended as warranted by the child's clinical condition. Because of vascular access (central lines are always used), chronic therapy in young children is used only when either no other therapy is available or the side effects of other therapy becomes unacceptable. In our experience, the frequency with which chronic PE must be performed varies from weekly to biweekly, based on the clinical condition and level of mediator.

PLASMA EXCHANGE

The beneficial effects of PE are due to the removal of toxic substances (i.e., antibodies, immune complexes, paraproteins, the provision of normal plasma constituents, or both). Because removal often does not slow the rate of synthesis of these factors, therapeutic effects are often transient. PE is unique as an immunosuppressive agent in that it has the ability to produce a significant and immediate reduction in the level of antibodies, immune complexes, and inflammatory mediators. This is in contrast to cytotoxic and anti-inflammatory agents, which may require days to weeks to achieve maximal therapeutic effect. In pediatrics, as in adult medicine, combined therapy is often the treatment of choice. It is used to produce a rapid remission, thus avoiding prolonged hospitalization and, in our experience, has been proved to be valuable in less emergent situations.

Individual disorders in childhood for which apheresis treatment is commonly utilized are discussed in the following sections. The role of apheresis must be considered in view of the natural history of the disorder. One cannot extrapolate data obtained from studies in adults. Table 33-1 lists the conditions treated and the number of plasma ex-

Table 33-1. Intensive Plasma Exchanges Performed at the Children's Hospital From October 1979 Through January 1994

Condition	Number of Patients	Number of Procedures
Hypercholesterolemia	8	405
Paraproteinemia		
Hyper-IgE	6	538
Hyper-IgM	1	287
Renal diseases		
Focal segmental glomerulosclerosis	5	83
Hemolytic uremic syndrome	24	205
Goodpasture's complex	2	27
Liver disease		
Acute hepatic failure	56	257
ABO incompatibility	4	4
Disseminated intravascular coagulation and Sepsis	11	14
ECMO support	13	21
Bone marrow transplant ABO incompatibility	6	21
Acquired hemolytic anemia	1	39
Delayed transfusion reaction	2	7
Guillain-Barré syndrome	11	89
Systemic lupus erythematosus		
Renal disease	1	9
Central nervous system disease	1	11
Staphylococcal A columns	2	11
	154	2,028

Abbreviation: ECMO, extracorporeal membrane oxygenation.

changes performed at Children's Hospital from 1979 to 1994.

Familial Hypercholesterolemia

This term applies to an inborn error of metabolism, with both homozygous and heterozygous patients having demonstrable symptoms. Therapy for homozygous patients involves lowering plasma low-density lipoprotein (LDL) levels by combining diet and medical and surgical approaches. PE with 5 percent albumin as replacement has been commonly utilized in homozygous patients, particularly in children when the other approaches did not lower LDL. Our experience is comparable to that of others in that there has been success in treating cutaneous and tendinous xanthomas and slowing the progression of atheromatous lesions.[20,21] The effect of PE is temporary; patients require treatment on a continuing basis, usually every 2 weeks. In young children, less than 2 to 3 years of age, rapid lowering of LDL levels improves response to medical therapy. There is some evidence that long-term survival is improved. All our patients have lived 5 to 15 years longer than their affected untreated siblings. The use of selective plasma filtration with hollow-fiber membrane machines and return of the patient's high-density lipoproteins offer hope for a more efficient therapeutic modality. Dextran sulfate columns have been used extensively in adults in both homozygous and heterozygous patients with excellent results, although anaphylactoid reactions have been reported.[22,23]

Paraproteinemia

The paraproteinemias are extremely rare in childhood, except for hyperimmunoglobulinemia E (HIE) and a hyper-IgM syndrome, which is often associated with ataxia telangiectasia.

HIE or Job's syndrome consists of chronic atopic dermatitis, defective neutrophil chemotaxis, recurrent severe pyogenic infection (primarily pulmonary), and the ocular finding of vernal conjunctivitis and atopic keratoconjunctivitis often complicated by herpetic or staphylococcal infection.[24,25] During the past 9 years, we have treated six such patients with 538 PEs in whom all forms of conventional medical therapy failed. The IgE levels before PE averaged 17,121 international units/ml (6,210 to 30,200) and were maintained at an average of 2,956 international units/ml (1,665 to 3,746) after chronic therapy. One and one-half plasma volumes were replaced with 5 percent albumin during each procedure. During severe exacerbation of symptoms, procedures were performed every other day for four to six times followed by weekly treatments. This has resulted in clearing of ocular manifestations, normal neutrophil chemotaxis, and control of pulmonary complications. PE in such instances is utilized with appropriate systemic antibiotic therapy. Two of our patients are under maintenance therapy.

Ataxia telangiectasia is often accompanied by both

an immunodeficiency syndrome and hyper-IgM. The latter is associated with high levels of immune complex, which targets the bone marrow and lung. Chronic PE with 5 percent albumin as replacement fluid in conjunction with steroids has eliminated pulmonary symptoms, maintained IgM levels in the high normal range, and resulted in absent immune complex levels. One of the patients we treated has had two CVL line infections during a 9-year period.

Guillain-Barré Syndrome

Although Guillain-Barré syndrome (GBS) is more common in adults, it is frequently rapidly progressive in childhood.[26,27] GBS is generally considered an autoimmune disorder, as evidenced by the demonstration of lymphocytic infiltration in proximal nerve routes, antibodies to peripheral nerve myelin, and circulating immune complexes.[28]

Early diagnosis is essential; if the neurologic findings are minimal, the patients can be hospitalized in the general pediatric nursing divisions. If there is evidence of rapidly progressive muscle weakness or a suggestion of respiratory compromise, the child is admitted to the intensive care unit. PE is instituted promptly with 5 percent albumin as the replacement solution. Before 1993, our approach was to exchange a 1.5 to 2.0 plasma volumes daily for 2 to 4 treatments, depending on the severity of the neurologic findings. This was followed by alternate-day therapy over a period of 10 to 14 days.[29] As previously mentioned, cryoprecipitate (autologous or homologous) is almost always required during the period of daily therapy because of depressed fibrinogen levels (less than 100 mg/dl) after PE.

The use of IVIG has been reported to be as effective as PE in controlled studies.[30] Combined PE and IVIG, although not thoroughly studied, is theoretically a logical approach. We have undertaken this approach in four patients. Table 33-2 summarizes our hospital's experience during the past 19 years. The patients grouped under historical controls were admitted to neurologic divisions and were treated conservatively (steroids) until 1992 and with IVIG since that time (three patients). The numbers are too small to draw any definitive conclusions. The patients receiving combined therapy required an average of four consecutive exchanges followed by two infusions of IVIG at a dose of 400 mg/kg. There were

Table 33-2. Results of Three Therapeutic Options for the Treatment of Guillain-Barré Syndrome

	"Historical" Controls[a] 1975–94 (n = 11)	PE 1980–92 (n = 8)	PE and IVIG 1992–94 (n = 4)
Mortality rate	1	0	0
Ventilator	4	0	0
Long-term disability	3	1	0
Hospital stay (days)	43 (26–73)	9 (7–10)	8 (6–9)

Abbreviations: PE, plasma exchange; IVIG, intravenous immune globulin.
[a] Patients were not admitted to the Intensive Care Unit but instead were treated conservatively.

no relapses in the latter group, which is not an uncommon occurrence in GBS of childhood. However, the decreased hospitalization rate and number of PEs in the combined therapy group are highly suggestive.

Renal Disease

The utilization of PE for renal disorders is age dependent. Adolescents and young adults have conditions similar to older patients and respond to PE in like manner. Recent reviews discuss the management of those disorders.[31–34] The subsequent sections emphasize those conditions that occur in childhood.

Hemolytic Uremic Syndrome

Hemolytic uremic syndrome (HUS) in childhood, although it often mimics TTP, tends to occur after episodes of bacterial gastroenteritis caused by a particular strain of *Escherichia coli* (O15:H7) that produces a verotoxin. HUS in children requires supportive care, including temporary hemodialysis, with spontaneous resolution in 80 to 85 percent of cases within 3 weeks.[35,36] A small percentage of patients have life-threatening symptoms, including coma, seizures, and a degree of obtundation beyond that expected for their renal status.[37] Our guidelines for the introduction of PE into their management include two or more of the following: seizures, neurologic findings, platelet count less than 30,000/μl lactate dehydrogenase (LDH) level greater than 400 units, severe anemia, and a low calcium level. PE, equivalent to 1.5 to 2 plasma volumes, is performed daily with fresh frozen plasma as the replacement fluid. The cell separator is primed with leukodepleted red cells; platelets are administered toward the end of the procedure. Anticoagulation is kept to a minimum, as judged by the patient's ACT. Patients with severe azotemia who receive fresh frozen plasma as replacement are extremely prone to hypocalcemia. An ionized calcium level is obtained after completion of the first 10 percent of the exchange. If replacement is necessary, based on a decrease of 20 percent from the normal, it is made with a 10 percent calcium chloride solution. This enables us to determine at what intervals calcium replacement will be required. Our end point for termination therapy is the maintenance of a platelet count of 100,00/µl and or an LDH finding of 100 units for 48 hours. Nine of the 24 patients treated during the past 15 years died. None of the survivors required chronic dialysis or transplantation.

Focal Segmental Glomerulosclerosis

Steroid-resistant nephrotic syndrome with focal segmental glomerulosclerosis (FSGS) and its recurrence after transplantation is mainly seen in children. The recurrence rate after transplantation approximates 30 percent, with more than one-half losing their graft. The risk of recurrent FSGS in subsequent transplants is 50 to 80 percent, and the overall mortality rate is 10 percent.[38] The appearance of proteinuria shortly after transplantation suggests that circulating factor(s) may be present. Multiple therapeutic regimens have been tried, including immunoadsorption, high-dose cyclosporine, and pulse methylprednisolone alone or with cyclophosphamide with poor results.[38,39]

Reports that indicate success with a regimen of high-dose steroids, cyclophosphamide, and plasma exchange prompted us to establish a protocol consisting of steroids, cyclosporine, and PE.[38,39] To date, we have treated four patients with recurrent FSGS after transplantation, and one patient with FSGS who was being maintained on dialysis. The patients ranged in age from 4 to 11 years; had nephrotic-range proteinuria, hypoalbuminemia, and elevated serum creatinine level; and were undergoing dialysis for varying lengths of time. PE was instituted once the diagnosis of recurrent disease was confirmed by biopsy. It was performed every other day for 10 procedures and then once a week for 2 to 6 weeks. All patients underwent 1.5 plasma volume exchanges with 5 percent albumin as replacement.

The grafts are functioning 11 to 45 months after transplantation in three of the four patients, and their serum chemical values are now normal. The one patient who was not transplanted is maintaining normal renal function without medication 1 year after his last PE. Based on this experience and that of others, PE in conjunction with steroids and cyclophosphamide should be tried in pre- and post-transplant FSGS.

Goodpasture's Syndrome Complex

This condition, although relatively rare in early childhood, presents as an acute emergency. Patients that were originally followed with a diagnosis of idiopathic pulmonary hemosiderosis are often in this category. During late childhood and early adolescence, they may develop mild to severe renal disease with associated antineutrophil cytoplasmic antibodies. Chronic immunosuppressive therapy with combinations of cyclophosphamide and steroids is most often used.[40]

Historically, the mortality rate was high with patients dying of pulmonary hemorrhage and renal failure. Acute episodes, manifested primarily by severe pulmonary hemorrhage, respond well to immunosuppressive regimens supplemented by PE. Our approach is to perform daily 1.5 volume plasma exchanges with 5 percent albumin as replacement. The duration of therapy is based primarily on the control of the pulmonary signs and symptoms. The patients are gradually weaned from PE by extending the interval between procedures to weekly and re-establishing control with immunosuppressive agents.

Liver Failure

Before transplantation, hepatic failure (HF) had a poor prognosis, with mortality rates exceeding 80 to 90 percent in patients with acute or advanced disease in spite of a variety of therapies. Many pediatric patients die of HF waiting for an organ, become too ill to qualify or survive surgery, or die of delayed onset of graft function or rejection. During the period of 1984 to 1994, 57 children with HF have undergone 257 PEs. The criteria utilized for PE in our hospital

Table 33-3. Criteria Used as an Indication for Plasma Exchange in Patients With Severe Liver Disease or Fulminant Hepatic Failure

Support began when one or more conditions were met.
   Required support with plasma products and albumin on 3 consecutive days
   Impending or actual fluid overload
   Developed clinically significant complications bleeding or change in mental status
   ABO incompatibility (an IgM isohemagglutinin titer of the recipient against the donor organ of 1:8 or greater)
   Elective transplant with coagulopathy if the preoperative coagulation profile showed
      PT >20 sec
      PTT >45 sec
      Fibrinogen <150 mg/dl or factors II, V, VII <20%
   Combinations of the above

Abbreviations: PT, prothrombin time; PTT, partial thromboplastin time.

for this group of patients are shown in Table 33-3. Thirty-nine of the 56 patients were transplanted; in 17 patients, support was withdrawn for a variety of reasons, primarily the underlying disease (i.e., generalized herpetic infection, malignancy, or veno-occlusive disease) or death. Four patients were exchanged because their plasma was ABO incompatible with the donor liver. Only one patient who underwent PE recovered without undergoing HT.

In general, the technique utilized for the exchange is identical for all patients. The replacement fluid consists of a mixture of fresh frozen plasma and cryoprecipitate. The number of units of cryoprecipitate added to the plasma depends on the patient's pre-exchange fibrinogen level. The degree of the coagulation abnormality determines the volume of the exchange (2 to 4 plasma volumes). The separator is primed with leukodepleted red cells; platelets are administered during the latter stage of the exchange. PE was performed once or, on occasion, twice daily until HT or support was withdrawn.

In patients with severe coagulopathy, ACT more than 300 seconds and markedly abnormal PT and PTT, anticoagulation is not utilized throughout most of the procedure. Low-dose heparin (10 to 15 units/kg) is administered by bolus if the ACT is less than 150 seconds. Because the separator has been

primed with red cells, clotting of the circuit is not a problem but does indicate that the coagulopathy has been corrected.

If the patient is fluid overloaded because of previous fresh frozen plasma administration, the exchange is performed at minus 1 to 5 ml/min. The child's blood pressure must be monitored carefully because both intravascular volume changes and an abnormal ionized calcium level can result in hypotension. Children with HF are markedly sensitive to the citrate load present in fresh frozen plasma. Calcium is administered as a 10 percent calcium chloride solution in a dose of 0.1 to 0.3 ml/kg over a period of 1 to 2 minutes. Ionized calcium levels must always be obtained from a peripheral site.

In chronically treated patients, fluid overload, coagulopathy, and metabolic abnormalities were either prevented or minimized by daily exchanges for up to 23 days. The improvement in coagulation factor levels after PE in the 123 instances in which they were measured is shown in Figure 33-1. The concentration of factor VIII, which is an acute-phase reactant and made by endothelial cells, was elevated in all but one instance. The mean PT fell from 27.9 to 14.4 seconds, with the PTT changing from 53.2 to 36.8 seconds, and the mean fibrinogen rose from 97 mg/dl to 184/dl in the same patients. The improvement in coagulation factors is transient, 18 to 32 hours. A return of the hepatic enzyme concentrations toward normal in the face of coagulation factor levels that remain persistently abnormal is indicative of a liver that is beyond repair. This has been repeatedly confirmed histologically at the time of transplant. Excluded from this group are those patients who underwent PE if the donor liver was an ABO mismatch with their plasma because their coagulation status was not markedly abnormal.[41,42] Fifty-nine percent of the patients transplanted are alive and well.

Kim et al.[43] reported anhepatic survival for 60 hours by the use of PE after liver graft failure. The patient subsequently underwent a successful second transplant. This approach is significant in view of the fact that four of our patients who died underwent PE after hepatic transplant as a result of liver graft failure. The condition rapidly deteriorated before another organ could be obtained. It obviously is

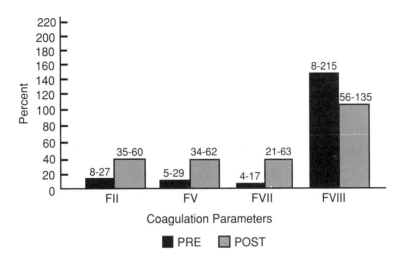

Fig. 33-1. Improvement in coagulation factor levels after a 1.5 to 2.0-volume plasma volume exchange in 29 patients with hepatic failure.

more efficacious to remove a dead organ than to leave it in situ.

Disseminated Intravascular Coagulation and Sepsis

Purpura fulminans is a life-threatening condition that can rapidly progress to shock and death within a few hours. Although primarily associated with meningococcal infection, it can also occur with gram-positive and viral infections. A potent inflammatory response is elicited whereby cytokines, including tumor necrosis factor and interleukin-1 are released and the complement cascade is activated.[44,45] The resultant endothelial damage initiates disseminated intravascular coagulation (DIC).

Recent reports suggest that PE, in combination with antibiotic and inotropic therapy, markedly reduces the mortality rate.[46,47] Natanson et al.,[48] utilizing a canine model that simulates some of the clinical and cardiovascular abnormalities of human septic shock, suggested that PE is associated with an increased mortality rate. However, in those experiments, continuous inotropic and ventilatory support was not provided.

McManus and Churchwell[49] demonstrated that coagulopathy was an excellent predictor of outcome in purpura fulminans. Standard therapy with fresh frozen plasma and cryoprecipitate requires administration of large fluid volumes, which is unacceptable because of the expansion of third-space volume and acute renal failure in many of these patients. This was confirmed by the postmortem findings of fluid overload and lungs that weighed more than two to three times normal for age. This was apparent clinically by the need to increase pressures on the ventilators markedly to ensure adequate oxygen delivery because of decreased pulmonary compliance in many patients.

In our institution, we have used PE in a variety of conditions as a means of rapidly correcting coagulopathy isovolemically. Eleven patients with purpura fulminans and DIC were treated with supportive therapy and PE from February 1990 to July 1994. All PEs were performed within 7 hours of admission. The separators were primed with leukodepleted red cells; replacement consisted of a mixture of fresh frozen plasma and cryoprecipitate. Platelets were administered at the end of the procedure. Anticoagulation, if needed during PE, was accomplished with heparin. Boluses of up to 250 units were initially administered, and/or a continuous heparin infusion of 2 to 10 units/min was titrated to maintain the ACT in the 150- to 180-second range. During the procedure, inotropic support and ionized calcium levels were (and must be) closely monitored. Three of the 11 patients required more than one PE.

All patients achieved a two- to threefold rise in

coagulation factor levels; the fibrinogen level increased from a mean of 65.2 to 207.1 mg/dl. The PT decreased from a mean of 38.3 to 15.4 seconds, and the mean PTT from 87.4 to 42.1 seconds. There was only one death in this group. PE in patients with purpura fulminans rapidly improves coagulopathy isovolemically and can be safety performed in the most unstable pediatric patient with proper techniques. The potential to improve survival has not been proved statistically.

Extracorporeal Membrane Oxygenation Support

Exclusion criteria for extracorporeal membrane oxygenation (ECMO) support have included neonates with evidence of intracranial hemorrhage or patients with any significant systemic bleeding or coagulopathy. A protocol was established with the ECMO support team based on our experience utilizing PE for the management of the coagulopathy associated with HF and DIC and our experience performing hand exchanges for patients undergoing ECMO.

During a 34-month period, 11 patients ranging in weight from 2.6 to 15 kg underwent 17 PEs while undergoing ECMO support. All patients were coagulopathic, as evidenced by the fact that their heparin requirement was minimal or nonexistent, their ACTs were more than 240 seconds, (ECMO range 160 to 180 seconds), their fibrinogen levels were low, or they had vasomotor instability beyond that usually observed in patients undergoing ECMO. Among the diagnoses were *E. coli* and group B streptococcal sepsis and postoperative cardiac surgery.

There are specific modifications necessary to perform the procedure. The separator circuit is primed in the usual manner with leukodepleted red cells. The volume to be exchanged is calculated based on the blood volume of the patient and that of the ECMO circuit, which can vary from 300 (neonate) to 2,000 ml (adolescent to adult). The replacement solution is a mixture of fresh frozen plasma and cryoprecipitate. Platelets, if necessary, must always be administered through a peripheral line, never by PE. As shown in Figure 33-2, the draw line is connected to a site before the oxygenator membrane and the

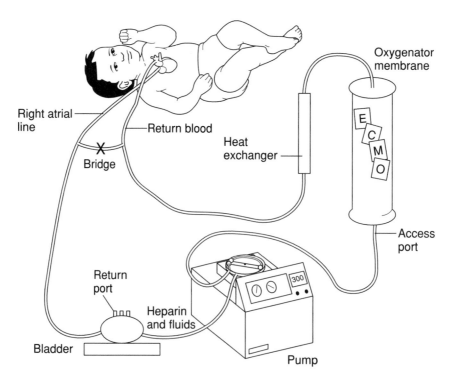

Fig. 33-2. Schematic of the ECMO system demonstrating the sites for access and return during PE.

return line, to the ECMO bladder with Luer-lock connectors. It is essential that the connections be made as indicated because the flow from the patient into the ECMO circuit bladder is by gravity. The separator is run in the manual mode. Inlet flows ranged from 25 to 50 ml/min, which requires a concomitant increase of blood flow in the ECMO circuit. Anticoagulation is adjusted according to the ACT, which is determined every 10 to 15 minutes. Heparin is administered as a bolus through the ECMO circuit. On initiation of the PE, small transient changes occurred in mean arterial pressure and pulse rate in most treatments, which resolved without therapy in all but one instance. All patients required supplemental calcium based on their ionized calcium level, the test sample for which must always be obtained from a peripheral site. Improvement of the coagulopathy was demonstrated by a decrease in the ACT, a decrease in PT, an increase in fibrinogen and coagulation factor levels, and an initiation or increase in heparin requirement. Eight of the 11 patients survived. One of the four patients with sepsis died, as did two of the three postcardiac surgical patients.[50]

Autoimmune Disorders

The immunologic features of these disorders include a variety of circulating antibodies and immune complexes, tissue deposition of antibodies, and low complement levels. The indications for PE depend on the severity of the particular illness; most are usually successfully treated with immunosuppression using a combination of steroids and cytotoxic drugs.[51] The use of PE in the management of these diseases is rare in childhood. Adolescents follow a pattern similar to that of adults.

Systemic Lupus Erythematosus

The indications for PE in systemic lupus erythematosus (SLE) are limited to patients with severe disease activity who are not responsive to drug therapy.[51,52] In childhood, these are most frequently limited to patients with central nervous system disease and rapidly progressive renal disease.

Patients should be treated daily with a 1.5 volume PE. Replacement fluid should be 5 percent albumin. There should be concomitant administration of immunosuppressive therapy. Many of these patients have very high fibrinogen levels (acute-phase reac-

tant) before the start of therapy; therefore, cryoprecipitate is often not required despite the fact that five to six consecutive procedures are performed. Daily treatments are recommended until there is objective clinical evidence of improvement and the laboratory parameters tend to normalize. Treatment can then be tapered over a 4- to 6-week period, as the patient resumes a normal medication schedule.

Juvenile Rheumatoid Arthritis

The use of PE in this disorder is highly controversial; most pediatric tertiary care centers with large arthritis clinics have never had a patient requiring PE, although there have been several reports of its use.[53,54] These patients usually have a macrophage adherence syndrome, which results in "hepatitis" and DIC.

Poisonings

Poisonings in childhood account for more than 400 deaths annually.[55] Most childhood poisonings occur by ingestion and involve pharmaceuticals.

Theoretically, PE can be an advantage in the treatment of poisons tightly bound to albumin (i.e., paraquat and the mushroom toxin α-amanitin). The evidence for its use is largely based on case reports.[55–57] The criteria for the use of PE include progressive clinical deterioration, coma, and decreased renal function. A general recommendation is to exchange 1.5 to 2 plasma volumes with 5 percent albumin as replacement. The frequency depends on the pharmacokinetic properties of the drug or poison.

Miscellaneous Conditions

ABO-Incompatible Marrow Transplantation

Patients who are to receive ABO-incompatible marrow are at risk for a severe hemolytic reaction to the red cells in the marrow harvest. There are two approaches to minimize either a severe hemolytic transfusion reaction or delayed engraftment of red cells. This can be accomplished by either removing the incompatible cells from the marrow or by markedly lowering the titer of isoagglutinins in the recipient's marrow.[58–60] Children have relatively low titers of isoagglutinins; titers less than 1:8 can easily be achieved by PE. However, like most centers, we have completely switched to red cell depletion of the marrow.

Hemophilia With Inhibitors

Children with inhibitors have the need to both control bleeding episodes and suppress the synthesis of antibody. Those with low levels of inhibitor (5 Bethesda units or less) can be treated with high doses of factor VIII, which is usually reserved for serious or life-threatening bleeding episodes. Moderate success has been achieved with the administration of porcine factor VIII and the activated coagulation factor concentrates. Obviously, the ideal treatment would be to suppress inhibitor synthesis. Attempts along these lines include the use of immunosuppressive agents, including steroids, cyclophosphamide, and cyclosporine.

The most promising results include the induction of tolerance after PE with daily infusion of large doses of factor VIII.[61,62] This program has been enhanced by the addition of the Excorim AB (Immunosorba protein A column) (COBE, BCT, Lakewood, CO) to the PE system.[63]

CYTOPHERESIS

The ability to remove cellular blood components selectively is an essential part of therapeutic apheresis. Stem cell collection for autologous use can also be considered "therapeutic." Table 33-4 lists the conditions treated and the number of cytopheresis procedures performed at Children's Hospital from 1979 to 1994.

Erythrocytopheresis

Flowing blood is a suspension of cells in plasma and has an anomalous viscosity; as flow decreases, viscosity increases. Fluids that behave in this manner are known as non-newtonian fluids. They do not have a constant viscosity, as do newtonian fluids. This physical property of blood is significant in the small vessels leading to the capillary circulation.[64] In the absence of hyperproteinemia, the chief determinant of whole blood viscosity is the hematocrit. In pediatric patients, polycythemia is most often secondary to cyanotic congenital heart disease. These patients have varying degrees of secondary polycythemia resulting from chronic hypoxemia.[65] The symptoms of hyperviscosity usually develop with hematocrits greater than 55 percent. These include headache, decreased exercise tolerance, lethargy and in many cases stroke.[65,66] Such patients may also have increased operative morbidity rates.[67] In the absence of a surgically completely correctable lesion, the only therapy for this form of polycythemia is red cell removal while maintaining cardiac output. This results in hemodynamic and symptomatic improvement.[66,67]

We have utilized both the Cobe 2997 and the Cobe Spectra continuous-flow separator as an alternative to manual phlebotomy. Our indications for treatment are symptomatic hyperviscosity with a hematocrit greater than 55 percent, asymptomatic polycythemia with a hematocrit greater than 65 percent, and prophylactic treatment in patients with a previous history of stroke. In the latter instance, we keep the hematocrit below 65 percent or lower, based on the hematocrit level at which the stroke occurred. It should be noted that iron deficiency in association with polycythemia increases the viscosity significantly at hematocrits greater than 55 percent (Fig. 33-3).[68]

All our procedures are now performed with the Cobe Spectra utilizing the "red cell exchange" disposables. The separator is run in the manual mode, and the centrifuge speed is set at 2,400 rpm. This allows one to remove the red cells at a hematocrit of 75 to 85 percent. If the machine is run in the automatic mode, the cells are removed at a hematocrit or 53 to 57 percent.

Table 33-4. Cytophresis Procedures Performed at Children's Hospital From October 1979 Through January 1994[a]

Conditions/Procedure	Number of Patients	Number of Procedures
Erythrocytopheresis		
Cyanotic congenital heart disease	47	510
Red cell exchange		
Sickle cell exchange		
Acute chest syndrome	51	57
Stroke	8	9
Priapism	7	7
Preoperative	39	39
Leukocytopheresis		
Acute leukemia	9	9
	161	631

[a] Several patients have had multiple erythrocytopheresis procedures during a 15-year period.

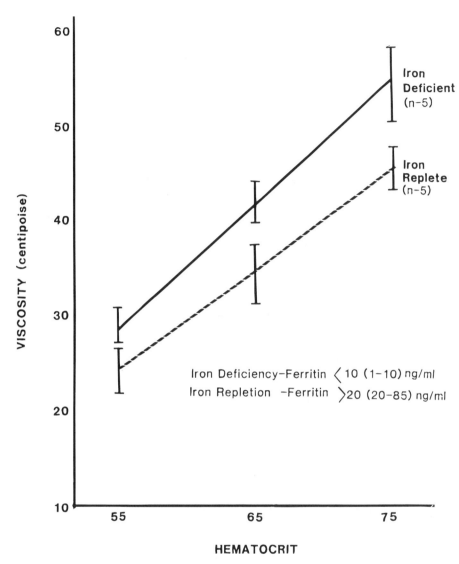

Fig. 33-3. Increase in viscosity of blood from polycythemic iron deficient patients compared with that from iron replete patients at hematocrits greater than 55 percent.

The treatment is designed to lower the hematocrit by 10 to 15 points. Patients receive the saline priming volume of the separator as their blood enters the extracorporeal circuit. The volume of red cells to be removed can be estimated based on the desired hematocrit, the patient's red cell volume, the decrease in hematocrit after the saline prime, and the hematocrit of the red cells removed. Spun hematocrits are monitored serially during the procedure be-

cause the red cell volume required to lower the hematocrit may differ from the calculated volume. Isovolemia is maintained with 5 percent albumin as the replacement solution. The blood is left in the separator on completion of the procedure; do not rinse back.

The interval between therapy for an individual patient varies from months to years. Those with iron deficiency have lower hematocrits and longer intervals between procedures. As noted above, however, their blood is more viscous at a given hematocrit. In patients with compromised flow to the microcirculation, simple phlebotomy, even with isovolemic replacement, can result in cardiovascular instability.[64,69] Manual methods are cumbersome; erythrocytapheresis can be accomplished in less than 1 hour.

Sickle Cell Disease

The transfusion management of sickle cell disease (SCD) has recently been reviewed in detail.[70] However, there are complications of SCD that are best treated by removing the patient's sickled cells and by replacing them with normal red cells utilizing a cell separator. Theoretically, sickling crises might be interrupted before tissue damage becomes irreversible. Our present policy is to perform red cell exchange when restoration of circulation is vital to preserving life or organ function and, prophylactically, before major surgery. Decreasing the hemoglobin S level results in improvement in the rheologic state, oxygen delivery, and clinical condition.[71,72] All patients are closely matched for all the Rh antigens, K, S, and if possible, Fy and Jk antigens to minimize alloimmunization.[73]

At the present time, all of our procedures are performed on the Cobe Spectra in the automatic mode utilizing red cell disposables. The volume of red cells required to complete the procedure is determined by entering the patient's blood volume, hematocrit, hematocrit of the red cell units, and the desired hemoglobin S level (FCR) on completion of the procedure. We aim for a hemoglobin S level after exchange of 20 to 30 percent and a hematocrit of approximately 35 percent (Fig. 33-4). The separator is primed with leukodepleted red cells for patients who are small (less than 20 kg), unstable, or severely anemic.

Acute Chest Syndrome

This syndrome is characterized by a combination of respiratory symptoms, thoracic pain, fever, and an abnormal chest examination, which is eventually confirmed by chest radiography.[74,75] There is great variability in severity; mortality rates as high as 14 percent have been reported.[64,66] There are numerous causes of acute chest syndrome; the underlying pathophysiology, however, involves pulmonary vaso-occlusion.

Our initial approach is to manage patients with hydration, supplemental oxygen to maintain an oxygen saturation above 95 percent, antibiotics, analgesics, and antipyretics. Red cell exchange is implemented if there is progressive respiratory deterioration. This is a clinical decision based on oxygen requirement and arterial blood gas analysis. Eighteen of our patients received a simple transfusion before red cell exchange. Patients were hospitalized on an average of 2 days (0 to 13 days) before

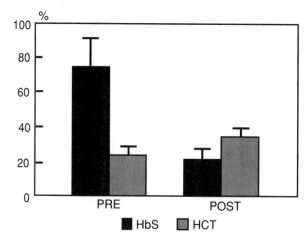

Fig. 33-4. Hemoglobin S and hematocrit levels before and after red cell exchange in 65 patients.

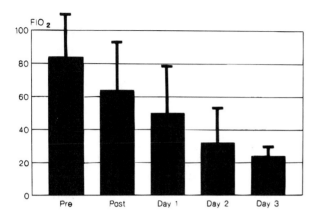

Fig. 33-5. FIO$_2$ levels required to maintain an oxygen saturation of ± 97 percent before and after red cell exchange.

exchange. The patient treated 13 days after the onset of symptoms was transferred to our hospital after intubation and simple transfusion on day 11. He died of progressive respiratory failure.

All but 3 of our 51 patients (one died, as noted above) responded dramatically to red cell exchange. Patients were weaned from oxygen within an average of 3 days and discharged in less than 1 week. Figure 33-5 demonstrates the fraction of inspired oxygen (FIO$_2$) required to maintain oxygen saturation in 47 of the patients treated by red cell exchange. Eight of the nine patients who required ventilatory support before the exchange were extubated within 72 hours.

Red cell exchange was performed in the most severely ill patients, some of whom received a prior simple transfusion, which may have had a salutary effect.

The wide variability in clinical definition, severity, and outcome of acute chest syndrome makes generalization difficult. Nonetheless, we suggest that exchange be considered for those with evidence for diffuse pulmonary involvement.

Cerebrovascular Disease

Acute or impending cerebrovascular episodes, whether caused by infarction, hemorrhage, hypoxemia, or transient ischemia, are absolute indications for exchange transfusion.[75] Furthermore, most patients will require chronic transfusion. Exchange is the safest way to initiate such therapy because it

avoids hyperviscosity and volume perturbation, which might exacerbate the situation. Our approach in these instances is to utilize a combination of ACD and low-dose bolus heparin or ACD alone for anticoagulation to prevent extension of any associated hemorrhage. The presenting symptom in all patients was severe headache. Four of the eight patients had hemiparesis; one had vision impairment. The findings were confirmed by computed tomographic scan. All patients recovered completely after physical therapy. A chronic transfusion program is instituted after hospital discharge. One patient who was not compliant with this program had a second episode of stroke. Several centers recommend red cell exchange before angiography to avoid intravascular sickling induced by intravenous hyperosmolar contrast agents. Although the newer nonionic contrast agents are associated with fewer overall side effects, they may carry a higher risk of thrombosis. Until their use is proved to be safe in SCD, we will continue to perform preangiographic exchange, even when these newer agents are used.

Priapism

Refractory priapism is associated with significant morbidity, most notably impotence.[76] There is a theoretical role for exchange transfusion. Anecdotal success with red cell exchange has been reported.[77,78] We routinely offer this modality to patients who demonstrate minimal response to 12 to 24 hours of conservative management with hydration, narcotics, and supplemental oxygen. The response to therapy varies at least in part with the duration of symptoms at the time of exchange. All patients treated within the first few days of onset gradually improved over 2 to 7 days. This, in our experience, is comparable to that observed in patients treated conservatively.

Preoperative Preparation

There is controversy over the optimal preoperative hematologic management of SCD. Historically, general anesthesia and surgery have been associated with significant perioperative morbidity and mortality rates. Virtually all of the problems occur in the postoperative period, especially after procedures that prevented the patient from breathing normally. There is still potential for severe sickle-related complications, and most centers recommend preoperative lowering of levels of hemoglobin S.[75,79,80] There are centers where preoperative transfusion therapy or erythrocytopheresis is not undertaken. However, there was a complication rate of 25 percent.[81] A prospective study is currently underway to evaluate the role and various methods of preoperative transfusion in SCD.[82]

Our approach is to offer chronic (during a 1-month period) or exchange transfusion to lower the hemoglobin S level to about 30 percent in preparation for major surgical procedures. Of the 35 patients we have treated with exchange, 33 underwent the planned procedure. There were no intraoperative complications, and postoperative recovery was uneventful in all but three. Two patients sustained wound infections, and one had pyelonephritis develop in the setting of nephrostomy drainage. None of these complications could directly be related to SCD or the exchange. We have treated two patients for acute chest syndrome in the postoperative period, one of whom was transferred to our hospital after laproscopic cholecystectomy. None of these patients was exchanged preoperatively. A preliminary report regarding the preoperative management of SCD indicates that there is a 13 percent incidence of acute chest syndrome in nontreated patients.[82]

Leukocytopheresis

There are situations in slowly proliferating leukemias in which, owing to side effects from or resistance to chemotherapy, intermittent leukocytopheresis can be used to control symptoms caused by a high number of circulating blasts.

The major use of leukocytopheresis is in the hyperviscosity state caused by extreme leukocytosis. With peripheral blast counts greater than 100,000 blasts/μl, the packed leukocyte volume ("leukocrit") may at times reach 25 percent, which results in dramatically increased whole blood viscosity.[83,84]

The organ systems most susceptible to toxic effects of extreme leukocytosis are the lungs and central nervous system. Pulmonary symptoms range from tachypnea to overt pulmonary failure; leukostasis in the nervous system can lead to hemorrhage, infarction, or both. The risk of developing symptomatic leukostasis is greater with myelogenous leukemia than with lymphocytic leukemia. Symptomatic leukostasis constitutes a medical emergency. The object of therapy is to reduce the white count as quickly as possible and follow with appropriate chemotherapy.

Our approach to therapy and utilization of the cell separator differs from that reported by others.[83,84] We maintain normovolemia or slight hypervolemia throughout the exchange.

The Cobe Spectra is run in the manual mode with an average centrifuge speed of 1,000 rpm (400 to 1,100) utilizing plasma exchange disposables. Because most if not all patients are anemic, the machine is primed with a mixture of leukodepleted red cells and fresh frozen plasma. The hematocrit of the prime is higher than that of the patient, but not so high as to raise the hematocrit significantly, which could increase viscosity.

At this centrifuge speed, the leukocytes are removed by allowing white cells to "spill" into the plasma layer. This allows one to supply fresh frozen plasma, platelets, and/or packed red blood cells as replacement for the removed plasma to correct the anemia, thrombocytopenia, and consumption coagulopathy that frequently accompany extreme leukocytosis.

The rate of leukocyte removal can be followed at the bedside by obtaining serial leukocrits. Blood is spun in a microcentrifuge tube, as with hematocrits. The leukocrit is the "crit" of the buffy coat layer. Therapy should continue until the white blood cell count is reduced by about 50 percent. If symptoms continue, therapy may be repeated up to twice daily. Because these patients frequently have coagulopathy and hypocalcemia, anticoagulation is best achieved using low doses of both heparin and acid-citrate dextrose formula A (ACD-A). The smallest child we have treated utilizing this technique weighed 4.5 kg.

STEM CELL COLLECTION

The technology of peripheral stem cell collection is a by-product of extracorporeal component separation. It was shown that primitive hematopoietic stem cells in peripheral blood separate with lymphocytes and monocytes on density and centrifugal gradients.[82]

Peripheral blood stem cells have been used in lieu of marrow as autologous cellular support after marrow-ablative radio/chemotherapy. Autologous marrow support allows the use of higher, more effective doses of therapy. Peripheral blood stem cells (PBSC) offer the potential for this form of "transplant" in patients with marrow involved with disease. PBSC use also allows the avoidance of marrow harvest under general anesthesia. There is also the advantage of earlier engraftment and decreased platelet utilization.[85,86]

Mobilization of PBSC into the circulating blood is accomplished by either chemotherapy, hematopoietic growth factors, or both, before leukocytopheresis.[87,88] Our current criteria are to start apheresis when white blood cell counts are greater than 1,000/μl and absolute neutrophil counts are greater than 200. PBSC are collected until 2.5×10^6/kg CD34 or 2×10^5/kg granulocyte-macrophage, colony-forming unit (CFU-GM) is reached. A complete blood count is obtained before treatment and a platelet count, after treatment.

If the platelet count is low, a platelet transfusion may be given before or after treatment. The anticoagulation used is a combination of heparin (25 to 40 units/kg) by intravenous bolus and ACD-A (1:20 to 1:30). To reduce the risk of volume overload and to maintain isovolemia in small children, the anticoagulant and the collection rates are kept equal.

RISKS AND COMPLICATIONS

The number of therapeutic plasma exchange and cytopheresis procedures performed in children has increased during the past 5 years. Associated with this growth is the potential for complications. Serious complications and deaths attributed to apheresis have been reported in adults.

A report from The Canadian Apheresis Study Group noted side effects in 12 percent of 5,235 procedures.[89] Most reactions were related to citrate or allergic reactions to plasma replacement solutions. A total of 0.5 percent of patients had severe reactions, including hypotension, arrhythmias, angina, seizures, respiratory arrest (two patients), and central nervous system bleeding (one patient). Approximately 50 deaths associated with apheresis have been reported, for an estimated fatality rate of 3 per 10,000 procedures.[90] The causes of death included arrhythmias, anaphylaxis, thromboembolism, vascular perforation, and hepatitis. In most reports, it is

not possible to determine whether the side effects were due to the procedure, the underlying disease, or a combination of both factors. Notably, most morbidity has been associated with the use of discontinuous devices, fresh frozen plasma replacement, or catheter placement.[91]

As previously noted, vascular access has been considered a major obstacle to apheresis in childhood. Problems include thrombosis, local and systemic infection, and the need for surgical procedures. The latter should not be a deterrent, even in the most seriously ill child. All CVLs in our patients were placed by members of the intensive care unit or the surgical service. In the more than 400 CVLs placed, the only complications were three line infections, two in the same child who has had his CVL in place for more than 10 years.

Apheresis is associated with a variety of potential complications; many, if not all, can be avoided. In pediatric patients, we recommend the use of continuous-flow devices, heparin alone or in combination with ACD-A, avoidance of fresh frozen plasma when possible, frequent monitoring of ionized calcium and ACT levels, close monitoring of fluid and electrolyte balance and hematocrit, and close attention to placement and care of vascular catheters. Patients with a borderline respiratory status should be electively intubated and stabilized on a ventilator before initiating apheresis.

EXTRACORPOREAL MEMBRANE OXYGENATION

ECMO is a modification of cardiac bypass for the support of respiratory failure. The membrane oxygenator used in ECMO circuits consists of a rectangular silicon membrane encased in rigid plastic (Sci-Med Life Systems, Inc, Minneapolis, MN). Blood and oxygen flow countercurrent on opposite sides of the membrane, which permits oxygen to diffuse from the gas phase into the blood while carbon dioxide diffuses from the blood into the gas phase.[92]

The initial ECMO trials with both bubble and membrane oxygenators were disastrous because the systemic heparinization required resulted in intracranial bleeding in most of the infants and children treated.[93] However, oxygenation was improved, which supported the tenet than an artificial lung was feasible.

Bartlett et al. were the first to utilize ECMO successfully in neonates with reversible respiratory failure.[94] Subsequent studies in neonates with attempts at randomization demonstrated greatly improved survival over the expected mortality rate.[95-98] The primary diagnoses for which ECMO support utilized for the neonate have changed during the past 4 years with the improvement in medical management of infants with congenital diaphragmatic hernia, persistent pulmonary hypertension of the newborn, and meconium aspiration syndrome. This is primarily due to the use of high-frequency oscilatory ventilation and nitric oxide.[99-102] In our center, the incidence of neonates with these conditions requiring ECMO has decreased by 30 percent, whereas there has been a fourfold increase in patients with cardiac disease and older children with reversible acute respiratory disease who have required ECMO support.

Selection criteria for ECMO support in our institution are based on historical "control" data used to determine which neonates and older children would not respond to conventional medical management. Among the major inclusion criteria are (1) an alveolar-arterial difference ($AaDO_2$) of greater than 610 on several determinations and (2) an oxygen index of greater than 40 after attempts at conventional management. Other centers utilize an arterial partial oxygen tension (PaO_2) of less than 50 mmHg for 4 hours as a criterion. This was based on a retrospective analysis that demonstrated that the PaO_2 was more sensitive and specific (96 percent) compared with $AaDO_2$ for predicting the mortality rate.[103,104]

The essential components of the ECMO system are shown in Figure 33-2. The circuit is primed with a blood mixture that is adjusted to a pH of 7.35 to 7.45. Under fentanyl anesthesia and paralysis, the right internal jugular and right common carotid arteries are catheterized using 12- to 14-French and 8- to 10-French polyvinylchloride catheters. The jugular catheter is advanced into the right atrium and the carotid to the beginning of the aortic arch. The catheter position changes if venovenous ECMO is used. Catheters are then connected to the circuit as quickly as possible. Circuit flow is gradually increased until approximately 60 percent of the cardiac output flows through the circuit. The partial oxygen pressure is maintained at 75 to 80 mmHg and the partial carbon dioxide tension at 40 to 50

mmHg. The infant is allowed to awaken and breathe on low ventilator settings. Anticoagulation is achieved with heparin administered as a bolus of 100 to 125 units/kg during cannulation, and a drip of 40 to 80 units/kg/hr is used to maintain the ACT at 180 to 200 seconds.

Hemorrhage is among the most frequent and devastating complications encountered in the use of ECMO. The reported incidence of intracranial hemorrhage during ECMO ranges from as high as 52 percent in early studies to approximately 15 percent today.[49,105]

Predisposition to hemorrhage in patients undergoing ECMO is presumed to be substantially related to heparin anticoagulation, yet factors including pre-existing hypoxia, acidosis, carotid ligation, and impaired cerebral autoregulation may contribution.[106] Neonates, the most frequent recipients of ECMO, possess coagulation factor levels substantially below adult levels.[107] This is also true of neonates requiring ECMO support after cardiac surgery.[108]

We examined the hypothesis that critically ill patients undergoing ECMO have reduced clotting factor levels, which may contribute to the risk of hemorrhagic complications. Blood samples were obtained before and 1 hour after initiation of ECMO. Heparin present in samples was removed by ECTEOLA cellulose resin adsorption (Sigma Diagnostics, St. Louis, MO). Factor deficiency was defined as levels greater than or equal to two standard deviations below published age-adjusted reference values. Sixty-eight percent of patients were found to have deficiencies of two or more factors before ECMO. Despite inclusion of some factor-containing blood products in the prime solution, 53 percent were found to have deficiencies of two or more factors after initiation of ECMO. Four patients had intracranial hemorrhages and were distinguished from those without hemorrhage by the presence of multiple factor deficiencies.[109]

Table 33-5 illustrates the current composition of our prime solution for neonatal and older pediatric patients. The red cell units have a hematocrit of ± 75 percent, are no more than 7 days old, and are sickle negative and leukodepleted. A recent survey of 79 active ECMO centers in the United States (69 responded) revealed that, currently, 79 percent of centers do not add coagulation factor-containing so-

Table 33-5. Neonatal and Childhood Extracorporeal Membrane Oxygenation Prime and Equipment Guidelines

Patient Weight	2–6 kg	6–10 kg	11–20 kg	21–35 kg	35–60 kg	60 kg +
Circuit (inch)	$\frac{1}{4}$ neonatal	$\frac{1}{4}$ neonatal	$\frac{3}{8}$ pedi	$\frac{3}{8}$ pedi	$\frac{1}{2}$ child	$\frac{1}{2}$ adolescent
Raceway (inch)	$\frac{3}{8}$	$\frac{3}{8}$	$\frac{3}{8}$	$\frac{3}{8}$	$\frac{1}{2}$	$\frac{1}{2}$
Oxygenator (m)	1.5	1.5	2.5	3.5	(2) 3.5	(2) 4.5
Bladder	RV30	RV30	RV50	RV50	RV50	RV50
Prime						
RBCs (ml)	500	500	900	1,050	1,300	1,600
FP (ml)	250	250	500	500	750	750
Cryo (units)	2	2	3	3	4	4
Platelets (units)	4	4	4–5	6	6	6
Drugs						
Heparin (units)	500	500	500		800	800
Calcium gluconate (mg)	500	500	3,000		4,000	4,000
Tham (ml)	100	100	300		300	300
Membrane volume (ml)	174	174	455	575	575 (2)	665 (2)
Premembrane pressure	350–400	350–400	350–400	350–400	350–400	350–400
Maximal blood flow rate (4 min)	1.8	1.8	4.5	5.5	5.5 each	6.5 each
Minimal blood flow rate (ml/min)	100	100	200	250	500	600

Abbreviations: RBCs, red blood cells; FFP, fresh frozen plasma; Cryo, cryoprecipitate; RV, reservoir volume (ml).

lutions to their prime.[110] Throughout the course of the ECMO run, we strive to maintain the platelet count in the 150,000/μl range, the fibrinogen level at 200 mg/dl, and the PT within normal limits.

As noted in a previous section, patients with severe coagulopathy undergo plasma exchange rather than infusion of plasma products to prevent fluid overload. Patients at high risk for bleeding complications (pre-existing or anticipated surgical procedures, pre-existing intracranial hemorrhage, profound hypoxia and acidosis, or prematurity) are given aminocaproic acid during the first 72 hours of the run or for an equivalent time period after surgery.[111]

CONCLUSIONS

PE and cytopheresis are valuable and sometimes life-saving tools in clinical conditions refractory to other therapeutic modalities. The future obviously lies in our ability to produce devices that function as true artificial internal organs. This would include the ability to grow and maintain hepatocytes, islet cells, and so forth on hollow fibers to ensure metabolic homeostases while awaiting solid organ transplants.

Other areas on the horizon include immunomodulation toward xenotransplantation. Several investigators have also proposed photopheresis for graft failure/rejection in cardiac transplantation.[112,113,114] Staphylococcal protein A immunoadsorption columns will undoubtedly be improved. Their success has been limited, with the reported reaction rate high.[115,116,117] The other area of growth will be in stem cell collection, both as adjunctive support to marrow transplantation, or even as its replacement.

Vascular access will remain a limiting factor but one that can be overcome. Children and many adults have small veins. Unfortunately, this problem has not been a major focus for those investigators interested in angiogenesis.

ECMO has matured beyond the neonatal period. Its future lies in the development of a surface that will inhibit or prevent coagulation. Extensive transfusion service support will be required as the number of older children and adults are supported through episodes of potentially reversible pulmonary failure.

REFERENCES

1. Freireich EJ, Judson G, Levin RH: Separation and collection of leukocytes. Cancer Res 25:1516, 1965
2. Jones AL: The IBM blood cell separator and blood cell processor: a personal prospective. J Clin Apheresis 4:171, 1988
3. Fosburg M, Dolan M, Kevy S: Intensive plasma exchange in small and critically ill pediatric patients: techniques and clinical outcome. J Clin Apheresis 1:215, 1983
4. Leitman SF, Smith JW, Gregg RE: Homozygous hypercholesterolemia: selective removal of low density lipoproteins by secondary membrane filtration. Transfusion 29:341, 1989
5. Malchesky PS, Nose Y: Biomodulation effects of extracorporeal circulation in apheresis. Semin Hematol, suppl. 1, 26:42, 1989
6. Gurland HJ: Therapeutic apheresis update. Adv Exp Med Biol 260:193, 1989
7. Lauterburg BH, Pineda AA, Burgstaler EA et al: Treatment of pruritus of cholestasis by plasma perfusion through USP charcoal coated glass beads. Lancet 1:53, 1980
8. Kevy S, Fosburg M: Therapeutic apheresis in childhood. J Clin Apheresis 5:87, 1990
9. Morse EE, Hohnadel DC et al: Decreased ionized calcium during therapeutic plasma exchange pheresis and platelet pheresis. Johns Hopkins Med J 146:260, 1980
10. Mollison PL, Engelfriet CP, Contreras M: Blood Transfusion in Clinical Medicine. 8th Ed. Blackwell Scientific Publications, Oxford, 1987
11. Dzik WH, Kirkley SA: Citrate toxicity during massive blood transfusion. Transfusion Med Rev 2:76, 1988
12. McCullough J, Bussell A: What are the established clinical indications for therapeutic plasma exchange and how important is the choice of replacement fluid? Vox Sang 43:270, 1982
13. Alung BM, Mojuma Y: Hypotension associated with prekallikrein (Hageman factor fragments) in plasma protein fraction. N Engl J Med 299:66, 1978
14. Rock GA, Shumak KH et al: Comparison of plasma exchange with plasma infusion in the treatment of thrombotic thrombocytopenic purpura. N Engl J Med 325:393, 1991
15. Ruggenenti P, Remuzzi G: Thrombotic thrombocytopenic purpura and related disorders. Hematol Oncol Clin North Am 4:219, 1990
16. Moake JL: TTP—desperation, empiricism, progress. N Engl J Med 325:426, 1991
17. Urbaniak SJ, Robinson FA: Therapeutic apheresis. BMJ 300:662, 1990
18. Chopek M, McCullough J: Protein and biochemical changes during plasma exchange. p. 133. In Therapeutic Hemapheresis: Technical Workshop (AABB). American Association of Blood Banks, Arlington, 1980
19. Keller AJ, Chirnside A, Urbaniak SJ: Coagulation abnormalities produced by plasma exchange on the cell separator with special reference to fibrinogen and platelet levels. Br J Haematol 42:593, 1979
20. Thompson GR, Miller JP, Breslow JL: Improved survival of patients with homozygous familial hypercholesterolemia treated with plasma exchange. BMJ 201:167, 1985
21. Borberg H, Gaczkowski A, Hombach V, Oette K: Regression of atherosclerosis in patients with familial hypercholesterolemia under LDL apheresis. Prog Clin Biol Res 255:317, 1988
22. Olbricht CJ, Schaumann, Fisher D: Anaphylactoid reactions, LDL apheresis with dextran sulfate, and ACE inhibitors. Lancet 340:980, 1992
23. Keller C, Grutzmacher P, Bahr F, Schwarzbeck A: LDL—apheresis with dextran sulfate-cellulose column and anaphylactoid reactions to ACE inhibitors. Lancet 341:60, 1993
24. Geha R, Leung D: Hyperimmunoglobulin E syndrome. Immunodefic Rev 1:155, 1989
25. Butrus S, Leung D, Gellis S et al: Vernal conjunctivitis in the hyperimmunoglobulinemia E syndrome. Ophthalmology 91:1213, 1984
26. Morris JH: The peripheral nervous system. p. 1444. In Cotran RS, Kumar V, Robbins SL (eds): Robbins Pathologic Basis of Disease. WB Saunders, Philadelphia, 1989
27. McKhann GM: Guillain-Barré syndrome: clinical and therapeutic observation. Ann Neurol, suppl. 27:513, 1990
28. Asbury AK, Cornblath DR: Assessment of current diagnostic criteria for Guillain-Barré syndrome. Ann Neurol, suppl. 27:S21, 1990
29. French Cooperative Group on Plasma Exchange in Guillain-Barré Syndrome: Role of replacement fluids. Ann Neurol 22:753, 1987
30. vander Meché FGA, Schmitz PIM, The Dutch Guillain-Barré Study Group: A randomized trial comparing intravenous immune globulin and plasma exchange in Guillain-Barré syndrome. N Engl J Med 326:1123, 1992
31. Balow JE, Austin HA, Tskos GC: Plasmapheresis therapy in immunologically mediated rheumatic and renal diseases. Clin Immunol Rev 3:225, 1984
32. Ferri C, Moriconi L, Gremignai G, Migliorini P: Treatment of the renal involvement in mixed cryog-

lobulinemia with prolonged plasma exchange. Nephrologic 43:246, 1986

33. Bell WR, Braine HG, Ness PM, Kickler TS: Improved survival in thrombotic thrombocytopenic purpura-hemolytic uremic syndrome. N Engl J Med 325:398, 1991

34. Glockner WM, Sieberth HG, Wichmann HE et al: Plasma exchange and immunosuppression in rapidly progressive glomerulonephritis: a controlled multi-centre study. Clin Nephrol 29:1, 1988

35. Cleary TG, Lopez EL: The Shiga-like toxin producing *Escherichia coli* and hemolytic uremia syndrome. Pediatr Infect Dis J 8:720, 1989

36. Milford DV, Taylor CM, Guttridge B et al: Haemolytic uraemic syndromes in the British Isles 1985–8: association with verotoxin producing *Escherichia coli*: part 1: clinical and epidemiological aspects. Arch Dis Child 65:716, 1990

37. Havens PL, O'Rourke PP, Hahn et al: Laboratory and clinical variables to predict outcome in hemolytic-uremic syndrome. Am J Dis Child 142:961, 1988

38. Ingulli E, Tegani: Incidence, treatment and outcome of recurrent focal glomerulosclerosis posttransplantation in 42 allografts in children. Transplantation 51:401, 1991

39. Cochat P, Kassier A, Colon S et al: Recurrent nephrotic syndrome after transplantation: early treatment with plasmapheresis and cyclophosphamide. Pediatr Nephrol 7:50, 1993

40. McCarthy LJ, Cotton J, Danielson C et al: Goodpasture's syndrome in childhood: treatment with plasmapheresis and immunosuppression. Clin Apheresis 9:116, 1994

41. Lund DP, Lillehei CW, Kevy SV et al: Liver transplantation in newborn liver failure: treatment for neonatal hemachromatosis. Transplant Proc 25:1068, 1993

42. Kevy S, Galacki D, Humphreys D et al: Intensive plasma and whole blood exchange in the management of hepatic failure—Ab. 69. J Clin Apheresis 9:57, 1994

43. Kim HC, Dugan N, Maller E, Lau HT: Prolongation of an hepatic survival by the use of therapeutic plasma exchange. Ab 71. J Clin Apheresis 9:57, 1994

44. Brandtzaeg P, Mollnes T, Kierulf P: Complement activation and endotoxin levels in systemic meningococcal disease. J Infect Dis 160:58, 1989

45. Girardin E, Grau G, Dayer J et al: Tumor necrosis factor and interleukin-1 in the serum of children with severe infectious purpura. N Engl J Med 319:397, 1988

46. van Deuren M, Santman F, van Dalen R et al: Plasma and whole blood exchange in meningococcal sepsis. Clin Infect Dis 15:424, 1992

47. Brandtzaeg P, Sirnes K, Folsland B et al: Plasmapheresis in the treatment of severe meningococcal or pneumococcal septicaemia with DIC and fibrinolysis. Scand J Clin Lab Invest, suppl. 178, 45:53, 1985

48. Natanson C, Hoffman W, Koev L et al: Plasma exchange does not improve survival in a canine model of human septic shock. Transfusion 33:243, 1993

49. McManus M, Churchwell K: Coagulopathy as a predictor of outcome in meningococcal sepsis and the systemic inflammatory response syndrome with purpura. Crit Care Med 21:706, 1993

50. Humphreys D, Galacki D, Kent P et al: Automated plasma exchange for the coagulopathic neonate on extracorporeal membrane oxygenation. J Clin Apheresis 8:42, 1993

51. Condemi JJ: The autoimmune diseases. Systemic lupus erythematosus. JAMA 268:282, 1992

52. Dau PC, Callahan J, Parker R, Golbus: Immunologic effects of plasmapheresis synchronized with pulse cyclophosphamide in systemic lupus erythematosus. J Rheumatol 18:270, 1991

53. Condemi JJ: The autoimmune diseases. Juvenile RA. JAMA 268:2887, 1992

54. Brewer EJ, Nickeson RW, Rossen RD et al: Plasma exchange in selected patients with juvenile rheumatoid arthritis. J Pediatr 98:194, 1991

55. Lovejoy FH, Linden CH: Acute poison and drug overdosage. p. 2163. In Wilson JD, Braunwald E, Isselbacher KJ (eds): Harrison's Principles of Internal Medicine. Vol. 2. McGraw-Hill, New York, 1991

56. Merciriali R, Sirchia G: Plasma exchange for mushroom poisoning. Transfusion 17:644, 1977

57. Miller J, Sanders E, Webb D: Plasmapheresis for paraquat poisoning. Lancet 1:875, 1978

58. Bensinger WI: Selective removal of A and B isoagglutinins in bone marrow transplant. p. 105. In Pineda AA (ed): Selective Plasma Component Removal. Futeir Publishing, Mount Kisco, NY, 1984

59. Braine HB, Sensebrenner LL, Wright SK et al: Bone marrow transplantation with major ABO incompatibility using erythrocyte depletion of marrow prior to infusion. Blood 60:420, 1982

60. Jin N, Hill R, Segal G: Preparation of red blood cell depleted marrow for ABO incompatible marrow transplantation by density-gradient separation using the IBM (Cobe) 2991 blood cell processor. Exp Hematol 15:93, 1987

61. Uehlinger J, Button GR, McCarthy JM et al: Immunoadsorption for coagulation factor inhibitors. Transfusion 31:265, 1991

62. Nilsson IM, Berntorp E, Zettervoll O: Induction of

immune tolerance in patients with hemophilia and antibodies to factor VIII by combined treatment with intravenous IgG, cyclophosphamide and factor VIII. N Engl J Med 318:947, 1988

63. Watt RM, Bunitsky K, Faulkner EB et al: Hemophilia Study Group. Treatment of congenital and acquired hemophilia patients by extracorporeal removal of antibodies to coagulation factors. Transfusion Sci 13: 233, 1992

64. Putnam TC, Kevy SV, Replogle RL: Factors influencing the viscosity of blood. Surg Gynecol Obstet 124: 547, 1967

65. Rosenthal A, Nathan DG, Nadas AS: Acute hemodynamic effects of red cell volume reduction in polycythemia of cyanotic congenital heart disease. Circulation 42:297, 1970

66. Oldershaw PJ, St. John Sutton MG: Haemodynamic effects of haematocrit reduction in patients with polycythemia secondary to cyanotic congenital heart disease. Br Heart J 44:584, 1980

67. Wedemeyer AL, Lewis JH: Improvement in hemostasis following phlebotomy in cyanotic patients with heart disease. J Pediatr 83:46, 1973

68. Fosburg M, Jacobson M et al: Red cell exchange for polycythemia in congenital heart disease: techniques and the effect of iron status on hematocrit and blood viscosity. p. 132. In Procedures of the International Society of Blood Transfusion, Munich, 1984

69. Harrison BD, Gregory RJ et al: Exchange transfusion in polycythemia secondary to hypoxic lung disease. BMJ 2:713, 1971

70. Wayne AS, Kevy SV, Nathan DG: Transfusion management of sickle cell disease. N Engl J Med 81:1109, 1993

71. Schmalzer EA, Lee JO, Brown AK et al: Viscosity of mixtures of sickle and normal red cells at varying hematocrit levels: implications for transfusion. Transfusion 27:228, 1987

72. Sprinkle RH, Cole T, Smith S, Buchanan GR: Acute chest syndrome in children with sickle cell disease: a retrospective analysis of 100 hospitalized cases. Am J Pediatr Hematol Oncol 8:105, 1986

73. Rosse WF, Gallagher D, Kinney TR et al: Transfusion and alloimmunization in sickle cell disease. Blood 76: 1431, 1990

74. Charache S, Scott JC, Charache P: Acute chest syndrome in adults with sickle cell anemia: microbiology, treatment and prevention. Arch Intern Med 139:67, 1979

75. Charache S, Lubin B, Reid CD: Management and Therapy of Sickle Cell Disease. Publication no. (NIH)

92-2117. US Department of Health and Human Services, Washington, DC, 1992

76. Emond AM, Holman R, Hayes RJ, Serjeant GR: Priapism and impotence in homozygous sickle cell disease. Arch Intern Med 140:1434, 1980

77. Walker EM, Mitchum EN, Rous SN et al: Automated erythrocytopheresis for relief of priapism in sickle cell disease. J Urol 130:912, 1983

78. Kleinman SH, Hurvitz CG, Goldfinger D: Use of erythrocytopheresis in the treatment of patients with sickle cell anemia. J Clin Apheresis 2:170, 1984

79. Fullerton MW, Philippart AL, Sarnaik S, Lusher JM: Preoperative exchange transfusion in sickle cell anemia. J Pediatr Surg 16:297, 1981

80. Bhattacharyya N, Wayne AS, Kevy SV, Shamberger RC: Perioperative management for cholecystectomy in sickle cell disease. J Pediatr Surg 28:72, 1993

81. Griffin TC, Buchanan GR: Elective surgery in children with sickle cell disease without preoperative blood transfusion. J Pediatr Surg 28:681, 1993

82. National SCA Preoperative Transfusion Study Group: Preoperative transfusion in sickle cell anemia, abstracted. Blood 74:184a, 1989

83. Bunin NJ, Pui C: Differing complications of hyperleukocytosis in children with acute lymphoblastic or acute nonlymphoblastic leukemia. J Clin Oncol 3: 1590, 1985

84. Lane TA: Continuous flow leukopheresis for rapid cytoreduction in leukemia. Transfusion 20:455, 1980

85. Lichtman MA, Row JM: Hyperleukocytic leukemias: rheological, clinical and therapeutic considerations. Blood 60:279, 1982

86. Bensinger W, Singer J, Appelbaum F et al: Autologous transplantation with peripheral blood mononuclear cells collected after administration of recombinant granulocyte stimulating factor. Blood 81:3158, 1993

87. Kessinger A, Armitage JO, Landmark JD et al: Autologous peripheral hematopoietic stem cell transplantation restores hematopoietic function following marrow ablative therapy. Blood 71:723, 1988

88. Sienna S, Bregni M, Brando B et al: Circulation of CD34 + hematopoietic stem cells in the peripheral blood of high-dose cyclophosphamide-treated patients: enhancement by intravenous recombinant human granulocyte-macrophage colony-stimulating factor. Blood 74:1905, 1989

89. Bender JG, To LB, Williams S, Schwartzberg L: Defining a therapeutic dose of peripheral blood stem cells. J Hematother 1:329, 1992

90. Sutton DMC, Nair RC, Rock G: Canadian Apheresis

Study Group: complications of plasma exchange. Transfusion 29:124, 1989

91. Huestis DW: Adverse reactions associated with hemapheresis. p. 40. In McPherson JL, Kasprisin DO (eds): Therapeutic Hemapheresis. CRC Press, Boca Raton, 1985

92. Couriel D, Weinstein R: Complications of therapeutic plasma exchange: a recent assessment. J Clin Apheresis 9:1, 1994

93. Luban NLC: Extracorporeal membrane oxygenation in the neonate. In Sacher RA, Strauss R (eds): Contemporary Issues in Pediatric Transfusion Medicine. American Association of Blood Banks, Arlington, 1989

94. Short BL, Pearson GD: Neonatal extracorporeal membrane oxygenator, a review. J Intensive Care Med 1:45, 1986

95. Bartlett RH, Andrews AF, Toomasian JM et al: Extracorporeal membrane oxygenation for newborn respiratory failure: forty-five cases. Surgery 92:425, 1982

96. Bartlett RH, Roloff DW, Cornell RG et al: Extracorporeal circulation in neonatal respiratory failure: a prospective randomized study. Pediatrics 76:479, 1985

97. Ware JH, Epstein MF: Extracorporeal circulation in neonatal respiratory failure: a randomized study. Pediatrics 76:849, 1985

98. Paneth N, Wllenstein S: Extracorporeal membrane oxygenation and play the winner rule. Pediatrics 76:622, 1985

99. Stolar CJ, Snedecor SM, Bartlett RH: Extracorporeal membrane oxygenation and neonatal respiratory failure: experience from the extracorporeal life support organization. J Pediatr Surg 26:563, 1991

100. HIFO Study Group: Randomized study of high-frequency oscillatory ventilation in infants with severe respiratory distress syndrome. J Pediatr 122:609, 1993

101. Bower LK, Betit P: Extracorporeal life support and high-frequency oscillatory ventilation: alternatives for the neonate in severe respiratory failure. Respir Care 40:61, 1995

102. Wessel DL, Adatia I, Thompson JE, Hickey PR: Delivery and monitoring of inhaled nitric oxide in patients with pulmonary hypertension. Crit Care Med 22:930, 1994

103. Adatia I, Wessel DL: Therapeutic use of inhaled nitric oxide. Curr Opin Pediatr 6:583, 1994

104. Cole CH, Jillson E, Keller D: ECMO: regional evaluation of need and applicability of selection criteria. Am J Dis Child 142:1320, 1988

105. Marsh TD, Wilkerson S, Cook LN: Extracorporeal membrane oxygenation selection criteria: partial pressure of arterial oxygen versus alveolar-arterial oxygen gradient. Pediatrics 82:162, 1988

106. Extracorporeal Life Support Organization (ELSO): International ECMO Registry Report. May 1994

107. Short BL, Walker LK, Traysman RJ: Impaired cerebral autoregulation in the newborn lamb during recovery from severe, prolonged hypoxia, combined with carotid artery and jugular vein ligation. Crit Care Med 22:1262, 1994

108. Andrew M, Paes B, Johnston M: Development of the hemostatic system in the neonate and young infant. Am J Pediatr Hematol Oncol 12:95, 1990

109. Kern FH, Morana NJ, Sears JJ, Hickey PR: Coagulation defects in neonates during cardiopulmonary bypass. Ann Thorac Surg 54:541, 1992

110. McManus ML, Kevy SV, Bower LK, Hickey PR: Coagulation factor deficiencies during initiation of extracorporeal membrane oxygenation. J Pediatr in press

111. Bower LK, Kevy SV, McManus ML: Survey of ECLS Centers: circuit priming practices (in preparation)

112. Wilson JM, Bower LK, Fackler JC, Kevy SV: Aminocaproic acid decreases the incidence of intracranial hemorrhage and other hemorrhagic complication of EMCO. J Pediatr Surg 28:536, 1993

113. Wieland M, Thiede VL, Strauss RG et al: Treatment of severe cardiac allograft rejection with extracorporeal photochemotherapy. J Clin Apheresis 9:171, 1994

114. Rose EA, Barr ML, Xu H et al: Photochemotherapy in human heart transplant recipients at high risk for fatal rejection. J Heart Lung Transplant 111:746, 1992

115. Morrison FS, Huestis DW: Toxicity of the staphylococcal protein A immunoadsorption column. J Clin Apheresis 7:171, 1992

116. Huestis DW, Rifkin RM, Durie BGM et al: An unexpected complication following immunoadsorption with a staphyloccal protein A column. J Clin Apheresis 7:75077, 1992

117. Smith RE, Gottschall JL, Pisciotta AV: Life-threatening reaction to staphylococcal protein A immunomodulation. J Clin Apheresis 7:4, 1992

Chapter 34

Bone Marrow Transplantation

Lawrence D. Petz

Advances in bone marrow transplantation (BMT) have depended to a significant degree on the striking improvements in transfusion medicine that have allowed for more effective supportive care. The ability to provide adequate blood component support is essential for the care of BMT recipients. Many patients require both red blood cell (RBC) and platelet transfusions prior to BMT as a result of their disease. In addition, recipients of marrow grafts receive intensive immunosuppressive therapy, chemotherapy, and/or radiotherapy prior to BMT, which results in severe pancytopenia. During this period, RBC and platelet transfusions are necessary, and granulocyte transfusions are sometimes needed.

In addition, there are a number of highly specialized considerations relating to the transfusion of BMT patients, such as the relationship of transfusion to graft rejection, the use of irradiated blood products, prevention of cytomegalovirus (CMV) infection, transfusion of the marrow donor, transfusion requirements of the patient, and the immunohematologic problems that arise when the marrow donor and recipient are of different blood groups. Finally, a unique consequence of allogeneic BMT is the development of mixed hematopoietic chimeras—that is, patients who have a mixture of both donor and recipient hematopoietic cells after BMT.

BLOOD TRANSFUSION AND GRAFT REJECTION

Research in the field of experimental and clinical BMT has indicated that sensitization of the transplant recipient via transfusions prior to BMT may jeopardize the success of BMT even when the marrow donor is genotypically identical with the recipient for the known human leukocyte antigens (HLAs).[1]

Experimental Data

Experimental studies concerning the effect of blood transfusion on subsequent marrow grafts were first performed in animals not matched for the major histocompatibility antigens. In mice, engraftment of allogeneic marrow was prevented when the recipients were given several whole-blood transfusions from the prospective marrow donors before conditioning of the recipients by total body irradiation (TBI).[2] Similar results were obtained in experiments in rhesus monkeys[3] and dogs[4] after transfusions of whole blood from the marrow donor or from unrelated donors. Transfusions were harmful regardless of whether they were given 3 minutes, 24 hours, or 10 days before BMT.[5] Further experiments in mice and dogs convincingly demonstrated that even minor antigenic differences are of importance. Loutit and Micklem[6] showed that injections prior to transplantation of spleen cells from allogeneic H_2-

compatible donors caused increased mortality in x-irradiated recipient mice after marrow grafting.

Storb and coworkers[7,8] performed a series of experiments with canine littermates matched for DLA (dog leukocyte antigen, analogous to HLA) and reported that 58 of 59 untransfused dogs successfully engrafted littermate marrows. In contrast, the graft rejection rate was 71 percent in dogs that had received one transfusion from the DLA-matched marrow donor 10 days before grafting. The rejection rate reached 100 percent when a DLA-matched donor transfusion was given three times prior to BMT. However, when transfusions were given from three random dogs on each of 3 days, the rejection rate was only 27 percent. The more pronounced effect of transfusions from the intended marrow donor as compared with random-donor transfusions has led to the practice of avoiding pretransplantation family member transfusions to prevent sensitization to the minor histocompatibility antigens that cause graft rejection. Because these minor histocompatibility antigens are inherited but are not on the same chromosome as the major histocompatibility locus, any transfusion from a family member would lead to a high probability of exposure to the relevant antigens as compared with the more diffuse distribution and therefore a lower risk of sensitization within a random population.[9]

Human Bone Marrow Transplantation

Graft rejection in patients with aplastic anemia has been a major problem in multiply transfused patients given marrow grafts from HLA-identical siblings. The results of allogeneic BMT in 30 patients with aplastic anemia who had received either no previous transfusions or transfusions only within 3 days of receiving immunosuppressive cyclophosphamide as their pretransplantation conditioning therapy were evaluated. Twenty-seven of 30 untransfused patients (90 percent) sustained marrow engraftment as compared with a reported engraftment rate of only 41 to 75 percent in transfused aplastics.[10] An extension of this study, with 50 untransfused patients, showed 42 patients still living, with an actuarial survival rate of 82 percent at 10 years.[11]

For reasons that are not entirely clear, graft rejection was only a minor problem in patients with acute leukemia or other hematologic malignancies prior to the use of T-cell-depleted marrow grafts. The dif-

ference in rejection rate between patients with aplastic anemia and hematologic malignancies has been attributed to the fact that blood product support for patients with acute leukemia is usually necessary during remission induction chemotherapy at a time when immunosuppression may be severe enough to prevent sensitization.[1,12] Indeed, Ho et al.[13] reviewed the outcome of BMT in 18 patients with leukemia who were transfused prior to BMT with platelets and/or leukocytes from related family members. In 15 cases in which the outcome could be evaluated, engraftment was rapid, and graft failure did not occur. Nevertheless, some investigators suggest that family member transfusions should probably be avoided even for patients with leukemia.[1,9,14] The only exception to this policy is for thrombocytopenic patients with life-threatening bleeding who are refractory to both random donor and HLA-matched community donor platelets and for whom HLA-matched family member platelet transfusions may be life-saving.[14]

Ho et al.[13] also pointed out that since recipients of T-cell-depleted transplants are at an increased risk of graft rejection, it may be wise to avoid family member transfusions in this setting. Such caution is also logical for all allogeneic marrow transplants when the donor is anyone other than an HLA-matched sibling.

Other Approaches to the Prevention of Alloimmunization and Graft Rejection

Storb et al.[15] studied the effectiveness of unirradiated buffy coat cells obtained from the marrow donor and given to the transplant recipient for 3 to 5 days after BMT. The rationale for using donor buffy coat cells was to enhance bone marrow engraftment. It was believed that graft enhancement could result from increasing the number of pluripotent stem cells infused. An alternative or additional mechanism that was suggested by studies in experimental animals was the facilitation of marrow engraftment by donor lymphocytes.[15] The rejection rate of 14 percent in transfused patients given an additional 5 days of unirradiated buffy coat transfusions from their marrow donor after grafting was less than the 38 percent rejection rate previously observed. Furthermore, the survival of patients who received buffy coat cells was also improved to 70 percent, as compared with 43 percent in a control group. However, the incidence of chronic graft-versus-host disease (GVHD) was 50 percent in recipients of buffy coat cells, as compared with 20 percent in patients who did not receive them.

Other groups have reported comparable rejection rates and a lower incidence of chronic GVHD when using conditioning regimens that did not include the use of buffy coat cells. This was accomplished with conditioning regimens that included cyclosporine with or without TBI. However, the survival rates were similar, and there is concern about using TBI because it may result in the development of post-transplantation malignancies.[16]

A more recent analysis of risk factors associated with graft rejection in patients with aplastic anemia showed a marked decrease—to 11 percent—in the rejection rate in transfused patients.[17] However, a large number of pretransplant platelet transfusions (> 40 units) were still strongly correlated with graft rejection. Also, Arranz et al.[18] reported that all 21 patients with aplastic anemia engrafted regardless of prior transfusions. Patients with more than 30 transfusions prior to BMT showed a trend toward a poorer outcome, although this was not statistically significant.

There is also experimental evidence indicating that the use of leukocyte-poor blood products can reduce the incidence of graft rejection in dogs.[19] In addition, exposing donor blood to ultraviolet light prevented transfusion-induced sensitization; 0 of 10 dogs given blood so treated rejected their grafts.[20]

SPECIALIZED CONSIDERATIONS REGARDING TRANSFUSION

Irradiated Blood Products

GVHD is a potentially lethal complication of BMT. GVHD is observed in allogeneic BMT recipients even when donor–recipient pairs are HLA-matched siblings. The basic requirements for the initiation of the graft-versus-host reaction are (1) genetically determined histocompatibility differences between the graft donor and the recipient, (2) the presence of immunocompetent cells in the graft that can recognize the foreign histocompatibility antigens of the host and mount an immunologic reaction against them, and (3) the inability of the host to react against and reject the donor graft.[21] Cellular immune mechanisms appear to be of critical importance in human GVHD; the generation of alloreactive T lymphocytes that recognize antigenic differences of the host is followed by lymphocyte-mediated damage to host target cells or organs. Thus, in the setting of BMT, GVHD may occur as a result of the engrafted donor marrow cells and could also occur as a result of the transfusion of viable lymphocytes in blood products given during the period of severe immunosuppression that results from the pretransplantation conditioning regimen. No completely effective means of preventing or treating GVHD caused by the engrafted marrow has been developed.

The approach taken to prevent the transfusion of viable lymphocytes in the post-transplantation period is the irradiation of blood products (see Ch. 42) Transfusion-associated GVHD has been caused by transfusions of whole blood, packed RBCs, buffy coats, granulocyte concentrates, fresh plasma, platelet concentrates, and chronic myelogenous leukemia leukocytes, but not as a result of transfusion of frozen-thawed RBCs, fresh frozen plasma, cryoprecipitate, or washed RBCs.[9] Irradiation of all cellular blood products is often recommended for BMT recipients, the only exception being for buffy coats from the marrow donor that are given to enhance engraftment in transfused aplastic anemia patients.[9]

The American Association of Blood Banks standards[22] state that the dose of γ-radiation delivered shall be a minimum of 25 Gy (2,500 cGy) targeted to the central portion of the container. A minimum dose of 15 Gy (1,500 cGy) shall be delivered to all other parts of a component.

The use of irradiated blood products is begun at the initiation of the pretransplantation conditioning regimen.[23] An unresolved question concerns the duration of time after BMT during which they should be administered. It seems logical to extend their use during the period of post-transplantation immunodeficiency. This may persist for 2 years and may be present even longer in patients who have GVHD.

Cytomegalovirus-Seronegative Blood Products

CMV infection is a major cause of morbidity and mortality after allogeneic BMT[24] (see Ch. 39). The cause of CMV infection in patients who are seropositive at the time of BMT appears to be primarily the reactivation of latent virus, whereas seronegative patients acquire primary CMV infection from the donor marrow or from blood transfusions. Evidence of active CMV infection after BMT developed in 69 percent of 258 patients who were seropositive at the time of BMT, compared with 28 percent in 208 seronegative patients with seronegative marrow donors ($P < .00005$), emphasizing the significance of the patient's baseline CMV status on post-BMT CMV infection.[14] All of these patients received blood products from donors not screened for their CMV status.

The effectiveness of CMV-seronegative blood products in preventing CMV infection in seronegative patients receiving allogeneic BMTs has been documented in two randomized prospective trials.[25,26] Overall, among recipients with a CMV-seronegative marrow donor, only 3 of 75 (4 percent) recipients of CMV-seronegative blood seroconverted, versus 22 of 69 (32 percent) who received CMV-unscreened blood products. If the marrow donor was CMV-seropositive, the provision of CMV-seronegative blood products was not helpful.

In contrast, there are no data to show that patients who are CMV-seropositive derive benefit from the provision of CMV-seronegative blood products.[14] Although the possibility of acquiring a new strain of CMV cannot be excluded when CMV-seropositive blood is given to a CMV-seropositive recipient, the frequency with which this occurs does not justify giving CMV-seronegative blood to BMT candidates who are already CMV-seropositive.[14] Also, the lower incidence of CMV pneumonia in autologous and syngeneic marrow transplant recipients indicates that receipt of CMV-seronegative blood will not improve survival in these patient groups.[9]

Accordingly, present concepts suggest that if the patient is CMV-seropositive or if the intended marrow donor is CMV-seropositive, the use of CMV-seronegative blood products offers no benefit in preventing CMV infection.[9] On the other hand, if the patient and the marrow donor are both CMV-seronegative, the patient is a candidate for CMV-seronegative blood products both before and after transplantation.[9,14]

Measures for Preventing Transfusion-Transmitted Cytomegolovirus Infection

A number of measures have been used to prevent or minimize transfusion-transmitted CMV infection. These are reviewed in detail in Chapter 39 and include (1) the adherence to appropriate indications for transfusion, (2) donor screening to provide seronegative blood products, (3) reduction of the white blood cell (WBC) content of blood and components, (4) immunoprophylaxis and antiviral agents, and (5) vaccination.

The provision of blood from CMV-seronegative donors is the only technique of donor selection that has been shown to reliably prevent CMV transmission by transfusion.[14] However, since leukocytes are thought to harbor latent CMV viruses and because fresh frozen plasma, cyroprecipitate, gammaglobulin, or clotting factors concentrates do not transmit CMV, there has been much interest in the use of leukodepleted blood products as a means of preventing CMV transmission. A number of studies have already been reported that indicate the effectiveness of leukodepleted blood products in preventing transmission of CMV,[27-33] and prospective trials comparing filtered blood products with products from CMV screened donors are underway. The data look promising that CMV transmission can be prevented by leukodepletion,[14] and some authorities believe that there is already sufficient evidence accumulated to show that CMV-seronegative components and third-generation filtered RBCs and platelets are equivalent in their ability to reduce the risk of transfusion-transmitted CMV infection.[34]

TRANSFUSION SUPPORT OF THE MARROW DONOR

BMT puts the marrow donor as well as the recipient at risk. Many marrow donors require transfusion support because of the volume of marrow that is required to provide an adequate dose of marrow cells for engrafting. Since the risks of transfusion are reduced by using autologous blood, every effort should be made to collect sufficient autologous units to support the donor's transfusion requirements. In one study of 1,160 donors, transfusion requirements were met for 86 percent of the men, 76 percent of the women, and 62 percent of the children under 10 years of age by collecting only 1 unit of autologous blood or the weight-adjusted equivalent for donors weighing less than 55 kg.[35]

When it can be estimated how much blood a bone marrow donor may require, an appropriate number

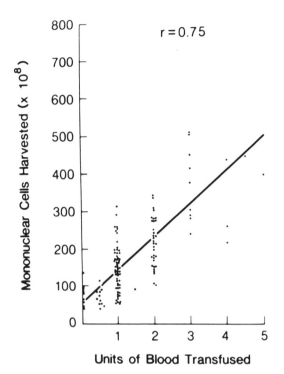

Fig. 34-1. Relationships of bone marrow collection to blood transfusion in 129 donors. (From Thompson and McCullough,[36] with permission.)

Table 34-1. Units of Red Blood Cells Transfused After HLA-Identical Marrow Transplantation

Diagnosis (No. Patients)	No. Units of RBCs	
	Mean	Range
Aplastic anemia (20)	15.7	3–37
Acute leukemia in remission (20)	10.5	3–25
Acute leukemia in relapse (20)	15.4	4–28
Chronic myelogenous leukemia[a] (12)	18.2	7–42

[a] Three of the patients with chronic myelogenous leukemia were in the chronic phase, two in the "accelerated" phase, and seven in blast crises. The somewhat larger of RBC transfusions required by patients with chronic myelogenous leukemia reflects a single patient with massive gastrointestinal bleeding.
(Data from Storb and Weiden.[37])

of autologous units can be collected prior to bone marrow harvest, and the use of allogeneic blood can be eliminated in most cases. Because the average number of mononuclear cells collected per volume of marrow aspirated has been determined, it is possible to construct a nomogram to calculate the amount of marrow needed and the corresponding number of transfusions that the marrow donor will require.[36] (Fig. 34-1).

If transfusion of homologous blood should be necessary before completion of the harvesting of the donor marrow, the blood products should be irradiated.

BLOOD COMPONENT REQUIREMENTS
Red Blood Cells

In one study, an average of about 15 units of RBCs (range, 3 to 42) was required to maintain hematocrit levels at 25 to 30 percent after allogeneic BMT for aplastic anemia, acute leukemia in remission or relapse, and chronic myelogenous leukemia[37] (Table 34-1). In another report, an average of 16 RBC transfusions and 37 platelet transfusion events, with the equivalent of 4 to 6 units of platelet concentrates per transfusion (median, 24; range, 1 to 223), were required to support the 390 patients given transplants by the Seattle team in 1990.[14] A need for increased numbers of units of RBCs in ABO-incompatible transplantation has been reported by several BMT groups.[23,38–40] Although the patient's ABO blood group antibodies that react with the donor's RBCs and their precursors do not preclude engraftment, they may cause a delay in donor RBC production, thereby necessitating more RBC transfusions (see the section below on increased transfusion requirements in major ABO-incompatible marrow transplants).

Platelets

The demand for platelet transfusions to support a BMT program has a significant impact on a transfusion service. In Seattle, a 1-year survey indicated that BMT patients received 21 percent of the random-donor platelet concentrates and over 85 percent of the HLA-selected single-donor apheresis platelet products prepared at the Puget Sound Blood Center.[9] During a 5-year period at the University of Minnesota the transplantation bed capacity increased 250 percent, the number of transplantations increased by nearly 300 percent, and the number of plateletphereses increased 1,450 percent. During this same period of time, the use of plateletpheresis products for other reasons did not change substantially.[41]

Although pooled random-donor platelet concentrates are frequently used until patients become refractory to platelet transfusion,[9] there is an increasing interest in the more widespread use of single-donor platelets obtained by plateletpheresis. The use of single-donor platelets has the potential for decreasing the number of donors to whom the recipient is exposed and thus decreasing the probability of transmission of infectious diseases.

Furthermore, leukocyte filters can be used to produce leukodepleted platelets that have a residual WBC of less than 1×10^6 per product. A number of reports indicate that the use of such leukodepleted blood products can decrease the incidence of alloimmunization and refractoriness to platelet transfusion. However, two editorials have suggested caution in interpreting data from these trials of leukodepleted products owing to the small numbers of patients and the conflicting data on the levels of leukocytes that either produce or prevent platelet alloimmunization or platelet refractoriness.[42,43] In spite of these views, the use of leukodepleted blood products for patients receiving chronic transfusion therapy and who are not yet alloimmunized has become widespread. One hopes that definitive data will be forthcoming since the filters add significant expense that would not be justified without commensurate benefit (see Chs. 16 and 32).

The principles of platelet transfusion for BMT recipients are generally similar to those with thrombocytopenia due to decreased marrow production, as described in Chapter 16. When HLA-matched platelets are used, a significant proportion can often be provided by family members,[9,14] with the remainder by a community donor panel.

Granulocytes

During the first weeks after BMT, there is a high probability of bacterial and fungal infection until the engrafted marrow functions adequately. A prospective study of the effectiveness of prophylactic granulocyte transfusions indicated that the incidence of septicemia episodes was lower in the granulocyte transfusion group, as compared with the control group.[44] However, overall mortality in both groups was not different.

In addition, difficulties in documenting effectiveness of therapeutic granulocyte transfusions, coupled with significant advances in antibiotic therapy, have led to a markedly reduced use of granulocyte transfusions in BMT patients.

Nevertheless, interest in granulocyte transfusions has been renewed in part because of the ability to provide a substantially higher dose of granulocytes than had been possible previously as a result of the administration of granulocyte colony-stimulating factor (G-CSF) to leukocyte donors[45,46] (see Ch. 17).

The indications for therapeutic granulocyte transfusions in BMT patients are similar to those in other patients with severe granulocytopenia and infection unresponsive to antibiotics. In general, granulocyte transfusions are indicated in patients with severe granulocytopenia (< 200 granulocytes/μl) and who have documented bacterial or fungal infections not responding rapidly to appropriate antibiotic therapy. Persistent high fever unresponsive to antibacterial and antifungal therapy and without culture proof of infection is also an indication for therapeutic granulocyte transfusions, particularly if accompanied by clinical deterioration. Once initiated, therapeutic granulocyte transfusions are continued until the marrow graft sustains the granulocyte count at greater than 200/μl[9,14] (see Ch. 17).

IMMUNOHEMATOLOGIC PROBLEMS UNIQUE TO MARROW TRANSPLANTATION

Several immunohematologic problems, some of which are unique to transplantation, are associated with BMT. Since the inheritance of blood group antigens is independent of the HLA gene complex, the RBCs of the donor and recipient will be of different genotypes even when the donor and recipient are HLA matched. The most important of these blood group incompatibilities are those within the ABO blood group system. This may be a "minor" incompatibility in which the donor possesses hemagglutinins capable of reacting with ABO antigens on the recipient's RBCs (e.g., group O donor and group A recipient) or a "major" incompatibility in which the recipient possesses hemagglutinins capable of reacting with ABO antigens on the surface of the donor's

Table 34-2. Potential Immunohematologic Consequences of ABO-Incompatible Bone Marrow Transplantation[a]

Minor ABO incompatibility
  Graft-versus-host disease
  Immune hemolysis at the time of infusion of the donor marrow caused by anti-A and anti-B in the plasma of the marrow product
  Immune hemolysis of delayed onset caused by red blood cell antibodies produced by the donor marrow
Major ABO incompatibility
  Failure of stem cell engraftment
  Delay in onset of hematopoiesis, especially erythropoiesis
  Acute hemolysis at the time of infusion of the donor marrow
  Delayed onset of hemolysis associated with persistence of anti-A and/or anti-B after transplantation
    Hemolysis of infused red blood cells of donor type
    Hemolysis of red blood cells produced by the engrafted marrow
  Mixed hematopoietic chimerism

[a] See text for details.

RBCs (e.g., group A donor and group O recipient). For other blood group systems, analogous definitions may be used. For example, a minor Rh_o (D) incompatibility is one in which the donor is able to make an antibody against antigens on the recipient's RBCs (i.e., an Rh-negative donor and an Rh-positive recipient). In some instances, both major and minor incompatibilities exist simultaneously, such as when the donor is group B and the recipient is group A.

The potential immunohematologic complications of ABO-incompatible transplants are listed in Table 34-2.

MAJOR ABO-INCOMPATIBLE TRANSPLANTATION

Immune Hemolysis at Time of Infusion of Donor Marrow

The donor marrow product ordinarily contains approximately the same volume of RBCs as a unit of whole blood. It is therefore evident that the RBC mass that is transfused is sufficient to precipitate a severe hemolytic transfusion reaction with the attendant hazards of disseminated intravascular coagulation, renal failure, and death. A number of pretransplantation maneuvers have been used in an attempt to circumvent this problem. These have involved removal of anti-A and anti-B antibodies from the patient or removal of RBCs from the donor marrow product.

Intensive Plasma Exchange and In Vivo Antibody Absorption

The quality of the marrow inoculum is obviously of extreme importance, and accordingly, early investigators preferred to reduce the anti-A and/or anti-B titers in the recipient before the transplantation rather than to manipulate the marrow product. One approach was the use of intensive plasma exchange (PE).[35,47] Buckner et al.[35] described 13 patients who underwent intensive PE equivalent to a median of 7.6 plasma volumes (2.8 to 10.6) over a 1- to 3-day period. After the exchanges, antibody persisted in 8 of the 13 patients. In these patients, infusion or exchange of 0.75 to 7.5 L of incompatible donor-type whole blood was carried out in an attempt to further reduce the titer by absorbing the remaining antibody onto the incompatible RBCs. Marrow was subsequently transfused in all patients without evidence of hemolysis at the time of the infusion. An additional method used by some investigators to reduce the anti-A or anti-B titers was the infusion of A or B substance.[47,48]

The large-volume PEs resulted in significant morbidity, including fatigue, dyspnea, hives, paresthesias, fluid management problems, and the risk of disease transmission. Titers were only transiently reduced[35,48–51] owing to equilibration from the extravascular compartment and/or continued antibody production by residual host cells. The rebound in antibody levels resulted in immune hemolysis of delayed onset in a number of patients (see Delayed Onset of Immune Hemolysis, below).

Extracorporeal Immunoadsorption

Bensinger et al.[52] reported the use of synthetic human blood group A or B antigen as an immunoadsorbent for the extracorporeal removal of antibodies in 11 patients. All patients also had a whole-blood exchange with donor-type RBCs after the immunoadsorption. The immunoadsorption procedure was tolerated better than PE was, and platelet decrements, although significant (10 to 72 percent), were less severe than were those usually seen with large-volume PE.

Subsequently, Bensinger et al.[53] reported a comparison of plasma immunoadsorption (PIA), whole blood immunoadsorption (WBIA), and PE in 140 marrow transplants in which a major ABO incompatibility between donor and recipient existed. Immunoadsorption columns were about 14 to 24 percent less efficient at removing antibody from patients than was PE, which is in keeping with the experience of others.[54] In a few instances, PIA or WBIA removed little or no antibody. In most situations in which immunoadsorption was ineffective, the patients were of blood group O, and most of these patients' plasma contained antibody of relative low affinity for the synthetic antigen used on the immunoadsorbent columns even though it was still capable of binding to group-specific RBCs.

Although immunoadsorption techniques are less efficient than plasma exchange, the latter technique has several disadvantages, including the cost of plasma, potential changes in electrolyte balance, the risk of transfusion-transmitted diseases, allergic reactions, immunoglobulin and coagulation factor depletion, and nonspecificity.

Since manipulation of the donor marrow (e.g., for removal of RBCs) has the potential to jeopardize engraftment because of a loss of stem cells, removal of isohemagglutinins by PE or by immunoadsorption is an appealing approach to prevention of hemolysis at the time of the marrow infusion. However, there is little evidence that techniques of RBC depletion of the donor marrow do lead to a lack of marrow engraftment.

Red Blood Cell Depletion of the Bone Marrow Product

An alternative method that is now used by most transplant centers to avoid hemolysis at the time of the marrow infusion is to deplete the donor marrow product of RBCs by using one of a number of methods. Several groups have reported the use of gravity sedimentation after the addition of hydroxyethyl starch (HES).[51,55–57] Ho et al.[56] used 6 percent HES, which was added in a ratio of 1:8 by volume; the marrow cells were allowed to settle under gravity for 30 to 45 minutes with visual monitoring. The dependent erythrocytes were evacuated from a port in the lower end of the inverted bag, and the supernatant plasma and buffy coat layer were resuspended and infused. The authors reported a median recovery of 70 percent of nucleated cells and 55 percent of colony-forming units in culture. The hematocrit of the marrow inoculum after separation was 1 to 2 percent, with the total volume of residual erythrocytes ranging from 3.1 to 12.0 ml. No evidence of hemolysis was noted after intravenous administration of the separated marrow.

Other sedimenting agents such as Plasmagel, Dextran, and Ficoll-Hypaque have proven to be less effective in this procedure.[58]

An alternative method is differential centrifugation using a COBE-2991 cell processor or discontinuous flow cell separators (H-30 or V-50 models Haemonetics, Inc, Braintree, MA). Centrifugation using these instruments yields a buffy coat concentrate containing 75 percent of the original nucleated cells and 57 to 83 percent of the colony-forming units. The average volume of the RBCs remaining in the concentrate varies from 8 to 38 ml.[58] This method is less time-consuming than the gravity sedimentation technique. In addition, it provides a better closed processing system and a more objective and reproducible separation.

It is important that the final volume of RBCs be small since the infusion of even rather small volumes of ABO-incompatible RBCs has led to hemolytic transfusion reactions with chills, fever, hypertension, bradycardia, and transient hemoglobinuria.[55,57,59] The total volume of RBCs in the marrow product that is infused is likely to determine the frequency of adverse reactions because several authors who reported maximum volumes of residual RBCs of 10 ml or less stated that the infusions caused no clinical symptoms or evidence of hemolysis.[60–63]

Delayed Onset of Immune Hemolysis

It was hoped that pre-BMT treatment with large-volume PE, in vivo antibody adsorption, and high-dose cytoreductive therapy with ablation of the patient's marrow would be adequate to eliminate the recipient's isohemagglutinins and thereby prevent hemolysis. However, these measures did not prove to be uniformly successful; a rebound of antibody occurred after BMT in some patients. Particularly severe complications have been reported in BMT recipients when incompatible RBCs were used prior to BMT for in vivo absorption and incompatible RBCs were also transfused as part of the marrow inoculum.

Lasky et al.[51] reported that seven of nine major ABO-incompatible BMT recipients who received incompatible donor-type RBCs before BMT developed hemolysis 6 to 10 days after BMT. In one patient the isohemagglutinins that had been reduced by PE reappeared on the sixth post-transplant day. His hematocrit dropped from 37 to 18 percent, the direct antiglobulin test was positive for IgG and complement, and anti-A and anti-B were eluted from his RBCs. He improved rapidly after therapy with fluids, corticosteroids, and the transfusion of several units of group O RBCs. Buckner et al.[35] and Bensinger et al.[64] reported similar patients who developed acute massive hemolysis and renal failure. Other patients have had less severe hemolysis[50] or merely positive direct antiglobulin test results.[35,57,59]

Less severe delayed hemolytic episodes have been reported in patients who received transplants with RBC-depleted marrow products. Hemolysis in this setting was rather unexpected since the only source of significant volumes of incompatible RBCs would be erythropoiesis by the newly engrafted marrow unless RBC transfusions of the donor type were used in the post-transplant period, as was sometimes done.[64] In addition, the patient's isohemagglutinins generally diminish in titer soon after BMT and usually become undetectable during the second month after major ABO-incompatible BMT. Nevertheless, Sniecinski et al.[65] reported that 5 of 58 evaluable patients developed overt evidence of hemolysis that was manifested by a sudden drop in hemoglobin of 1.5 to 4 g/dl (median, 2.5 g/dl), increases in bilirubin and lactic dehydrogenase, and decreases in serum haptoglobin concentrations (Table 34-3). Hemolysis occurred only among the 28 of the 58 evaluable patients who received cyclosporine-prednisone for prophylaxis and did not occur among patients who received methotrexate-prednisone instead. The hemolysis was managed with transfusions of group O RBCs and, in some instances, by an increase in the dose of prednisone.

Delayed Onset of Hematopoiesis

A number of groups have reported that there is a delay in the onset of hematopoiesis, especially erythropoiesis, in some patients with major ABO-mis-

Table 34-3. Laboratory Data in Five Patients Who Received a Marrow Transplant from a Major ABO-Incompatible Donor and Who Developed Hemolysis of RBCs Produced by the Engrafted Marrow

Onset of hemolysis	Day +37 to +105 (median, +65)
Severity of hemolysis	Drop in hemoglobin of 1.5 to 4.0 g/dl (median, 2.5 g/dl)
Duration of hemolysis	10 to 94 days (median, 36 days)
Isohemagglutinin titers at onset of hemolysis	IgG: 1:1 to 1:4 IgM: 1:1 to 1:2
Antibody in RBC eluate	Anti-A or anti-B

(From Petz,[62] with permission.)

matched marrow transplants. Braine et al.[59] indicated that major ABO-incompatible transplantation patients achieved a reticulocyte count of over 1 percent on day 37 ($\pm$ 15) after BMT, whereas ABO-compatible patients achieved greater than 1 percent reticulocytes on day 25 ($\pm$ 10). Bone marrow examination revealed that erythroid differentiation was markedly reduced in over 70 percent of ABO-incompatible transplantation patients at a time when myeloid differentiation had achieved greater than 1,000 leukocytes/μl in the peripheral blood. In general, those patients with the highest pretransplantation hemagglutinin titers manifested the longest delay in reticulocyte recovery. In marrow recipients with high-titer isohemagglutinins, reticulocytosis did not occur until there had been a substantial reduction in titer to about a level of 4 or less.

Further reports have indicated impaired or failed engraftment of all cell lineages in some patients when there is major ABO incompatibility between donor and recipient.[61,66,67] Figure 34-2 illustrates the findings in a patient with high anti-A titers who had detectable antibody until 15 weeks after BMT and who had delayed engraftment of RBCs, neutrophils, and platelets[61] (the latter is not illustrated).

Sniecinski et al.[68] reported that 10 of 66 evaluable patients had persistence of anti-A or anti-B isohemagglutinins beyond day 120. The isohemagglutinin titers in five of these patients are illustrated in Figures 34-3 and 34-4. The persistence of high titers of isohemagglutinins was associated with a correspond-

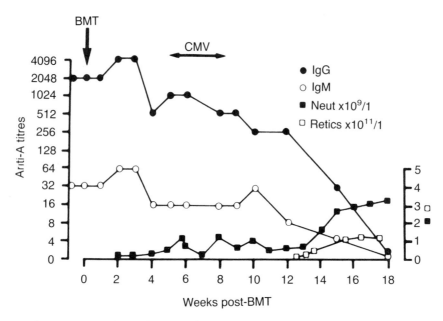

Fig. 34-2. Serial anti-A titers and reticulocyte and neutrophil counts during the weeks after bone-marrow transplantationin a major ABO-incompatible transplant. CMV, cytomegalovirus infection. (From Blacklock et al.,[40] with permission.)

ing delay in the onset of erythropoiesis to beyond day 40. In five of the patients, erythropoiesis, as defined by a reticulocyte count of at least 0.5 percent, was markedly delayed to 170 days or more. In comparison, the onset of erythropoiesis in 378 ABO-identical or minor-mismatched transplants ranged from post-transplant day 16 to 36, with a median of day 26. One of the patients (unique patient number [UPN] 279) remained dependent on RBC transfusions for 5 years before the onset of erythropoiesis

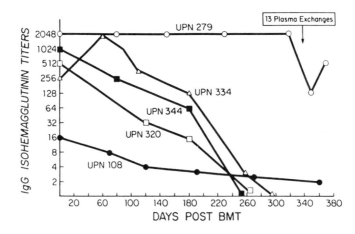

Fig. 34-3. IgG-isohemagglutinin titers in five patients whose antibodies persisted for more than 255 days. (From Sniecinski et al.,[65] with permission.)

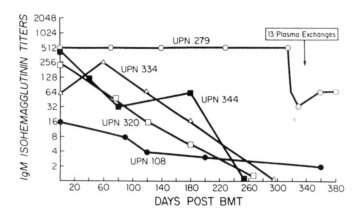

Fig. 34-4. IgM-isohemagglutinin titers in five patients whose antibodies persisted for more than 255 days. (From Sniecinski et al.,[65] with permission.)

even though adequate WBC and platelet production occurred on post-transplant days 11 and 20, respectively. The isohemagglutinins persisted in spite of PEs that were performed on 13 occasions in a 6-week period beginning 10 months after BMT in an unsuccessful attempt to reduce the anti-A titer. Also, because of a suspicion that cyclosporine administration might have been contributing to the patient's exceptional course, treatment with the drug was discontinued at 150 days post-BMT without change in her condition.

Increased Transfusion Requirement

As might be expected as a result of a delayed onset of erythropoiesis in recipients of major ABO-mismatched transplants, there is an increased requirement for RBC transfusion in this group of patients as compared with ABO-compatible transplants.[14,60,65] Jin et al.[60] found that the median number of RBC units transfused post-transplant to 19 evaluable ABO-incompatible patients was 95 as compared with 13 units in ABO-compatible patients ($P = .02$). Prior to post-transplant day 28, RBC transfusion requirements were not significantly different between the two groups. After day 28, ABO-incompatible patients received a median of 14 RBC transfusions as compared with 6 for the ABO-compatible group ($P = .03$). The median day to the last RBC transfusion for ABO-incompatible patients was day 93 (range, 18 to 177) as compared with day 73 (range, 12 to 101) ($P < .005$) for the ABO-compatible group. The

number of RBC units given and the days to achievement of RBC independence were not different for ABO-incompatible patients who received transplants of RBC-depleted marrow as compared with patients who underwent depletion of isohemagglutinins by immunoadsorption columns.

Characteristic Course

Several patients exhibited a characteristic course[65] as illustrated in Figure 34-5. Early in the post-transplant period, isohemagglutinin titers remained high (i.e., above 16) and the engrafted marrow did not produce RBCs (reticulocyte count < 0.5 percent), although WBCs and platelets were produced. Subsequently, the titers fell to a low level, and during this time the engrafted marrow produced RBCs that were hemolyzed to a variable extent by the persisting antibody. Still later, the isohemagglutinins became undetectable, hemolysis ceased, and adequate erythropoiesis occurred.

MANAGEMENT OF MAJOR ABO-INCOMPATIBLE MARROW TRANSPLANTS

Pretransplantation Measures

PE followed by in vivo absorption of the remaining low levels of antibody by transfusion of incompatible RBCs successfully circumvents acute hemolysis at the time of infusion of the marrow product. However, the procedure causes significant morbidity and uses

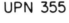

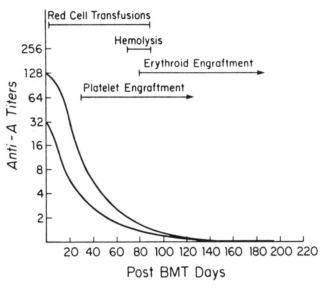

Fig. 34-5. Post-transplant course in a patient with a bone marrow transplant from a major ABO-incompatible donor (patient, group O; donor, group A). There was no RBC production while isohemagglutinin titers remained high. Hemolysis occurred while titers were low (≤ 4). Resolution of hemolysis occurred when hemagglutinins became undetectable. Findings of hemolysis were present even though donor marrow–derived RBCs were undetectable, which suggests intramedullary hemolysis. The upper curve represents IgG isohemagglutinins and the lower curve, IgM isohemagglutinins. (From Sniecinski et al.,[65] with permission.)

large volumes of blood products, and severe hemolysis of transfused cells can occur when there is a rebound of the patient's antibody after BMT. Moreover, the infusion of incompatible RBCs after lowering of isohemagglutinin titers by PE appears to be unnecessary, as indicated by Bensinger[53,64] who reported that when titers are 1:16 or less, marrow may be safely infused. Thus the transfusion of incompatible RBCs for in vivo absorption of isohemagglutinins has been abandoned as unnecessary.[64]

Blacklock et al.,[66] favor the use of RBC-depleted marrow but also suggest some form of antibody depletion in those patients with high titers of isohemagglutinins because the majority of delayed problems have been reported in patients with high and persistent anti-A titers, predominantly of the IgG class. Specifically, they recommend that recipients with high-titer IgG anti-A, particularly with A₁ donors, should have some form of antibody depletion, perhaps before marrow infusion but particularly

after BMT if marrow development is not proceeding.[61,66] However, there are no reports of the effectiveness of this policy and, in reports to date, there has been no serious morbidity related to the delayed onset of erythropoiesis and the transient episodes of delayed hemolysis that have occurred following the use of RBC-depleted marrow. These facts suggest that adding the morbidity of high-volume PE or other means of antibody removal to the morbidity of the preparative regimen does not seem warranted. In addition, high-volume PE has not been helpful in more than transiently reducing antibody in a patient in whom isohemagglutinins were present in high titer and erythropoiesis still absent more than 600 days post-BMT.[65,68]

Thus, presently available information suggests that the optimal approach in major ABO-mismatched transplants is to use RBC-depleted marrow; to anticipate possible delayed erythropoiesis and immune hemolysis as possible sequelae of BMT, especially in patients with high titers of isohemagglutinins; and to manage these problems appropriately when they occur.[62]

Blood Component Therapy

From the onset of the preparative regimen, it is advisable to use group O RBCs when transfusion is necessary. Also, the transfusionist should minimize the volume of any plasma products that contain isohemagglutinins that will react with RBCs of the donor type. This policy is advisable because at least a small concentration of such cells will be in the donor marrow product and such RBCs will be produced by the newly engrafted marrow. Minimizing the volume of plasma that is transfused can be accomplished by giving platelets of the donor type or, when not readily available, by removing some of the plasma from the platelet product by centrifugation.

Although both packed RBCs and centrifuged platelet components do contain some plasma, it is generally unnecessary to use washed cells.

MINOR ABO-INCOMPATIBLE TRANSPLANTS

The Role of the ABO System as Transplantation Antigens

Early investigators in BMT reasoned that if the ABO system is an important transplantation antigen system, there might be an increased incidence and/or severity of GVHD in recipients receiving transplants from donors with minor ABO incompatibilities. Buckner et al.[35] analyzed the results of BMT in regard to graft rejection, incidence and severity of GVHD, and survival in 46 evaluable patients who had minor ABO mismatches with their donors. Only patients who were genotypically HLA matched at the A, B, and D loci with a sibling donor were included in the analysis; 246 patients with ABO-identical donors were available for comparison. Results indicated that there was no effect of minor ABO incompatibility on graft rejection or on the incidence or severity of GVHD. Also, survival times of patients having compatible or incompatible transplants were not significantly different. Other investigators have reached similar conclusions.[47,51]

More recently, Bacigalupo et al.[69] reported an analysis of 174 patients who received a BMT from an HLA-identical sibling for severe aplastic anemia, acute lymphoblastic leukemia, or chronic granulocytic leukemia. Twenty-three transplants were ABO major-mismatched, 27 were ABO minor-mismatched, and 124 were ABO matched. Double mismatched grafts (A to B and B to A) were excluded from their analysis. They concluded that ABO compatibility was clearly associated with a different risk of grade II to IV acute GVHD. Recipients of ABO minor-mismatched grafts had the highest incidence of GVHD, recipients of ABO-identical grafts had an intermediate risk, and patients given an ABO major-mismatched BMT had the lowest incidence of GVHD. To explain the low incidence of GVHD in ABO major-mismatched BMT, the authors suggested that donor lymphocytes may absorb ABO antigens and then become the target for immune destruction by anti-A/B antibodies, thus contributing to a low incidence of GVHD.

Immune Hemolysis Caused by Isohemagglutinins in the Marrow Product

Lasky et al.[51] reported 13 patients who received bone marrow from a donor with a minor ABO incompatibility. One patient was managed with exchange transfusion before BMT by using RBCs of the donor's type in order to prevent hemolysis caused by isohemagglutinins in the marrow product. Five were managed by centrifuging the bone marrow to remove plasma and thus reduce the amount of antibody. Two of the seven patients who received uncentrifuged bone marrow experienced minimal hemolysis on the first transplantation day (indirect bilirubin level, 0.9 to 1.1 mg/dl). However, one of the patients who received centrifuged marrow also developed hemolysis; this occurred on the sixth post-transplant day, at which time there was a decrease in the patient's hemoglobin concentration of 4 g/dl. This was attributed to the post-BMT transfusion of 2,000 ml of plasma of the donor's type to the patient who was a child with an estimated plasma volume of only 1,565 ml. Although the transfused plasma may have caused the hemolysis in this child or contributed to its pathogenesis, subsequent reports of patients who did not receive incompatible plasma products but who developed post-transplant immune hemolytic anemia indicate that immune hemolytic anemia in ABO minor-mismatched transplants is primarily caused by other mechanisms (see the following section).

Delayed Hemolysis Caused by Antibodies Produced by Cells of the Donor Marrow

Rowley and Braine[70] described six group A patients and one group AB patient who received transplants from group O donors. Five of the group A patients showed evidence of hemolysis between post-transplantation days 6 and 10. Two patients developed renal failure, and one of these required hemodialysis. All of the patients received incompatible plasma in association with platelet transfusions, but no similar episodes of hemolysis were noted in patients who received ABO-compatible transplants and who also received incompatible plasma products. This suggested that transfused plasma was not the source of the anti-A that caused the hemolysis.

Hows et al.[71] reported five cases of immune hemolytic anemia that were attributed to donor-derived RBC antibodies after ABO minor-mismatched transplants (Table 34-4). Severe intravascular hemolysis with hemoglobinuria was seen in two of the patients, and one of these patients was treated by PE. The hemolysis was frequently abrupt in onset and appeared unexpectedly. All the patients required increased RBC transfusion in the post-transplant period, as compared with recipients of ABO-compatible transplants. In all instances, anti-A or anti-B was first detected 4 to 10 days after BMT.

The direct antiglobulin test was positive, and eluates made from the recipients' RBCs showed the same specificity as the serum antibody. Hemolysis ceased as hemolyzed RBCs of the marrow recipient were replaced by transfused group O erythrocytes. The patients were generally transfused with packed group O RBCs. However, the transfusion of some group A or B RBCs may have contributed to the severity of the hemolytic episodes in patients 1, 2, 4, and 5. The course of one patient is illustrated in Figure 34-6.

Several findings indicate that the hemolysis was not caused by passive administration of antibody in donor plasma. No hemolysis occurred at the time of the marrow infusion, the direct antiglobulin test did not become positive until 4 or more days post-BMT, and the hemolysis did not reach its maximum intensity until 10 to 16 days post-BMT (Table 34-4). These findings, coupled with the fact that none of the six patients received significant volumes of incompatible plasma in blood products in the post-BMT period, indicate that active production of antibody by donor lymphocytes is the most likely source of antibody.

All the patients who developed hemolysis were receiving cyclosporine to prevent GVHD. To determine the significance of cyclosporine administration and the frequency of hemolysis in minor ABO-mismatched transplants, Hows et al.[71] retrospectively analyzed 16 consecutive cyclosporine-treated pa-

Table 34-4. Clinical and Laboratory Data in Patients Who Had Immune Hemolysis of Delayed Onset Following a Minor ABO-Incompatible Marrow Transplantation

Case No.	ABO and Rh Type		Day Post-BMT DAT Became Positive	Details of Hemolysis and RBC Transfusion Needs
	D	R		
1	O+	A−	+18	Severe IVH: hemoglobinuria; maximum hemolysis, day +15; treated with PE; 9 U RBCs required days +10 to +15
2	O+	A+	+15	Moderate hemolysis, maximum on day +16; 6 U RBCs required days +16 to +22
3	O+	B+	+10	Severe hemolysis; hemoglobinuria; maximum hemolysis, day +10; 14 U RBCs required days +10 to +19
4	O+	A+	+14	Moderate hemolysis, maximum on day +10; 7 U RBCs required days +9 to +18
5	B+	AB+	+9	Moderate hemolysis, maximum, day +12; 6 U RBCs required days +11 to +14

Abbreviations: DAT, direct antiglobulin test; D, donor; R, recipient; IVH, intravascular hemolysis; PE, plasma exchange; RBCs, red blood cells. (From Petz,[62] with permission.)

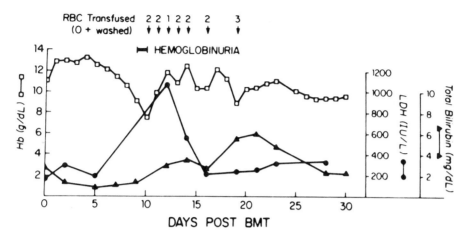

Fig. 34-6. Minor ABO-mismatched bone marrow transplantation (BMT) (donor group O, recipient group B). The flow chart shows hematologic and biochemical evidence for hemolysis. Fourteen units of packed group O RBCs were required to maintain the hemoglobin level between day 10 and day 19 post-BMT. Note that the hemoglobin, the lactic dehydrogenase (LDH), and the total bilirubin levels were normal for the first 5 days post-BMT. During the hemolytic episode, no incompatible isohemagglutinins were infused; transfused RBCs were washed group O, and platelets were group B or washed and resuspended in fresh AB plasma. (From Petz,[62] with permission.)

tients and compared this group with 13 patients in whom methotrexate was used in the postgraft period for GVHD prophylaxis. Six of the 16 patients in the cyclosporine group developed a positive direct antiglobulin test result, and 2 of these developed clinically significant hemolysis. In contrast, no instance of hemolysis was found among the 13 patients treated with methotrexate.

Hazelhurst et al.[72] described hemolysis after T cell–depleted BMT involving minor ABO incompatibility. Of particular interest is the fact that none of the patients reported had received cyclosporine. Nine consecutive recipients (8 group A and 1 group AB) of T cell–depleted bone marrow from group O donors were studied. Ten to 19 days after BMT, 8 of the 9 patients developed isohemagglutinins. Seven patients had a rise in bilirubin content, and 2 of these had decreases in hemoglobin concentration up to 2 g/dl. No positive direct antiglobulin test results or evidence of hemolysis occurred in any of 4 group AB patients who received transplants of group O marrow that was not T-cell depleted.

Gajewski et al.[73] reported extraordinary degrees of hemolysis in a series of patients receiving minor ABO-incompatible marrow grafts that were not T-

cell depleted but were from unrelated donors. In three consecutive patients excessive hemolysis was observed that required the transfusion of 26 units of group O RBC between days 5 and 20. These transfusion requirements (4,680 ml of RBC) were greater than the patient's total RBC volume before the onset of hemolysis. Such findings indicate that, in addition to hemolysis of the patient's RBC by the donor-derived antibody, transfused group O RBC are also hemolyzed by a process that is defined as bystander immune hemolysis.[74]

All patients with excessive hemolysis had received cyclosporine without post-transplant methotrexate. In contrast, no hemolysis was observed in similar patients who received cyclosporine and also received methotrexate, although weakly positive tests for anti-A or anti-B were found in two of seven patients so treated. The authors suggested that post-transplant immunosuppression with methotrexate may prevent the passenger lymphocyte syndrome from occurring even in patients receiving cyclosporine. Indeed, methotrexate has been shown to be cytotoxic for B lymphocytes and may prevent the antibody production necessary for the passenger lymphocyte syndrome to occur.[75,76]

Additional reports have described the development of anti-Jk[b77] and anti-A[78] in recipients of T cell–depleted marrow transplants, the latter antibody resulting in hemolysis.

Isohemagglutinins in the Post-Transplant Period

Of particular interest are the post-transplant isohemagglutinin titers in patients in whom these were determined 1 year or more after BMT. Buckner et al.[35] reported eight instances in which the donor was group O. Six of the recipients were group A, and all of these patients had anti-B (IgG titers of 16 to 128), but none had anti-A. Two recipients were group AB, and neither of these had detectable anti-B, but both had anti-A, in one instance only detectable in undiluted serum and in the other case present at a titer of 2. Neither of the patients developed clinical manifestations of GVHD or had any other evident adverse effects related to the presence of anti-A. Lasky et al.[51] also reported the presence of ABO isohemagglutinins more than 1 year after BMT in three of five recipients of minor ABO-incompatible transplants who survived longer than 5 months after BMT. The isohemagglutinins were first detected at 10 months (anti-A in an AB recipient, B donor) and 21 and 27 months following BMT (anti-A in A recipients, O donors). No adverse effects of the antibodies were discernible.

MINOR RH-INCOMPATIBLE TRANSPLANTATION

The development of RBC alloantibodies by the engrafted marrow owing to minor incompatibility between donor and recipient in blood group systems other than ABO had also been reported.

Lasky et al.[51] reported that two of four Rh-positive recipients who received marrow from an Rh-negative donor developed anti-D. The patients had received at least four Rh-positive platelet concentrates within the first month after BMT. Anti-D apparently developed 1 year or more after the most recent exposure to the D antigen. Because the anti-D became apparent long after the time that the recipient's RBC type would have changed from Rh-positive to Rh-negative, it would not be capable of causing adverse consequences unless the patient were to be transfused with Rh-positive blood. This is similar to the pattern of development of anti-A in minor ABO-mis-matched transplants described by the same authors (see the section above immune hemolysis).

Hows et al.[71] reported a patient who developed immune hemolysis caused by anti-D in an Rh-positive recipient who received a marrow transplant from an Rh-negative donor. Anti-D first became detectable in the recipient's serum 13 days after BMT and rose to a titer of 256 on day 70. The patient received cyclosporine for post-BMT GVHD prophylaxis and developed moderate hemolysis that was maximum on day 13. Anti-D was present in the donor's serum, thus indicating that the donor had been sensitized to the D antigen. The anti-D produced in the patient after BMT was therefore the result of a secondary immune response to the D antigen by the donor lymphocytes, which is analogous to the production of anti-A and anti-B in minor ABO-incompatible cases.

On retrospective analysis of six additional minor Rh-incompatible transplants,[71] two were found to have produced donor-derived anti-D. Of particular interest was the fact that in one of these patients there was no evidence for donor presensitization to rhesus antigens. Indeed, the donor was a 15-year-old boy who had not been transfused, which suggested that in this case the production of antibody after BMT was due to a primary immune response by the donor lymphocytes. In addition to anti-D, this patient also produced anti-C and anti-E.

Management

If the marrow donor has a high isohemagglutinin titer (e.g., higher than 1:128 to 1:256), it is reasonable to remove much of the plasma from the marrow product to minimize the possibility of an immediate hemolytic reaction. Lasky et al.[51] centrifuged marrow in 600-ml plastic bags at 4,500 g for 10 minutes at 22°C. Supernatant plasma was expressed into sterile 300-ml plastic transfer packs until 2 cm remained above the cell mass. Bone marrow cells were resuspended in the remaining autologous plasma. The original marrow volume was reduced 54 percent by plasma removal, and the plasma volume was reduced by 71 percent. The transfused marrow contained a mean of 99.5 percent of the original nucleated cells present and 203 ml (5 ml/kg) of donor plasma. Recovery of colony-forming units in culture after plasma removal averaged 95.2 percent. No pa-

Table 34-5. Management of Minor ABO- or RH-Incompatible Bone Marrow Transplants

Remove plasma from marrow product if donor has high-titer isohemagglutinins (e.g., 128 or greater)

All plasma products (e.g., platelet transfusions) should be of the recipient's type. If platelets of appropriate type are not available, use concentrated or washed platelets

Red blood cell transfusions, beginning at the onset of the preparative regimen, should be group O (and/or Rh-negative) and given as packed (or washed) cells

Anticipate the possibility of hemolysis in all minor ABO- or Rh-mismatched transplants, especially in association with cyclosporine and/or the use of T-cell-depleted marrow

Perform direct antiglobulin tests and antibody screening tests every 2 or 3 days during the second and third weeks post-BMT

Management hemolysis with red blood cell transfusions, corticosteroids, and supportive care. More aggressive measures such as red blood cell exchange or plasma exchange are ordinarily not necessary

(From Petz,[62] with permission.)

tient had hemolysis at the time of the marrow infusion.

Additional blood products that contain plasma, such as platelet concentrates, should preferably be of the recipient's group in order to avoid infusion of isohemagglutinins in ABO-incompatible plasma. When this is not feasible, transfusion of significant volumes of plasma can be avoided by using platelet preparations concentrated by centrifugation.

Additional aspects of management are indicated in Table 34-5.

DONOR-DERIVED LEWIS ANTIBODIES

Two patients have been reported who developed donor-derived Lewis antibodies in the post-transplantation period.[79,80] In one patient, the onset of renal failure was associated with the demonstration of Lewis antibodies, which could only have been derived from donor lymphocytes.[79] In the other patient,[80] results of post-transplantation lymphocytotoxicity testing revealed strong reactivity only in Le(a+) panel members and was neutralized with commercial Lewis substance. The patient began experiencing renal and gastrointestinal difficulties by

day 48 and died on day 60. It was suggested that it is possible that incompatibility associated with determinants present on renal cells may account for other instances of acute renal failure after allogeneic BMT.[79] Indeed, the significance of a Lewis phenotype in cadaveric renal allografts has been supported by observations of a number of investigators who noted decreased survival in recipients lacking the Lewis gene (thus expressing the [a−, b−] phenotye.[81,82] However, other data suggest that *Le*-gene incompatibility has no influence on renal graft survival or the frequency of chronic rejections.[83,84]

PLATELET- AND GRANULOCYTE-SPECIFIC ANTIBODIES AFTER TRANSPLANTATION

Minchinton et al.[85] have reported the presence of antibodies reacting with circulating platelets and/or granulocytes in 16 of 19 patients studied. In some cases, the presence of antibody coincided with a decrease in the peripheral cell count, while in others there was no noticeable effect. Because 7 of these patients received autologous marrow grafts, the antibodies were considered to be autoantibodies. In the patients receiving allografts, the authors were not able to determine whether the antibodies were auto- or alloantibodies.

POST-TRANSPLANTATION CHIMERISM

In Greek mythology, Chimera was a creature that, according to one description, was a lion in front, a goat in the middle, and a snake in the back (Fig. 34-7). She devoured many men and animals and was ultimately killed by consent of the gods.

In medical science, the term *chimera* is used to designate an organism whose body contains cell populations derived from different individuals of the same or different species,[86] occurring spontaneously or produced artificially. The term *radiation chimera* was introduced in 1956 by Ford et al.[87] to designate an animal that carries a foreign hematopoietic system as a result of whole-body irradiation followed by transplantation of hematopoietic cells derived from another animal. Humans who receive transplants of allogeneic marrow are chimeras since their hematopoietic cells are derived from the donor's marrow.

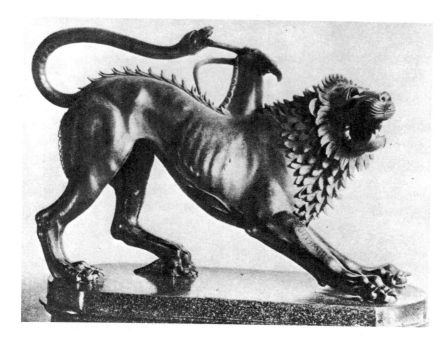

Fig. 34-7. Chimera, the Greek mythologic creature.

Some patients have mixtures of hematopoietic cells of donor and recipient origins for varying lengths of time after BMT. The term *mixed chimera* is frequently used to distinguish these individuals from "complete chimeras" (only cells of donor origin detectable) and from those unusual patients who develop entirely autologous marrow recovery.

A large number of methods have been used to document and characterize chimerism after BMT.[88] These are reviewed below, and an example of the results of various genetic marker studies in a patient who is a mixed hematopoietic chimera after BMT is given in Table 34-6.

Cytogenetic Markers

Sex chromosomes are commonly used to document the type of chimerism that is present after BMT. This method is, of course, applicable only when the donor and recipient are of different sex.

Even when the sex of donor and recipient are the same, polymorphic differences revealed by various banding techniques[89] or constitutional chromosomal abnormalities may be useful in determining the source of cells.

Also, if chromosome abnormalities are present that are markers of the malignant clone, such as the Philadelphia chromosome (Ph) in chronic myeloid leukemia, the remission status of the patient can be monitored.[90-94]

Chromosome analyses have also been used to document leukemic transformation of engrafted human marrow cells and for the identification of persisting host cells after BMT that lacked any cytogenetic abnormalities, suggesting that they were members of residual normal clones not involved in the leukemic process.[93,95,96]

Cellular Genetic Markers

Post-transplantation chimerism can be documented with a number of cellular genetic markers, including RBC and white cell antigens and intracellular enzymes. HLA typing has limited applicability after BMT in humans since most transplantations have been carried out using HLA-matched sibling donors. However, with an increasing number of transplantations performed using donors mismatched for at least one HLA locus,[97] HLA typing for documentation of chimerism may be appropriate more frequently.

In patients who are mixed hematopoietic chimeras, RBC antigen typing reveals various percentages of RBCs derived from the donor and from the

Table 34-6. Mixed Hematopoietic Chimera

Patient data	
Diagnosis	Acute nonlymphoblastic leukemia
Number of days post-BMT	680
Clinical condition	Complete remission; no acute or chronic GVHD
Age at time of transplantation	25 yr
Pre-BMT conditioning regimen	Ara-C; Cytoxan; 10 Gy TBI
RBC antigens	
Donor	Group O; Fy^a-negative
Recipient pre-BMT	Group O; Fy^a-positive
Recipient post-BMT (days 87, 122, 281, 362, 456, 602)	40% of RBCs are Fy^a-positive
Donor	XX
Recipient	XY
Post-BMT (day 650)	[6 donor metaphases; 9 recipient metaphases 15 metaphases analyzed
Total	
Immunoglobulin allotypes	
Donor	G2m(23)-negative
Recipient pre-BMT	G2m(23)-positive (pretransplantation)
Recipient post-BMT (day 447)	G2m(23)-positive
Granulocyte antigens	
Donor	NA1-negative
	NA2-positive
	NB1-positive
	NB2-positive
	NC1-positive
Recipient (day 608)	NA1-positive
	NA2-positive
	NB1-positive
	NB2-positive
	NC1-positive

Abbreviations: BMT, bone marrow transplantation, GVHD, graft-versus-host disease, TBI, total body irradiation.

recipient marrow. This is in contrast to "complete chimeras," who have only cells of donor-marrow origin. In order to be able to detect small percentages of donor or host RBCs with confidence after BMT, it is important to do extensive RBC phenotyping on both the donor and the recipient before BMT. This is done with the aim of identifying both donor and recipient markers (i.e., antigens present on donor but not on recipient RBCs, and vice versa). It useful to type for the following antigens: A$_1$, B, A, C, E, c, e, K, k, Fy^a, Fy^b, Jk^a, Jk^b, P$_1$, M, S, and s.[98]

When mixed chimerism is present after BMT, "mixed-field" reactions are observed when testing for antigens that have been identified as donor- or recipient-specific markers.[98] It is important to identify both recipient- and donor-specific markers before to BMT because both are necessary to document engraftment and exclude mixed chimerism. If donor markers are merely identified among hematopoietic cells in the post-transplant period, engraftment has been documented but it has not been demonstrated that host hematopoietic cells are no longer present.

Documentation of post-transplant chimerism is complicated by the fact that patients may receive RBC transfusions prior to BMT and very frequently receive them in the post-transplant period. In some instances, reticulocyte enrichment of the patient's RBCs[99] can aid in establishing the correct RBC phenotype. Nevertheless, the necessity for blood transfusions after BMT results in the major disadvantage of RBC antigen typing for documentation or exclusion of mixed chimerism; that is, it is often difficult, if not impossible, to provide definitive results until about 5 months after BMT. On the other hand, for patients who are chronic mixed chimeras, RBC antigens are sensitive and frequently informative as genetic markers.

In situ hybridization for the Y chromosome has been used to monitor engraftment[100–104] and a Y chromosome–specific DNA probe has been used for Southern hybridization or dot blot analysis of DNA.[105]

Other Methods: Immunoglobulin Allotypes and Persisting RBC Antibodies

Immunoglobulin allotype analysis is a very sensitive method to document mixed chimerism.[106] However, informative markers are not present as frequently as with other techniques, and the procedure is not widely performed.

The persistence of RBC antibodies longer than 6 months after transplantation has been used as an indication of persistence of the recipient's B lymphocytes.[106] Antibodies of the ABO blood group system may be used when there is a blood group incompatibility between donor and recipient. A 6-month period seems appropriate since studies have indicated that patients' RBC alloantibodies ordinarily persist for no longer than 120 days after BMT.[107] Immunoglobulin allotyping was performed in two patients with persistent RBC antibodies and confirmed mixed chimerism of B lymphocytes.[106] In two other patients, RBC alloantibodies persisted even though cytogenetic analyses failed to reveal recipient-type karyotypes. Occasionally, Rh antibodies or RBC autoantibodies may be present and may serve as markers.

DNA Polymorphisms

The use of DNA-sequence polymorphisms is an informative and versatile method of distinguishing patient and donor cells.[108,109] After digestion with restriction endonucleases, variations in DNA sequences among individuals result in DNA fragments of differing lengths known as restriction fragment-length polymorphisms (RFLPs). "Conventional" RFLP may be created by either loss or gain of a restriction enzyme cleavage site or by insertion or deletion of DNA between restriction sites. RFLPs are inherited as codominant mendelian traits and can be identified in Southern transfer hybridizations using cloned DNA probes.[109] RFLP analysis is applicable to all hematopoietic cells except fully differentiated erythrocytes, in aggregate or in sorted cell fractions. In addition to "conventional" RFLP, DNA polymorphisms also occur as a result of variation in the number of tandemly repeated sequences in different alleles at hypervariable regions in the human genome. These are called minisatellite or variable number of tandem repeat loci.

Changes in relative concentration of donor and recipient cells can be assessed in serial studies[108,109] and an increasing concentration of DNA of recipient origin associated with a recurrence of leukemia suggests that the recurrence is in cells of host origin.[108] This can be documented more definitively by demonstrating only recipient-type DNA in purified blast cell preparations.[110–112]

Amplification by the Polymerase Chain Reaction of Hypervariable Regions of the Human Genome

Introduction of the polymerase chain reaction (PCR) as a method for rapid amplification of DNA in vitro has provided a powerful tool for analysis of human polymorphisms.[113–115] The PCR technique allows the selective amplification of a particular DNA region while it is still incorporated in total genomic DNA.

The major advantage of using a PCR-based analysis is increased sensitivity (i.e., it is possible to detect a very small proportion of DNA of donor or recipient origin). In addition, only small amounts of DNA are required, there is no need for restriction enzyme digestion, and the analysis can be performed more rapidly than traditional RFLP analysis.[116]

PCR primers have been synthesized for the amplification of a Y chromosome expressed sequence[100,117] and for a number of highly polymorphic loci[118–123] including variable number of tandem repeat loci.[116,119,124] Ugozzoli et al.[116] designed locus-specific oligonucleotides for hybridization probes that were complementary to tandem repeat sequences and were highly informative. Using a set of 6 PCR primer pairs and locus-specific oligonucleotide probes, all 13 patients studied had recipient- and donor-specific fragments. A minor population of DNA could be detected even when its concentration was as low as 0.1 percent of the total. They demonstrated the utility of the method for detecting mixed chimerism, complete chimerism, recurrent leukemia, and endogenous repopulation of marrow.

Applications of Genetic Marker Studies

Although originally used primarily to document engraftment of the donor marrow, studies of chimerism after BMT also have the potential to (1) better our understanding of mechanisms of graft rejection and marrow failure, (2) detect the recurrence of leukemia and evaluate whether recurrent leukemia occurs in donor or recipient cells, (3) determine the clinical significance of mixed chimerism, (4) provide insights regarding the mechanisms of tolerance and GVHD, (5) provide information concerning the kinetics of engraftment in various disease states or after different preparative regimens, and (6) determine the origin of tissue macrophages and the cells of the marrow microenvironment.[88]

Significance of Mixed Hematopoietic Chimerism

Using various genetic markers, several early reports indicated that mixed chimerism after BMT for hematologic malignancy may exist even in patients in continuous complete remission.[125–127] Singer et al.[125] reported a patient who had stable mixed hematopoietic chimerism in both lymphoid and myeloid cell lines but remained in complete remission for over 5 years after BMT for acute lymphoblastic leukemia. Reports by Branch et al.[126] and Petz et al.[127] described eight patients transplanted for acute leukemia who were mixed chimeras but who were in continuous complete remission for periods of 673 to 1,499 days after BMT.

The existence of mixed hematopoietic chimeras who are in long-term continuous complete remission indicates that the mechanism by which remission is produced after BMT is not simply that of marrow ablation followed by rescue with donor marrow. A graft-versus-leukemia effect[128,129] may contribute to the maintenance of remission after BMT.

There are conflicting data in the literature concerning the influence of mixed chimerism on the risk of leukemic relapse, and this question is currently being further evaluated using specific markers of clonality.[88,130]

A number of investigators have found, in agreement with results in animal models,[131] that there is an increased incidence of GVHD in patients with complete chimerism, compared to mixed chimerism.[132–136] Thus, the absence of GVHD (i.e., tolerance), may be responsible for the persistence of host hematopoietic cells[134,135] or, alternatively, mixed chimerism may play a role in the development of tolerance. In accord with the latter possibility, some investigators have studied mixed allogeneic chimerism in animal models as an approach to transplantation tolerance.[137,138]

REFERENCES

1. Storb R, Kolb HJ, Graham TC et al: The effect of prior blood transfusions on hemopoietic grafts from histocompatible canine littermates. Transplantation 14:248, 1972
2. Barnes DWH, Loutit JF: What is the recovery factor in spleen? Nucleonics 12:68, 1954
3. van Putten LM, van Bekkum DW, de Vries MJ, Balner H: The effect of preceding blood transfusions on the fate of homologous bone marrow grafts in lethally irradiated monkeys. Blood 30:749, 1967
4. Storb R, Floerscheim GL, Weiden PL et al: Effect of prior blood transfusions on marrow grafts: abroga-

5. Weiden PL, Storb R, Kolb JH et al: Effect of time on sensitization to hemopoietic grafts by preceding blood transfusion. Transfusion 19:240, 1975
6. Loutit JF, Micklem HS: Active and passive immunity to transplantation of foreign bone marrow in lethally irradiated mice. Br J Exp Pathol 42:577, 1961
7. Storb R, Epstein RB, Rudolph RH, Thomas ED: The effect of prior transfusion on marrow grafts between histocompatible canine siblings. J Immunol 105:627, 1970
8. Storb R, Weiden PL, Deeg HJ et al: Rejection of marrow from DLA-identical canine littermates given transfusions before grafting: antigens involved are expressed on leukocytes and skin epithelial cells but not on platelets and red blood cells. Blood 54:477, 1979
9. Slichter SJ: Transfusion and bone marrow transplantation. Transf Med Rev 2:1, 1988
10. Storb R, Thomas ED, Buckner CD et al: Marrow transplantation in thirty "untransfused" patients with severe aplastic anemia. Ann Intern Med 92:30, 1980
11. Anasetti C, Doney KC, Storb R et al: Marrow transplantation for severe aplastic anemia: Long term outcome in fifty "untransfused" patients. Ann Intern Med 104:461, 1986
12. Holohan TV, Terasaki PI, Deisseroth AB: Suppression of transfusion-related alloimmunization in intensively treated cancer patients. Blood 58:122, 1981
13. Ho WG, Champlin RE, Winston DJ, et al: Bone marrow transplantation in patients with leukaemia previously transfused with blood products from family members. Br J Haematol 67:67, 1987
14. Slichter SJ: Principles of transfusion support before and after bone marrow transplantation. p. 273. In Forman SJ, Blume KG, Thomas DE (eds): Bone Marrow Transplantation. Boston, Blackwell Scientific, 1994
15. Storb R, Doney KC, Thomas ED et al: Marrow transplantation with or without donor buffy coat cells for 65 transfused aplastic anemia patients. Blood 59:236, 1982
16. Deeg HJ, Sanders J, Martin P et al: Secondary malignancies after marrow transplantation. Exp Hematol 12:660, 1984
17. Deeg HJ, Self S, Storb R et al: Decreased incidence of marrow graft rejection in patients with severe aplastic anemia: changing impact of risk factors. Blood 68:1363, 1986
18. Arranz R, Otero MJ, Ramos R et al: Clinical results in 50 multiply transfused patients with severe aplastic

anemia treated with bone marrow transplantation or immunosuppressive therapy. Bone Marrow Transplant 13:383, 1994

19. Storb R, Deeg HJ: Failure of allogeneic canine marrow grafts after total-body irradiation: allogeneic "resistance" versus transfusion-induced sensitization. Transplantation 42:571, 1986

20. Deeg HJ, Aprile J, Graham TC et al: Ultraviolet irradiation of blood prevents transfusion-induced sensitization and marrow graft rejection in dogs. Blood 67:537, 1986

21. Tsoi MS: Immunological mechanisms of graft-versus host disease in man. Transplantation 33:459, 1982

22. Klein HG: Standards for Blood Banks and Transfusion Services. American Association of Blood Banks, Bethesda, MD, 1994

23. Brand A, Claas FHJ, Falkenburg JHF et al: Blood component therapy in bone marrow transplantation. Semin Hematol 21:141, 1984

24. Wallington TB: Cytomegalovirus and transfusion. p. 26. In Cash JD (ed): Progress in Transfusion Medicine. Vol. 2. Churchill Livingstone, New York, 1987

25. Bowden RA, Sayers M, Flournoy N et al: Cytomegalovirus immune globulin and seronegative blood products to prevent primary cytomegalovirus infection after marrow transplantation. N Engl J Med 314:1006, 1986

26. Miller WJ, McCullough J, Balfour HH Jr et al: Prevention of cytomegalovirus infection following bone marrow transplantation: a randomized trial of blood product screening. Bone Marrow Transplant 7:227, 1991

27. Verdonck LF, de Graan-Hentzen YC, Dekker AW et al: Cytomegalovirus seronegative platelets and leukocyte-poor red blood cells from random donors can prevent primary cytomegalovirus infection after bone marrow transplantation. Bone Marrow Transplant 2:73, 1987

28. Gilbert GL, Hayes K, Hudson IL, James J: Prevention of transfusion-acquired cytomegalovirus infection in infants by blood filtration to remove leucocytes. Neonatal Cytomegalovirus Infection Study Group [see comments]. Lancet 1:1228, 1989

29. de Graan-Hentzen YC, Gratama JW, Mudde GC et al: Prevention of primary cytomegalovirus infection in patients with hematologic malignancies by intensive white cell depletion of blood products. Transfusion 29:757, 1989

30. Murphy MF, Grint PC, Hardiman AE, Lister TA, Waters AH: Use of leucocyte-poor blood components to prevent primary cytomegalovirus (CMV) infection in patients with acute leukaemia. Br J Haematol 70:253, 1988

31. De Witte T, Schattenberg A, Van Dijk BA et al: Prevention of primary cytomegalovirus infection after allogeneic bone marrow transplantation by using leukocyte-poor random blood products from cytomegalovirus-unscreened blood-bank donors. Transplant 50:964, 1990

32. Eisenfeld L, Silver H, McLaughlin J et al: Prevention of transfusion-associated cytomegalovirus infection in neonatal patients by the removal of white cells from blood. Transfusion 32:205, 1992

33. Bowden RA, Slichter SJ, Sayers MH et al: Use of leukocyte-depleted platelets and cytomegalovirus-seronegative red blood cells for prevention of primary cytomegalovirus infection after marrow transplant. Blood 78:246, 1991

34. Hillyer CD, Emmens RK, Zago-Novaretti M, Berkman EM: Methods for the reduction of transfusion-transmitted cytomegalovirus infection: filtration versus the use of seronegative donor units. Transfusion 34:929, 1994

35. Buckner CD, Clift RA, Sanders JE et al: Marrow harvesting from normal donors. Blood 64:430, 1984

36. Thompson HW, McCullough J: Use of blood components containing red cells by donors of allogeneic bone marrow. Transfusion 26:98, 1986

37. Storb R, Weiden PL: Transfusion problems associated with transplantation. Semin Hematol 18:163, 1981

38. Wulff JC, Santner TJ, Storb R et al: Transfusion requirements after HLA-identical marrow transplantation in 82 patients with aplastic anemia. Vox Sang 44:366, 1983

39. McCullough J, Lasky LC, Warkentin PI: Role of the blood bank in bone marrow transplantation. p. 379. In McCullough J, Sandler SF (eds): Advances in Immunobiology. Blood Cell Antigens and Bone Marrow Transplantation. Alan R Liss, New York, 1984

40. Blacklock HA, Prentice HG, Evans JPM et al: ABO-incompatible bone-marrow transplantation: Removal of red blood cells from donor marrow avoiding recipient antibody depletion. Lancet 2:1061, 1982

41. McCullough J, Steeper TA, Connelly DP et al: Platelet utilization in a university hospital. JAMA 259:2414, 1988

42. Schiffer CA: Prevention of alloimmunization against platelets [editorial]. Blood 77:1, 1991

43. Snyder EL: Clinical use of white cell-poor blood components. Transfusion 29:568, 1989

44. Clift RA, Sanders JE, Thomas ED et al: Granulocyte transfusions for the prevention of infection in pa-

tients receiving bone-marrow transplants. N Engl J Med 298:1052, 1978

45. Caspar CB, Seger RA, Burger J, Gmur J: Effective stimulation of donors for granulocyte transfusions with recombinant methionyl granulocyte colony-stimulating factor. Blood 81:2866, 1993

46. Bensinger WI, Price TH, Dale DC et al: The effects of daily recombinant human granulocyte colony-stimulating factor administration on normal granulocyte donors undergoing leukapheresis. Blood 81: 1883, 1993

47. Gale RP, Feig S, Ho W: ABO blood group system and bone marrow transplantation. Blood 50:185, 1977

48. Bleyer WA, Blaese RM, Bujak JS et al: Long-term remission from acute myelogenous leukemia after bone marrow transplantation and recovery from graft-versus-host reaction and prolonged immunoincompetence. Blood 45:171, 1975

49. Hershko C, Gale RP, Ho W et al: ABH antigens and bone marrow transplantation. Br J Haematol 44:65, 1980

50. Curtis JE, Messner HA: Bone marrow transplantation for leukemia and aplastic anemia: management of ABO incompatibility. Can Med Assoc J 126:649, 1982

51. Lasky LC, Warkentin PI, Kersey JH et al: Hemotherapy in patients undergoing blood group incompatible bone marrow transplantation. Transfusion 23: 277, 1983

52. Bensinger WI, Baker DA, Buckner CD et al: Immunoadsorption for removal of A and B blood-group antibodies. N Engl J Med 304:160, 1981

53. Bensinger WI, Buckner CD, Clift RA, Thomas ED: Plasma exchange and plasma modification for the removal of anti-red cell antibodies prior to ABO-incompatible marrow transplant. J Clin Apheresis 3: 174, 1987

54. Bussel A, Schenmetzler C, Gluckman E, Reviron J: Removal of recipient allo-agglutinins in ABO-incompatible bone marrow transplantation. Comparative study between plasma exchange and immunoadsorption. Plasma Ther Transf Technol 6:461, 1985

55. Dinsmore RE, Reich LM, Kapoor N et al: Transplantation of ABH incompatible bone marrow: removal of erythrocytes by starch sedimentation. Br J Haematol 54:441, 1984

56. Ho WG, Champlin RE, Feig SA et al: Transplantation of ABH incompatible bone marrow: gravity sedimentation of donor marrow. Br J Haematol 57:155, 1984

57. Warkentin PI, Hilden JM, Kersey JH, et al: Transplantation of major ABO-incompatible bone marrow depleted of red cells by hydroxyethyl starch. Vox Sang 48:89, 1985

58. Sniecinski I: Management of ABO incompatibility in allogeneic bone marrow transplantation. p. 497. In Forman SJ, Blume KG, Thomas DE (eds): Bone Marrow Transplantation. Blackwell Scientific, Boston, 1994

59. Braine HG, Sensenbrener LL, Wright SK et al: Bone marrow transplantation with major ABO blood group incompatibility using erythrocyte depletion of marrow prior to infusion. Blood 60:420, 1982

60. Jin N-R, Hill R, Segal G et al: Preparation of red-blood-cell depleted marrow for ABO-incompatible marrow transplantation by density-gradient separation using the IBM 2991 blood cell processor. Exp Hematol 15:93, 1987

61. Blacklock HA, Prentice HG, Evans JPM et al: ABO-incompatible bone-marrow transplantation: removal of red blood cells from donor marrow avoiding recipient antibody depletion. Lancet 2:1061, 1982

62. Petz LD: Immunohematologic problems associated with bone marrow transplantation. Transfus Med Rev 1:85, 1987

63. Sniecinski I, Henry S, Ritchey B et al: Erythrocyte depletion of ABO-incompatible bone marrow. J Clin Apheresis 2:231, 1985

64. Bensinger WI, Buckner CD, Thomas ED et al: ABO-incompatible marrow transplants. Transplant 33: 427, 1982

65. Sniecinski IJ, Oien L, Petz LD, Blume KG: Immunohematologic consequences of major ABO-mismatched bone marrow transplantation. Transplant 45:530, 1988

66. Blacklock HA, Katz F, Michalevicz R et al: A and B blood group antigen expression on mixed colony cells and erythroid precursors: relevance for human allogeneic bone marrow transplantation. Br J Haematol 58:267, 1984

67. Graw RS, Krueger GRD, Yankee RA et al: ABO blood group system and bone marrow transplantation in acute leukaemia employing cyclophosphamide. Exp Hematol 22:118, 1972

68. Sniecinski IJ, Petz LD, Oien L, Blume KG: Immunohematologic problems arising from ABO incompatible bone marrow transplantation. Transplant Proc 19:4609, 1987

69. Bacigalupo A, Van Lint MT, Occhini D et al: ABO compatibility and acute graft-versus-host disease following allogeneic bone marrow transplantation. Transplant 45:1091, 1988

70. Rowley S, Braine H: Probable hemolysis following minor and incompatible marrow transplantation (IMT) (abstract). Blood 60 (suppl. 1):171, 1982

71. Hows J, Beddow K, Gordon-Smith E, et al: Donor-

derived red blood cell antibodies and immune hemolysis after allogeneic bone marrow transplantation. Blood 67:177, 1986

72. Hazelhurst GR, Brenner MK, Wimperis JZ, et al: Haemolysis after T-cell depleted bone marrow transplantation involving minor ABO incompatibility. Scand J Haematol 37:1, 1986

73. Gajewski JL, Petz LD, Calhoun L et al: Hemolysis of transfused group O red blood cells in minor ABO-incompatible unrelated-donor bone marrow transplants in patients receiving cyclosporine without posttransplant methotrexate. Blood 79:3076, 1992

74. Petz LD: The expanding boundaries of transfusion medicine. p. 73. In Nance SJ (ed): Clinical and Basic Science Aspects of Immunohematology. American Association of Blood Banks, Arlington, VA, 1991

75. Kazmers IS, Daddona PE, Dalke AP, Kelley WN: Effect of immunosuppressive agents on human T and B lymphoblasts. Biochem Pharmacol 32:805, 1983

76. Rosenthal GJ, Weigand GW, Germolec DR et al: Suppression of B cell function by methotrexate and trimetrexate. Evidence for inhibition of purine biosynthesis as a major mechanism of action. J Immunol 141:410, 1988

77. Robertson V, Hill M, Bryant J, Dickson L: Anti-Jk^b identified in Jk^b positive recipient following T-cell depleted bone marrow transplant (abstract). Transfusion 27:5254, 1987

78. Robertson V, Hill M, Henslee J et al: Hemolysis post transplant in ABO minor incompatible T-cell depleted bone marrow recipients (abstract). Transfusion 27:525, 1987

79. Blajchman MA, King DJ, Heddle NM et al: Association of renal failure with Lewis incompatibility after allogeneic bone marrow transplantation. Am J Med 79:143, 1985

80. Myser T, Steedman M, Hunat K et al: Lymphocytotoxic anti-Le^a as seen in a bone marrow transplant patient. Transfusion 25:445, 1985

81. Oriol R, Cartron J, Yvart J, et al: The Lewis system: new histocompatibility antigens in renal transplantation. Lancet 1:574, 1978

82. Pfaff WW, Howard RJ, Ireland J, Scornik J: The effect of Lewis antigen and race on kidney graft survival. Transplant Proc 15:1139, 1983

83. Posner MP, McGeorge MB, Picon-Mendez G et al: The importance of the Lewis system in cadaver renal transplantation. Transplantation 41:474, 1986

84. Rydberg L, Samuelson BE, Brynger H: Influence of Lewis incompatibility in living donor kidney transplantation. Transplant Proc 27:2292, 1985

85. Minchinton RM, Waters AH, Malpas JS et al: Platelet and granulocyte-specific antibodies after allogeneic and autologous bone marrow grafts. Vox Sang 46: 125, 1984

86. Tippett P: Blood group chimeras: a review. Vox Sang 44:333, 1983

87. Ford CE, Hamerton JL, Barnes DWH, Loutit JF: Cytological identification of radiation chimeras. Nature 177:452, 1956

88. Petz LD: Documentation of engraftment and characterization of chimerism following marrow transplantation. p. 136. In Forman SJ, Blume KG, Thomas DE (eds): Bone Marrow Transplantation. Blackwell Scientific, Boston, 1994

89. Sparkes RS: Cytogenetic analysis in human bone marrow transplantation. Cancer Genet Cytogenet 4:345, 1981

90. Thomas ED, Clift RA, Fefer A et al: Marrow transplantation for the treatment of chronic myelogenous leukemia. Ann Intern Med 104:155, 1986

91. Graham DL, Tefferi A, Letendre L et al: Cytogenetic and molecular detection of residual leukemic cells after allogeneic bone marrow transplantation in chronic granulocytic leukemia. Mayo Clin Proc 67: 123, 1992

92. Arthur CK, Apperley JF, Guo AP et al: Cytogenetic events after bone marrow transplantation for chronic myeloid leukemia in chronic phase. Blood 71:1179, 1988

93. Alimena G, De Cuia MR, Mecucci C et al: Cytogenetic follow-up after allogeneic bone-marrow transplantation for Ph^1-positive chronic myelogenous leukemia. Bone Marrow Transplant 5:119, 1990

94. Sessarego M, Frassoni F, Defferrari R et al: Cytogenetic follow-up after bone marrow transplantation for Philadelphia-positive chronic myeloid leukemia. Cancer Genet Cytogenet 42:253, 1989

95. Schmitz N, Godde-Salz E, Loffler H: Cytogenetic studies on recipients of allogeneic bone marrow transplants after fractionated total body irradiation. Br J Haematol 60:239, 1985

96. Becher R, Beelen DW, Graeven U et al: Case report: triple chimaerism after allogeneic bone marrow transplantation for Philadelphia chromosome positive chronic granulocytic leukaemia. Br J Haematol 67:373, 1987

97. Stroncek DF: Results of bone marrow transplants from unrelated donors. Transfusion 32:180, 1992

98. Petz LD: Immunohematologic problems unique to bone marrow transplantation. p. 195. In Garratty G (ed): Red Cell Antigens and Antibodies. American Association of Blood Banks, Arlington, VA, 1986

99. Griffin GD, Lippert LE, Dow NS et al: A flow cytome-

tric method for phenotyping recipient red cells following transfusion. Transfusion 34:233, 1994

100. Hutchinson RM, Pringle JH, Potter L et al: Rapid identification of donor and recipient cells after allogeneic bone marrow transplantation using specific genetic markers. Br J Haematol 72:133, 1989

101. Durnam DM, Anders KR, Fisher L et al: Analysis of the origin of marrow cells in bone marrow transplant recipients using a Y-chromosome-specific in situ hybridization assay. Blood 74:2220, 1989

102. Przepiorka D, Ramberg R, Thomas ED: Host metaphases after chemoradiotherapy and allogeneic bone marrow transplantation for acute nonlymphoblastic leukemia. Leuk Res 13:661, 1989

103. Przepiorka D, Gonzales-Chambers R, Winkelstein A et al: Chimerism studies using in situ hybridization for the Y chromosome after T cell-depleted bone marrow transplantation. Bone Marrow Transplant 5: 253, 1990

104. Przepiorka D, Thomas ED, Durnam DM, Fisher L: Use of a probe to repeat sequence of the Y chromosome for detection of host cells in peripheral blood of bone marrow transplant recipients. Am J Clin Pathol 95:201, 1991

105. Morisaki H, Morisaki T, Nakahori Y et al: Genotypic analysis using a Y-chromosome-specific probe following bone marrow transplantation. Am J Hematol 27: 30, 1988

106. Petz LD, Yam P, Wallace B et al: Mixed hematopoietic chimerism following bone marrow transplantation for hematologic malignancies. Blood 70:1331, 1987

107. Witherspoon RP, Rainer S, Ochs HD et al: Recovery of antibody production in human allogenic marrow graft recipients: influence of time posttransplantation, the presence or absence of chronic graft-versus-host disease, and antithymocyte globulin treatment. Blood 58:360, 1981

108. Yam PY, Petz LD, Knowlton RG et al: Use of DNA restriction fragment length polymorphisms to document marrow engraftment and mixed hematopoietic chimerism following bone marrow transplantation. Transplantation 43:399, 1987

109. Knowlton RG, Brown VA, Braman JC et al: Use of highly polymorphic DNA probes for genotypic analysis following bone marrow transplantation. Blood 68: 378, 1986

110. Ginsburg D, Antin JH, Smith BR et al: Origin of cell populations after bone marrow transplantation. Analysis using DNA sequence polymorphisms. J Clin Invest 75:596, 1985

111. Biondi A, Norman C, Messner HA, Minden MD: Re-

striction fragment length polymorphism analysis of hematopoietic cells following successful treatment of relapsed acute lymphoblastic leukemia following bone marrow transplantation. Bone Marrow Transplant 4:705, 1989

112. Minden MD, Messner HA, Belch A: Origin of leukemic relapse after bone marrow transplantation detected by restriction fragment length polymorphism. J Clin Invest 75:91, 1985

113. Saiki RK, Scharf SJ, Faloona F et al: Enzymatic amplification of β-globin genomic sequences and restriction site analysis for diagnosis of sickle cell anaemia. Science 230:1350, 1985

114. Macintyre EA: The use of the polymerase chain reaction in haematology. Blood 3:201, 1989

115. Sklar J: Polymerase chain reaction: the molecular microscope of residual disease. J Clin Oncol 9:1521, 1991

116. Ugozzoli L, Yam P, Petz LD, Ferrara GB et al: Amplification by the polymerase chain reaction of hypervariable regions of the human genome for evaluation of chimerism after bone marrow transplantation. Blood 77:1607, 1991

117. Lawler M, McCann SR, Conneally E, Humphries P: Chimerism following allogeneic bone marrow transplantation: detection of residual host cells using the polymerase chain reaction. Br J Haematol 73:205, 1989

118. Chalmers EA, Sproul AM, Mills KI et al: Use of the polymerase chain reaction to monitor engraftment following allogeneic bone marrow transplantation. Bone Marrow Transplant 6:399, 1990

119. Roth MS, Antin JH, Bingham EL, Ginsburg D: Use of polymerase chain reaction-detected sequence polymorphisms to document engraftment following allogeneic bone marrow transplantation. Transplantation 49:714, 1990

120. Jeffreys AJ, Wilson V, Neumann R, Keylte J: Amplification of human minisatellites by the polymerase chain reaction: towards DNA fingerprinting of single cells. Nucleic Acids Res 16:10953, 1988

121. Boerwinkle E, Xiong WJ, Fourest E, Chan L: Rapid typing of tandemly repeated hypervariable loci by the polymerase chain reaction: application to the apolipoprotein B 3′ hypervariable region. Proc Natl Acad Sci USA 86:212, 1989

122. Bowcock AM, Ray A, Erlich H, Sehgal PB: Rapid detection and sequencing of alleles in the 3′ flanking region of the interleukin-6 gene. Nucleic Acids Res 17:6855, 1989

123. Horn GT, Richards B, Klinger KW: Amplification of a highly polymorphic VNTR segment by the polymerase chain reaction. Nucleic Acids Res 17:2140, 1989

124. Nakao S, Nakatsumi T, Chuhjo T et al: Analysis of late graft failure after allogeneic bone marrow transplantation: detection of residual host cells using amplification of variable number of tandem repeats loci. Bone Marrow Transplant 9:107, 1992

125. Singer JW, Keating A, Ramberg R et al: Long term stable hematopoietic chimerism following marrow transplantation for acute lymphoblastic leukemia: a case report with in vitro marrow culture studies. Blood 62:869, 1983

126. Branch DR, Gallagher MT, Forman SJ et al: Endogenous stem cell repopulation resulting in mixed hematopoietic chimerism following total body irradiation and marrow transplantation for acute leukemia. Transplantation 34:226, 1982

127. Petz LD, Branch RD, Stock AD et al: Endogenous stem cell repopulation after high-dose pretransplant radiochemotherapy. Transplant Proc 27:432, 1985

128. Bertheas MF, Maraninchi D, Lafage M et al: Partial chimerism after T-cell depleted allogeneic bone marrow transplantation in leukemic HLA matched patients: a cytogenetic documentation. Blood 72:89, 1988

129. Roy DC, Tantravahi R, Murray C et al: Natural history of mixed chimerism after bone marrow transplantation with CD6-depleted allogeneic marrow: A stable equilibrium. Blood 75:296, 1990

130. Negrin RS, Cleary ML: Laboratory evaluation of minimal residual disease. p. 179. In Forman SJ, Blume KG, Thomas DE (eds): Bone Marrow Transplantation. Blackwell Scientific, Boston, 1994

131. Ildstadt ST, Sachs DH: Reconstitution with syngeneic plus allogeneic or xenogeneic bone marrow leads to specific acceptance of allografts or xenografts. Nature 307:168, 1984

132. Schattenberg A, De Witte T, Salden M et al: Mixed hematopoietic chimerism after allogeneic bone marrow transplantation with lymphocyte-depleted bone marrow is not associated with a higher incidence of relapse. Blood 73:1367, 1989

133. Bertheas MF, Lafage M, Levy P et al: Influence of mixed chimerism on the results of allogeneic bone marrow transplantation for leukemia. Blood 78:3103, 1991

134. Frassoni F, Strada P, Sessarego M et al: Mixed chimerism after allogeneic marrow transplantation for leukaemia: correlation with dose of total body irradiation and graft-versus-host disease. Bone Marrow Transplant 5:235, 1990

135. Hill RS, Petersen FB, Storb R et al: Mixed hematologic chimerism after allogeneic marrow transplantation for severe aplastic anemia is associated with a higher risk of graft rejection and a lessened incidence of acute graft-versus-host disease. Blood 67:811, 1986

136. Sykes M, Sachs DH: Mixed allogeneic chimerism as an approach to transplantation tolerance. Immunol Today 9:23, 1988

137. Sharabi Y, Sachs DH: Mixed chimerism and permanent specific transplantation tolerance induced by a nonlethal preparative regimen. J Exp Med 169:493, 1989

138. Bretagne S, Vidaud M, Kuentz M et al: Mixed blood chimerism in T cell depleted bone marrow transplant recipients: evaluation using DNA polymorphisms. Blood 70:1692, 1987

Chapter 35

Solid Organ Transplantation

Walter H. Dzik

Dramatic progress has been made in the application of solid organ transplantation to the treatment of disease. The growth of programs in renal, liver, heart, pancreas, and lung transplantation not only have brought requests for greater transfusion support but also have provided new insights into the basic biology of the allogeneic response. Improved pharmacologic immunosuppression has been an important key to the increased use of transplantation. Currently, the demand for transplantation outstrips the supply of suitable organs. For example, the United Network for Organ Sharing (UNOS) reports that in 1993 there were 8,168 cadaver kidney transplantations and 2,752 living related donor kidney transplantations performed in the United States. However, 33,538 patients were on the UNOS waiting list for kidney transplantation.[1] In 1993, the number of individuals on UNOS waiting lists for some form of solid organ transplantation was over 50,000, nearly twice the number on the waiting list in 1988. Solid organ transplantation is likely to remain a focus in the debate to allocate expenditures for health care.

TOLERANCE, ANERGY, AND IMMUNOSUPPRESSION

The induction of immune acceptance of the allograft is a requirement for successful organ transplantation. Research in the prevention of allograft rejec-

tion has continued to advance our understanding of the basic biology of immune tolerance.[2] Allograft acceptance can result from three broad categories of immune intervention: central tolerance, peripheral anergy, and pharmacologic immunosuppression.

Central Tolerance

Central tolerance refers to tolerance induced by the thymus. The thymus ordinarily induces nonresponsiveness to self-antigens. The biology of thymic education of T cells is a fundamental area of immunologic investigation.[3-5] The thymus gland is functionally and anatomically divided into cortex and medulla. T cell precursors phenotypically characterized as CD3+; CD4-; CD8- cells enter the thymic cortex. Within the cortex, they develop into CD3+; CD4+; CD8+ (double-positive) T cells and undergo rearrangement of the αβ genes resulting in low-level expression of the T cell receptor (TCR) on the cell surface. The double-positive TCR-low cells come into contact with two classes of cells to which they may respond—thymic epithelial cells and bone marrow–derived cells. These two cell populations both strongly express major histocompatibility complex (MHC) antigens and can be distinguished by the radioresistance of the former. The traditional view of thymic education links T cell selection in the thymus to the affinity of the TCR with MHC antigens expressed on thymic epithelial cells.

As the double-positive TCR-low precursors encounter these thymic cells, one of three possible affinities may be present. T cell precursors with high affinity to self-MHC are given a signal to undergo apotosis, resulting in clonal deletion of cells that are strongly self-reactive to MHC.[6] This process is called negative selection and is a fundamental property of self-tolerance. Precursor cells with very low affinity to the thymic cells also undergo destruction. Precursors that react with midrange affinity to self-MHC on thymic cells are positively selected and allowed to undergo continued maturation within the thymic medulla. This results in MHC restriction. The developing cells then increase expression of their TCR and ultimately differentiate into either CD3+; CD4−; CD8+ T-cytotoxic cells or CD3+; CD4+; CD8− T-helper cells.

Newer theories regarding the education of T cells have placed less emphasis on specialized thymic stromal cells. Instead, it has been suggested that properties of the developing T cells themselves may control positive versus negative selection[2,7] (Fig. 35-1). According to this hypothesis, when the T cell precursor is at an early stage of development with low TCR expression, positive interaction with MHC-bearing cells in the thymic cortex is required to sustain continued maturation. This process represents positive selection and fosters MHC restriction of the eventual mature T cell. At a latter stage of T cell development within the thymus (perhaps within the medulla), strong positive interaction with MHC-bearing cells results in apoptosis. Under normal circumstances, this serves to clonally delete self-reactive T cells. These newer theories of T cell selection are of direct relevance to central tolerance in organ transplantation. They suggest that the "decision" regarding positive and negative selection results from different outcomes when the TCR reacts with MHC antigen at different stages of T cell development. Although under normal conditions, developing T cells would encounter only self-MHC, it might be expected that if allogeneic cells were introduced into the thymus, any developing T cells destined to react strongly with the MHC antigen expressed on those allogeneic cells would be clonally deleted. Thus, the insertion of donor MHC cells into a thymus may be expected to induce central tolerance to that MHC prior to

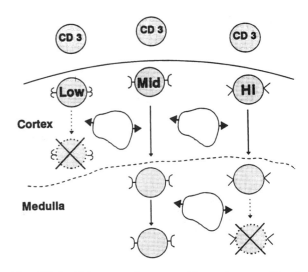

Fig. 35-1. Schematic of one possible mechanism of T cell development in the thymus. Early CD3+ prothymocytes enter the thymus and undergo gene rearrangement of the T-cell receptor genes. During early development in the cortex, cells require positive signaling to survive. In the absence of positive signaling, cells with low affinity for major histocompatibility complex (MHC) antigens (left) undergo apoptosis (dotted cell outline). Later in thymic development, cells with strong interaction with MHC (right) undergo apoptosis as a means of deleting self-reactive clones. Cells with midrange affinity for self-MHC survive as MHC-restricted T cells.

transplantation. Exactly this outcome has been observed in the animal models described below.

Two different experimental systems have been used to demonstrate induction of central transplantation tolerance. In the 1980s, central tolerance was investigated using an experimental model of mixed bone marrow chimeras in which the animal is given a lethal dose of total body irradiation and then infused with a mixture of donor and recipient bone marrow cells. The animals repopulate their thymus glands with both donor and recipient cells and appear to develop central tolerance toward the donor MHC.[8] More recently, a direct demonstration of central tolerance has been demonstrated by injecting donor cells into recipient thymus glands.[9] The original model injected pancreatic islet cells in a rodent model.[10] Within the injected thymus, developing T cells whose TCR reacts strongly with donor MHC undergo clonal deletion. The thymic injection model has been extended to injection of donor spleen cells, marrow cells, and kidney cells.[11–14]

Peripheral Anergy

Peripheral anergy refers to the induction of tolerance outside the thymus. There are a number of mechanisms by which an individual might become nonreactive (anergic) as a result of nonthymic immune forces. For humoral immunity, the development of anti-idiotypes is likely to play an important role in the disappearance of anti-human leukocyte antigen (HLA) antibodies. Detectable anti-HLA antibody results from the clonal expansion and immunoglobulin secretion of B cells committed to the production of the antibody. As the titer of antibody rises, the new antibody itself may be seen in some instances as a new antigen. Although the constant region, hinge region, and light chain region of the new antibody would not represent new protein, the hypervariable tip at the Fab combining site might be regarded as unique. Other B cells that recognize this new protein as foreign will produce an antibody (termed an anti-idiotype or Ab2) directed against the hypervariable region of the original antibody (Ab1). Because Ab2 recognizes and attaches directly to the combining site on Ab1, many Ab2 antibodies are capable of neutralizing the action of Ab1. To the extent that Ab2 antibodies bind to surface immunoglobulin on the B cells secreting Ab1, the Ab2 antibodies may also promote destruction of the Ab1 B cell clones.

Peripheral anergy may also develop for T cells. Among the many proposed mechanisms for peripheral anergy, two are under current active investigation—second signal anergy and the veto phenomenon. In order for allorecognition to occur, the responding T cell must bind via its TCR to the MHC-peptide complex on the target. This interaction is referred to as the first signal. Evidence has accumulated that allorecognition also requires interaction of other T cell structures with the target, referred to as the second signal. Several ligand-receptor interactions are candidates for the second signal. These include CD80/CD28 (B7/BB1), LFA-1/ICAM-1, and CD2/LFA-3. Blocking the second signal prevents an adequate T cell response. Studies have suggested that stimulation of the TCR by antigen (first signal) in the absence of a second signal can induce nonresponsiveness of that T cell to future encounters with

the antigen.[15–18] Because foreign antigens are presented by CD80 positive antigen presenting cells, whereas most self-tissue does not express CD80, this has been proposed as one mechanism underlying the development of peripheral anergy to self. Blockade of the second signal might be used to induce peripheral anergy to allografts. For example, investigators have been able to induce peripheral tolerance in animal cardiac or xenograft models by blocking CD80/CD28 interaction via infusion of a soluble form of an alternative ligand for CD80, known as CTLA-4.[19,20] Peripheral tolerance has also been induced by blockade of other second-signal ligands.[2] Physical damage to second-signal cell surface molecules may underlie the mechanism by which ultraviolet B light appears to block alloantigenicity in both transplantation and transfusion experiments.

A second mechanism of peripheral T cell anergy relies on the veto phenomenon. Within the thymus, central tolerance results when cells are eliminated if they react strongly with self-MHC. A similar process directed against mature circulating T cells is suggested by the veto hypothesis.[21,22] A veto cell is a functional designation assigned to a cell that induces inactivation of T-cytotoxic cells that recognize it ("recognize me and you die"). Under normal circumstances, veto cells may play a backup role to the thymus to inactivate autoimmune T cells that have escaped clonal deletion in the thymus. Because of the normal involution of the thymus with aging, it is possible that veto cells play a greater role in prevention of autoreactive T cells among adults compared with children. The concept of veto-cell activity is of direct relevance to transplantation tolerance. If veto cells of donor origin can be allowed to circulate in the recipient, they may be able to induce peripheral anergy toward donor MHC. Preliminary experimental evidence in animals has suggested that veto cell activity mediated by donor cells is detectable and can account for donor-specific tolerance and allograft survival. For example, Thomas et al. have studied veto cell activity in a rhesus monkey model.[23] Animals received kidney transplants from mixed lymphocyte culture strongly reactive donors. Recipient animals were first made lymphopenic by infusion of rabbit antimonkey thymocyte globulin. After this conditioning, recipient animals were infused with donor bone marrow containing veto cells prior to renal transplantation. No further immunosuppression was given. Animals so treated displayed prolonged allograft survival (20 percent allograft survival for 1 year after transplantation) compared with animals treated with antimonkey thymocyte globulin alone (0 percent allograft survival at 1 year). Recipient animals treated with veto cells developed a decrease in in vitro measured T-cytotoxic precursors directed at donor antigen but not at third-party antigens (donor-specific nonresponsiveness). In vitro veto cell activity was demonstrated using a three-cell coculture system in which veto cells were shown to decrease recipient T cell lysing of donor target cells. This in vitro veto activity required cell-to-cell contact and was removed if the veto cells were separated from the T-cytotoxic cells by a semipermeable membrane. Ultraviolet B or γ-irradiation of the donor marrow prevented the demonstration of the veto cell effect and resulted in poor allograft survival.

Pharmacologic Immunosuppression

The last decade has witnessed tremendous progress in the understanding and application of pharmacologic immunosuppression for the maintenance of solid allograft survival. The use of cyclosporine A (CyA) beginning in the 1980s and the development of FK-506 and rapamycin have been the foundation of this approach. Unlike the more donor-specific mechanism of central tolerance and peripheral anergy, pharmacologic immunosuppression is nonspecific, placing recipients at increased risk of infection.

The mechanism of action of CyA, FK-506, and rapamycin has been under intense experimental investigation.[24,25] Cyclosporine and FK-506 are taken up by all cells within the body, including erythrocytes. Although these agents have been shown experimentally to affect B cell and macrophage function, the predominant action is directed against T cells. The drugs interrupt intermediate steps between signal transduction of the T cell receptor and transcriptional activation of the interleukin 2 (IL-2) gene. Signal transduction of the T cell receptor results in activation of membrane-associated phospholipases, which results in a rise in intracellular Ca^{++}. This in turn activates Ca^{++}-dependent kinases and phosphatases, which serve as intermediate steps toward production of nuclear transcription factors that initiate IL-2 gene transcription. Once inside T lympho-

cytes, CyA, FK-506, and rapamycin bind to a family of cytosolic proteins that include the cyclophilins and FK binding protein. The drug–protein complex exhibits activity not found in either alone. This complex is capable of binding calcineurin, a calcium-calmodulin–dependent protein phosphatase. Binding to calcineurin disrupts the action of this phosphatase, thereby interrupting a principal intermediate step of IL-2 gene activation.[25] In vitro observations of IL-2 down-regulation by these agents have shown that alternate pathways of T cell activation exist. For example, stimulation of T cells by phorbol esters plus anti-CD28 is not sensitive to inhibition by CyA or FK-506.[26] Such observations highlight the complexity of T cell signal–response coupling and suggest a mechanism by which these potent immunosuppressive agents can blunt but not completely destroy host immunity.

IMMUNOMODULATORY EFFECT OF ALLOGENEIC TRANSFUSION

The most commonly recognized immune response to allogeneic transfusion is immune stimulation and the development of an alloimmune response. However, it has been postulated for decades that under some circumstances allogeneic transfusion may result in a immunosuppressive effect. In the setting of organ transplantation, this effect might serve to condition the recipient for subsequent allograft acceptance.

Evidence for a tolerogenic effect of transfusion was widely recognized after the publications by Opelz et al. that reported that pretransplantation blood transfusion conferred benefit on subsequent renal allograft survival.[27,28] They observed the renal allograft survival had declined with the switch from unmodified blood components to frozen deglycerolized blood. Pretransplantation transfusion of unmodified red blood cells (RBCs) resulted in a dose-dependent improvement in renal allograft survival.[29] Pretransplantation transfusions were not always beneficial, however. Some patients became sensitized to HLA alloantigens, reducing the number of available crossmatch-compatible kidney donors. Although occasional reports suggested a benefit even if transfusion were given perioperatively, most studies found the transfusion effect was maximal if the transfusions were given weeks to months prior to transplantation.[30]

Initially, it was believed that pretransplantation transfusions were little more than a means to "weed out" immunologic responders and identify nonresponders. This was referred to as the selection hypothesis. Because individuals who were able to make HLA antibodies would do so in response to transfusions and because pretransplantation crossmatching eliminates patients who have formed class I antibodies against the donor, immunologic responders would be less likely to be accepted for transplantation. However, it was found that even among patients who did not form HLA antibodies, transfused individuals maintained allograft acceptance better than nontransfused patients.

For patients awaiting kidney transplantation from living related donors, it was found that pretransplantation transfusions were most effective if the future kidney donor was also used as a blood donor—a technique termed *donor-specific transfusions* (DSTs). DSTs were usually administered as three fresh-blood transfusions (200 ml whole blood) given at 1- to 3-week intervals. Approximately 30 percent of recipients became alloimmunized to HLA antigens of the DST donor, which often resulted in elimination of that person as a kidney donor. Because of this serious down side, some DST programs administered oral immunosuppressives to the patient in order to decrease alloimmunization during the period of DSTs. Using this approach, DSTs proved even more successful than random transfusion for the induction of allograft tolerance.[31]

Three changes in the clinical care of transplantation patients contributed to a decreased use of deliberate random pretransplantation blood transfusions. First, with the advent of cyclosporine and FK-506, the beneficial effect of pretransplantation blood transfusions became increasingly more difficult to demonstrate.[32] Because transfusion added little to the excellent allograft survival achieved by modern immunosuppressives, there was little advantage to offset the potential for HLA sensitization.[33] Second, the heightened awareness of the infectious complications of transfusion resulted in a more conservative transfusion policy in general. Third, the nearly universal application of recombinant erythropoietin for the treatment of the anemia associated with end-stage renal disease significantly reduced the need for RBC transfusions among patients on dialysis. Deliberate pretransplantation transfusion protocols that use donor-specific transfusions are still in use in some centers.

In addition to the effect of pretransplantation blood transfusions on allograft survival, it has been suggested that transfusions result in an increased rate of postoperative bacterial infections among surgical patients and an increased risk of tumor recurrence among patients who have undergone surgical resection of a primary malignancy (see Ch. 4).[34] Thus, exploration of the transfusion effect remains an area of active clinical and biologic investigation. A very large body of experimental work has been done to investigate the mechanism underlying the transfusion effect in transplantation.[35] The observed immunosuppressive effects of transfusion may be attributed to more than one mechanism.

Early Hypotheses for the Transfusion Effect

A theory of clonal deletion was proposed by Terasaki.[36] He reasoned that patients undergoing transfusion would in fact be stimulated to undergo primary alloimmunization to MHC antigens presented at the time of transfusion. At the time of the transplantation, recipient immune cells would undergo a secondary immune reaction to the MHC antigens on the transplanted kidney. This burst of secondary clonal response would occur in the immediate postoperative period just at the time when the highest doses of clonally deleting immunosuppressive medicines (azathioprine and prednisone) were being given. In contrast, nontransfused patients would have not had previous exposure to the MHC antigens of the kidney donor. Therefore, in the immediate postoperative period, nontransfused patients underwent a slower primary immune response with less rapid clonal expansion and correspondingly less susceptibility to the effects of azathioprine and prednisone. The clonal deletion model fit extremely well with the observed success of DSTs and also was consistent with a transfusion effect that was more pronounced during the azathioprine and prednisone era, compared with the cyclosporine era. However, the hypothesis was difficult to substantiate experimentally and did not account for the immunosuppressive effect of transfusion observed among individuals who were not given immunosuppressive medication.

T-suppressor cells induced by transfusion have been the subject of much experimental investigation. Leivestad and Thorsby studied one-way mixed lymphocyte reactions (MLRs) between transfusion recipient and donor before and after a series of pretransplantation DSTs.[37] Pretransfusion recipient cells responded strongly to donor stimulation. After transfusion, however, there was marked suppression of the MLR response to donor cells but not to third-party stimulators. Of interest, using a three-cell MLR, the investigators showed that the pretransfusion MLR response to donor cells could be decreased by the presence of post-transfusion recipient cells. The results of this and other studies[38] were interpreted to indicate the presence of T-suppressor cells in the post-transfusion blood. Other attempts to conclusively demonstrate T-suppressor cells as a result of transfusion have yielded conflicting results. An important difference among these studies may result from the HLA similarity between blood donor and recipient. In the report by Leivestad et al., donor and recipient were one-haplotype matched.

The production of anti-idiotypes (Ab2) acting as HLA-blocking antibodies was demonstrated by Reed et al.,[39] who used a relatively simple laboratory assay for Ab2 in which serums of recipients who had formed anti-HLA antibodies (Ab1) in response to transfusion were saved. After at least 6 months, each recipient's serum was tested for its ability to inhibit reactivity between the Ab1 serum and donor target lymphocytes. The inhibitory activity of the Ab2 serum localized to the immunoglobulin fraction and was donor-antigen specific. In a retrospective analysis of renal transplant recipients, they reported that 9 of 10 patients with allograft survival longer than 1 year had detectable Ab2, whereas Ab2 were found in none of 10 patients whose bodies rejected transplants within 1 month.[39]

Recipient Exposure to Allogeneic Donor Leukocytes and the Transfusion Effect

The original observation of the transfusion effect occurred during the change from unmodified blood to frozen blood prior to kidney transplantation. This change represented not only leukocyte depletion but also plasma removal. Most subsequent studies of the immunomodulatory effect of transfusion have focused attention on donor leukocytes. A large number of different animal models have used purified suspensions of donor mononuclear cells to induce transfusion effects. Human studies have demonstrated pretransplantation tolerance by transfusion of buffy coat,[40,41] absence of increased cancer recurrence by transfusion of buffy coat–depleted plasma–containing components,[42] and correlation of postoperative infection with the presence or absence of donor leukocytes.[43]

However, recipient exposure to a factor present in the plasma of blood components has also been suggested as the cause of the transfusion effect. Interest in a plasma-based effect was increased by the observation in retrospective studies of tumor recurrence that transfusion of whole blood or plasma-containing components appeared to be more highly correlated with tumor recurrence than transfusion of RBC concentrates.[35] One nonrandomized study found lower levels of skin test response among individuals transfused with whole blood, compared to those transfused with additive solution blood.[44] No completely cohesive mechanism by which plasma factors would induce immunosuppression has been studied. Candidate factors responsible for recipient immunomodulation include soluble histocompatibility antigens, immune complexes, and release of prostaglandins.[35,45]

HLA Similarity Between Donor and Recipient and the Transfusion Effect

Animal and human studies suggest that the transfusion effect occurs when the donor-recipient pair share some degree of HLA similarity. Both Quigley et al.[46] (rodent model) and Leivestad and Thorsby[37] (human DST model) showed transfusion-induced decline in MLRs, provided that donor and recipient were a one-haplotype HLA match. Lagaaij et al. observed improved allograft survival among individuals transfused with blood from unrelated donors provided that the donor-recipient pair shared one HLA-DR antigen.[47] van Twuyer et al. studied 23 patients given deliberate transfusions prior to renal transplant. T cell anergy toward donor cells developed in 10 of 23 patients. Anergy developed only if the blood donor and recipient were a one HLA haplotype match or if they shared one HLA-B plus one HLA-DR antigen.[48]

Recent Theories of the Transfusion Effect

Two recent proposed mechanisms for the transfusion effect involve regulation of natural killer (NK) cell function and the development of mononuclear microchimerism. Downregulation of NK cells has been proposed as a consequence of transfusion. Abnormalities in NK cell function among heavily transfused individuals have been recognized for some time. However, these changes may have reflected the influence of iron overload or transfusion-acquired chronic viral infection. An acute decline in NK cell function directly attributable to transfusion was reported by Jensen et al.[43] In their randomized clinical trial, patients transfused with leukodepleted allogeneic blood developed a transient decline in NK cell activity at the time of surgery that quickly returned to preoperative baseline levels. This pattern of NK function was also seen in untransfused controls. In contrast, among patients randomized to receive unmodified allogeneic transfusions, a more persistent decline in in vitro NK cell activity was observed. Because the transfusion effect has been implicated in host immune functions ranging from allograft rejection to resistance to postoperative infection and tumor recurrence, NK cells are an intellectually appealing target of investigation for the transfusion effect.

Recently, the development of donor mononuclear cell microchimerism as been documented after solid organ transplantation. Starzl et al.[49,50] and others[51] have examined a variety of recipient tissues, including blood, lymph node, skin, heart, and liver, for the presence of donor cells. Using polymerase chain reaction (PCR) to amplify genes of organ donor origin and immunohistochemistry to stain for antigens of donor origin, they have demonstrated persistence of donor mononuclear cells for several years after transplantation. According to Starzl, patients who demonstrate microchimerism also demonstrate tolerance toward the allograft and require lower doses of pharmacologic immunosuppression. The development of transient donor leukocyte microchimerism following transfusion is consistent with a number of observations of the transfusion effect.[52,53] These include the importance of leukocyte expo-

sure, the need for HLA similarity between donor and recipient, the experimental observation in animals of the correlation between tolerance and microchimerism, and the use of donor stem cell infusions in both animals[23] and humans[54] as a means to achieve microchimerism and tolerance. Whether transient mononuclear microchimerism among HLA-similar blood donor-recipient pairs will be shown to contribute to immunomodulation by transfusion awaits further research.

PREVENTION OF HLA SENSITIZATION BY LEUKOCYTE DEPLETION OF BLOOD COMPONENTS

Numerous studies of oncology patients have demonstrated that the use of leukodepleted cellular components can decrease the incidence of primary HLA sensitization. Leukodepletion is unlikely to prevent an anamnestic alloimmune response among previously sensitized individuals. The utility of leukodepletion filters has not been documented by clinical trials in patients awaiting renal transplantation. However, a nonrandomized trial by Fisher et al. suggested that leukodepleted blood might be expected to decrease the incidence of HLA alloimmunization.[55] Because the development of HLA class I alloantibodies reactive in a warm T cell crossmatch decreases the available donor pool for renal transplantation patients, strategies designed to limit HLA alloimmunization through the use of erythropoietin and leukodepleted blood are rational. Because the immunomodulatory effect of pretransplantation transfusions probably depends upon recipient exposure to allogeneic leukocytes, the potential benefit of leukodepleted blood for prevention of sensitization needs to be weighed against the loss of this immunologic effect. Some programs also provide leukodepleted blood for renal transplantation patients during the intraoperative and postoperative periods in order to prevent primary alloimmunization to HLA should a subsequent renal transplantation be needed.

CMV INFECTION AND DISEASE IN SOLID ORGAN ALLOGRAFT RECIPIENTS

Primary cytomegalovirus (CMV) infection and reactivation infection are important potential complications for all transplantation patients. Although the morbidity and mortality associated with CMV among solid organ transplant recipients is not as severe as in allogeneic bone marrow transplant recipients,[56] CMV still represents a common serious infectious complication of solid organ transplantation. A clinical distinction is drawn between CMV infection and disease. CMV infection is defined by laboratory evidence of viral infection, whereas CMV disease refers to symptomatic infection.

In addition to the direct morbidity resulting from CMV disease, concern has existed for years that CMV infection is associated with dysfunction of the allograft. The allograft is the most common site of recognized disease when recipients of kidney, liver,[56,57] or heart transplants[58] develop primary or reactivation CMV. In the setting of allograft dysfunction, rejection versus CMV infection is a differential diagnosis common to all three solid organ transplants. Glomerulopathy,[59] vanishing bile duct syndrome,[60] accelerated atherosclerosis,[61] and obliterative bronchiolitis have been proposed to occur in renal, hepatic, cardiac, and lung allografts, respectively, as a result of CMV infection. However, despite repeated attempts to document a direct causal role between CMV infection and allograft dysfunction, the connection remains unproven. One possible common link may be that local cytokine elaboration resulting from host immune response to the allograft fosters viral activation and replication in endothelial cells, thereby promoting a vasculopathy.[62,63]

Numerous studies have documented that the dominant factors controlling the development of CMV after transplantation are the serologic status of the organ donor and recipient and the degree of immunosuppression given to the recipient.[56,58,64–66] Table 35-1 shows the general incidence of CMV infection and CMV disease among kidney, heart, or liver recipients as a function of the serostatus of the donor-recipient pair. Patients at greatest risk are CMV-seronegative recipients (no immunologic protection) who receive organs from CMV-seropositive donors. In contrast, infection rates are far lower among CMV-seronegative recipients of CMV-seronegative organs. These two categories of patients document that the infectiousness of unmodified cellular blood components is far less than that of the organ allograft.

Use of CMV-Safe Blood Components in Solid Organ Transplantation

Although no randomized trials exist to document the clinical outcomes of solid organ transplantation patients who are supported with leukodepleted blood compared with CMV-seronegative blood, either product would be expected to be highly effective in preventing transfusion-transmitted CMV infection (see Ch. 39). In this chapter, these products are referred to as CMV-safe components.

Recipient CMV-Seronegative and Donor CMV-Seronegative

The risk for acquiring CMV infection from blood transfusion is highest when both donor and recipient are CMV-seronegative. Patients in this setting derive the greatest benefit from the use of CMV-safe blood components. For transplantations requiring low volumes of transfusion, it is reasonable to provide exclusively CMV-safe components. Because liver transplantation patients often require massive transfusion support, a rational strategy is to reserve a number of CMV-safe units for initial blood support (e.g., 20 units) and then transfuse blood without regard to

Table 35-1. Estimates of the Incidence of CMV Infection and CMV Disease Among Different Categories of Solid Organ Allograft Patients

CMV Serostatus	Kidney[65,69]		Liver[56,64]		Heart[58]	
	Infection	Disease	Infection	Disease	Infection	Disease
Recipient negative, donor negative	0–10%	<1%	0–20%	10–20%	20–25%	5–15%
Recipient negative, donor positive	70–90%	50–70%	75–90%	60–80%	80–85%	25–40%
Recipient positive, donor negative	25–55%	0–40%	50–70%	10–30%	40–50%	10–30%
Recipient positive, donor positive	50–80%	20–40%	65–100%	25–55%	60–100%	20–40%

CMV reactivity for patients whose transfusion needs are greater.[56]

One liver transplantation program found that the intraoperative RBC transfusion requirement did not have a significant impact on the incidence of CMV disease. The mean ($\pm$ SD) intraoperative packed RBC transfusion requirement in adults and children was 15.0 $\pm$ 12.8 and 3.7 $\pm$ 3.1 units, respectively. Massive transfusions ($>$ 20 units in adults, $>$ 5 units in children) did not place patients at a higher risk of developing CMV disease (P = .20).[56]

Although the use of CMV-safe blood products might be expected to be a critical consideration when both the patient and the donor are seronegative, one study has demonstrated that the deliberate use of CMV-untested, nonleukodepleted blood in CMV-seronegative patients receiving a CMV-seronegative liver allograft resulted in only a 10 percent incidence of CMV disease, with no deaths attributed to CMV (unpublished data, Deaconess Hospital, Boston). This finding is consistent with the fact that, in contrast to transfusion of blood from donors who are positive for anti-human immunodeficiency virus, anti-human T cell leukemia virus I/II, HB$_s$Ag, or anti-Hepatitis C virus (HCV), there is a low rate of CMV transmission by blood transfusion even with transfusion of CMV-seropositive blood. Preiksaitis et al.[67] have estimated that the risk of CMV transmission is 0.38 percent of seropositive cellular blood products transfused, and Bowden[68] has pointed out that bone marrow transplantation patients who are transfused with 80 to 100 units of unscreened blood may remain seronegative and without any evidence of infection.

Recipient CMV-Seronegative and Donor CMV-Seropositive

CMV-seronegative patients who receive CMV-seropositive donor organs are at the greatest risk of CMV disease and acquire their infection chiefly from the allograft itself (Table 35-1). Because CMV is a latent virus, it is not surprising that continued survival of the allograft in an immunosuppressed host would result in a high frequency of CMV infection. Studies in different solid organ settings have suggested that infection of the seronegative patient by the seropositive donor organ leads to more severe clinical infection than reactivation infection.[58,64,69] Although some authors have suggested that CMV-negative recipients be restricted to CMV-negative donor organs

("protective organ matching"), the scarcity of solid organs suitable for transplantation has limited the application of this approach. The use of CMV-safe blood components in this category of patients is of little or no utility. Patients susceptible to the more limited burden of virus provided by blood are also susceptible to the presumably greater burden of virus provided by the allograft. There is no clinical evidence that the subset of recipients who fail to acquire CMV disease from the CMV-positive allograft would be susceptible to infection and disease from blood components. Using DNA typing of CMV strains, one could collect data on the actual incidence of transfusion-transmitted CMV in this category. Until such data become available, the use of CMV-safe blood components for this category of patients should not be regarded as standard care.

Recipient CMV-Seropositive and Donor CMV-Seronegative

CMV-seropositive patients who receive CMV-seronegative donor organs are principally subject to disease resulting from reactivation of endogenous infection. The development of reactivation infection depends primarily on the degree of host immunosuppression required for maintenance of the allograft. Some immunosuppressive regimens appear to be more likely to allow CMV reactivation than others. For example, immunosuppression protocols involving antilymphocyte globulin, antithymocyte globulin, or OKT3 have been shown to have the greatest incidence of reactivation disease.[56,65] Although the degree of host immunosuppression dominates the risk of reactivation, other factors may possibly play a role. Among these is the presence of allogeneic tissue, which, by stimulating activation of the host immune system, might also stimulate CMV to move from latency to active replication. Although a theoretic role for leukodepletion exists to prevent activation of host-infected cells by allogeneic donor leukocytes, organ allograft patients have a much larger and more persistent allogeneic stimulus represented by the allograft itself. Thus, the role of blood donor leukocytes in promoting reactivation of latent host CMV infection is currently unsubstantiated.

In theory, patients in this category may also acquire second-strain primary infection from transfused blood. However, no studies have demonstrated second-strain infection resulting from blood components. Because patients in this category have some preformed immunity to CMV, it is possible that the viral burden presented by transfusion is insufficient to result in second-strain infection except in rare instances of intense preoperative host immunosuppression. Currently, the theoretic risk of second-strain CMV infection transmitted by blood components among solid organ allograft patients is not sufficient to merit the use of CMV-safe blood.

Recipient CMV-Seropositive and Donor CMV-Seropositive

CMV-seropositive patients who receive CMV-seropositive donor organs can both develop reactivation CMV disease and acquire second-strain infection from the allograft. Although it might be expected that these patients would have the highest incidence of CMV disease, the data (Table 35-1) demonstrate this is not the case, presumably as a result of some degree of host preformed immunity. Second-strain infections can be documented by DNA typing of PCR-amplified CMV genomic material obtained from the host. The nucleic acid sequence of the newly acquired strain (not present preoperatively) can then be matched to the donor source. This approach has been used to document second-strain CMV infections resulting from the allograft.[69–71] The frequency of second-strain infections of graft origin is not known, but at least one study has estimated that second-strain infection from the allograft is more common than reactivation of host infection.[69] The potentially higher incidence of second-strain infection may have an immune basis. Recipient humoral immunity may not neutralize the particular CMV strain of the donor. Recipient cell-mediated immunity may be less effective against donor second-strain virus owing to the lack of MHC restriction between recipient T-cytotoxic cells and donor tissue. Finally, cytokine activation as part of rejection may provoke local release of donor strain virus. Because of the presence of CMV in both the donor and recipient and the lack of evidence of second-strain infection resulting from transfusion, the use of CMV-safe blood components is not currently indicated.

TRANSFUSION SUPPORT OF LIVER TRANSPLANTATION

Of all solid organ transplantations, orthotopic liver transplantation (OLT) has placed the greatest demands on clinical transfusion services. In the early to mid-1980s, patients undergoing OLT frequently required very large quantities of transfusion support. Although blood use steadily declined with the refinement of surgical technique during the last decade,[72] OLT still frequently demands transfusion equal to one blood volume (massive transfusion) and occasionally demands blood support equal to five or more blood volumes of the patient (ultramassive transfusion). The intraoperative RBC transfusions required for adult liver transplantations at our hospital during the last decade are shown in Figure 35-2. These data demonstrate three common findings in other programs: a decline in median blood use per operation during the 1980s, the plateau that has been reached, and the continued occurrence of massive transfusion. Because the transfusion needs during hepatic transplantation are unpredictable, transfusion services must remain prepared to effectively deliver massive transfusion support.[73–75] Lessons learned in the care of liver transplant patients have immediate application to other adult patients requiring massive blood transfusion.[76–78]

Liver transplant surgery is divided into three phases: (1) the recipient hepatectomy, (2) the anhepatic phase, and (3) the postreperfusion phase. During phase 1, the patient's diseased liver and its vessels are dissected free, and surgical tapes are placed around four major vessels: the inferior vena cava above the liver, the inferior vena cava below the liver, the portal vein, and the hepatic artery. The donor liver is prepared for implantation. An extracorporeal, nonanticoagulated veno-venous bypass circuit is often used to provide venous return to the heart and is usually instituted at the end of phase 1. This circuit drains venous blood from the portal circulation and from one of the femoral veins, passes the blood through a pump, and returns the blood into the axillary vein while the inferior vena cava is clamped. The anhepatic phase begins with the clamping of the four vessels that isolate the liver: the inferior vena cava above and below the liver, the portal vein, and the hepatic artery. The vessels are cut and the patient's liver is removed. Any residual air and preservative solution is flushed out of the donor liver and it is inserted into the patient by connecting the donor-recipient inferior vena cava above and below the donor liver, and then connecting the donor-recipient portal vein. Opening the clamps of

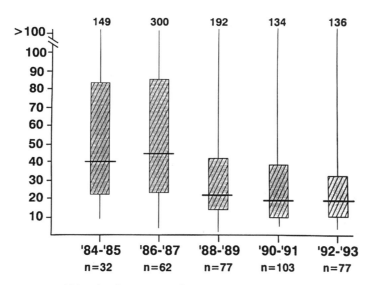

Fig. 35-2. Intraoperative red blood cell (RBC) use from 1983 to 1993 for 351 adult liver transplantation, Deaconess Hospital, Boston. The number of units (both banked RBCs and salvaged RBCs) is shown on the y axis. The range is represented by the vertical line, the box encompasses the middle two quartiles of RBC use, and the central horizontal bar is the median.

these major vessels is referred to as reperfusion and is a particularly dangerous moment in the procedure when hemodynamic, metabolic, and hemostatic abnormalities can arise. After reperfusion the veno-venous bypass circuit is removed. The third phase of surgery involves creating the hepatic arterial anastamosis, preparing a form of biliary drainage for the new liver, obtaining good surgical hemostasis, and closing.

Causes of Excessive Blood Loss

Technical skill, experience, and judgment are required by surgeons performing liver transplantation and are reflected in the blood requirements for this procedure. Improvements in preoperative preparation under evaluation include preoperative magnetic resonance imaging, the use of distal-splenorenal shunts, and transjugular intraportal shunts instead of protocaval shunts. Intraoperative techniques include the use of veno-venous bypass, use of argon-directed photocoagulation, and preparation of the graft arterial supply before the recipient hepatectomy. Although the skills of the surgeon are of paramount importance, proper patient selection, skilled anesthesia practice, recognition and treat-

ment of the unique coagulopathy of OLT, and prevention of dilution coagulopathy are also important contributors to clinical success.

The selection of patients and the timing of surgery during the course of their liver disease play dominant roles in the incidence of disastrous operations that consume large quantities of blood components. During periods of high demand, less suitable cadaver donors may be tried and long waiting lists may result in deterioration of the patient's clinical status. As a result, patients may not always have surgery at the optimum time in the course of their disease.

OLT is associated with several hemostatic defects that contribute to the risk of massive blood loss. These result from both the preexisting coagulopathy of terminal liver disease and the unique coagulopathy that accompanies some liver transplantations. Patients with advanced liver disease may suffer from one or more of the hemostatic defects listed in Table 35-2. Although the preoperative prothrombin time (PT), partial thromboplastin time (PTT), fibrinogen, D-dimer, and platelet count serve as rough guides to the severity of liver disease, these tests cannot be relied upon to predict the expected blood requirements during surgery.[79]

Table 35-2. Preoperative Hemostatic Defects in Patients Awaiting Liver Transplantation

Poor nutritional state with friable vessels

Large collateral veins due to portal hypertension

Thrombocytopenia due to splenomegaly

Platelet dysfunction (drugs, circulating fibrin degradation products)

Decreased synthesis of coagulation factors in liver

Decreased γ-carboxylation of factors II, VII, IX, and X

Dysfibrinogenemia

Increased levels of fibrin(ogen) breakdown products due to decreased hepatic clearance

Low-grade fibrinolysis (decreased clearance of tissue plasminogen activator, decreased synthesis of antiplasmin)

Disordered thrombin regulation (decreased AT-3)

During surgery, marked changes in coagulation can occur.[80] These may result from hemodilution, platelet consumption, disordered thrombin regulation, and fibrinolysis. Some patients develop an especially severe coagulopathy during the anhepatic and early postreperfusion phase of OLT. This coagulopathy is characterized by a burst of fibrinolysis, which results in excessive lysis of previously formed clots in the surgical field, diffuse bleeding, and a rapid fall in fibrinogen and rise in PT and PTT. The fibrinolysis appears to be mediated by the combination of a sudden release of tissue plasminogen activator (tPA) and the inability of the absent liver to clear tPA from the bloodstream[81,82] (Fig. 35-3). More research is needed to understand the triggers for the release of tPA. Once fibrinolysis has begun, infusions of fresh frozen plasma (FFP) are often ineffective and may simply represent a source of exogenous plasminogen substrate for the excess tPA. Antifibrinolytic therapy with ε-aminocaproic acid (Amicar)[83] or with aprotinin (Trasylol)[84] is the most effective therapy for this coagulopathy. Failure to recognize and promptly treat fibrinolysis during OLT can result in dramatic and excessive blood use.

Dilution coagulopathy can occur in any patient receiving massive transfusion, but it is easily avoided with proper laboratory monitoring and if the blood component resuscitation mixture provides a sufficient quantity of coagulation factors and platelets.[85] As long as an agreed-upon clinical protocol (see below) is used, dilution coagulopathy should not occur except during unusual blood shortages or in patients with platelet refractoriness. I believe it is much easier to prevent dilution coagulopathy than it is to recover from it.

Considerations of ABO and Rhesus Factor

Except in emergencies, donor livers are ABO-compatible with the recipient. ABO-identical RBCs and FFP are generally used for transfusion support for group O and group A recipients. Group B recipients who need large quantities of RBCs are switched to group O packed RBCs. Group AB recipients receiving massive transfusion are usually switched to group A packed RBCs to conserve group O RBCs for other patients. If a sufficient quantity of AB FFP is not expected to be available, early use of group A RBCs and then a switch to group A FFP is appropriate. As a general rule in massive transfusion, first switch RBCs and then switch FFP, reversing the order when returning to the patient's original blood group. The more desperate use of group A RBCs for group O patients during extreme shortages of group O blood has been described.[86]

The recipient of an ABO-compatible but not ABO-matched liver transplant deserves special consideration for RBC support. Transplantation of ABO-compatible unmatched grafts is common and occurred in 20 percent of group B and 50 percent of group AB recipients in our program during the 1980s. Such patients may develop postoperative hemolysis due to the production of ABO antibodies by lymphocytes of donor origin.[87] In a large series, Ramsey found a 40 percent incidence of donor-derived ABO antibodies and a 30 percent incidence of passenger lymphocyte hemolysis.[87] Either recipient RBCs or transfused RBCs or both may be hemolyzed by the passenger lymphocyte antibodies. Although passenger lymphocyte hemolysis may occur in any ABO-compatible unmatched combination, significant hemolysis is usually restricted to the group A_1 recipient of a group O liver.[87,88] For this particular combination, three possible strategies for the use of group O RBCs are possible: (1) transfusing exclusively group A RBCs and switching to group O RBCs if the postoperative direct antiglobulin test results become positive and/or if clinical hemolysis occurs; (2) transfusing group A RBCs at the beginning of surgery and switching to group O cells for the final third

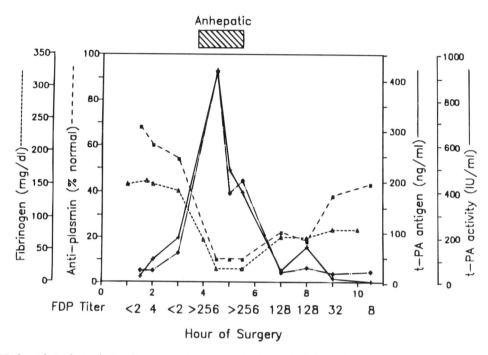

Fig. 35-3. Fibrinolysis during liver transplantation. At the end of the anhepatic phase and during the early reperfusion phase of surgery, tissue plasminogen activator (tPA) is released and poorly cleared by the liver. The resulting fibrinolysis consumes fibrinogen and free antiplasmin, and releases fibrin degradation products (FDP). A dramatic coagulopathy can ensue.

of surgery and for the immediate postoperative period; or (3) transfusing exclusively group O RBCs from the beginning of surgery. Option three is considered too wasteful of group O resources and either of the other options is more appropriate.

Transfusion support of Rh-negative patients who lack anti-D is not standardized. Since successful pregnancy has occurred after liver transplantation, transfusionists in most programs would consider providing a limited number of D-negative units to D-negative premenopausal females not expected to require large quantities of blood support. Should massive blood loss occur, the patients would then be switched intraoperatively to D-positive blood. Other programs offer a greater fixed amount of D-negative blood to all D-negative patients (without anti-D) in order not to sensitize them in case a second transplantation is required. However, perhaps because of postoperative immunosuppression, D-negative liver transplantation patients exposed to the D antigen appear not to form anti-D with the same frequency as

other D-negative patients.[89] Ramsey reported results for 19 D-negative liver, heart, and heart-lung transplant recipients who received 3 to 153 (median 10) units of D-positive RBCs during surgery and who were then tested for anti-D more than 2 months later. An anamnestic response to previous sensitization occurred in 3 patients. None of the other 16 patients made anti-D, including 13 who were tested more than 11 months after transplantation.[89] Some transplantation programs use D-positive blood for D-negative OLT patients without anti-D because of the frequent requirement for large-volume blood support, the low probability of anti-D plus pregnancy after liver transplantation, and the needs of other D-negative patients. In our program, D-negative males and postmenopausal D-negative women without anti-D are transfused exclusively with D-positive blood.. For premenopausal females without anti-D, 10 initial units of D-negative RBCs are reserved. If more than 10 units are required, we switch to D-positive blood. Once transfusion support has switched to D-positive RBCs, we do not switch back until the second or third postoperative day after all transfusion need has ceased.

Red Blood Cell Alloantibodies

Liver transplantation patients with clinically significant RBC alloantibodies can represent a special challenge to the blood bank.[90,91] Studies have shown that the prevalence of clinically significant RBC alloantibodies in the OLT patient population is reasonably high (14 percent).[91] Three different strategies can be used to provide compatible RBCs. First, a sufficient quantity of antigen-negative blood can be secured before surgery. This is the best approach and is most practical when dealing with antibodies to relatively low incidence antigens, such as anti-K_1. A second approach is to reserve a limited number of antigen-negative units for use at the beginning and end of surgery. This strategy can be used for patients with alloantibodies of midrange titer (e.g., < 1:16). Antigen-negative units (antihuman globulin [AHG]-compatible) are used in the beginning of surgery when the alloantibody is present. Depending on the initial titer, a repeat antibody screen obtained during surgery will be no longer reactive due to washout of the alloantibody after one or more blood volumes of transfusion. When the antibody screen becomes nonreactive, antigen-positive units (immediate spin-compatible) are used. At the very end of surgery, 6 to 8 antigen-negative units are transfused in order to prevent significant postoperative hemolysis. During the first postoperative week, additional antigen-negative units can be secured for support should delayed hemolysis occur. The third strategy is to use preoperative plasmapheresis to remove clinically significant low-titer alloantibodies, particularly if the antibody is directed against high-frequency antigens (e.g., anti-e, anti-s). We have successfully used all three of these approaches alone and in various combinations to support patients with single or multiple RBC alloantibodies.

Human Leukocyte Antigen Sensitization

Patients with high-titer, broadly reacting anti-HLA antibodies are usually refractory to random platelet transfusions during surgery. As a result, preoperative thrombocytopenia due to splenomegaly and intraoperative dilution thrombocytopenia may not be correctable by transfusion. As expected, studies have documented that patients refractory to platelet support (panel reactive antibodies > 70 percent) often require a considerably greater number of blood components during liver transplantation.[92] We identify such patients during our preoperative serologic workup. The surgeons and anesthesiologists are informed of patients with strongly reacting antibodies to a high percentage of panel lymphocytes. If thrombocytopenia develops during surgery, these patients are given a trial transfusion of 10 units of platelet concentrates with an immediate post-transfusion platelet count. If no increment is obtained, we withhold transfusion of platelet concentrates until the postreperfusion phase.

Intraoperative Transfusion Protocols

The use of both a laboratory protocol and a clinical transfusion protocol is required for the smooth delivery of massive transfusion support. The laboratory staff is an excellent source of ideas for streamlining the workload to a productive and efficient state. In our program, patients with a negative antibody screen are given immediate-spin crossmatch units from the beginning of surgery. Blood requisition slips are stamped with the patient's demographic information in advance. RBCs are crossmatched and tagged in batches of 10. A specific plan for anticipatory thawing of FFP and for pooling platelet concentrates is established. The blood bank physician or designate is responsible for the coordination of the blood support with the operating room (OR) during the operation. By frequent communication between OR and blood bank, this individual can match the demands of the case with the supply of the laboratory. For particularly difficult cases, the blood bank physician may intermittently visit the OR to assess the progress of the transplantation, the basic clinical status of the patient, the progression of laboratory monitoring, and the existing supply of components. The information is used to predict anticipated blood support. While in the OR, the blood bank physician and the anesthesiologist can teach each other a great deal about what each needs in order to deliver smooth and expert care. In the laboratory, the blood bank physician can directly communicate to the charge technologist the current status in the OR as well as the anticipated blood need, can assist the staff to speed accomplishment of their tasks, and can directly observe the functioning of the laboratory at peak workload to identify areas for improvement.

A clinical protocol for the delivery of blood support under massive transfusion conditions is an important way to deliver consistent care. Although the details of these protocols undoubtedly vary greatly from one institution to another, all include (1) an adequate mix of components, (2) guidance provided by periodic laboratory monitoring, and (3) the need for flexibility and good communication. The protocol used in our institution is shown in Table 35-3. This clinical protocol was established by consensus agreement among the transplant surgeons, the assistant chief of anesthesia, and the blood bank director. Several clinical scenarios common to my experience are described in the Appendix.

Intraoperative Coagulation Monitoring

The coagulation status of the patient can be monitored intraoperatively by the use of either traditional coagulation tests or the thromboelastogram. Our program uses the following traditional laboratory tests as a guide to component support: hematocrit, platelet count, PT, PTT, and fibrinogen. The hematocrit guides the mix of RBCs and crystalloid/colloid; the platelet count guides transfusion of platelet concentrates; the PT and PTT guide FFP use; and the fibrinogen guides the use of cryoprecipitate and antifibrinolytic agents.[93] Rapid turnaround of these five tests is of critical importance. Laboratory directors should take an active role in devising systems of rapid laboratory turnaround to assist in massive transfusion. In our hospital, rapid results depend on an intact chain of the following: a plentiful supply of the appropriate blood collection tubes and stamped requisitions near the anesthesiologist, a simple system for labeling specimen tubes, clear and assigned responsibilities for specimen transport to a stat laboratory located near the OR, a laboratory protocol for prioritization of massive transfusion samples arriving in the laboratory, the use of small-volume aliquots that permit rapid centrifugation of whole blood, redundant centrifuges, automated analyzers, a clear policy to "accept" abnormal results and report them, and electronic result reporting directly into the OR. We also consider it critically important that the serially obtained results of these tests be recorded on a flowsheet in the OR. The flowsheets

Table 35-3. One Clinical Protocol Used for Transfusion in Liver Transplantation[a]

RBCs, FFP, and crystalloid are given in the rapid transfusion device and in the intravenous lines according to the following mix: 2 units of RBCs (banked plus salvaged added) + 1 unit of FFP (200 ml) + 200 ml of crystalloid. This mixture will generate Hct > 30%, PT in the range of 14–18 seconds, and fibrinogen >100 mg/dL in most patients.

RBCs, FFP, and volume:
1. Each salvaged unit counts as a unit of RBCs.
2. Switch from crystalloid to a mixture of crystalloid and 5% albumin if the patient requires a cumulative total of 125 ml/kg crystalloid from all sources.
3. Avoid prolonged periods when blood recirculates in the rapid-transfusion device without transfusion. This increases the risk of bacterial overgrowth.
4. Toward the end of surgery, allow the blood reserve in the rapid-transfusion device to drain down and switch to transfusion via intravenous sets. This will prevent blood wastage.

FFP—increase or decrease the proportion of FFP added to the transfusion mix depending on the results of serial PT and PTT:
1. In the presence of active fibrinolysis and fibrinogen <70 mg/dl, the PT/PTT will overestimate the degree of hemodilution.
2. Mild to moderate prolongations of the PT need not be corrected. In the absence of active fibrinolysis or a surgical bleeder, an INR <2.5 is adequate.

Platelet concentrates:
1. The platelet count will halve from dilution with each blood volume transfused.
2. In nonrefractory patients, maintain platelet count >75,000/μl for patients without severe splenomegaly and >50,000 for those with splenomegaly.
3. For refractory patients, do not transfuse for numbers. Consult with blood bank physician.
4. There is no evidence for a benefit from DDAVP.

Cryoprecipitate and Amicar:
1. Most patients do not require cryoprecipitate.
2. For fibrinolysis (fibrinogen <100 mg/dl) with bleeding, give 5 g intravenous Amicar infusion. If lysis continues after 1 hour, reload Amicar and begin drip of 1 g/h.
   Transfuse 10 units cryoprecipitate. Consult with transplantation surgeon and blood bank physician.

Laboratory monitoring:
1. Check Hct, platelet count, PT, and fibrinogen at least hourly. Check half-hourly during periods of extreme bleeding.

[a] Adjust these guidelines according to the clinical situation.

Abbreviations: RBC, red blood cell; FFP, fresh frozen plasma; Hct, hematocrit; PT, prothrombin time; PTT, partial thromboplastin time; INR, international normalized ratio.

are an indispensable way to ensure the proper mix of components, tailor the clinical transfusion protocol to the case, and document the care. Blood component therapy is guided by the results of these laboratory tests as described in Table 35-3.

In the absence of rapid turnaround systems of coagulation monitoring, many liver transplantation programs have established coagulation monitoring within the OR via the use of the thromboelastogram.[94] The thromboelastogram coagulation analyzer (Haemoscope Corp., Morton Grove, IL) allows bedside monitoring of whole-blood coagulation. The device uses a stainless steel piston and cuvette. Whole blood is placed in the cuvette and maintained at 37°C. The cuvette oscillates through a 4-degree, 45-minute angle. As the blood coagulates, it entraps the piston and transfers the oscillation to the piston, which is attached to a recording device. The oscillatory tracings made over time by the torsion on the piston, produce the thromboelastograph. Several aspects of the time and width of the recorded tracings can be interpreted. The time to the initial oscillations (reaction time) and the time to maximum oscillations are considered to reflect the activity of coagulation factors, platelets, and fibrinogen. The maximum width of the tracing is said to reflect function of fibrinogen, platelets, and factor XIII. The slope of the increase in width of the oscillations represents the speed of coagulation and is affected by the quality of fibrinogen and platelets. Whole-blood fibrinolytic activity is measured by the time from maximum tracing width to zero oscillations and can be estimated by the decline in amplitude that occurs in the tracing during the first hour. Kang et al.[94] have found the thromboelastogram a useful guide to intraoperative blood therapy. For example, they transfuse 2 units of FFP when the reaction time is longer than 15 minutes, 10 units of platelets when the maximum amplitude is less than 40 mm, and 6 units of cryoprecipitate when the other treatments do not improve the tracing or when the slope of increase in tracing width is persistently less than 40 degrees.[94] Disadvantages of the thromboelastogram are its low specificity, lack of any standards or controls, and the long time required (1 hour) for complete interpretation.

Rapid-Infusion Device and Blood Warmer

Some form of rapid-infusion device is commonly used in liver transplantation.[95] Both commercially

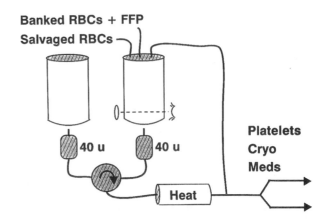

Fig. 35-4. Rapid transfusion device. Banked red blood cells (RBCs), salvaged RBCs, and FFP are added to a canister reservoir and infused through a filter and a heat exchanger. A second reservoir is used as a backup in case of filter failure, suspected bacterial contamination, or other mishap.

available and inhouse devices are used. Although several variations of configuration exist, the devices consist of one or two sterile holding reservoirs (cardiotomy reservoirs) to which banked RBCs, washed salvaged RBCs, FFP, crystalloid, and colloid are added. An example of one configuration is shown in Figure 35-4. Although only one reservoir is used at any time, some programs install a second reservoir as an immediately available backup. Banked RBCs are generally filtered as they are added to the reservoir. Blood exits the reservoir via tubing that leads to a high-volume microaggregate blood filter, through a roller pump, and then through a high-capacity blood warmer. Blood can either be directed toward the patient or diverted by a recirculation line back to the top of the canister. The recirculation line allows the blood to be continuously mixed during periods of no transfusion. If the blood is pumped toward the patient, the blood line divides via a Y connector into two lines that are attached to large-bore angiocatheters placed in central and/or peripheral lines. To prevent air embolus, a light detector is fitted to the bottom of the reservoir and automatically shuts off the roller pump if the reservoir empties. This system allows blood to be delivered at rates of 5 L/min without difficulty. Platelets, cryoprecipitate, and medications are delivered "downstream" and not put into the reservoir.

Intraoperative Salvage

Intraoperative blood salvage is now routinely used by many centers for OLT.[96,97] Several different protocols exist. In our hospital, we collect salvaged blood exclusively in citrate anticoagulant, centrifuge the salvaged blood, and wash 250 ml of packed cells with 500 to 1,500 ml saline. The washed RBCs are then pumped from the machine to either a transfer pack or (more commonly) directly into the sterile reservoir of the rapid-transfusion device (Fig. 35-4). We use intraoperative blood salvage for all patients except those who are known to have bacterial infection of the liver or biliary tree or those in whom there is inadvertent colonic injury during surgery. Because large numbers of units can be salvaged, a continuous running tally of the number of units returned to the patient must be kept in order to follow the clinical protocol of component therapy during massive transfusion (Table 35-3). Not all liver transplantation programs use intraoperative salvage.

Metabolic Complications of Massive Transfusion During Surgery

Dramatic and life-threatening metabolic complications can accompany liver transplantation and massive transfusion. Serial laboratory monitoring of key metabolic values (pH, PCO_2, HCO_3^-, K^+, ionized Ca^{++}, and glucose) is an invaluable aid to the anesthesiologist faced with massive transfusion. These results must be quickly correlated with the clinical situation and the continuous monitoring of blood pressure, heart rate, body temperature, urine output, cardiac filling pressures, and cardiac output.

Although hepatic failure alone may result in dramatic metabolic disarray, patients with concomitant renal failure due to hepatorenal syndrome or other causes have severely limited metabolic reserve. Patients with renal insufficiency may come to surgery with preexisting cardiac congestion, acidosis, and increased total body K^+. In the absence of good urine output, it is more difficult to control the acute hyperkalemia that develops in response to acidemia. Impaired renal excretion of metabolic acids and a decreased buffering capacity are present in renal failure. Because a proportion of the citrate load of banked blood is excreted in the urine, renal failure also increases the risk of citrate toxicity.

It has long been recognized that a decline in cardiac contractility may accompany massive transfusion. Poor cardiac contractility, decreased tissue perfusion, and the development of shock with ischemic tissue metabolism are dire signals during OLT that, if not quickly corrected, lead on to a downward spiral to arrhythmia and death. Several factors interfere with cardiovascular performance during massive transfusion. These include fluctuating preload and afterload, cold toxicity, acidemia, hyperkalemia, hypocalcemia, hypomagnesemia, and a dramatic loss of vascular tone somewhat unique to liver transplantation. During difficult resections of the patient's liver or during resections of very large livers (as occurs in polycystic liver disease) manipulation of the liver by the surgeon can compress the inferior vena cava and obstruct venous return to the heart. Poor flow through the veno-venous bypass circuit during the anhepatic phase can lead to shock despite volume overload. Although massive infusion of blood components without a blood warmer would certainly provoke hypothermia and poor cardiac contractility, this is rare in the era of blood warmers. Rather, the extensive and prolonged exposure of the body cavity to room temperature and the insertion of an iced liver result in dramatic heat loss during surgery. The use of heated respiratory gases, high ambient room temperature, and convective air heating devices are important means to combat heat loss.

Acidemia and hyperkalemia often occur together as release of intracellular K^+ occurs in response to low pH. Both metabolic derangements depress cardiac performance. In addition, hyperkalemia increases the chance of cardiac arrhythmia, especially if there is coexisting hypocalcemia. Acidemia during liver transplantation is dangerous and demands immediate attention. Reports suggest that acidemia during OLT does not result from blood infusion, but rather from lactic acid release from poor perfusion.[98] Patients who do not experience shock or develop tissue ischemia can receive phenomenal quantities of stored blood components and not develop acidemia.

The plasma of stored RBCs does represent an acute K^+ load that must be internalized into cells or excreted in the urine. Hyperkalemic cardiac standstill has been attributed to extremely rapid infusion of large volumes of banked blood.[99] However, the quantity of K^+ presented by transfusion is only a small percentage of the K^+ releasable by the patient's ischemic tissues. Patients who do not experience shock develop hypokalemia after massive transfusion.[100,101] Hypokalemia results not only from the alkalemia of citrate metabolism but also from the reuptake of K^+ into transfused RBCs that had lost K^+ during storage.

Citrate toxicity and hypocalcemia are a recognized risk of massive transfusion during OLT.[73,102–104] Although any cell with mitochondria can metabolize citrate via the Krebs cycle, the liver is the major organ for citrate metabolism and the kidney is the major organ for citrate excretion. FFP and platelet concentrates have the highest citrate content.[102] Because liver transplantation patients often require rapid infusions of large quantities of FFP and RBCs, the rate of citrate infusion can exceed the ability of the recipient to metabolize and excrete citrate. As a result, the concentration of citrate may become 100 times greater than preoperative levels.[105] As the level of ionized Ca^{++} begins to drop, the patient releases parathormone in an attempt to mobilize bone resources of Ca^{++}.[102] Some patients—such as those with renal failure or with hepatic osteodystrophy—may be less able to mobilize Ca^{++} stores.[106] Although mild to moderate depressions of the ionized Ca^{++} level are of little consequence to the patient, severe depression of the ionized Ca^{++} level leads to a decline in cardiac contractility, followed by the development of widening of the QRS complex, bizarre T-wave changes, and arrhythmias. Frequent monitoring of the ionized Ca^{++} level using an ion-selective electrode and done by a laboratory with rapid result turnaround is essential for proper management of massive transfusion in liver transplantation. Supplements of calcium chloride or calcium gluconate may be given either as repeated small injections or continuous by infusion, the infusion rate being adjusted based on the rate of FFP transfused and the laboratory Ca^{++} values. In our program, we attempt to maintain the ionized Ca^{++} above at least 50 percent of its normal value. If given in equivalent molar doses of calcium, each calcium preparation is equally effective.[107] Calcium should not be administered according to a fixed schedule of blood administration. Excessive calcium injections and inattention to monitored levels of the ionized Ca^{++} can result in life-threatening hypercalcemia.[102,106] After successful implantation of a viable new hepatic graft, the new organ is able to metabolize citrate and the need for supplemental calcium usually ends. As the citrate is metabolized in the Krebs cycle, bicarbonate is generated. As a result, alkalemia is often seen after massive transfusion and liver transplantation.[108]

Magnesium may also be chelated as a result of citrate toxicity. Blood Mg^{++} levels are not usually monitored during transplantation, and one study suggested that Mg^{++} levels may not drop as much as Ca^{++} levels during massive transfusion.[109] However, severe hypomagnesemia can depress myocardial function[110] and may result in a characteristic tachyarrhythmia termed *torsade des pointes* that is difficult to treat.[111]

At the time when either the vena cava or the portal vein is unclamped and blood is allowed to drain from the newly revascularized allograft into the systemic circulation, up to 30 percent of patients may develop some degree of hypotension and bradycardia.[112] In some patients, the vasodepression is severe and cardiac arrest occurs.[113] The effect has been attributed to the sudden release from the allograft of blood and flushing solution, which is cold and rich in potassium. One report suggested that the risk of the reperfusion syndrome could be decreased by discarding the initial 500 to 600 ml that drains from the newly revascularized allograft.[112] Some patients experience a more prolonged and profound loss of vascular tone after reperfusion, particularly in the setting of primary graft nonfunction. Although the cause remains mysterious, the effect is obvious: the patient develops hypotension with almost complete loss of systemic vascular resistance that is nearly unresponsive to high doses of pressors such as norepinephrine, phenylephrine, and dopamine. The condition may be related in part to excess release of nitric oxide, a potent vasodilator synthesized from L-arginine.[114] Nitrous oxide may be directly released by the nonfunctioning graft or the graft may release other factors that stimulate recipient vessels to synthesize nitrous oxide.

Massive Transfusion by Itself Does Not Produce Coagulopathy

If the patient does not have strong coagulation inhibitors or high-titer anti-HLA or antiplatelet antibodies and if care is taken to avoid dilution of plasma coagulation factors and platelets, massive blood transfusion by itself will not produce a serious coagulopathy. In the absence of shock, tissue hypoperfusion, or damage to vital organs and in the presence of a properly functioning hepatic graft, OLT patients can sustain very large volume blood support and reach the recovery area with excellent hemostasis. After several blood volumes of transfusion, nearly all the circulating platelets in the patient have been supplied from the blood bank. These platelets may demonstrate mild functional defects typical of stored platelet concentrates, but a clinically important platelet defect is usually not present. However, the life span of the transfused platelets is fixed, and during the first few postoperative days, massively transfused patients will predictably demonstrate a dramatic drop in their platelet count as the life span of transfused platelets comes to an end. This sudden drop in the platelet count may be misunderstood and attributed to other causes.

The Need for Markers to Identify Patients at High Risk of Massive Transfusion

There is good evidence that in general patients who require massive blood support have a higher mortality than those requiring less transfusion.[115–117]

Among 68 adult OLT patients in Pittsburgh, 28 percent (15 of 54) of patients died if 70 or fewer units of RBCs were required for surgery. By contrast, among those who required more than 70 units of RBCs, 64 percent (9 of 14) died ($X^2_{Yates} = 4.9$; $P < .05$).[116] A smaller study from the Mayo Clinic reported that 14 percent (13 of 94) OLT patients receiving 50 or fewer units of RBCs died, in comparison with 33 percent (2 of 6) who received more than 50 units of RBCs.[115] A report from Minnesota also found a significant inverse correlation between blood transfusion requirements and survival.[117] Data collected from a larger number of patients in our own program are shown in Figure 35-5. Kaplan-Meier survival curves were prepared according to RBC requirements. Three categories of blood use were established prior to examination of the data. The results illustrate two points: (1) there is a clear decline in survival in association with massive transfusion; and (2) the increased mortality associated with massive transfusion is not restricted to the immediate postoperative period. Rather, massively transfused patients continue to experience higher death rates during the first post-transplantation year. By the third post-transplantation year, the survival

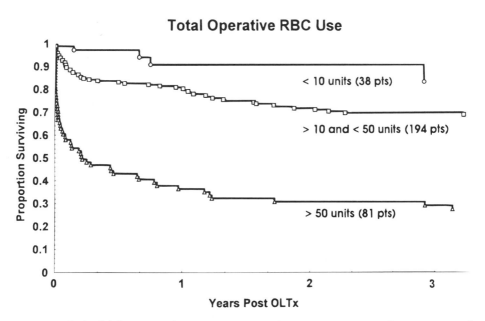

Fig. 35-5. Survival of adult liver transplantation patients at the Deaconess Hospital in Boston as a function of the number of intraoperative red blood cells transfused.

curve appears to plateau. These observations underscore the value of more research being done on developing clinical and laboratory indicators that can identify preoperatively those patients likely to require massive transfusion support.

In the United States, the problem of high-risk patients is exacerbated by the serious shortage of donor livers. Allocation of solid organs has become an extremely complex topic.[118,119] Organs are allocated to the sickest patients and to those who have been on the waiting list for the longest period of time. If the imbalance between demand and supply worsens and the waiting period grows longer, more patients may slip from low-risk to high-risk clinical status.[118,120]

Deciding When Withdraw Blood Support

Because liver transplantation can require extraordinary quantities of medical resources, those involved in liver transplantation programs must reach some decision regarding the limits of support that are appropriate for any single patient. Open-ended, unlimited blood support is unjustifiable. Blood resources are limited and other patients with a better chance for survival have a legitimate claim to blood support should complications arise during their surgery. From a physiologic standpoint, there is little value in continued transfusion to a patient with severe acidemia, uncorrectable shock, uncontrolled bleeding, and diffuse uncorrectable coagulopathy. Physicians in our liver transplantation program believe it is best to decide in advance what should be an acceptable upper limit of blood support. This decision should be made by consensus of the surgical team, the director of transfusion medicine, a patient advocate, and other interested individuals. Two basic strategies can be used: a single-rule approach that sets a single upper limit for any liver transplantation, or a patient-tailored approach that sets a limit for each patient.

The patient-tailored approach has the advantage of extending or limiting the resources offered to match the physiologic chance of recovery. Using this approach, a surgeon would assign a higher upper limit of blood support to a low-risk patient than to a poor-risk patient. However, the patient-tailored approach may place too much emphasis on physiologic risk assessment, which is inexact and may limit or extend blood resources based on incorrect judg-

ments about individual patients. We believe that a single-rule approach is more appropriate. Since the 1980s, our liver transplantation program has functioned under the guideline that allocates up to 100 units of banked RBCs per patient. We recognize that although this limit may be too low for some patients and too high for others, it is well beyond the cutoff for decreased survival found in other studies.[115–117] Since the 1980s, we have occasionally encountered patients who exhausted their blood allocation while actively bleeding in the OR and were considered unsalvageable. In the now unusual circumstance of ultramassive transfusion, 100 units of banked RBCs may be supplemented with 80 to 150 additional RBCs collected by intraoperative blood salvage and combined with 80 units of FFP, 50 units of platelets, and 20 units of cryoprecipitate, for a total of over 300 units of component support. During periods of regional blood shortages, our transfusion medicine service has reserved the right to reduce the allocation given to liver transplantation. During such times, clear and careful dialogue with the attending surgeon is required before making the difficult decision to embark on liver transplantation with decreased blood resources.

BLOOD SERVICES AND THE SHORTAGE OF SOLID ORGAN DONORS

With continuing advances in solid organ transplantation, the imbalance between supply and demand for donated solid organs widens. The legal, ethical, moral, and religious issues surrounding the selection and consent for solid organ donation by heart-beating cadavers are complex issues.[119] Proponents of the expansion in solid organ allografting point to the need for greater public education about the utility of transplantation. The responsibility for this educational effort has fallen to organ procurement societies. Although such programs as the national bone marrow donor registry have enrolled over one million individuals who are HLA typed, these individuals have not as yet been the focus of education efforts concerning solid organ donation after death. The question of whether blood services should play a role in the education of the general public about organ donation is not resolved. Because blood services have established contacts with the general public regarding altruistic donation during life, it is possible that these services are well suited to education about organ donation. Indeed, blood donors may be more inclined than nondonors to participate in solid organ donation after death.[121]

REFERENCES

1. United Network for Organ Sharing Update. Richmond. 10:25, 1994
2. Charlton B, Auchincloss H, Fathman CG: Mechanisms of transplantation tolerance. Ann Rev Immunol 12:707, 1994
3. van Rood JJ, Claas FH: The influence of allogeneic cells on the human T and B cell repertoire. Science 248:1388, 1990
4. von Boehmer H, Kisielow P: Self-nonself discrimination by T cells. Science 248:1369, 1990
5. Boyd R, Tucek CL, Godfrey DI et al: The thymic microenvironment. Immunol Today 14:445, 1993
6. Swat W, Ignatowicz L, von Boehmer H, Kisielow P: Clonal deletion of immature CD4 + 8 + thymocytes in suspension culture by extrathymic antigen-presenting cells. Nature 351:150, 1991
7. Pawlowski TJ, Staerz UD: Thymic education—T cells do it for themselves. Immunol Today 205:205, 1994
8. Ildstad ST, Sachs DH: Reconstitution with syngeneic plus allogeneic or xenogeneic bone marrow leads to specific acceptance of allografts or xenografts. Nature 307:168, 1984
9. Posselt AM, Campos L, Mayo GL et al: Selective modulation of T-cell immunity by intrathymic cellular transplantation. Transplant Rev 7:200, 1993
10. Posselt AM, Barker CF, Tomaszewski JE et al: Induction of donor-specific unresponsiveness by intrathymic islet transplantation. Science 249:1293, 1990
11. Ohzato H, Monaco AP: Induction of specific unresponsiveness (tolerance) to skin allografts by intrathymic donor-specific splenocyte injection in antilymphocyte serum-treated mice. Transplantation 54:1090, 1992
12. Goss JA, Makafusa Y, Flye MW: MHC class II presenting cells are necessary for the induction of intrathymic tolerance. Ann Surg 217:217, 1993
13. Remuzzi G, Rossini M, Imberti O, Perico N: Kidney graft survival in rats without immunosuppressants after intrathymic glomerular transplantation. Lancet 337:750, 1991
14. Campos L, Alfrey EJ, Posselt AM et al: Prolonged survival of rat orthotopic liver allografts after intrathymic inoculation of donor-strain cells. Transplantation 55:866, 1993
15. Lenschow DJ, Blueston JA: T cell co-stimulation and in vivo tolerance. Curr Opin Immunol 5:747, 1993
16. Wood KJ: The induction of tolerance to alloantigens using MHC class I molecules. Curr Opin Immunol 5:759, 1993
17. Mueller DL, Jenkins MK, Schwartz RH: Clonal expansion versus functional clonal inactivation. Ann Rev Immuol 7:445, 1989
18. Fuchs EJ, Matzinger P: B cells turn off virgin but not memory T cells. Science 258:1156, 1992
19. Turka LA, Linsley PS, Lin H et al: T-cell activation by the CD28 ligand B7 is required for cardiac allograft rejection in vivo. Proc Natl Acad Sci USA 89:11102, 1992
20. Linsley PS, Ledbetter JA: Ann Rev Immunol 11:191, 1993
21. Heeg K, Wagner H: Induction of peripheral tolerance to class I major histocompatibility complex (MHC) alloantigens in adult mice: transfused class I MHC-incompatible splenocytes veto clonal responses of antigen-reactive Lyt-2 + T cells. J Exp Med 172:719, 1990
22. Rammensee HG: Veto function in vitro and in vivo. Int Rev Immunol 4:175, 1989
23. Thomas JM, Carver FM, Kasten-Jolly J et al: Further studies of veto activity in rhesus monkey bone marrow in relation to allograft tolerance and chimerism. Transplantation 57:101, 1994
24. Sigal NH, Dumont FJ: Cyclosporin A, FK-506, and rapamycin: pharmacologic properties of lymphocyte signal transduction. Ann Rev Immunol 10:519, 1992
25. Liu J: FK506 and cyclosporin, molecular probes for studying intracellular signal transduction. Immunol Today 14:290, 1993
26. Kay JE, Benzie CR: T lymphocyte activation through the CD28 pathway is insensitive to inhibition by the immunosuppressive drug FK-506. Immunol Lett 23:155, 1989
27. Opelz G, Sengar D, Mickey M, Terasaki P: Effect of blood transfusions on subsequent kidney transplants. Transplant Proc 5:253, 1973
28. Opelz G, Terasaki P: Improvement of kidney graft survival with increased numbers of blood transfusions. N Engl J Med 299:799, 1978
29. Horimi T, Terasaki P, Chia D, Sasaki N: Factors influencing the paradoxical effect of transfusions on kidney transplants. Transplantation 35:320, 1983
30. Hourmant M, Soulillou J, Bui-Quang D: Beneficial effect of blood transfusion: role of the time interval between the last transfusion and transplantation. Transplantation 28:40, 1979

31. Salvatierra O: Donor-specific transfusions in living related transplantation. World J Surg 10:361, 1986

32. Opelz G: Effect of HLA matching, blood transfusions, and presensitization in cyclosporine treated kidney transplant recipients. Transplant Proc 17:2179, 1985

33. Kerman R, van Buren C, Lewis R, Kahan B: Successful transplantation of 100 untransfused cyclosporine-treated primary recipients of cadaveric renal allografts. Transplantation 45:37, 1988

34. Triulzi DJ, Heal JM, Blumberg N: Transfusion-induced immunomodulation and its clinical consequences. p. 1. In Nance SJ (ed): Transfusion Medicine in the 1990's. American Association of Blood Banks, Bethesda, MD, 1990

35. Blumberg N, Heal JM: Transfusion-induced immunomodulation. p. 580. In Anderson KC, Ness PM (eds): Scientific Basis of Transfusion Medicine: Implications for Clinical Practice. WB Saunders, Philadelphia, 1994

36. Terasaki PI: The beneficial effect on kidney graft survival attributed to clonal deletion. Transplantation 37:119, 1984

37. Leivestad T, Thorsby E: Effects of HLA-haploidentical blood transfusions on donor-specific immune responsiveness. Transplantation 37:175, 1984

38. Hutchinson IV: Suppressor T cells in allogeneic models. Transplantation 41:547, 1986

39. Reed E, Hardy M, Benvenisty A et al: Effect of antiidiotypic antibodies to HLA on graft survival in renal allograft recipients. N Engl J Med 316:1450, 1987

40. Takahashi H, Iwaki Y, Terasaki P et al: Deliberate buffycoat transfusions and the risk of antibody formation. Transplant Proc 14:302, 1982

41. Norman D, Barry J, Durr M, Wetzsteon P: A preliminary analysis of a randomized study of buffy coat transfusions in renal transplantation. Transplant Proc 17:2335, 1985

42. Busch ORC, Hop WCJ, Hoynck van Papendrecht MAW et al: Blood transfusions and prognosis in colorectal cancer. N Engl J Med 328:1372, 1993

43. Jensen LS, Andersen AJ, Christiansen PM et al: Postoperative infection and natural killer cell function following blood transfusion in patients undergoing elective colorectal surgery. Br J Surg 79:513, 1992

44. Nielsen JH, Hammer JH, Moesgaard F, Kehlet H: Comparison of the effects of SAGM and whole blood transfusion on postoperative suppression of delayed hypersensitivity. Can J Surg 34:146, 1991

45. Shelby J, Marushack MM, Nelso EW: Prostaglandin production and suppressor cell induction in transfusion-induced suppression. Transplantation 43:113, 1987

46. Quigley RL, Wood KJ, Morris PJ: The relative roles of major and minor histocompatibility antigens in the induction of immunologic unresponsiveness by blood transfusion. Transfusion 29:789, 1989

47. Lagaaij EL, Hennemann PH, Ruigrok M et al: Effect of one-HLA-DR antigen matched and completely HLA-DR-mismatched blood transfusions on survival of heart and kidney allografts. N Engl J Med 321:701, 1989

48. van Twuyer E, Mooijaart RJD, ten Berge UM et al: Pretransplant blood transfusions revisited. N Engl J Med 325:1210, 1991

49. Starzl TE, Demetris AJ, Trucco M et al: Cell migration, chimerism, and graft acceptance. Lancet 339:1579, 1992

50. Starzl TE, Demetris AJ, Trucco M et al: Chimerism and donor-specific nonreactivity 27 to 29 years after kidney allotransplantation. Transplantation 55:1272, 1993

51. Schlitt JH, Kanehiro H, Raddatz G et al: Persistence of donor lymphocytes in liver allograft recipients. Transplantation 56:1001, 1993

52. Dzik WH: Mononuclear cell microchimerism and the immunomodulatory effect of transfusion. Transfusion 34:1007, 1994

53. deWaal LP, van Twuyver E: Blood transfusion and allograft survival: is mixed chimerism the solution for tolerance induction in clinical transplantation? Crit Rev Immunol 10:417, 1991

54. Monaco AP, Wood ML, Maki T et al: The use of donor-specific antigen for the induction of immunologic unresponsiveness to experimental and clinical allografts. Transplant Proc 20:122, 1988

55. Fisher M, Chapman JR, Ting A, Morris PJ: Alloimmunization to HLA antigens following transfusion with leukocyte-poor and purified platelet suspensions. Vox Sang 49:331, 1985

56. Stratta RJ, Shaefer MS, Markin RS et al: Cytomegalovirus infection and disease after liver transplantation: an overview. Dig Dis Sci 37:673, 1992

57. Paya CV, Hermans PE, Wiesner RH et al: Cytomegalovirus hepatitis in liver transplantation: prospective analysis of 93 consecutive orthotopic liver transplantation. J Infect Dis 160:752, 1989

58. Wreghitt TG, Hakim M, Gray JJ et al: Cytomegalovirus infections in heart and heart and lung transplant recipients. J Clin Pathol 41:660, 1988

59. Richardson WP, Colvin RB, Cheeseman SH et al: Glomerulopathy associated with cytomegalovirus viremia in renal allografts. N Engl J Med 305:57, 1981

60. Arnold JC, Portmann BC, O'Grady JG et al: Cytomegalovirus infection persists in the liver graft in the

vanishing bile duct syndrome. Hepatology 16:285, 1992

61. Grattan MT, Moreno-Cabral CE, Starnes VA et al: Cytomegalovirus infection is associated with cardiac allografts rejection and atherosclerosis. JAMA 261: 3561, 1989

62. Rubin RH: Infectious disease complications of renal transplantation. Kidney Int 44:221, 1993

63. Kendall TJ, Wilson JE, Radio SJ et al: Cytomegalovirus and other herpesviruses: do they have a role in the development of accelerated coronary arterial disease in human heart allografts? J Heart Lung Transpl 11:S14, 1992

64. Wiesner RH, Marin E, Porayko MK et al: Advances in the diagnosis, treatment, and prevention of cytomegalovirus infections after liver transplantation. Gastroenterol Clin North Am 22:351, 1993

65. Farrugia E, Schwab TR: Management and prevention of cytomegalovirus infection after renal transplantation. Mayo Clin Proc 67:879, 1992

66. Gorensek MJ, Stewart RW, Keys TF et al: A multivariate analysis of the risk of cytomegalovirus infection in heart transplant recipients. J Inf Dis 157:515, 1988

67. Preiksaitis JK, Brown L, McKenzie M: The risk of cytomegalovirus infection in seronegative transfusion recipients not receiving exogenous immunosuppression. J Infect Dis 157:523, 1988

68. Bowden RA: Cytomegalovirus infections in transplant patients: methods of prevention of primary cytomegalovirus. Transplant Proc 23:136, 1991

69. Grundy JE, Lui SF, Super M et al: Symptomatic cytomegalovirus infection in seropositive kidney recipients: reinfection with donor virus rather than reactivation of recipient virus. Lancet 2:132, 1988

70. Chou SW: Acquisition of donor strains of cytomegalovirus by renal transplant recipients. N Engl J Med 314:1418, 1986

71. Morris DJ, Longson M, Poslethwaite RJ et al: Donor seropositivity and prednisolone therapy as risk factors for cytomegalovirus infection and disease in cyclosporin-treated renal allograft recipients. Q J Med 77:1165, 1990

72. Lewis JH, Bontempo FA, Cornell F et al: Blood use in liver transplantation. Transfusion 27:222, 1987

73. Seaman MJ, Culank LS, Price CP: Perioperative laboratory support. p. 199. In Calne R (ed): Liver Transplantation: The Cambridge–King's College Hospital Experience. 2nd Ed. Grune & Stratton, Orlando, FL, 1987

74. Lake JR: Advances in liver transplantation. Gastroenterol Clin North Am 22:213, 1993

75. Danielson CF: Transfusion support and complicating coagulopathies in solid organ transplantation. p. 43. In Hackel E, Aubuchon J (eds): Advances in Transplantation. American Association of Blood Banks, Bethesda, MD, 1993

76. Marco AP, Furman WR: Anesthetic problems: venous air embolism, airway difficulties and massive transfusion. Surg Clin North Am 73:213, 1993

77. Dzik WH: Massive transfusion. p. 211. In Churchill H, Kurtz S (eds): Transfusion Medicine. Blackwell Scientific, Boston, 1988

78. Hathaway WE, Goodnight SH: Disorders of Hemostasis and Thrombosis. McGraw-Hill, New York, 1993

79. Ritter DM, Rettke SR, Lunn RJ et al: Preoperative coagulation screen does not predict intraoperative blood product requirements in orthotopic liver transplantation. Transplant Proc 21:3533, 1989

80. Lewis JH, Bontempo FA, Awad SA et al: Liver transplantation: intraoperative changes in coagulation factors in 100 first transplants. Hepatology 9:710, 1989

81. Dzik WH, Arkin CF, Jenkins RL, Stump DC: Fibrinolysis during liver transplantation in humans: role of tissue-type plasminogen activator. Blood 71:1090, 1988

82. Porte RJ, Bontempo FA, Knot EAR et al: Systemic effects of tissue plasminogen activator-associated fibrinolysis and its relation to thrombin generation in orthotopic liver transplantation. Transplantation 47: 978, 1989

83. Kang Y: Clinical use of synthetic antifibrinolytic agents during liver transplantation. Sem Thromb Hemost 19:258, 1993

84. Welte M, Groh J, Azad S et al: Effect of aprotinin on coagulation parameters in liver transplantation. Semin Thromb Hemost 19:297, 1993

85. Leslie SD, Toy PTCY: Laboratory hemostatic abnormalities in massively transfused patients given red blood cells and crystalloid. Am J Clin Pathol 96:770, 1991

86. Yang SL, Ballas S, Angstadt J et al: Using ABO-incompatible blood in massive transfusion in orthotopic liver transplantation. Transplant Proc 20: 295, 1988

87. Ramsey G: Red cell antibodies arising from solid organ transplants. Transfusion 31:76, 1991

88. Triulzi DJ, Shirey RS, Ness PM, Klein AS: Immunohematologic complications of ABO-unmatched liver transplants. Transfusion 32:829, 1992

89. Ramsey G, Hahn LF, Cornell FW et al: Low rate of rhesus immunization from Rh-incompatible blood transfusions during liver and heart transplant surgery. Transplantation 47:993, 1989

90. Ramsey G, Cornell FW, Hahn LF et al: Incompatible blood transfusions in liver transplant patients with

significant red cell alloantibodies. Transplant Proc 21:3531, 1989

91. Ramsey G, Cornell FW, Hahn LF et al: Red cell antibody problems in 1000 liver transplants. Transfusion 29:396, 1989

92. Weber T, Marino IR, Kang Y et al: Intraoperative blood transfusions in highly alloimmunized patients undergoing orthotopic liver transplantation. Transplantation 47:797, 1989

93. Dzik WH: Blood component therapy during liver transplantation in adults. Immunohematology Check Sample 31:1, American Society of Clinical Pathologists, 1988

94. Kang Y: Monitoring and therapy of coagulation. p. 151. In Winter PM, Kang Y (eds): Hepatic transplantation: Anesthetic and Perioperative Management. Praeger, New York, 1986

95. Sassano JJ: The rapid infusion system. p. 120. In Winter PM, Kang Y (eds): Hepatic Transplantation: Anesthetic and Perioperative Management. Praeger, New York, 1986

96. Dzik WH, Jenkins R: Use of intraoperative blood salvage during orthotopic liver transplantation. Arch Surg 120:946, 1985

97. Williamson KR, Taswell HF, Rettke SR, Krom RA: Intraoperative autologous transfusion: its role in orthotopic liver transplantation. Mayo Clin Proc 64:340, 1989

98. Fath J, Estrin J, Belani K et al: Lactate metabolism during hepatic transplantation: evidence for a perfusion-sensitive patient population. Transplant Proc 17:284, 1985

99. Jameson LC, Popic PM, Harms BA: Hyperkalemic death during use of a high-capacity fluid warmer for massive transfusion. Anesthesiology 73:1050, 1990

100. Carmichael D, Hosty T, Kastl D et al: Hypokalemia and massive transfusion. South Med J 77:315, 1984

101. Linko K, Saxelin I: Electrolyte and acid base disturbances caused by blood transfusion. Acta Anaesthesiol Scand 30:134, 1986

102. Dzik WH, Kirkley S: Citrate toxicity in massive transfusion. Transfus Med Rev 2:76, 1988

103. Marquez JM: Citrate intoxication during hepatic transplantation. p. 110. In Winter PM, Kang Y (eds): Hepatic Transplantation: Anesthetic and Perioperative Management. Praeger, New York, 1986

104. Wu AHB, Bracey A, Bryan-Brown CW et al: Ionized calcium monitoring during liver transplantation. Arch Pathol Lab Med 111:935, 1987

105. Gray TA, Buckley BM, Sealey MM, Smith SCH, Tomlin P et al: Plasma ionized calcium monitoring during liver transplantation. Transplantation 41:335, 1986

106. Munoz SJ, Nagelberg SB, Green PJ et al: Ectopic soft tissue calcium deposition following liver transplantation. Hepatology 8:476, 1988

107. Martin TJ, Kang Y, Robertson KM et al: Ionization and hemodynamic effects of calcium chloride and calcium gluconate in the absence of hepatic function. Anesthesiology 73:62, 1990

108. Driscoll DF, Bistrian BR, Jenkins RL et al: Development of metabolic alkalosis after massive transfusion during orthotopic liver transplantation. Crit Care Med 15:905, 1987

109. Lieberman N, Plevak D, Moyer T et al: Is it important to measure magnesium concentrations during and immediately after liver transplantation? Transplant Proc 25:1826, 1993

110. Chernow B, Smith J, Rainey RG, Finton C: Hypomagnesemia: implications for the critical care specialist. Crit Care Med 10:193, 1982

111. Kulkarni P, Bhattacharya S, Petros AJ: Torsade de pointes and long QT syndrome following major blood transfusion. Anaesthesia 47:125, 1992

112. Brems JJ, Takiff H, McHutchison J et al: Systemic versus nonsystemic reperfusion of the transplanted liver. Transplantation 55:527, 1993

113. Aggarwal S, Kang Y, Freeman J et al: Postreperfusion syndrome: cardiovascular collapse following hepatic reperfusion during liver transplantation. Transplant Proc 19:54, 1987

114. Moncada S, Higgs A: The L-arginine-nitric oxide pathway. N Engl J Med 329:2002, 1993

115. Motschman TL, Taswell HF, Brecher ME et al: Intraoperative blood loss and patient and graft survival in orthotopic liver transplantation: their relationship to clinical and laboratory data. Mayo Clin Proc 64:346, 1989

116. Butler P, Israel L, Nusbacher J et al: Blood transfusion in liver transplantation. Transfusion 25:120, 1985

117. Stock PG, Estrin JA, Fryd DS et al: Factors influencing early survival after liver transplantation. Am J Surg 157:215, 1989

118. Lake JR: Changing indications for liver transplantation. Gastroenterol Clinics North Am 22:213, 1993

119. Keown PA: Proceedings of the 2nd International Congress of the Society for Organ Sharing. Transplant Proc 25:2983, 1993

120. Dzik WH: Ethical problems in liver transplantation: who should decide which patients are candidates for transplantation. Transplantation 53:712, 1992

121. Szuflad P, DeSantis D, Dzik W: Attitudes toward solid organ donation: blood donors vs non-blood donors, abstracted. Transfusion (suppl.) 33:S93, 1993

Appendix
Clinical Scenarios of Massive Transfusion and Liver Transplantation

Case 1. Thirty units of banked RBCs have been given and the patient is still in phase 1 of surgery. Whatever the preoperative assessment, this case is not going well. There may be multiple adhesions around the liver in a patient with sclerosing cholangitis, friable collaterals in a patient with severe portal hypertension, or an inadvertent tear in the inferior vena cava during mobilization of the liver. Attention must be paid to avoid dilution coagulopathy, avoid shock and hypoperfusion, and increase resources assigned to this patient.

Case 2. During the anhepatic phase, surgical blood loss and a period of hypotension occurred—this has been corrected. About 30 minutes after opening the portal vein, the patient began bleeding diffusely, including bleeding from cut surfaces that were previously clotted. The PT has jumped in the last hour from 17 to 28 seconds and the fibrinogen has fallen from 130 to less than 40 mg/dL. The rapid-transfusion device is pumping blood rapidly, and up to this point, the patient has received 30 RBCs, 10 salvaged RBCs, 20 FFP, and 10 platelets.

This situation is typical of the hyperfibrinolysis of liver transplantation. This condition peaks at the end of the anhepatic phase, is more common in patients with shock, and results in lysis of previously clotted sites and a dramatic fall in the concentration of fibrinogen, which cannot be attributed to dilution. At my institution, we would give 5 g Amicar intravenously now and repeat it at hourly intervals until under control. Additional units of RBCs, FFP, and platelets will be needed. We would transfuse cryoprecipitate, although FFP has sufficient fibrinogen to restore the situation to normal, provided the fibrinolysis is stopped.

Case 3. The patient suffers a cardiac arrest shortly after opening the vena cava.

The two most likely possibilities are (1) an air embolus from the vena cava or from the new liver and (2) arrhythmia caused by hyperkalemia. If air is not sufficiently flushed out of the new liver or if air enters the vena cava during the anastomoses, a pulmonary air embolus may occur. A rapid drop in end-tidal CO_2 may be a clue to the sudden decrease in pulmonary perfusion. Residual storage solution and the initial blood draining the new liver are rich in K^+. If the patient was hyperkalemic prior to opening the vena cava and is also hypocalcemic from citrate toxicity, the additional K^+ load may precipitate a fatal arrhythmia. The anesthesia team must give particular attention to the pH, K^+, and Ca^{++} in preparation for the opening of the vena cava. If this patient is resuscitated, major fibrinolysis and massive bleeding is highly likely.

Case 4. The patient's platelet count is 40,000/μl and does not increase with platelet transfusion.

This patient may be refractory owing to anti-HLA antibodies. If the patient is not bleeding, there is no need to raise his platelet count, and platelet concentrates should be reserved for later, in case a dilution coagulopathy develops and in case the anti-HLA antibodies have also been diluted. This is not a good time to argue with the anesthesiologists. The institution's approach to this problem should be discussed in advance.

Case 5. The OR calls the blood bank to say, "Send us everything you've got."

This is a sign of failure. The panic request may have resulted from (1) an unexpected major surgical mishap, (2) an inexperienced anesthesiologist, or (3) a breakdown in the continuous communication needed between the OR and the blood bank to provide the smooth delivery of the proper mix of components. When the surgery is over, it is time to review protocols.

Case 6. The patient is in the third phase of surgery and so far has used a total of 10 units banked RBCs, 3 units salvaged RBCs, 6 units FFP, and no platelets. Continuous bleeding is present from behind the liver. In the last hour, the PT has increased from 16 to 18 seconds with a fibrinogen of 180. The blood pressure is 80/50 and pressors have been started. One hour later, after 5 additional units RBCs, 3 units salvaged RBCs, 20 units platelets and 12 units FFP, the PT is 22 seconds with a fibrinogen of 180. Despite increased pressors, the blood pressure is still 80/50. The new liver appears swollen. There is minimal urine output, no bile formation by the new liver, and increased bleeding.

This patient likely has primary graft nonfunction.

Although this may be seen in ABO-incompatible donor-recipient pairs or in the setting of other undefined immunologic incompatibilities, the condition most likely occurs because of damage to the donor liver during the illness that resulted in the death of the donor, during the organ harvesting, or during the storage period before transplantation. Although some livers recover after a rocky period of initial nonfunction, it is likely that this patient's new liver will never work. Relisting the patient with the organ bank for an emergency retransplantation is usually tried with poor success. If the decision is made to sustain this patient and go on with an emergency retransplantation, this patient may ultimately stress the limits of blood resources allocated to him.

Chapter 36

General Overview of Transfusion-Transmitted Infections

Steven Kleinman and Michael P. Busch

Since the discovery of transfusion-transmitted acquired immunodeficiency syndrome (AIDS), interest in accurately quantifying the risks of transfusion-transmitted infection and of developing policies to reduce these risks has dramatically increased. This chapter elucidates and clarifies many of the issues common to various transfusion-transmitted infections; details pertinent to specific agents such as human immunodeficiency virus (HIV), human T-cell lymphotropic virus (HTLV), hepatitis B virus (HBV), hepatitis C virus (HCV), cytomegalovirus (CMV), and bacterial and parasitic infections can be found in Chapters 37 to 40.

ASSESSING RISKS OF TRANSFUSION

Accurate estimates of transfusion-transmitted risk are important to enable patients and physicians to make informed decisions about whether to receive an allogeneic transfusion or to select another therapeutic option. These risk estimates are also important to enable policy makers to evaluate the expected benefits and costs of proposed interventions to reduce the transfusion-transmitted infection risk further.

Although each donated unit of blood is tested for markers of viral infection, there are at least three reasons why transmission of viral agents still occurs. The primary reason is the lack of a positive screening test result during the early stages of infection, known as the window period. For example, an individual exposed to HIV does not have HIV antibody develop until some defined period has elapsed. However, if such an individual were to donate blood during this HIV antibody-negative window period (estimated to be approximately 22 days with current HIV antibody tests),[1] the transfused unit would be capable of transmitting HIV infection. A second factor contributing to the risk of transfusion-transmitted infection for some agents is the existence of a chronic carrier state in which a donor persistently tests negative on donor screening assays. For example, there is evidence that some HCV-infected individuals may carry the virus but be undetectable by current HCV antibody tests.[2] Similarly, some chronic HTLV-II carriers are not detected by current HTLV-I antibody tests.[3] A third factor that theoretically contributes to transfusion-transmitted infection is laboratory error in performing screening tests; however, given the low prevalence of infected donors and the high accuracy of automated testing, the occurrence of such errors is thought to be extremely rare.

The most scientifically accurate method of establishing transfusion-transmitted infection risk is to perform a prospective controlled study of transfusion recipients. In this type of study, samples are obtained before transfusion and at periodic intervals after transfusion; such studies are further strengthened when serum samples from recipients and/or donors are frozen so that they may be re-evaluated when more sensitive blood screening tests become available. Since the mid 1970s, the National Heart, Lung and Blood Institute (NHLBI) has funded three such studies: the Transfusion Transmitted Virus Study (TTVS, recipients transfused from 1974 through 1979), the Transfusion Safety Study (TSS, recipients transfused in 1984 and 1985), and the Frequency of Agents Communicated by Transfusion Study (FACTS, recipients transfused from 1985 to 1991).[4-6] In addition, investigators at the National Institutes of Health Clinical Center have performed ongoing studies of the incidence of post-transfusion hepatitis for the past two decades.[7]

A second direct method of determining risk involves screening of donor units with sensitive laboratory tests that are not utilized routinely in donor testing. One such study was performed in San Francisco in which, over a several-year interval, approximately 200,000 blood donor samples were screened for HIV nucleic acid.[8,9]

Given the current low risks of transfusion-transmitted infection and the consequent need for very large sample sizes to determine risks accurately, it is unlikely that prospective studies will be funded in the future. It is therefore necessary to rely on other methods to determine risk. These approaches usually involve the evaluation of a limited data set and the use of reasonable assumptions that model the data to generate an estimate of risk. A recent approach, utilized by investigators from the Retrovirus Epidemiology Donor Study (REDS) and independently by the Centers for Disease Control and Prevention, was to estimate risk by measuring the incidence of new infection (seroconversion) in a blood donor population over a specific time interval and then multiplying this incidence by the average time interval that a seroconverting donor would be expected to be able to transmit infection (i.e., length of time in the window period).[10,11] This approach requires that the number of seroconverting donors be accurately measured and that a variable be defined to account for different intervals of observation (interdonation intervals) by nonseroconverting donors in the data set. The incidence model approach has several limitations. First, it is only fully applicable to agents that do not establish chronic nondetect-

able carrier states. Second, it is difficult to evaluate the contribution of single-time donors to the model. Third, the preseroconversion window period of infection for each agent may itself be an estimate rather than a measured parameter. Nevertheless, this approach has the distinct advantages of not requiring funding of special research studies for determination of risk, of being able to show changes in risk over time, and of being able to generate risk estimates for multiple agents using the same data set.

One limitation of all risk estimates is that, in addition to yielding a single best estimate of risk (known as the point estimate), they usually include wide ranges or confidence limits. These wide ranges result from the very low rates of risk being measured and the need to estimate certain variables (as discussed above). Unfortunately, confidence intervals often confuse physicians, patients, and the media, all of whom want to quote a single best number. Therefore, the risk estimates provided in Table 36-1 omit confidence intervals and give only the point estimate. Other limitations of risk estimates are that they become obsolete when newer more sensitive donor screening or laboratory testing protocols are adopted and that they may have been obtained in particular geographic areas, which restricts their generalizability to other locations.

Early studies expressed infection risk on a per-recipient basis. This method of reporting data made it difficult to compare the risk for patients receiving different numbers of transfusion. More recently, it has become standard practice to express the risk of infection on a per-unit or per-blood component basis (i.e., the risk per unit is a given percentage such as

Table 36-1. Per-Unit Risk of Infection From Screened Blood Units in the United States

Agent	1992 Published Estimate	1994 Estimate
HCV	1 in 3,300	1 in 5,000
HTLV[a]	1 in 50,000	1 in 100,000
HBV	1 in 200,000	1 in 200,000
HIV	1 in 225,000	1 in 410,000

Abbreviations: HCV, hepatitis C virus; HTLV, human T-cell lymphotropic virus; HBV, hepatitis B virus; HIV, human immunodeficiency virus.

[a] Only platelets and red cells stored less than 14 days will transmit infection to recipients.

0.001 percent or 1 in a given number such as 1 in 100,000). It is important to remember that when such per-unit risk estimates are presented to an individual patient or a physician, the risk needs to be adjusted for the number of units to be received by that particular patient. Because transfusion risks are of such a small magnitude, the per-patient risk can be approximately obtained by multiplying the per-unit risk by the number of units transfused. The mathematically correct way to determine per-patient risk is as follows, where p represents the probability of infection with a given blood unit and n represents the number of units transfused. The probability that a single unit is free of infection is $(1 - p)$, the probability that all n units that the recipient receives would be infection free is $(1 - p)^n$, and therefore, the probability that a recipient would get infected would be one minus the probability that the recipient would not get infected or $1 - (1 - p)^n$. For small risks, this formula can be ignored, and the direct multiplication described above can be performed.

RISK ESTIMATES FOR SPECIFIC AGENTS

Table 36-1 shows the estimates for transfusion-transmitted infection published in a 1992 *New England Journal of Medicine* editorial[12] and compares these with 1994 estimates derived from more recent data and from mathematic modeling techniques.

For HIV and HCV, the per-unit risk is the same for each type of blood component transfused (i.e., red blood cells, platelets, fresh frozen plasma [FFP], and cryoprecipitate). Furthermore, recipients who receive a component from donors infected with one of these agents have an 80 to 90 percent likelihood of acquiring the infection.[13,14] Although data are not available for HBV, it is likely that similar rates apply, given the high transmission rate from needlestick injury.[15] The situation is different for HTLV because there is no risk of transmission from acellular components (such as FFP or cryoprecipitate) as a result of the required cell association of the virus.[16] Furthermore, transmission rates of HTLV from cellular products obtained from infected donors vary with the length of storage of the blood components; although overall transmission rates in the United States are 33 percent from red cells or platelets,

there has been no transmission from red cell units stored greater than 14 days.[17]

The 1992 estimate for HCV transmission in Table 36-1 was derived before blood was being screened by more sensitive second-generation assays. More recently, it has been estimated that the risk of transfusion-transmitted HCV infections is approximately 1 in 5,000 with the introduction of this improved testing.[18,19] This estimate is based on the observation that, in approximately 10 percent of post-transfusion hepatitis cases, testing of frozen donor sera by second-generation anti-HCV assays did not detect an implicated donor.[19,20] These data are further corroborated by the results of a study of community-acquired hepatitis in which 10 percent of HCV-infected patients were not detected by anti-HCV second-generation antibody testing.[1] Thus, the estimate for transfusion-transmitted HCV risk is based on data that indicate the existence of a chronic, undetectable carrier state. If future data do not corroborate these initial observations, HCV transfusion risk would be confined only to newly infected donors, and the overall risk estimate would be much lower. Incidence data from REDS suggest that window-period HCV transmission may occur at a rate of about 1 per 62,500 units.[10]

HTLV transmission can be expected to occur for the following two reasons: (1) current anti-HTLV-I screening tests do not detect some HTLV-II-infected donors and (2) some donors are newly infected with HTLV-I or HTLV-II. The 1992 estimate for HTLV infection (1 in 50,000 units) was based on the results of a post-transfusion recipient follow-up study performed in two cities in the United States.[6] Newer data provide an alternative method to estimate HTLV risk. The risk from undetected HTLV-II carriers associated with failures of HTLV-I screening assays can be estimated from data on New Mexican blood donors, which indicate that approximately 22 percent of HTLV-II-infected donors were missed by current assays.[3] These data can be combined with the current HTLV-II seroprevalence rate in blood donors in the United States to yield a risk estimate of HTLV-II infection of 0.00084 percent per unit. Incidence data from the REDS indicate that newly acquired HTLV infection (i.e., window period donations) may contribute a risk of 0.00025 percent per unit.[10] The overall risk, which is the sum of these two estimates, is 0.00099 percent or 1 in 100,000 units.

The risk of HBV infection from blood transfusion is extremely low because of the simultaneous use of both hepatitis B surface antigen and hepatitis B core antibody (anti-HB^c) screening assays. By using these two tests, HBV transmission is prevented unless the donor is in the early incubation (window) phase of infection. Based on the incidence of reported cases of symptomatic post-transfusion hepatitis, the risk of HBV is currently estimated to be 1 in 200,000 units; this risk is similar to that of nosocomial HBV transmission.[12,21]

Since 1992, risk estimates for HIV infection have decreased by almost 50 percent from 1 in 225,000 units to 1 in 410,000 units[11,12]; this decreased risk is primarily due to the improved sensitivity of the anti-HIV screening assay, which has decreased the length of the window period by approximately 50 percent (from 45 days to 22 days).[1,22]

Recently, there has been renewed concern about the risk of transmitting bacterial infection by blood transfusion.[23] It is known that septic transfusion reactions are more frequent with transfused platelet concentrates than with red cells; platelets are stored for up to 5 days at room temperature and provide a better growth medium for bacteria than do refrigerated red cells. Data indicate that reported fatal transfusion reactions caused by bacterial sepsis occur at a rate of approximately 1 in 6 million.[24] It has not been possible, however, to assess the rate of significant morbidity from bacterially infected units. Although laboratory data indicate that bacteria can be cultured from up to 0.3 percent of platelet concentrates, the significance of these findings is unclear.[24,25] It is unknown whether these in vitro data represent true contamination of the unit; furthermore, it is not known whether small amounts of transfused bacteria cause recipient morbidity.

PROGRESSION OF TRANSFUSION-TRANSMITTED INFECTION TO DISEASE

Because both HIV and HCV infection ordinarily take years to develop into clinical disease, the impact of transfusion transmission of these agents will not be apparent unless the patient survives for a long period after transfusion. Therefore, the transfusion of many infected components will never produce any clinical effects. Data from look-back studies have indicated that there is approximately a 50 percent likelihood that a specific blood component will have been transfused to an individual who will die within 1 year.[26] (This should not be misinterpreted to indicate that 50 percent of blood recipients die within 1 year but rather that large-volume users with poor prognoses receive a high percentage of transfused blood components).

Recipients who acquire HIV infection from blood transfusion progress to AIDS at a rate similar to that of other infected individuals, now estimated to occur with a mean incubation period of 10 years[27]; therefore, virtually all persons infected with HIV from blood transfusion will eventually have AIDS develop if they survive the underlying disease that necessitated their transfusion. Disease associations arising from HTLV-I or -II infection are much less frequent than HIV. It has been estimated that 4 percent of individuals infected with HTLV-I at birth may progress to adult T-cell leukemia-lymphoma (ATL) during their lifetime, usually after an incubation period of at least 20 to 30 years.[28] A neurologic syndrome, HTLV-I-associated myelopathy has been estimated to occur in 0.25 percent of persons infected with this virus after an incubation period of months to years.[29] A neurologic syndrome similar to that caused by HTLV-I has been documented as a result of HTLV-II infection[30] however, there is no evidence linking HTLV-II infection with ATL.

The natural history of transfusion-acquired HCV is similar to that of HCV acquired through other modes of transmission. Approximately 50 percent of patients will have chronic elevations of liver enzymes, and 20 percent of these will have microscopic evidence of cirrhosis. Although case reports of significant morbidity and deaths have been published, only a small percentage of chronically infected patients (estimated at 1.5 to 5 percent) are likely to become significantly symptomatic.[26,31] An extensive study did not document any excess deaths at 18 years of follow-up in patients with documented post-transfusion HCV infection.[32]

Most transfusion recipients who acquire HBV have the initial infection resolve and immunity develop; in the TTVS, only 1 of 15 HBV-seroconverting recipients had their disease progress to a chronic carrier state.[33] Moreover, additional evidence makes it unlikely that the long-term outcome of transfusion-acquired chronic HBV infection is highly significant. A long-term follow-up study of patients who acquired HBV in adulthood from exposure to contaminated yellow fever vaccine demonstrated lack of serious sequelae and no progression to liver cancer.[34]

Although the risks of acquiring transfusion-transmitted HCV infection are estimated to be 80-fold higher than those of acquiring HIV, the adverse long-term disease outcomes of HIV are probably 20- to 100-fold higher; hence, when both these estimates are considered, it is likely that these viral agents make comparable contributions to long-term morbidity and mortality rates.

In 1992, Dodd[12] concluded that, when the data for all transfusion-transmitted agents are taken into account, it is reasonable to suggest that about 3 in 10,000 blood recipients contract serious or fatal transfusion-transmitted disease. He contrasted this with the results of a study of hospitalized patients in which 60 of 10,000 patients died of accidental or preventable causes other than their underlying disease, a risk that is 20-fold higher than that from blood transfusion.[35]

RISK PERCEPTION

Although it is important that transfusion medicine specialists attempt to quantify risk, it should also be recognized that patients and their families tend to be influenced by psychological and/or emotional factors when they assess risk. Consequently, perceived risk may differ substantially from actual risk, and presentation of quantitative estimates of risk may do little to change the perception of individual patients or the lay public. One approach to understanding factors involved in the public's risk perception is a conceptual model designated as the risk grid.[36] The grid consists of two axes that divide risk into four quadrants. One axis assesses increasing amount of dread, and the other axis plots the degree to which the true risk is unknown or unclear. Studies have revealed that elements that contribute to increased dread include the assessment that the event is uncontrollable, involuntary, unjust, or unfair and that the outcome of the event is catastrophic or fatal. Studies have also concluded that events scoring high on the

dread scale and low on the "clear" knowledge scale will be perceived as riskier than predicted by quantitative estimates; as a consequence, the public will make a greater effort to avoid these situations and will expect government or industry regulators to adopt policies to decrease these risks.[36] The conceptual model discussed above seems to explain clearly the public's considerable fear of acquiring AIDS from blood transfusion; this fear still persists despite good data showing the very small risk of such an occurrence.[37] Additional contributing factors to a higher perception of risk occur when there is not a significant perceived benefit that warrants the risk taking and when the person has little choice but to participate in the risky event.[38]

Public fear about HIV infection from transfusion was heightened in the mid-1980s by the lack of scientific knowledge about the actual risk. Medical experts quoted risks that reflected the number of known transfusion-associated AIDS detected at that time. When it was discovered that the actual risks were far greater than had been stated, the public lost faith in the credibility of the estimates provided by the experts. Many people have remained suspicious and distrustful of subsequent statements about risk made by transfusion medicine specialists.[37,39]

These concepts may explain some aspects of transfusion recipient behavior. For example, some patients still refuse transfusions, continuing to focus on their perceived risk rather than their risk-benefit ratio. As a second example, many people choose to receive blood from a directed donor, despite statistics that show no lowering of risk, perhaps because they believe that they gain control over an otherwise uncontrollable situation.

RISK REDUCTION GOALS

In establishing policies for decreasing the risk of infectious disease transmission by blood transfusion, it is important to define the target goal. The three possibilities are zero risk, minimal risk, and minimal risk at an acceptable cost. With heightened public concern about transfusion safety in the middle to late 1980s, policy formation was driven by an attempt to reduce the risk of blood transfusion to zero.[39] However, because blood transfusion involves a biologic material collected from a human source, it is unlikely that this risk will ever be reduced to zero.[39,40] In considering and evaluating interventions to improve the safety of blood, it appears that certain theoretic principles will hold.[41] First, in a biologic system, it is unlikely that any method can be 100 percent effective. Therefore, if we desire to approach zero risk, multiple overlapping methods are required. Second, when multiple methods are used, procedures become administratively more complex and the potential for error increases. Third, successive risk reductions achieve less but cost more. Fourth, if the risk is already low, it will be extremely difficult to measure the effect of adding additional procedures that are designed to provide further safeguards.

More recently, with the diminished risk of transfusion-associated infection, the pendulum has swung back toward attempting to assess the efficacy and cost impact of an intervention before its implementation. Rather than striving for zero risk, decision making for agents other than HIV is now more likely to be based on minimizing risk at an acceptable cost. With regard to HIV, public concern may still influence policymakers to adopt zero risk as a target goal.[26]

It is useful to review the usual sequence of events that occurs when it is suspected that an infectious disease is transmitted by blood transfusion. To be cautious, safety measures may be implemented even at this initial hypothesis or discovery stage, despite the absence of data proving transmission or quantifying the risk. For example, based on the epidemiologic pattern of the disease, a hypothesis is formulated as to which group in the population is most likely to contain asymptomatic carriers. Criteria may then be adopted for selection of acceptable donors, and appropriate questions may be added to the donor health history. If there is enough interest generated, prototype laboratory tests will be developed. Large-scale prospective seroepidemiologic studies of blood donors or retrospective testing of linked donor and recipient repository samples will be performed. Such studies may influence manufacturers to develop serologic screening tests for Food and Drug Administration (FDA) licensure. Depending on the results of these studies and the deliberations of the FDA and expert blood bank advisory committees, these licensed tests may or may not be implemented for routine blood donor screening.[41]

RISK REDUCTION METHODS

Because of the inherent variability of biologic systems, it is necessary to use multiple methods to minimize the risk of transmitting infection. These methods include the minimizing of unnecessary transfusion, minimizing exposures to multiple donors, donor selection and screening procedures (see Ch. 10), laboratory testing, and modification of the blood unit after collection either by removal of infectious cells or by inactivation of infectious agents.

MINIMIZING ALLOGENEIC EXPOSURE

The fact that recipient risk will be reduced if fewer allogeneic transfusions are administered has prompted changes in transfusion practice over the last decade.[42,43] Some patients receive fewer transfusions as a result of more conservative transfusion criteria being utilized for red cells, platelets, and FFP.[42,44,45] Allogeneic blood requirements for other patients have been reduced by the increased use of autologous blood, through predeposit autologous donation for patients undergoing elective surgery, and/or by intra- and postoperative reinfusion of shed blood.[42,46,47] Many patients can now avoid transfusion as a result of administration of pharmacologic agents that stimulate the coagulation system (desmopressin) or endogenous blood cell production (erythropoetin).[48,49]

The second approach to reduce transfusion risk is to minimize the number of different donors to which the recipient is exposed. Methods to accomplish this include the use of single-donor plateletapheresis products rather than pools of platelet concentrates from six to eight donors, the use of sterile connecting devices to produce small-aliquot components and thereby support neonatal transfusion needs from one rather than many donors, and the collection of multiple blood units for a given recipient from a single dedicated donor at an interval that is shorter than the usual 56-day allogeneic requirement.[42,50–52] These approaches are summarized in Table 36-2 and discussed in detail in various chapters of this textbook; they are mentioned here to illustrate that one driving force in many of the far-reaching changes in transfusion medicine during recent years has been the concern for minimizing in-

Table 36-2. Strategies to Minimize Allogeneic Donor Exposure

Minimize transfusion
    Application of conservative transfusion criteria
    Use of pharmacologic agents
Minimize allogeneic exposures
    Use of autologous blood
    Plateletapheresis therapy
    Sterile connecting devices in neonatal transfusion
    Multiple units from a single dedicated donor

fectious risk associated with exposure to allogeneic blood units from different donors.

LABORATORY TESTING

In 1994, seven screening tests (Table 36-3) are routinely performed on pilot tubes that accompany each donated unit of blood.[53] Five of these seven tests use the enzyme-linked immunosorbent assay method and follow the same general protocol, that is, if the initial optical density of the sample is below the cutoff, the sample is classified as negative for that agent, and the unit is released for transfusion. If the optical density value of the sample exceeds that of the cutoff, the result is classified as initially reactive. These initially reactive samples are retested in duplicate, usually on the next working day, using the original pilot tube and a sample obtained from a second source (another pilot tube or a segment from the unit). If one or both of the duplicate tests are also reactive, the sample is classified as repeat reactive and is, by definition, positive. A positive screening test results in the destruction of the unit. If both repeat test re-

Table 36-3. Routine Laboratory Testing of Donated Blood

Infection or Disease	Test
AIDS	Anti-HIV-1/HIV-2 combo
Hepatitis B	HBsAg, anti-HBc
Hepatitic C	Anti-HCV, anti-HBc, ALT
Syphilis	STS
HTLV*	Anti-HTLV-I

Abbreviations: HTLV, human T-cell lymphotropic virus; AIDS, acquired immunodeficiency syndrome.

sults are negative, the initially reactive result is equivalent to a negative result, and the unit is released from quarantine and transfused. Such an approach is scientifically sound because of the known problems with nonspecific binding resulting in initially positive enzyme immunoassay results that cannot be duplicated on careful repeat testing.

Figure 36-1 details the dates of introduction of various blood donor screening tests in the United States.[53] The introduction of such a large number of tests in a short time interval has introduced several additional challenges to blood donor centers. Because the expansion of testing could be expected to increase the potential for error, blood centers have needed to develop more sophisticated computer systems to handle the complexity of information. This, in turn, has prompted the need for quality assurance programs to validate computer function. This complexity is leading to the development of centralized testing laboratories using automated sampling and testing systems that directly transmit data to appropriately validated computer systems.[39,54]

For any transfusion-transmitted infectious agent, the agent will be of low prevalence in the asymptom-

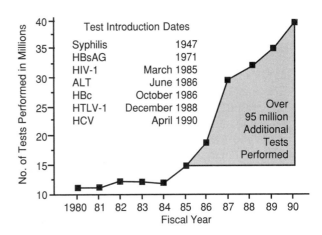

Fig. 36-1. Dates of implementation of donor screening assays and number of tests carried out by American Red Cross Blood Services during the 1980s, by fiscal year (July 1 to June 30). HBsAg, hepatitis B surface antigen; HIV-1, human immunodeficiency virus antibody; ALT, alanine aminotransferase; HBc, hepatitis B core antibody; HTLV-1, human T-cell lymphotropic virus; HCV, hepatitis C virus antibody. (Adapted from McCullough,[53] with permission.)

atic donor population. Therefore, the predictive value of a positive screening test result will be low; in other words, a positive screening test finding will usually be a false-positive result.[55] For this reason, it is essential that screening tests be followed with a more specific supplementary or confirmatory test before notifying donors of their test results. Such tests are often complex and expensive and may need to be performed in reference laboratories. The results of supplemental testing may indicate either that the donor is infected, the result is false positive, and the donor is not infected or they may be inconclusive (indeterminate).

DONOR NOTIFICATION AND DONOR ELIGIBILITY

Blood centers have developed notification and counseling procedures for each type of result for each tested agent.[56] The basic principles of donor notification for confirmed seropositive donors involve providing information to the donor accurately, confidentially, as quickly as possible, and in a manner that alleviates anxiety and promotes understanding. Seropositive donors need to be informed of their ineligibility as donors, the medical significance of their test result, the need to see a physician (if appropriate), and the possible modes of transmission of the agent. Because of the significance of the findings, most blood centers conduct in-person notification of HIV-seropositive donors. Most other notifications are conducted by letter, with the donor being given an opportunity to telephone an appropriate person at the blood center to obtain further information.

Decisions as to the future eligibility of the donor must also be made.[56] For HIV and HCV, donors are ineligible for future donation regardless of confirmatory test results unless they choose to participate in a formal re-evaluation known as re-entry.[56,57] In brief, re-entry involves retesting a blood sample collected at least 6 months subsequent to the repeat reactive screening results, obtaining negative screening and supplemental test results, reviewing all other donor history and test records, and finally deleting the donor's name from a computerized list of deferred donors. In contrast, donors with repeat reactive anti-HBc or anti-HTLV test results (that are not confirmed as positive by supplemental testing) are allowed by FDA regulations to continue donating until a second such occurrence; there are no re-entry programs once these donors are deferred.

MODIFICATION OF BLOOD COMPONENTS AND BLOOD DERIVATIVES

Plasma derivatives are preparations of purified plasma proteins that have therapeutic effect; these derivatives include antihemophilic factor or factor VIII concentrate, factor IX concentrate, albumin, plasma protein fraction (PPF), intravenous immunoglobulin (IVIG), and intramuscular immunoglobulin. Historically, some of these plasma-derived protein products have had a significantly higher infectious disease risk than individual blood components. Because the preparation of plasma derivatives involves the pooling of plasma from thousands of donors, there is a significant likelihood that the pool includes plasma from at least one infectious donor, even if the prevalence of the infectious agent in the donor population is low.[58,59]

Plasma derivatives are manufactured by a process known as Cohn alcohol fractionation. This process has been shown to result in partitioning of viruses into different plasma products and is hypothesized to be one of the reasons why preparations of albumin, PPF, and intramuscular immunoglobulin have been free of the risk of infectious disease transmission. In addition, albumin and PPF are also subjected to a pasteurization step. In contrast, factor VIII and IX preparations have historically shown high rates of disease transmission.[59]

Over the last decade, heat treatment and chemical inactivation techniques have been routinely applied in the manufacture of coagulation factor concentrates and have resulted in dramatically improved safety of these products.[59] Experimentally, the currently used techniques of solvent detergent treatment or wet heating (pasteurization) have been shown to inactivate high titers of viruses; however, solvent detergent treatment is ineffective against nonlipid-enveloped viruses.[60-62] Coagulation factor products prepared by these methods have not been shown to transmit HIV, HBV, or HCV to recipients, whereas transmission was documented from dry-heated products; these particular implicated products were withdrawn from the market after such transmissions were identified.[58] Recent reports have documented several outbreaks of hepatitis A (a non-enveloped virus) in recipients of particular batches of virally inactivated coagulation factors.[63]

Several preparations of IVIG used in Europe have been documented to transmit non-A, non-B hepatitis.[58,64] Furthermore, a recent report documented HCV transmission from a particular preparation of FDA-licensed IVIG despite a long history of safety of similarly prepared intramuscular immunoglobulin preparations licensed in the United States.[58] These events illustrate that continued monitoring of recipients of plasma derivatives is necessary to detect possible transmission of infectious agents; these transmissions may result from failures in the manufacturing process or for unknown reasons.

Over the last several years, investigators have studied many procedures for removal, depletion, or inactivation of viruses and other pathogens from single-donor blood components.[66,67] These approaches include physical modification of components by elaborate filtration and washing procedures and chemical or photochemical treatment of the component. To date, the most success has been obtained with viral inactivation of FFP for which considerations of preserving the functionality of blood cells do not pertain. Three processes, pasteurization (heat treatment), solvent detergent treatment, and photosensitization with methylene blue have all been clinically evaluated in Europe.[66–70] Extensive clinical trials have established that solvent detergent-treated plasma can be safely transfused to patients and has an efficacy similar to FFP. The solvent detergent process is similar to that used for the treatment of plasma derivatives. Briefly, frozen plasma is thawed, multiple ABO identical units are pooled, and the plasma is treated with a mixture of tri-n-butyl phosphate (solvent) and Triton X-100 (detergent) for several hours. The chemicals are then removed by chromatography, and the plasma is filtered and refrozen.[69] In the United States, a license application for solvent detergent-treated plasma is under review by the FDA. Even though this product has been shown to be free of the risk of transmitting lipid-enveloped viruses, risks of transmitting nonenveloped viruses such as hepatitis A and parvovirus B19 still remain.[62] Recently, a cost-benefit analysis modeling the use of solvent detergent-treated plasma in the United States indicated that increased safety will be achieved at a very considerable cost.[71] Thus, even if licensure were forthcoming, it still remains to be determined to what extent this type of plasma will replace FFP in clinical practice.

Modification of cell-containing blood components such as red cells and platelets poses the additional problem of preserving cell function while inactivating viruses and other pathogens. The most promising approach to date involves the use of photosensitization in which chemicals are added to individual blood components, which are then exposed to particular wavelengths of light to activate the chemicals biologically. Virus kill is achieved either by alteration of viral nucleic acid and/or envelope lipoprotein.[66,67] To date, platelet concentrates have been treated with various psoralen compounds with good in vitro results; the results of similar approaches to the treatment of red cells have been more variable.[72–76] Future studies will need to demonstrate preservation of cell function and to establish that infusion of components treated with these chemicals will not adversely affect other genetic material of the host.

One successful modification of cell-containing components is leukocyte reduction using leukocyte depletion filters that remove between 10^3 and 10^4 leukocytes. Numerous studies have shown that this approach significantly reduces the risk of transfusion-transmitted CMV, which is known to be obligatorily associated with leukocytes.[66]

MAINTAINING VIGILANCE FOR "NEW" INFECTIOUS AGENTS

As recent events have illustrated, transfusion medicine specialists must be on guard against the possibility that previously unknown or underappreciated infectious agents may be transmitted by transfusion. Aspects of this vigilance include careful attention to basic research on animal and human infectious diseases and participation in epidemiologic and molecular investigations attempting to find new agents. On the other hand, it is important not to overreact to reports of new "sightings," as the past shows clearly that only the minority stand the test of scientific validation. For example, early claims of retroviruses (and hence transfusion risk) associated with multiple sclerosis, mycosis fungoides, chronic fatigue syndrome, and idiopathic T-cell lymphocytopenia were all false.[77–81]

Once a "new" human retrovirus or infectious agent is found, the transfusion medicine community must work with test manufacturers to develop sensitive and specific serologic screening and confirmation assays. We must then quickly determine the prevalence of the agent among contemporary donors and recipients, its transmissibility by transfusion, its disease consequences, and the incidence of disease among infected donors and recipients. This will require rapid access to large numbers of donor and recipient specimens. In preparation for this scenario, the NHLBI REDS group has built a several repository of several hundred thousand donor samples collected from five geographically diverse blood centers. Previous NHLBI-supported repositories (i.e., TTVS, TSS, and FACTS) represent similar resources, which also include recipient samples.[4–6] Testing of these repositories will enable determination of the retrospective prevalence of the agent among donors, its transmissibility to recipients, and its long-term disease consequences. Some of these repositories include cellular material that can be evaluated by DNA technology. Continued government support and blood center and hospital cooperation in building such repositories are important to ensure that we are prepared to react appropriately in protecting transfusion recipients from newly discovered retroviruses or other infectious agents.

REFERENCES

1. Busch MP, Lee LLL, Satten GA et al: Time course of detection of viral and serological markers preceding HIV-1 seroconversion; implications for blood and tissue donor screening. Transfusion 35:91, 1995
2. Alter MJ, Margolis HS, Krawczynski K et al: The natural history of community-acquired hepatitis C in the United States. N Engl J Med 327:1899, 1992
3. Hjelle B, Wilson C, Cyrus S et al: Human T-cell leukemia virus type II infection frequently goes undetected in contemporary U.S. blood donors. Blood 81:1641, 1993
4. Aach RD, Szmuness W, Mosley JAW et al: Serum alanine aminotransferase of donors in relation to the risk of non-A, non-B hepatitis in recipients. The Transfusion-Transmitted Viruses Study. N Engl J Med 304:989, 1981
5. Kleinman SH, Niland JC, Azen SP et al: Prevalence of antibodies to human immunodeficiency virus type 1 among blood donors prior to screening: the Transfusion Safety Study/NHLBI Donor Repository. Transfusion 29:572, 1989
6. Nelson KE, Donahue JG, Munoz A et al: Transmission of retroviruses from seronegative donors by transfusion during cardiac surgery; a multicenter study of HIV-1 and HTLV-I/II infections. Ann Intern Med 117:554, 1992
7. Alter HJ, Purcell RH, Holland PV et al: Donor transaminase and recipient hepatitis. Impact on blood transfusion services. JAMA 246:630, 1981
8. Busch MP, Eble BE, Khayam-Bashi H et al: Evaluation of screened blood donations for human immunodeficiency virus type 1 infection by culture and DNA amplification of pooled cells. N Engl J Med 325:1, 1991
9. Vyas GN, Rawal BP, Babu G, Busch MP: Diminishing risk of acquiring HIV infection from transfusion of seronegative blood. Transfusion, suppl. 34:S250, 1994
10. Schreiber GB, Busch MP, Gilcher RO et al: Transfusion, suppl S292, 1994
11. Lackritz EM, Satten GA, Raimondi VP et al: Estimated risk of HIV transmission by screened blood in the United States. Program and Abstracts of the Second National Conference on Human Retroviruses and Related Infections, Washington, DC, January 1995, p. 50
12. Dodd RY: The risk of transfusion-transmitted infection. N Engl J Med 327:419, 1992
13. Donegan E, Stuart M, Niland JC et al: Infection with human immunodeficiency virus type 1 (HIV-1) among recipients of antibody-positive blood donations. Ann Intern Med 113:733, 1990
14. Alter HJ, Purcell RH, Shih JW et al: Detection of antibody to hepatitis C virus in prospectively followed transfusion recipients with acute and chronic non-A, non-B hepatitis. N Engl J Med 321:1494, 1989
15. Masuko K, Mitsui T, Iwano K et al: Factors influencing postexposure immunoprophylaxis of hepatitis B virus infection with hepatitis B immune globulin. High deoxyribonucleic acid polymerase activity in the inocula of unsuccessful cases. Gastroenterology 82:502, 1982
16. Okochi K, Satao H, Hinuma Y: A retrospective study on transmission of adult T cell leukemia virus by blood transfusion: seroconversion in recipients. Vox Sang 46:245, 1984
17. Donegan E, Lee H, Operskalski EA et al: Transfusion transmission of retroviruses: human T-lymphotropic viruses types I and II compared with human immunodeficiency virus type 1. Transfusion 34:478, 1994
18. Kleinman S, Busch J, Holland P: Post-transfusion hep-

atitis C virus infection (letter to the editor). N Engl J Med 327:1601, 1992

19. Kleinman S, Alter H, Busch M et al: Increased detection of hepatitis C virus (HCV)-infected blood donors by a multiple-antigen HCV enzyme immunoassay. Transfusion 32:805, 1992

20. Aach RD, Stevens CE, Hollinger FB et al: Hepatitis C virus infection in post-transfusion hepatitis—an analysis with first- and second-generation assays. N Engl J Med 325:1325, 1991

21. Centers for Disease Control: Public Health Service inter-agency guidelines for screening donors of blood, plasma, organs, tissues, and semen for evidence of hepatitis B and hepatitis C. MMWR Morb Mortal Wkly Rep 40 (RR-4):1, 1991

22. Petersen LR, Satten GA, Dodd R et al: Duration of time from onset of development of detectable antibody. Transfusion 34:283, 1994

23. Blajchman MA: Transfusion-associated bacterial sepsis: the phoenix rises yet again. Transfusion 34:940, 1994

24. Wagner SJ, Friedman LI, Dodd RY: Transfusion-associated bacterial sepsis. Clin Microbiol Rev 7:290, 1994

25. Goldman M, Blajchman MA: Blood product-associated bacterial sepsis. Transfusion Med Rev 5:73, 1991

26. Dodd RY: Adverse consequences of blood transfusion: quantitative risk estimates. p. 1. In Nance ST (ed): Blood Supply Risks, Perceptions and Prospects for the Future. American Association of Blood Banks, Bethesda, 1994

27. Brookmeyer R: Reconstruction and future trends of the AIDS epidemic in the United States. Science 253: 37, 1991

28. Murphy EL, Hanchard B, Figueroa JP et al: Modeling the risk of adult T-cell leukemia/lymphoma in persons infected with human T-lymphotropic virus type I. Int J Cancer 43:250, 1980

29. Kaplan JE, Osame M, Kubota H et al: The risk of development of HTLV-I-associated myelopathy/tropical spastic paraparesis among persons infected with HTLV-I. J Acquir Immune Defic Syndr Hum Retrovirol 3:1096, 1990

30. Murphy EL, Fridey J, Smith JW et al: High prevalence of HTLV-associated myelopathy in a cohort of HTLV-I and HTLV-II infected blood donors. Ann Neurol 1995 (submitted)

31. Alter HJ: You'll wonder where the yellow went: a 15-year retrospective of post-transfusion hepatitis. p. 53. In Moore SB (ed): Transfusion Transmitted Viral Diseases. American Association of Blood Banks, Arlington, 1987

32. Seeff LB, Buskell-Bales Z, Wright EC et al: Long-term mortality after transfusion-associated non-A, non-B hepatitis. N Engl J Med 327:1906, 1992

33. Mimms LT, Mosley JAW, Hollinger FB et al: Effect of concurrent acute infection with hepatitis C virus on acute hepatitis B virus infection. BMJ 307:1095, 1993

34. Seeff LB, Beebe GW, Hoofnagle JH et al: A serologic follow-up of the 1942 epidemic of post-vaccination hepatitis in the United States Army. N Engl J Med 316:965, 1991

35. Leape LL, Brennan TA, Laird N et al: The nature of adverse events in hospitalized patients—results of the Harvard Medical Practice Study II. N Engl J Med 324: 377, 1991

36. Slovic P: Perception of risk. Science 236:280, 1987

37. Menitove JE: Perception of risk. p. 45. In Nance ST (ed): Blood Supply Risks, Perceptions and Prospects for the Future. American Association of Blood Banks, Bethesda, 1994

38. Gregory R, Mendelsohn R: Perceived risk, dread, and benefits. Risk Anal 13:259, 1993

39. Perkins HA: Safety of the blood supply: making decisions in transfusion medicine. p. 125. In Nance SJ (ed): Blood Safety: Current Challenges. American Association of Blood Banks, Bethesda, 1992

40. Zuck TF: Greetings: a final look back with comments about a policy of a zero-risk blood supply. Transfusion 27:47, 1987

41. Kleinman S: Donor screening procedures and their role in enhancing transfusion safety. p. 207. In Smith D, Dodd RY (eds): Transfusion Transmitted Infection. American Society of Clinical Pathologists, Chicago, 1991

42. AuBuchon JP: Minimizing donor exposure in hemotherapy. Arch Pathol Lab Med 118:380, 1994

43. Soumerai SB, Salem-Schatz SR, Avorn J et al: A controlled trial of educational outreach to improve blood transfusion practice. JAMA 270:961, 1993

44. Office of Medical Application of Research, National Institutes of Health: Perioperative red cell transfusion. JAMA 260:2700, 1988

45. Gmur J, Burger J, Schanz U et al: Safety of stringent prophylactic platelet transfusion policy for patients with acute leukemia. Lancet 338:1223, 1991

46. Hallett JAW, Popovsky MA, Ilstrup D: Minimizing blood transfusions during abdominal aortic surgery: recent advances in rapid autotransfusion. J Vasc Surg 5:601, 1987

47. Giordano GF, Rivers SL, Chung GKT et al: Autologous platelet-rich plasma in cardiac surgery: effect on intraoperative and postoperative transfusion requirements. Ann Thorac Surg 46:416, 1988

48. Salzman EW, Weinstein MJ, Weintraub RM et al:

Treatment with desmopressin acetate to reduce blood loss after cardiac surgery. N Engl J Med 341:1402, 1986

49. Eschbach JW, Adamson JW: Guidelines for recombinant human erythropoietin therapy. Am J Kidney Dis 14:2, 1989

50. Shah VP, Applel SA: Limiting neonatal donor exposure by using assigned red blood cell units up to 24 days. Transfusion, suppl 32:11S, 1992

51. Brecher ME, Taswell HF, Clare DE et al: Minimal-exposure transfusion and the committed donor. Transfusion 30:599, 1990

52. Strauss RG, Wieland MR, Randels MJ, Koerner TA: Feasibility and success of a single-donor red cell program for pediatric elective surgery. Transfusion 32:747, 1992

53. McCullough J: The nation's changing blood supply system. JAMA 269:2239, 1993

54. Barbara JAJ: Challenges in transfusion microbiology. Transfusion Med Rev 7:96, 1993

55. Kaplan H, Kleinman SH: AIDS: Blood donor studies and screening programs. p. 297. In Dodd RY, Barker LF (eds): Infection, Immunity and Blood Transfusion. Alan R. Liss, New York, 1985

56. Bianco C, Kessler D: Donor notification and counseling management of blood donors with positive test results. Vox Sang 67:255, 1994

57. Center for Biologics Evaluation and Research, FDA: Revised Recommendations for the Prevention of Human Immunodeficiency Virus (HIV) Transmission by Blood and Blood Products. April 23, 1992, Rockville, MD

58. Epstein J, Fricke W: Current safety of clotting factor concentrates. Arch Pathol Lab Med 114:335, 1990

59. Suomela H: Inactivation of viruses in blood and plasma products. Transfusion Med Rev 7:52, 1993

60. Pollard E: Theory of the physical means of the inactivation of viruses. Ann N Y Acad Sci 83:654, 1960

61. Prince A, Horowitz B, Brotman B: Sterilization of hepatitis and HTLV-III viruses by exposure to tri (n-butyl)-phosphate and sodium cholate. Lancet 1:706, 1986

62. Horowitz B, Wiebe M, Lippin A et al: Inactivation of viruses in labile blood derivatives. Transfusion 25:516, 1985

63. Mannucci PM, Gdovin S, Gringeri A et al: Transmission of hepatitis A to patients with hemophilia by factor VIII concentrates treated with organic solvent and detergent to inactivate viruses. The Italian Collaborative Group. Ann Intern Med 120:1, 1994

64. Bjorkander J, Cunningham-Rundles C, Lundin P et al: Intravenous immunoglobulin prophylaxis causing liver damage in 16 of 77 patients with hypogammaglo-bulinemia or IgG subclass deficiency. Am J Med 84:107, 1988

65. Centers for Disease Control: Outbreak of hepatitis C associated with intravenous immunoglobulin administration—United States, October 1993-June 1994. Morb Mortal Wkly Rep 43:505, 1994

66. Friedman LI, Stromberg RR, Wagner SJ: Reducing the infectivity of blood components—what we have learned. In Nance ST (ed): Blood Supply: Risks, Perceptions and Prospects for the Future. American Association of Blood Banks, Bethesda, 1994

67. Pehta JC: Viral inactivation of blood components. Lab Med 25:102, 1994

68. Burnouf-Radosevich M, Burnouf T, Haurt J: A pasteurized therapeutic plasma. Infusionsther Transfusionsmed 19:91, 1992

69. Horowitz B, Bonomo R, Prince A et al: Solvent/detergent-treated plasma: a virus-inactivated substitute for fresh frozen plasma. Blood 79:826, 1992

70. Lambrecht B, Mohr H, Knuver-Hopf J et al: Photoinactivation of viruses in fresh plasma by phenothiazine dyes in combination with visible light. Vox Sang 60:207, 1991

71. AuBuchon JP, Birkmeyer JD: Safety and cost-effectiveness of solvent-detergent-treated plasma: in search of a zero-risk blood supply. JAMA 272:1210, 1994

72. O'Brien J, Montgomery R, Burns W et al: Evaluation of merocyanine 540-sensitized photoirradiation as a means to inactivate enveloped viruses in blood products. J Lab Clin Med 116:439, 1991

73. Horowitz B, Rywkin S, Margolis-Nuno H et al: Inactivation of viruses in red cell and platelet concentrates with aluminum phthalocyanine sulfonates. Blood Cells 18:141, 1991

74. Margolis-Nunno H, Williams B, Rywkin S et al: Virus sterilization in platelet concentrates with psoralen and ultraviolet light in the presence of quenchers. Transfusion 32:541, 1991

75. Lin L, Wieshahn G, Morel P et al: Use of 8-methoxy psoralen and long-wavelength ultraviolet radiation for decontamination of platelet concentrates. Blood 74:517, 1989

76. Corash L, Lin L, Wiesehahn G: Use of 8-methoxy psoralen and long-wavelength ultraviolet radiation for decontamination of platelet concentrates. Blood 82:292, 1993

77. Reddy EP, Sandberg-Wollheim M, Mettus R et al: Amplification and molecular cloning of HTLV-I sequences from DNA of multiple sclerosis patients. Science 243:529, 1989

78. Richardson JH, Wucherpfenning KW, Endo N et al:

PCR analysis of DNA from multiple sclerosis patients for the presence of HTLV-I. Science 246:821, 1989

79. Zucker-Franklin D, Coutaves EE, Rush MG, Zouzias DC: Detection of human T-lymphotropic virus-like particles in cultures of peripheral blood lymphocytes from patients with mycosis fungoides. Proc Natl Acad Sci U S A 88:7630, 1991

80. Busch MP, Murphy EL, Nemo G for the REDS Study Group: More on HTLV tax and mycosis fungoides (comments on Pancake, Zucker-Franklin). N Engl J Med 329:2035, 1993

81. Heredia A, Hewlett IK, Soriano V, Epstein JS: Idiopathic CD4 + T lymphocytopenia: a review and current perspective. Transfusion Med Rev 7:223, 1994

Retroviral Infections

Michael P. Busch

This chapter reviews those aspects of human retrovirus epidemiology and pathophysiology of greatest relevance to specialists in transfusion medicine. First, the molecular characteristics and life cycle of retroviruses and the evolution of our understanding of their role in human diseases is briefly reviewed. The four major known pathogenic human retroviruses (human immunodeficiency virus types 1 and 2 [HIV-1, HIV-2] and human T cell leukemia/lymphoma viruses [HTLV-I, HTLV-II]) are discussed next, beginning with a hindsight view of the epidemiology of each virus in blood donor and recipient populations prior to implementation of routine donor screening. Next, data on transmissibility of each agent by transfusions and on the disease consequences of infection in donors and recipients is reviewed. The sections focused on each agent conclude with an outline of the current testing algorithm used in blood banks and a review of the current risk of viral transmission by screened blood transfusions. The final section of the chapter addresses the need for additional donor screening procedures, as well as efforts directed at detection of as yet unrecognized retroviruses in the blood supply.

DEFINITION, LIFE CYCLE, AND DISTRIBUTION OF RETROVIRUSES

Retroviruses comprise a major class of membrane-coated, single-stranded RNA viruses. They are characterized by their distinct genomic organization, the presence of viral particle (virion)-associated reverse transcriptase, and a unique replication cycle (Fig. 37-1). After entry into a host cell, typically by fusion of the virion and host cell membranes, the reverse transcriptase enzyme copies viral RNA into complementary double-stranded DNA (cDNA). Virion-associated integrase then mediates integration of this cDNA into random sites in the host cell's chromosome, forming integrated viral cDNAs termed *proviruses*. Subsequent transcription, processing, and translation of viral genes are mediated principally by host cell enzymes, although both viral and host cell regulatory gene products influence the level and pattern of viral gene expression and replication. The classic retrovirus life cycle is completed when nascent particles associate and bud from the plasma membrane to form progeny virions, which can then infect other cells and other organisms. Retroviruses can also spread horizontally by fusion of infected and uninfected cells, or vertically by replication of integrated viral DNA along with cellular DNA during mitosis or meiosis. Indeed, integrated proviruses have evolved that are passed congenitally through the germ line; these so-called endogenous retroviral elements (as contrasted with vertically transmitted exogenous retroviruses) are present in many species, including humans, and in some species account for up to 10 percent of total genomic DNA[1].

Retroviruses are distributed widely in nature; examples exist in genera ranging from insects to rep-

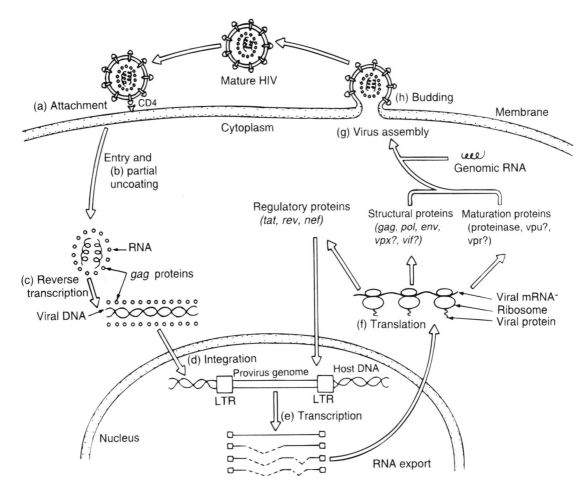

Fig. 37-1. Replication cycle of human immunodeficiency virus type 1. *(a)* After attachment of virus particles to the CD4-receptor molecule, virus enters the cell by a pH-dependent mechanism and/or endocytosis. *(b)* The outer lipid envelope of the virus is removed when the particle undergoes fusion with cytoplasmic vacuoles. *(c)* The core particle that remains is the site for reverse transcription of the virion RNA into DNA. *(d)* After translocation into the nucleus, integration into the DNA of the cell occurs. *(e)* The integrated provirus genome is transcribed by cellular RNA polymerase II. *(f)* Translation of viral messenger (m)RNA produces regulatory proteins, which stimulate synthesis of maturation proteins and the structural proteins of the virion. *(g)* Accumulation of structural proteins in the cell membrane permits the assembly of virus particles. *(h)* Maturation and release from the cell by budding. (From Mayer and Busch,[149] with permission.)

tiles to virtually all mammals.[1] Animal retroviruses have highly variable disease manifestations. Many species harbor exogenous or endogenous retroviruses that appear to be benign, and may in fact be beneficial in restricting infection by related pathogenic retroviruses. On the other hand, retroviruses became the focus of intense research in the 1960s and 1970s because of their capacity to induce malig-

nancies in a wide range of species. The demonstration that certain retroviruses (termed *acute RNA tumor viruses*) rapidly transform target cells in vitro and induce tumors within days to weeks of inoculation into animals greatly facilitated experimental investigation of viral carcinogenesis.[2] Studies of the molecular differences between these acute retroviruses and genetically related slow viruses (which failed to transform cells in vitro and only occasionally caused tumors many months after inoculation) led to the discovery of viral oncogenes, which were responsible for tumorigenesis. This was followed by the revolutionary discovery that these viral oncogenes had in fact arisen by recombination events between slow viruses and key cellular genes termed *proto-oncogenes*.[2] Thus, investigation of retrovirus-induced cancers in animals led to unparalleled insights into normal cell biology and disease pathogenesis in humans.

Despite intense research throughout the 1960s and 1970s directed at isolating human retroviruses from patients with a wide variety of diseases, exogenous human retroviruses remained elusive. Several early reports of human retroviruses isolated from brain and mammary neoplasms proved to be due to contaminating animal viruses.[1] Other claims of human retrovirus detection by electron microscopy, reverse transcriptase assays, and DNA hybridization or immunologic techniques could not be replicated. The first report of successful isolation and characterization of a bonafide human retrovirus (later termed HTLV-I) occurred in 1980 and involved a patient with a rare type of leukemia (now termed adult T cell leukemia [ATL]).[3] A series of follow-up studies in the early 1980s failed to show any serologic association between this virus and other human diseases.[4] (See below for subsequent developments.) A second, closely related human retrovirus (HTLV-II) was isolated in 1982 from a patient with a somewhat more common type of leukemia (hairy cell leukemia)[5]; however, further surveys failed to show a relationship between HTLV-II and either hairy cell leukemia or any other diseases.[4,6] Thus, in the early 1980s it appeared as if humans had been essentially spared the ravages of this unique class of infectious agents. Then in 1984, HIV was established as the cause of acquired immune deficiency syndrome (AIDS).

HUMAN IMMUNODEFICIENCY VIRUS TYPE 1

Risk of Transfusions Before Discovery and Donor Anti-HIV-1 Screening

The HIV-1 epidemic presents an excellent example of how an infectious agent with a prolonged clinical incubation period (i.e., the interval between initial infection and clinically apparent disease) can spread silently within a population (and its blood donor base) for years before recognition.[7] In the United States, this early phase was localized primarily to homosexual and bisexual men, groups who were eligible blood donors at the time. Although we now know that the virus began to spread at an exponential rate in these men in the late 1970s, it was not until 1981 that clusters of Kaposi's sarcoma and pneumocystis pneumonia were first recognized among homosexual men in New York and Los Angeles. In late 1982, descriptions of AIDS-like illnesses in hemophiliacs and recipients of blood components first appeared.[8,9] With these reports, a blood-borne infectious etiology for AIDS became probable, and efforts were initiated to exclude from blood donation persons with symptoms of or risk factors associated with AIDS.[10] Approximately a year later HIV-1 was discovered, followed rapidly by development of the anti-HIV-1 tests, which were licensed for donor screening in March 1985.

Although over a decade has passed since the first cases of AIDS were reported in hemophiliacs and transfusion recipients, we continue to learn about the scope of the HIV-1 epidemic among these patient groups during the prescreening era and about the effectiveness of measures to reduce transmission. The Transfusion Safety Study (TSS) was able to piece together an accurate picture of the risk of a transfusion recipient having been infected with HIV-1 between 1978 and 1985 in San Francisco by combining seroprevalence data from local studies involving the rate of infection among homosexual men with data from the TSS Donor Repository collected in San Francisco in late 1984[11] (Fig. 37-2). This analysis showed that the risk of transfusion-associated (TA) HIV-1 infection rose rapidly from its first occurrence in 1978 to a peak risk of approximately 1.1 percent per transfused unit in late 1982. Beginning in early 1983 and continuing through implementation of anti-HIV-1 screening, there was marked, progressive decline in risk as a result of declining number of blood donations from at-risk or infected individuals. This decline was directly attributable to increasing awareness of the infectious nature of AIDS in the homosexual community and to implementation and refinement of donor education and deferral measures by blood banks.[11,12] In fact, in San Francisco,

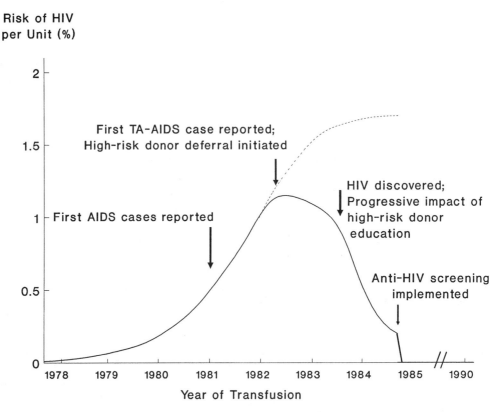

Fig. 37-2. Risk of human immunodeficiency virus (HIV-1) infections from transfusions in San Francisco before anti-HIV screening. Solid line represents estimated risk of recipient infection per unit transfused. Dashed line indicates what the risk would have been if high-risk donor deferral measures had not been implemented. The risk in the United States as a whole probably trailed that in San Francisco by approximately 1 year, and the peak risk was of lower magnitude. (Modified from Busch et al.,[11] with permission.)

we estimated that approximately 90 percent of high-risk men who were donors between 1980 and 1982 self-deferred prior to implementation of the anti-HIV-1 test in early 1985.[11] These data illustrate dramatically the effectiveness of donor education and self-deferral measures.

Kroner et al. recently reported a similar analysis of incidence of HIV-1 seroconversion over time among hemophiliacs.[13] These investigators compiled incidence and prevalence data from 1978 through 1990 for 16 hemophiliac cohorts in the United States and Europe. They estimated the overall hazard of HIV-1 infection over time, as well as the variation in risk according to geographic region and type and dose of factor concentrate. Infections began in 1978, peaked in October 1982 at 22 infections per 100 person-years

at risk, and declined to 4 per 100 person-years by July 1984 (Fig. 37-3). Although few new infections occurred among hemophiliacs after 1986, by that time, 50 percent of subjects in the combined cohort were infected. Median seroconversion dates for infected hemophiliacs in U.S. cohorts ranged from July 1980 for those treated with high doses of factor VIII, to December 1983 for those treated with low doses of factor IX; corresponding dates for European cohorts were approximately 1 year later, reflecting the delay in importation and use of products manufactured from American plasma. The decline in incidence from the infection peak in late 1982 coincided with health interventions introduced to reduce transmission, including recommendations for reduction in use of factor concentrates in 1982, voluntary donor deferral in

1983, availability of heat-treated factor VIII in 1984, and HIV-1 screening in 1985.

This temporal profile for the risk of HIV from blood components and derivatives was further corroborated in a recent report from the Centers for Disease Control and Prevention (CDC),[14] in which 4,619 TA AIDS cases reported from 1982 through 1991 were reviewed. (These cases represented 2 percent of the 222,418 overall U.S. AIDS cases reported over that period.) When these same cases were analyzed by year of AIDS diagnosis (with adjustment for delay between diagnosis and report), the number of TA AIDS cases climbed steeply from 14 in 1982 to 824 in 1987, and subsequently remained relatively stable through 1991 (hatched bars in Fig. 37-4). In contrast, when these same cases were plotted by year of implicated transfusion that led to HIV infection, the number of cases rose from 56 in 1978 to 714 in 1984, dropped sharply to 288 by 1985 when screening for antibody began, and fell to a mean of 20 per year from 1986 through 1991 (solid bars in Fig. 37-4). This difference reflects the incubation period between infection (transfusion) and diagnosis of clinical AIDS (see below). For example, over 95 percent of TA AIDS cases diagnosed in 1991 were attributable to transfusions received before implementation of anti-HIV screening in early 1985. Upon further

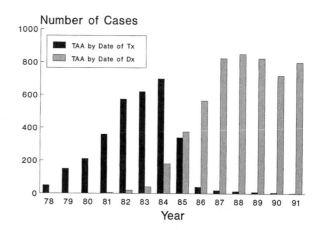

Fig. 37-4. Distribution of 5,058 transfusion-associated cases of acquired immunodeficiency syndrome reported to the Centers for Disease Control and Prevention as of June 30, 1992, plotted both according to year of transfusion (solid bars) and year of diagnosis (hatched bars). (Adapted from Selik et al.,[14] with permission.)

investigation, the patients in many of the cases diagnosed from post-1985 transfusions were found to be infected from sources other than HIV seronegative blood transfusions[14] (see below).

Rate of Transmission by Transfusion

Clinical, virologic, and immunologic studies of exposed transfusion recipients and hemophiliacs have yielded a number of insights into the significance of factors that might influence transmission of HIV-1 infection and disease course. The TSS, which is unique in being the only study that traced and enrolled recipients of known seropositive units,[15,16] offers some of the clearest data addressing these issues. In the TSS, 111 (89.5 percent) of 124 enrolled recipients transfused with anti-HIV-1–positive blood components seroconverted to anti-HIV-1 positivity.[16] Neither characteristics of the donor's infection nor inherent recipient susceptibility factors significantly influenced transmission of HIV-1 by transfusions.[17] The only variables that have been identified to correlate with likelihood of HIV-1 transmission are the type of blood component transfused and its duration of storage.[18] Washed red blood cell (RBC) units and RBC units stored more than 26 days had lower transmission rates than other components. This suggests that component manipulations that reduce the num-

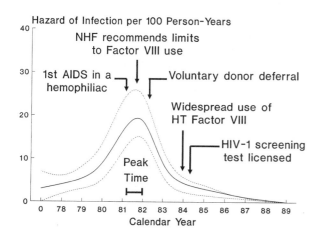

Fig. 37-3. Estimates of human immunodeficiency virus type 1 infection rate (risk among susceptibles) from 1978 to 1989 for a five-center cohort of 636 hemophiliacs. ---, 95 percent confidence interval. (From Kroner et al.,[13] with permission.)

ber of viable leukocytes and/or free virus in plasma may reduce but not eliminate infectiousness. Indeed, subsequent studies have demonstrated reduction in HIV infectiousness (and that of other viruses) by filtration of leukocytes from blood components,[19] and routine filtration has been proposed as an ancillary measure to further reduce infectious risks of transfusion.[20]

With regard to recipients of clotting factor concentrates, an average of approximately 50 percent of hemophiliacs treated with factor VIII in the early 1980s seroconverted.[13,21] However, those hemophiliacs treated with very high doses of factor VIII (> 500,000 units) seroconverted to anti-HIV-1 positivity at a rate approaching 100 percent.[13] This indicates that no one is resistant to HIV-1 infection given a large enough inoculum and repeated exposures. Although there was early hope that a proportion of seropositive hemophiliacs might have seroconverted as a result of exposure to denatured HIV-1 proteins rather than infectious virus, several large studies have confirmed persistent HIV-1 infection in 100 percent of seropositive hemophiliacs using sensitive viral culture and polymerase chain reaction (PCR) techniques.[22,23] On the other hand, while several early studies using PCR reported detection of HIV-1 DNA in a subset of seronegative-exposed hemophiliacs,[24] recent studies have refuted these reports[25,26] as well as the general concept of seronegative (so-called immunosilent) HIV-1 infections.[27]

Clinical Course of Infection in Transfusion Recipients and Hemophiliacs

Studies of the outcome of HIV-1 infection in transfusion recipients are of particular interest because the date of infection/transfusion is precisely known, and because recipients lack many cofactors (e.g., other sexually transmitted diseases or intravenous drug use) that might influence disease course in other infected cohorts. In addition, the transfusion setting is unique in that disease course in the recipient can be compared to that in a linked donor, thus allowing the study of whether a relationship exists between disease progression in a donor and his or her recipients.[17,28,29]

Of the 112 infected recipients enrolled in the TSS, 37 had progressed to AIDS (CDC's 1987 revised definition) by 7 years of post-transfusion follow-up.[30]

Based on Kaplan-Meyer analysis, the actuarial risk of AIDS at 7 years was 51 percent. This rate is faster than the rate of progression observed for the infected donors and hemophiliacs followed in parallel in that study.[30,31] As observed by others,[32] an effect of age on rate of disease progression was noted in all three TSS groups, with older patients manifesting symptoms of AIDS earlier than younger individuals. Once age and underlying disease were controlled for, progression rates to clinical AIDS were virtually identical for TSS recipients and hemophiliacs, whereas the rate of AIDS diagnosis was slightly higher for enrolled donors (most of whom were homosexual men).[30] This suggests that factors such as route of infection, inoculum size, and proposed cofactors, such as other viral infections (e.g., cytomegalovirus or hepatitis B virus), are not highly significant in determining HIV disease course. Continuing study of linked donors and recipients enrolled in TSS (so-called transmission clusters), including detailed comparisons of genetic evolution of viral genes over time (so-called quasispecies analysis), should contribute significantly to our understanding of the relative importance of viral strain versus host factors in HIV pathogenesis.[28,29,33–35]

HUMAN IMMUNODEFICIENCY VIRUS TYPE 2

HIV-2, discovered in 1985 in several countries in West Africa, was initially called HTLV-IV and lyphadenopathy-associated virus type 2. More recently, HIV-2 has spread throughout Western Europe, where a substantial number of infected blood donors have been detected and where cases of transfusion transmission have been documented.[36] HIV-2 is transmitted in the same manner as HIV-1 (i.e., by sexual contact, intravenous drug use, and, at a lower rate than for HIV-1, from mother to child). HIV-2 causes progressive immunodeficiency, with susceptibility to a similar array of opportunistic infections, as seen with HIV-1. Recent studies indicate that rates of disease progression and secondary viral transmission are lower in persons infected with HIV-2 as compared to HIV-1, possibly due to lower viral burden in HIV-2 infection.[37]

HIV-1 and HIV-2 are highly (> 50 percent) homologous at the nucleic acid sequence level, and they cross-react immunologically to a great extent (particularly the core and polymerase antigens). For this reason, up to 90 percent of sera from HIV-2-infected persons have been found to test positive on U.S. Food and Drug Administration (FDA)-licensed anti-HIV-1 assays, with variable reactivity on HIV-1 Western blots.[38,39] This cross-reactivity undoubtedly prevented transfusion-transmission of HIV-2 by anti-HIV-1-screened blood in areas where the virus was present prior to implementation of combination HIV-1/HIV-2 screening tests. This high-level cross-reactivity has also facilitated surveillance for HIV-2 in regions where it is currently rare or absent.[40,41]

In a comprehensive review of the extent of HIV-2 in the United States through the end of 1991, CDC identified 17 case reports with confirmed HIV-2 infection.[36] Of these 17 cases, 13 had immigrated to the United States from West Africa, a fact that formed the basis for the geographic exclusion from donation of sub-Saharan Africans prior to implementation of improved HIV-2-sensitive screening assays in early 1992. One of the case reports was an American woman identified as reactive on anti-HIV-1 enzyme immunoassay (EIA) screening (indeterminate Western blot) after a volunteer blood donation in New York City in 1986; she had recently traveled to Africa but denied specific risk factors for infection.[42] She remains the only U.S. blood donor identified as infected with HIV-2 (through mid-1994). To date, no cases of HIV-2-infected transfusion recipients have been reported in the United States.

Serologic surveys of over 40,000 samples from high-risk persons (homosexual men, intravenous drug users, and sexually transmitted disease clinic patients) in U.S. cities that are frequent destinations of immigrants from West Africa have uncovered 2 additional probable cases of HIV-2 infection.[36] An additional 11 probable cases were found by testing 2,771 HIV-1 Western blot–indeterminate samples from New York and Maryland HIV-1 testing sites. In contrast, retrospective analysis of 35,000 HIV-1 EIA-reactive donor sera identified through screening of over 24 million donations through 1991 has failed to uncover any additional HIV-2 infected blood donors.[36,40,41]

Based on these data, the CDC estimated the current prevalence of HIV-2 in U.S. blood donors at less than 3 infected units per 10 million screened donations.[36] Although these data indicate a very low

prevalence of HIV-2 in the United States, the virus will almost certainly increase in prevalence over time. For this reason, combination HIV-1/2 assays were developed,[43–45] and mandatory implementation of either a combination test or a separate anti-HIV-2 test in the donor screening setting was required by the FDA effective June 1, 1992.[46] As of August 1994, prospective donor screening with either anti-HIV-2 or anti-HIV-1/2 reagents has failed to detect any additional infected donors.

CURRENT HIV-1/2 TESTING ALGORITHM USED BY BLOOD BANKS

Routine serologic screening of blood donors for antibodies to HIV-1 and HIV-2 is carried out according to the scheme shown in Figure 37-5. All units of blood are now screened using licensed enzyme immunoassays that are sensitive to both anti-HIV-1 and

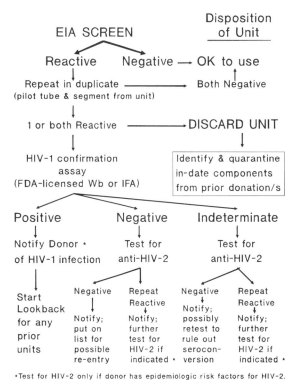

Fig. 37-5. Algorithm for current routine screening and supplemental testing of blood donors. (From Schochetnan and George,[52] with permission.)

anti-HIV-2.[43–46] Initial testing is performed on serum or plasma from "pilot" tubes collected at the time of donation. If this initial test is reactive, repeat testing is performed on both the originally tested pilot tube serum/plasma and either a second pilot tube or an aliquot of plasma obtained from segmented tubing attached to the blood components. This element of the algorithm is designed as an additional safeguard to identify and resolve possible specimen labeling errors. If one or both repeat tests are reactive, the unit is designated "repeat reactive" and discarded. A process is also initiated to identify and quarantine all in-date components from any prior donation(s) from that donor.[47]

Supplemental testing must use FDA-licensed reagents, and rule out both HIV-1 and HIV-2 infection.[46] Although combination HIV-1/HIV-2 supplemental assays using recombinant DNA-derived or synthetic peptide antigens have been developed that appear to accurately detect and discriminate anti-HIV-1 and anti-HIV-2,[48] these are not yet approved by FDA. Therefore, current confirmatory algorithms in U.S. blood banks employ HIV-1 viral lysate-based Western blots or immunofluorescence assays, in combination with a licensed anti-HIV-2 EIA and unlicensed HIV-2 supplemental assays.[46] Interpretive criteria for Western blots have evolved over time as tests have improved and our understanding of the meaning of various banding patterns has increased. For currently licensed assays, a positive interpretation requires antibody reactivity to 2 of the following 3 HIV antigens: p24 (the major *gag* protein), gp41 (transmembrane *env* protein) or gp120/160 (external *env* protein/*env* precursor protein). While these criteria are generally very accurate, recent reports indicate that some donors who show antibody reactivity only to the envelope glycoproteins are not infected with HIV-1.[49] It is important, therefore, that all initial positive Western blot results are confirmed using a separate follow-up sample, both to rule out specimen mix-up or testing errors and to discriminate nonspecific patterns from early seroconversion.[44,45,48,49] A negative test result on Western blot is, by definition, the absence of any bands. Any other pattern of reactivity is classified as indeterminate. Only a very small proportion of donors who test indeterminate on Western blot are infected with HIV-1.[50,51] Detailed discussion of interpretive criteria

and review of recent developments in HIV supplemental test technology can be found in Schochetman and George.[52]

All repeat-reactive donors are deferred from further blood donations and notified of their screening and supplemental test results. For confirmed positive donors, recipients of prior donations are traced in a process called "lookback."[47,53] Donors whose supplemental test results are completely negative are eligible for possible reentry into the donor pool according to an FDA-specified protocol.[46] Critical aspects of the reentry protocol include a 6-month interval between the initial repeat-reactive donation and a reentry sample, both of which must test negative on reentry testing using two licensed EIAs (at least one of which is viral lysate based) and a licensed supplemental assay. Although donors with persistent indeterminate Western blot patterns are currently ineligible for re-entry, this policy is presently under review by the FDA, and it is possible that such donors will be allowed to donate in the future if they test negative by EIA on follow-up.

PERFORMANCE OF HIV SCREENING TESTS OVER TIME

Developments in test methodology have occurred at a rapid rate, and blood banks have implemented improved assays as soon as possible after FDA licensure. The evolution of antibody assays has been achieved by improvements in the antigens on the solid phase, and in assay formats. From crude viral lysates, production moved to viral lysate assays spiked with purified HIV-1 antigens, and then on to use of cloned (recombinant DNA [rDNA]-derived) and synthetic peptide antigens. Although concerns have been raised regarding sensitivity of rDNA and peptide antigen-based EIAs to immunologically variant strains,[54] these assays have been "engineered" to include highly selected antigenic regions of HIV-1 and HIV-2 that maximize sensitivity to infected subjects from around the world. Consequently, rDNA-derived and synthetic peptide antigen-based assays are now in wide use in U.S. blood banks. Test manufacturers have also developed new assay formats that have increased capacity to detect low-titer IgM antibody produced during early seroconversion. For example, the recombinant "antigen sand-

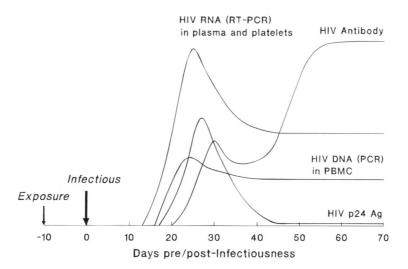

Fig. 37-6. Sequence of virologic events during primary human immunodeficiency virus (HIV) infection: hematologic dissemination consistent with an infectious blood donation (defined as day 0) occurs 1 to 2 weeks after HIV exposure; viremia is first detectable by reverse-transcription (RT)-PCR for HIV-RNA in plasma or platelets on days 14 to 16, with viral RNA and p24 antigen levels peaking between days 20 and 30; infected (DNA PCR-positive) leukocytes are detected subsequent to free virus at stable, low levels at approximately days 17 to 20; earliest detectable anti-HIV appears between days 20 and 25, with an early IgM spike followed by high-titer IgG; seroconversion induces clearance of viremia to "set-points" that correlate with long-term outcome of disease, and with probability of secondary transmission of the virus. (Adapted from Busch,[150] with permission.)

wich" EIA format employed in Abbott's anti-HIV-1/HIV-2 EIA allows use of lower dilutions of donor sera and detects IgM with improved sensitivity.[44,48] The progressive introduction of assays with increased sensitivity to early infection has led to significant narrowing of the seroconversion window (Fig. 37-6), with concomitant reductions in the risk of screened blood transfusions[44,45,48,55] (see below).

The results of anti-HIV donor testing at Irwin Memorial Blood Centers in San Francisco from 1985 through 1992 are illustrated in Figure 37-7. Note the declining rate of Western blot–positive donations over time (see below). Note also the marked decline in the rate of false positive (EIA-reactive, Western blot–negative) results from 1985 through 1990, which resulted from exclusion of false-positive donors from the repeat donor pool, and the improved specificity of EIAs. The increased rate of false-positive results observed in the second half of 1991 was partially attributable to nonspecific reactivity observed in donors who received influenza vaccines. The further increase in false-positive results

in mid-1992 coincided with implementation of anti-HIV-1/HIV-2 combitests. These recombinant DNA-antigen–based tests appear to have detected a new subpopulation of donors as falsely reactive; as these donors are culled from the donor base, reactive rates should continue to decline. This effect of increased false reactive rates after introduction of a new test shows how changing tests in the donor setting can result in significant additional unit loss and donor deferral.

RISK OF HIV FROM SCREENED TRANSFUSIONS

After implementation of anti-HIV-1 screening in 1985, there was initial hope that the blood supply had become essentially risk-free.[56] The rate of confirmed positive infections among donors was observed to decline markedly over the first several years of screening[31,57] (Fig. 37-7). This was attributed in part to notification and exclusion of repeat donors who had tested positive. In addition, interviews of seropositive donors led to insights regarding

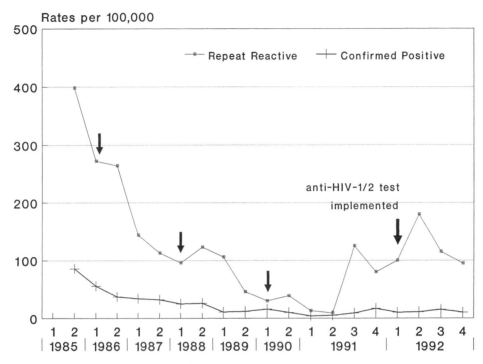

Fig. 37-7. Rate of anti-HIV EIA repeat reactivity and confirmed positivity among volunteer blood donations to Irwin Memorial Blood Centers, San Francisco. Arrows indicate dates new versions of anti-HIV enzyme immunoassays were implemented.

why some infected individuals with established risk factors failed to self-defer, which in turn led to modifications of donor informational documents and interview questions.[57,58] For example, the rate of anti-HIV-1 positivity among donors in San Francisco declined from 0.1 percent when screening began in 1985 to 0.008 percent in 1993, which is 0.1 percent of the estimated 4 percent infection rate in the general population in San Francisco. On a national level, Cumming et al.[59] estimated that the HIV infection rate among first-time blood donors is less than 2 percent of the background prevalence of the virus in the general population.

However, in the late 1980s well-documented cases of HIV-1 transmission from screened blood transfusions were reported.[60] These early cases were traced to donors who had given blood during the window period between infection and seroconversion. Through June 1992, the CDC had received 201 AIDS case reports in which the only acknowledged mode of HIV exposure was one or more transfusions

received from 1986 through 1991 (Fig. 37-4).[14] On reinvestigation of 106 of these cases, 55 (52 percent) were reclassified as *not* transfusion associated, either because no transfusion was received or another, more probable mode of HIV exposure existed; an additional 34 cases (32 percent) involved persons who had also received earlier transfusions of unscreened blood or who were transfused in foreign countries. Thus, only 14 (13 percent) of the cases initially reported as due to infections from screened blood transfusions were confirmed. After adjustment for noninvestigated cases, and assuming an equal distribution of infections from 1986 through 1991, the CDC investigators estimated that approximately 5 TA AIDS cases have occurred per year due to infections from anti-HIV–screened blood transfusions.[14]

Of course, owing to the long incubation period from infection to clinical AIDS and the relatively high underlying mortality of transfused patients, monitoring TA AIDS case reports represents an insensitive and inadequate approach for assessing the residual risk of HIV transmission from screened transfusions. Two prospective studies were initiated in 1986 that were specifically designed to acquire data for defining this risk. The first study, carried out in the Baltimore and Houston areas, involved testing patients for anti-HIV-1 before and after cardiac surgery.[61] Observed seroconversions were investigated to rule out other risk factors, and donors in those cases were traced so as to document their seroconversion. Two cases of HIV-1 infection were documented after the transfusion of 120,000 units of blood. In the other study,[62,63] conducted in San Francisco, viral culture and PCR analyses were used to detect HIV-1 in pooled peripheral blood mononuclear cells derived from 200,000 anti-HIV-negative donations; only a single infected donation was identified. These studies' findings are summarized in Table 37-1.

Because of their high cost, the two prospective studies discussed above were discontinued in 1992. This has led to the need for an alternative, more practical approach for estimating the risk of HIV infection from transfusions on an ongoing basis. The approach that has evolved uses data from "lookback" investigations to estimate the number of HIV-1 transmissions that occur from donors who donate in the "window period" preceding detectable antibody. By tracing recipients of earlier seronegative donations given by repeat donors who seroconverted to anti-HIV-1 positivity, the rate of recipient infection by these pre-seroconversion transfusions can be determined, and then the duration of the seronegative "infectious" window can be estimated. The risk of HIV-1 transmission from repeat donors, and, with some adjustments, from first-time donors can then be calculated.

This approach was recently employed by CDC investigators,[64] who traced previous recipients of blood from 701 donors who had seroconverted to anti-HIV positivity prior to 1991. One or more recipients of preseroconversion donations were identified and tested for 179 seroconverting donors. The most recent seronegative donation resulted in infection in 36 (20 percent) of the cases. The recipient infection rate correlated with the time interval between the seropositive and seronegative donations (e.g., interval < 90 days, 76 percent; 91 to 180 days, 28 percent; > 180 days, 11 percent). Mathematic modeling of these data indicated a median 45-day infectious window period (95 percent confidence interval: 34 to 55 days) for the overall period (1985 to 1990). Separate analysis of donations given prior and subsequent to March 1987 (when improved sensitivity EIAs were implemented in U.S. donor centers) indicated a reduction in the median infectious seronegative window from 55 to 42 days. With routine introduction in 1992 of new format anti-HIV-1/HIV-2 "combi-tests," which detect HIV-specific IgM antibody 10 to 15 days earlier than previously available assays,[44,45,48] the residual infectious window has likely been narrowed further to approximately 22 to 25 days (Figure 37-6).

By combining the 25-day window estimate with data on the frequency of HIV seroconversions in the donor setting, the CDC estimated the risk of HIV-1 from transfusion in 1992 at 1 infection for every 420,000 units transfused[65] (Table 37-1). By multiplying this risk estimate by 18 million transfused components per year in the United States, the CDC projected that approximately 43 recipients per year are transfused with HIV-1 infected blood. Only 5 to

Table 37-1. Risk for Transfusion-Transmitted HIV-1 from Anti-HIV Screened Blood Transfusions

Study Design	Period of Study	No. Infections Found	No. Units Studied	Risk (%)	Upper 95% Confidence Limit (%)
Recipient seroconversion[61]	1985–1991	2	120,301	1/60,000 (0.0017)	1/19,245 (0.0053)
Donation PCR/ Culture[62,63]	1987–1992	1	200,000	1/160,000 (0.0053)	1/28,000 (0.0108)
Incidence X SC Window Model[64,65]	1992–1993	NA	NA	1/420,000 (0.00023)	1/200,000 (0.0005)

Abbreviations: PCR, polymerase chain reaction; SC, seroconversion; NA, not applicable (see text); HIV, human immunodeficiency virus.

10 of these infected recipients would be expected to develop AIDS-related diseases prior to dying from other causes, consistent with the report by Selik et al.[14] discussed above. The risk of HIV-2 transmission has been estimated at less than 1 in 10 million,[36] with other rare subtypes (e.g., HIV-1 subtype O)[54] being of even lesser concern. These combined risks are 2,000-fold lower than that existing at the peak of the transfusion-AIDS epidemic between 1982 and 1984.[11]

HUMAN T CELL LEUKEMIA/LYMPHOMA VIRUSES

Prevalence and Epidemiology in the Donor Setting

Within several years after the first report of isolation of HTLV-I in 1980 from an American patient with an atypical cutaneous T cell neoplasm,[3] investigators in Japan established a strong epidemiologic linkage between HTLV-I and an endemic form of leukemia in southern Japan termed ATL.[66,67] Molecular studies of leukemia cells from a number of ATL patients confirmed that HTLV-I DNA was clonally integrated in the tumor cells,[68] thus establishing a direct causal relationship between HTLV-I infection and malignant transformation. In the mid-1980s, studies conducted in Japan and in the Caribbean region, where a second endemic focus of HTLV-I was discovered, established a convincing association between HTLV-I infection and a chronic and progressive neurologic disease termed *tropical spastic paraparesis* or *HTLV-I-associated myelopathy* (TSP/HAM).[69,70]

Data from Japan and the Caribbean conclusively documented that HTLV-I could be transmitted by transfusion,[71,72] and several cases of probable post-transfusion TSP/HAM were reported.[73,74] Based on these findings, the American Red Cross initiated a study to determine the prevalence of the virus among U.S. blood donors.[75] Between October 1986 and January 1987, 39,898 donors in eight regions of the country were tested, and 10 donors (.025 percent) were confirmed to be infected. Assuming that HTLV-I seropositivity equated to HTLV-I infection, and that transmission by transfusion was comparable to the 60 percent rate reported from Japan (see below), the Red Cross investigators estimated that approximately 2,800 new HTLV-I infections were

occurring annually in the United States as a result of transfusions. Based on these data, U.S. blood banks began screening donated blood for HTLV-I antibodies shortly after the FDA licensed test kits on November 29, 1988.

When confirmed anti-HTLV-positive donors were notified, interviewed, and further tested, some surprising epidemiologic and virologic findings were made. First, there was a significant increased relative risk of infection among females and for nonwhite and Hispanic donors of both sexes.[75-78] As expected, significant risk factors for seropositivity included Japanese or Caribbean birth or sexual contact with someone from those areas, but unexpected were high infection rates associated with intravenous drug use or sexual contact with an intravenous drug-using partner,[75-78] and, in several southwestern states, Native American Indian ancestry.[79] Even more surprising, when PCR and, more recently, peptide-based serologic HTLV typing were performed on specimens from seropositive donors, over half proved to be infected with the closely related virus HTLV-II rather than HTLV-I.[77-83] Most of the donors infected with HTLV-I had links to regions known to be endemic with that virus. In contrast, HTLV-II infection was found to be highly associated with intravenous drug use or sexual contact with an intravenous drug-using partner[77]; in addition, the virus was found to be endemic in several Indian tribes in New Mexico,[79] as well as in regions of Central and South America.[84,85]

Given the many changes in donor-selection criteria and laboratory screening implemented in the mid- to late 1980s to address concerns over TA AIDS, it is possible that the rates of HTLV-I and HTLV-II infection observed at the time screening of donors was begun in late 1988 may have underestimated the risk to transfusion recipients in the preceding decade. Two lines of evidence suggest that this was not the case. First, when 200,000 donor sera in the TSS repository, collected in 1984, were tested using HTLV-I antibody assays, the rate of confirmed positivity was essentially identical to those found in the participating centers when screening began in 1989 (0.06 to 0.1 percent).[76] Second, retrospective seroepidemiologic studies of HTLV-I and HTLV-II prevalence in intravenous drug users[86,87] and of HTLV-II in endemic Native American populations indicate that these viruses have been present at relatively stable rates in this country for the past several decades.

Transmission Rate by Blood

Early studies of recipients of HTLV-I antibody positive transfusions in Japan and the Caribbean indicated that HTLV-I was transmitted by cellular blood components at rates of 63 and 45 percent, respectively.[71,72] Noncellular blood components (i.e., fresh frozen plasma and cryoprecipitate) were not associated with transmission. Whereas several U.S. studies have confirmed the absence of transmission by fresh frozen plasma or cryoprecipitate, they have found significantly lower rates of transmission by cellular products than suggested by the earlier studies.[88–90] For example, only 33 percent of recipients of cellular components from HTLV-seropositive donors in the TSS seroconverted (PCR has confirmed that seronegative recipients of seropositive blood are not infected).[88] The rate of HTLV transmission documented in two retrospective Red Cross studies was even lower (12.8 and 26 percent, respectively).[89,90]

Several explanations have been proposed for the reduced rates of transmission of HTLV by transfusions in the United States. One consideration was that HTLV-II, which accounts for the majority of U.S. HTLV infections, could have a significantly lower rate of transmission than HTLV-I. However, both TSS data and data from a Red Cross lookback study indicate comparable rates of transmission for HTLV-II and HTLV-I.[88,90] Second, all investigators have observed an inverse relationship between HTLV transmission and duration of storage of units in the blood bank. This effect is much more marked than with HIV, with virtual absence of HTLV-I or -II transmission by units stored more than 14 days.[71,88–91] Blood in the United States is typically stored longer prior to transfusion than blood from Japan or the Caribbean, so this storage effect probably explains much of the difference in transmission rates.

HTLV-I Disease Associations

HTLV-I was first isolated from patients with cutaneous T cell lymphoma similar to mycosis fungoides. It later became apparent that these American patients actually had ATL, an aggressive leukemia described in detail in the Japanese literature.[92] Patients typically have a rapidly progressing clinical course with lymphadenopathy, dermal involvement, lytic bone lesions (with associated hypercalcemia), and involvement of liver, spleen, and meninges.[92,93] The peripheral blood of ATL patients contains circulating neoplastic cells with convoluted or lobular nuclei (termed *flower cells*). Variant forms of HTLV-I-associated T cell lymphoproliferative disease have also been described, including non-Hodgkin's lymphomas without leukemic manifestations, and pre- or smoldering ATL syndromes with either normal white blood cell counts and skin infiltrates or low-grade atypical lymphocytosis without systemic manifestations.[94] There is also one report of a chronic lymphocytic leukemia of B cell origin in which the tumor cells were shown to be clonally reactive to HTLV-I antigenic determinants.[95]

In studies from Japan and Jamaica, it has been estimated that the lifetime risk of developing ATL or a related neoplasm is 4 percent or less for persons infected with HTLV-I in childhood.[96] Because only two cases of ATL have been reported in persons who may have acquired HTLV-I from a transfusion in endemic regions,[97] it is difficult to calculate a disease incidence estimate for persons infected as adults. In nonendemic areas such as the United States, HTLV-I-associated leukemia/lymphomas are so rare that incidence estimates are not available. For example, in one study of 2,583 plasma samples from 1,053 leukemia/lymphoma patients treated in New York, none were positive for HTLV antibodies.[98] No cases of ATL have been reported to date in the United States among transfusion recipients.

An association between HTLV seropositivity and an endemic form of neurologic disease called either TSP or HAM was first reported in 1985.[99,100] TSP/HAM is characterized by a chronic progressive course with loss of pyramidal function, spastic paralysis, sphincter dysfunction, and sensory neuropathy. The clinical features, pathology, and laboratory diagnosis of this disorder have been reviewed recently.[101] HTLV-I seropositivity has been detected in 75 to 90 percent of patients with TSP/HAM in endemic areas, and virus has been isolated from both blood and spinal fluid of TSP/HAM patients.[69,70] Virologic studies have now established that ATL and TSP/HAM are different manifestations of infection with the same virus.[102] In addition to demyelination and atrophy of the spinal cord, some patients with TSP/HAM have symptoms of polymyositis, characterized by muscle pain, weakness, and an elevated erythrocyte sedimentation rate.[103]

The prevalence and incidence of TSP/HAM among HTLV-I infected individuals is not well known because most published reports of the disease have consisted of case series. Published estimates from Japanese population-based surveys have ranged from 1/1,464 (0.068 percent) to 1/1,309 HTLV-I (0.076 percent) seropositives.[104,105] In contrast, two population-based surveys in endemic regions of Zaire reported neurologic disease in 0.5 percent[106] and 1.5 percent[107,108] of HTLV-I infected persons, and a cohort study of HTLV-I seropositives in Jamaica found a disease prevalence of 0.5 percent.[109] The lifetime incidence of myelopathy in persons infected with HTLV-I was recently estimated by Kaplan et al. at 0.25 percent.[110] In the Retrovirus Epidemiology Donor Study 4 (2.4 percent) of 166 HTLV-I infected donors have been diagnosed with TSP/HAM.[111]

Several reports have linked HTLV-I with multiple sclerosis, based on weak serologic reactivity or detection of HTLV-I-related DNA by PCR.[112] However, these data have been refuted by other groups,[113,114] and the current weight of evidence indicates no relationship, aside from an overlapping clinical spectrum necessitating careful differential diagnosis. Preliminary associations between HTLV-I infection and some cases of mycosis fungoides,[115] arthritis,[116] lymphocytic pulmonary disease,[117] and bacterial dermatitis in childhood[118] have also been described but not confirmed in prospective cohort studies.[119] Laboratory abnormalities such as atypical lymphocytosis,[94] activated T cells detected by flow-cytometric analysis,[120] spontaneous lymphocyte proliferation,[121] and suppressed tuberculin skin reactivity[122] have also been reported. The prevalence and significance of these findings and their predictive value vis-à-vis more serious HTLV-I-associated disease outcomes have yet to be established.

HTLV-II Disease Associations

The initial isolations of HTLV-II from two patients with hairy cell leukemia appear to have been coincidental, since the tumor cells were negative for HTLV-II DNA, and larger surveys of hairy cell leukemia patients have not revealed increased rates of HTLV-II antibody.[6] Subsequent isolations of HTLV-II from patients with atypical chronic lymphocytic leukemia, large granular lymphocytic leukemia, prolymphocytic leukemia, erythroderma, thrombocytopenia, and aplastic anemia all also appear anecdotal.[123] Thus, to date there does not appear to be a significant relationship between HTLV-II infection and either neoplastic or hypoproliferative hematologic disorders.

In contrast, evidence is accumulating supporting an association with neurologic diseases similar to TSP/HAM. For example, 2 out of 404 HTLV-II positive donors in the REDS study have been diagnosed with TSP/HAM.[111] Two HTLV-II-infected New Mexico Indian sisters were also reported with spastic paraparesis.[124] At least five additional case reports of neurologic disease among HTLV-II infected patients have appeared over the past 2 years. Subtle laboratory and clinical abnormalities similar to those reported with HTLV-I have also been observed in several studies.[111,125–127] In summary, the evidence to date supports a significant risk of neurologic disease for HTLV-II, albeit at a lower rate than for HTLV-I. Therefore, discrimination of virus type using HTLV-I and -II-specific peptide EIAs[106–109] is recommended as a routine element of HTLV confirmatory testing for counseling purposes.[128]

LABORATORY TESTING ALGORITHMS FOR HTLV

Donor serum specimens are currently screened for antibody to HTLV-I using licensed enzyme immunoassays prepared from HTLV-I whole-virus lysate antigens. These assays vary in their sensitivity to detect antibodies to HTLV-II (see below). As summarized above for HIV (Fig. 37-5), initially reactive specimens are retested in duplicate to minimize the chance that reactivity is due to technical error. Units corresponding to specimens that are repeatedly reactive are discarded. Donor eligibility is determined by results of supplemental tests. Donors whose supplemental tests are positive are permanently deferred, whereas donors with negative or indeterminate supplemental test results are allowed to continue donating until a second repeat-reactive (EIA) result is obtained. There is no FDA-approved reentry protocol for donors deferred as a result of HTLV test results.

Although additional supplemental tests are required and employed routinely to establish if EIA reactivity is due to true HTLV-I/II infection and to discriminate HTLV-I from HTLV-II infection, no supplemental tests for HTLV-confirmatory testing are licensed by the FDA to date. According to Public Health Service consensus criteria, supplemental tests must be capable of identifying antibodies to both core (p24 *gag* antigen) and envelope (gp21, gp46, and/or gp61/68) proteins of HTLV-I/II.[128] Because of the virtual absence of envelope antigens in viral lysate Western blots, early confirmatory algorithms involved parallel performance of a Western blot (to detect *gag* reactivity) and a radioimmunoprecipitation assay (RIPA) to detect *env* reactivity, followed by HTLV-I and -II-specific peptide EIA analysis of confirmed positive samples. Follow-up studies of HTLV-I EIA-reactive donors tested using these algorithms established that these algorithms can be highly accurate.[128,129] For example, Table 37-2 summarizes the results of a study of 699 donors by the REDS,[129] in which very few false-positive or false-negative results were observed. Although a large proportion (over 50 percent) of EIA-reactive donor specimens test indeterminate using these algorithms, follow-up studies indicate that only a small percentage of these donors are infected (usually with

Table 37-2. Results of HTLV-I and HTLV-II PCR Assays on 699 HTLV EIA Repeat-Reactive Donations According to Serologic Classification of Specimens by Supplemental Antibody Assays at Blood Center Laboratories

Anti-HTLV-I/II Supplemental Serology (WB/RIPA/p21e EIA)	PCR Results			
	No. Donations	HTLV-I	HTLV-II	Negative
Positive	115	34	69	12[a]
Indeterminate	425	1	5	419
Negative	159	0	0	159

[a] Ten of 12 HTLV-I/II-seropositive, PCR-negative donors enrolled in follow-up studies; 7 were positive for HTLV-II and 1 for HTLV-I by PCR on freshly separated peripheral blood mononuclear cells.

Abbreviations: PCR, polymerase chain reaction; HTLV, human T cell leukemia virus; WB, Western blot; RIPA, radioimmunoprecipitation assay; EIA, enzyme immunoassay.

HTLV-II); such donors should therefore be counseled similarly to supplemental test–negative donors.[128,129]

Because of the complexity and expense of performing both Western blot and RIPA, as well as type-specific EIAs, manufacturers have recently developed so-called spiked HTLV Western blot assays.[130,131] These tests contain recombinant envelope antigens (rp21, rgp46-I, and rpg46-II) in addition to the HTLV-I viral lysate antigens. They therefore allow for simultaneous detection of antibodies to *gag* and *env* antigens, as well as differentiation of HTLV-I from HTLV-II. Preliminary studies indicate that with proper interpretive criteria, these tests are highly accurate.[131] Several of these assays are now being used by blood bank reference laboratories, and are pending licensure at the FDA.

RISK OF HTLV TRANSMISSION BY SCREENED TRANSFUSIONS

Data on the current risk of acquiring HTLV-I or -II from transfusions are limited. The best estimate is based on testing of specimens collected during the course of the HIV recipient seroconversion study carried out in Baltimore and Houston between 1987 and 1991.[61] In that study, post-transfusion specimens were tested by anti-HTLV-I EIA, and those that were reactive were confirmed using HTLV-I Western blots and RIPAs, with subsequent peptide EIA analysis of confirmed positive specimens to differentiate HTLV-I from -II reactivity. Of 5,908 patients transfused with 50,650 units collected prior to anti-HTLV screening, 2 were determined to have seroconverted to anti-HTLV-I positivity, while 4 seroconverted to anti-HTLV-II. Based on these data, Nelson, et al., calculated the risk of HTLV-I/II transmission before donor anti-HTLV-I screening to be 0.02 percent (1/5000) per unit. This rate is consistent with the rate of infection observed among donors from these regions (0.05 percent) at the time screening was implemented, and the 20 to 30 percent virus transmission rate discussed above. Recipients of 69,000 units transfused after implementation of anti-HTLV-I screening were later tested, and only 1 patient, transfused 5 months after initiation of screening, seroconverted to HTLV-II positivity. Thus, the risk of HTLV infection from transfusion was reduced 10-

Table 37.3 Risk of Transfusion-Transmitted HTLV-I or HTLV-II in Relation to Serologic Screening of Donors[a]

Relation to Donor Screening	HTLV-I		HTLV-II	
	Before[a]	After[a]	Before[a]	After[a]
No. seroconvertors	2	0	4	1
No. units transfused	51,026	69,272	51,036	69,272
Risk (%)	0.0039	0	0.0078	0.0014
Upper 95% confidence limit, (%)	0.0123	0.0042	0.0180	0.0068

[a] Transfused before or after December 1988 when specific serologic screening of donors for HTLV-I was initiated.
Abbreviation: HTLV, human T cell leukemia lymphoma virus.
(From Nelson et al.,[61] with permission.)

fold after screening to 0.0016 percent (1/50,000) per unit (Table 37-3).

There is concern, however, that because we are employing anti-HTLV-I based EIAs (both for donor screening and recipient monitoring), we may be missing a significant proportion of HTLV-II infected donors and recipients. Several investigators have reported detection of a small number of HTLV-II-infected persons, using HTLV-II PCR or HTLV-II based serologic assays, who test consistently negative on FDA-licensed HTLV-I-based EIAs.[12,132–134] Given the relatively high prevalence of HTLV-II versus HTLV-I in the United States (particularly among intravenous drug users and Native American populations), it would seem appropriate to develop and implement combination HTLV-I/II assays optimized with regard to sensitivity of detection of persons infected with either virus. Reagent manufacturers have begun development of such combination HTLV-I/II screening assays, and it is likely that they will be licensed and implemented (in place of the current anti-HTLV-I–based EIAs) within the next several years.

HOW THE RISK OF ACQUIRING RETROVIRUS TRANSMISSION BY TRANSFUSIONS CAN BE FURTHER REDUCED

Although the likelihood of acquiring a retrovirus infection from a screened blood transfusion is exceedingly small, there continues to be strong political and regulatory pressure to further reduce the risk in any way possible, seemingly at all costs. This has led to continued research into approaches for identifica-

tion and selective recruitment of "safer" donor populations, and to considerations of new or improved methods for screening donors for retrovirus-related risk factors.[135] For example, because of the disproportionate impact of the HIV epidemic on poor urban racial minorities and the known higher prevalence of HIV among minority donors, some have argued for what has been termed "demographic recruitment." However, this concept fails to recognize the critical need for a genetically diverse donor base to support the transfusion needs of a similarly diverse recipient population. Others have proposed expanding or modifying the risk factor interview process (e.g., by adding questions on recent heterosexual activity [see below], using cartoon depictions of risk behaviors to increase understanding by less-educated donors, or implementing computer-based interview strategies to enhance confidentiality).[136] Convincing data to support these proposals have not been generated, however.[137]

Risk-factor profiles of seropositive donors have changed over time. For example, Petersen et al.[138] recently compared HIV risk factors among 508 seropositive donors identified at 20 blood centers between May 1988 and August 1989, with those of 472 seropositive donors identified from January 1990 through May 1991. The overall rate of seropositive donations declined slightly over time (from 0.021 to 0.018 percent), primarily as a result of a decrease in infected donations by homosexual and bisexual men. In contrast, the rate of infected donations by persons likely exposed by heterosexual contact remained stable. During the most recent period, 56 percent of infected female and 12 percent of infected male donors had seropositive heterosexual partners, while an additional 41 percent of women and 29 percent of heterosexual men were likely infected by heterosexual contact (based on serologic studies for sexually transmitted disease markers), even though specific infected sex partners could not be identified. These authors rejected the option of deferring donors based on recent or lifetime number of heterosexual partners because numeric cutoffs that would capture only half of the seropositive heterosexual donors would result in loss of 7 to 13 percent of all donations. This illustrates the significant trade-offs required to maintain an adequate as well as safe blood supply.

There continues to be great interest in tests that might detect HIV-infected persons earlier than current antibody assays, particularly those targeting viral antigens or nucleic acids. Although large studies conducted between 1989 and 1990 found no p24-antigen-positive/antibody-negative donations in over a million donations in the United States,[139,140] there is renewed interest in antigen screening for several reasons. First, antigen assays have been developed that are increasingly sensitive and are compatible with more rapid turn-around times required for donor screening. Second, antigen-positive/antibody-negative blood donations have been detected at moderate rates in Thailand (where the prevalence of HIV-1 among donors in some cities is 100-fold that in the United States), and antigen screening of blood donors is now routine in this setting.[141,142] Similarly, studies in certain U.S. settings such as emergency rooms have indicated a possible role for antigen screening as a supplement to antibody screening for detection of window-phase infections.[143] Third, recent studies of seroconverting plasma donors indicate that p24 antigen testing would reduce the average infectious preseroconversion window by 5 to 8 days[44,45,48]; based on this window-reduction and current HIV incidence estimates in U.S. donors, antigen screening would theoretically detect and prevent transfusion of approximately 1 HIV-infectious donation per 1.6 million screened donations,[48] thereby reducing the risk of HIV from transfusions by about one quarter. The net yield would be interdiction of approximately 7 p24 antigen-positive/antibody-negative units per year in the United States, at a cost of $50 million to $100 million and up to 12,000 p24 antigen false-positive donations.[139] The decision for or against p24 antigen screening will probably be reviewed by the FDA.

The development of techniques for sensitive detection of HIV nucleic acids holds promise for even more sensitive donor screening in the future. Considerable research has been devoted to simplification of nucleic acid extraction, amplification, and detection methods. There has been substantial recent progress in development of HIV DNA and RNA PCR test kits using 96-well–format thermocyclers and microplate-based calorimetric readers rather than gel electrophoresis and radioactive probe detection systems.[144–146] Several significant problems and questions must be resolved, however, before PCR or alternative nucleic acid amplification techniques are seriously considered for donor screening. For example, although the problem of frequent false-positive PCR results due to "carryover" of amplified product from positive to negative samples has been reduced through implementation of stringent technical precautions and strategies for sterilization of amplified product,[144] false-positivity due to blood cross-contamination may present a problem when thousands of samples are processed per day.[147] Furthermore, whereas the cost of adding nucleic acid detection assays to donor screening would clearly be substantial, the incremental safety benefit that would be achieved is unclear. Recent studies suggest that cell-associated HIV DNA and cell-free HIV RNA are detected no more than several weeks prior to development of detectable anti-HIV.[48,148–150] Decisions on further development and implementation of nucleic acid screening systems of donors will likely be determined to a great extent by the success of parallel developments in artificial blood substitutes and viral inactivation techniques.

REFERENCES

1. Levy JA (ed): The Retroviridae. Plenum Publishers, New York, 1994
2. Bishop JM: The molecular genetics of cancer. Science 235:305, 1987
3. Poiesz BJ, Ruscetti FW, Gazdar AF et al: Detection and isolation of type C retrovirus particles from fresh and cultured lymphocytes of a patient with cutaneous

T-cell lymphoma. Proc Natl Acad Sci USA 77:7415, 1980

4. Blattner WA (ed): Human Retrovirology: HTLV. Raven Press, New York, 1990

5. Kalyanaraman VS, Sarngadharan MG, Robert-Groff M et al: A new subtype of human T-cell leukemia virus (HTLV-II) associated with a T-cell variant of hairy cell leukemia. Science 218:571, 1982

6. Rosenblatt JD, Chen IS, Golde DW: HTLV-II and human lymphoproliferative disorders. Clin Lab Med 8:85, 1988

7. Kilbourne ED: New viral diseases: a real and potential problem without boundaries. JAMA 264:68, 1990

8. Centers for Disease Control: Update on acquired immune deficiency syndrome (AIDS) among patients with hemophilia A. MMWR 31:644, 1982

9. Centers for Disease Control: Possible transfusion-associated acquired immune deficiency syndrome (AIDS)—California. MMWR 31:652, 1982

10. American Association of Blood Banks (AABB), Council of Community Blood Centers (CCBC), American Red Cross (ARC): Joint statement on acquired immune deficiency syndrome (AIDS) related to transfusion. Transfusion 23:87, 1983

11. Busch MP, Young MJ, Samson SM et al and the Transfusion Safety Study Group: Risk of human immunodeficiency virus transmission by blood transfusions prior to the implementation of HIV antibody screening in the San Francisco Bay Area. Transfusion 31:4, 1991

12. Perkins HA, Samson S, Busch MP: How well has self-exclusion worked? Transfusion 28:601, 1988

13. Kroner BL, Rosenberg PS, Aledort LM et al, for the Multicenter Hemophilia Cohort Study: HIV-1 infection incidence among persons with hemophilia in the United States and western Europe, 1978–1990. J Acquir Immune Defic Syndr 7:279, 1994

14. Selik RM, Ward JW, Buehler JW: Trends in transfusion-associated acquired immune deficiency syndrome in the United States, 1982 through 1991. Transfusion 33:890, 1993

15. Kleinman SH, Niland JC, Azen SP et al and the Transfusion Safety Study Group: Prevalence of antibodies to human immunodeficiency virus type 1 among blood donors prior to screening: the Transfusion Safety Study/NHLBI donor repository. Transfusion 29:572, 1989

16. Donegan E, Stuart M, Niland JC et al and the Transfusion Safety Study Group: Infection with human immunodeficiency virus type 1 (HIV-1) among recipients of antibody-positive blood donations. Ann Intern Med 113:733, 1990

17. Busch M, Donegan E, Stuart M, Mosley JW, for the Transfusion Safety Study Group: Donor HIV-1 p24 antigenaemia and course of infection in recipients. Lancet i:1342, 1990

18. Donegan E, Lenes BA, Tomasulo PA, Mosley JW and the Transfusion Safety Study Group: Transmission of HIV-1 by components type and duration of shelf storage before transfusion. Transfusion 30:851, 1990

19. Rawal BD, Busch MP, Endow R et al: Reduction of human immunodeficiency virus-infected cells from donor blood by leukocyte filtration. Transfusion 26: 460, 1989

20. Rawal BD, Davis RE, Busch MP, Vyas GN: Dual reduction in the immunologic and infectious complications of transfusion by filtration/removal of leukocytes from donor blood soon after collection. Transfus Med Rev 4(suppl. 1):36, 1990

21. Kim HC, Nahum K, Raska K Jr et al: Natural history of acquired immunodeficiency syndrome in hemophilic patients. Am J Hematol 24:168, 1987

22. Jackson JB, Sannerud KJ, Hopsicker JS et al: Hemophiliacs with HIV antibody are actively infected. JAMA 260:2236, 1988

23. Jackson JB, Kwok SY, Sninsky JJ et al: Human immunodeficiency virus type 1 detected in all seropositive symptomatic and asymptomatic individuals. J Clin Microbiol 28:16, 1990

24. Hewlett IK, Laurian Y, Epstein J et al: Assessment by gene amplification and serological markers of transmission of HIV-1 from hemophiliacs to their sexual partners and secondarily to their children. J Acquir Immun Defic Syndr 3:714, 1990

25. Jason J, Ou C-Y, Moore JL et al and the Hemophilia-AIDS Collaborative Study Group: Prevalence of human immunodeficiency virus type 1 DNA in hemophilic men and their sex partners. J Infect Dis 160: 789, 1989

26. Gibbons J, Cory JM, Hewlett IK et al: Silent infections with human immunodeficiency virus type 1 are highly unlikely in multitransfused seronegative hemophiliacs. Blood 76:1924, 1990

27. Sheppard HW, Busch MP, Louie PH et al: HIV-1 PCR and isolation in seroconverting and seronegative homosexual men: absence of long-term immunosilent infection. J Acquir Immun Defic Syndr 6:1339, 1993

28. Ward JW, Bush TJ, Perkins HA et al: The natural history of transfusion-associated infection with human immunodeficiency virus. N Engl J Med 321: 947, 1989

29. Ashton LJ, Learmont J, Luo K et al: HIV infection in recipients of blood products from donors with known duration of infection. Lancet 344:718, 1994

30. Operskalski EA, Stram DO, Lee H et al and the Transfusion Safety Study Group: Human immunodeficiency virus-1 infection: relationship of risk group and age to rate of progression to AIDS. J Infect Dis 1995 (in press)

31. Busch MP, Operskalski EA, Mosley JW et al and the Transfusion Safety Study Group: Epidemiologic background and long-term course of disease in human immunodeficiency virus type 1-infected blood donors identified before routine laboratory screening. Transfusion 34:858, 1994

32. Bluxhelt A, Granath F, Lidman K, Giesecke J: The influence of age on the latency period to AIDS in people infected by HIV through blood transfusion. AIDS 4:125, 1990

33. Balfe P, Simmonds P, Ludlam CA et al: Concurrent evolution of human immunodeficiency virus type 1 in patients infected from the same source: rate of sequence change and low frequency of inactivating mutations. J Virol 64:6221, 1990

34. Simmonds P, Beatson D, Cuthbert RJG et al: Determinants of HIV disease progression: six-year longitudinal study in the Edinburgh haemophilia/HIV cohort. Lancet 338:1159, 1991

35. Diaz R, Sabino EC, Mayer A et al: Dual human immunodeficiency virus type 1 infection and recombination in a dually-exposed transfusion recipient. J Virol 69:3273, 1995

36. O'Brien TR, George JR, Holmberg SD: Human immunodeficiency virus type 2 infection in the United States: epidemiology, diagnosis, and public health implications. J Am Med Assoc 267:2775, 1992

37. Marlink R, Kanki P, Thior I et al: Reduced rate of disease development after HIV-2 infections as compared to HIV-1. Science 265:1587, 1994

38. George JR, Rayfield MA, Phillips S et al: Efficacies of U.S. Food and Drug Administration licensed HIV-1-screening enzyme immunoassays for detecting antibodies to HIV-1. AIDS 4:321, 1990

39. de Cock KM, Porter A, Kouadio J et al: Cross-reactivity on Western blots in HIV-1 and HIV-2 infection. AIDS 5:859, 1991

40. Busch MB, Petersen L, Schable C, Perkins HA: Monitoring blood donors for HIV-2 infection by testing anti-HIV-1 reactive sera. Transfusion 30:184, 1990

41. Centers for Disease Control. Surveillance for HIV-2 infection in blood donors—United States, 1987–1989. MMWR 39:829, 1990

42. O'Brien T, Polon C, Schable C: HIV-2 infection in an American. AIDS 5:85, 1991

43. Parry JV, McAlpine L, Avillez MF: Sensitivity of six commercial enzyme immunoassay kits that detect both anti-HIV-1 and anti-HIV-2. AIDS 4:355, 1990

44. Gallarda JL, Henrard DR, Liu D et al: Early detection of antibody to HIV-1 using an antigen conjugate immunoassay correlates with the presence of IgM antibody. J Clin Microbiol 30:2379, 1992

45. Zaaijer HL, v Exel-Oehlers P, Kraaijeveld T et al: Early detection of antibodies to HIV-1 by third-generation assays. Lancet 340:770, 1992

46. Center for Biologics Eval and Research, FDA: Revised recommendations for the prevention of human immunodeficiency virus (HIV) transmission by blood and blood products. April 23, 1992, Rockville, MD

47. FDA: Proposed change to 21 CFR Parts 606, 610 (Docket No. 91N-0152). Current good manufacturing practices for blood and blood components; notification of consignees receiving blood and blood components at increased risk for transmitting HIV infection. Fed Reg 58:34962, -70, 1993

48. Busch MP, Lee LLL, Satten GA et al: Time course of detection of viral and serological markers preceding HIV-1 seroconversion; implications for blood and tissue donor screening. Transfusion 35:91, 1995

49. Healey DS, Bolton WV: Apparent HIV-1 glycoprotein reactivity on Western blot in uninfected blood donors. AIDS 7:655, 1993

50. Eble BE, Busch MP, Khayam-Bashi H et al: Resolution of infection status of HIV-seroindeterminate and high-risk seronegative individuals using PCR and virus-culture: absence of persistent silent HIV-1 infection in a high-prevalence area. Transfusion 32:503, 1992

51. Jackson JB: Human immunodeficiency virus (HIV)-indeterminate Western blots and latent HIV infection. Transfusion 32:497, 1992

52. Schochetman G, George JR (eds): AIDS Testing: Methodology and Management Issues. 2nd Ed. Springer-Verlag, New York, 1994

53. Busch MP: Let's look at human immunodeficiency virus lookback before leaping into hepatitis C virus lookback! Transfusion 31:655, 1991

54. Loussert-Ajaka I, Ly TD, Chaix ML et al: HIV-1/HIV-2 seronegativity in HIV-1 subtype O infected patients. Lancet 343:1393, 1994

55. Busch MP: Retroviruses and blood transfusions: the lessons learned and the challenge yet ahead. p. 1. In Nance SJ (ed): Blood Safety: Current Challenges (transcription of the Emily Cooley Award/AABB 1992 Annual Seminar). American Association of Blood Banks, Bethesda, MD, 1992

56. Bove JR: Transfusion-associated hepatitis and AIDS: what is the risk? N Engl J Med 317:242, 1987

57. Leitman SF, Klein HG, Melpolder JJ et al: Clinical implications of positive tests for antibodies to human immunodeficiency virus type 1 in asymptomatic blood donors. N Engl J Med 321:917, 1989

58. Petersen LR, Doll L and the HIV Blood Donor Study Group: HIV-1 infected blood donors: epidemiologic, laboratory, and donation characteristics. Transfusion 31:698, 1991

59. Cumming PD, Wallace EL, Schorr JB, Dodd RY: Exposure of patients to human immunodeficiency virus through the transfusion of blood components that test antibody-negative. N Engl J Med 321:941, 1989

60. Ward JW, Holmberg SD, Allen JR et al: Transmission of human immunodeficiency virus (HIV) by blood transfusions screened as negative for HIV antibody. N Engl J Med 318:473, 1988

61. Nelson KE, Donahue JG, Munoz A et al: Transmission of retroviruses from seronegative donors by transfusion during cardiac surgery; a multicenter study of HIV-1 and HTLV-I/II infections. Ann Intern Med 117:554, 1992

62. Busch MP, Eble BE, Khayam-Bashi H et al: Evaluation of screened blood donations for human immunodeficiency virus type 1 infection by culture and DNA amplification of pooled cells. N Engl J Med 325:1, 1991

63. Vyas GN, Rawal BP, Babu G, Busch MP: Diminishing risk of acquiring HIV infection from transfusion of seronegative blood. Transfusion 34(suppl.):63S, 1994

64. Petersen LR, Satten GA, Dodd R et al and the HIV Seroconversion Study Group: Duration of time from onset of human immunodeficiency virus type 1 infectiousness to development of detectable antibody. Transfusion 34:283, 1994

65. Lackritz EM, Satten GA, Raimondi VP et al: Estimated risk of HIV transmission by screened blood in the United States. Abstract 9. p. 56. 2nd National Conference on Human Retroviruses and Related Infections, Washington, D.C., Jan-Feb 1995

66. Hinuma YK, Nagata K, Hanoaka M et al: Adult T-cell leukemia: antigen in an ATL cell line and detection of antibodies to the antigen in human sera. Proc Natl Acad Sci USA 78:6476, 1981

67. Hinuma YK, Komoda H, Chosa T et al: Antibodies to adult T-cell leukemia-virus-associated antigens (ATLA) in sera from patients with ATL and controls in Japan: a nationwide seroepidemiologic study. Int J Cancer 29:631, 1982

68. Seiki M, Eddy R, Shows TB, Yoshida M: Non-specific integration of the HTLV provirus into adult T-cell leukemia cells. Nature 309:640, 1984

69. Jacobson S, Raine CS, Mingioli ES, McFarlin DE: Isolation of an HTLV-I-like retrovirus from patients with tropical spastic paraparesis. Nature 331:540, 1988

70. Bhagavati S, Ehrlich G, Kula R et al: Detection of human T-cell lymphoma/leukemia virus type I DNA and antigen in spinal fluid and blood of patients of chronic progressive myelopathy. N Engl J Med 318:1141, 1988

71. Okochi K, Satao H, Hinuma Y: A retrospective study on transmission of adult T cell leukemia virus by blood transfusion: seroconversion in recipients. Vox Sang 46:245, 1984

72. Kamihira S, Nakasima S, Oyakawa Y et al: Transmission of human T-cell lymphotropic type I by blood transfusion before and after mass screening of sera from seropositive donors. Vox Sang 52:43, 1987

73. Kurosawa M, Machii T, Kitani T et al: HTLV-I associated myelopathy (HAM) after blood transfusion in a patient with CD2 + hiry cell leukemia. Am J Clin Pathol 95:72, 1991

74. Gout O, Baulac M, Gessain A et al: Rapid development of myelopathy after HTLV-I infection acquired by transfusion during cardiac transplantation. N Engl J Med 322:383, 1990

75. Williams AE, Fang CT, Slamon DJ et al: Seroprevalence and epidemiologic correlates of HTLV-I infection in U.S. blood donors. Science 240:643, 1988

76. Operskalski EA, Schiff ER, Kleinman SH et al and the Transfusion Safety Study Group: Epidemiologic background of blood donors with antibody to human T-cell lymphotropic virus. Transfusion 29:746, 1989

77. Lee HH, Swanson P, Rosenblatt JD et al: Relative prevalence and risk factors of HTLV-I and HTLV-II infection in US blood donors. Lancet 337:1435, 1991

78. Taylor PE, Stevens CE, Pindyck J et al: Human T-cell lymphotropic virus in volunteer blood donors. Transfusion 30:783, 1990

79. Hjelle B, Mills R, Swenson S et al: Incidence of hairy cell leukemia, mycosis fungoides, and chronic lymphocytic leukemia in first known HTLV-II-endemic population. J Infect Dis 163:435, 1991

80. Hjelle B, Cyrus S, Swenson S, Mills R: Serologic distinction between human T-lymphocyte virus (HTLV) type I and HTLV type II. Transfusion 31:731, 1991

81. Lal RB, Heneine W, Rudolph DL et al: Synthetic peptide-based immunoassays for distinguishing between human T-cell lymphotropic virus type I and type II infections in seropositive individuals. J Clin Microbiol 29:2253, 1991

82. Lal RB, Rudolph DL, Lairmore MD et al: Serologic discrimination of human T cell lymphotropic virus

infection by using a synthetic peptide-based enzyme immunoassay. J Infect Dis 163:41, 1991

83. Viscidi RP, Hill PM, Li S et al: Diagnosis and differentiation of HTLV-I and HTLV-II infection by enzyme immunoassays using synthetic peptides. J Acquir Immun Defic Syndr 4:1190, 1991

84. Centers for Disease Control: Human T-lymphotropic virus type II among Guaymi Indians—Panama. MMWR 41:209, 1992

85. Reeves WC, Cutler JR, Gracia F et al: Human T cell lymphotropic virus infection in Guaymi Indians from Panama. Am J Trop Med Hyg 43:410, 1990

86. Khabbaz RF, Hartel D, Lairmore M et al: Human T lymphotropic virus type II (HTLV-II) infection in a cohort of New York intravenous drug users: an old infection? J Infect Dis 163:252, 1991

87. Khabbaz RF, Onorato IM, Cannon RO et al: Seroprevalence of HTLV-I and HTLV-II among intravenous drug users and persons in clinics for sexually transmitted diseases. N Engl J Med 326:375, 1992

88. Donegan E, Lee H, Operskalski EA et al and the Transfusion Safety Study Group: Transfusion transmission of retroviruses: human T-lymphotropic viruses types I and II compared with human immunodeficiency virus type 1. Transfusion 34:478, 1994

89. Kleinman S, Allain JP, Lee H: HTLV transmission by transfusion: serology and PCR results. (Abstract) Transfusion 31(suppl.):41S, 1991

90. Sullivan MT, Williams AE, Fang CT et al (The American Red Cross HTLV-I/II Collaborative Study Group): Transmission of human T-lymphocyte virus types I and II by blood transfusion. A retrospective study of recipients of blood components (1983 through 1988). Arch Intern Med 151:2043, 1991

91. Manns A, Wilks RJ, Murphy EL et al: A prospective study of transmission by transfusion of HTLV-I and risk factors associated with seroconversion. Int J Cancer 51:886, 1992

92. Uchyama T, Yodoi J, Sagawa K et al: Adult T-cell leukemia: clinical and hematological features of 16 cases. Blood 50:481, 1977

93. Bunn PA, Schechter GP, Jaffe E et al: Clinical course of retrovirus-associated adult T-cell lymphoma in the United States. N Engl J Med 309:258, 1983

94. Kinoshita K, Amagasaki T, Ikeda S et al: Preleukemic state of adult T cell leukemia: abnormal T lymphocytosis induced by human adult T cell leukemia-lymphoma virus. Blood 66:120, 1985

95. Mann DL, DeSantis P, Mark G et al: HTLV-I-associated B-cell CLL: indirect role for retrovirus in leukemogenesis. Science 236:1103, 1987

96. Murphy EL, Hanchard B, Figueroa JP et al: Model-ing the risk of adult T-cell leukemia/lymphoma in persons infected with human T-lymphotropic virus type I. Int J Cancer 43:250, 1989

97. Chen Y-C, Wang C-H, Su I-J et al: Infection of human T-cell leukemia virus type I and development of human T-cell leukemia/lymphoma in patients with hematologic neoplasms: a possible linkage to blood transfusion. Blood 74:388, 1989

98. Srivastave BIS, Gonzales C, Loftus R et al: Examination of HTLV-I ELISA-positive leukemia/lymphoma patients by Western blotting gave mostly negative or indeterminate reaction. AIDS Res Hum Retroviruses 6:617, 1990

99. Gessain A, Vernant JC, Sonan T et al: Antibodies to human T-lymphotropic virus type-I in patients with tropical spastic paraparesis. Lancet ii:407, 1985

100. Osame M, Usuku K, Izumo S et al: HTLV-I associated myelopathy, a new clinical entity. Lancet i:1031, 1986

101. Gessain A, Gout O: Chronic myelopathy associated with human T-lymphotropic virus type I (HTLV-I). Ann Intern Med 117:933, 1992

102. Yoshida M, Osame M, Usuku K et al: Viruses detected in HTLV-I-associated myelopathy and adult T-cell leukaemia are identical on DNA blotting. Lancet i: 1085, 1987

103. St Claire Morgan O, Mora C, Rodgers-Johnson P, Char G: HTLV-I and polymyositis in Jamaica. Lancet ii:1184, 1989

104. Osame M, Janssen R, Kubota H et al: Nationwide survey of HTLV-I-associated myelopathy in Japan: association with blood transfusion. Ann Neurol 28: 50, 1990

105. Kawai H, Nishida Y, Sano Y et al: HTLV-I-associated myelopathy (HAM) in Tokushima prefecture—geographical and clinical studies in an area between endemic and non-endemic areas of HTLV-I infection. Japan J Med 30:534, 1991

106. Jeannel D, Garin B, Kazadi K et al: The risk of tropical spastic paraparesis differs according to ethnic group among HTLV-I carriers in Inongo, Zaire. J Acquir Immun Defic Syndr 6:840, 1993

107. Kayembe K, Goubau P, Desmyter J et al: A cluster of HTLV-I associated tropical spastic paraparesis in Equateur (Zaire): ethnic and familial distribution. J Neurol Neurosurg Psychiatry 53:4, 1990

108. Goubau P, Carton H, Kazadi K et al: HTLV seroepidemiology in a central African population with high incidence of tropical spastic paraparesis. Trans R Soc Trop Med Hyg 84:577, 1990

109. Murphy EL, Wilks R, Morgan OS et al: A case-control study of HTLV-I in Jamaica: modes of transmission and health outcomes. Abstract T-IX-2, presented at

IV Annual Conference on Human Retrovirology: HTLV, Montego Bay, Jamaica, February 1991

110. Kaplan JE, Osame M, Kubota H et al: The risk of development of HTLV-I-associated myelopathy/tropical spastic paraparesis among persons infected with HTLV-I. J Acquir Immun Defic Syndr 3:1096, 1990

111. Murphy EL, Fridey J, Smith JW et al and the REDS Investigators. High prevalence of HTLV-associated myelopathy in a cohort of HTLV-I and HTLV-II infected blood donors. Ann Neurol 1995 (submitted)

112. Reddy EP, Sandberg-Wollheim M, Mettus R et al: Amplification and molecular cloning of HTLV-I sequences from DNA of multiple sclerosis patients. Science 243:529, 1989

113. Madden DL, Mundon FK, Tzan NR et al: Serologic studies of MD patients, controls, and patients with other neurologic diseases: antibodies to HTLV-I, II, III. Neurol 38:81, 1988

114. Richardson JH, Wucherpfennig KW, Endo N et al: PCR analysis of DNA from multiple sclerosis patients for the presence of HTLV-I. Science 246:821, 1989

115. Zucker-Franklin D, Coutaves EE, Rush MG, Zouzias DC: Detection of human T-lymphotropic virus-like particles in cultures of peripheral blood lymphocytes from patients with mycosis fungoides. Proc Natl Acad Sci USA 88:7630, 1991

116. Kitajima I, Maruyama I, Maruyama Y et al: Polyarthritis in human T lymphotropic virus type I-associated myelopathy. Arthritis Rheum 32:1342, 1989

117. Sugimoto M, Nakashima H, Watanabe S et al: T-lymphocyte alveolitis in HTLV-I-associated myelopathy. Lancet ii:1220, 1987

118. LaGrenade L, Hanchard B, Fletcher V et al: Infective dermatitis of Jamaican children: A marker for HTLV-I infection. Lancet 336:1345, 1990

119. Busch MP, Murphy EL, Nemo G for the REDS Study Group: More on HTLV tax and mycosis fungoides. (Comments on Pancake, Zucker-Franklin) N Engl J Med 329:2035, 1993

120. Fletcher MA, Hassett J, Donegan E et al: Lymphocyte phenotypes in HTLV seropositive blood donors and recipients. Abstract, presented at III International Retrovirology Conference, Maui, HI, March 1990

121. Kramer A, Jacobson S, Reuben JF et al: Spontaneous lymphocyte proliferation in symptom-free HTLV-I positive Jamaicans. Lancet ii:923, 1989

122. Tachibana N, Okayama A, Ishizaki J et al: Suppression of tuberculin skin reaction in healthy HTLV-I carriers from Japan. Int J Cancer 42:829, 1988

123. Hjelle B: Human T-cell leukemia/lymphoma viruses. Arch Pathol Lab Med 115:440, 1991

124. Hjelle B, Appenzeller O, Mills R et al: Chronic neurodegenerative disease associated with HTLV-II infection. Lancet 339:645, 1992

125. Prince H, Kleinman S, Doyle M et al: Spontaneous lymphocyte proliferation in vitro characterizes both HTLV-I and HTLV-II infection. J Acquir Immun Defic Syndr 3:1199, 1990

126. Wiktor SZ, Jacobson S, Weiss SH et al: Spontaneous lymphocyte proliferation in HTLV-II infection. Lancet 337:327, 1991

127. Murphy E, Miller K, Sacher R et al and the Retrovirus Epidemiology Donor Study: A multicenter study of HTLV-I and -II health effects. Abstract, presented at V International Conference on Human Retrovirology: HTLV, Kumamoto, Japan, May 1992

128. Centers for Disease Control and Prevention (CDC) and the US PHS Working Group: Guidelines for counselling persons infected with human T-lymphotropic virus type I (HTLV-I) and type II (HTLV-II). Ann Intern Med 118:448, 1993

129. Busch MP, Laycock M, Kleinman SH et al and the Retrovirus Epidemiology Donor Study (REDS): Accuracy of supplementary serological testing for human t-lymphotropic virus (HTLV) types I and II in US blood donors. Blood 83:1143, 1994

130. Lal RB, Brodine S, Kuzura J et al: Sensitivity and specificity of a recombinant transmembrane glycoprotein (rgp21)-spiked Western immunoblot for serologic confirmation of human T-cell lymphotropic virus type I and type II infection. J Clin Microbiol 30:296, 1992

131. Brodine SK, Kaime EM, Roberts C et al: Simultaneous confirmation and differentiation of human T-lymphotropic virus types I and II infection by modified Western blot containing recombinant envelope glycoproteins. Transfusion 33:925, 1993

132. Ehrlich GD, Glaser JB, LaVigne K et al: Prevalence of human T-cell leukemia/lymphoma virus (HTLV) type II infection among high-risk individuals: type-specific identification of HTLVs by polymerase chain reaction. Blood 74:1658, 1989

133. Hjelle B, Wilson C, Cyrus S et al: Human T-cell leukemia virus type II infection frequently goes undetected in contemporary U.S. blood donors. Blood 81:1641, 1993

134. Gallo D, Khashe S, Hoffman M: Comparison of sensitivity of two new commercial HTLV enzyme immunoassays for the detection of HTLV-I and HTLV-II antibody. Abstract 735, p. 187. Presented at 1st National Conference on Human Retroviruses and Related Infections, Washington D.C., Dec 1993

135. Kleinman S: Donor selection and screening procedures. In Nance SJ (ed): Blood Safety: Current Chal-

lenges. p. 169. American Association of Blood Banks, Bethesda, MD, 1992

136. Mayo DJ, Rose AM, Matchett SE et al: Screening potential blood donors at risk for human immunodeficiency virus. Transfusion 31:466, 1991

137. Johnson ES, Doll LS, Satten GA et al: Direct oral questions to blood donors: the impact on screening for human immunodeficiency virus. Transfusion 34: 769, 1994

138. Petersen LR, Doll LS, White CR et al and the HIV Blood Donor Study Group: Heterosexually acquired human immunodeficiency virus infection and the United States blood supply: considerations for screening of potential blood donors. Transfusion 33: 552, 1993

139. Alter HJ, Epstein JS, Swenson SG et al and the HIV-Antigen Study Group: Prevalence of human immunodeficiency virus type 1 p24 antigen in U.S. blood donors—an assessment of the efficacy of testing in donor screening. N Engl J Med 323:1312, 1990

140. Busch MP, Taylor PE, Lenes BA et al and the Transfusion Safety Study Group: Screening of selected male blood donors for p24 antigen of human immunodeficiency virus type 1. N Engl J Med 323:1308, 1990

141. Chiewsilp P, Isarangkura P, Poonkasem A et al: Risk of transmission of HIV by seronegative blood. (letter) Lancet 338:1341, 1991

142. Mundee Y, Kamtorn N, Chaiyaphruk S et al: Prevalence of HIV antibodies and p-24 antigen among blood donors in northern Thailand. Transfusion 34(suppl.):63S, 1994

143. Clark SJ, Kelen GD, Henrard DR et al: Unsuspected primary human immunodeficiency virus type 1 infection in seronegative emergency department patients. J Infect Dis 170:194, 1994

144. Wolcott MJ: Advances in nucleic acid-based detection methods. Microbiol Rev 5:370, 1992

145. Jackson JB, Ndugwa G, Mmiro F et al: Non-isotopic polymerase chain reaction methods for the detection of HIV-1 in Ugandan mothers and infants. AIDS 5: 1463, 1991

146. Mulder J, McKinney N, Christopherson C et al: A rapid and simple PCR assay for quantitation of HIV-1 RNA in plasma: application to acute retroviral infection. J Clin Microbiol 32:292, 1994

147. Sabino EC, Delwart E, Lee T-H et al: Identification of low-level contamination of blood as basis for detection of human immunodeficiency virus (HIV) DNA in anti-HIV-negative specimens. J Acquir Immun Defic Syndr 7:853, 1994

148. Farzadegan H, Vlahov D, Solomon L et al: Detection of human immunodeficiency virus type 1 infection by polymerase chain reaction in a cohort of seronegative intravenous drug users. J Infect Dis 168:327, 1993

149. Mayer A, Busch MP: Human immune deficiency viruses. p. 654. In Anderson KC, Ness P (eds): The Scientific Basis of Transfusion Medicine: Implications for Clinical Practice. WB Saunders, Philadelphia, 1994

150. Busch MP: HIV and blood transfusions: focus on seroconversion. Vox Sang 67(suppl. 3):S13, 1994

Hepatitis

Roger Y. Dodd

The transmission of hepatitis by human blood was recognized well before the widespread use of transfusion, but by the 1940s, hepatitis was acknowledged to be a major and intractable complication of transfusion. Not only did this problem stimulate and support much of the subsequent research on viral hepatitis, but it also laid the groundwork for dealing with other infectious outcomes of transfusion. Selection of safe donor populations, screening by medical history and risk factors, and the use of both specific and nonspecific laboratory tests all had their genesis in the management of post-transfusion hepatitis. These measures also helped to show that *viral hepatitis* has turned out to be a deceptively simple term, since it is now clear that there are five well-characterized hepatitis viruses and perhaps others yet to be discovered, in addition to a number of other agents, such as cytomegalovirus (CMV), which may also affect the liver. Resolution of the problem of post-transfusion hepatitis has been an incremental process, with each advance leading to the recognition of additional agents or difficulties. However, at the time of writing, it does appear that the major causes of post-transfusion hepatitis have been identified and that effective interventions have been put into place. Indeed, it is now possible to ask whether some measures could be relaxed.

HISTORICAL REVIEW

The first well-documented study of hepatitis transmission by blood was probably the outbreak described by Lürman in 1885.[1] Hepatitis was observed among a population of shipyard workers who had received a human lymph-derived product used as a smallpox vaccine; coworkers who had not been treated were not affected. In retrospect, this almost certainly represented transmission of hepatitis B virus (HBV). During the early part of the twentieth century, hepatitis was noted in association with a variety of injection-based therapies; these infections were most probably a result of multiple use of hypodermic equipment. Subsequently, a very large outbreak of hepatitis occurred in 1942, as a result of the use of a yellow fever vaccine that had been stabilized with pooled human plasma. Around this time, it also became apparent that hepatitis was a frequent adverse outcome of transfusion of blood itself. In the absence of any other measures that could be taken, attempts were made to control this transmission by asking potential donors about a prior history of hepatitis, and rejecting those with such a history. At least in part, this approach recognized the fact that some hepatitis viruses are very likely to result in chronic infection; it failed to recognize the tendency of such infections to be asymptomatic.

During the 1950s and 1960s, epidemiologic and transmission studies established two broad categories of viral hepatitis. They were infectious, or type A, hepatitis (HAV), characterized by a fecal-oral transmission route, and serum, or type B, hepatitis, characterized by a parenteral transmission route.

Even then, however, there were hints that there might be additional agents, since some individuals were known to have had three or more separate bouts of hepatitis. At that time, post-transfusion hepatitis was considered to be exclusively type B. During the same period, it also became increasingly apparent that some donor populations offered a significantly increased risk of hepatitis transmission. Allen performed pioneering studies on transfusion associated hepatitis, concluding that prison donors were particularly risky, leading to the eventual abandonment of blood collection in prisons.[2] Similar findings also resulted in avoidance of collections from paid blood donors.

Such epidemiologically based approaches were not successful in eliminating post-transfusion hepatitis, although it is now well known that they did achieve a greater risk reduction than other subsequent measures. Some effort had been made to identify potentially infectious donors by liver function tests, but those measures were not widely adopted. Others looked for immunologic markers of infection. Prince, in particular, had observed a serum antigen that was associated with transfusion-transmissible hepatitis.[3] His work was overshadowed by Blumberg's prior serendipitous recognition of the so-called Australia antigen (now known as hepatitis B surface antigen [HBsAg]) and London's finding that this antigen was in fact clearly associated with hepatitis B.[4,5] These observations rapidly led to universal blood donor screening for HBsAg, albeit using insensitive gel immunoprecipitation procedures. Perhaps not unexpectedly, the initial testing failed to eliminate post-transfusion hepatitis. What was more surprising was the fact that the much more sensitive radioimmunoassay procedure also failed to eliminate post-transfusion hepatitis, despite the fact that it appeared to detect many more antigenemic donors; however, the majority of these were false-positives.

Feinstone and colleagues, working at the National Institutes of Health (NIH), identified the hepatitis A virus and its corresponding antibody in 1975.[6] Application of this antibody test, along with one for hepatitis B virus, revealed that neither agent was the cause of the residual cases of post-transfusion hepatitis. This led directly to the term *non-A, non-B hepatitis* (NANBH). Numerous studies were performed in

order to identify the causative agent of NANBH, or at least to develop a means for identifying and interdicting infectious blood donations. These studies all followed the same general protocol: patients were identified and pretransfusion blood samples were obtained. At transfusion, a sample of each transfused product was retained. The transfused patients were then followed for about 6 months. Samples were taken, usually at 2- to 4-week intervals and subjected to tests for alanine aminotransferase (ALT) levels. Two successive ALT elevations (one of which generally had to be greater than about two times the upper limit of normal) were defined as evidence of hepatitis. In the majority of these studies, about 95 percent of such events were unaccompanied by any evidence of infection with HAV or HBV and were thus defined as NANBH. Such outcomes were observed in 4 to 12 percent of all recipients. Analysis of donor samples in these studies failed to identify any specific immunologic or virologic marker for NANBH infectivity, but two major studies showed that donors with ALT elevations were more likely to be associated with recipient NANBH than were those with normal ALT levels.[7,8] Interestingly, and paradoxically, both of these studies subsequently showed a similar but nonoverlapping relationship between the presence of antibodies to the hepatitis B core antigen (anti-HBc) in the donor and NANBH in the recipient.[9,10] These observations led directly to the implementation of so-called surrogate testing for NANBH, in which all donors were tested for ALT levels and anti-HBc in order to reduce (but not eliminate) the incidence of post-transfusion NANBH.

Work to try to identify the causative agent of NANBH continued; a combination of painstaking transmission studies in chimpanzees and heroic molecular biology was eventually successful. The infectious agent for NANBH was passaged in chimpanzees until one animal with a very high infectiousness titer was identified. Large quantities of plasma were obtained from this animal and ultracentrifugal pellets were treated on the assumption that they contained a virus. Other evidence suggested that the virus was likely to be an RNA virus. Consequently, a nucleic acid preparation was made and reverse-transcribed to DNA. Fragments of the resultant DNA were incorporated into an expression vector, which was grown in *Escherichia coli*. After investigation of millions of clones, a single colony was found that expressed a protein that reacted with convalescent serum from a patient with NANBH.[11,12] As a result of this finding, it eventually became possible to sequence the entire genome of the virus, which was named hepatitis C virus (HCV).[13] Initially, a single expressed protein (C100-3) was used as the capture reagent in an enzyme immunoassay (EIA) test for antibodies to HCV: this test was uniformly implemented in 1990. The test demonstrably reduced the risk of transfusion-transmitted HCV infection. Subsequently, tests of improved sensitivity have been introduced, as more viral antigens have been expressed and incorporated into the assays.

As a result of these advances, there are now questions as to whether there are additional viruses that are responsible for post-transfusion hepatitis. There is certainly information that suggests that transfused patients may develop hepatitis in the absence of any serologic signs of infection with HAV, HBV, or HCV. Intriguingly, such events may also be seen with a similar frequency among individuals who have received autologous transfusions, suggesting that the etiology is likely to be nonviral. Also, this form of hepatitis does seem to be mild and self-limited.

As a consequence of all of these measures, it is reasonable to suggest that the problem of post-transfusion HBV and HCV among recipients of single-donor products has essentially been resolved, although in common with other infectious agents, it is clear that zero risk has not been achieved. In addition, the development and implementation of a variety of inactivation procedures has resulted in a very high degree of safety for labile factor concentrates prepared from pooled plasma. It appears that such inactivation procedures will also be applied to fresh frozen plasma. At the same time, there has been increased recognition that hepatitis A virus, which is not readily inactivated by current procedures, may offer some risk to recipients, particularly of pooled products.

HEPATITIS A

Disease

Epidemics of hepatitis have been noted almost from the beginning of recorded history. It is more than likely that these epidemics, associated as they were with crowded, unsanitary conditions or military actions, were caused by HAV. It is indeed a typical epidemic disease, often with point-source outbreaks, traceable to food or water that was presumably fecally contaminated.

Infection with HAV is characteristically acute and self-limited. As is common with other hepatitis viruses, symptoms range from inapparent to severe, although the mortality rate for HAV is 0.2 percent or less.[14] In fact, the course of disease is normally mild to moderate, and seroprevalence studies suggest that many cases must go unrecognized, since 5 to 74 percent of the U.S. population has antibodies to HAV, depending upon age.[15] The average incubation period for HAV is 25 to 30 days, with a range of about 15 to 45 days. In symptomatic infection, there may be a relatively short prodromal phase of 2 to 10 days, which may involve fever, chills, malaise, and arthralgias. In some cases, these flulike symptoms may be the only outcome of infection. During this phase, serum transaminase levels rise, peaking shortly after the appearance of typical hepatitis symptoms, including anorexia, nausea and vomiting, and epigastric tenderness. Serum bilirubins may increase, peaking around 8 to 10 days after onset of illness and, where levels are high enough, leading to jaundice. The disease usually resolves over a period of 4 to 6 weeks. There is no evidence of chronic hepatitis due to HAV infection, although unapparent infection accompanied by viral shedding may be seen in neonates.

Laboratory diagnosis of HAV is usually based upon evaluation of serum transaminase levels plus immunoassay for IgM antibodies to HAV in an acute-phase sample; in fact, diagnosis of infection may be made solely upon the presence of IgM anti-HAV. IgG antibodies may develop shortly after the acute phase, but unless an increasing titer is seen in successive samples, they have little diagnostic significance. It is important to note that high titers of virus are shed in the feces starting during the prodromal phase. In addition, virus particles may be present in the blood during some part of this period, including the day or so before any signs or symptoms become apparent. It is this viremic period that accounts for the occasional transmission of HAV by blood transfusion.

Virus

HAV was first recognized in the 1970s as a result of animal transmission studies and, more importantly, by visualization of viral particle in fecal samples, using immune electronmicroscopy.[6] Subsequently, and uniquely for human hepatitis viruses, HAV has been successfully propagated in a variety of tissue culture systems. HAV is a small, spherical, nonenveloped virus with a single positive-stranded RNA genome. Its diameter is about 27 nm and the capsid comprises 60 copies each of four structural proteins, VP1 to VP4. It is loosely classified as an enterovirus: more formally, it is classified in the family Picornaviridae, genus Hepatovirus.

Epidemiology

As noted above, HAV is predominantly transmitted enterically. Typical sources of infection are contaminated water supplies, uncooked shellfish taken from contaminated waters and consumption of food contaminated by an infected handler. Often, this will result in a typical point-source outbreak. Outbreaks have also been noted in day-care establishments that look after diapered children.[15,16] Again, it is reasonable to suggest that the infection was transmitted by the fecal-oral route. These findings suggest a clear potential for secondary infection, and such secondary infections have been noted in a nursery population as a result of at least one transfusion-transmitted HAV case.

In 1992, 23,112 cases of HAV were reported in the United States, reflecting a rate of 9.06/100,000.[15] Serologic studies have shown that the prevalence of HAV antibodies varies extensively with age and sociodemographic status, but not race or sex. Ten to twenty percent of the population has antibodies to HAV by age 20, and 50 percent by age 50.[17] HAV infection does occur among children and infants; indeed, in the United States, almost all viral hepatitis occurring before the age of 11 is due to HAV. Consequently, it is now considered appropriate in the United States to accept individuals with a history of viral hepatitis as blood donors, provided that the hepatitis occurred prior to the age of 11. Some other countries, including the United Kingdom, no longer ask donors about a history of hepatitis. Among blood donor populations, 10 to 20 percent are seropositive. A recent small study indicates donor seroprevalence rates of 12.3 percent among donors in St. Louis and 41 percent among donors in San Bernadino, California.[18]

Transfusion Risk

Infection with HAV is not considered to be a significant risk of transfusion with single-donor products. About 25 cases of post-transfusion HAV had been reported in the literature by 1989; overall, these reports suggest that the risk of symptomatic infection among recipients is considerably less than one case per million component units transfused.[19] In some cases, these have been accompanied by an outbreak of secondary infections.[20] In particular, transfusion-associated cases in neonatal units were observed to lead to secondary cases in the same units.[19,21,22] In addition, a puzzling series of HAV infections have been reported among recipients of pooled plasma products in Europe in 1993.[23] These events are discussed in more detail below.

Interventions

Although donors are currently deferred on the basis of a history of viral hepatitis (occurring after the age of 10), this measure is unlikely to have any value in preventing the transmission of HAV by transfusion, since there is no long-term carrier state for HAV. In addition, transmission occurs as a result of collection of blood during the preacute phase of the infection. Donors who report a history of close contact with a case of viral hepatitis (including the sharing of kitchen and/or toilet facilities) are routinely deferred for 12 months. It seems likely that this practice could prevent transmission of HAV in some limited circumstances. Occasionally, it becomes known after collection that a donor or donor group may have been exposed to a source of HAV (for example, an infectious food handler). In these circumstances, careful judgment is required: it may be appropriate to recall products if it is apparent that the donors were at risk of infection and that they gave blood during a period when they were themselves potentially infectious.

Clearly, it is inappropriate to consider any form of donor testing, since it is unlikely that any serologic test has the capability of identifying a donor during the viremic phase. In addition, the frequency of post-transfusion HAV is extremely low. Some concern has been expressed about the potential for transmission of HAV from pooled plasma or plasma products subject to inactivation by the solvent-detergent process. As a result, there is interest in developing or validating inactivation methods with the capability of eliminating nonenveloped viruses. Additionally, safe, effective HAV vaccines are now becoming available; they may be used to protect populations at particular risk of HAV infection.[24,25]

HEPATITIS B

Disease

The manifestations of hepatitis B vary widely in both severity and duration. Many cases of hepatitis B infection are asymptomatic, but some lead to serious disease or death. Similarly, infection and disease may be acute, chronic, or even lifelong. In general, after infection with HBV, about 60 to 70 percent of individuals do not manifest any disease, or have anicteric or subclinical disease. Overall, about 90 percent of cases recover completely. Some 2 to 10 percent of infections become chronic in adults, but the frequency of chronicity is much higher among those infected early in life, occurring among 90 percent of infants born to chronically infected mothers.[26]

The incubation period ranges from 45 to 120 days. There appears to be an inverse relationship between the inoculum and the incubation period. It is also known that prophylaxis with HBV immunoglobulin can increase the incubation period, a finding that resulted in extension of the period of deferral for potential donors who have been exposed to HBV infection. The onset of acute disease may be heralded by a prodromal phase lasting for a few days. The symptoms include mild fever, malaise, muscle aches, loss of appetite, nausea and vomiting, and tiredness. In some cases, there may hepatomegaly, with attendant tenderness and pain. Icteric disease, if it occurs, has an insidious onset, usually occurring within 10 days of the initial symptoms. Bilirubin levels in the serum and urine increase, followed in a few days by discoloration of the skin and the whites of the eyes, if serum levels exceed 2 to 4 mg/dl. The liver becomes enlarged and tender. In some cases, fulminant hepatitis develops, with more extensive necrosis and profound loss of liver function. This is

accompanied by severe symptoms and may lead to hepatic coma and death.[26] It has been estimated that 0.2 to 0.5 percent of those infected and 0.5 to 1.5 percent of icteric cases may develop fulminant disease, which has 70 to 90 percent mortality. The risk of dying increases with age.[14]

As pointed out above, some 2 to 10 percent of adult cases become chronic, whether or not acute symptoms are seen. Overall, chronic hepatitis may remain mild or may evolve toward life-threatening illness. Even in the absence of clear symptoms, patients may have histologic evidence of chronic persistent hepatitis, or the more serious chronic active hepatitis. A proportion of chronic cases will lead to cirrhosis; this proportion is less than 10 percent for those with chronic persistent hepatitis, but may be much higher among those with chronic active hepatitis, particularly if it is symptomatic. In addition, some patients may develop primary hepatocellular carcinoma. This may occur after the development of cirrhosis, but it is also clear that liver cancer can develop directly as a result of HBV infection in the absence of cirrhosis. Symptoms of chronic hepatitis vary: in some cases, there may be series of relapses. Symptoms, particularly of chronic active hepatitis, include fatigability, anxiety, anorexia, and malaise. In more severe cases, there may be ascites and edema and gastrointestinal (esophageal) bleeding.

Chronic HBV infection is clearly a risk factor for the development of primary hepatocellular carcinoma, as shown by epidemiologic studies in the Far East, Africa, Europe, and the United States.[27–29] It seems likely that infection early in life is a prerequisite for development of liver cancer, since liver cancer was not observed among a large cohort of individuals who were infected with HBV as a result of the use of a yellow fever vaccine in the 1940s.[30] HBV is directly oncogenic, probably as a result of integration of its genome into that of the host cell.

One other clinical aspect of HBV infection is the occurrence of extrahepatic manifestations of disease, which may be seen in approximately 10 to 20 percent of patients.[26] Most of these manifestations are believed to be related to circulating immune complexes of HBsAg and its corresponding antibody. The disease states include a transient serum-sickness–like syndrome, polyarteritis nodosa, and glomerulonephritis. These symptoms or disease states may occur a matter of days or weeks before jaundice or may be the only manifestation of disease.

Diagnosis

As with any other form of hepatitis, preliminary diagnosis of hepatitis B is based upon symptoms and routine liver function tests, with particular reference to serum transaminase and perhaps bilirubin levels. There is an extensive battery of serologic tests that may be used to define whether the disease is caused by HBV; in some cases, these tests may also be used to define the stage of disease or infection. As indicated in Figure 38-1, HBsAg is the first serologic marker to appear after infection, usually some days before the development of symptoms. Anecdotal data suggest that there may be a brief viremic period prior to the development of detectable levels of HBsAg. This is not unreasonable, since the analytic sensitivity of current immunoassays is 0.2 to 0.5 ng/ml, or about 3×10^7 HBsAg particles/ml. In fact, in both acute and chronic infection, there may be up to 10^{13} particles/ml. Soluble HBe antigen (HBeAg) may be found in the serum after about 10 days, although this is not a reliable marker of infection. On the other hand, the presence of HBeAg is often associated with high viral titers, thus representing an indicator of high infectivity. Antibodies to HBc appear about 2 weeks after detectable HBsAg and persist for many years thereafter in both acute and chronic cases. Although both IgG and IgM anti-HBc are formed, the IgM does not seem to be present significantly in advance of IgG, although this may be a function of the analytic sensitivity of the available tests. Specific tests for IgM anti-HBc are commer-

cially available and are of considerable value for diagnosing acute or recent HBV infection, since they generally give positive results for up to 6 months after initial detection. Subsequently, at least in the case of acute infection, detectable levels of HBeAg are likely to be lost and potentially replaced by the corresponding antibody. HBsAg also declines, usually over a period of weeks to 2 months or so. During this period, it is very likely that there are circulating immune complexes, since loss of detectable HBsAg is fairly rapidly followed by the appearance of detectable levels of anti-HBs. This is thought to represent resolution of infection and absence of circulating virus. Anti-HBs is a protective antibody.

Chronic HBV infection is serologically indistinguishable from acute infection during the early stages, but HBsAg does not decline, and detectable levels of anti-HBs are not found (Fig. 38-2). Anti-HBc persists and HBeAg may persist. Ultimately, levels of these markers may decline with time. The appearance of anti-HBe may, however, indicate that an integration event has occurred, at which point the chronically infected individual may be at more risk of development of liver cancer.[26,31]

Virus

The human HBV is the prototype virus of the family Hepadnaviridae, genus Orthohepadnavirus. In common with other hepatitis viruses, HBV is highly species-specific, infecting only humans and chimpanzees. There are other HBVs that infect rodents and ducks, and these have proven to be useful models for at least some aspects of the virology of human HBV. The HBV is relatively small (42 to 47

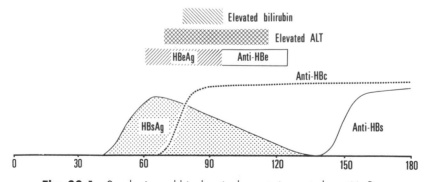

Fig. 38-1. Serologic and biochemical events in acute hepatitis B.

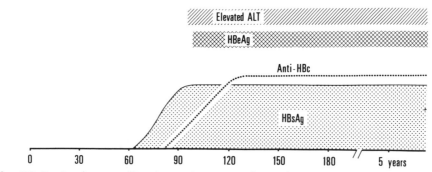

Fig. 38-2. Serologic and biochemical events in chronic hepatitis B/HBsAG carrier state.

nm in diameter). The virus is sensitive to lipid solvents and the envelope incorporates the antigenically characteristic HBsAg peptides. The DNA genome is packaged within an inner capsid or core with its own antigenic specificity. The genome structure is unique: it is circular and partially double-stranded and has overlapping reading frames (Fig. 38-3). The longer strand (which is nicked) is classified as a negative strand inasmuch as it is transcribed to RNA, which can act as a messenger. In addition, the virion has a DNA polymerase that, when active, "fills in"

the single-stranded component of the genome. Replication of the viral genome is extremely unusual, since the DNA viral genome is synthesized by reverse transcription of a more than full-length RNA transcript of about 3,400 bases, which is longer than the approximately 3,200-base DNA genome.

A number of peptides are encoded by the viral genome. There are multiple initiation sites, so the sequences for different peptides actually overlap. The S gene, which includes the pre-S1 and pre-S2 regions, codes for the surface antigen peptides that are incorporated in the outer envelope of the virus and that define its surface antigens. S peptides also self-assemble, generating the noninfectious HBsAg particles and tubules that are so characteristic of HBV infection. The C (core) gene also has two initiation sites; the full-length translation is about 22 kd and 183 to 185 amino acids long. This core peptide is a component of the inner capsid of the virus. A smaller 16-kd peptide may also be expressed; it lacks the 34 C-terminal amino acids that are the DNA binding site. This peptide is released in soluble form as HBeAg. The epitopes that represent the *e* antigenicity are masked in the full-length core protein, which is confined to the virion.

The initial characterization of the virus and of its immune response was by serologic techniques. HBsAg was the first serologic marker of HBV infection to be described, as Australia antigen, by Blumberg. The circulating antigen was recognized as a result of the presence of antibodies to HBsAg in the serum of multiply transfused individuals.[4] Subsequently, core antigen was recognized by Almeida as a result of immune electronmicroscopic studies on

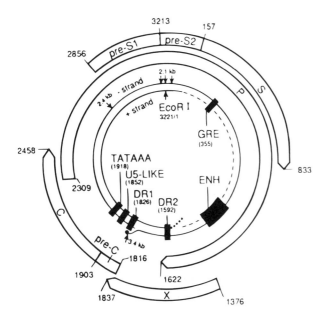

Fig. 38-3. Circular map of the hepatitis B virus genome. (From Robinson,[131] with permission.)

virions which had been lysed with detergents.[32] Further serologic studies upon different populations revealed that HBsAg was antigenically diverse, and a number of subtypes of HBsAg have been described. Basically, a common antigen (*a*) is found on all HBsAg particles. In addition, there are two pairs of antigens that act like mutually exclusive alleles (*d,y* and *w,r*). Consequently, the major subtypes are *adw*, *adr*, *ayw*, and *ayr*. Additional subspecificities of the *w* antigen have also been described. For a time, these subtypes proved useful in epidemiologic tracing. Since they tend to be geographically restricted, they have also been evaluated in the context of population movements. Modern techniques have revealed that the antigenic subtypes of HBsAg are, as might be expected, based upon variations in genomic sequences and usually represent simple, single-amino acid substitutions in key epitopes. At this time, there is relatively little interest in serologic aspects of HBsAg subtypes, since direct studies on genomic sequences are more precise.

It is now clear that there are HBV mutants that have direct implications for transfusion medicine. Pre-S mutants are a class of mutants that appear to affect the expression of the *a* determinant of HBsAg. As a consequence, HBV infection occurs without the expression of readily detectable circulating antigen, although the virus does appear to be replication-competent. Consequently, individuals without detectable HBsAg may, nevertheless, be infectious for HBV; they could be missed in laboratory screening.[33] Those infected with pre-S mutant strains of HBV do, however, develop anti-HBc, so would be detected in circumstances where anti-HBc testing is used. Pre-S mutants seem to be rare and should not be the focus of excess concern at this time. Such mutants may eventually become somewhat more frequent, since they may arise as escape mutants in the face of HBV vaccination or the use of HBV immunoglobulin.[33]

Another class of mutants are the precore mutants, which are base substitutions that insert a stop codon into the C region open reading frame. As a result, the soluble *e* antigen is not expressed during infection. It is thought that the soluble *e* antigen may affect the host immune response, leading to induction of cellular tolerance to *e* antigen expressed upon the surface of infected hepatocytes. This is thought to be the mechanism that leads to the high frequency of persistent infection in infants born to *e*-positive HBV-infected mothers, since the *e* antigen can cross the placenta. Conversely, precore mutants have been found to be significantly associated with fulminant HBV infection, presumably reflecting the inability of the host to eliminate infected hepatocytes that fail to express the antigen. In some cases, these mutants can arise during chronic infection, whereas in other situations, the infecting virus itself is the mutant.[33,34]

Finally, it has been reported that there may be a second strain of HBV, termed HBV-2, which is characterized by the absence of anti-HBc or anti-HBe in infected patients, although HBsAg is expressed.[33]

Epidemiology

HBV infection occurs worldwide. It is considered to be a global problem, with an estimated 250 million HBsAg carriers. On an international basis, the prevalence and incidence of HBV infection vary extensively. In parts of Asia and Oceania, population prevalence rates for serologic markers of HBV may exceed 90 percent, whereas the corresponding figure for the United States or Northern Europe is 5 percent or less. The predominant, if not the only, transmission route for HBV is parenteral. Because of the potential for extremely high viral titers, the actual transmission mechanism is not always apparent or readily understood. For example, it does not appear that HBV can be transmitted via the enteric route. However, entry of the virus through the oral mucous membrane is possible, thus generating the appearance of infection via the gut. Broadly speaking, HBV transmission is characterized by two major routes: (1) the perinatal route, in which an infected mother transmits the virus to her baby at or around the time of birth; and (2) horizontal transmission by a number of routes, but particularly during sexual intercourse. Taken together, these two broad transmission routes tend to stabilize the overall population prevalence of infection. Thus, children born to infected mothers are most likely to become long-term infectious carriers who may transmit the infection to others later in life.

In addition to birth to an infected mother, there are a number of well-established behavioral and environmental risk factors for HBV infection that reflect the transmission routes. These risk factors include intravenous drug use, sexual exposure to infected partners (particularly for male homosexuals), exposure to nonsterile skin-piercing instruments, and employment in a health-care environment. In addition, close exposure to other cases, particularly in an institutional setting, has been cited as a risk factor. In the past, it was clear that a history of blood transfusion or of treatment with clotting factor concentrates was also a risk factor. Fortunately, recognition of the threat of HBV transmission, along with the implementation of appropriate interventions, has significantly reduced the impact in many of these areas.[35,36] For example, the proper use of HBV vaccine and universal handling precautions have significantly reduced the transmission of HBV in the health-care workplace. Cosmetologists and practitioners of ear-piercing and tattooing have accepted the need to use sterile or single-use devices. All labile clotting factor concentrates are subjected to one or more inactivation procedures.

A wide variety of unusual transmission routes for HBV have been described, but all seem to be explainable by the transfer of small volumes of blood or body fluids. There may be a risk of infection of up to 27 percent in the case of a needlestick if the needle has been contaminated with blood from an HBsAg-positive individual.[37] The virus is relatively stable on surfaces and is thus transmitted by a number of fomites, including such unexpected items as file cards (in association with paper cuts), shared razors and toothbrushes, and so on. It should also be noted that contamination of the mucous membranes with droplets of infected fluids may lead to infection, as may entry of the virus through even extremely minor skin wounds and abrasions. Conversely, the virus may be transmitted in exudates from wounds or skin irritations.

The number of reported cases of HBV in the United States has been declining since 1985. In 1992, a total of 16,126 cases were reported to the Centers for Disease Control and Prevention (CDC) through the states, for an overall incidence of 6.32/ 100,000. The majority of cases were among those aged 20 to 40, and 57.8 percent of cases were among males. There was an over-representation of nonwhite individuals. Among a subset of 4,562 reported cases, the following possible exposure factors were reported in the 6 weeks to 6 months prior to disease:

multiple sex partners (20.2 percent), close personal contact with a patient (19.2 percent), drug use (13.1 percent). Although 15.1 percent of patients reported dental work, this was also true of 10.5 percent of those who contracted HAV. Homosexual activity was reported among 8.4 percent of those with HBV. Only 1.4 percent of cases reported having received a blood transfusion, compared to 0.5 percent for HAV and 4.3 percent for NANBH.[15]

A seroepidemiologic assessment of HBV infection in the United States has been reported for a representative population sample collected from 1976 to 1980.[38] In brief, the overall prevalence rate for HBV infection markers was 5.67 percent, based upon the cumulative presence of HBsAg, anti-HBs, or anti-HBc. Adjusted seroprevalence rates for whites and blacks were 3.2 percent and 13.7 percent, respectively. In both groups, there was little infection among children, and seroprevalence rates began to increase in the teenage years. Prevalence rates increased with age, with the most marked increase among blacks. Other independent predictors of HBV seropositivity included male sex, residence in the South, Northeast, or West, residence in cities with a population of 250,000 or greater, living below the poverty level, and having a positive treponemal test for syphilis. It is not clear whether these patterns are still true in 1994, since there have been substantial changes in the overall epidemiology of HBV infection in the United States.[35] The epidemiologic patterns of HBV infection in the donor population have not been comprehensively reviewed recently. Overall prevalence rates for HBsAg are on the order of 0.03 percent and are between 1 and 2 percent for anti-HBc. In some part at least, these figures reflect the impact of continued testing on the repeat donor population. Frequencies of HBV markers are higher among autologous donors.[39]

Transfusion Risk

In the past, blood transfusion offered significant risk of transmission of HBV. However, at this time, the actual risk of transmission appears to be very low, if not negligible. This is a result of steadily increasing attention to donor selection and laboratory screening. Reporting rates for clinically apparent, acute transfusion-associated HBV are fewer than 100 cases per year for the American Red Cross system, representing about half of the single-donor products transfused in the United States. This figure may be compared with the CDC reports, indicating that 1.4 percent, or 225 of the 16,126 cases reported in 1992, might have been associated with transfusion. At the same time, it should be recognized that about 230 clinical cases of acute HBV would be expected to occur in a population of 4 million individuals (which is the size of the transfused patient population) in the absence of transfusion, if the incidence rate is 6.3/100,000.[15] Consequently, it is reasonable to suppose that some cases of HBV that occur among transfusion recipients may not actually have been transmitted by the blood components. At the same time, there are certainly anecdotal reports of cases of HBV in blood recipients in which a blood donor has subsequently been shown to have seroconverted. It is thought that, in these circumstances, transmission of HBV occurred at a time prior to the appearance of detectable levels of HBsAg. This emphasizes the continuing value of recalling implicated donors for serologic testing and implies that there is an ongoing need for donor screening to identify those at risk of early infection. It is also thought that there may be situations in which there may be continuing low-level infection with circulation of virus, but undetectable levels of HBsAg. It should be noted that some of the mutants of HBV might also offer risk of transmission, although this seems unlikely in the face of both HBsAg and anti-HBc testing. There are no contemporary measures of the residual risk of HBV infectivity among blood donors in the United States. At least one estimate has been made, however. Alter has suggested that the residual infectivity of the fully screened blood supply is about 1/200,000 components, translating to a potential of some 100 infections per year in the United States.[40,41] This estimate was based upon the frequency of positive test results for HBsAg and anti-HBc among donors and some assumptions about the sensitivity of those tests.

For many years, it has been recognized that circulating HBV DNA may be found in the presence of other markers of infection. The availability of sensitive means for detecting such DNA, such as the polymerase chain reaction (PCR), has extended these studies. In particular, there have been a number of publications suggesting that HBV DNA may be found in a significant proportion of individuals with-

out serologic markers of HBV infection, or in those with presumptive indicators, such as ALT elevations.[42–45] A number of these studies claimed to show an unexpectedly high prevalence of HBV DNA, frequencies that were clearly not commensurate with the residual frequency of HBV transmission. More recently, essentially negative findings have been reported,[46] suggesting that studies of this type should be interpreted with caution.

Interventions

Screening

Many of the measures now used to select blood donors resulted from earlier efforts to reduce the incidence of post-transfusion hepatitis. In particular, the avoidance of paid donors and donors from penal institutions was based upon data that demonstrated that such donor populations offered increased risk of infection.[2] Donor history questions relating to a past history of viral hepatitis reflected recognition of the persistent nature of HBV (and, in retrospect, HCV) infection, although it is now clear that such measures could have had only limited value, given the high frequency of clinically mild or inapparent hepatitis virus infection. In the United States, it is now permissible to accept individuals as donors if they had viral hepatitis prior to the age of 11. This reflects the virtual absence of HBV infection in this age group: viral hepatitis before the age of 11 is almost invariably due to HAV. Some countries, such as the United Kingdom, have abandoned deferring donors on the basis of a history of hepatitis. Nevertheless, a number of studies do show that individuals reporting a history of prior viral hepatitis do indeed have an elevated prevalence of markers for −HAV, HBV, or HCV.[47,48]

Questioning donors and inspecting their forearms for evidence of intravenous drug use also reflects a clear recognition of the connection between needle-sharing and hepatitis infection. Also, questioning for a history of transfusion, use of clotting factor concentrates or other parenteral exposures, or close contact with a hepatitis-infected person all reflected known risks for HBV infection. The attendant deferral periods have been modified from time to time. In particular, early experience with the use of hepatitis B immunoglobulin indicated that it could extend the incubation period for HBV beyond the normal 6 months, resulting in a one-year deferral for those receiving this product as a result of presumed HBV exposure. Subsequently, additional screening questions have been introduced in order to attempt to reduce the risk of human immunodeficiency transmission. It is likely that some of these questions, particularly those that deal with sexual exposure, may have further reduced the proportion of donors who are potentially infectious for HBV.

Testing

Specific testing for HBV infectiousness has been uniformly in place in the United States since 1971. The testing was based upon the recognition of HBsAg and its relationship to HBV infectivity by Prince and Blumberg, et al.[3,5] HBsAg was first detected by diffusion and precipitation in agar gels (Ouchterlony technique), using serum from multiply transfused individuals as a source of antibody. This procedure was insensitive and impractical for routine use; indeed, only a few establishments used it. It was rapidly replaced by facilitated gel precipitation techniques, in which an electrical field (counterimmunoelectrophoresis) or evaporative solvent flow (rheophoresis) drove the antigen and antibody reactants together. These methods were cumbersome and highly subjective. The development and commercialization of solid-phase radioimmunoassay (RIA) procedures for HBsAg by Ling and Overby led to an operational revolution in blood testing.[49] In brief, a solid-phase capture reagent (originally a plastic test tube, but subsequently plastic beads, microplate wells, or particulate substrates were also used) was coated with antibodies to HBsAg. The sample was added to the solid phase, allowed to incubate, then washed out. HBsAg, if present, was bound by the antibodies. The presence of this antigen was detected by a probe reagent, which was a purified anti-HBs labeled with [125]I. After incubation, excess probe was washed out and residual reactivity was measured using a scintillation counter. This procedure became the standard of practice and remained so for a number of years. The analytic sensitivity of RIA was on the order of 1 to 2 ng/ml, an improvement of several orders of magnitude. Nevertheless, as pointed out above, RIA had relatively little impact upon residual post-

transfusion hepatitis (which was, of course, mainly NANBH).

RIA was markedly less specific than gel diffusion. There was a high frequency of nonrepeatable reactive results that were usually attributable to minor contamination of the reaction tube with radioactive label. These events were identified and corrected by replicate retesting of samples with initially reactive readings, a practice that continues to date for enzyme immunoassays. It was also found that there were significant numbers of repeatedly reactive samples that did not seem to be associated with any other evidence of HBV infection or infectivity. As a result, confirmatory procedures were developed for RIA. The approach taken was to use a human antibody to HBsAg to block the binding of HBsAg to the anti-HBs capture reagent and to compare the signal from such a blocked test with one from a test using normal human serum. Samples were considered to be confirmed if the use of anti-HBs resulted in at least a 50 percent inhibition of signal relative to the control.

Subsequently, RIA was replaced by EIA, which is currently the method of choice. The principle is exactly the same as that for RIA, except the probe reagent is labeled with an enzyme, such as alkaline phosphatase or horseradish peroxidase. In order to detect bound probe reagent, one further step is required: a chromogenic substrate for the enzyme is added to the washed solid phase, and after reaction, the assay is evaluated spectrophotometrically. A number of modifications have been introduced, including the use of monoclonal antibodies, which may permit the simultaneous addition of sample and probe. The current analytic sensitivity of EIA procedures is on the order of 0.5 ng/ml or less.

Other test methods for HBsAg have been used in the past; some are still in use in some parts of the world. In particular, reversed passive hemagglutination is a relatively simple procedure, although it is probably about one order of magnitude less sensitive than EIA. Unlike EIA, this method is not licensed for use in the United States.

As discussed elsewhere in this chapter, blood donations are routinely tested for anti-HBc in the United States and in a number of other countries. For a number of years after the original recognition of anti-HBc, there were suggestions that some cases of transfusion-associated HBV infection were associated with donations that were positive only for anti-HBc. It was thought likely that these donations were made during the HBsAg-negative "window" during acute infection.[50] Anti-HBc testing of blood donations was not introduced until 1986–87, when it was adopted as a surrogate test for NANBH infectivity in donors. There is some indirect evidence that this test may also have had some impact upon the overall incidence of posttransfusion HBV infection, although such evidence is confounded by changes in the underlying epidemiology of HBV.[51] Nevertheless, the anti-HBc test was subsequently licensed as a biologic by the United States Food and Drug Administration (FDA), and was specifically recommended as a measure to reduce the incidence of post-transfusion HBV.

In contrast to tests for HBsAg, and indeed for most other donor screening tests, the most common format for anti-HBc tests is as an inhibition test. The solid-phase capture reagent bears anti-HBc and the probe is an enzyme- or radionuclide-labeled anti-HBc. The test sample competes with the probe, so that a positive result is defined by a reduced signal, relative to a negative control. Unfortunately, this approach is much more subject to procedural error than are direct-binding assays, since the final signal is directly influenced by the accuracy of pipetting and the cutoff value is on the steepest part of the assay response curve. At least one manufacturer has developed a direct antiglobulin test for anti-HBc, however. Testing for anti-HBc identifies all donors with this antibody, but many such individuals are also positive for anti-HBs. Since anti-HBs signifies a resolved infection, such donors do not offer increased risk of HBV infection. Thus, the positive predictive value of anti-HBc for those at risk of transmitting HBV is extremely low. The FDA does not require or recommend anti-HBc testing for source plasma—in fact, this would reduce the titers of protective anti-HBs in plasma pools and immunoglobulin preparations.[52]

In general, implementation of current regulatory requirements leads to the policy that blood donors with repeatedly reactive test results for HBsAg or for anti-HBc (on the second occasion) are no longer acceptable for further donations. Such deferral policies provide backup in the event that a donor presents again but the laboratory fails to detect a positive result. Owing to the significant rate of false-positivity for anti-HBc, donors who have repeat reactive results on a single donation are still eligible for future donation. Furthermore, in the case of a reactive HBsAg test result that cannot be confirmed by neutralization, or for which a neutralization result is not available, the donor may be accepted for a future donation, provided that at least 8 weeks have passed since the last donation, that the current donation is nonreactive on an EIA for HBsAg, and that the current donation is nonreactive on an EIA test for anti-HBc.

Prophylaxis

Anti-HBs appears to be a protective antibody for HBV infection or disease. Consequently, passive administration of anti-HBs or active vaccination with HBsAg are used as interventions to prevent transmission of, or infection with, the virus. In the past, there were extensive trials of the use of specific hepatitis B immunoglobulin (HBIG), usually prepared by conventional techniques from pools of plasma with high titers of anti-HBs; such products are available commercially. HBIG treatment proved efficacious for postexposure prophylaxis, particularly in cases of needlestick exposure to infectious blood. Data were not as convincing in other settings, with the possible exception of newborn infants of mothers with HBsAg.[53]

Subsequently, an inactivated subunit HBV vaccine was prepared from purified HBsAg obtained from naturally infected humans. In meticulous studies, Szmuness and colleagues definitively demonstrated the safety and efficacy of this vaccine in populations of at-risk homosexual men. Subsequently, the vaccine was licensed and recommended for use in all populations at elevated risk of HBV infection, including health-care workers and recipients of labile clotting factor concentrates prepared from pooled plasma.[54] The vaccine was, and is, considered particularly appropriate for the prevention of infection in infants of HBsAg-positive mothers; interruption of such transmission is eventually expected to have a major impact upon the prevalence of the HBsAg carrier state. In the United States, vaccination of infants was originally proposed only in cases in which the prospective mother was HBsAg-positive. This approach was not found to provide a broad enough coverage, and vaccination of all infants is now recommended. Although plasma-derived vaccines were safe and effective, they have now been supplanted by recombinant vaccines prepared from yeast-derived HBsAg peptides. In some circumstances, such as postexposure prophylaxis, the use of both HBIG and vaccine is recommended.

A final aspect of HBV vaccine that is relevant to transfusion medicine is the impact of the vaccine upon donors. The vaccine itself is noninfectious, and there is no safety reason to defer a recently vaccinated prospective donor. Yeast-derived recombinant vaccines are used in a higher dosage than the plasma-derived vaccine, and in a number of instances, detectable levels of HBsAg have been found in the blood of individuals who received vaccine in the preceding 24 hours. Such HBsAg positivity is, of course, confirmable by neutralization, making the donor unsuitable for future donations, at least from a regulatory perspective. Consequently, it makes sense to temporarily defer prospective donors for a few days after receipt of HBV vaccine. It should also be remembered that there may be cause for a more lengthy deferral period if the vaccine has been given as a result of explicit risk of HBV infection.

HEPATITIS C

Disease

It is now clear that the majority of cases of the disease previously termed NANBH are due to infection with HCV. Indeed, in reevaluation of earlier post-transfusion hepatitis studies, at least 85 percent of cases of NANBH were shown to be due to HCV infection.[55,56] In general, the acute manifestations of HCV infection are less severe than those of HBV. HCV infection is characterized by a very high rate of chronicity, and the long-term effects may be quantitatively and qualitatively more serious than those associated with other hepatitis viruses.

The average incubation period for HCV is 7 to 8 weeks, although a wide range has been noted. It has been estimated that 25 percent of cases may be acutely symptomatic, although it appears that such symptoms are mild, and rarely lead to hospitalization. In addition, peak aminotransferase levels tend to be lower than those observed in HBV infection.

Symptoms, if present, include fatigue, anorexia, abdominal pain, and weight loss. A proportion of patients may become jaundiced. In acute disease, symptoms may persist for up to 10 weeks. Fulminant disease is rare, and the mortality rate for acute disease is less than 1 percent.[14] In almost all cases of HCV infection, viral nucleic acid is persistently present. Furthermore, about 70 percent of infections lead to chronic liver dysfunction or disease, as demonstrated by persistent or fluctuating transaminase levels for longer than 1 year. There appears to be no relationship between the development of chronic disease and the presence or absence of acute disease. Biopsy studies show that some 60 percent of these individuals with persistent transaminase elevations have microscopic evidence of chronic persistent or chronic active hepatitis or cirrhosis.[57–60] Despite this evidence of disease, most such patients appear to be asymptomatic. Seeff and colleagues showed no increased mortality among about 500 transfused individuals with post-transfusion hepatitis relative to those who did not have hepatitis, even after about 20 years' follow-up, but there was some evidence of increased liver disease among this group.[61] Similar long-term follow-up of 80 patients by Koretz et al. suggested evidence of overt liver failure among about 20 percent of those with chronic post-transfusion HCV, with an overall death rate of about 5 to 6 percent.[59] In addition, prolonged observation of individuals with post-transfusion HCV in Japan has shown occasional progression to cirrhosis and liver cancer over a period of 23 years or more.[62] In some parts of the world, a high proportion of patients with HBV-negative primary hepatocellular carcinoma have evidence of HCV infection. Since HCV is a positive-strand RNA virus, it seems unlikely that it is directly oncogenic. Rather, liver cancer may reflect progression from cirrhosis, presumably as a result of uncontrolled liver cell regeneration.

Diagnosis

As with other forms of hepatitis, diagnosis of HCV disease is based upon symptoms and liver function tests, particularly serum transaminase levels. Serologic diagnosis may be made on the basis of the presence of anti-HCV in the absence of other markers of acute viral hepatitis. At the time of publication of this book, there is no commercially available IgM specific test for anti-HCV, but research studies have shown the presence of IgM antibodies during the early stages of HCV infection. It has been suggested that this marker may thus be of value, but its expression may be variable.[63,64] Thus, serodiagnosis is best achieved by recognition of seroconversion. The EIA test for HCV is not really quantitative, so it is not strictly possible to look for rising antibody titers. As discussed below, the EIA test should preferably be confirmed using a supplementary test procedure. Most such confirmatory tests are based upon immunoblot procedures that permit the identification of antibodies to separate viral peptides. There is, however, no definitive pattern of the order of appearance of antibodies to different peptides, so these confirmatory assays do not necessarily add a great deal of information. Active infection is usually accompanied by serum RNA detectable by PCR, but such findings are also present in many individuals with chronic infection.

Virus

NANBH was recognized as a separate entity in 1975.[6] Extensive epidemiologic and animal model studies (in chimpanzees) clearly demonstrated that the disease had a viral etiology. Laboratory manipulation of infectious inocula also provided hints about the nature of the putative virus, indicating that it was enveloped, that it was probably about 60 nm in diameter, and that it was most probably an RNA virus. As with most other hepatitis viruses, it proved recalcitrant to growth in tissue culture systems and still has not been conventionally isolated. Nevertheless, a combination of skillful animal work and molecular biology led to cloning and expression of a portion of the genome of what is now known as HCV. More specifically, Bradley and colleagues at the CDC repeatedly passaged the infectious agent in chimpanzees, until they were able to identify an animal with a persistent high titer of circulating virus. An ultracentrifugal pellet derived from the plasma of this animal was reverse-transcribed and cloned into *E. coli,* using an expression vector, by Houghton and colleagues at Chiron. After examining millions of bacterial colonies, one was found to express a protein that reacted with serum from an individual who had diagnosed NANBH.[11,12] This clone, termed 5-1-1, was shown to express a protein that was re-

active with presumed antibodies from patients with NANBH, but not with other forms of hepatitis.[55] As discussed below, the ability to express antigenic peptides from the viral genome led directly to the development of immunoassays for HCV infection. In addition, the isolation of a single clone led rapidly to a sequence for the entire genome of HCV.[13]

The genome of HCV is a single positive strand of RNA of approximately 9,400 bases (Fig. 38-4). Its functional organization and sequence homologies suggest that it is related to the flaviviruses and pestiviruses; it has been suggested that it should be classified as a new genus of the Flaviviridae. At the 5' end of the genome, there is a highly conserved untranslated region. Sequences in this region are commonly used as target sequences for genome detection by PCR. The open reading frame is comprised of regions that translate to structural proteins at the 5' end; the nonstructural region is toward the 3' end of the genome. The C region codes for the capsid protein, followed by the E1 and E2/NS1 regions, coding for envelope peptides. The NS2 region is thought to code for a membrane-binding function, the NS3 for helicase/protease function, NS4 for membrane-binding, and NS5 for polymerase. The initially isolated clone, 5-1-1, is located in the NS4 region. Subsequently, the larger C100-3 clone was expressed, which included the 5-1-1 sequence; this peptide became the basis for the initial anti-HCV test. Eventually, antigenic peptides have been expressed from the C region (core, or C22c), from E2, from NS3 (C33c), and from NS5. In addition, a clone termed C200 includes the C33c and C100-3 sequences.[13] Some of the genomic sequences show significant sequence variation, and six major genotypes have been identified.[65] These genotypes seem to have differing geographic distributions, and there are hints that some of them may be associated with somewhat differing clinical outcomes.[66]

As indicated above, HCV is known to be lipid-enveloped, and careful filtration studies suggest a diameter of 60 nm or less; both of these characteristics would be anticipated for a flavivirus. As an enveloped virus, HCV is susceptible to inactivation by solvent-detergent procedures, so that clotting factor concentrates treated with the solvent-detergent procedure are now considered to be safe from risk of HCV infectivity. This is also true of products that

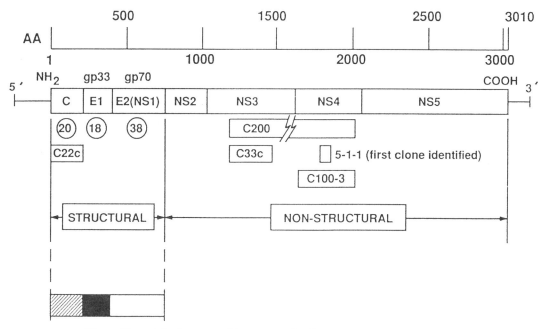

"Target" protein for recombinant vaccine?

Fig. 38-4. Hepatitis C virus: genome organization and location of expressed proteins. (From Bradley,[13] with permission.)

have been treated by the more intensive heating protocols. There have been a few reports that HCV has been visualized, and the electronmicroscopic appearance of the candidate particles is consistent with the expected morphology.[67] Virus usually appears to circulate at low titer, and direct detection by immunologic methods is difficult. On the other hand, viral genomic material is readily detected in serum or plasma by reverse-transcription PCR technology.[68–72] Indeed, many studies suggest unexpectedly high genome copy numbers in the circulation.

HCV is thought to replicate in the liver, as do other hepatitis viruses. In addition, there are a number of studies reporting that HCV sequences, including replicative forms, may be found in peripheral blood monocytes from infected individuals. As with HBV, the significance of this finding is unclear at this time.[73,74]

Epidemiology

The availability of tests for antibodies to HCV has resulted in a much clearer picture of the descriptive epidemiology of NANBH. During 1992, the CDC reported 6,010 cases of clinically recognized acute NANBH, rather more than in preceding years. Some of the increase in the reported number appeared to reflect fewer cases reported as "unspecified." The reporting rate for 1992 was 3.36/100,000.[15] Active surveillance suggests that the true frequency is about twofold greater.[75] Overall, it has been estimated that there may be as many as 170,000 NANBH infections annually in the United States, of which the great majority are due to HCV.[76] NANBH is clearly parenterally transmitted, but sporadic or community-acquired cases also occur. Overall, 85 percent or more of cases are due to infection with HCV. The natural history of HCV disease does not seem to differ on the basis of transmission route, with sporadic cases having similar outcomes to transfusion-associated cases.

Seroprevalence studies show an unusual consistency in prevalence rates for HCV infection worldwide, with about 0.5 to 1.5 percent of the general population found positive for HCV antibodies.[14] There is a characteristic age-specific prevalence pattern, with the highest rates in the 20 to 40 age group.

There are reports of clusters of high prevalence, but these usually seem to be attributable to readily recognizable factors, such as needle-sharing or similar exposures. Overall, however, the similar seroprevalence rates imply some common, underlying transmission mechanism. The sexual route would appear to be a good candidate, but the available data tend to be contradictory. In particular, the frequency of HCV antibodies among male homosexuals is around 4 to 5 percent, much lower than that for human immunodeficiency virus (HIV) or HBV.[77,78] Similarly, patients at sexually transmitted disease clinics have HCV seroprevalence rates of 8 to 10 percent.[79,80] A number of studies on sexual partners of HCV-infected intravenous drug users or hemophiliacs similarly suggest infrequent transmission.[81–85] Additionally, epidemiologic studies on community-acquired HCV identify sexual contact with an infected person as a risk factor, but only for 6 percent of cases.[58] In contrast, however, two recent studies from Japan and Italy report anti-HCV among 27 percent of spouses of HCV-infected individuals.[86,87] Interestingly, in both of these reports, the frequency of infection was correlated with the length of the exposure; in fact, Akahane et al.[86] report no apparent transmission between individuals married for less than 10 years. It is unclear whether the clinical status of an individual, the infecting strain of virus, or indeed any other factors influence infectivity.[88] Overall, however, the data suggest that sexual transmission of HCV does occur, but that such transmission is inefficient. Nevertheless, this does not eliminate this vector as the predominant one by which HCV infection is maintained within the population.

Surveillance studies on acute NANBH cases reveal that, in 1992, the major risk factor was illicit intravenous drug use, with 21.4 percent of cases reporting it prior to illness. Dental work, multiple sex partners, personal contact with an infected person, and surgery were respectively reported in 15.5 percent, 12.4 percent, 12.0 percent, and 10.2 percent of cases, respectively. Blood transfusion was reported in only 4.3 percent of cases.[15] Once again, this is generally consistent with current reports of around 100 cases per year of HCV among recipients of blood components from the American Red Cross system. Over the past 15 years, the frequency of cases with drug use as a risk factor has increased, while that for trans-

fusion has decreased markedly. Studies on risk factors among HCV-seropositive blood donors have yielded generally similar results.[89] As with HBV and a number of other infections, a significant proportion of cases (about 40 percent) do not report readily identifiable risk factors.[75]

It is thought that the titer of circulating HCV is usually relatively low, with about 100 infectious doses per milliliter, although much higher levels (around 10^6 infectious doses per milliliter) have been documented. This probably accounts for the relative inefficiency of transmission by some routes, compared to HBV. For example, it appears that only about 3 percent of needlestick exposures (in the health-care setting) result in HCV infection, compared to 30 percent for HBV.[90] Transmission by intravenous drug use is probably more efficient because larger volumes of blood are generally exchanged by this route. There is some evidence of transmission from mother to child, with infection reported in 5.6 percent of infants born to HCV RNA-positive mothers, but unlike HBV, this also seems to be an inefficient transmission route.[87,91,92]

As discussed extensively above, most infection with HCV is persistent, with long-term circulation of potentially infectious virus, as indicated by viral RNA detectable by PCR.[93,94] Such infected individuals must be the major reservoir for transmission of the virus.

Transfusion Risk

The risk of transmission of HCV by transfusion has declined markedly over the years, largely—but not entirely—as a result of enhanced donor screening and the sequential implementation of a number of laboratory tests. In addition, the underlying epidemiology of HCV has itself changed, resulting in decreased rates of transfusion-associated infection (at least in Canada) in the absence of overt interventions.[95] Certainly in the late 1970s, a high proportion of transfusion recipients (8 to 12 percent or more) developed post-transfusion hepatitis, as demonstrated by serum transaminase elevations. Some 95 percent of these cases were NANBH, and more than 50 percent of them became chronic. Reanalysis of these studies shows that at least 85 percent of these cases were caused by HCV infection.[55,56] The impact of successive measures to reduce this risk was demonstrated by Donahue and colleagues, who evaluated the frequency of HCV seroconversion among a large population of blood recipients. When first published, the study used the first-generation, single-antigen (C100-3) test for anti-HCV to define the frequency of infection among recipients. As a result, they showed that the per-unit risk of transmission was 0.45 percent immediately before initiation of surrogate testing. After surrogate testing was implemented, the risk declined to 0.19 percent per unit. After first-generation HCV testing was implemented, the per-unit risk dropped to 0.03 percent.[96] There were no data representing rates after the implementation of second- or third-generation tests. This group did subsequently reevaluate infection rates from blood screened with first-generation HCV tests using second-generation tests to detect HCV seroconversion in recipients. They identified 11 HCV seroconversions among 1,122 patients who had received a total of 18,392 units of blood, for a rate of 1 infection per 1,672 units.[97]

Kleinman et al. reviewed the increased detection rates achieved by second-generation tests for anti-HCV among donors, and came to the conclusion that the residual risk of HCV infection among current, fully tested units lay between 1 in 2,000 and 1 in 6,000 per component unit.[98] A number of post-transfusion studies performed outside the United States have found no infections among recipients of anti-HCV–tested products; these studies were all relatively small, and the results are compatible with Kleinman's estimate. Not incidentally, these studies also invariably show that surrogate testing does not appear to have any significant additional contribution to the prevention of HCV infection, once anti-HCV testing has been implemented. Interestingly, in an interim report on his long-standing study of post-transfusion hepatitis at the NIH, Harvey Alter reported that he had observed no cases of post-transfusion hepatitis among 300 recipients transfused since the implementation of sensitive tests for anti-HCV.[99]

Unfortunately, at this time, there are no means of estimating the infectious window period for HCV, and information on seroconversion rates among donors is very limited. Consequently, other approaches to estimation of risk are not available. Miriam Alter has suggested that there may now be somewhat fewer

than 170,000 HCV infections per year in the United States[76]; if 2 to 3 percent of these are transfusion-associated, then there would be 3,000 to 4,500 infections annually—a figure that is entirely compatible with the risk figures presented above.

Interventions

Screening

A number of screening questions that were introduced as a general measure to reduce post-transfusion hepatitis (see above) probably did have some limited impact upon the incidence of post-transfusion HCV infection. For example, although the majority of cases of acute HCV infection are subclinical or asymptomatic, there is an excess prevalence of HCV antibodies among those reporting a history of viral hepatitis.[48] Such seropositive individuals have a high likelihood of being infectious. Similarly, prohibition of donation by intravenous drug users probably prevented cases of HCV transmission, as did the move to an all-volunteer donor population. In fact, clinical trials of HCV antibody tests in the United States did reveal higher frequencies of seropositivity among paid plasma donors.[100]

It is also thought that additional screening measures that were introduced to reduce the risk of transmission of HIV by transfusion may also have impacted HCV transmission. At the same time, it should be recognized that the prevalence of HCV antibodies among homosexual men has been found to be unexpectedly low,[77,78] so that interventions directed against sexually transmitted HIV may have had relatively little overall effect.

Testing

Recognition of NANBH in 1975 led to extensive and ongoing efforts to identify serologic markers that could be used to identify donations that would be likely to transmit the agent. In retrospect, it is clear that in the absence of any ability to isolate the virus and grow it in laboratory culture, and because of the low titer of virus in the circulation, such attempts were doomed to failure. Nevertheless, post-transfusion studies, notably the Transfusion-Transmitted Viruses (TTV) and NIH studies, showed a clear association between elevations in donor ALT levels and increased risk of recipient hepatitis. Data from both of these studies, published in the early 1980s, suggested that screening blood donations for ALT and discarding those with elevated levels would be expected to reduce the incidence of post-transfusion hepatitis by about 30 percent. On the basis of these data, a limited number of blood-collection establishments in the United States did implement such screening. Others did not; there was some controversy about the cost-effectiveness of this approach, along with some concern that prospective studies had not defined its efficacy.[101]

ALT is an enzyme that catalyzes the transfer of an amino group from alanine to pyruvic acid to generate glutamate. ALT is found within a number of cells, including red blood cells and muscle cells. Release of ALT into the circulation is a sensitive, if not a specific, measure of liver damage. The enzyme is routinely measured by the reverse of its physiologic reaction. Samples are exposed to glutamate and 2-oxo-glutarate in conditions that generate a pseudo-first-order reaction. The pyruvate that is generated is measured by a secondary reaction in which the pyruvate is reduced to lactate by lactate dehydrogenase, linked to the oxidation of nicotinamide adenine dinucleotide (NADH). The overall reaction rate is monitored by following the loss of absorbance at 340 nm, reflecting the consumption of NADH. The level of enzyme in the original sample is proportional to the rate of change of absorbance. Enzyme levels are generally expressed in units, or international units, per liter (at least in the United States). Although the distribution of values is somewhat dependent upon the measurement system, the upper limit of normal (i.e., the 97.5 percentile value) for a test performed at 37°C generally falls into the range 40 to 55 IU/L. The conversion factor for SI units is 0.01667: that is, 1 IU/L is equivalent to 0.01667 μkat/L.

A key issue in implementing ALT testing was (and is) the definition of a cutoff, since ALT levels are distributed continuously. Publications from the TTV Study group noted that risk of infectivity appeared to be proportional to ALT levels, and recommended the use of the upper limit of normal as a cutoff.[7] This would be expected to result in a discard rate of about 2.5 percent. However, the upper limit of normal is usually calculated upon specially selected populations, along with elimination of outliers, so the actual impact was often greater. Alter, on the other hand,

determined that the optimum cutoff, based upon efficacy of prevention and economy of the donor resource, was achieved with a cutoff reflecting 2.25 standard deviations from the mean of the logarithmically transformed ALT distribution. This translated to about the 98.4 percentile value for the donor population.[8]

ALT distributions are affected by many factors, including age, sex, and race, along with body weight and use of medications, alcohol, and so forth. Additionally, technical factors, such as the reagent and instrument system, also impact the data. Accordingly, there have been attempts to standardize ALT testing by assigning a single cutoff value to multiple sites with standardized equipment, or by normalizing different systems to a secondary standard.[102]

Although ALT testing was not uniformly adopted in the early 1980s, subsequent recognition of the potential severity of chronic post-transfusion NANBH led to its uniform implementation in the United States in 1986. At essentially the same time, tests for anti-HBc were also implemented, because further evaluations of the TTV and NIH post-transfusion hepatitis studies had suggested that anti-HBc testing would have efficacy similar to that of ALT testing in preventing post-transfusion hepatitis, and that these two measures were additive.[9,10] The nature and impact of anti-HBc testing has been described above.

Retrospective evidence suggesting the efficacy of these two surrogate testing procedures has been derived not only from changes in reporting and seroconversion rates for HCV among blood recipients, but also from the finding that a significant proportion of HCV-positive donations at the initiation of testing were also positive for anti-HBc, or had ALT elevations, or both.[55,103,104] At least for first-generation tests, there was evidence that ALT elevations could be identified well before the appearance of anti-HCV; this apparent window period appears to be greatly reduced by the use of the more sensitive tests. Currently, there seems to be little if any residual value for surrogate testing in the face of second- and third-generation tests for anti-HCV.[99]

The first available test for anti-HCV was a direct antiglobulin EIA. The solid-phase capture reagent was the c100-3 peptide expressed from the HCV genome. The probe was an enzyme-labeled antiglobulin. This test was reactive on about 0.7 percent of donations at the initiation of testing. Although there was no licensed confirmatory test, a strip immunoblot assay, based upon viral peptides, was available as a research reagent. Its use suggested that about 50 percent of repeat reactive samples actually contained antibodies to HCV. Subsequently, second-generation tests were developed, including the C100-3, C22, and C33 antigens as capture reagents, which resulted in increased sensitivity. Further development has led to so-called third-generation tests, with additional expressed antigens, including those from the NS-5 region. At the same time, at least some manufacturers have modified or even eliminated some of the original peptides, in order to increase the inherent sensitivity of the test.[105] Also, confirmatory assays have been improved alongside the primary test. In general, the confirmatory procedures are strip or dot-blot immunoassays with separately identifiable peptides in specific locations.[106,107] The presence of antibody reactivity to two such peptides, in the absence of reactivity to expression proteins (such as superoxide dismutase) is interpreted as positive. Currently, about 0.3 percent of blood donations are confirmed positive to anti-HCV. There are still some difficulties in interpreting indeterminate results in confirmatory assays (usually reflecting weak reactivities, or reactivities to a single band), as these samples are occasionally found to be positive for HCV RNA in PCR.[68,108]

Prophylaxis

There are no clear data about the value of immunoglobulin preparations in protecting against infection with HCV. Needlestick and post-transfusion studies, taken overall, have not been definitive in this regard. Now that the HCV genome has been expressed, attention has turned toward the development of a vaccine for HCV. At the time of writing, the prospects for early availability of such a vaccine are remote, given the evidence that the coding sequence for the viral envelope is very variable. As with HIV, it appears that this variability may be expressed not only between individuals, but also over time in the same individual. Since this sequence variability appears to be expressed in the epitopes, which are susceptible to antibody neutralization, it will be difficult to design an effective vaccine.[109,110]

OTHER HEPATITIS VIRUSES

At least two additional hepatitis viruses have been definitively described, and there continues to be some concern about the possibility of additional transfusion-transmissible forms of viral hepatitis. The available data indicate, however, that there does not appear to be a great deal of cause for concern.

Hepatitis D Virus

Hepatitis D virus (HDV) originally termed *delta,* or the *delta agent,* is an extremely unusual virus. It is a defective virus, and can only infect in the presence of HBV. It was first recognized by detection of an intranuclear antigen in liver biopsies from individuals with chronic HBV infection. It is now known that the virus RNA and capsid are, in fact, released in an envelope consisting of HBsAg derived from the co-infecting HBV. The virus itself is about 35 nm in diameter. The genome consists of a single-stranded RNA molecule, which is circular, although it has significant and unusual secondary structure, so that it appears as a rodlike form. The genome is 1,700 nucleotides long. It is encapsulated with the only known protein transcript, the delta antigen (which was the originally identified nuclear antigen). HDV is unlike any other known animal virus, but is strikingly similar to plant accessory viruses or viroids. Because of its dependence upon HBV, it can only be found in association with HBV infection, although animal model studies have shown that it can also use other hepadnaviruses, such as the woodchuck hepatitis virus.[14,111]

HDV may be transmitted along with HBV, resulting in co-infection, but it may also be transmitted to an individual who already has chronic HBV infection. In the latter case, the superinfecting HDV uses the HBsAg encoded by the existing chronically infecting HBV. The long-term clinical outcomes of co-infection and superinfection appear to differ, although the acute manifestations do not. Although the actual acute illness does not differ extensively from other forms of hepatitis, there is a tendency toward a biphasic pattern, with 2 to 5 weeks between the phases. Co-infection leads to fulminant hepatitis more often than does infection with HBV. Although it is rare for coinfection to lead to an HBsAg carrier state (HDV infection appears to suppress HBV), when this does occur, the patient may progress rapidly to cirrhosis. Thus, acute disease is more severe overall than with hepatitis B, and is more often fatal. Although the acute outcomes of superinfection with HDV do not differ from those associated with co-infection, it is much more likely that chronic HDV infection will be established, with attendant progression to chronic active hepatitis and cirrhosis in 20 to 60 percent of patients.[111]

Because of its association with HBV, the epidemiology, transmission, and preventive measures for HDV do not differ significantly from those for HBV. There are about 250 million HBV carriers worldwide, and it is thought that about 5 percent of these are also infected with HDV. There do appear to be variations in the global distribution of HDV, with areas of very low, low, moderate, or high endemicity. In high-endemicity areas, transmission is thought to be via person-to-person contact, whereas in low-endemicity areas such as the United States, HDV may be transmitted predominantly by exposure to blood. In the United States, only 1.4 to 12.4 percent of HBsAg carriers have evidence of HDV infection.[111] Measures to prevent the transmission of HBV by blood should also prevent HDV transmission, so this virus does not offer any independent risk. In the past, there was considerable concern about the possibility of transmitting HDV to recipients of pooled plasma products who were already infected with HBV. Indeed, studies in 1987 to 1988 showed that 35 percent of HBsAg-positive hemophiliacs were infected with HDV in the United States.[111] Since pooled plasma products are now inactivated and unable to transmit HBV, it is reasonable to assume that these products no longer offer risk of HBV/HDV co-infection. More recently, in a multicenter study on 727 hemophiliacs in the United States, it was shown that 39 (12.1 percent) of the 321 patients with positive HBV serology were also seropositive for HDV. The majority (286) of the HBV-seropositive patients were found among the 382 who were also HIV-infected.[112] It also seems likely that solvent-detergent treatment would be effective in disrupting the HDV virions, thus preventing superinfection.

Hepatitis E Virus

The hepatitis E virus (HEV) is a nonenveloped RNA virus that appears to be similar to the caliciviruses. It is typically responsible for waterborne outbreaks of hepatitis; as such, its mode of spread is similar to that for HAV. Its distribution appears to be restricted to central and southeast Asia (including India), northern and western Africa, and parts of Mexico. The incubation period is about 40 days and the associated disease is mild to moderate, with a normal mortality rate of 0.2 to 1 percent, although it is unusually severe in pregnancy, with a mortality rate increasing with the length of pregnancy (up to 20 percent in the third trimester). A single experimental enteric transmission of HEV has been reported; there was a viremic phase first recognized about 1 week prior to disease, implying that infection could be transmitted by transfusion in the same manner as HAV.[113] There is no chronic carrier state and it seems to have little current relevance to transfusion medicine, particularly in the United States.[14] Nevertheless, a significant seroprevalence rate of 2.1 percent for HEV antibodies using newly developed reagents has been observed in 386 randomly selected U.S. blood donors.[114] It will be critical to confirm this preliminary observation, given the apparent near-absence of HEV disease in the United States. In common with a number of other transfusion-transmissible agents, the major risk in the United States may result from infected travelers returning from endemic areas.

Is There Another Parenterally Transmitted Hepatitis Virus?

Although the actual and potential causes of post-transfusion hepatitis are very well understood, there continues to be concern about the possibility that there may be additional as yet uncharacterized hepatitis viruses with a parenteral transmission mechanism. The major focus of this concern derives from the finding that a proportion of post-transfusion hepatitis cases do not have serologic evidence of infection with any of the known hepatitis viruses.[55,56,115–118] In addition, studies on community-acquired NANBH also reveal disease in the absence of serologic markers. The epidemiologic pattern of this disease has been interpreted as being consistent with parenteral spread.[75] Finally, there have been reports (which do not appear to have been confirmed by other workers) that different preparations that are infectious for NANBH have markedly different physicochemical properties, such as buoyant density and susceptibility to lipid solvents.[119]

On the other hand, Alter reported that at least some hepatitis in his studies appeared to be due to infection with CMV, although this particular etiology is no longer seen in his series.[120] More recently, some cases of post-transfusion hepatitis in Taiwan appear to have been associated with CMV infection.[121] In the TTV Study, a significant proportion of nontransfused controls were found to have post-operative ALT elevations, which would have qualified as hepatitis in that study.[10] Perhaps more startling was a report of a major post-transfusion study in Canada, in which the incidence of this so-called non-A, non-B, non-C hepatitis was equivalent among recipients of allogeneic and autologous blood.[121a] Thus, while there may be little doubt that liver dysfunction may occur postoperatively, it is by no means clear that this represents the outcome of an infection. Nevertheless, by the middle of 1995, two groups had reported on the identification of additional, parenterally transmitted flavi-like viruses.

Clinical data about these cases of hepatitis that lack known serologic markers indicate that, for the most part, the disease is mild, with comparatively low peak ALT levels and a low frequency of symptoms. In addition, it appears to be self-limited, although there may be a few cases of chronic disease. Overall, this phenomenon, although it bears careful scrutiny, may be of little or no relevance to transfusion safety.

HEPATITIS AND PRODUCTS MANUFACTURED FROM POOLED PLASMA

In the past, recipients of selected pooled plasma products were at greatly increased risk of infection with hepatitis viruses. This was due to the large number of separate donations (perhaps tens of thousands) that constituted a single pool. Obviously, even a very low overall prevalence of infectivity could result in almost all pools being contaminated. In addition, the Cohn ethanol procedures used to prepare most plasma products (with the possible exception of immunoglobulins) did not affect the infectiousness of hepatitis viruses to any great extent. However, risks did vary with products, as discussed below. In fact, the very poor safety record of fibrinogen products resulted in a decision, by the then equiva-

lent of the FDA, to remove that product from the market. The introduction and continued improvement of viral inactivation procedures has resulted in a situation where pooled plasma products are now generally regarded as being safer than the corresponding single-donor products.[122]

Albumin

Albumin has always been regarded as a safe product, and no cases of hepatitis infection have been attributed to properly manufactured albumin preparations. This safety record is largely attributable to the fact that albumin preparations are routinely pasteurized by heating to 60°C for 10 hours in the liquid state. This process is more than adequate to inactivate the levels of virus that may be present in the final product. The long safety record for albumin led to attempts to apply inactivation procedures to other pooled plasma products.

Clotting Factor Concentrates

Although the development of lyophilized clotting factor concentrates revolutionized life for hemophiliacs, these products were almost invariably infectious for HBV and HCV, and the vast majority of treated patients were found to have evidence of infection and also, in many cases, of chronic liver damage. Tragically, many of them also eventually became infected with HIV, as inactivation procedures did not become available until well after the introduction of this virus into the blood supply. Some improvement in safety was achieved by donor screening and testing, at least for HBV. Straightforward pasteurization could not be used for clotting factors because the proteins are inherently labile and procedures necessary to inactivate viruses also destroyed the biologic activity of the clotting factors. In order to use heat for inactivation, it was necessary to protect the proteins in some way; unfortunately, some protective compounds also stabilize the virus. Perhaps most successful were procedures that relied upon heating the lyophilized product in the dry state. Although the initial procedures appeared to result in products that were safe from infection by HIV, and perhaps from HBV (although most hemophiliacs were receiving the HBV vaccine by that time), there was clear evidence that these initial products continued to transmit HCV.[123] Subsequently, more rigorous heating protocols were developed that were able to re-move the risk of HCV infection. Another highly suc-cessful inactivation procedure is the use of an organic solvent, such as tributyl phosphate, along with a detergent, such as Tween 80 or Triton X-100.[124] This procedure dissolves the lipid envelope of the virus, rendering it unable to infect. Since both HBV and HCV are enveloped, they are rapidly and extensively inactivated by this procedure. The sol-vent and detergent are removed by hydrophobic chromatography. Additional safety has been ob-tained by the use of a monoclonal antibody-based immunoabsorption step for further purification of factors VIII or IX. Virally inactivated clotting factor concentrates are regarded as extremely safe, and have been recommended in preference to single-donor products.[125] Recombinant products are also available; they are, of course, free of the risk of trans-mission of human viruses.

Unexpectedly, there have been a number of out-breaks of HAV infection among European recipients of factor VIII concentrates that have been inactivated with a solvent-detergent procedure.[23] HAV is not en-veloped and is thus not susceptible to this approach. There does not seem to be a significant history of HAV infection among recipients of earlier products. Studies on these recent outbreaks clearly show that the concentrates were the source of the infection. It is possible that virus entered the pool from one or more infected donors, although there has also been a suggestion that there may have been some break-down in appropriate manufacturing practice. Frac-tionation procedures used in the United States are reported to have a high level of attenuation of infec-tiousness from nonenveloped as well as enveloped viruses, although there have been calls for the use of procedures specifically designed to inactivate non-enveloped viruses. The outbreaks appear to have been confined, and at the time of this publication, there have been no reports of additional cases.

Immunoglobulins

Immunoglobulin preparations have, for many years, been regarded as essentially safe, even though, until recently, no specific measures were undertaken to inactivate them. Standard immunoglobulin is usu-ally prepared by the Cohn-Oncley procedure and is exposed to relatively high concentrations of ethanol,

which may be responsible, at least in part, for the safety of this product. Consequently, there was con-cern about the safety of immunoglobulin prepara-tions designed for intravenous use (IVIG), since at least some of these IVIG products were purified by alternate methods that did not involve significant ethanol concentrations. There were indeed some re-ports of infection from a number of these products, but for many years, there was no evidence of infec-tion from licensed products prepared in the United States. It seemed possible that any viruses present in the pools were neutralized or immunoprecipi-tated by the corresponding antibodies also present in the pool.

In 1993 and 1994, a number of cases of HCV infec-tion were found among recipients of an IVIG prepa-ration.[126] The infections were indeed traced to the product, which was subsequently withdrawn from the market and replaced by a solvent-detergent treated IVIG. The reasons for this unexpected outbreak are unclear. One possible explanation is that the intro-duction of HCV antibody screening reduced or elim-inated protective antibodies in the pool, thus permit-ting the HCV, which was clearly present, to express its infectiousness. It is of interest that the FDA ex-pressed concern about this possibility when tests for anti-HCV became available, recommending against testing of source plasma. Subsequently, animal stud-ies were performed that indicated that pooled, anti-HCV–negative plasma could be infectious, but that immunoglobulins prepared from such pools did not transmit HCV to chimpanzees.[127] In vitro studies did show that HCV RNA could be detected in immuno-globulins (and other fractions) prepared from HCV-positive starting material.[128]

Fresh Frozen Plasma

One potential advance in transfusion safety is the development of procedures to inactivate viruses in single-donor products. At this time, no method has been developed for cellular products, but there are procedures that can be used on fresh frozen plasma. In the United States, clinical trials have been com-pleted on a solvent-detergent–treated fresh frozen plasma product that is prepared in small, ABO type–specific pools.[129] It is anticipated that this product will become available in the near future, subject to licensure by the FDA. This method has also been used in Europe, as have procedures based upon heat, and photoinactivation using methylene blue.[130] In fact, by the end of 1994, the use of such inactivated fresh frozen plasma products was routine in a number of European countries, and many hundreds of thousands of units had been transfused. It does not appear that there has been any overall effort to gather data on outcomes of such treatment.

FUTURE PROSPECTS

It is apparent that great strides have been made in improving the safety of blood transfusion with respect to transmission of hepatitis viruses. Indeed, it seems that very large, complex, and expensive studies would be needed in order to measure the residual risk of transfusion-transmitted infection with HBV and HCV. It is unlikely that such studies will be funded in the near future. Although it is doubtful that there will be any major improvements in testing for HBV infection, it should be recognized that concerted efforts to establish universal HBV vaccination may eventually be expected to reduce or eliminate this disease. Significant increments of sensitivity in tests for HCV appear to be unlikely, as most of the antigenic components of the virus have been expressed or synthesized. It would be desirable to understand more about the seronegative window period for HCV, since this is likely to be the most significant source of donor infectiousness in the future. It is also necessary to make accurate assessments of the incidence of new HCV infections in the donor population, since this will be needed to define the actual risk of transmission. Available data suggest that true seroconversion is relatively rare in the donor population. It is reasonable to suppose that resolution of the problems of HBV and HCV will focus more attention upon other forms of hepatitis; the most important question is whether uncharacterized diseases such as non-A, non-B, non-C hepatitis do have an infectious etiology. Finally, tools are now available to assess the efficacy of earlier measures, such as surrogate testing, which were introduced to reduce the risk of post-transfusion hepatitis. It will be desirable to examine these procedures carefully, with a view to eliminating them if they no longer serve any useful purpose.

REFERENCES

1. Lürman A: Eine Icterusepidimie. Berlin Klin Wochenschr 22:20, 1885
2. Allen JG: The epidemiology of posttransfusion hepatitis. Basic blood and plasma tabulations. p.1. Commonwealth Fund, Stanford, CT, 1972
3. Prince AM: An antigen detected in the blood during the incubation period of serum hepatitis. Proc Natl Acad Sci USA 60:814, 1968
4. Blumberg BS, Alter HJ, Visnich S: A "new" antigen in leukemia sera. JAMA 191:541, 1965
5. Blumberg BS, Gerstley BJS, Hungerford DA et al: A serum antigen (Australia antigen) in Down's syndrome, leukemia and hepatitis. Ann Intern Med 66:924, 1967
6. Feinstone SM, Kapikian AZ, Purcell RH et al: Transfusion-associated hepatitis not due to viral hepatitis type A or B. N Engl J Med 292:767, 1975
7. Aach RD, Szmuness W, Mosley JW et al: Serum alanine aminotransferase of donors in relation to the risk of non-A, non-B hepatitis in recipients. The Transfusion-Transmitted Viruses Study. N Engl J Med 304:989, 1981
8. Alter HJ, Purcell RH, Holland PV et al: Donor transaminase and recipient hepatitis. Impact on blood transfusion services. JAMA 246:630, 1981
9. Koziol DE, Holland PV, Alling DW et al: Antibody to hepatitis B core antigen as a paradoxical marker for non-A, non-B hepatitis agents in donated blood. Ann Intern Med 104:488, 1986
10. Stevens CE, Aach RD, Hollinger FB et al: Hepatitis B virus antibody in blood donors and the occurrence of non-A, non-B hepatitis in transfusion recipients. An analysis of the Transmission-Transmitted Viruses Study. Ann Intern Med 101:733, 1984
11. Choo Q-L, Kuo G, Weiner AJ et al: Isolation of a cDNA clone derived from a blood-borne non-A, non-B viral hepatitis genome. Science 244:359, 1989
12. Kuo G, Choo Q-L, Alter HJ et al: An assay for circulating antibodies to a major etiologic virus of human non-A, non-B hepatitis. Science 244:362, 1989
13. Bradley DW: Virology, molecular biology, and serology of hepatitis C virus. Transfus Med Rev 6:93, 1992
14. Purcell RH: Hepatitis viruses: Changing patterns of human disease. Proc Natl Acad Sci USA 91:2401, 1994
15. CDC: Hepatitis Surveillance Report No. 55, p. 1.

Centers for Disease Control and Prevention, Atlanta, 1994

16. Hadler SC, Webster HM, Erben JJ et al: Hepatitis A in day-care centers: a community-wide assessment. N Engl J Med 302:1222, 1980

17. Lemon SM: Type A viral hepatitis. New developments in an old disease. N Engl J Med 313:1059, 1985

18. Robbins DJ, Krater J, Kiang W et al: Detection of total antibody against hepatitis A virus by an automated microparticle immunoassay. J Virol Methods 32:255, 1991

19. Giacoia GP, Kasprisin DO: Transfusion-acquired hepatitis A. South Med J 82:1357, 1989

20. Hollinger FB, Khan NC, Oefinger PE et al: Posttransfusion hepatitis type A. JAMA 250:2313, 1983

21. Noble RC, Kane MA, Reeves SA et al: Posttransfusion hepatitis A in a neonatal intensive care unit. JAMA 252:2711, 1984

22. Azimi PH, Roberto RR, Guralnick J et al: Transfusion-acquired hepatitis A in a premature infant with secondary nosocomial spread in an intensive care nursery. Am J Dis Child 140:23, 1986

23. Mannucci PM, Gdovin S, Gringeri A et al: Transmission of hepatitis A to patients with hemophilia by Factor VIII concentrates treated with organic solvent and detergent to inactivate viruses. Ann Intern Med 120: 1, 1994

24. Westblom TU, Gudipati S, DeRousse C et al: Safety and immunogenicity of an inactivated hepatitis A vaccine: Effect of dose and vaccination schedule. J Infect Dis 169:996, 1994

25. Innis BL, Snitbhan R, Kunasol P et al: Protection against hepatitis A by an inactivated vaccine. JAMA 271:1328, 1994

26. Hollinger FB: Hepatitis B virus. p. 217. In Fields BN, Knipe DM, Chanock RM et al (eds): Virology. 2nd Ed. Raven Press, New York, 1990

27. Feitelson M: Hepatitis B virus infection and primary hepatocellular carcinoma. Clin Microbiol Rev 5:275, 1992

28. McMahon BJ, London T: Workshop on screening for hepatocellular carcinoma. J Natl Cancer Inst 83:916, 1991

29. Di Bisceglie AM, Order SE, Klein JL et al: The role of chronic viral hepatitis in hepatocellular carcinoma in the United States. Am J Gastroenterol 86:335, 1991

30. Seeff LB, Beebe GW, Hoofnagle JH et al: A serologic follow-up of the 1942 epidemic of post-vaccination hepatitis in the United States Army. N Engl J Med 316:965, 1990

31. Heyward WL, Lanier AP, McMahon BJ et al: Serological markers of hepatitis B virus and alpha-fetoprotein levels preceding primary hepatocellular carcinoma in Alaskan Eskimos. Lancet 2:879, 1982

32. Almeida JD, Rubenstein D, Stott EJ: New antigen-antibody system in Australia-antigen positive hepatitis. Lancet 2:1225, 1971

33. Brown JL, Carman WF, Thomas HC: The clinical significance of molecular variation within the hepatitis B virus genome. Hepatology 15:144, 1992

34. Liang TJ, Hasegawa K, Munoz SJ et al: Hepatitis B virus precore mutation and fulminant hepatitis in the United States. A polymerase chain reaction-based assay for the detection of specific mutation. J Clin Invest 93:550, 1994

35. Margolis HS, Alter MJ, Hadler SC: Hepatitis B: evolving epidemiology and implications for control. Semin Liver Dis 11:84, 1991

36. Alter MJ, Hadler SC, Margolis HS et al: The changing epidemiology of hepatitis B in the United States. Need for alternative vaccination strategies. JAMA 263:1218, 1990

37. Owens DK, Nease RF Jr: Occupational exposure to human immunodeficiency virus and hepatitis B virus: a comparative analysis of risk. Am J Med 92:503, 1992

38. McQuillan GM, Townsend TR, Fields HA et al: Seroepidemiology of hepatitis B virus infection in the United States: 1976 to 1980. Am J Med 87(Suppl.): 5S, 1989

39. Starkey JM, Macpherson JL, Bolgiano DC et al: Markers for transfusion-transmitted disease in different groups of blood donors. JAMA 262:3452, 1989

40. Dodd RY: The risk of transfusion-transmitted infection. N Engl J Med 327:419, 1992

41. CDC: Public Health Service inter-agency guidelines for screening donors of blood, plasma, organs, tissues, and semen for evidence of hepatitis B and hepatitis C. MMWR 40:1, 1991

42. Shih L-N, Sheu J-C, Wang J-T et al: Detection of hepatitis B viral DNA by polymerase chain reaction in patients with hepatitis B surface antigen. J Med Virol 30:159, 1990

43. Jackson JB: Polymerase chain reaction assay for detection of hepatitis B virus. Am J Clin Pathol 95:442, 1991

44. Douglas DD, Taswell HF, Rakela J et al: Absence of hepatitis B virus DNA detected by polymerase chain reaction in blood donors who are hepatitis B surface antigen negative and antibody to hepatitis B core antigen positive from a United States population with

a low prevalence of hepatitis B serologic markers. Transfusion 33:212, 1993

45. Liang TJ, Bodenheimer HC Jr, Yankee R et al: Presence of hepatitis B and C viral genomes in US blood donors as detected by polymerase chain reaction amplification. J Med Virol 42:151, 1994

46. Sankary TM, Yang G, Romeo JM et al: Rare detection of hepatitis B and hepatitis C virus genomes by polymerase chain reaction in seronegative donors with elevated alanine aminotransferase. Transfusion 34:656, 1994

47. Tabor E, Hoofnagle JH, Barker LF et al: Antibody to hepatitis B core antigen in blood donors with a history of hepatitis. Transfusion 21:366, 1981

48. Tegtmeier GE, Parks LH, Blosser JK et al: Hepatitis markers in blood donors with a history of hepatitis or jaundice. Transfusion 31(suppl.):64, 1991

49. Ling CM, Overby LR: Prevalence of hepatitis B virus antigen as revealed by direct radioimmune assay with 125-I-antibody. J Immunol 109:834, 1972

50. Hoofnagle JH, Seeff LB, Bales ZB et al: Type B hepatitis after transfusion with blood containing antibody to hepatitis B core antigen. N Engl J Med 298:1379, 1978

51. Chambers LA, Popovsky MA: Decrease in reported posttransfusion hepatitis: contributions of donor screening for alanine aminotransferase and antibodies to hepatitis B core antigen and changes in the general population. Arch Intern Med 151:2445, 1991

52. Zuck TF, Sherwood WC, Bove JR: A review of recent events related to surrogate testing of blood to prevent non-A, non-B posttransfusion hepatitis. Transfusion 27:203, 1987

53. CDC: General recommendations on immunization. Recommendations of the Advisory Committee on Immunization Practices (ACIP). MMWR 43:1, 1994

54. Szmuness W, Stevens CE, Harley EJ et al: Hepatitis B vaccine: demonstration of efficacy in a controlled clinical trial in a high-risk population in the United States. N Engl J Med 303:833, 1980

55. Alter HJ, Purcell RH, Shih JW et al: Detection of antibody to hepatitis C virus in prospectively followed transfusion recipients with acute and chronic non-A, non-B hepatitis. N Engl J Med 321:1494, 1989

56. Aach RD, Stevens CE, Hollinger FB et al: Hepatitis C virus infection in post-transfusion hepatitis—an analysis with first- and second-generation assays. N Engl J Med 325:1325, 1991

57. Di Bisceglie, Goodman ZD, Ishak KG et al: Long-term clinical and histopathological follow-up of chronic posttransfusion hepatitis. Hepatology 14:969, 1991

58. Alter MJ, Margolis HS, Krawczynski K et al: The natural history of community-acquired hepatitis C in the United States. N Engl J Med 327:1899, 1992

59. Koretz RL, Abbey H, Coleman E et al: Non-A, non-B post-transfusion hepatitis: looking back in the second decade. Ann Intern Med 119:110, 1993

60. Cuthbert JA: Hepatitis C: Progress and problems. Clin Microbiol Rev 7:505, 1994

61. Seeff LB, Buskell-Bales Z, Wright EC et al: Long-term mortality after transfusion-associated non-A, non-B hepatitis. N Engl J Med 327:1906, 1992

62. Kiyosawa K, Sodeyama T, Tanaka E et al: Interrelationship of blood transfusion, non-A, non-B hepatitis and hepatocellular carcinoma: Analysis by detection of antibody to hepatitis C virus. Hepatology 12:671, 1990

63. Clemens JM, Taskar S, Chau K et al: IgM antibody response in acute hepatitis C viral infection. Blood 79:169, 1992

64. Zaaijer HL, Mimms LT, Cuypers HTM et al: Variability of IgM response in hepatitis C virus infection. J Med Virol 40:184, 1993

65. McOmish F, Yap PL, Dow BC et al: Geographical distribution of hepatitis C virus genotypes in blood donors: an international collaborative survey. J Clin Microbiol 32:884, 1994

66. Dusheiko G, Schmilovitz-Weiss H, Brown D et al: Hepatitis C virus genotypes: an investigation of type-specific differences in geographic origin and disease. Hepatology 19:13, 1994

67. Kaito M, Watanabe S, Tsukiyama-Kohara K et al: Hepatitis C virus particle detected by immunoelectron microscopic study. J Gen Virol 75:1755, 1994

68. Bresters D, Zaaijer HL, Cuypers HTM et al: Recombinant immunoblot assay reaction patterns and hepatitis C virus RNA in blood donors and non-A, non-B hepatitis patients. Transfusion 33:634, 1993

69. Zaaijer HL, Cuypers HTM, Reesink HW et al: Reliability of polymerase chain reaction for detection of hepatitis C virus. Lancet 341:722, 1993

70. Kurosaki M, Enomoto N, Sato C et al: Correlation of plasma hepatitis C virus RNA levels with serum alanine aminotransferase in non-A, non-B chronic liver disease. J Med Virol 39:246, 1993

71. Young KKY, Resnick RM, Myers TW: Detection of hepatitis C virus RNA by a combined reverse transcription-polymerase chain reaction assay. J Clin Microbiol 31:882, 1993

72. Silva AE, Hosein B, Boyle RW et al: Diagnosis of chronic hepatitis C: Comparison of immunoassays and the polymerase chain reaction. Am J Gastroenterol 89:493, 1994

73. Wang J-T, Sheu J-C, Lin J-T et al: Detection of replicative form of hepatitis C virus RNA in peripheral blood mononuclear cells. J Infect Dis 166:1167, 1992

74. Bouffard P, Hayashi PH, Acevedo R et al: Hepatitis C virus is detected in a monocyte/macrophage subpopulation of peripheral blood mononuclear cells of infected patients. J Infect Dis 166:1276, 1992

75. Alter MJ, Hadler SC, Judson FN et al: Risk factors for acute non-A, non-B hepatitis in the United States and association with hepatitis C virus infection. JAMA 264:2231, 1990

76. Alter MJ: Hepatitis C: A sleeping giant? Am J Med 91(suppl.)112S, 1991

77. Esteban JI, Esteban R, Viladomiu L et al: Hepatitis C virus antibodies among risk groups in Spain. Lancet 2:294, 1989

78. Osmond DH, Charlebois E, Sheppard HW et al: Comparison of risk factors for hepatitis C and hepatitis B virus infection in homosexual men. J Infect Dis 167:66, 1993

79. Weinstock HS, Bolan G, Reingold AL et al: Hepatitis C virus infection among patients attending a clinic for sexually transmitted diseases. JAMA 269:392, 1993

80. Thomas DL, Cannon RO, Shapiro CN et al: Hepatitis C, hepatitis B, and human immunodeficiency virus infections among non-intravenous drug-using patients attending clinics for sexually transmitted diseases. J Infect Dis 169:990, 1994

81. Kolho E, Naukkarinen R, Ebeling F et al: Transmission of hepatitis C virus to sexual partners of seropositive patients with bleeding disorders: a rare event. Scand J Infect Dis 23:667, 1991

82. Brettler DB, Mannucci PM, Gringeri A et al: The low risk of hepatitis C virus transmission among sexual partners of hepatitis C-infected hemophilic males: an international, multicenter study. Blood 80:540, 1992

83. Hallam NF, Fletcher ML, Read SJ et al: Low risk of sexual transmission of hepatitis C virus. J Med Virol 40:251, 1993

84. Pachucki CT, Lentino JR, Schaaff D et al: Low prevalence of sexual transmission of hepatitis C virus in sex partners of seropositive intravenous drug users. J Infect Dis 164:820, 1991

85. Everhart JE, Di Bisceglie AM, Murray LM et al: Risk for non-A, non-B (type C) hepatitis through sexual or household contact with chronic carriers. Ann Intern Med 112:544, 1990

86. Akahane Y, Kojima M, Sugai Y et al: Hepatitis C virus infection in spouses of patients with type C chronic liver disease. Ann Intern Med 120:748, 1994

87. Coltorti M, Caporaso N, Morisco F et al: Prevalence of hepatitis C virus infection in the household contacts of patients with HCV-related chronic liver disease. Infection 22:183, 1994

88. Seeff LB, Alter HJ: Spousal transmission of the hepatitis C virus. Ann Intern Med 120:807, 1994

89. van der Poel C, Cuypers H, Reesink H et al: Risk factors in hepatitis C virus-infected blood donors. Transfusion 31:777, 1991

90. Kiyosawa K, Sodeyama T, Tanaka E et al: Hepatitis C in hospital employees with needlestick injuries. Ann Intern Med 115:367, 1991

91. Oshita M, Hayashi N, Kasahara A et al: Prevalence of hepatitis C virus in family members of patients with hepatitis C. J Med Virol 41:251, 1993

92. Ohto H, Terazawa S, Sasaki N et al: Transmission of hepatitis C virus from mothers to infants. N Engl J Med 330:744, 1994

93. Romeo R, Thiers V, Driss F et al: Hepatitis C virus RNA in serum of blood donors with or without elevated transaminase levels. Transfusion 33:629, 1993

94. Zhang HY, Kuramoto IK, Mamish D et al: Hepatitis C virus in blood samples from volunteer donors. J Clin Microbiol 31:606, 1993

95. Blajchman MA, Feinman SV, Bull SB: The incidence of post-transfusion hepatitis. N Engl J Med 328:1280, 1993

96. Donahue JG, Muñoz A, Ness PM et al: The declining risk of post-transfusion hepatitis C virus infection. N Engl J Med 327:369, 1992

97. Nelson KE, Ahmed F, Ness P et al: The incidence of post-transfusion hepatitis. Reply. N Engl J Med 328:1280, 1993

98. Kleinman S, Alter H, Busch M et al: Increased detection of hepatitis C virus (HCV)-infected blood donors by a multiple-antigen HCV enzyme immunoassay. Transfusion 32:805, 1992

99. Alter HJ: Transfusion transmitted hepatitis C and non-A, non-B, non-C. Vox Sang 67(suppl.):19, 1994

100. Dawson GJ, Lesniewski RR, Stewart JL et al: Detection of antibodies to hepatitis C virus in U.S. blood donors. J Clin Microbiol 29:551, 1991

101. Hornbrook MC, Dodd RY, Jacobs P et al: Reducing the incidence of non-A, non-B post-transfusion hepatitis by testing donor blood for alanine aminotransferase. Economic considerations. New Engl J Med 307:1315, 1982

102. AuBuchon JP, Wilkinson JS, Kassapian SJ et al: Establishment of a system to standardize acceptability criteria for alanine aminotransferase activity in donated blood. Transfusion 29:17, 1989

103. Stevens CE, Taylor PE, Pindyck J et al: Epidemiology of hepatitis C virus. A preliminary study in volunteer blood donors. JAMA 263:49, 1990

104. Richards C, Holland P, Kuramoto K et al: Prevalence of antibody to hepatitis C virus in a blood donor population. Transfusion 31:109, 1991

105. Uyttendaele S, Claeys H, Mertens W et al: Evaluation of third-generation screening and confirmatory assays for HCV antibodies. Vox Sang 66:122, 1994

106. van der Poel CL, Cuypers HTM, Reesink HW et al: Confirmation of hepatitis C virus infection by new four-antigen recombinant immunoblot assay. Lancet 337:317, 1991

107. Evans CS, Tobler L, Polito A et al: Comparative evaluation of supplemental hepatitis C virus antibody test systems. Transfusion 32:408, 1992

108. Tobler LH, Busch MP, Wilber J et al: Evaluation of indeterminate c22-3 reactivity in volunteer blood donors. Transfusion 34:130, 1994

109. Farci P, Alter HJ, Govindarajan S et al: Lack of protective immunity against reinfection with hepatitis C virus. Science 258:135, 1992

110. Farci P, Alter HJ, Wong DC et al: Prevention of hepatitis C virus infection in chimpanzees after antibody-mediated in vitro neutralization. Proc Natl Acad Sci 91:7792, 1994

111. Polish LB, Gallagher M, Fields HA et al: Delta hepatitis: Molecular biology and clinical and epidemiological features. Clin Microbiol Reviews 6:211, 1993

112. Troisi CL, Hollinger FB, Hoots WK et al: A multicenter study of viral hepatitis in a United States hemophilic population. Blood 81:412, 1993

113. Chauhan A, Jameel S, Dilawari JB et al: Hepatitis E virus transmission to a volunteer. Lancet 341:149, 1993

114. Dawson GJ, Chau KH, Cabal CM et al: Solid-phase enzyme-linked immunosorbent assay for hepatitis E virus IgG and IgM antibodies utilizing recombinant antigens and synthetic peptides. J Virol Methods 38:175, 1992

115. Hibbs JR, Frickhofen N, Rosenfeld SJ et al: Aplastic anemia and viral hepatitis: non-A, non-B, non-C. JAMA 267:2051, 1992

116. Koretz RL, Brezina M, Polito AJ et al: Non-A, non-B posttransfusion hepatitis: comparing C and non-C hepatitis. Hepatology 17:361, 1993

117. Azar N, Valla D, Lunel F et al: Post-transfusional anti-HCV-negative, non-A, non-B hepatitis. (I) A prospective clinical and epidemiological survey. J Hepatol 18:24, 1993

118. Thiers V, Lunel F, Valla D et al: Post-transfusional anti-HCV-negative non-A, non-B hepatitis. (II) Serological and polymerase chain reaction analysis for hepatitis C and hepatitis B viruses. J Hepatol 18:34, 1993

119. Bradley DW, Maynard JE, Popper H et al: Posttransfusion non-A, non-B hepatitis: physicochemical properties of two distinct agents. J Infect Dis 148:254, 1983

120. Alter HJ: You'll wonder where the yellow went: a 15-year retrospective of posttransfusion hepatitis. p. 53. In Moore SB (ed): Transfusion-Transmitted Viral Diseases. American Association of Blood Banks, Arlington, VA, 1987

121. Huang YY, Yang SS, Wu CH et al: Impact of screening blood donors for hepatitis C antibody on posttransfusion hepatitis: a prospective study with a second-generation anti-hepatitis C virus assay. Transfusion 34:661, 1994

121a. Blajchman MA, Bull SB, Feinman SV: Post-transfusion hepatitis: impact of non-A non-B hepatitis surrogate tests. Lancet 345:21, 1995

122. Fricke WA, Lamb MA: Viral safety of clotting factor concentrates. Semin Thromb Hemost 19:54, 1993

123. Epstein JS, Fricke WA: Current safety of clotting factor concentrates. Arch Pathol Lab Med 114:335, 1990

124. Horowitz MS, Rooks C, Horowitz B et al: Virus safety of solvent/detergent-treated antihaemophilic factor concentrate. Lancet 2:186, 1988

125. Suomela H: Inactivation of viruses in blood and plasma products. Transfus Med Rev 7:42, 1993

126. CDC: Outbreak of hepatitis C associated with intravenous immunoglobulin administration-United States, October 1993–June 1994. MMWR 43:505, 1994

127. Biswas RM, Nedjar S, Wilson LT et al: The effect on the safety of intravenous immunoglobulin of testing plasma for antibody to hepatitis C. Transfusion 34:100, 1994

128. Yei S, Yu MW, Tankersley DL: Partitioning of hepatitis C virus during Cohn-Oncley fractionation of plasma. Transfusion 32:824, 1992

129. Horowitz B, Bonomo R, Prince AM et al: Solvent/detergent-treated plasma: a virus-inactivated substitute for fresh frozen plasma. Blood 79:826, 1992

130. Lambrecht B, Mohr H, Knüver-Hopf J et al: Photoinactivation of viruses in human fresh plasma by phenothiazine dyes in combination with visible light. Vox Sang 60:207, 1991

131. Robinson WS: Hepadnaviridae and their replication. p. 2141. In Fields BN, Knipe DM et al (eds): Virology. 2nd Ed. Raven Press, New York, 1990

Chapter 39

Cytomegalovirus and Other Herpesviruses

Merlyn H. Sayers

THE BIOLOGY OF HUMAN HERPESVIRUSES

The Herpesviridae include five human herpesviruses. They are herpes simplex type 1 (HSV-1), herpes simplex type 2 (HSV-2), varicella zoster virus (VZV), Epstein Barr virus (EBV), and cytomegalovirus (CMV). An alternative nomenclature for the group is human herpesvirus 1 through 5, respectively. A sixth human herpesvirus, human B cell lymphotropic virus, has also been promoted as a member of the family,[1] and more recently, a seventh human herpesvirus has also been proposed.[2]

These viruses share a number of features. They are large, enveloped, double-stranded DNA viruses that are highly cell-associated, producing infections that are described as primary, reactivation, or reinfection. Primary infections occur in individuals who have never been exposed to the virus before. The majority of primary infections are asymptomatic, but they do leave serologic evidence by provoking an IgM followed by an IgG antibody response. A consequence of primary infection, shared by all of the human herpesviruses, is latent infection that persists for the lifetime of the host. Latency can be interrupted with periods of intermittent reactivation that are frequently triggered by immunosuppression in the infected individual. Reinfection with some herpesviruses, such as CMV, can occasionally occur. Under these circumstances, a second strain becomes established in an individual already latently infected with a different strain. As with primary infection, reactivation or reinfection are usually asymptomatic, provided the host is immunocompetent. On the other hand, significant mobidity and mortality may be an outcome in immunocompromised patients. Immunocompromise develops for a number of reasons. For example, the immune response is immature in premature infants, and individuals with the acquired immunodeficiency syndrome (AIDS) also have a blunted response. Other common causes of compromise are iatrogenic, occurring in tissue and organ transplant recipients where successful regimens rely on aggressive pharmacologic immunosuppression to facilitate engraftment.

The human herpesviruses can be subdivided into groups depending on their site of predilection for latency and the attendant clinical manifestations. HSV-1 and HSV-2, along with VZV, are cytolytic viruses that establish latency in neurons. HSV-1 and HSV-2 most often cause vesicular lesions of the oropharynx, eye, skin, and genitalia. Primary VZV infection is common in children and presents as chickenpox. In adults, reactivation of VZV manifests as shingles. CMV has a predilection for glandular and renal tissue, and during viremia, it is excreted in saliva, breast milk, cervical secretions, semen, and urine. Congenital CMV infection, resulting from primary or reactivated maternal infection, can cause intrauterine death, and neonatal fatalities are com-

875

mon in severely infected infants. While the majority of congenital infections are ostensibly asymptomatic, up to 10 percent of infected infants subsequently show subtle evidence of neurosensory impairment. As far as adults are concerned, primary infection with CMV usually goes undetected except in occasional individuals who develop a syndrome clinically similar to infectious mononucleosis. Although there is incontrovertible evidence that CMV can be transmitted by transfusion, it has yet to be established which cells in the mononuclear cell fraction are latently infected. The sites of latency for EBV are lymphocytes. In children, primary EBV infection is often asymptomatic, but in young adults it can give rise to infectious mononucleosis. In addition, this virus is associated with the pathogenesis of African Burkitt's lymphoma and nasopharyngeal carcinoma. Not only do patients with these malignancies have high concentrations of EBV antibodies, but the virus is readily detected in tumor cells. T lymphocytes have been proposed as the site of latency for human herpesvirus type 6; infection presents as roseola infantum in children.

PATIENT GROUPS AT RISK OF TRANSFUSION-TRANSMITTED CYTOMEGALOVIRUS INFECTION

CMV was first recognized as an infectious complication of blood transfusion in the 1960s, when it was shown to be the cause of the postperfusion or "pump" syndrome. This infection, which was frequently seen in patients undergoing cardiopulmonary bypass, was marked by fever, atypical lymphocytosis, and splenomegaly.[3,4] Although the incidence of this syndrome has declined recently, probably because cardiac surgery patients today require less blood and because the old insistence that transfusions must be "fresh" has been dropped,[5] there are special categories of patients in whom transfusion-acquired CMV infection is an important cause of morbidity and mortality.

As has been emphasized, the majority of primary CMV infections, as well as reinfections or reactivations, are inapparent in immunocompetent hosts, but the same cannot be said for individuals who are immunocompromised. In this category are premature infants, patients whose underlying disease is associated with immune dysfunction, and patients whose immune response is impaired by therapy. Pri-

Table 39-1. Patients at Risk of Transfusion-Transmitted Cytomegalovirus Infection

Patients for whom the risk is well established:
  Cytomegalovirus-seronegative pregnant women
  Premature infants (<1,200 g) born to cytomegalovirus-seronegative mothers
  Cytomegalovirus-seronegative recipients of allogeneic bone marrow transplants from cytomegalovirus-seronegative donors
  Cytomegalovirus-seronegative patients with evidence of infection with human immunodeficiency virus type 1
  Intrauterine transfusions
Patients for whom the risk is less well established but sufficient to merit consideration:
  Cytomegalovirus-seronegative patients receiving tissue transplants (renal, heart, liver, lung) from cytomegalovirus-seronegative donors
  Cytomegalovirus-seronegative patients who are potential candidates for bone marrow transplantation (allogeneic or autologous)
  Cytomegalovirus-seronegative autologous bone marrow transplant recipients
  Cytomegalovirus-seronegative patients undergoing splenectomy
  Cytomegalovirus-seronegative recipients of bone marrow from cytomegalovirus-seropositive donors
Patients for whom the risk is not established:
  Cytomegalovirus-seropositive recipients of bone marrow transplants
  Full-term neonates
  Cytomegalovirus-seropositive recipients of solid organ allografts (e.g., heart, kidney)

mary CMV infection under these circumstances can be associated with pneumonitis, hepatitis, gastroenteritis, retinitis, and disseminated disease.[6] Since transfusion support provided by a donor latently infected with CMV could be the source of viral infection in these patients, it is essential that physicians know what individuals are at particular risk so that blood products that are less likely to be infectious for CMV can be ordered for them. While the risk has been clearly defined for some groups, evidence on risk for other groups is still emerging. Table 39-1 summarizes current understanding.

Pregnant Women

Although primary CMV infection seldom has any clinical sequelae in the mother, there may be serious, even fatal outcomes for congenitally infected infants.

CMV is the most common congenital viral infection; up to 1.0 percent of newborns are infected.[6] Some 7 percent of these neonates have symptoms of the cytomegalic inclusion disease syndrome, which can include fever, rash, jaundice, thrombocytopenia, intracerebral calcifications, and microcephaly.[7,8] Long-term outcomes of congenital CMV infection include mental retardation, deafness, and behavioral complications.[9]

The likelihood that a CMV-seronegative woman would become infected with CMV during pregnancy is only between 1 and 3 percent.[10] Furthermore, the contribution of transfusion-transmitted CMV infection to this incidence is presumed to be small. It would seem prudent, however, to avoid using blood products that could transmit CMV infection to pregnant women who have never been exposed to CMV. A similar caution should be extended in the choice of blood products for intrauterine transfusion.

Neonates

The majority of CMV infections acquired during the first few months of life are unapparent. However, some infants develop pneumonitis, lymphadenopathy, splenomegaly, and hemolytic anemia. Insights into the circumstances posing the greatest risk of symptomatic CMV infection in newborn infants have been provided by a couple of studies.[11,12] For example, nearly a quarter of infants born to mothers who had not been previously exposed to CMV acquired CMV infection when their transfusion requirements (at least 50 ml red blood cells [RBCs]) exposed them to a CMV-seropositive donor. Half of the infected infants experienced substantial morbidity, with the brunt of disease being borne by infants weighing less than 1,200 g. In another study,[12] the particular vulnerability of underweight infants was confirmed when it was shown that all neonates acquiring CMV infection weighed less than 1,050 grams. By contrast, birth weight was not a factor that influenced the course of acquired CMV infection in infants born to CMV-seropositive mothers. Fifteen percent of these infants became infected after transfusion with RBCs that in some cases were provided by seropositive donors. No fatal or serious symptoms due to CMV occurred in these infants.

Although the risk of primary transfusion-transmitted CMV infection in low–birth weight infants is not disputed, opinion varies about the prevalence of infection and the severity of the disease in this group. Recent studies[13,14] reveal a much lower rate of infection and less attendant morbidity and mortality by comparison with earlier published reports. The reasons for the changing patterns have not been defined, but they may be the result of the use of rigorous donor screening procedures and sensitive serologic tests for other transfusion-transmittable diseases, which may serve as a surrogate means of excluding donors capable of transmitting CMV.

The routine provision of transfusion products that would not transmit CMV infection to low–birth weight infants of unknown serologic status has been questioned. Seropositive infants in this category are potentially at risk for losing their maternally derived antibody, as well as the protection against CMV infection that it affords, if continuing transfusion support is provided using antibody-negative products. Clinical CMV disease has been described in infants whose passive humoral immunity was lost when transfusion support was provided exclusively with seronegative blood products.[15]

Although much attention has been paid to the transfusion requirement of low–birth weight neonates and the role of blood products screened for CMV, debate has now been extended to include the appropriateness of the products for infants in general. Recognizing that CMV infection in neonates can cause clinical sequelae, it has been recommended that all newborns, regardless of CMV serology and birth weight, receive CMV-seronegative products if they are going to require multiple transfusions.[16] While the evidence supporting the general use of these products in all infants has yet to be presented, it is generally agreed prudent to provide seronegative blood for seronegative infants of low weight.

Recipients of Bone Marrow Transplants

CMV infection causes substantial morbidity and mortality in the recipients of allogeneic bone marrow transplants. Two different circumstances may prevail. First, reactivation of latent virus may occur in transplant recipients who were seropositive prior to transplantation. Second, primary infection may occur in seronegative patients from either marrow or blood products provided by seropositive donors.

The incidence of CMV infection is 70 percent and 40 percent in seropositive and seronegative patients, respectively.[17] Clinical symptoms of CMV infection, when present, are variable, and they include fever, arthralgia, myalgia, abnormal liver function tests, and enterocolitis. The most serious complication of CMV infection in the post-transplantation setting is interstitial pneumonia, which carries a mortality of 85 percent. CMV enteritis, hepatitis, and leukopenia also contribute substantially to post-transplantation morbidity.[18] It has also been suggested that transplantation patients who escape CMV infection enjoy a faster immunologic recovery.[19]

With regard to factors that influence the outcome of CMV infection in bone marrow transplant recipients, it is recognized that irradiation and drugs used in preliminary conditioning regimens play a role. The degree of immunosuppression in the patient may also be influenced, not only by the preexisting disease, but also by the therapy that was indicated in the treatment of that disease. CMV pneumonia was twice as common in patients who received transplants for hematologic malignancies than in patients who received transplants for aplastic anemia.[20] Differences also emerge when the incidence of CMV pneumonia is compared among recipients of syngeneic, autologous, and allogeneic bone marrow transplants. Although the risk for CMV infection is similar for recipients of allogeneic, syngeneic, and autologous marrow transplants,[19,21] CMV pneumonia is most common after allogeneic transplantation and more common still when the recipient's course is complicated by graft-versus-host disease. It has been postulated that this higher frequency of CMV pneumonia reflects the harmful effect of graft-versus-host disease on immune competence.[22]

For seronegative recipients of allogeneic bone marrow from seronegative donors, the use of seronegative blood products is effective for preventing CMV infection.[23] CMV-seronegative recipients of bone marrow from CMV-seropositive donors may also benefit from the use of seronegative blood products because the bone marrow may not transmit CMV even though it is seropositive. However, one study concluded that the use of seronegative blood products did not appear to prevent CMV infection among patients with seropositive donors.[23]

CMV seronegative recipients of autologous marrow can also be protected from transfusion-transmitted CMV infection by the use of seronegative products.[24] Although the probability of CMV infection is lower in autologous transplant recipients by comparison with recipients of allogeneic bone marrow, the risk remains. The recommendation that CMV-seronegative blood products or their equivalent be used in these patients was contrary to the conclusion from an earlier study that the routine provision of CMV-seronegative blood products for seronegative recipients of autologous marrow transplants was inappropriate.[25] The reasons for the differing rates of CMV infection in the two studies are unclear, but they may relate to differences in treatment, particularly the use of total body irradiation for conditioning and the use of 4-hydroperoxycyclophosphamide for marrow purging. Although more information needs to be gathered about the pathogenesis of CMV in this setting, it would seem prudent to recommend that CMV-seronegative products be used for all seronegative recipients of autologous bone marrow transplants.

It should be noted that while the provision of CMV-seronegative blood components reduces the risk of transfusion-acquired infection in these categories of patients, the risk is not reduced to zero. Two investigations reported an incidence of three percent and six percent, respectively, of "breakthrough" infection in the marrow transplant setting.[26,27] This failure rate has been attributed to a combination of the high volume of blood support required by marrow transplant patients and the limited sensitivity of the tests used to distinguish CMV-seronegative from CMV-seropositive blood donors.[28] By the same token, these tests may falsely identify some patients as seronegative, thereby prompting a subsequent diagnosis of primary CMV infection rather than reactivation.

Recipients of Renal Transplants

The pathogenesis of CMV infection in renal transplant recipients is similar to that in bone marrow transplant recipients. Seronegative patients may acquire primary infection from the donor organ or transfusion products, and seropositive patients may experience a reactivation of latent CMV infection. Reinfection with a new CMV strain has also occasionally been described in recipients of kidneys from seropositive donors.[29] CMV infection is less often associated with substantial morbidity and mortality in renal transplant recipients than in bone marrow transplant recipients; infection is subclinical in about 50 percent of patients.[30] In symptomatic patients, several syndromes, including fever, pneumonia, and a mononucleosis-like disease, have been described. Only two or three percent of infected patients die of disseminated CMV disease.

The contribution of transfusion to primary CMV infection has been studied in CMV-seronegative recipients of organs from CMV-seronegative donors. A 10 percent prevalence of primary infection has been reported in patients whose only source of CMV infection was transfusion with unscreened blood in one study[31] and 20 percent in another.[32] As has been the experience of marrow transplant teams, primary CMV infection can be prevented by using transfusion products from CMV-seronegative donors, and many authorities recommend this practice.[33] There is, however, one subset of renal transplant candidates where different considerations apply. Seronegative patients who are scheduled to receive seropositive allografts may not be candidates for CMV-safe blood products. This is because data on renal transplant patients suggest the risk of CMV infection and disease is much lower when patients acquire infection prior to transplantation and therefore are seropositive at the time of allografting.[28]

Recipients of Heart, Heart-Lung, and Liver Transplants

While the postoperative transfusion requirements of renal transplantation patients are usually limited, the needs of heart, heart-lung, and liver transplant recipients can make dramatic demands on a blood center's inventory, especially if products screened for CMV are indicated. Despite the greater transfusion requirements of these patients, the incidence of CMV infection in seronegative recipients of hearts from seronegative donors is 20 percent, a figure similar to that seen in renal transplant recipients.[34]

As in renal transplant recipients, CMV infection rarely causes mortality in heart transplant recipients, but infection may cause fever, hepatitis, chorioretinitis, and atypical lymphocytosis.[35] Although the use of screened blood products to prevent primary CMV infection has been advised,[36] this practice for trans-

plant recipients may not be feasible in most blood programs, especially in those geographic areas where the seronegativity rate in the donor community is low. However, because the provision of CMV-seronegative blood for CMV-seronegative recipients of livers from CMV-seronegative donors has been shown to eliminate postoperative CMV infection,[37] it might be reasonable to provide, when indicated, screened products for liver transplant recipients if it can be predicted that their transfusion needs will be small (see Ch. 35).

Patients with Acquired Immunodeficiency Syndrome

CMV infection in patients with AIDS may be associated with hepatitis, chorioretinitis, pneumonitis, and central nervous system involvement. Since CMV infection is highly prevalent in persons at the greatest risk of developing AIDS, namely homosexual/bisexual men, intravenous drug abusers, and recipients of clotting factor concentrates, most CMV infections in patients with AIDS are caused by reactivation. Although there are no data from prospective studies to support the use of screened blood products in AIDS patients, the risk for primary CMV infection should be avoided. It would seem prudent to provide transfusion products from screened donors for both CMV-seronegative patients with AIDS and CMV-seronegative patients who have evidence of human immunodeficiency virus type 1 (HIV-1) infection, regardless of the presence of disease. In emphasizing this recommendation, it has been pointed out[38] that only 57 percent of HIV-infected hemophiliacs were seropositive for CMV, implying that many patients were at risk of primary CMV infection. Furthermore, it is likely that the proportion of HIV-infected patients requiring transfusion will increase as the use of the marrow-suppressing agent azidothymidine becomes more common.

Patients with Malignancy

Although patients undergoing treatment for malignancy account for the use of about 20 percent of the nation's annual blood supply, it is not clearly understood which, if any, of these patients are at risk of transfusion-transmitted CMV infection. In general, it is felt that the transfusion needs of most patients with malignancy can be met without resorting to the use of screened products.[39] Although underlying disease and chemotherapy impair immunocompetence, the impairment may not be sufficient to increase the risk of developing CMV disease. Before this position is adopted with confidence, however, more information is needed about the risks for transfusion-transmitted CMV infection in some specific settings. For example, it has been reported[40] that an increasing proportion of children treated for acute lymphoblastic leukemia and non-Hodgkin's lymphoma are CMV-seropositive. In some of these children, symptomatic disease, especially hepatitis, caused postponement of chemotherapy. If this observation is confirmed, then it may be appropriate to provide screened products for selected patients with cancer. The purpose would be twofold: to reduce the risk for relapse during any delay in treatment prompted by the intervening CMV infection and to ensure that an uninfected patient does not become infected and then risk the reactivation of infection during a future transplantation.

Surgical Patients

About 20 percent of patients needing transfusion during surgery develop primary CMV infection.[41,42] Since this infection is not associated with morbidity in immunocompetent patients, the practice of not routinely providing blood products screened for CMV to surgery patients is appropriate.

There is, however, some evidence that splenectomy alters the course of CMV infection. Although published evidence is limited,[43,44] severe primary CMV infection has been reported in previously healthy young male victims of trauma who underwent splenectomy. These observations have prompted the suggestion[44] that antibody-negative, or leukodepleted, blood be used for CMV-seronegative patients undergoing splenectomy, provided a controlled, prospective study confirms the limited observations concerning the likelihood that primary CMV disease is more common and more severe in patients having such surgery.

LABORATORY TESTS FOR CYTOMEGALOVIRUS

Laboratory testing for CMV infection takes two approaches: serologic tests to detect CMV antibodies, and culture techniques to identify virus in secretions or in specimens taken at biopsy or autopsy. Depend-

ing on the circumstances, either or both of these methods need to be invoked.

A positive test for CMV antibodies identifies individuals who have been previously exposed to CMV. There are a number of different assays that are useful for this purpose, including enzyme-linked immunosorbent assays (ELISA), latex agglutination tests, and immunofluorescence assays. Older assays that have fallen out of favor because of relative insensitivity include complement fixation and hemagglutination inhibition tests. Since CMV infection is associated with life-long infection and latency, individuals who seroconvert after primary infection usually maintain a detectable antibody concentration for life. Seropositivity does not imply active infection. Moreover, positive serologic test results for CMV antibodies do not confirm the diagnosis of CMV in patients with clinical features of viral disease, and serologic tests cannot distinguish reactivation after primary infection from reinfection with a different strain of virus. Recent CMV infection is, however, likely in an individual who seroconverts from negative to positive or who experiences a fourfold or greater rise in antibody titer. Additionally, tests that permit detection of CMV-specific IgM antibody also suggest recent infection. Serologic tests find their greatest use in three settings: blood donor screening (to identify donors with latent and potentially transmissible virus), testing pregnant women, and in the workup of patients who are transplantation candidates. In the latter two groups, the role of serologic testing is to identify those individuals at risk of primary CMV infection and, consequently, significant morbidity and mortality. It should be noted that in the clinical setting, CMV antibody assays are difficult to interpret in patients who have received passively acquired CMV antibody, either from intravenous immunoglobulin or from blood products, such as plasma, provided by donors who are themselves CMV-seropositive.

Most blood programs screen some of their donors for individuals who are CMV-seronegative, relying on their donations for the transfusion needs of immunocompromised patients in whom there is a risk of primary CMV infection. Whereas the exclusion of CMV-seropositive donors in general does reduce the incidence of transfusion-transmitted CMV, this serologic screening does not distinguish the small subset of donors who are potentially infectious. The size of this subgroup may be small. Published evidence has suggested that the percentage of individuals capable of transmitting the virus is between only 1 and 3.5 percent.[39] A more efficient way of identifying the infectious donor, as opposed to identifying all donors who have ever been infected, has yet to be defined.

Because of the shortcomings inherent in using antibody assays for the diagnosis of active infection, virus isolation by culture is the test of choice when viral syndromes are being investigated. Many different specimens are suitable including urine, saliva, semen, vaginal secretions, milk, peripheral blood leukocytes, bronchial washings, and amniotic fluid. One of the drawbacks to viral culture as a diagnostic tool is the sluggish in vitro growth of CMV. Depending on the viral content of the innoculum, the cytopathic effects of CMV may take up to 6 weeks to appear. Furthermore, a positive culture does not distinguish between asymptomatic shedding, which can occur in the urine and saliva of renal and marrow transplant patients without systemic disease, and invasive disease. There is, however, a good correlation between the recovery of virus from peripheral blood leukocytes and either active or impending disease.[45]

Recent modifications of viral culture methods have sought to expedite the procedure.[46] One method, shell vial centrifugation culture, can provide results in 24 to 48 hours. The technique relies on a combination of tissue culture isolation and direct CMV antigen detection. The specimen is inoculated onto cells that have been grown on a coverslip contained in a small "shell" vial. The vial is then centrifuged at low speed for 45 minutes. The centrifugation step alters the cell membranes, rendering the cells more sensitive to viral attachment and penetration. At 16 hours and again at 72 hours after inoculation, the cell monolayer is stained with monoclonal antibody to a CMV-specific early nuclear protein. The sensitivity of this technique has been shown to be comparable to conventional culture for most specimens. Electron microscopy and histologic methods to look for viral inclusions have also been described, but they have low sensitivity when compared to culture for many clinical applications. Direct CMV antigen detection, using fluorescein-labeled monoclonal antibodies has proven useful in preparations from lung biopsy or bronchial lavage. This method is also less sensitive than culture, but has the advantage of providing results within 24 hours. More recently, the polymerase chain reaction (PCR), which promises dramatically enhanced sensitivity and a rapid turn-around, has been invoked in tests for CMV.[47] This technique has been shown to detect as little as 0.001 pg of viral nucleic acid in less than 10 hours.

MEASURES FOR PREVENTING TRANSFUSION-TRANSMITTED CYTOMEGALOVIRUS INFECTION

Adhering to Appropriate Indications for Transfusion

Although the section above discussing those categories of patients most at risk of transfusion-transmitted infection makes frequent reference to the use of screened donors found negative for antibodies to CMV, there are other approaches to consider.

Recent reappraisals of "transfusion triggers" for a number of components, including RBCs, platelets, and fresh frozen plasma, have emphasized an emerging conservatism in transfusion practice. Against this background, it is essential that the decision to transfuse reflects not only an evaluation of the clinical circumstances, but also an evaluation of laboratory test results that are much less generous than they have been. For example, the transfusion trigger for RBCs was generally regarded as an hematocrit below 30. With a better understanding of the effectiveness of compensatory mechanisms, such as increased cardiac output and elevated oxygen extraction ratio, rigid adherence to this trigger is now regarded as inappropriate, especially if the patient does not have ischemic heart disease, pulmonary disease, or cerebrovascular disease (see Chs. 7 and 21).

Whereas most of the infectious morbidity associated with inappropriate transfusions is attributable to the most common transfusion-transmitted pathogen, namely the hepatitis C virus, many studies have shown that the risk of transfusion-transmitted CMV infection increases with the number of transfusions. For example, it was found that there was a threefold increase, from 7 percent to 21 percent, in the incidence of primary CMV infection when patients receiving more than 15 units of blood were compared with those receiving 15 or fewer units.[48] In other studies of seronegative pediatric patients undergoing cardiac surgery, the risk for acquiring primary CMV infection by transfusion was calculated at about 2.7 percent per unit.[49]

Donor Screening to Provide a Cytomegalovirus-Seronegative Blood and Component Inventory

With regard to blood and component support for those individuals with an established indication for transfusion, most experience in providing CMV-safe products has come from the use of inventories provided by donors screened negative for CMV antibodies. Although CMV seropositivity in a donor does indicate previous infection, it is not possible to identify which positive donors are actually infectious. Older estimates suggested that about 10 percent of donors who are antibody-seropositive are capable of transmitting infection, but more recent reports indicate that the risk of CMV transmission is 0.38 percent of seropositive cellular blood products.[50–52] Since there are no tests to identify this subset of donors, screening relies on the use of tests that measure CMV-specific IgG or total antibodies. The most popular methods are ELISAs and latex agglutination tests. Blood and components negative in these assays are used to provide transfusion support for patients at risk of transfusion-transmitted CMV infection.

Although a more efficient donor screening strategy that identifies only the infectious CMV-seropositive donors has yet to be identified, some new approaches hold promise. For example, in a study of patients who had cardiac surgery,[53] post-transfusion infection was more often associated with lower CMV antibody titers in donors. Patients who were not infected were found to have received transfusions with blood from donors with high antibody titers. There is also evidence that the infectious CMV-seropositive donors are those with CMV-specific IgM antibodies.[54] More experience is required with these approaches before they can be regarded as an alternative to or a substitute for providing inventories from CMV-seronegative donors. The effectiveness of providing transfusion support from donors who have been screened for CMV antibodies in reducing the risk for primary CMV infection in patients needing transfusion has emerged in a number of different studies, including investigations of infants born to seronegative mothers[11,12] and seronegative recipients of seronegative bone marrow.[23,24]

Although providing screened blood for selected categories of patients is a satisfactory approach, maintaining an inventory of blood and platelets is a difficult task for some blood programs. This is particularly true when the prevalence of CMV-seropositivity in the donor community is high. Whereas blood programs in areas with a high seroprevalence are at a theoretic advantage because patients are also more likely to be seropositive, there may be problems providing screened products when more intense support is needed than that required by premature infants and renal transplantation patients. For example, maintaining an inventory for occasional CMV-seronegative patients undergoing organ or marrow transplantation could present insurmountable problems. Even when the prevalence of CMV-seropositivity in the community is low, blood programs may be confronted with an increasing requirement for screened products as the number of solid organ and marrow transplantations increases. In addition, new categories of patients who are candidates for CMV-screened blood are likely to emerge. For example, some physicians believe that CMV-seronegative patients with malignancies—if there is even a slight possibility that they are candidates for marrow transplant—should receive blood from seronegative donors.

REDUCING THE WHITE BLOOD CELL CONTENT OF BLOOD AND COMPONENTS

Because of the limited availability of CMV-seronegative blood and platelets, attention has been turned to alternative methods for decreasing CMV transmission by transfusion. Approaches to reducing the risk of transfusion-transmitted CMV that do not depend on selecting donors without evidence of CMV infection rely on reducing the concentration of leukocytes in transfusion products. As has been pointed out, while it has yet to be established with confidence which cells carry CMV, there is evidence that granulocytes are the vehicles for replicating virus.[55] It is also unclear as to the extent to which the concentration of white blood cells (WBCs) in transfusion products needs to be reduced to eliminate the risk of CMV infection. A unit of packed RBCs contains, on average, 1×10^9 leukocytes, and a single platelet unit contains about 1×10^8. Recent developments in filtration technology have made possible increasingly efficient removal of leukocytes. For example, the new third-generation filters achieve 99 percent, or a two-log removal, leaving fewer than 1×10^6 leukocytes in a unit of packed RBCs or platelets.[56]

Investigations relying on less efficient means of leukoreduction have also met with some success. Conventional centrifugation and removal of the buffy coat reduces the number of WBCs by 60 to 80 percent.[57] This combination was shown to reduce the risk of CMV infection in cardiac surgery patients.[58] The fact that this maneuver was only partially successful was attributed to the incomplete removal of leukocytes from the transfused RBCs that still contained about 40 percent of their original number of WBCs. The addition of saline washing after the centrifugation step results in a much more efficient removal of leukocytes, with only 10 percent of the original number remaining.[59] A combination of centrifugation and washing has been shown to be associated with a low rate of transfusion-transmitted CMV in transfusion-dependent neonates.[60]

It has been recognized for some time that the risk of transfusion-transmitted CMV is reduced in patients requiring frozen deglycerolized RBCs. The risk reduction, which has been shown in hemodialysis patients and low–birth weight neonates, has been attributed to the reduction in the number of WBCs in frozen deglycerolized units.[61,62]

While centrifugation and washing, either alone or in combination, have been shown to reduce the number of WBCs in units of blood; they are labor-intensive and inefficient. Filtration offers a much more attractive alternative, both in terms of the reduction in the number of contaminating WBCs and also convenience, since some filters can be used at the bedside. New filters also offer versatility, since both platelet and RBC units can be subjected to this procedure.

The filters that are currently used to remove WBCs represent a third-generation development. First-generation filters, with a pore size of 170 to 260 μm^3, are the standard blood filters that are mandatory for all transfusions. Whereas they remove gross debris, they play no specific role in leukoreduction of components for transfusion. Second-generation, or mi-croaggregate, filters were developed in the hope that their smaller screen size, 20 to 40 μm^3, would ensure the removal of particles that were thought to contribute to the development of adult respiratory distress syndrome in multiply transfused patients. Although this role for second-generation filters has not been established, these filters, while unsuitable for platelet transfusions, can remove up to 85 percent of leukocytes from units of RBCs. This reduction is sufficient, for some patients, to forestall the development of febrile transfusion reactions. Microaggregate filters are more effective if the RBC unit is specially prepared before filtration. Up to 90 percent leukocyte removal can be achieved by centrifuging the RBCs before filtration. An additional small increment in leukoreduction is achieved by the spin, cool, and filter procedure, which involves a 3- to 4-hour period of refrigeration after the initial centrifugation.

In spite of the general interest in filtration of blood products, published experience with third-generation filters in reducing transfusion-transmitted CMV infection is limited. Many studies lack control groups, and the experimental groups are small. In addition, filtration is often used, in the same study, in combination with a different approach, also designed to reduce the risk of transfusion-transmitted CMV infection. Only a few studies on at-risk patients requiring both platelets and RBCs have relied on filtration for both components. These concerns aside, filtration with third-generation filters has been shown to be effective in the recipients of autologous bone marrow transplants who are at risk for primary CMV infection,[63] in neonates requiring RBCs,[64] and in patients with leukemia or non-Hodgkin's lymphoma undergoing induction therapy.[65,66]

Although filtration technology has gained wide use, particularly in transplantation and oncology settings, the evidence for its superiority over donor screening is lacking. Under well-controlled conditions, many of the third-generation filters are certainly capable of effective leukodepletion. Whether this translates to similar performance in the component preparation department at a blood center or in the hospital ward during bedside filtration has yet to be shown. It is not known whether filters have their own failure rate, either because of malfunction or misuse, or if the salutory effect of filtration in the transplantation setting is to be expected in all other settings in which transfusion-transmitted CMV infections should be avoided. It is also not known if there are circumstances whereby the retention of RBCs and platelets on filters is sufficiently large such that additional transfusions, and thereby donor exposure, are necessary to achieve the intended therapeutic effect.

Although prospective trials comparing filtered blood products with blood products from CMV-screened donors are underway, some authorities believe that there is sufficient evidence already accumulated to show that CMV-seronegative components and third-generation filtered RBCs and platelets are equivalent in their ability to reduce the risk of transfusion-transmitted CMV infection.[67]

Immunoprophylaxis and Antiviral Agents

Several approaches have been suggested for preventive therapy in settings in which donations from screened volunteers are unavailable or leukodepletion is impractical. Experience with CMV immunoglobulin has been mixed. Although one study suggested that bone marrow recipients at risk of primary infection from transfusion were protected by an intramuscular preparation,[68] the same investigators could not show a similar benefit using an intravenous product.[20] On the other hand, studies of intravenous immunoglobulin in CMV-seronegative recipients of kidneys from CMV-seropositive donors did reveal a reduction in the incidence of CMV disease from 60 to 21 percent.[69] Although the findings are not directly applicable to prophylaxis for recipients of CMV-seropositive bone marrow or blood products, the possibility deserves investigation. Studies suggest that intravenous immunoglobulin is ineffective for treating recurrent CMV infection in seropositive recipients of bone marrow transplants.[70] Reasons for the inconsistencies in experience with passive immunoprophylaxis probably relate to differences in antiviral titers in various preparations and differing dosage regimens.

There is encouraging early experience with three antiviral agents—acyclovir, ganciclovir, and phoscarnet.[71] When acyclovir was administered intravenously to bone marrow transplant recipients who were seropositive for CMV, the risk of CMV pneumonia and all CMV disease was substantially reduced.[72] Early treatment with ganciclovir to prevent CMV dis-

ease after allogeneic marrow transplantation has also been shown to be effective.[73] In this double-blind placebo-controlled trial, patients who were CMV-seropositive or patients who were recipients of seropositive marrow were screened by surveillance culture. Treatment was started as soon as cultures became positive, regardless of whether symptoms of disease were present. CMV disease developed in 15 of 35 placebo recipients and in 1 of 37 ganciclovir recipients during the first 100 post-transplant days. All patients in the treatment arm were culture-negative by day 21, compared with the majority of patients in the placebo group, who remained culture-positive. Ganciclovir apparently reduced the incidence of CMV disease and improved survival, at 100 days and 180 days, after allogeneic marrow transplantation. In another study, 40 allogeneic bone marrow transplant recipients at risk of CMV disease underwent bronchoscopy and bronchioalveolar lavage on day post-transplant 35.[74] Patients with evidence of pulmonary CMV infection were then randomized into two groups. No treatment was provided the one group; the other received ganciclovir. Four of 20 patients in the treatment group and 14 of 20 patients in the "observation only" group developed interstitial pneumonia. Although the study was not blinded, it was concluded that the incidence of CMV disease was significantly lower in the group treated with ganciclovir. Ganciclovir has also been shown to reduce the overall incidence of CMV disease in heart transplant recipients at risk of reactivation of primary CMV infection. Twelve of 76 patients receiving ganciclovir, as opposed to 31 of 73 placebo control patients, developed CMV disease during the post-transplant period.[75]

Although the use of antiviral agents effective against CMV has become routine and highly effective in selected transplantation patients, these strategies have not been studied for a specific role in reducing the contribution of transfusion-associated CMV infection to post-transplantation morbidity and mortality.

Vaccination

Whereas there are no human herpesvirus vaccines available in the United States, a live attenuated VZV strain has been licensed in Japan, where it has been used in vaccination programs for children with normal immune responses. As far as CMV is concerned, live attenuated viruses have also been studied in both renal transplantation and in mothers whose children attended day-care centers.[76] Results were variable. Although the incidence of infection was unaltered by vaccination in either group, vaccinated renal transplant recipients who developed primary infection were much less likely to develop severe disease. More recent CMV vaccination studies have relied on the fact that the viral genome has been sequenced. As a result, it has been possible to select promising subunits for use as vaccination studies. For example, an envelope glycoprotein has been shown to provoke cytotoxic T lymphocyte responses and neutralizing antibody production in animal and human experiments. The gene encoding this glycoprotein has also been inserted into a mutant adenovirus,[77] a strategy prompted by evidence that attenuated strains that do not replicate fail to immunize.

Although the major goal in the development of a CMV vaccine is the prevention of congenital CMV disease, it is tempting to speculate that once a safe, effective vaccine is developed, its indications could be extended beyond use in seronegative pregnant women to include individuals at risk of transfusion-transmitted CMV disease.

Human Herpesvirus 6 Infection

Human herpesvirus 6 (HHV-6) is genomically and epidemiologically similar to CMV. It was originally isolated from the peripheral blood leukocytes of a small group of patients with either lymphoma or HIV infection.[1] Since the virus selectively targeted B cells, it was initially named human B lymphotropic virus. The nomenclature was changed when it was discovered that the virus also has affinity for CD4-positive T lymphocytes and genetic and physical properties that place it in the herpesvirus family. It has also been established that HHV-6 has tropism for monocytes, macrophages, and megakaryocytes. Infection with HHV-6 is common, in that 60 to 85 percent of healthy adults have antibodies to the virus.

Primary HHV-6 generally causes an acute febrile illness in young children. The virus is also responsible for exanthem subitum (roseola), which is characterized by fever and short-lived maculopapular rash that starts on the trunk and spreads to the extremi-

ties. In a recent study of emergency-department admissions for the investigation of fever in children younger than 2 years of age, 14 percent were attributed to HHV-6 infection.[78] There is also evidence that HHV-6 is frequent cause of febrile seizures in infants and young children.[79] Rare instances of benign liver disease have also been attributed to HHV-6 in both adults and infants.[80,81] By the age of 3 years, most children have been infected with HHV-6, as evidenced by positive serologic test results.

It is suspected that the virus can persist in a latent form after primary infection, and there are reports of reactivation of infection in immunocompromised patients undergoing bone marrow or solid organ transplantation.[82,83] In recipients of bone marrow transplants, the virus has been implicated in interstitial pneumonitis.[84] However, the patients whose cases were reported were seropositive before receiving transplants and it is likely that reactivation of HHV-6 accounted for their clinical picture. Since the patients showed poor graft function, the authors suggested that a HHV-6 had the potential to infect marrow cells and interfere with their function. A mechanism for this effect proposes that HHV-6 infection provokes the production of mediators that impede marrow responses to growth factors.[85] As far as transfusion medicine is concerned, there is insufficient evidence to decide if special steps need to be taken in meeting the transfusion requirements of patients who are seronegative for antibodies to HHV-6. If it emerges that precautions are necessary, it could be that immunocompromised patients at risk of primary infection will be candidates. Before this claim can be made, the anecdotal information about HHV-6 infection needs to be augmented by larger studies that formally disclose the relevance of HHV-6 infection to clinical disease in general, and transfusion-associated disease in particular.

EPSTEIN-BARR VIRUS INFECTION

EBV, or human herpesvirus 4, is ubiquitous; more than 90 percent of blood donors have EBV antibodies.[86] Infection with the agent, which has tropism for B lymphocytes, is common during childhood, and spread occurs by the oropharyngeal route. In young children, primary infection may pass unnoticed. In adults, however, the disease presents as infectious mononucleosis, with its characteristic features of fever, pharyngitis, tonsillitis, lymphadenopathy, and lymphocytosis. There may also be an associated splenomegaly and elevated liver enzyme concentrations. In addition, it has been postulated that EBV infection accounts for some cases of chronic fatigue syndrome, a disease of young adults who experience recurring bouts of debilitating fatigue, myalgia, cervical lymphadenopathy, and pharyngitis.[87]

The EBV is also occasionally involved in the pathogenesis of lymphomas of the small noncleaved type that are endemic in some parts of Africa (Burkitt's lymphoma) and in nasopharyngeal carcinoma. The association with lymphoma may be more extensive, since EBV has also, rarely, been implicated in the development of lymphoma in patients with heart and kidney transplants receiving continuous immunosuppression and in patients with AIDS. Some patients with AIDS have also developed interstitial pneumonia as a result of reactivation of latent EBV.

Regarding transfusion-acquired EBV infection, two early case reports[88,89] showed that the virus could be transmitted in units provided by ostensibly healthy donors who were nonetheless viremic for EBV. The EBV has also been implicated in the postperfusion syndrome and in infectious mononucleosis-like viral illness in patients who undergo cardiac surgery, usually developing 4 to 6 weeks after transfusion. Although the disease is more often caused by CMV, there is evidence that EBV can also account for the syndrome.[90,91]

Another group of heavily transfusion-dependent patients, namely recipients of bone marrow transplants, have high rates of active EBV infection. In one study, 60 percent had evidence of EBV infection.[92] While 90 percent of these infections appeared to represent reactivation, primary infection can occur when the virus is acquired from the bone marrow or blood of an infected donor. However, when infection occurs under these circumstances, it is usually mild or inapparent. This could be due to the beneficial effect of transfusion-acquired EBV antibodies provided by seropositive donors.

Because transfusion-transmitted EBV infections are frequently asymptomatic, no recommendations have been made to provide blood products from donors screened negative for evidence of infection. It is also worth noting that since the virus is cell-associated, patients managed with leukoreduced components might also be at less risk of transfusion-related primary EBV infection.

REFERENCES

1. Salahuddin SZ, Abalashi DV, Markham PD et al: Isolation of a new virus, HBLV, in patients with lymphoproliferative disorders. Science 234:596, 1986
2. Frenkel N, Schirmer EC, Wyatt LS et al: Isolation of a new herpesvirus from human CD4+ T cells. Proc Natl Acad Sci USA 87:748, 1990
3. Kreel I, Zaroff LI, Canter JW et al: A syndrome following total body perfusion. Surg Gynecol Obstet 111:317, 1960
4. Kaariainen L, Kemola E, Paloheimo J: Rise of cytomegalovirus antibodies in an infectious mononucleosis-like syndrome after transfusion. Br Med J 1:1270, 1966
5. Tegtmeier GE: Blood transfusion and the transmission of cytomegalovirus. p. 87. In Moore SB (ed): Transfusion-Transmitted Viral Diseases. American Association of Blood Banks, Arlington, VA, 1987
6. Ho M: Cytomegalovirus, Biology and Infection. p. 171. Plenum, New York, 1982
7. Weller TH: The cytomegalovirus: ubiquitous agents with protean clinical manifestations. N Engl J Med 285:203, 1971
8. Stagno S, Pass RF, Dworsky ME et al: Congenital cytomegalovirus infection: the relative importance of primary and recurrent maternal infection. N Engl J Med 306:945, 1982
9. Kumar ML, Nankervis GA, Jacobs IB et al: Congenital and postnatally acquired cytomegalovirus infections: long-term follow-up. J Pediatr 104:674, 1984
10. Onorato IM, Morens DM, Martone WJ, Stansfield SK: Epidemiology of cytomegalovirus infections: recommendations for prevention and control. Rev Infect Dis 7:479, 1985
11. Yeager AS, Grumet FC, Hafleigh EB et al: Prevention of transfusion-acquired cytomegalovirus infections in newborn infants. J Pediatr 98:281, 1981
12. Adler SP, Chandrika T, Lawrence L, Baggett J: Cytomegalovirus infections in neonates acquired by blood transfusions. Pediatr Infect Dis 2:114, 1983
13. Preiksaitis JK, Brown L, McKenzie M: Transfusion-acquired cytomegalovirus infection in neonates. A prospective study. Transfusion 28:205, 1988
14. Lamberson HV Jr, McMillan JA, Weiner LB et al: Prevention of transfusion-associated cytomegalovirus (CMV) infection in neonates by screening blood donors for IgM to CMV. J Infect Dis 157:820, 1988

15. Yeager AS, Palumbo PE, Malachowski N et al: Sequelae of maternally derived cytomegalovirus infections in premature infants. J Pediatr 102:918, 1983

16. Adler SP: Cytomegalovirus and transfusion. Transfus Med Rev 2:235, 1988

17. Meyers JD: Infection in recipients of marrow transplants. p. 261. In Remington JS, Swartz MN (eds): Current Clinical Topics in Infectious Diseases. McGraw-Hill, New York, 1985

18. Bowden RA, Meyers JD: Transfusion-associated cytomegalovirus infection. In Dutcher JP (ed): Modern Transfusion Therapy. Vol. 2. CRC Press, Inc., Boca Raton, FL, 1990

19. Verdonck LF, van der Linden JA, Bast BJ, Gmelig Meyling FH: Influence of cytomegalovirus infection on the recovery of humoral immunity after autologous bone marrow transplantation. Exp Hematol 15:864, 1987

20. Meyers JD, Flournoy N, Thomas ED: Nonbacterial pneumonia after allogeneic marrow transplantation: a review of ten years' experience. Rev Infect Dis 4:1119, 1982

21. Appelbaum RF, Meyers JD, Fefer A et al: Nonbacterial pneumonia following marrow transplantation in 100 identical twins. Transplantation 33:265, 1982

22. Santos GW, Hess AD, Vogelsang GB: Graft-versus-host reactions and disease. Immunol Rev 88:169, 1985

23. Bowden RA, Sayers M, Flournoy N et al: Cytomegalovirus immune globulin and seronegative blood products to prevent primary cytomegalovirus infection after marrow transplantation. N Engl J Med 314:1006, 1986

24. Reusser P, Fisher LD, Buckner CD et al: Cytomegalovirus infection after autologous bone marrow transplantation: occurrence of cytomegalovirus disease and effect on engraftment. Blood 75:1888, 1990

25. Wingard JR, Chen DY, Burns WH et al: Cytomegalovirus infection after autologous bone marrow transplantation with comparison to infections after allogeneic bone marrow transplantation. Blood 71:1432, 1988

26. Bowden RA, Sayers M, Gleaves CA et al: Cytomegalovirus-seronegative blood components for the prevention of primary cytomegalovirus infection after marrow transplantation. Transfusion 27:478, 1987

27. Miller WJ, McCullough J, Balfour HH Jr et al: Prevention of CMV infection following bone marrow transplantation: a randomized trial of blood product screening. Bone Marrow Transplant 7:227, 1991

28. Bowden RA: Cytomegalovirus: transmission by blood components and measures of prevention. p. 201. In Nance SJ (ed): Blood Safety: Current Challenges. American Association of Blood Banks, Bethesda MD, 1992

29. Chou SW: Acquisition of donor strains of cytomegalovirus by renal-transplant recipients. N Engl J Med 314:1418, 1986

30. Glen J: Cytomegalovirus infections following renal transplantation. Rev Infect Dis 3:1151, 1981

31. Fryd DS, Peterson PK, Ferguson RM et al: Cytomegalovirus as a risk factor in renal transplantation. Transplantation 30:436, 1980

32. Rubin RH, Tolkoff-Rubin NE, Oliver D et al: Multicenter seroepidemiologic study of the impact of cytomegalovirus infection on renal transplantation. Transplantation 40:243, 1985

33. Kurtz JB, Thompson JF, Ting A et al: The problem of cytomegalovirus infection in renal allograft recipients. Q J Med 53:342, 1984

34. Preiksaitis JK, Rosno S, Grumet C, Merigan TC: Infections due to herpesvirus in cardiac transplant recipients: role of the donor heart and immunosuppressive therapy. J Infect Dis 147:974, 1983

35. Rand KH, Rasmussen LE, Pollard RB et al: Cellular immunity and herpesvirus infections in cardiac-transplant patients. N Engl J Med 296:1372, 1976

36. Adler SP: Transfusion-associated cytomegalovirus infections. Rev Infect Dis 5:977, 1983

37. Rakela J, Wiesner RH, Taswell HF et al: Incidence of cytomegalovirus infection and its relationship to donor-recipient serologic status in liver transplantation. Transplant Proc 19:2399, 1987

38. Jackson JB, Erice A, Englund JA et al: Prevalence of cytomegalovirus antibody in hemophiliacs and homosexuals infected with human immunodeficiency virus type 1. Transfusion 28: 187, 1988

39. Tegtmeier GE: Cytomegalovirus infection as a complication of blood transfusion. Semin Liver Dis 6:82, 1986

40. Kornhuber B, Gerein V: Transfusion-transmitted CMV infections. Clinical importance and means of prevention? Vox Sang 46:387, 1984

41. Preiksaitis JK, Grumet FC, Smith WK, Merigan TC: Transfusion-acquired cytomegalovirus infection in cardiac surgery patients. J Med Virol 15:283, 1985

42. Wilhelm JA, Matter L, Schopfer K: The risk of transmitting cytomegalovirus to patients receiving blood transfusion. J Infect Dis 154:169, 1986

43. Baumgartner JD, Glauser MP, Burgo-Black AL et al: Severe cytomegalovirus infection in multiply transfused, splenectomized, trauma patients. Lancet 2:63, 1982

44. Drew WL, Miner RC: Transfusion-related cytomegalovirus infection following noncardiac surgery. JAMA 247:2389, 1982

45. Griffiths PD: Diagnostic techniques for cytomegalovirus infection. Clin Hematol 13:631, 1984

46. Gleaves CA, Smith TF, Shuster EA et al: Comparison of standard tube and shell vial culture techniques for the detection of cytomegalovirus in clinical specimens. J Clin Microbiol 21:217, 1985

47. Hsia K, Spector DH, Lawrie J et al: Enzymatic amplification of human cytomegalovirus sequences by polymerase chain reaction. J Clin Microbiol 27:1802, 1989

48. Prince AM, Szmuness W, Millian SJ, David DS: A serologic study of cytomegalovirus infections associated with blood transfusions. N Engl J Med 284:1125, 1971

49. Armstrong JA, Tarr GC, Youngblood LA et al: Cytomegalovirus infection in children undergoing open-heart surgery. Yale J Biol Med 49:83, 1975

50. Adler SP, Chandrika T, Lawrence L, Baggett J: Cytomegalovirus infections in neonates acquired by blood transfusions. Pediatr Infect Dis J 2:114, 1983

51. Diosi P, Moldovan E, Tomescu N: Latent cytomegalovirus infection in blood donors. Br Med J 4:660, 1969

52. Preiksaitis JK, Brown L, McKenzie M: The risk of cytomegalovirus infection in seronegative transfusion recipients not receiving exogenous immunosuppression. J Infect Dis 157:523, 1988

53. Beneke JS, Tegtmeier GE, Alter HJ et al: Relation of titers of antibodies to CMV in blood donors to the transmission of cytomegalovirus infection. J Infect Dis 150:883, 1984

54. Burns WH, Saral R: Opportunistic viral infections. Br Med Bull 41:46, 1985

55. Hersman J, Meyers JD, Thomas ED et al: The effects of granulocyte transfusions on the incidence of cytomegalovirus infection after allogeneic marrow transplantation. Ann Intern Med 96:149, 1982

56. Lane TA, Anderson KC, Goodnough LT et al: Leukocyte reduction in blood component therapy. Ann Intern Med 117:151, 1992

57. Brand A: White cell depletion: why and how? In Nance SJ (ed): Transfusion Medicine in the 1990's. American Association of Blood Banks, Arlington, VA, 1990

58. Lang DJ, Ebert PA, Rodgers BM et al: Reduction of postperfusion cytomegalovirus infections following the use of leukocyte depleted blood. Transfusion 17:391, 1977

59. Demmler GJ, Brady MT, Bijou H et al: Posttransfusion cytomegalovirus infection in neonates: role of saline-washed red blood cells. J Pediatr 108:762, 1986

60. Luban NL, Williams AE, McDonald MG et al: Low incidence of cytomegalovirus infection in neonates transfused with washed red blood cells. Am J Dis Child 141:416, 1987

61. Betts RF, Cestero RV, Freeman RB, Douglas RG Jr: Epidemiology of cytomegalovirus infection in end stage renal disease. J Med Virol 4:89, 1979

62. Taylor BJ, Jacobs RF, Baker RL et al: Frozen deglycerolized blood prevents transfusion-acquired cytomegalovirus infections in neonates. Pediatr Infect Dis 5:188, 1986

63. Verdonck LF, de Graan-Hentzen YC, Dekker AW et al: Cytomegalovirus seronegative platelets and leukocyte-poor red blood cells from random donors can prevent primary cytomegalovirus infection after bone marrow transplantation. Bone Marrow Transplant 2:73, 1987

64. Gilbert GL, Hayes K, Hudson IL, James J: Prevention of transfusion-acquired cytomegalovirus infection in infants by blood filtration to remove leucocytes. Neonatal Cytomegalovirus Infection Study Group. Lancet i:1228, 1989

65. de Graan-Hentzen YCE, Gratama JW, Mudde GC et al: Prevention of primary cytomegalovirus infection during induction treatment of acute leukemia using at random leukocyte-poor blood products. Br J Haematol 66:421, 1987

66. Murphy MF, Grint PC, Hardiman AE et al: Use of leukocyte-poor blood components to prevent primary cytomegalovirus (CMV) infection in patients with acute leukemia. Br J Haematol 70:253, 1988

67. Hillyer CD, Emmens RK, Zago-Novaretti M, Berkman EM: Methods for the reduction of transfusion-transmitted cytomegalovirus infection: filtration versus the use of seronegative donor units. Transfusion 34:929, 1994

68. Meyers JD, Leszczynski J, Zaia JE et al: Prevention of cytomegalovirus infection by cytomegalovirus immune globulin after marrow transplantation. Ann Intern Med 98:442, 1983

69. Snydman DR, Werner BG, Heinze-Lacey B et al: Use of cytomegalovirus immune globulin to prevent cytomegalovirus disease in renal-transplant recipients. N Engl J Med 317:1049, 1987

70. Ringden O, Pihlstedt P, Volin L et al: Failure to prevent cytomegalovirus infection by cytomegalovirus hyperimmune plasma: a randomized trial by the Nordic Bone Marrow Transplantation Group. Bone Marrow Transplant 2:299, 1987

71. Bowden RA, Meyers JD: Prophylaxis of cytomegalovirus infection. Semin Hematol 27(suppl.):17, 1990

72. Meyers JD, Reed AC, Shepp DH et al: Acyclovir for prevention of cytomegalovirus infection and disease after allogeneic bone marrow transplantation. N Engl J Med 318:70, 1988

73. Goodrich JM, Mori M, Gleaves CA et al (Fred Hutchinson Cancer Research Center, Seattle; Syntex Research, Palo Alta, Calif): Early treatment with ganciclovir to prevent cytomegalovirus disease after allogeneic bone marrow transplantation. N Engl J Med 325:1601, 1991

74. Schmidt G, Horak D, Niland JC et al: A randomized, controlled trial of prophylactic ganciclovir for cytomegalovirus primary infection in recipients of allogeneic bone marrow transplants. N Eng J Med 15:1005, 1991

75. Merigan TC, Renlund DG, Keay S et al: A controlled trial of ganciclovir to prevent cytomegalovirus disease after heart transplantation. N Engl J Med 326:1182, 1992

76. Plotkin SA, Starr SE, Friedman HM, Gonczol K: Vaccines for the prevention of human cytomegalovirus infection. Rev Infect Dis 12(suppl.):S827, 1990

77. Marshall GS, Ricciardi RP, Rando RF et al: An adenovirus recombinant that expresses the human cytomegalovirus major envelope glycoprotein and induces neutralizing antibodies. J Infect Dis 162:1177, 1990

78. Pruksananonda P, Hall CB, Insel RA et al: Primary human herpesvirus 6 infection in young children. N Engl J Med 326:1445, 1992

79. Segondy M, Astruc J, Atoui N et al: Herpesvirus 6 infection in young children. N Engl J Med 327:1099, 1992

80. Dubedat S, Kappagoda N: Hepatitis due to human herpesvirus-6. Lancet ii:1463, 1989

81. Tajiri H, Nose O, Baba K, Okada S: Human herpesvirus-6 infection with liver injury in neonatal hepatitis. Lancet 335:863, 1990

82. Yosikawa T, Suga S, Asano Y et al: Human herpesvirus-6 infection in bone marrow transplantation. Blood 78:1381, 1991

83. Okuno T, Higashi K, Shiraki K et al: Human herpesvirus 6 infection in renal transplantation. Transplantation 49:519, 1990

84. Carrigan DR, Drobyski WR, Russler SK et al: Interstitial pneumonitis associated with human herpesvirus-6 infection after marrow transplantation. Lancet 338:147, 1991

85. Burd EM, Knox K, Carrigan DR: Human herpesvirus-6-associated suppression of growth factor-induced macrophage maturation in human bone marrow cultures. Blood 81:1645, 1993

86. Henle W, Henle G: Immunology of Epstein-Barr virus. p. 209. In Roizman B (ed): The Herpesviruses. Plenum Press, New York, 1982

87. Dubois RE, Seeley JK, Brus I et al: Chronic mononucleosis syndrome. South Med J 77:1376, 1984

88. Solem JH, Jörgensen W: Accidentally transmitted infectious mononucleosis. Acta Med Scand 186:433, 1969

89. Turner AR, McDonald RN, Cooper BA: Transmission of infectious mononucleosis by transfusion of pre-illness blood. Ann Intern Med 77:751, 1972

90. Gerber P, Walsh JH, Roseblum EN, Purcell RH: Association of EB-virus infection with the post-perfusion syndrome. Lancet i:593, 1969

91. Henle W, Henle G, Scriba M et al: Antibody responses to the Epstein-Barr virus and cytomegalovirus after open-heart and other surgery. N Engl J Med 282:1068, 1970

92. Burns WH, Saral R: Opportunistic viral infections. Br Med Bull 41:46, 1985

Bacterial and Parasitic Infections

Kaaron Benson

BACTERIAL INFECTIONS

Etiology

In the early days of blood transfusion therapy, risks of transfusion-transmitted disease were high and a multitude of infections could be transmitted. Transfusion-transmitted sepsis due to bacterial contamination during processing or contamination by donor skin bacterial flora was not uncommon. The introduction of closed collection systems, improved sterilization techniques, and refrigerated storage of red blood cell (RBC) components dramatically reduced the risk of receiving bacterially contaminated blood.

While the total annual number of bacterial contamination cases associated with blood transfusion has decreased over the past 30 years, the number of cases identified with platelets has increased in recent years.[1] This is due to the continuing rise in numbers of platelets transfused, storage of platelets at the warmer temperatures that most bacteria prefer, and transfusion to a largely immunocompromised patient population.

In Goldman and Blajchman's review[2] of culture surveillance studies, bacteria were identified in 0 to 7 percent of platelet concentrates, 0 to 3.2 percent of apheresis platelets, and 0 to 0.2 percent of frozen deglycerolized RBCs when a minimum of 100 units were cultured. The Blood Transfusion Service of the Canadian Red Cross Society samples over 4,000

RBC and platelet units annually as part of their quality control program. From 1980 to 1990, over 47,000 units were tested; 0.3 percent had positive bacterial cultures.[2] These figures do not translate, however, into an equal number of septic transfusion recipients. Studies have shown that the incidence of bacterial contamination is higher in sampled units than in transfusion recipients. Some false-positive cultures will be found owing to contamination at the time of sampling, and some organisms will not ultimately survive refrigerated storage or the bactericidal activities of plasma and white blood cells (WBCs).[3] It has been estimated that the risk of fatal bacterial contamination is approximately 1 in 6 million; from 1986 through 1988, 10 septic fatalities were reported to the U.S. Food and Drug Administration (FDA) at a time when approximately 60 million blood components were transfused.[4] While the true risk of a nonfatal case is not known, estimates have ranged from 1/1,000 to 7/1,000.[5]

The bacteria implicated in cases of transfusion-induced sepsis are primarily endotoxin-producing, gram-negative bacilli that can be found in soil, water, and feces; and that grow slowly at 4 to 8°C, rapidly at 25 to 30°C and, typically, not at all at 37°C. They are described as psychrophilic, capable of growing in temperatures of less than 5°C. Most of these organisms can use citrate as a source of carbon[1] as they multiply during storage. The most common organisms involved in bacterially contaminated RBCs have been *Yersinia enterocolitica* and psychrophilic pseudomonades, such as *Pseudomonas fluorescens* and *P. cepacea.*[2] *Salmonella* species have also been responsible for some cases. Bacteria commonly associated with contaminated platelets have been the gram-positives, *Staphylococci* and *Streptococci* species, and a variety of gram-negative organisms.[6] Symptoms of septic platelet transfusions may result either from endotoxin production or as a direct reaction to proliferation of large numbers of bacteria during in vitro storage.

Diagnosis and Treatment

In many cases, the presence of bacterial endotoxin has been implicated as the source of the "warm shock" that develops in recipients; high fever and profound hypotension occur rapidly. Since up to half of such affected patients can die,[7] early diagnosis and treatment is essential. In suspected cases, a sample from both the blood bag and patient should be cultured. Simple direct inspection of the bag or a gram stain of its contents are generally not productive. Cultures from a RBC unit should be placed at 37°C, 25 to 30°C, and 1 to 6°C. When culturing a platelet unit, the 1 to 6°C incubation can be eliminated. Samples should be taken directly from the bag and not from a segment, to avoid a false-negative result. If a culture remains sterile, bacterial contamination can usually be discounted. A positive culture result should be compared to the patient's blood culture result, to reduce the risk of overinterpreting contamination at the time of sampling.

Initial treatment involves managing the septic shock manifestations and initiating empiric antibiotics. Coverage for both gram-positive and -negative organisms should be started. Culture results and sensitivities may mandate a change in antibiotics. Factors that appear to affect the severity of the patient's reaction include the number and type of organism involved, the patient's immune status and concurrent antibiotic therapy.

Whereas a variety of etiologies may be responsible for blood and blood component contamination, asymptomatic donor bacteremia is frequently implicated (Table 40-1). When carefully questioned, some donors may recall recent episodes of diarrhea or mild abdominal pain, findings that have been associated with *Y. enterocolitica* or *Salmonella* infection.[2,8] Often, though, no such history can be obtained, even

Table 40-1. Factors Associated with Bacterial Contamination

Donor bacteremia

Prolonged storage interval of unit

Temperature favorable for bacterial growth

Contamination at time of blood collection: skin flora organisms, poor skin cleansing, skin core in needle hub, contaminated solutions or equipment

Contamination at time of blood processing: open system created and contaminated during pooling, contaminated water bath

though resampling of the donor may provide serologic evidence of a bacterial infection.[2]

Bacterial contamination of a unit can also occur during the blood collection process. Inadequate cleansing of the donor's skin, contaminated solutions or equipment, or capturing a skin core in the needle hub can result in bacterial growth within the bag. The organisms involved will generally be normal skin flora. Contamination at the time of processing may involve an unsanitary water bath and unprotected ports on the unit or improper pooling technique. Once an open system is created, the shelf life must be reduced to 24 hours because of the risk that microorganisms may have been introduced.

Preventive Measures

Methods employed to decrease the risk of bacterial contamination focus on the factors that are associated with contamination. (Table 40-2). Donors are asked if they feel well and current users of antibiotics will be questioned as to possible recent infection. The donor must appear to be in good health and the temperature must not be greater than 37.5°C. Pitting of the skin should alert the phlebotomist to more carefully cleanse the antecubital fossa.

Autologous donors should be carefully questioned about potential bacteremia, since bacterial contamination of autologous blood is one of the few hazards associated with receiving one's own blood; such an occurrence has been reported.[9] Autologous donors are more likely than allogeneic donors to be bacteremic owing to factors such as recent hospitalization, current use of antibiotics for recent infection, and current catheter placement. Donors with intravenous catheters are at even higher risk since microor-

Table 40-2. Methods Used to Decrease Bacterial
Contamination Risk

Donor history questions:
     Feeling well?
     Antibiotic use?

Donor examination:
     Temperature at time of donation
     Skin pits/adequate cleansing

Proper storage and shipping:
     Maintain proper temperatures
     Maintain proper storage intervals

Appropriate handling of unit:
     Maintain closed system
     Sterile technique during pooling procedures
     Protection of ports during thawing procedures

Visual inspection of the unit:
     Color change
     Clots
     Gas
     Hemolysis

Transfuse promptly:
     Do not keep RBC unit on floor unrefrigerated

Monitor for early signs and symptoms of sepsis

ganisms may gain direct access to the venous system. Furthermore, autologous donors may have diseases that confer some degree of immunosuppression, rendering them less able to fend off invading bacteria.

Maintaining blood and blood components at the proper temperatures and storage intervals will reduce the risk of proliferation of small numbers of bacteria that may be present in the collected unit. The storage interval for platelets was once 3 days, was lengthened to 5 days in 1983 with the introduction of new gas-permeable plastic bags, and was then further extended to 7 days in December 1984.[1] With reports of a number of fatal and life-threatening bacterial contamination cases due to platelets stored 6 and 7 days, the storage interval was reduced to 5 days in 1986. Most often, cases of platelet-associated bacterial contamination involve older platelets (i.e., those stored for 5 days)[6] (Fig. 40-1).

Any processing of the unit should be done in a manner that will avert the introduction of microor-

ganisms, such as maintaining a closed system, using sterile technique during pooling procedures, and protecting the unit's ports during thawing. Prior to transfusion, there should be a visual inspection of the unit; specifically, one should look for a color change, clots, gas, or hemolysis, all of which can occur owing to presence of bacteria. All units should be transfused promptly, as small numbers of bacteria in RBC units may proliferate as the component warms. Finally, all transfusionists should recognize that they are the last ones capable of stopping a potential fatality by closely monitoring the recipient for early manifestations of sepsis and taking appropriate action if those signs and symptoms appear.

Cases of bacterial contamination continue to occur despite the measures used to decrease the risk. Additional measures have been proposed to further decrease the risk of this potentially fatal occurrence (Table 40-3). Donors could be specifically questioned about a history of recent abdominal pain or diarrhea or recent dental work or other invasive procedure.[10,11] However, these questions are not specific for bacteremic individuals; many healthy donors would be deferred.

The majority of RBC units implicated in bacterial contamination cases have been stored for a minimum of 25 days prior to transfusion.[12,13] Therefore, small numbers of bacteria introduced at the time of collection have an opportunity to multiply over time.

Table 40-3. Proposed Methods to Additionally
Decrease the Risk of Bacterial
Contamination

More donor history questions

Reduction of red blood cell storage interval

Antibiotic additives to blood bag

Bacteriologic screening:
     Gram's stain—false-negatives and false-positives
     Culture all or selected (older) units—false-negatives
          and false-positives, risk of introducing bacteria dur-
          ing sampling
     Radiometric technique
     Detect microbial CO_2 production
     RNA probes

Leukoreduction of unit

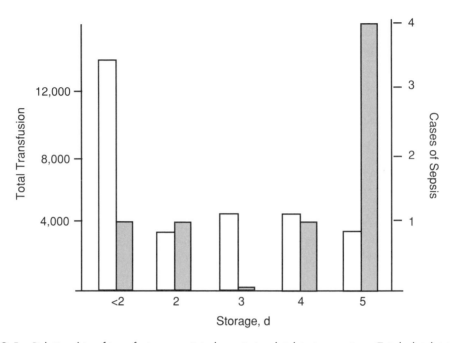

Figure 40-1. Relationship of transfusion-associated sepsis to platelet storage time. Total platelet transfusions are shown in open bars in left-hand scale. Numbers of cases of transfusion-associated sepsis are shown in cross-hatched bars in right-hand scale. (From Morrow et al.,[80] with permission.)

In vitro studies suggest a basis for these in vivo observations, in that RBC units deliberately inoculated with gram-negative organisms showed significant growth and endotoxin production only after a 2- to 3-week lag.[14–16] Due to these findings, it has been suggested by the Centers for Disease Control and Prevention (CDC) that RBC storage be reduced to a maximum of 25 days or that older RBC units be screened for endotoxin and/or the presence of bacteria.[12] However, this would not eliminate all cases of *Y. enterocolitica* sepsis, as some have occurred within 3 weeks of storage. This measure would also severely hamper transfusion services and would likely decrease an already limited blood supply. An alternate strategy, introducing antibacterial additives to RBC and platelet units would reduce the risk of sepsis,[17,18] but would also introduce problems such as allergic and toxic reactions to the transfused antibiotics.

Screening units for either bacteria or endotoxin would be ideal, as only hazardous units would be destroyed. Unfortunately, a method such as Gram staining a sample from each unit is generally unsuit-

able since a false-negative result can occur owing to low numbers of organisms and a false-positive result can occur when debris is interpreted as bacteria. Nevertheless, one study found Gram staining to be effective in identifying contaminated platelets that had been stored for 4 and 5 days.[19] Culturing units is also problematic, owing to the lengthy incubation time, false-negative results when bacteria fail to grow, and false-positive results due to contaminated samples. Current research is directed toward identifying techniques that are highly sensitive, rapid, and noninvasive; however, no such current methodology has been validated. Techniques under evaluation include the use of rapid automated blood culturing systems and the use of a chemiluminescence-linked recombinant RNA gene probe system.[20,21]

Leukoreduction of cellular blood components prior to storage appears to offer promise in reducing the risks of bacterial contamination. In experiments with in vitro inoculation of units with *Y. enterocolitica*, leukoreduction by filtration decreased or eliminated bacterial growth.[15,22,23] Filtration was performed soon after collection and prior to storage. Leukocyte phagocytosis of small numbers of bacteria may occur if these WBCs are allowed to remain in the unit for a few hours after collection.[22] The risk of contamination may then be reduced by filtering out those possibly bacteria-laden phagocytes. It is not yet known whether these in vitro bacterial inoculation experiments accurately simulate donor bacteremia. Leukoreduction by filtration is expensive and bacterial contamination is rare; it is not known whether this would be a cost-effective approach to preventing transfusion-associated (TA) sepsis.

Whereas it is rare, bacterial contamination of blood and blood components remains a life-threatening event. Sepsis due to *Y. enterocolitica*–contaminated RBCs is an infrequent but widely recognized threat; to better understand this phenomenon, both fatal and nonfatal cases should be reported to the CDC, through state health departments.[12]

PARASITIC INFECTIONS

Syphilis

Syphilis is caused by the coiled anaerobic microorganism *Treponema palladium*. TA syphilis is a very rare occurrence, in part due to the relative fragility of the spirochete; it does not survive prolonged storage in refrigerated temperatures. A review of the literature by De Schryver[24] showed that viable organisms do not persist beyond 48 to 72 hours under usual RBC storage conditions, although heavy inoculations of treponemes can survive up to 120 hours in refrigerated storage. Owing to the rarity of TA syphilis, the need to continue using a serologic test for syphilis for all donors has been questioned.

Proponents for abandoning the serologic test for syphilis (Table 40-4) argue that mandatory testing was established at a time when the risk of TA syphilis was significant owing to the high prevalence of syphilis in the general population, the use of paid blood donors, and the frequent use of blood that was transfused fresh or after limited storage. There is now a volunteer blood donor system, the incidence and prevalence of syphilis markedly dropped with the advent of penicillin, and current anticoagulants allow for prolonged RBC storage. The risk of TA

Table 40-4. Serologic Testing for Syphilis in Blood Donors

Reasons to discontinue testing:
    Organism nonviable in refrigerator
    Transfusion-associated syphilis rare
    False-negative test result can occur
    Biologic false-positive test result can occur
    Recipients often on spirochetocidal antibiotics

Reasons to continue testing:
    Incidence of syphilis rising recently
    Surrogate test for human immunodeficiency virus and hepatitis
    Increasing use of fresh blood and platelets
    Low cost of test
    Identification of undiagnosed cases/contacts

syphilis probably dropped further still with screening measures for hepatitis and human immunodeficiency virus (HIV)-infected donors. An infectious unit may pose little risk today, as many transfused patients are also receiving spirocheticidal antibiotics. While in recent years there has been increasing use of components, such as platelets and fresh blood, which could transmit viable treponemes from an infectious donor, there has not been a parallel increase in reported TA syphilis.

The serologic screening tests for syphilis are problematic. Infectious donors with early primary and even tertiary syphilis may be seronegative (false-negative). Biologic false-positives, using nonspecific screening tests such as Venereal Disease Research Laboratory (VDRL) or rapid plasma reagin (RPR), are common and can occur in donors after recent viral or bacterial infections, immunizations, and in those with autoimmune diseases. Most confirmed seropositive donors have already undergone treatment for syphilis; finding undiagnosed syphilis is rare. Only seven donors with active syphilis were identified over a 10-year period at a major blood center in London.[25] More recently, automated direct treponemal antibody tests have been introduced in many centers. These newer tests detect a significant number of donors whose syphilis occurred in the remote past and has been adequately treated.[26]

Those that argue that testing for syphilis should continue cite the rising incidence of the disease as one motivator. An epidemic of syphilis developed in the late 1980s; in 1990, the number of reported cases of primary and secondary syphilis was the highest since 1948.[27] It has been argued that serologic screening for syphilis also serves as a surrogate test for HIV-infected donors. Donors with a history of syphilis or gonorrhea in the last 12 months are now deferred, per an FDA recommendation,[28] in an effort to exclude persons at increased risk of HIV infection by heterosexual transmission. Syphilis is more likely to be transmitted in fresh blood and platelets, components that are being transfused with greater frequency. Screening tests for syphilis are relatively inexpensive (10 cents per test for the VDRL screening test in 1982)[24] and have recently been automated, using equipment that performs other necessary blood donor screening tests. Last, testing for syphilis benefits the community as a whole by identifying undiagnosed infectious individuals and, through the local health department, their sexual contacts. Syphilis is readily treated with penicillin; undiagnosed cases may be infectious for long intervals and these persons may suffer significant morbidity.

In the current transfusion safety climate, there does not appear to be any likelihood that the FDA will alter its long-standing requirement to perform syphilis testing of all donated units.

TA syphilis, though rare, can still occur today when an asymptomatic infectious donor is nonreactive on serologic testing and fresh blood or platelets are transfused. The disease has been reported to have an incubation of 1 to 4 months; secondary syphilis develops, but may be atypical if the patient is receiving antibiotics.[29] While syphilis should pose only a minor threat since it is readily cured with penicillin, transfusion-associated syphilis is so rare that few might consider the diagnosis in a transfusion recipient with the fever and rash associated with secondary syphilis.

Malaria

Malaria is a rare TA disease in the United States; an average of 3 cases were reported annually from 1972 to 1988, a rate of 0.25 cases per million blood units collected.[30] Numbers of post-transfusion malaria cases may increase, though, as malaria eradication programs in endemic areas have not been successful and as travel to and immigration from endemic areas continues.

The four malaria species that infect humans, *Plasmodium falciparum*, *P. malariae*, *P. ovale*, and *P. vivax*, can all be transfusion-transmitted. It is the asexual forms of this intraerythrocytic parasite that are responsible for post-transfusion disease. All RBC-containing components can transmit the organism; whole blood, RBCs, platelets,[31] leukocytes,[32] and fresh plasma[33] have been implicated as sources of infection. Malaria parasites can easily survive refrigerated storage for several days.

Diagnosis and treatment of TA malaria can be problematic. Physicians in nonendemic countries may not recognize the early manifestations and post-transfusion cases may appear atypical. Fever may not be present or may lack the characteristic periodicity. Malaria can be a life-threatening disease, particularly in asplenic and other immunosuppressed patients.[34] Increasing numbers of drug-resistant cases may complicate the management of infected patients.

Preventing infectious units from entering the blood supply is crucial. Two preventative methods predominate—oral donor questioning and/or serologic testing. In the United States, oral questioning of donors is used; from 1974 to 1994, the American Association of Blood Banks (AABB) Standards[35] required deferral of visitors to endemic areas for 6 months after their return, provided they had been asymptomatic. For visitors who had taken antimalarial chemoprophylaxis, residents of endemic areas, and those with a history of malaria, the deferral interval was 3 years after arrival in a nonendemic area or after cessation of symptoms. These standards apply only to donors of components containing intact RBCs. The 3-year interval was used since *Plasmodia* organisms, with the exception of *P. malariae*, will have died off in that period of time. *P. malariae* can survive for decades within a human host.

These malaria deferral criteria were established in an effort to balance the post-transfusion risk, though small, of malaria with the need for blood donors. Some have proposed liberalizing existing regulations to make more units available for transfusion with a minimal increase in the risk of post-transfusion malaria.[30] Others, in an effort to attain a "zero-risk" blood supply, have proposed deferring all potential donors with a history of malaria[36] or identifying a donor's country of birth as means of finding those at greater risk of transmitting disease.

Recently, donor deferral criteria for malaria have been changed in the United States.[37,38] The FDA and AABB have both indicated that visitors to endemic areas be deferred for 1 year. There is no longer a requirement to defer such donors for differing length of times based on whether they have taken malaria chemoprophylaxis. The new criteria maintain the 3-year deferral for residents or immigrants from an endemic area who arrive in the United States. The new criteria indicate that prospective donors who have had malaria should be deferred for 3 years after becoming asymptomatic.

In the United States, many donors implicated in post-transfusion malaria cases should have been eliminated by current screening measures.[30] A quality donor interview is imperative for malaria prevention. Having maps and lists of countries with endemic areas is important in helping donors recognize endemic foci.

In many European countries, potentially infectious donors are identified via oral questioning and then serologically tested. Antimalarial antibodies can be identified prior to or concurrent with parasitemia.[39] Indirect immunofluorescence with *P. falciparum* antigen is the most common serologic method employed.[39] Although this method optimally detects *P. falciparum* antibodies, some cross-reactivity with antibodies directed against the other species occurs. Detection of *P. falciparum* infected donors is critical owing to the high morbidity associated with this species. Serologic testing is also problematic in that it is costly and laborious to perform.

Reports of serologic screening in Europe have shown that approximately 5 percent of donors are tested and more than 70 percent of those tested are seronegative.[40] Oral questioning alone, therefore, may eliminate considerable numbers of potentially healthy donors. In Los Angeles in the late 1980s, 0.75 percent of donors were deferred because of potential malaria risk.[41] If this figure applies nationwide, and if each donor only donated 1 unit, with 14,229,000 units collected in 1989 in the United States,[42] a minimum of 107,000 units were lost due to malaria deferrals. Serologic testing would almost

certainly show that a highly significant percentage of these units were free of malaria risk.

Eliminating infectious donors in endemic countries is difficult. Direct microscopic examination of blood smears has been tried, but is of little value, since most infectious donors have levels of parasitemia too low to be detected in this fashion. Serologic screening is not practical because of large numbers of seropositive donors. Medicating potential donors or recipients at the time of transfusion can also be done.[43] Testing for malarial antigen may prove to be the best approach. In India, detection of *P. falciparum* antigen using a monoclonal antibody has been beneficial in identifying infectious individuals, who are subsequently treated.[44]

Chagas Disease

Chagas disease or American trypanosomiasis is caused by the parasite *Trypanosoma cruzi* and is usually transmitted by the bite of an infected triatomine insect (reduviid bug). Parasitized blood-sucking insects come in contact with humans in the rural areas of South and Central America. The second most common means of transmission of *T. cruzi* is by blood transfusion. The implicated donor is asymptomatic, yet has chronic, low-grade parasitemia. Chagas disease is a major TA disease in endemic countries, as migration from rural to urban areas brings infected populations and the lure of paid blood donations attracts poor, infected people to blood collection facilities.

TA Chagas disease is threatening North America owing to continuing immigration from endemic areas. It has been estimated that there are 16 to 18 million infected people worldwide,[45] with approximately 100,000 of them now in the United States.[46] Three cases of TA Chagas disease in North America have been recognized,[46] and it is speculated that many more may have occurred. These 3 patients were immunosuppressed and presented with acute Chagas disease. Many acute infections may remain subclinical or are not accurately diagnosed by physicians in nonendemic countries.

Components that have transmitted the parasite include RBCs, platelets, WBCs, fresh frozen plasma, and cryoprecipitate.[45] Using older generations of antibody screening tests, data indicate that approximately 15 to 50 percent of recipients of seropositive units may become infected.[45]

Acute disease manifestations usually present in 20 to 40 days. Fever, lymphadenopathy, and hepato-splenomegaly can occur and typically resolve without treatment. Diagnosis can be made with direct visualization of the parasites on peripheral smear; the yield can be increased by examining the buffy coat. Without trypanocidal therapy, infection is thought to remain throughout life.

Chronically infected individuals are generally asymptomatic and are the source of TA disease. Clinical manifestations, cardiomyopathy and/or gastrointestinal disease, may develop in some chronically infected individuals, years after the initial infection. Cardiac arrhythmias may cause sudden death. Dilation of the esophagus (megaesophagus) and colon (megacolon) is debilitating and life-threatening. Diagnosis is made based on clinical findings and presence of antitrypanosomal antibodies.

In endemic countries, prevention of transmission involves serologic testing of donors and destruction of seropositive units. In areas where seropositivity rates are very high, parasites are inactivated with trypanocidal chemicals. The dye crystal violet is nontoxic and trypanocidal, but causes transient bluish discoloration of recipients' skin.

In nonendemic countries, some institutions have made efforts to identify infected individuals by oral questioning. Prospective donors who have the appropriate risk factors may be deferred and offered serologic testing for *T. cruzi* antibodies.[47] Such questioning is not required by the AABB Standards; however, any donor with a history of Chagas disease must be permanently deferred from blood donation.[38] Serologic tests have moderately high sensitivity but low specificity, and in nonendemic areas a greater number of false-positives can occur.

Babesiosis

Babesiosis, formerly known as piroplasmosis, is a rare, malaria-like illness caused by a protozoan parasite that also invades erythrocytes. The parasite responsible for human disease in the United States is *Babesia microti*.[48] Humans are an accidental host when they are bitten by an infected vector, which is the deer tick, *Ixodes dammini*. The usual hosts for the vector are the white-footed mouse and the white-

tailed deer. Cases of babesiosis in the United States have occurred primarily in the Northeast, where the vector and hosts flourish. Endemic foci of the organism exist in Massachusetts and New York, especially on offshore islands. There is a seasonal predilection for the infection, with most cases occurring during summer months,[48] when humans are more likely to receive tick bites.

Whereas the tick is the usual carrier, asymptomatic infected individuals can also serve as vectors when they donate blood, resulting in TA babesiosis. Absence of symptoms is not uncommon; one study[49] found 68 percent of seropositive persons were asymptomatic. As babesiosis is an uncommon infection, transmission by blood transfusion has been quite limited. Fewer than 10 cases have been reported in the English literature.[50–57] Transmission has occurred in units stored as long as 35 days.[54] RBC-containing components are responsible for transmitting the organism; liquid RBCs,[54,57] frozen deglycerolized RBCs,[50] and platelets[52] have been linked with transmission. As most infections with *B. microti* are mild,[56] many more TA cases may not have been recognized.

Whereas there have been few reported cases of babesiosis transmitted by transfusion, the numbers can be expected to increase. The tick vector has been identified outside of endemic areas owing to the expanding range of the deer population.[58,59] Babesiosis is a disease well known to veterinary medicine specialists, as it is life-threatening in cattle. The first published case of babesiosis in man occurred in 1956,[60] with the first U.S. case reported in 1968.[61] Most of the transfusion-transmitted disease cases were reported in the 1980s. More cases will be identified as clinicians consider babesiosis in the differential diagnosis of febrile hemolytic anemia.[48] Cases of TA disease have already been identified in areas not previously considered endemic.[54,55]

The clinical manifestations of symptomatic babesiosis can include fever (spiking or persistent), headaches, shaking chills, thrombocytopenia, and hemolytic anemia that ranges from mild to severe. Unlike other tick-borne illnesses, there are no characteristic skin lesions.[48] Diagnosis can be delayed when the findings are misdiagnosed as malaria, owing to the similarity in symptomatology and similar appearance of intraerythrocytic parasites (Fig. 40-2). The

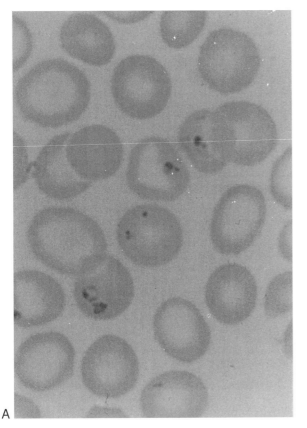

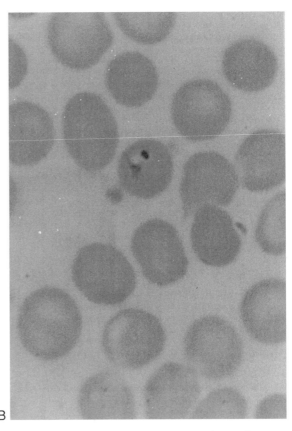

A   B

Figure 40-2. *(A) Babesia microti:* one intact ring form present within red blood cell; other nonintact forms also present. (Giemsa stain, oil immersion.) *(B) Plasmodium malariae:* intraerythrocytic ring form. (Giemsa stain, oil immersion). Note the similarities between ring forms of *B. microti* and *P. malariae.*

two can be distinguished by the lack of gametocytes and absence of intracellular pigment in babesia infections on peripheral smears. Serologic testing can confirm the diagnosis, by detecting raised titers of IgG antibody to *B. microti.*[59] Hamster inoculation with patient blood can also be helpful in proving the diagnosis. Failure to diagnose the disease and treat promptly can result in renal failure, disseminated intravascular coagulation, shock, and death.[62] The greatest morbidity occurs in immunocompromised, asplenic, and elderly individuals.[63] If treatment is required, exchange transfusion and/or antibiotic therapy (clindamycin and oral quinine) may prove beneficial.[52,57,63] Pentamidine has been shown to decrease the parasitemia, but not to eliminate the organism.[64]

Methods recommended to curtail TA disease were issued in a 1989 AABB bulletin[65] and include the deferral of all donors with a history of babesiosis (though plasma should not pose a risk). Patients with babesiosis need to be questioned about having served as blood donors and a "lookback" should be performed when previous donation has occurred. Any units available in inventory need to be identified and destroyed. It was recommended that additional questions or serologic testing not be added to the current donation procedure. Current donor screening will eliminate those carriers that are febrile or anemic. Eliminating blood collections from endemic areas during summer months has not been shown to be effective.[66]

Lyme Disease

Borrelia burgdorferi, the spirochetal bacterium responsible for causing Lyme disease, has received much media attention, due to the difficulty in diagnosing this chronic debilitating disease. Its rising incidence has made it the most common tick-borne infection in the United States.[67] *B. burgdorferi* is transmitted by the same tick vector that causes babesiosis, *I. dammini*. With the spread of the tick's animal hosts, Lyme disease is being diagnosed in areas far outside the Connecticut town it was originally recognized in.

Lyme disease has not been reported to be transmitted by blood transfusion, but it is suspected that blood-borne spread can occur. During the early infection, *Borrelia* organisms can sometimes be isolated from the blood by using specialized media.[68] The organisms have also been shown to survive up to 6 weeks in RBCs,[69] 6 days in platelets, and 45 days in fresh frozen plasma[70] in inoculated specimens.

Perhaps TA Lyme disease will never occur, since patients with spirochetemia have been symptomatic and would be deferred from blood donation due to the associated fever, skin lesions, and other clinical manifestations. At least two blood donors, diagnosed with Lyme disease soon after donation, failed to transmit the infection to the recipients available for testing.[67,71]

In 1989, the AABB recommended[72] that no additional questions or testing be performed for Lyme disease and that a history of a tick bite was not a cause for deferral. Asymptomatic donors with a history of Lyme disease may donate after completing a course of antibiotics. Medical staff should continue to search for possible TA Lyme disease by questioning infected patients about having been a blood donor or transfusion recipient. Identifying TA cases may prove difficult, since the tick bite and characteristic rash would be absent.[67]

OTHER BACTERIAL AND PARASITIC INFECTIONS

Whereas there are a multitude of other real and potential bacterial and parasitic infections that can or could be transmitted by transfusion, these other infectious agents present a low risk in the United States and in other developed countries.

The potential transmission of *Leishmania tropica* was an issue that received much attention after the U.S. involvement in the Desert Storm conflict in Kuwait. This protozoal parasite was found to be responsible for visceral leishmaniasis in seven members of the military who had served in the Persian Gulf.[73] Visceral leishmaniasis has been transmitted by transfusion and *L. tropica* has been shown to survive in refrigerated components and retain its infectivity.[74] In November 1991, the U.S. Department of Defense recommended that all individuals who had traveled to the Persian Gulf after August 1, 1990, be deferred as blood donors. The ban was lifted in December 1993, as none of the donors identified with potential risk of infection were subsequently diagnosed with infection.[75] Transmission of leishmanial organisms continues to be a real, though very rare, risk of blood transfusion in the countries where it is endemic.

Transmission of *Toxoplasma gondii*, the etiologic agent of toxoplasmosis, has occurred in immunocompromised recipients of leukocyte transfusions.[76] This protozoal organism has worldwide endemicity; up to half of American adults have been found to be potentially capable of transmitting this parasite.[77] The trophozoite may circulate in infected individuals and can survive in refrigerated blood.[78] Owing to the high seroprevalence, there are probably many infectious donors and, yet, there has been only very rare clinically evident TA disease. Therefore, there is probably little need for donor screening measures at the current time. Most clinically significant toxoplasmosis is believed to be due to reactivation of a patient's latent infection.[77]

Microfilarial infections generally do not occur in developed countries. Current donor questions regarding travel and potential malaria exposure are probably sufficient to prevent TA infection in the United States.[79]

Rickettsia are intracellular parasites that resemble bacteria. Although TA rickettsial disease can occur, the risk is extremely remote, as it is an uncommon infection and there is only a brief asymptomatic period, prior to the onset of manifestations that would defer an individual from donating. There is no evidence that screening donors for rickettsial infections is indicated at the current time.

African trypanosomiasis, also known as sleeping sickness, can be transmitted by transfusion. Immigrants from and travelers to endemic areas should be screened out by donor questions currently used to decrease the risk of malaria transmission.

Whereas TA bacterial and parasitic infections are rare events, we must remain vigilant to recognize any change in the current rates of infection and take additional measures to protect the blood supply when necessary.

REFERENCES

1. Wallis CH: Transfusion of blood components contaminated with bacteria. p. 195. In Smith DM, Dodd RY (eds): Transfusion Transmitted Infections. American Society of Clinical Pathologists Press, Chicago, 1991
2. Goldman M, Blajchman MA: Blood product-associated bacterial sepsis. Transfus Med Reviews 5:73, 1991
3. Rawal BD, Vyas GN: Complement-mediated bactericidal action and the removal of Yersinia enterocolitica by white cell filters (letter). Transfusion 33:536, 1993
4. Wagner SJ, Friedman LI, Dodd RY: Transfusion-associated bacterial sepsis. Clin Microbiol Rev 7:290, 1994
5. Hamill TR: The 30-minute rule for reissuing blood: are we needlessly discarding units? Transfusion 30:58, 1990
6. Morrow JF, Braine HG, Kickler TS et al: Septic reactions to platelet transfusions. JAMA 266:555, 1991
7. Aber RC: Transfusion-associated Yersinia enterocolitica. Transfusion 30:193, 1990
8. Heal JM, Jones ME, Forey J et al: Fatal Salmonella septicemia after platelet transfusion. Transfusion 27:2, 1987
9. Richards C, Kolins J, Trindade CD: Autologous transfusion-transmitted Yersinia enterocolitica. JAMA 268:1541, 1992
10. Ness PM, Perkins HA: Transient bacteremia after dental procedures and other minor manipulations. Transfusion 20:82, 1980
11. Grossman BJ, Kollins P, Lau PM et al: Screening blood donors for gastrointestinal illness: a strategy to eliminate carriers of Yersinia enterocolitica. Transfusion 31:500, 1991
12. MMWR: Yersinia enterocolitica bacteremia and endotoxin shock associated with red blood cell transfusion—United States, 1991. MMWR 40:176, 1991
13. Tipple MA, Bland LA, Murphy JJ et al: Sepsis associated with transfusion of red cells contaminated with Yersinia enterocolitica. Transfusion 30:207, 1990
14. Arduino MJ, Bland LA, Tipple MA et al: Growth and endotoxin production of Yersinia enterocolitica and Enterobacter agglomerans in packed erythrocytes. J Clin Microbiol 27:1483, 1989
15. Hogman CF, Gong J, Hambraeus A et al: The role of white cells in the transmission of Yersinia enterocolitica in blood components. Transfusion 32:654, 1992
16. Peitersz RNI, Reesink HW, Pauw W et al: Prevention of Yersinia enterocolitica growth in red-blood-cell concentrates. Lancet 340:755, 1992
17. Novak M: Preservation of stored blood with sulfanilamide. JAMA 113:2227, 1939
18. Sloand E, Pierce P, Tuerner J, Klein HG: Vancomycin inhibits bacterial growth in platelet concentrate (PC's) while maintaining platelet integrity and function (abstracted). Blood 1(suppl.):1587, 1993
19. Yomtovian R, Lazarus HM, Goodnough LT et al: A prospective microbiologic surveillance program to detect and prevent the transfusion of bacterially contaminated platelets. Transfusion 33:902, 1993
20. Nolte FS, Williams RC, Jerris JA et al: Multicenter clinical evaluation of a continuous monitoring blood culture system using fluorescent-sensor technology (BACTEC 9240). J Clin Microbiol 31:552, 1993
21. Hogan J, Curry B, Brecher M et al: Detection of bacterially contaminated platelet units with an all-bacterial DNA probe test (abstract S152). Transfusion 33S:40S, 1993
22. Buchholz DH, AuBuchon JP, Snyder EL et al: Removal of Yersinia enterocolitica from AS-1 red cells. Transfusion 32:667, 1992
23. Kim DM, Brecher ME, Bland LA et al: Prestorage removal of Yersinia enterocolitica from red cells with white cell-reduction filters. Transfusion 32:658, 1992
24. De Schryver A, Meheus A: Syphilis and blood transfusion: a global perspective. Transfusion 30:844, 1990
25. Barbara JAJ, Hewitt P, Enright S: Routine blood donor screening for syphilis can reveal recent infection. Vox Sang 65:243, 1993
26. Strauss D, Del Valle C, Valinsky JE et al: Donor screening for syphilis using the Olympus PK-TP assay-implications for donor notification and reentry. Transfusion 33(suppl.):42S, 1993
27. CDC: Surveillance for primary and secondary syphilis—United States, 1991. MMWR 42:13, 1993
28. Food and Drug Administration: Clarification of FDA recommendation for donor deferral and product distribution based on the results of syphilis testing. Bethesda, MD, Dec. 12, 1991
29. Chambers RW, Foley HT, Schmidt PJ: Transmission of syphilis by fresh blood components. Transfusion 9:32, 1969
30. Nahlen BL, Lobel HO, Cannon SE, Campbell CC: Reassessment of blood donor selection criteria for

United States travelers to malarious areas. Transfusion 31:798, 1991

31. Garfield MD, Ershler WB, Maki DG: Malaria transmission by platelet concentrate transfusion. JAMA 240: 2285, 1978

32. Dover AS, Guinee VF: Malaria transmission by leukocyte component therapy. JAMA 217:1701, 1971

33. Dike AE: Two cases of transfusion malaria. Lancet 1: 72, 1970

34. Walzer PD, Gibson JJ, Schultz MG: Malaria fatalities in the United States. Am J Trop Med Hyg 23:328, 1974

35. Widmann FK: Standards for Blood Banks and Transfusion Services. 15th Ed. American Association of Blood Banks, Bethesda, MD, 1993

36. BPAC considers malaria deferral, ICL study, source plasma. Blood Bank Week 10:1, 1993

37. FDA memorandum dated July 26, 1994: "Recommendations for deferral of donors for malaria risk"

38. Klein HG: Standards for Blood Banks and Transfusion Services. 16th Ed. American Association of Blood Banks, Bethesda, MD, 1994

39. Ambroise-Thomas P: International forum: which are the appropriate modifications of existing regulations designed to prevent transmission of malaria by blood transfusion, in view of the increasing frequency of travel to endemic areas? Vox Sang 52:138, 1987

40. Masure R: International forum: which are the appropriate modifications of existing regulations designed to prevent transmission of malaria by blood transfusion, in view of the increasing frequency of travel to endemic areas? Vox Sang 52:138, 1987

41. Kleinman S: Donor screening procedures and their role in enhancing transfusion safety. p. 207. In Smith DM, Dodd RY (eds): Transfusion-Transmitted Infections. American Society of Clinical Pathologists Press, Chicago, 1991

42. Wallace EL, Surgenor DM, Hao HS et al: Collection and transfusion of blood and blood components in the United States, 1989. Transfusion 33:139, 1993

43. Turc JM: Malaria and blood transfusion. p. 31. In Westphal RG, Carlson KB, Turc JM (eds): Emerging Global Patterns in Transfusion Transmitted Infections. American Association of Blood Banks, Arlington, VA, 1990

44. Choudhury N, Jolly JG, Mahajan RC et al: Selection of blood donors in malaria-endemic countries. Lancet ii:972, 1988

45. Schmunis GA: Trypanosoma cruzi, the etiologic agent of Chagas' disease: status in the blood supply in endemic and nonendemic countries. Transfusion 31: 547, 1991

46. Kirchhoff LV: American trypanosomiasis (Chagas' disease)—a tropical disease now in the United States. N Engl J Med 329:639, 1993

47. Appleman MD, Shulman IA, Saxena S, Kirchhoff LV: Use of a questionnaire to identify potential blood donors at risk for infection with Trypanosoma cruzi. Transfusion 33:61, 1993

48. Dammin GJ, Spielman A, Benach JL, Piesman J: The rising incidence of clinical Babesia microti infection. Hum Pathol 12:398, 1981

49. Ruebush TK, Juranek DD, Chisholm ES et al: Human babesiosis on Nantucket Island. Evidence for self-limited and subclinical infections. N Engl J Med 297:825, 1977

50. Grabowski EF, Giardina PJV, Goldberg D et al: Babesiosis transmitted by a transfusion of frozen-thawed blood. Ann Intern Med 96:466, 1982

51. Healy GR, Walzer PD, Sulzer AJ: A case of asymptomatic babesiosis in Georgia. Am J Trop Med Hyg 25: 376, 1976

52. Jacoby GA, Hunt JV, Kosinski KS et al: Treatment of transfusion-transmitted babesiosis by exchange transfusion. N Engl J Med 303:1098, 1980

53. Marcus LC, Valigorsky JM, Fanning WL et al: A case report of transfusion-induced babesiosis. JAMA 248: 465, 1982

54. Mintz ED, Anderson JF, Cable RG, Hadler JL: Transfusion-transmitted babesiosis: a case report from a new endemic area. Transfusion 31:365, 1991

55. Reddy RL, Dalmasso AP: Transfusion acquired babesiosis in Minnesota (abstracted). p. 112. In: ISBT and AABB 1990 Joint Congress Abstract Book. American Association of Blood Banks, Arlington, VA, 1990

56. Smith RP, Evans AT, Popovsky M et al: Transfusion-acquired babesiosis and failure of antibiotic treatment. JAMA 256:2726, 1986

57. Wittner M, Rowin KS, Tanowitz HB et al: Successful chemotherapy of transfusion babesiosis. Ann Intern Med 96:601, 1982

58. Spielman A, Wilson ML, Levine JF, Piesman J: Ecology of Ixodes dammini-borne human babesiosis and Lyme disease. Annu Rev Entomol 30:439, 1985

59. Gadbaw JJ, Anderson JF, Cartter ML, Hadler JL: Babesiosis—Connecticut. MMWR 38:649, 1989

60. Skrabalo Z, Deanovic Z: Piroplasmosis in man: report on a case. Doc Med Geogr Trop 9:11, 1957

61. Scholtens RG, Braff EH, Healy GR, Gleason N: A case of babesiosis in man in the United States. Am J Trop Med Hyg 17:810, 1968

62. Gombert ME, Goldstein EJC, Benach JL et al: Human babesiosis: clinical and therapeutic considerations. JAMA 248:3005, 1982

63. Rosner F, Zarrabi MH, Benach JL, Habicht GS: Babesiosis in splenectomized adults. Review of 22 reported cases. Am J Med 76:696, 1984

64. Francioli PB, Keithly JS, Jones TC et al: Response of babesiosis to pentamidine therapy. Ann Intern Med 94:326, 1981

65. American Association of Blood Banks bulletin: Recommendations regarding babesiosis and potential transmission by blood transfusion. American Association of Blood Banks, Arlington, VA, July 29, 1989

66. Popovsky MA, Lindberg LE, Syrek AL, Page PL: Prevalence of Babesia antibody in a selected blood donor population. Transfusion 28:59, 1988

67. Aoki SK, Holland PV: Lyme disease—another transfusion risk? Transfusion 29:646, 1989

68. Benach JL, Bosler EM, Hanrahan JP et al: Spirochetes isolated from the blood of two patients with Lyme disease. N Engl J Med 308:740, 1983

69. Nadelman RB, Sherer C, Mack L et al: Survival of Borrelia burgdorferi in human blood stored under blood banking conditions. Transfusion 30:298, 1990

70. Badon SJ, Fister RD, Cable RG: Survival of Borrelia burgdorferi in blood products. Transfusion 29:581, 1989

71. Halkier-Sorensen LH, Kragballe K, Nedergaard ST, Hansen K: Lack of transmission of Borrelia burgdorferi by blood transfusion. Lancet 1:550, 1990

72. American Association of Blood Banks bulletin: Recommendations regarding Lyme disease and potential transmission by blood transfusion. American Association of Blood Banks, Arlington, VA, July 29, 1989

73. Magill AJ, Grogl M, Gasser RA et al: Viscerotropic leishmaniasis caused by Leishmania tropica in soldiers returning from Operation Desert Storm. N Engl J Med 328:1383, 1993

74. Grogl M, Daugirda JL, Hoover DL et al: Survivability and infectivity of viscerotropic Leishmania tropica from Operation Desert Storm participants in human blood products maintained under blood bank conditions. Am J Trop Med Hyg 49:308, 1993

75. American Association of blood Banks: Defense department drops question on Leishmania for blood donors. Blood Bank Week, Dec. 17, 1993

76. Siegel SE, Lunde MN, Gelderman AH et al: Transmission of toxoplasmosis by leukocyte transfusion. Blood 37:388, 1971

77. McCabe JR, Remington JS: Toxoplasmosis: the time has come. N Engl J Med 318:313, 1988

78. Miller MJ, Aronson WJ, Remington JS: Late parasitemia in asymptomatic acquired toxoplasmosis. Ann Intern Med 71:139, 1969

79. Westphal RG: Parasitic disease and blood transfusion. p. 97. In Nance SJ (ed): Blood Safety: Current Challenges. American Association of Blood Banks, Bethesda, MD, 1992

80. Morrow JF, Braine HG, Kickler TS et al: Septic reactions to platelet transfusions. JAMA 266:555, 1991

Chapter 41

Diagnosis and Management of Transfusion Reactions

Paul W. Jenner and Paul V. Holland

Although transfusion of blood and its components is usually a safe and effective form of therapy, there are risks of adverse effects. These adverse effects are often called *transfusion reactions,* but this term does not cover all potentially deleterious consequences that may accompany the administration of blood or blood components. Some of the adverse effects are preventable, but some cannot be completely avoided. Thus, every physician should be aware of the risks of blood transfusions and weigh these against the potential therapeutic benefits.

This chapter deals with transfusion reactions and adverse effects of transfusion. Infectious disease transmission, graft-versus-host disease (GVHD), and immunomodulation are covered in more detail in other chapters. The types of adverse reactions are subdivided here according to whether they are immediate or delayed and whether they are immunologically mediated. Each potential ill effect is discussed in terms of etiologic factors, diagnosis, treatment, and possible preventive measures. In addition, this chapter attempts to answer such questions as the following: what clinical findings merit a detailed workup? When should the blood transfusion be stopped, and can it be restarted? What are the relative merits of different modes of treatment for certain types of reactions?

When any unexpected or untoward sign or symptom occurs during or shortly after the transfusion of

blood or one of its components, consider that it might have been caused by the blood component until proven otherwise. Only a high index of suspicion allows transfusion reactions to be diagnosed.

DIFFERENTIAL DIAGNOSIS OF ACUTE (IMMEDIATE) TRANSFUSION REACTIONS

Transfusion reactions to blood or its components that occur during the infusion, or within 1 to 2 hours of its completion, are termed acute or immediate. When a patient experiences an acute transfusion reaction, the physician must first consider the differential diagnosis of possible causes. Once a diagnosis is made, appropriate treatment may be started to minimize the morbidity of the reaction, and steps may be taken to minimize the risk of subsequent, similar reactions. Table 41-1 lists some potential acute adverse reactions to transfusions. The reactions are categorized as immunologically or nonimmunologically mediated, and next to each is listed the most common causes. Figure 41-1 is a sample transfusion reaction form that lists the most common signs and symptoms of acute transfusion reactions.

A review of 256 transfusion-related deaths (excluding hepatitis and human immunodeficiency virus [HIV]-related deaths) reported to the United States Food and Drug Administration (FDA) from 1976 through 1985 showed that 61 percent resulted

REPORT OF A SUSPECTED TRANSFUSION REACTION

DATE & TIME STARTED   TIME OF REACTION   DIAGNOSIS   PHYSICIAN

BLOOD TYPE UNIT NUMBER   COMPONENT   VOLUME TRANSFUSED   NUMBER IN SERIES

PRE-TRANSFUSION   POST-TRANSFUSION

Temp____ BP____ Pulse ____   Temp____ BP____ Pulse____

CLINICAL SIGNS & SYMPTOMS

Check those which apply
- Hives (urticaria)
- Itching
- Increased pulse
- Chills
- Elevated temp. > 1°C
- Flushing
- Muscle aching
- Dark or red urine
- Decreased urine output
- Petechiae
- Failure to clot
- Jaundice
- Hypotension
- Anaphylaxis
- Dyspnea

SUGGESTED NURSING ACTION

PERFORM CLERICAL CHECK ON BLOOD BAG LABEL, PATIENT ARM BAND, AND PAPERWORK   ACCURATE____ INACCURATE____
PERFORMED BY ____

Allergic Reactions
1) Slow transfusion
2) Take vital signs q 30 min x 4
3) Notify physician

Acute Reactions Other than Allergic
1) Stop transfusion immediately, but keep IV open with saline drip using new saline and IV set
2) Send blood bag, saline, and set *intact* to lab
3) Take vital signs q 30 min x 4
4) Notify physician
5) Send first voided urine specimen to lab

LABORATORY INVESTIGATION

PERFORM LABORATORY CLERICAL CHECK ON ALL LABELS, TUBES, AND PAPERWORK   ACCURATE____ INACCURATE____
PERFORMED BY ____

Visual check for: Pre   Post
  Free hemoglobin
  Icterus

Appearance check of:
  Blood bag
  Saline
  Administration set

When Indicated:
  Gram stain
  Culture

	Pre	Post	Unit
Direct antiglobulin test			
ABO and Rh			
Antibody screen			
Plasma hemoglobin			
Major crossmatch			
Minor crossmatch			
Urine free hemoglobin			6 hr
Serum bilirubin			
Additional testing			

INTERPRETATION: ____

Technologist Signature   Pathologist Signature   Date

XYZ HOSPITAL TRANSFUSION SERVICE   PATIENT'S NAME ____

EXTENSION # ____   HOSPITAL # ____

Fig. 41-1. Form used to report a suspected transfusion reaction.

Table 41-1. Acute Adverse Effects of Transfusion

Types of Reactions	Usual Cause
Immunologic	
Hemolysis *with* symptoms	Red cell incompatibility
Anaphylaxis	Antibody to IGA in donor plasma
Febrile, nonhemolytic	Antibody to donor leukocyte antigens
Urticaria	Antibody to donor plasma proteins
Noncardiogenic pulmonary edema	Donor antibody to leukocytes of patient
Nonimmunologic	
Congestive heart failure	Volume overload
Marked fever with shock	Bacterial contamination
Hypothermia	Rapid infusion of cold blood
Hemolysis *without* symptoms	Physical or chemical destruction of blood (e.g., freezing, overheating, or addition of hemolytic drug or solution)
Air embolus	Air infusion in line
Hyperkalemia	Rapid infusion of multiple units of stored blood or packed red cells
Hypocalcemia	Massive transfusion of citrated blood

from acute immune-mediated hemolysis; 12 percent, from acute pulmonary edema; 10 percent, from bacterial contamination; 3 percent, from anaphylaxis, and 3 percent, from nonimmune hemolysis.[1] The possibility of an acute immune-mediated hemolytic reaction should always be considered in the differential diagnosis of an acute transfusion reaction.

Table 41-2 classifies adverse reactions to transfusion according to their clinical significance. Clinically significant reactions should be subsequently reviewed, in detail, by the hospital transfusion committee. An outline of treatment for the major types of acute transfusion reactions is given in Table 41-3.

Fever

Fever, defined as a rise of at least 1°C during the transfusion of blood or blood components, or within 1 or 2 hours thereafter, must be recognized and diag-

nosed as quickly as possible. Although the fever may be due to the patient's underlying condition, the fever might also be due to the transfusion.[2] If it is transfusion related, most often the cause of the fever is a reaction between the patient's antibodies and leukocytes in the donor's blood or a reaction to passively transfused cytokines (see Fever Without Hemolysis).[3,4] However, fever may be the presenting sign of an acute hemolytic transfusion reaction[2] or of infusion of bacteria (or endotoxin) in the blood or component.[5] Prompt recognition and appropriate management may prevent a fatal outcome. To rule out the potentially severe, transfusion-induced causes of fever, first, stop the transfusion, but keep the intravenous (IV) line open! Next, rule out a he-

Table 41-2. Adverse Reactions to Transfusion According to Clinical Significance[a]

Clinically significant reactions should always be reported to the transfusion committee
  Hemolytic
    Immune
      Acute
      Delayed
    Nonimmune (physical or chemical causes)
  Transfusion of blood or components containing infectious agents
    Bacteria
    Hepatitis viruses
    Retroviruses (e.g., HIV)
    Parasites (e.g., malaria)
  Anaphylactic reactions
  Severe febrile reactions
  Graft-versus-host disease
  Post-transfusion purpura
  Noncardiogenic pulmonary edema
Possibly clinically significant reactions that should often be reported to the transfusion committee, especially if investigation identifies improper procedures or poor transfusion practice
  Volume overload
  Massive transfusion effects
Reactions that are generally clinically insignificant
  Febrile nonhemolytic
  Allergic (e.g., urticaria or rash)
  Chills without fever

Abbreviation: HIV, human immunodeficiency virus.
[a] Note: Other adverse results include air embolism, microemboli, transmission of other infectious agents, and iron overload. These should be reported to the transfusion committee if they cause significant morbidity or if improper procedures or poor transfusion practices are identified.

Table 41-3. Treatment of Acute Transfusion Reactions

Sign or Symptom	Treatment
Congestive heart failure	Slow the transfusion and give diuretic (e.g. 40 mg of furosemide) Phlebotomize and transfuse packed cells as necessary
Urticaria	Diphenhydramine or tripelennamine 50 mg IM or PO May restart blood slowly after 15–30 min Consider prophylactic antihistamine before next transfusion
Fever *without* hemolysis	Acetaminophen 650 mg PO Do not restart transfusion/rule out sepsis Consider prophylactic antipyretic therapy next time and/or white cell-poor blood component (e.g., filtered to reduce leukocytes)
Anaphylaxis or asthma	Epinephrine 0.4 ml of 1:1,000 subcutaneously (or give 0.1 ml diluted in 10 ml saline over 5 min IV if in severe shock)
Acute hemolytic transfusion reaction	To prevent renal failure 1,000 ml 0.9% NaCl over 1–2 hr Diuretic therapy: furosemide 20–80 mg IV or ethacrynic acid Continue fluids and diuretics to maintain urine flow over 100 ml/hr Prevent overhydration If hypotension is present, consider dopamine (see text) If AO incompatibility and >200 ml of blood infused and/or evidence of diffuse bleeding, consider heparin (see text)

Abbreviations: IM, intramuscular; PO, oral; IV, intravenous.

molytic transfusion reaction by (1) determining whether the patient is receiving the blood intended (clerical check), (2) observing the patient's plasma for free hemoglobin, and (3) performing a direct antiglobulin (Coombs) test on a new sample of red cells (RBC) drawn from the patient. If no clerical error has occurred, the plasma is not pink or red, and the direct Coombs test finding on the patient's post-transfusion blood sample is negative, an acute hemolytic transfusion reaction, especially as a result of ABO incompatibility, is extremely unlikely.

Once an acute hemolytic transfusion reaction

caused by RBC antigen-antibody incompatibility has been ruled out, other potential causes of fever can be evaluated. If the transfusion-associated fever is accompanied by shock, hemoglobinuria, and/or a bleeding diathesis, sepsis caused by bacteria or bacterial toxins in the blood component should be suspected. The blood or component should be examined for evidence of bacterial growth (e.g., abnormal color, clots, hemolysis, or gas) and then stained for bacteria. If a bacterial stain preparation does not reveal bacteria, culture of both the patient's blood and the blood component may be necessary to prove the presence of bacteria. Treatment of the patient with broad-spectrum antibiotics should be started while awaiting culture results. Keep in mind that bacteremia during transfusion might also be due to contaminated IV solutions[6] or may be unrelated to the transfusion.

Fever without hemolysis or hypotension is most likely due to a reaction between leukocytes transfused with the blood component and antileukocyte antibodies (usually anti-HLA) in previously pregnant or multiply transfused recipients.[7] Thus, once an acute hemolytic transfusion reaction caused by sepsis or immune-mediated hemolysis is ruled out, antipyretic treatment of a febrile, nonhemolytic (FNH) transfusion reaction should be started.

Hemolysis

Hemoglobinuria or hemoglobinemia that occurs during the transfusion of blood or its components must be assumed to be due to an acute hemolytic transfusion reaction until proven otherwise. Fever, hypotension, flank pain, and/or a bleeding diathesis may accompany the hemolysis, particularly if ABO-incompatible or bacterially contaminated blood components were infused. These two diagnostic possibilities, despite their rarity, must be ruled out before searching for other causes of hemolysis. Thus, the transfusion should be stopped, keeping the IV line open, while a workup for these two possibilities proceeds, as described in the preceding section.

If hemolysis occurs during a transfusion without other signs or symptoms, nonimmunologic causes for the hemolysis should be sought. Infusion of blood that has been hemolyzed by freezing, overheating, or mixing with hypotonic solutions may produce hemoglobinemia and hemoglobinuria, which are generally benign clinical events in and of themselves.[8,9] Infusion of hypotonic IV solutions may cause intravascular hemolysis. Drugs administered at the time of transfusion may cause hemolysis of the patient's or the donor's blood on a nonimmune basis (e.g., glucose-6-phosphate dehydrogenase deficiency).[10] Drugs may also cause hemolysis on the basis of hypotonicity[11] and several well-defined immune mechanisms.[12]

Allergic Reactions: Urticaria to Anaphylaxis

Hives (urticaria) may occur during a transfusion. Generally, no other signs or symptoms are present, and serious sequelae seldom result. Slowing the transfusion or temporarily stopping it, while awaiting the effects of an administered antihistamine, effectively manage an urticarial reaction. Hives are generally attributed to an allergic, antibody-mediated response to a donor's plasma proteins but might be due to other substances in blood bags or components (such as residual ethylene oxide).[14]

Allergic reactions that proceed beyond urticaria with anaphylactoid symptoms, or full anaphylaxis, may be caused by an anti-IgA reaction to IgA in the donor's blood components. Abrupt hypertension followed by profound hypotension, asthma, and gastrointestinal symptoms, but no fever, should alert one to this type of reaction.[15] Immediate treatment with epinephrine may be indicated to avert a fatal outcome (Table 41-3).

Pulmonary symptoms of dyspnea and cyanosis without congestive heart failure may be due to a pulmonary hypersensitivity reaction caused by a transfusion.[16,17] Leukocyte antibodies in a donor's blood directed against a recipient's leukocytes can provoke leukoagglutination and leukostasis in the pulmonary microvasculature, with rapid onset of noncardiogenic pulmonary edema. This acute pulmonary hypersensitivity reaction, which is due to transfused donor antibodies to leukocytes, is uncommon. Most often, the congestive heart failure that occurs during a transfusion is due to volume overload and is not an immunologic reaction.[18] In the past, an air embolus was an unusual cause of acute cardiopulmonary dysfunction during transfusion. The use of plastic bags instead of glass bottles for blood has largely eliminated the occurrence of air embolism. However, if fluids and blood are being rapidly pumped into a patient, air may be infused from one of the containers, and an acute cardiopulmonary disaster might result (see Air Embolism section for treatment).

DIFFERENTIAL DIAGNOSIS OF DELAYED TRANSFUSION REACTIONS

Fever With Hemolysis

The onset of fever and anemia days to weeks after a transfusion may herald the onset of a delayed hemolytic transfusion reaction,[19,20] which is caused by RBC alloantibodies or by the transfusion of certain infectious agents, most notably the plasmodia of malaria.[21] In both situations, hemolysis accompanies the fever. Although fever is the most common symptom of a delayed hemolytic transfusion reaction, hemolysis may be asymptomatic, in which case, it must be diagnosed by an unexpected fall in hemoglobin or hematocrit level without evidence of bleeding. The hemolysis is generally extravascular; therefore hemoglobinemia and hemoglobinuria are rarely present.[2] Some delayed hemolytic transfusion reactions are accompanied by oliguria, but it is extremely uncommon for acute renal failure or disseminated intravascular coagulation (DIC) to be present.[19] Diagnosis is made by the finding of a positive direct antiglobulin (Coombs) test result (i.e., the presence of complement and/or antibody-coated donor RBC) or the appearance of previously undetected RBC antibodies and a rapid disappearance of transfused donor cells. If intravascular hemolysis (of both donor and recipient RBC) is evident, then transfusion-induced malaria or babesiosis[22] should be suspected. Thick films to search for parasites should be performed, and a rising antibody titer to Plasmodium species should be sought.

Fever Without Hemolysis

When fever without hemolysis occurs during the days, weeks, or months after a transfusion, transfusion-associated GVHD[23] and transmission of infectious agents should be considered.[24] Acute transfusion-induced GVHD begins with high fever, a diffuse rash, liver function test abnormalities, and gastrointestinal symptoms 4 to 30 days after transfusion of a lymphocyte-containing blood component in a susceptible recipient. GVHD caused by blood transfusion is usually fatal. Only about 10 percent of reported patients survive, and most of these have residual chronic GVHD.[23] Acute transfusion-mediated GVHD is usually accompanied by severe marrow suppression and pancytopenia, leading to death as a result of sepsis or bleeding. Chronic GVHD is manifested by fever, a scleroderma-like disease, sicca syndrome, interstitial pneumonitis, and malabsorption. Evidence supporting the diagnosis of GVHD after a transfusion may be made by the demonstration of circulating donor lymphocytes by HLA typing, cytogenetic studies, or DNA restriction fragment-length polymorphisms.[25,26] Characteristic findings of GVHD may be present in a skin biopsy specimen (see Ch. 42).[23]

If fever occurs several weeks after a transfusion and is accompanied by lymphadenopathy, arthralgias, fatigue, malaise, and other nonspecific symptoms, a transfusion-transmitted infectious disease should be suspected. An infectious mononucleosis-like syndrome may be the initial manifestation of infection with HIV[27] but is more likely due to infection with cytomegalovirus (CMV)[24] or, rarely, Epstein-Barr virus.[28] Seroconversion with appearance of antibodies to these viruses can establish these diagnoses. Fever that occurs 2 to 26 weeks after transfusion may also be due to transfusion-transmitted viral hepatitis agents.[24] Symptoms may be mild and nonspecific, such as anorexia, nausea, and loss of appetite, or severe, such as clinically evident jaundice. Liver tests, especially transaminase levels, reveal hepatic dysfunction and injury. Serologic tests for hepatitis A and B are usually negative because more than 90 percent of transfusion-transmitted viral hepatitis is due to hepatitis C virus (HCV), formerly referred to as non-A, non-B viral hepatitis.[24] If the infection is due to HCV, then seroconversion with the appearance of anti-HCV antibodies results.

Fevers and opportunistic infections that occur months to years after a transfusion may be due to acquired immunodeficiency syndrome (AIDS).[27] If there is no evident reason for immune deficiency or immune suppression and the patient has no other risk factors for AIDS, transfusion-transmitted HIV infection should be suspected.

ACUTE TRANSFUSION REACTIONS IMMUNOLOGICALLY MEDIATED

Acute Hemolytic Reactions

Hemolysis of transfused donor blood by antibodies present in a patient's plasma can have disastrous consequences for that patient. The patient may initially have no signs or symptoms when incompatible blood is being destroyed in the circulation. Usually, however, the transfusion recipient has at least some complaints—sometimes these are mild but often they are severe. There is no pathognomonic sign or symptom that accompanies a hemolytic transfusion reaction. Fever, however, is the most common initial manifestation of immune hemolysis; it was present in 35 of 47 cases reported by Pineda et al.[2] About 50 percent of the time, the fever is accompanied by chills. A patient often experiences a vague uneasiness, back pain, or chills during the early stages of a hemolytic transfusion reaction. Generalized flushing, nausea, dyspnea, chest pain, or lightheadedness occur less commonly. Red or dark urine caused by hemoglobinuria (not hematuria) may be the first sign noticed. Severe hemolytic transfusion reactions may begin with dyspnea, flank pain, and/or hypotension. These can progress to shock, with all of its consequences, including oliguria or complete renal shutdown. Rarely, generalized oozing or frank bleeding may be the first sign of DIC triggered by an incompatible transfusion. In patients who are anesthetized or unconscious for other reasons, shock, red urine, anuria, or a bleeding diathesis may be the presenting findings of a hemolytic transfusion reaction.

The pathophysiology of these signs and symptoms was recently reviewed.[29] The interaction of RBC antigens with antibodies of the IgM, IgG_1, or IgG_3 subclasses may lead to intravascular lysis by way of the complement cascade and result in the release of free hemoglobin and antigen-antibody complexes into the circulation. If the complement cascade does not proceed to completion, RBCs coated with IgG and/or C3b may undergo extravascular destruction by macrophages. The activation of complement leads to the formation of fragments C3a and C5a, which promote the release of histamine and serotonin from mast cells. These vasoactive amines may cause vasodilation and hypotension, bronchial and intestinal smooth muscle contraction, and flushing. Antigen-antibody complexes may lead to the release of bradykinin, resulting in vasodilation, hypotension, flushing, and localized pain. Norepinephrine release secondary to antigen-antibody complexes or hypotension may lead to vasoconstriction of renal and pulmonary vessels, tachycardia, nausea, and vomiting.

A number of cytokines have been implicated in the pathogenesis of hemolytic transfusion reactions. In vitro systems have demonstrated the production and release of tumor necrosis factor, interleukin-1β, interleukin-6, and interleukin-8 by human monocytes in response to sensitized (antibody-coated) RBC.[30,31] The in vitro production of interleukin-8 in whole blood after the addition of ABO-incompatible RBC has been demonstrated and shown to be inhibited by complement inactivation.[32] This work was the topic of a recent review article.[33] Tumor necrosis factor and interleukin-1β may act synergistically to cause shock and pulmonary hemorrhage.[29] Bleeding is caused by the consumption of clotting factors caused by the RBC antigen-antibody complexes and complement activation. Cytokines may also contribute to the initiation of DIC.

Renal failure is usually due to hypotensive shock. With hypotension, blood is shunted away from the kidneys, with resultant renal cortical ischemia.[34] Free hemoglobin can be found in the tubules of the kidneys but is not responsible for oliguria or anuria. Hemoglobin is not directly toxic to the kidneys (except in the presence of dehydration). Tumor necrosis factor, interleukin-1β and interleukin-8 are known endogenous pyrogens and may be involved in the pathogenesis of fever in hemolytic reactions.

Diagnosis

When a hemolytic transfusion reaction is suspected, immediate steps must be taken to diagnose it and minimize its consequences. As noted already, the infusion of blood should be stopped because the morbidity and mortality rates of a hemolytic reaction are roughly proportional to the amount of incompatible blood infused.[35] The risk of a severe reaction is much higher if more than 200 ml of incompatible blood has been transfused (proportionally less in children). However, marked symptoms and signs are often produced after the transfusion of as little as 5

to 20 ml of ABO-incompatible blood, and these have even been reported to occur after the transfusion of only 0.7 ml.[36] Because hypotension often accompanies a severe hemolytic reaction and may progress to frank shock, the IV line should be kept open with a saline infusion (0.9 percent normal saline).[37]

Next, check to see that the patient has been receiving the intended blood. One of the most common reasons for the transfusion of incompatible blood is a clerical error, which results in the infusion of the wrong patient's blood. Check the patient's name and blood group on the blood unit against the recipient's name and blood group. If the wrong unit of blood is transfused to a patient, there is a one-in-three chance of a major ABO incompatibility between patient and donor that may result in severe hypotension, acute renal shutdown, DIC, and death.[37] Once this "clerical" check has been performed, draw an anticoagulated (e.g., ethylenediaminetetraacetic acid) and an unanticoagulated sample of blood (clot) from the patient and send these, along with the clamped off (intact) unit of blood (include the IV tubing and infusion set) that was being transfused, to the blood bank for workup of a suspected hemolytic transfusion reaction. Draw the patient's samples carefully to avoid iatrogenic hemolysis. The anticoagulated specimen can be quickly evaluated visually for free plasma hemoglobin after centrifugation and for evidence of antiglobulin-coated RBC by the direct antiglobulin (Coombs) test. The clotted sample can be recrossmatched with the RBC from inside the bag of donor blood and can be used for baseline chemistry tests on the transfusion recipient, if desired. The blood bank can determine whether the unit of blood that was being transfused to the patient is incompatible with the postreaction patient's serum. If an incompatibility is found, one should crossmatch with the prereaction serum specimen to see whether an incompatibility was missed before the transfusion.

The most useful tests to document the occurrence of an immune-mediated hemolytic transfusion reaction are the plasma hemoglobin level and the direct antiglobulin test. As little as 50 mg/dl of free hemoglobin in plasma can be detected by the naked eye (Fig. 41-2). The direct antiglobulin (Coombs) test takes only minutes to perform and can detect the presence of antibody-coated RBC. If these two obser-

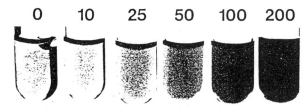

Fig. 41-2. Increasing levels of free hemoglobin (in milligrams per deciliter) in the plasma of patients with hemolytic transfusion reactions. The patient's postreaction plasma should be compared with the pretransfusion plasma specimen.

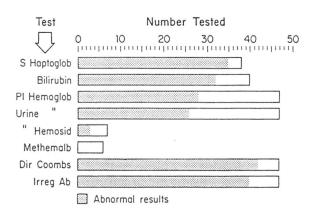

Fig. 41-3. Usefulness of tests for RBC destruction during an acute or a delayed hemolytic transfusion reaction. S Haptoglob, serum haptoglobin; Pl Hemoglob, plasma hemoglobin; Hemosid, hemosiderin; Methemalb, methemalbumin; Irreg Ab, irregular antibodies. (From Pineda et al.,[2] with permission.)

vations are negative, it is unlikely that a patient is undergoing a hemolytic reaction. If either test result is positive in this clinical setting, a hemolytic transfusion reaction has probably occurred, and one should begin appropriate treatment (Table 41-3).

A hemolytic transfusion reaction may still be suspected, even when the patient's plasma does not have free hemoglobin and the direct antiglobulin test finding is negative. The former may be due to rapid clearance of the free hemoglobin from the plasma, and the latter may be due to removal of all of the antibody-coated donor cells from the circulation by the reticuloendothelial system. With no free plasma hemoglobin, one may measure the patient's plasma haptoglobin level on the pretransfusion specimen and on a sample obtained as soon as practical after the suspected transfusion reaction. If the pretransfusion haptoglobin level is within the expected range (usually 100 to 150 mg/dl) and the post-transfusion level is negligible, hemolysis is likely to have occurred. After transfusion of several units of blood, even of banked blood close to its expiration date, the patient's plasma haptoglobin is usually more than 50 percent of its initial, pretransfusion level.[38] Remember, however, that nonimmunologically caused hemolysis (e.g., infusion of distilled water and large retroperitoneal hematomas) can lower the serum haptoglobin level significantly (to less than 50 percent of the expected value).

Additional confirmatory tests may also be used to verify a hemolytic transfusion reaction. Figure 41-3 illustrates laboratory tests that have been used when a hemolytic reaction, either acute or delayed, is sus-

pected and their frequency of yielding a useful result. One should also determine whether the patient's hemoglobin or hematocrit level has risen, as expected, after a transfusion (e.g., in a 70-kg adult, an increase of about 1 g/dl of hemoglobin should be expected when measured 24 hours [and in some cases as soon as 15 minutes] after transfusion for each unit of whole blood or packed cells transfused).[39] If the serum or plasma does not reveal evidence of hemolysis, a sample of urine may be tested for hemoglobinuria or breakdown products of hemoglobin.[2]

Treatment

Once it has been determined that a transfusion of incompatible blood has occurred, therapy should begin (Table 41-3). The morbidity and mortality rates of a hemolytic transfusion reaction are primarily due to acute renal failure (acute tubular necrosis) or a bleeding diathesis.

To prevent renal failure, therapy should be directed toward maintaining adequate perfusion of the kidneys. After an acute hemolytic transfusion reaction, the urine output must be monitored. If hypotension or shock can be adequately treated, renal perfusion can usually be maintained and renal failure prevented. Thus, fluid, primarily in the form of normal saline (0.9 percent NaCl), should be the first therapeutic modality used. Adequate hydration (but not overhydration) should be continued to keep the urine flow over 100 ml/hr in adults. Fluid therapy should be restricted after 1,000 ml of normal saline has been administered if urine output is poor.

Diuretic agents should be given concomitantly with fluids. Furosemide has been recommended[40,41] for this purpose, and it apparently increases renal cortical perfusion,[42] thus minimizing the likelihood of renal tubular ischemia and renal failure. This drug is satisfactory when used in conjunction with adequate IV fluid replacement.

Some authorities recommend the use of dopamine for shock caused by hemolytic transfusion reactions.[42] Dopamine possesses α-adrenergic vasopressor effects that support arterial blood pressure, β-adrenergic effects that increase the cardiac output, and unique "dopaminergic" renal vasodilatory effects that enhance renal cortical perfusion. Thus, dopamine combats both shock and renal failure. Dopamine administration requires careful monitoring of a patient's electrocardiogram, blood pressure, cardiac output, and urinary output.

If, in spite of these measures, progressive oliguria occurs, care should be taken to prevent overhydration of the patient. The management problem now becomes that of acute tubular necrosis with anuria, a problem that should be entrusted to a physician well versed in its management. Dialysis may be required acutely to correct fluid and electrolyte imbalance if these have developed and more chronically if the renal failure is of long duration.

DIC, with its potential for causing a bleeding diathesis, may result from a hemolytic transfusion reaction. The management of DIC is controversial. Many investigators argue against the use of heparin, despite a lack of published case reports or series in the literature regarding the adverse effects of heparin in DIC.[43] Similarly, many individuals strongly encourage the use of heparin, but there is also a surprising void of published reports authenticating the positive effects of this drug in patients with DIC.

Heparin itself can result in bleeding and may be contraindicated in a patient undergoing surgery or who is already bleeding because of the pre-existing condition for which the transfusion was being given. Thus, the decision to give heparin for an acute hemolytic transfusion reaction, which may or may not result

in DIC, is difficult. The factors to consider regarding heparinization are the severity of the reaction and the patient's clinical status. The most severe hemolytic transfusion reactions are those due to infusion of more than 200 ml of ABO-incompatible blood.[35] This is also the situation that is likely to result in DIC and death. In this clinical setting, Goldfinger[41] recommended the use of heparin to prevent DIC. For an adult, he recommends a loading dose of 5,000 units of heparin IV followed by a continuous infusion of 1,500 units/hr. This may be continued for 6 to 24 hours. In patients with relative contraindications to heparin therapy (e.g., postsurgical cases) one-half of this dose may be given. If bleeding develops, heparin reversal with protamine should be considered. This program of management is also appropriate for the patient in whom DIC has already developed. Because severe hemolytic transfusion reactions are rare, there are no controlled studies that indicate the effectiveness of heparin therapy in this setting. Other aspects of management of DIC must also be kept in mind, particularly blood component therapy when necessary to replenish depleted components.[43] A hemolytic transfusion reaction has reportedly been attenuated with the administration of high-dose methylprednisolone and immunoglobulin therapy.[44]

Consideration should be given to transfusion of the patient with compatible blood if, indeed, the patient was in need of transfusion in the first place. Many physicians are reluctant to do this. They are concerned about a second hemolytic episode. However, if the blood bank has resolved the cause of the donor-recipient incompatibility, a transfusion at this point is as safe as any transfusion. Platelets and fresh frozen plasma (FFP) may be useful if a coagulopathy develops, especially with bleeding.

Prevention

Acute hemolytic reactions occur rarely (approximately once for every 12,000 to 21,000 units of blood transfused),[45] but it is difficult to establish effective means to prevent them completely. Those reactions caused by errors, such as initially drawing a blood sample from the wrong patient for crossmatching or transfusion of blood intended for Mary Smith to John Jones, can only be prevented by careful attention to details (e.g., having two individuals check the patient's identification). Transfusion therapy should be used judiciously, only when absolutely needed, and then to stabilize the patient but *not* routinely to normalize the hemoglobin or hematocrit levels.

Each blood transfusion carries a risk of about 1 percent of immunizing a patient to one of the "minor" blood group factors.[46] Although antibody screening and crossmatching with a recently obtained blood sample from a patient usually identifies unexpected RBC antibodies, blood bank techniques are not perfect and do not identify all cases of incompatibility. Rarely, hemolytic reactions occur after a blood transfusion even when compatibility testing using all available methods indicated that the transfused RBC were compatible (see Ch. 9).[47] All clinicians who use transfusions should be aware of the manifold presentations of hemolytic transfusion reactions. Physicians should be prepared to diagnose this uncommon type of reaction quickly and should know how and when to institute therapy to minimize the severe complications that can result.

Anaphylactic Transfusion Reactions

Anaphylactic reactions are dramatic and can result in death unless recognized and treated promptly. The onset of shock, loss of consciousness, or severe gastrointestinal symptoms may occur after the infusion of only a few milliliters of blood or plasma. Few transfusion reactions are so quickly evident after the receipt of such small volumes. Symptoms usually begin with nausea, abdominal cramps, emesis, and diarrhea. Transient hypertension is followed by profound hypotension. Generalized flushing and, occasionally, chills may be present, but fever is virtually never found. In fact, the rapid onset of gastrointestinal symptoms and/or shock in the *absence* of fever often distinguishes the anaphylactic reaction from reactions caused by leukocyte incompatibility, hemolysis, or sepsis.[15]

Severe anaphylactic or anaphylactoid reactions may be caused by antibodies to IgA. Two types of anti-IgA have been identified.[13] Class-specific antibodies react by passive hemagglutination with all IgA proteins and are detected only in the sera of persons who lack IgA. Anti-IgA of limited specificity reacts with only a limited variety of IgA proteins and occurs in patients with normal levels of IgA. Class-specific IgA antibodies are thought to be responsible for IgA-mediated anaphylactic transfusion reactions,

whereas anti-IgA antibodies of limited specificity are of uncertain clinical significance.[48,49]

Although some anaphylactic reactions are apparently caused by anti-IgA antibodies, many such reactions have no apparent cause. Although extensive data are not available to indicate the percentage of anaphylactic reactions caused by anti-IgA compared with other causes, Laschinger et al.[48] reported that blood samples from 152 patients were referred to the national reference laboratory of the Canadian Red Cross Society because the referring hospitals had not been able to determine the cause of the patients' severe nonhemolytic transfusion reactions. Twenty-one patients were found to be IgA deficient, and 12 of these 21 samples (58 percent) had strong class-specific anti-IgA antibodies, which were presumed to have been responsible for the reactions. Thus, only 8 percent (12 of 152) of patients who had severe reactions were found to be IgA deficient and to have anti-IgA, although 58 percent of the 21 IgA-deficient patients had class-specific antibodies to IgA. In another study, Sandler et al.[50] found class-specific anti-IgA in 76.3 percent of 80 IgA-deficient patients with a history of an anaphylactic transfusion reaction.

The frequency of IgA-mediated anaphylactic reactions has been variously estimated. One estimate is that such a reaction occurs after 1 in 20,000 to 47,000 transfusions.[51] However, other data suggest that anaphylactic reactions caused by anti-IgA are much less common. In Canada, the frequency of anti-IgA-mediated anaphylactic transfusion reactions has been estimated to be 1.3 per 1,000,000 units of blood or blood products transfused.[48] Also, in a 10-year period from 1982 to 1992, during which time 297,190 blood components were transfused at Georgetown University Medical Center, approximately 0.9 percent of transfusions were investigated for adverse reactions, but no cases of anti-IgA-mediated anaphylactic reactions were identified.[50] Although anaphylactic reactions are alarming, only one case of a fatal anaphylactic transfusion reaction associated with anti-IgA has been reported.[51]

Diagnosis

To make the diagnosis of an anti-IgA reaction as the cause of an anaphylactic transfusion reaction, the most practical approach is to determine the patient's serum level of IgA. If IgA deficiency can be ruled out, other causes of anaphylactic transfusion reactions should be sought. Only about 1 in 700 individuals is IgA deficient. If the patient is IgA deficient, it is prudent to assume that the reaction was anti-IgA mediated and supply IgA-deficient blood products until arrangements can be made to determine whether anti-IgA is present. Unfortunately, few laboratories are equipped to measure anti-IgA.[50]

Even if one performs a test for anti-IgA, there are difficulties in interpreting this result. As indicated above, only 58 to 76 percent of patients who are IgA deficient and have anaphylactic reactions have class-specific anti-IgA. Sandler et al.,[50] using a passive hemagglutination inhibition assay, found that 1 in 1,200 blood donors is IgA deficient and also has class-specific anti-IgA. These investigators concluded that the relatively high frequency of class-specific anti-IgA detected by a standard passive hemagglutination assay in IgA-deficient donors compared with the rarity of anaphylactic reactions in transfusion recipients strongly suggests that tests for anti-IgA lead to an overestimation of persons who are presumed to be at risk for clinically significant anti-IgA-mediated anaphylactic reactions.

Furthermore, studies of anti-IgA antibodies of limited specificity indicate that they are of uncertain clinical significance.[48,49] Rivat et al.[49] screened 1,010 blood donors and found IgA antibodies of limited specificity in 59 percent, a frequency that did not differ significantly from that among patients with suspected anti-IgA-mediated anaphylactic reactions. Therefore, the presence of antibodies of limited specificity in reports of anaphylactoid reactions may be coincidental.[50]

Treatment

The immediate treatment of an anaphylactic reaction to blood or plasma is to stop the transfusion and administer epinephrine. Once again, keep the IV line open with normal saline because severe hypotension is the most significant manifestation of an anaphylactic transfusion reaction. Epinephrine, 0.4 ml of a 1:1,000 solution, should be given subcutaneously as quickly as possible. If tissue perfusion is already compromised by the presence of shock, give instead 0.1 ml of 1:1,000 epinephrine diluted in 10 ml with normal saline slowly IV (e.g., over 5 min-

utes). *Under no circumstances should the transfusion be restarted.*

Prevention

To prevent anaphylactic transfusion reactions in patients who have class-specific anti-IgA, the patients must be transfused with blood components that lack IgA. Whole blood and components may be obtained from IgA-deficient (less than 0.05 mg/dl) blood donors. Many regional blood centers have identified blood donors with selective IgA deficiency and maintain supplies of IgA-deficient plasma; in addition, registries of such donors are available. The American National Red Cross, the American Association of Blood Banks, and the Canadian National Red Cross maintain lists of donors with IgA deficiency as part of their rare donor files. It is more practical, however, to use RBC that have been completely freed of the IgA in the plasma. This may be accomplished by thorough "washing" of the RBC. Usually, extensive washing in a mechanical cell washer is adequate, but, rarely, frozen-thawed RBC are necessary.[15] The frozen-thawed RBC are essentially free of IgA by virtue of their method of preparation (glycerolization and then deglycerolization) and can be safely transfused to even highly immunized, IgA-deficient patients with antibodies to IgA.

IgA-deficient patients with anti-IgA can be their own "donors." For anticipated, elective transfusion (e.g., planned surgical procedures) IgA-deficient patients might donate blood preoperatively that can be stored for several weeks in the blood bank in a liquid state or frozen and held for years as frozen RBC and frozen plasma. If large quantities of plasma are required, plasma may be obtained by plasmapheresis even from anemic IgA-deficient patients. The autologous plasma may be stored in the frozen state (as FFP) and given later, for the patient who needs volume replacement.

Minute quantities of IgA are present in most albumin preparations, and even more IgA is present in plasma protein fraction (PPF). These plasma derivatives should not be given to highly sensitized, IgA-deficient patients.[15] In an emergency, crystalloid solutions may be necessary, along with frozen-thawed RBC, for the IgA-deficient patient in need of a blood transfusion who has not had the opportunity to set aside autologous blood or plasma. Patients with IgA deficiency who have class-specific antibodies to IgA should wear or carry some type of medical alert device to notify emergency room physicians of their condition.

Noncardiogenic Pulmonary Edema

Pulmonary edema that occurs during a blood transfusion is most frequently due to heart failure secondary to hypervolemia, especially in very young or very old patients or those with long-standing anemia. Rarely, however, transfusion can provoke a form of noncardiogenic pulmonary edema. In one study, noncardiogenic pulmonary edema occurred in association with 0.02 percent of transfused units.[16] Noncardiogenic pulmonary edema is characterized by acute respiratory distress, bilateral pulmonary edema, and severe hypoxemia. Fever and hypotension may be present. The reaction usually develops within 6 hours of transfusion and may occur after the infusion of relatively small quantities of blood or plasma. Symptoms usually resolve completely within 96 hours, provided there is prompt and adequate respiratory support. Death may occur, however, in up to 5 percent of cases.[17] Noncardiogenic pulmonary edema caused by a transfusion is usually due to passively transfused antibodies to leukocytes that have been induced by prior transfusions or pregnancy in the donor. Antibodies reactive with granulocytes were demonstrated in at least one donor in 32 of 36 cases.[16] To date, most antibodies have HLA rather than granulocyte-specific reactivities. The HLA specificity of the donor's antibody corresponded to the patient's HLA type in more than 50 percent of cases in one study.[52] Antigen-antibody reactions are thought to activate complement, resulting in the production of fragment C5a, which, in turn, promotes neutrophil aggregation and sequestration in the lung. The release of neutrophil granules leads to pulmonary vascular damage and extravasation of fluid into the alveoli and interstitium.

Diagnosis

Noncardiogenic pulmonary edema should be suspected if acute respiratory distress develops during or shortly after (usually within 6 hours of) a transfusion. Cardiogenic causes should be ruled out first. The identification of antileukocyte antibodies in donor plasma that react with recipient leukocytes provides strong support for the diagnosis of noncardiogenic pulmonary edema. These donor antibodies may have HLA- or neutrophil-specific reactivities and can be demonstrated in more than 50 percent of cases.[17] Patients with noncardiogenic pulmonary edema have normal or low pulmonary wedge pressures and normal central venous pressure.

Treatment

The treatment of noncardiogenic pulmonary edema begins with stopping the transfusion. Because of the rarity of this condition, therapy has been empiric, with respiratory support varying from oxygen by mask to intubation and mechanical ventilatory assistance when necessary. Most patients have resolution of their symptoms within 12 to 24 hours and clearance of the bilateral pulmonary infiltrates within a few days. The successful use of extracorporeal membrane oxygenation in one patient with inadequate oxygenation despite medical treatment has been reported.[53]

Prevention

HLA antibodies with a defined specificity are found in 1 to 2 percent of blood donors.[52] However, reports of noncardiogenic pulmonary edema are rare. The routine diversion of blood components from donors who have had three or more pregnancies from use as whole blood, FFP, and single-donor apheresis platelets has been recommended unless such donors have been found negative for HLA- or neutrophil-specific antibodies.[17] This approach would result in a significant cost and loss of donors, and the effectiveness of this approach is unclear. Recognition of the entity of noncardiogenic pulmonary edema and differentiation of it from hypervolemic cardiac failure are the most important aspects of this uncommon event.

Fever Without Hemolysis

Fever without hemolysis (also called an FNH transfusion reaction) is one of the most commonly recognized adverse effects of transfusion. Goldfinger and Lowe,[54] after careful evaluation of 6,359 reported transfusions, concluded that the incidence of non-RBC-mediated reactions was approximately 0.5 percent. Although the authors did not distinguish between FNH and other types of nonhemolytic reactions, most such reactions can be assumed to have been FNH. As the name implies, FNH reactions are manifested by fever with or without chills without RBC hemolysis. The fever may be mild to severe but does not usually occur until most of the unit of blood or component has been transfused and, sometimes, not for 1 to 2 hours after completion of the transfusion. FNH reactions appear more frequently in blood recipients who have been pregnant or transfused repeatedly with blood components. These individuals may have been sensitized to foreign leukocyte antigens.[3] In one study, white blood cell (WBC) antibodies were identified in approximately 70 percent of patients who experienced FNH transfusion reactions.[55] The reaction of patient's antibodies with donor WBCs or platelets may give rise to the characteristic febrile reaction by the release of pyrogens from patient macrophages or from donor WBC.[56] A second mechanism for FNH reactions is the accumulation of cytokines in blood units (especially platelet concentrates) during storage. Tumor necrosis factor-α and interleukins-1, -6, and -8 have been shown to increase over time in stored platelet concentrates.[57–59] In one study, the reaction rate to leukocyte-reduced platelet concentrates stored for less than 3 days was significantly less than the reaction rate to similar concentrates stored for 3 days or more (8.7 vs. 17.6 percent).[60] Heddle et al.[61] demonstrated that FNH reactions to platelet transfusions were more commonly associated with plasma supernatant than with platelets or cells.

Diagnosis

Fever is the hallmark and most important sign of an FNH transfusion reaction. Fever may, however, be an initial symptom of an immune-mediated hemolytic reaction or a response to a blood component contaminated with bacteria.[5] Thus, the transfusion should be stopped so that an investigation can be completed to rule in or out these more serious possibilities.

Treatment and Prevention

FNH reactions may be treated with antipyretics such as acetaminophen. The successful use of meperidine to control the manifestations of a febrile reaction in a patient who had had a recent myocardial infarction has been described.[62] The prevention of subsequent

FNH reactions, however, is usually a more important consideration than their immediate management. If a patient experiences one FNH reaction, the odds are one in eight that a similar reaction will occur to the next blood transfusion.[4] WBC reduction to a level of 5×10^8 or less in RBC components eliminates most FNH reactions.[8] This can be performed by the blood bank or at the bedside using special filters that have been designed to remove WBC and platelets without appreciable loss of RBC. Febrile reactions associated with platelet transfusions may be associated with alloimmunization and poor posttransfusion platelet recoveries.[63] Although different filters designed to remove WBC from platelets are available, they appear to be less effective in preventing febrile reactions in alloimmunized patients receiving platelet transfusions.[64,65] In one study, the rate of febrile reactions to platelet transfusions was reduced by using single-donor platelets versus pooled platelets (8.4 vs. 21.4 percent).[66] Prestorage leukocyte-reduced platelets may be available directly from the blood bank. This component may help reduce FNH mediated by cytokine release during storage.[67]

Urticaria

Although urticaria is one of the most frequent transfusion reactions, hives are generally only a mild and bothersome complication. This allergic reaction to blood or blood components may accompany 1 or 2 percent of transfusions.[7] This may be an underestimate, however, because hives are considered such a common and insignificant adverse effect of a transfusion that urticaria is often not reported to the blood bank.

Diagnosis

In most clinical situations, the cause of urticarial reactions is never ascertained. This type of reaction is mild and does not warrant a detailed investigation. Recurrent hives occasionally are due to antibodies in patients directed against antigenic determinants on donor serum proteins, such as IgA allotypes.[13]

Treatment and Prevention

Urticarial reactions, if they are unaccompanied by any other signs or symptoms, are the only type of transfusion reactions in which the blood component does not have to

be discontinued and discarded. Usually, an antihistamine is administered while the flow of blood is slowed or temporarily stopped. After 15 to 30 minutes, when the hives have faded, the blood may be slowly transfused once again. In patients who frequently experience urticarial reactions, pretreatment with an antihistamine is warranted before each transfusion. Alternatively, removal of plasma proteins from blood components may avert urticarial reactions (e.g., with saline washed or frozen and then deglycerolized RBC).

ACUTE TRANSFUSION REACTIONS: NONIMMUNOLOGIC

Congestive Heart Failure

Heart failure induced by the transfusion of blood or its components is a potentially serious adverse effect of a transfusion. Its true frequency in unknown because it is often not recognized and certainly rarely reported to the blood bank. Hypervolemia with secondary congestive failure can occur in any patient who is transfused too rapidly.[18] In practice, transfusion-induced heart failure occurs primarily in very young and elderly patients, those with established cardiac disease, and those with expanded plasma volumes (especially when associated with chronic, long-standing anemia). In these patients, the usual transfusion rate of about 200 ml/hr of blood may be excessive. They cannot accommodate this rapid expansion of their blood volume and may experience congestive heart failure.

Treatment and Prevention

The therapy for transfusion-induced congestive heart failure is essentially the same as that for congestive heart failure of any cause. The transfusion should be stopped or infused extremely slowly. Rapid-acting diuretics, such as furosemide or ethacrynic acid, should be given IV. At the same time, patients should be placed in a sitting position, provided oxygen by mask, and given IV morphine if necessary. If frank pulmonary edema has developed, phlebotomy of 200 to 400 ml of blood may be necessary, along with slow infusion of concentrated (packed) RBC.

Prevention is the key to handling transfusion-in-duced congestive heart failure. In susceptible patients, transfusions should be administered slowly (e.g., 1 ml/kg body weight/hr) and in the most concentrated form available.[18] Packed RBC or RBC suspended in a minimal amount of saline should be used to raise the hematocrit of infants, elderly patients, or those with chronic anemias. Plasmapheresis or partial exchange transfusion (removing whole blood and replacing with packed RBC) may also be considered at the time of transfusion to reduce the patient's expanded plasma volume and permit more rapid infusion of RBC.

Transfusion of Bacterially Contaminated Blood

It is possible for bacteria to enter a blood component through several mechanisms (see Ch. 40).[68] Today, most contaminants are thought to arise from the donor, either from the skin during venipuncture or from an unrecognized transient or chronic bacteremia at the time of blood donation. Accidental contamination during the collection or processing of blood is documented sporadically.[69] A small number of bacteria introduced at the time of blood collection can grow and divide in the stored blood and cause a subsequent septic transfusion reaction. When blood components are heavily contaminated with bacteria, a devastating transfusion reaction can occur. Patients may experience high fever, shock, hemoglobinuria, renal failure, and DIC.[5] Of note is the fact that the shock, when it occurs, is usually of the "warm" type, with flushing and dryness of the skin, and it may be accompanied by either abdominal pain with cramps and diarrhea or pain in the extremities with generalized muscle aches.

In two recent prospective studies, 6 of 14,481 random platelet concentrates (1 in 2,414)[70] and at least 7 of 15,838 (1 in 2,500)[71] were found by bacterial culture to be contaminated. In another recent study, the transfusion of 1 in 13,460 platelet concentrates resulted in a diagnosed septic reaction.[72] From 1986 through 1991, 16 percent of transfusion-associated fatalities reported to the FDA were caused by bacterial contamination. Of these fatalities, 72 percent were associated with platelet transfusions, and 28 percent were associated with RBC transfusions. Gram-negative organisms are more frequently recovered from RBC, whereas gram-positive organisms are more frequently recovered from platelet concentrates.[73] Many septic reactions may have previously gone unrecognized or were considered to be FNH type reactions.[71]

Diagnosis

Prompt recognition of a reaction caused by bacterially contaminated blood or components is essential. As soon as this possibility is considered, transfusion of the blood component should be stopped, and the component should immediately be examined for evidence of bacteria. This can be done either by gross observation, which may reveal an unusual color[74] of the blood component, gross hemolysis, or clots in the bag, or by a stain for bacteria of the bag's contents.[70,75] If the diagnosis of a septic transfusion is likely, both the patient's blood and the blood component should be cultured for both aerobic and anaerobic organisms. The IV solution should also be cultured because this, too, is a potential source of infused organisms.[6]

Treatment and Prevention

Broad-spectrum antibiotic coverage should be instituted for a septic transfusion reaction. Antibiotic(s), to cover a variety of organisms, are administered IV, pending a determination of the responsible organism(s) and its sensitivities. Fluids, including plasma volume expanders, and vasopressors should be used to maintain the blood pressure, if necessary. If DIC is evident, appropriate therapy should be considered.

Hemolysis Caused by Physical or Chemical Factors

RBC intended for transfusion may be inadvertently hemolyzed by physical or chemical means. Freezing of whole blood or packed cells without a cryoprotective agent such as glycerol and the heating of RBC to greater than 50°C will result in hemolysis. Drugs and hypertonic or hypotonic solutions, when mixed with or simultaneously infused with RBC, may also cause RBC lysis.[11]

Asymptomatic hemoglobinuria is the most usual result of transfusing hemolyzed but compatible RBC. Patients do not experience fever, chills, hypotension, or any of the other signs or symptoms associated with an immune hemolytic reaction or transfusion of bacterially hemolyzed blood. Examine the bag that contains the blood or packed cells for evi-

dence of free hemoglobin (centrifuge an aliquot and look for red or pink plasma or supernatant).

Most patients clear free hemoglobin without difficulty, but DIC is at least a theoretic possibility after the transfusion of lysed, compatible RBC. Shulman et al.[76] showed that infusions of compatible RBC stroma caused no problems in humans, but Quick[77] demonstrated that lysed erythrocytes can release procoagulant materials. Even hemolyzed autologous RBC could induce DIC. After infusion of lysed, compatible RBC, DIC has rarely been observed clinically. Thus, therapy for DIC should be withheld pending some evidence of intravascular clotting. Fluids should be given and careful observation maintained if hemolyzed blood has been administered. Hypotension or dehydration may predispose the patient to acute renal insufficiency, even when benign hemoglobinemia is present.

Clinicians should make every effort to prevent inadvertent hemolysis of RBC; when hemolysis caused by physical or chemical factors occurs, there is always the worry that the patient really has had an immune or septic hemolytic reaction. Documenting nonimmune hemolysis and ruling out an immune basis for it are two steps that should always be taken in these situations. Care to see that refrigerated blood is not accidentally placed in a freezer or heated excessively by a blood warmer will prevent most cases of physical hemolysis of blood.[9] A strict rule of never adding a drug or any IV solution to blood, unless these are known to be compatible with blood, will eliminate chemical or osmotic hemolysis.[8] Drugs infused into patients should be in isotonic solutions to prevent hemolysis.[11] Keep in mind that patients undergoing prostate surgery have inadvertently received distilled water IV from the bladder irrigation fluid with resultant intravascular hemolysis.[38]

Air Embolism

With the widespread use of plastic bags instead of glass bottles, the hazard of an air embolism from the transfusion of blood has virtually disappeared. Mechanical means of rapidly infusing blood work primarily by placing pressure on the outside of the blood bag, so an air embolism is not very likely. When air is pumped into the blood container to speed infusion, an air embolus is a distinct possibility; therefore, this should never be done.

Patients who receive air IV may experience acute cardiopulmonary insufficiency. The air tends to lodge in the right ventricle and prevents blood from entering the pulmonary artery. Acute cyanosis, pain, cough, dyspnea, shock, and cardiac arrhythmia may result. Death may supervene unless immediate action is taken. Having the patient lie head down on the left side usually displaces the air bubble away from the pulmonary valve. This also places the patient in an optimal position for removal of the air by aspiration using a transthoracic needle inserted below the second or third rib just to the right of the sternum.

Microemboli

Microaggregates form in blood while it is stored in the blood bank refrigerator.[78] WBC and platelets, plus some fibrin and entangled RBC, make up most of the microscopic debris that accumulates during the storage of blood despite the anticoagulant-preservative solution in which it is kept. These microaggregates can be demonstrated by using special filters with openings smaller than the usual blood filter of 170-μm pore size. Because most of the microaggregates pass through the standard blood bank filter, this material may be trapped in the lungs after transfusion and cause microemboli. The main questions, however, are how clinically important this is and what, if anything, should be done to prevent it. Although microaggregates do form in blood stored in the blood bank, there is little clinical information documenting their deleterious effect. Special "micropore" blood filters are on the market and can be shown to remove microaggregates missed by standard blood filters. Whether such filters are needed routinely, or are of significant benefit, remains to be shown. Some also remove platelets and thus should not be used with platelet transfusions.[78]

Massive Transfusion Effects

Patients who receive large volumes of blood may experience some untoward effects of these multiple transfusions, especially if the transfusions are given rapidly (see Chs. 25 and 35). "Massive transfusion" here refers to the infusion of a minimum of 10 units of blood in an adult or the replacement of at least one blood volume within a 24-hour period. Despite its anticoagulant-preservative, blood does age while

sitting in the blood bank refrigerator. As part of the aging process, the pH of the blood, already slightly acid as a result of the citrate added, falls somewhat, potassium leaks from the RBC, and some labile clotting components deteriorate.[79] In addition, the RBC 2, 3-diphosphoglycerate (2, 3-DPG) level falls. Thus, a massive transfusion can have physical, chemical, and physiologic effects on a patient.

A rapid transfusion of banked blood right out of the refrigerator (at 1 to 6°C) can cause hypothermia in patients and can have hypothermic effects on the heart.[80] To affect the heart adversely by lowering its temperature, a very rapid infusion of multiple units of cold blood is usually necessary (e.g., 50 to 100 ml/min of blood). If transfusion at this rapid pace is contemplated, then the blood should be warmed to body temperature (but not above 37°C) during the transfusion. The rapid infusion of cold blood may compound the cardiac effects of hypocalcemia and hyperkalemia of stored (more than 2 or 3 weeks in the refrigerator) blood and packed cells.

The chemical effects of a massive transfusion of stored blood can be due to its lack of ionized calcium (complexed by the citrate anticoagulant), acidity, and hyperkalemia. One unit of stored blood contains citrate levels ranging from approximately 175 mg in additive solution (AS)-1 RBCs to 600 mg in AS-3 RBCs. The citrate content of FFP units is approximately 385 mg/dl. Because citrate is normally rapidly metabolized in the body, it is difficult for a patient to have significant hypocalcemia develop. In adults, massive transfusion associated with severe hepatic ischemia or interrupted hepatic blood flow (e.g., liver transplantation) may result in clinically significant citrate toxicity.[81] Neonatal massive exchange transfusion may also result in citrate toxicity. Toxic effects may be seen on the electrocardiogram (e.g., prolongation of the QT interval) and result in decreased cardiac performance. Two-to-one electromechanical heart block has been reported as a result of citrate toxicity.[82] To minimize the possibility of transfusion-induced hypocalcemia, some clinicians recommend the infusion of 10 ml of 10 percent calcium chloride after every few units of banked blood. However, this is generally regarded as unnecessary, and extreme hypercalcemia has been induced by this means.[83] In settings in which citrate toxicity is a significant risk, the use of ionized calcium measurements has been recommended.[81]

The plasma level of potassium may increase 0.5 to 1 mEq/L/day of refrigerator storage.[84] Thus, another possible adverse effect during a massive transfusion is hyperkalemia from the rapid infusion of blood or packed RBC with an elevated potassium level caused by the potassium that has leaked from the RBC; however, this is rarely of clinical consequence, except perhaps in patients with renal insufficiency or pre-existing hyperkalemia (or neonates).[85] A massive transfusion may actually result in hypokalemia in a patient. This may be due to the fact that, in the circulation, the transfused RBC take up potassium to replace what has been lost during storage.

Additional effects of massive transfusion may result from (1) shifting of the oxygen dissociation curve of hemoglobin so that it binds oxygen more tightly or (2) depletion of labile clotting factors. A massive transfusion of stored blood (more than 2 weeks in the refrigerator) with low RBC 2, 3-DPG levels may, temporarily, impair tissue oxygenation. The 2, 3-DPG is regenerated in vivo by the RBC and is usually nearly normal within 24 hours of the transfusion. How real a problem this is at a clinical level remains unclear because there is little useful information on this point.

During refrigeration of blood, platelets rapidly become nonfunctional, the factor VIII (antihemophilic factor) level quickly falls, and factor V (labile factor) deteriorates.[79] Infusion of large quantities of banked blood may result in a deficiency of one or more of these coagulation components in massively transfused patients or those getting large quantities of their own intraoperatively salvaged RBC (washed free of plasma and debris with saline). The management of potential coagulation factor deficiencies occurring during a massive transfusion is discussed in Chapters 25 and 35.

A point to be kept in mind during massive transfusion is the possible adverse effect of a rapid infusion of PPF or, even more rarely, 5 percent albumin solution. Some lots of these purified plasma derivatives contain vasoactive substances that provoke hypotension.[86] This may not be immediately recognized in the urgency of the clinical situation because, often, the patient is already hypotensive as a result of blood loss. Slowing the infusion rate of the protein solution, which may, on occasion, have this hypotensive effect, is usually sufficient to handle this problem. Recently produced lots of PPF appear to be free of this undesirable property.

DELAYED TRANSFUSION EFFECTS

Transfusion reactions and other adverse effects of blood transfusions can occur some time after completion of the infusion. The delay can be days, months, or years later. Immunologic or nonimmunologic mechanisms may be responsible (Table 41-4). These potential, late hazards should always be

Table 41-4. Delayed Transfusion Reactions

Types of Reactions	Usual Etiology
Immunologic	
Hemolysis	Anamnestic antibody to RBC antigen
Serum sickness-like	Developing RBC antigen incompatibility
Graft-versus-host disease	Functional lymphocytes in blood or component transfused
Post-transfusion purpura	Development of antiplatelet antibody, usually anti-Pl^A1 (anti-HPA-1a)
Alloimmunization	Transfusion of RBC
Immunomodulation	Transfusion of leukocytes
Nonimmunologic	
Iron overload	Multiple transfusions (100+) in chronically anemic patients without blood loss
Disease transmission	
Hepatitis	Hepatitis C virus but occasionally type B (almost never type A)
AIDS	Human immunodeficiency virus
Cytomegalovirus infection	Cytomegalovirus
Protozoa	Malaria parasites (rarely Babesia)
Leukemia or TSPP	HTLV I/II

Abbreviations: AIDS, acquired immunodeficiency syndrome; TSPP, tropical spastic paraparesis; RBC, red blood cell; HTLV, human T-cell lymphotropic virus.

kept in mind after blood transfusions, even if no untoward effects occurred during the actual infusion.

Delayed Hemolytic Transfusion Reactions

Even though blood is usually crossmatched and given as ABO and Rh_O (D) compatible to a patient, a recipient may still subsequently have an antibody develop to any of hundreds of other RBC antigens.[46] Immunization to RBC antigens can also occur during pregnancy. If an RBC antibody is formed or recalled in an anamnestic fashion while there are circulating transfused donor RBC, a delayed hemolytic transfusion reaction can result. Most often, this is completely asymptomatic and only noted by a more rapid fall in the patient's hemoglobin level than expected and/or a low-grade fever. Occasionally, a patient exhibits symptoms similar to those of serum sickness. A delayed transfusion reaction can be documented in some cases by the presence of a mixed-field, positive direct antiglobulin (Coombs) test result, demonstrating antibody-coated donor, but not recipient, cells. Antibody is usually also demonstrated in the patient's serum by the indirect antiglobulin test. On occasion, the delayed hemolytic reaction can be so brisk as to evoke symptoms, usually significant fever and hemoglobinemia, and, rarely, it may even result in renal shutdown and death.[2,19,20] The clinical course of a patient who experienced a delayed hemolytic transfusion reaction with consequent renal failure is illustrated in Figure 41-4. An RBC antibody to one of the Kidd (Jk) antigens on donor cells (which the patient lacked) was the precipitating cause of the reaction. Delayed hemolytic transfusion reactions are of particular concern in patients with sickle cell anemia. After an RBC exchange, a sickle cell crisis might be suspected incorrectly instead of a delayed hemolytic transfusion reaction.[87] In addition, patients may become acutely ill with vaso-occlusive crises, bone infarction, biliary obstruction, renal insufficiency, and profound anemia, in part because their own marrow has been suppressed by the transfusions.[88]

Three things concerning delayed hemolytic transfusion reactions must be kept in mind. First, the risk of immunizing a recipient to a minor RBC antigen (not in the ABO system) is about 1 percent for each unit of blood transfused.[46] Second, the onset of a delayed hemolytic reaction is usually insidious, most often virtually unnoticed, save for the gradual recurrence of anemia (with or without fever). Third, when there are symptoms, fever is the most common sign and symptom of a delayed hemolytic transfusion reaction.[2] Fever and anemia that occur 10 to 14 days after a blood transfusion may, rarely, be due to transfusion-induced malaria[21] or acute GVHD,[23] but a delayed, immune-mediated hemolytic transfusion reaction is much more likely.

Alloimmunization/Immunomodulation

Because no two humans, except identical twins, have the same genetic makeup, a blood transfusion exposes a patient to numerous "foreign" antigens. Those antigens infused that the patient does not possess are potentially immunogenic. Antibodies in the recipient may be formed days, weeks, or months after a transfusion to any nonself antigens.

For patients in whom antibodies to multiple RBC antigens have developed, it may be difficult to find compatible blood that lacks these factors. Thus, the presence of irregular or unexpected antibodies induced by a prior transfusion may severely limit subsequent safe transfusion. Even blood components that contain only minimal RBC, such as platelet concentrates, can evoke antibodies to RBC antigens. This risk, however, is lower in immunosuppressed patients.[89]

Alloimmunization to antigens on platelets, WBC, and plasma proteins (and RBC antigens) may also occur after blood transfusions. Antibodies to platelets may cause not only febrile transfusion reactions but also immune-mediated destruction of transfused platelets.[90]

Post-Transfusion Purpura

Very rarely, post-transfusion purpura with severe thrombocytopenia has been induced by the transfusion of blood.[91,92] In this situation, which most often occurs in women who have been immunized to platelet antigens during pregnancy, an antibody to transfused platelets, most commonly anti-Pl^{A1} (anti-HPA-1a), causes thrombocytopenia even though the patient's platelets lack the Pl^{A1} (HPA-1a) antigen.[92] This may result from cross-reactivity of the antibody with the patient's own platelets or "nonspecific" destruction of the patient's Pl^{A1}-negative platelets. In some patients, thrombocytopenia is not profound,

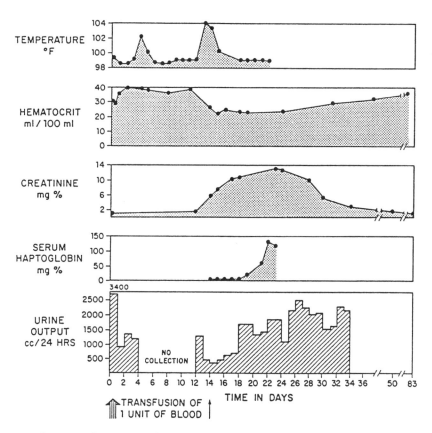

Fig. 41-4. Hospital course of a patient who experienced a delayed hemolytic transfusion reaction with acute renal failure caused by an anamnestic antibody response to the RBC antigen Jk^b. (From Holland and Wallerstein,[19] with permission.)

and no therapeutic intervention is necessary. In others, corticosteroids, plasma exchange, high-dose IV immunoglobulin, and transfusion of Pl^{A1}-negative platelets have all been used.[91–95] Plasma exchange (formerly a whole blood exchange) seems to be the most effective therapy,[92,93] although others recommend high-dose IV immunoglobulin (IVIG)[88] on the basis of a favorable response in a small number of patients, some of whom had shown no response to plasmapheresis.[95]

Neonatal Immune Thrombocytopenia

Immunization to platelet-specific antigens may also cause neonatal alloimmune thrombocytopenia (see Ch. 28), which may be managed by the transfusion of platelets from the mother or from other persons who lack the specific platelet antigen.[96,97]

Neonatal alloimmune thrombocytopenia must be distinguished from neonatal autoimmune thrombocytopenia;[96,97] the latter occurs in neonates born of mothers with autoimmune thrombocytopenia (e.g., idiopathic thrombocytopenic purpura [ITP]). In neonatal autoimmune thrombocytopenia, platelet transfusion is not likely to be successful. Optimal management consists of treatment of the mother during pregnancy.[98–100] Therapy of the pregnant woman with ITP usually does not differ significantly from that of nonpregnant individuals.[100] Prednisone remains the first line of therapy, and the response to therapy does not differ from that observed in nonpregnant individuals, with a response rate of 60 to 70 percent. For patients who do not respond adequately to prednisone, IVIG should be tried. For those who do not respond adequately to either or both of these modalities, splenectomy should be considered, especially during the second trimester.

Determination of the appropriate management for the fetus is more complex. McCrae et al.[100] recommend that patients with apparent incidental thrombocytopenia (no history of thrombocytopenia before pregnancy) and with a platelet count greater than 75,000/μl undergo routine vaginal delivery unless obstetric indications dictate otherwise and, second, that women with platelet counts of less than 75,000/μl be considered potentially to have ITP. Measurements of either platelet-associated IgG or circulating platelet antibodies alone should not be used in determining the mode of delivery of the fetus of a thrombocytopenic mother. Percutaneous umbilical blood sampling may be performed to determine the fetal platelet count. Those fetuses with platelet counts greater than 50,000/μl may be delivered vaginally, whereas those with lower counts should be delivered by cesarean section. McCrae et al. point out, however, that the risk of fetal blood sampling may, in fact, outweigh the risk of intracranial hemorrhage resulting from the trauma of vaginal delivery and that more data are required before definitive recommendations can be made.

Immune Modulation

It was once thought that blood transfusions, with their propensity to evoke alloimmunization might cause decreased survival of a kidney transplant. It has been well demonstrated that, as long as the donor kidney is ABO compatible with the recipient and a crossmatch between recipient serum and donor histocompatibility antigens is negative, blood transfusions can actually enhance the survival of a kidney transplant (see Chs. 4, 6, and 35).[101,102]

Graft-Versus-Host Disease

Transfusion-induced GVHD may occur in certain susceptible recipients as a result of viable lymphocytes in blood components. Except for FFP and cryoprecipitate (which are largely acellular and frozen without cryoprotective agents),[103] all blood components contain sufficient viable lymphocytes to initiate GVHD in patients. Whole blood, washed RBC, platelet concentrates, and especially granulocyte concentrates have all been associated with GVHD. WBC concentrates (including buffy coat infusions) are one of the most often implicated blood compo-

nents in transfusion-acquired GVHD.[104,105] Frozen-thawed RBC have not been implicated in GVHD but contain sufficient viable lymphocytes to initiate GVHD in high-risk patients, because 10^7 to 10^8 lymphocytes are present in frozen-thawed RBC, considerably more than 44×10^4 lymphocytes in fresh plasma that caused GVHD in three patients with severe combined immunodeficiency disorders.[103] "Fresh" blood may be more likely to cause GVHD than blood that has been stored for several days.[106] Acute GVHD has its onset 4 to 30 days after a transfusion; chronic GVHD usually begins more than 100 days after an implicated transfusion.[103] Few patients manifest acute GVHD first and then subsequent chronic GVHD because most die during the acute phase. The onset of GVHD in some patients is with the chronic form of the disease, however.

Acute GVHD begins with a high fever but is followed within 24 to 48 hours by a diffuse, erythematous, maculopapular rash. The eruption rapidly progresses to generalized erythroderma and often results in bullae and generalized desquamation. Gastrointestinal symptoms of anorexia, nausea, and vomiting are frequently accompanied by a profuse, watery diarrhea of 5 to 8 L/day. Liver enlargement and jaundice may or may not be evident, but markedly elevated transaminase values and hyperbilirubinemia are usually present. Pancytopenia is usually profound and is the primary finding that differentiates transfusion-induced GVHD[23] from that after marrow transplantation, which is less lethal and of more delayed onset (typically 35 to 70 days after a marrow transplant). The treatment of acute, transfusion-induced GVHD is usually ineffective, with more than 90 percent of those affected dying, usually of overwhelming sepsis.

Chronic GVHD after a transfusion has a more insidious onset than does acute GVHD. Beginning more than 100 days after an implicated transfusion, a scleroderma-like illness may herald chronic GVHD. Skin atrophy, tightening, and ulceration may occur, especially about the joints. Sicca syndrome, bronchitis, and interstitial pneumonitis may follow. Except for a slight elevation of liver function test values, liver disease may not be apparent. There may also be a malabsorption syndrome, with minimal diarrhea as the gastrointestinal manifestation of chronic GVHD.

Table 41-5. Patients at Risk of Transfusion-Induced Graft-Versus-Host Disease

High Risk	Relative Risk	Negligible Risk
Severe combined immunodeficiency disease	Wiskott-Aldrich syndrome	Aplastic anemia
	Intrauterine transfusion recipients	
Allogeneic or autologous bone marrow transplantation or peripheral stem cell infusion	Neonatal exchange transfusion recipients (especially after intrauterine transfusion)	Acquired immunodeficiency syndrome
		Humoral immunodeficiency states
		Granulocyte dysfunction syndromes
HLA-matched components, including those from blood relatives, even without immune compromise of patient	Acute leukemia and lymphoma during nadir of chemotherapy-induced marrow suppression	
	Solid tumors treated with chemotherapy or radiation therapy	

Prevention

Irradiation is the most feasible means to inactivate lymphocytes (without harming other constituents)[107] in blood components to obviate GVHD. A dose of 2,500 cGy is sufficient to inactivate the lymphocytes without harming the other cellular or humoral components of blood.[103] The types of patients at risk of transfusion-induced GVHD, and thus the indications for use of irradiated blood and components, are summarized in Table 41-5. This topic is covered in more detail in Chapter 42.

Other Delayed Immunologic Effects of Transfusions

Viable, mononuclear cells in donor blood may result in other immunologic effects in recipients besides GVHD. Donors who have had tuberculosis and/or are purified protein derivative positive can transfer delayed hypersensitivity to recipients by the lymphocytes in their blood.[108] If a patient has a positive skin test response develop to tuberculin, consider whether this might have been caused by a blood transfusion in the previous months. A blood donor's lymphocytes can react against those of a recipient and be the cause of a transient, atypical lymphocytosis after transfusion.[109]

Nonimmunologic Delayed Complications of Blood Transfusion

Disease Transmission

Blood donors may carry a variety of pathogens in their blood despite their apparent healthy status. Viral hepatitis, primarily due to HCV and hepatitis B virus, can be transmitted by asymptomatic blood donor carriers and is still the most significant risk of a transfusion, despite the best efforts of the blood bank. Transmission of HIV, the retrovirus responsible for AIDS, and other retroviruses continue to be a concern despite their minute risk after transfusions.[110–113] Transfusion-transmitted malaria and babesiosis occur rarely, and syphilis almost never occurs. CMV remains a concern in certain immunosuppressed patients. Transfusion-transmitted infectious diseases are discussed at length in Chapters 36 to 40.

Iron Overload: Transfusion Hemosiderosis Hemochromatosis

Every pint of blood contains approximately 200 mg of iron complexed with its hemoglobin. Although the iron in blood is not a problem for most transfused patients, it poses a threat to chronically transfused patients who do not have continuing blood losses. In individuals with congenital hemolytic anemias or long-standing aplastic anemia, the iron load of chronic transfusion therapy can become deleterious over time. Transfusion hemosiderosis may be manifested after the transfusion of as few as 100 units of blood in these chronically transfused patients. Unless some means is taken to remove the excess iron from the body, it accumulates in critical organs such as the liver, heart, and endocrine glands and eventually causes failure of these organs. Iron chelation therapy can be effective in reducing the accumulated body iron, but it is a slow, tedious process (see Ch.

25).[114] Oral iron chelators may be an effective and safe means of reducing body iron in the future.[115] Transfusion should be kept to a minimum in this patient population, specifically to reduce the likelihood of transfusion hemosiderosis. Transfusion with neocytes (young RBC) has been reported to be effective in decreasing the rate of iron accumulation,[116] as has the use of erythrocytopheresis.[117]

REFERENCES

1. Sazama K: Reports of 355 transfusion-associated deaths: 1976 through 1985. Transfusion 30:583, 1990
2. Pineda AA, Brzica SM, Taswell HF: Hemolytic transfusion reaction. Recent experience in a large blood bank. Mayo Clin Proc 53:378, 1978
3. Thulstrup H: The influence of leukocyte and thrombocyte incompatibility on nonhaemolytic transfusion reactions: a retrospective study. Vox Sang 21:233, 1971
4. Kevy SV, Schmidt PJ, McGinniss MH, Workman WG: Febrile, non-hemolytic transfusion reactions and the limited role of leukoagglutinins in their etiology. Transfusion 2:7, 1962
5. Braude AI: Transfusion reactions from contaminated blood: their recognition and treatment. N Engl J Med 258:1289, 1958
6. Elin RJ, Lundberg WB, Schmidt PJ: Evaluation of bacterial contamination in blood processing. Transfusion 15:260, 1975
7. Ahrons S, Kissmeyer-Nielsen F: Serological investigations of 1,358 transfusion reactions in 74,000 transfusions. Dan Med Bull 15:259, 1968
8. Ryder SW, Oberman HA: Compatibility of common intravenous solutions with CPD blood. Transfusion 15:250, 1975
9. Staples PJ, Griner PF: Extracorporeal hemolysis of blood in a microwave blood warmer. N Engl J Med 285:217, 1971
10. Sazama K, Klein H, Davey R, Corash L: Intraoperative hemolysis: the initial manifestation of glucose-6-phosphate dehydrogenase deficiency. Arch Intern Med 140:845, 1980
11. Davey R, Lee B, Coles S: Acute intraoperative hemolysis following rapid infusion of hypotonic solution. Lab Med 17:282, 1986
12. Petz LD: Drug-induced immune hemolytic anemia. p.53. In Nance ST (ed): Immune Destruction of Red Blood Cells. American Association of Blood Banks, Arlington, 1989
13. Vyas GN, Holmdahl L, Perkins HA, Fudenberg HH: Serologic specificity of human anti-IgA and its significance in transfusion. Blood 34:573, 1969
14. Dolovich H, Sagona M, Pearson F et al: Sensitization of repeat plasmapheresis donors to ethylene oxide gas. Transfusion 27:90, 1987
15. Miller WV, Holland PV, Sugarbaker E et al: Anaphylactic reaction to IgA: a difficult transfusion problem. Am J Clin Pathol 54:618, 1970
16. Popovsky MA, Moore SB: Diagnostic and pathogenetic considerations in transfusion-related acute lung injury. Transfusion 25:573, 1985
17. Popovsky MA, Chaplin HC, Moore SB: Transfusion-related acute lung injury: a neglected, serious complication of hemotherapy. Transfusion 32:589, 1992
18. Mariott HL, Kekwick A: Volume and rate in blood transfusion for the relief of anemia. BMJ 1:1043, 1940
19. Holland PV, Wallerstein RD: Delayed hemolytic transfusion reaction with acute renal failure. JAMA 204:1007, 1968
20. Pineda AA, Taswell HF, Brzica SM: Delayed hemolytic transfusion reaction: an immunologic hazard of blood transfusion. Transfusion 18:1, 1978
21. Bruce-Chwatt LJ: Transfusion-associated parasitic infections. p. 101. In Sandler SG, Nusbacher J, Shanfield MS (eds): Immunobiology of the Erythrocyte. Alan R. Liss, New York, 1985
22. Smith RP, Evans AT, Popovsky MA et al: Transfusion-acquired babesiosis and failure of antibiotic treatment. JAMA 256:2726, 1986
23. Holland PV: Transfusion-associated graft-versus-host disease: Prevention using irradiated blood products. p. 295. In Garratty G (ed): Current Concepts in Transfusion Therapy. American Association of Blood Banks, Arlington, 1985
24. Alter HJ, Purcell RH, Feinstone SM, Tegtmeier GE: Non-A, non-B hepatitis: its relationship to cytomegalovirus, to chronic hepatitis, and to direct and indirect test methods. p. 272. In Szmuness W, Alter HJ, Maynard JE (eds): Viral Hepatitis 1981 International Symposium. Franklin Institute Press, Philadelphia, 1982
25. Yam PY, Petz LD, Knowlton RG et al: Use of DNA restriction fragment length polymorphisms to document marrow engraftment and mixed hematopoietic chimerism following bone marrow transplantation. Transplantation 43:399, 1987
26. Petz LD, Calhoun L, Yam P et al: Transfusion-associated graft-versus-host disease in immunocompetent patients: report of a fatal case associated with transfusion of blood from a second-degree relative, and a

survey of predisposing factors. Transfusion 33:742, 1993

27. Peterman TA, Jaffe HW, Feorino PM et al: Transfusion-associated acquired immunodeficiency syndrome in the United States. JAMA 254:2913, 1985

28. Gerber P, Walsh JH, Rosenbloom E, Purcell RH: Association of EB virus infection with the post perfusion syndrome. Lancet 1:593, 1969

29. Beauregard P, Blajchman MA: Hemolytic and pseudo-hemolytic transfusion reactions: an overview of the hemolytic transfusion reactions and the clinical conditions that mimic them. Transfusion Med Rev 8: 184, 1994

30. Hoffman M: Antibody-coated erythrocytes induce secretion of tumor necrosis factor by human monocytes: a mechanism for the production of fever by incompatible transfusions. Vox Sang 60:184, 1991

31. Davenport RD, Burdick M, Moore SA, Kunkel SL: Cytokine production in IgG-mediated red cell incompatibility. Transfusion 33:19, 1993

32. Davenport RD, Strieter RM, Standiford TJ, Kunkel SL: Interleukin-8 production in red blood cell incompatibility. Blood 76:2439, 1990

33. Davenport RD, Kunkel SL: Cytokine roles in hemolytic and nonhemolytic transfusion reactions. Transfusion Med Rev 8:157, 1994

34. Schmidt PJ, Holland PV: Pathogenesis of the acute renal failure associated with incompatible transfusion. Lancet 2:1169, 1967

35. Heustis DW, Bove JR, Busch S: Practical Blood Transfusion. 2nd Ed. Little, Brown, Boston, 1976

36. Mollison PL, Englefriet CP, Contreras M: Blood Transfusion in Clinical Medicine. 9th Ed. Blackwell Scientific Publications, London, 1993

37. Schmidt PJ: The mortality of incompatible transfusion. p. 251. In Sandler SG, Nusbacher J, Shanfield MS (eds): Immunobiology of the Erythrocyte. Alan R. Liss, New York, 1980

38. Fink DJ, Petz LD, Black MD: Serum haptoglobin: a valuable diagnostic aid in suspected hemolytic transfusion reactions. JAMA 199:615, 1967

39. Wiesen AR, Hospenthal DR, Byrd JC et al: Equilibration of hemoglobin concentration after transfusion in medical inpatients not actively bleeding. Ann Intern Med 121:278, 1994

40. Barry KG, Crosby WH: The prevention and treatment of renal failure following transfusion reactions. Transfusion 3:34, 1963

41. Goldfinger D: Acute hemolytic transfusion reactions—a fresh look at pathogenesis and considerations regarding therapy. Transfusion 17:85, 1977

42. Smith DM, Jr: Management of transfusion reactions.

p. 121. In Judd WJ, Barnes A (eds): Clinical and Serological Aspects of Transfusion Reactions. American Association of Blood Banks, Arlington, 1982

43. Bick RL, Bennett JM, Brynes RK et al (eds): Hematology. Clinical and Laboratory Practice. CV Mosby, St. Louis, 1993

44. Woodcock BE, Walker S, Adams K: Haemolytic transfusion reaction—successful attenuation with methyprednisolone and high dose immunoglobulin. Clin Lab Haematol 15:59, 1993

45. Popovsky M: Immune mediated transfusion reactions. p. 205. In Nance SJ (ed): Immune Destruction of Red Blood Cells. American Association of Blood Banks, Arlington, 1989

46. Lostumbo MM, Holland PV, Schmidt PJ: Isoimmunization after multiple transfusions. N Engl J Med 175: 141, 1966

47. Stewart JW, Mollison PL: Rapid destruction of apparently compatible cells. BMJ 1:1247, 1959

48. Laschinger C, Shepherd FA, Naylor DH: Anti-IgA-mediated transfusion reactions in Canada. Can Med Assoc J 130:141, 1984

49. Rivat L, Rivat C, Daveau M, Ropartz C: Comparative frequencies of anti-IgA antibodies among patients with anaphylactic transfusion reactions and among normal blood donors. Clin Immunol Immunopathol 7:340, 1977

50. Sandler SG, Eckrich R, Mamamut D, Mallory D: Hemagglutination assays for the diagnosis and prevention of IgA anaphylactic transfusion reactions. Blood 84:2031, 1994

51. Pineda AA, Taswell HF: Transfusion reactions associated with anti-IgA antibodies: report of four cases and review of the literature. Transfusion 15:10, 1975

52. Popovsky MA, Abel MD, Moore SB: Transfusion-related acute lung injury associated with passive transfer of antileukocyte antibodies. Annu Rev Respir Dis 128:185, 1983

53. Worsley MH, Sinclair CJ, Campanella C et al: Noncardiogenic pulmonary edema after transfusion with granulocyte antibody containing blood: treatment with extracorporeal membrane oxygenation. Br J Anaesth 67:116, 1991

54. Goldfinger D, Lowe C: Prevention of adverse reactions to blood transfusion by the administration of saline-washed red blood cells. Transfusion 21:277, 1981

55. Brubaker DB: Clinical significance of white cell antibodies in febrile nonhemolytic transfusion reactions. Transfusion 30:733, 1990

56. Dzik WH: Is the febrile response to transfusion due

to donor or recipient cytokine? Transfusion 32:594, 1992

57. Muylle L, Joos M, Wouters E et al: Increased tumor necrosis factor α (TNF α), interleukin 1, and interleukin 6 (IL-6) levels in the plasma of stored platelet concentrates: relationship between TNFα and IL-6 levels and febrile transfusion reactions. Transfusion 33:195, 1993

58. Heddle NM, Klama LN, Griffith L et al: A prospective study to identify the risk factors associated with acute reactions to platelet and red cell transfusions. Transfusion 33:794, 1993

59. Stack G, Snyder EL: Cytokine generation in stored platelet concentrates. Transfusion 34:20, 1994

60. Muylle L, Wouters E, DeBock R, Peetermans ME: Reactions to platelet transfusion: the effect of the storage time of the concentrate. Transfusion Med 2: 289, 1992

61. Heddle NM, Klama L, Singer J et al: The role of the plasma from platelet concentrates in transfusion reactions. N Engl J Med 331:58, 1994

62. Friedlander M, Noble WH: Meperidine to control shivering associated with platelet transfusion reaction. Can J Anaesth 36:460, 1989

63. Herzig RH, Herzig GP, Bull MI et al: Correction of poor platelet transfusion responses with leukocyte-poor HLA-matched platelet concentrates. Blood 46: 743, 1975

64. Mangano MM, Chambers LA, Kruskall MS: Limited efficacy of leukopoor platelets for prevention of febrile transfusion reactions. Am J Clin Pathol 95:733, 1991

65. Goodnough LT, Riddell J, Lazarus H et al: Prevalence of platelet transfusion reactions before and after implementation of leukocyte-depleted platelet concentrates by filtration. Vox Sang 65:103, 1993

66. Chambers LA, Kruskall MS, Pacini DG, Donovan LM: Febrile reactions after platelet transfusion: the effect of single versus multiple donors. Transfusion 30:219, 1990

67. Muylle L, Peetermans ME: Effect of prestorage leukocyte removal of the cytokine levels in stored platelet concentrates. Vox Sang 66:14, 1994

68. Wagner SJ, Friedman LI, Dodd RY: Transfusion-associated bacterial sepsis. Clin Microbiol Rev 7:290, 1994

69. Heltberg O, Skov F, Gerner-Smidt P et al: Nosocomial epidemic of *Serratia marcescens* septicemia ascribed to contaminated blood transfusion bags. Transfusion 33:221, 1993

70. Yomtovian R, Lazarus HN, Goodnough LT et al: A prospective microbiologic surveillance program to detect and prevent the transfusion of bacterially contaminated platelets. Transfusion 33:902, 1993

71. Blajchman MA, Ali AM, Richardson HL: Bacterial contamination of cellular blood components. Vox Sang, suppl. 3:25, 1994

72. Ciavarella D: Sepsis after platelet transfusions. JAMA 267:1206, 1992

73. Sazama K: Bacteria in blood for transfusion. Arch Pathol Lab Med 118:350, 1994

74. Kim DM, Brecher ME, Bland LA et al: Visual identification of bacterially contaminated red cells. Transfusion 32:221, 1992

75. Morrow JF, Braine HG, Kickler TS et al: Septic reactions to platelet transfusion. JAMA 266:555, 1991

76. Shulman NR, Weinrach RS, Libre EP, Andrews HL: The role of the reticuloendothelial system in the pathogenesis of idiopathic thrombocytopenic purpura. Trans Assoc Am Physicians 78:374, 1965

77. Quick AJ: Influence of erythrocytes on the coagulation of blood. Am J Med Sci 239:101, 1960

78. Marshall BE, Wurzel HA, Ellison N et al: Microaggregate formation in stored blood: III. comparison of Bentley, Fenwal, Pall and Swank micropore filtration. Circ Shock 2:249, 1975

79. Counts RB, Haisch C, Simon TL et al: Hemostasis in massively transfused trauma patients. Ann Surg 190: 91, 1979

80. Boyan CP, Howland WS: Cardiac arrest and temperature of bank blood. JAMA 183:58, 1963

81. Dzik WH, Kirkley SA: Citrate toxicity during massive blood transfusion. Transfusion Med Rev 2:76, 1988

82. Doyle DJ, Livingston P: Transfusion-related 2-to-1 electromechanical block during surgery. Can J Anaesth 36:732, 1989

83. Wolf PL, McCarthy LJ, Hafleigh B: Extreme hypercalcemia following blood transfusion combined with intravenous calcium. Vox Sang 19:544, 1970

84. Bailey DN, Bove JR: Chemical and hematological changes in stored CPD blood. Transfusion 15:244, 1975

85. Hall TL, Barnes A, Miller JR et al: Neonatal mortality following transfusion of red cells with high plasma potassium levels. Transfusion 33:606, 1993

86. Alving BM, Hojima Y, Pisano JJ et al: Hypotension associated with prekallikrein activator (Hageman-factor fragments) in plasma protein fraction. N Engl J Med 299:66, 1978

87. Diamond WJ, Brown F, Bitterman P et al: Delayed hemolytic transfusion reaction presenting as sickle cell crisis. Ann Intern Med 93:231, 1980

88. Milner PF, Squires JE, Larison PJ et al: Posttransfusion crises in sickle cell anemia: role of delayed hemo-

lytic reactions to transfusion. South Med J 78:1462, 1985

89. Goldfinger D, McGinnis MH: Rh-incompatible platelet transfusions: risks and consequences of sensitizing immunosuppressed patients. N Engl J Med 284:942, 1971

90. Brittingham TE, Chaplin H: Febrile transfusion reactions caused by sensitivity to donor leukocytes and platelets. JAMA 165:819, 1957

91. Mueller-Eckhardt C, Lechner K, Heinrich D et al: Post-transfusion thrombocytopenia purpura: immunological and clinical studies in two cases and review of the literature. Blut 40:249, 1980

92. Shulman NR: Posttransfusion purpura: clinical features and the mechanism of platelet destruction. p. 137. In Nance SJ (ed): Clinical and Basic Aspects of Immunohematology. American Association of Blood Banks, Arlington, 1991

93. Gerstner JB, Smith MJ, David KD et al: Posttransfusion purpura: therapeutic failure of Pl^{A1}-negative platelet transfusion. Am J Hematol 6:71, 1979

94. Lippman SM, Lizak GE, Foung SKH, Grumet FC: The efficacy of Pl^{A1}-negative platelet transfusion therapy in posttransfusion purpura. West J Med 148:86, 1988

95. Mueller-Eckhardt C: Post-transfusion purpura. Br J Haematol 64:419, 1986

96. Kelton JG, Blanchette VS, Wilson WE et al: Neonatal thrombocytopenia due to passive immunization: prenatal diagnosis and distinction between maternal platelet alloantibodies and autoantibodies. N Engl J Med 302:1401, 1980

97. McGill M, Mayhaus C, Hoff R, Carey P: Frozen maternal platelets for neonatal thrombocytopenia. Transfusion 27:347, 1987

98. Karpatkin M, Porges RF, Karpatkin S: Platelet counts in infants of women with autoimmune thrombocytopenia: effect of steroid administration to the mother. N Engl J Med 305:936, 1981

99. Handin RI: Neonatal immune thrombocytopenia—the doctor's dilemma (editorial). N Engl J Med 305:951, 1981

100. McCrae KR, Samuels P, Schreiber AD: Pregnancy-associated thrombocytopenia: pathogenesis and management. Blood 80:2697, 1992

101. Opelz G, Terasaki PI: Improvements of kidney-graft survival with increased numbers of blood transfusion. N Engl J Med 299:799, 1978

102. Cats S, Terasaki P, Perdue S et al: Effects of HLA typing and transfusions on cyclosporin-treated renal allograft recipients. N Engl J Med 311:675, 1984

103. Leitman SF, Holland PV: Irradiation of blood products: indications and guidelines. Transfusion 25:293, 1985

104. Lowenthal RM, Goldman JM, Buskard NA et al: Granulocyte transfusions in treatment of infections in patients with acute leukemia and aplastic anemia. Lancet 1:353, 1975

105. Rosen RD, Heustis DW, Corrigan JJ: Acute leukemia and granulocyte transfusion: fatal graft-versus-host reaction following transfusion of cells obtained from normal donors. J Pediatrics 93:268, 1978

106. Petz LD, Calhoun L, Yam P et al: Transfusion-associated graft-versus-host disease in immunocompetent patients: report of a fatal case associated with transfusion of blood from a second-degree relative, and a survey of predisposing factors. Transfusion 33:742, 1993

107. Button LN, DeWolf WC, Newburger PE et al: The effects of irradiation upon blood components. Transfusion 21:419, 1981

108. Mohr JA, Killebrew L, Muchmore HG et al: Transfer of delayed hypersensitivity: the role of blood transfusion in humans. JAMA 207:517, 1969

109. Schechter JP, Soehnlen F, McFarland W: Lymphocyte response to blood transfusion in man. N Engl J Med 287:1169, 1972

110. Dodd RY: The risk of transfusion-transmitted infection (editorial). N Engl J Med 327:419, 1992

111. Cumming PD, Wallace EL, Schorr JB, Dodds RY: Exposure of patients to human immunodeficiency virus through the transfusion of blood components that test antibody-negative. N Engl J Med 321:947, 1989

112. Ward JW, Holmberg SD, Allen JR et al: Transmission of human immunodeficiency virus (HIV) by blood transfusions screened as negative for HIV antibody. N Engl J Med 318:473, 1988

113. Zuck TF: Transfusion-transmitted AIDS reassessed. N Engl J Med 318:511, 1988

114. Hoffbrand AV, Gorman A, Laulicht M et al: Improvement in iron status and liver function in patients with transfusional iron overload with long-term subcutaneous desferrioxamine. Lancet 1:947, 1979

115. Nathan DG, Piomelli S: Oral iron chelators. Semin Hematol 27:83, 1990

116. Propper RD, Button LN, Nathan DG: New approach to the transfusion management of thalassemia. Blood 55:1, 1980

117. Kim HC, Dugan NP, Silber JH et al: Erythrocytapheresis therapy to reduce iron overload in chronically transfused patients with sickle cell disease. Blood 83:1136, 1994

Graft-Versus-Host Disease

Ramesh A. Shivdasani and
Kenneth C. Anderson

Graft-versus-host disease (GVHD) is a frequent complication of allogeneic bone marrow transplantation (ABMT), in which setting viable lymphocytes derived from the donor bone marrow cannot be eliminated by an immunodeficient host. GVHD is mediated by the donor T lymphocytes that recognize host HLA antigens as foreign and mount a vigorous immune response, which is manifested clinically by the development of fever, a characteristic cutaneous eruption, diarrhea, and liver function abnormalities.[1] GVHD is also encountered, although less frequently, in the setting of solid organ transplantation, in which case it is mediated by T lymphocytes that may be present in the transplanted organ.[2] Along the same lines, GVHD can occur as a complication of transfusion of cellular blood components, which also usually contain donor T lymphocytes. A number of reports in the 1970s and 1980s served to establish transfusion-associated GVHD (TA-GVHD) as a distinct disease entity,[3–8] and the number of reported cases has been increasing. In addition to the aforementioned clinical features, TA-GVHD is further characterized by marrow aplasia, resulting in pancytopenia; in contrast to GVHD that develops in the setting of ABMT, TA-GVHD is notoriously resistant to treatment, almost always resulting in rapid death.

PATHOPHYSIOLOGY

The central issue in the pathogenesis of GVHD is the extent to which the recipient of a graft or transfusion is able to mount an immune response against donor T lymphocytes. The immune status of the host and the extent of HLA disparity between donor and recipient together determine the extent of any host-versus-graft reaction. Thus, Billingham[9] proposed three requirements for the development of GVHD: (1) differences in HLA between the donor and the recipient, (2) the presence of immunocompetent cells in the graft, and (3) inability of the host to reject these immunocompetent cells.

Because transfused cellular blood products are rarely tested for HLA antigens, the first of these requirements is almost always present in the circumstance of blood transfusion. TA-GVHD is mediated by the viable T lymphocytes that inevitably contaminate nonirradiated transfused cellular blood products. Congenital or acquired immunodeficiency states provide the most common and obvious basis for an individual's failure to reject donor-derived cells, and TA-GVHD has been described in a wide variety of patients with apparent immune compromise;[5] the naturally or iatrogenically immunosuppressed recipient has only a limited capacity to generate an effective host-versus-graft reaction. As in GVHD post-BMT, greater HLA disparity between the donor and the recipient confers increased probability that donor lymphocytes will attack host tissues.

Because immune cells in an immunocompetent host typically far outnumber donor-derived T cells, the latter are effectively eliminated by virtue of a host-versus-graft reaction. However, if an immunocompetent HLA-heterozygous individual is transfused with functional T lymphocytes derived from a donor who is homozygous for one of the recipient's HLA haplotypes, the recipient's immune system does not recognize the major histocompatibility antigens on these cells as being foreign and is therefore incapable of eliminating them. Conversely, some donor-derived T cells recognize those host HLA antigens that are encoded by the unshared haplotype as being foreign, undergo clonal expansion, and establish TA-GVHD.[10] The HLA relationship between such individuals is referred to as a "one-way HLA match," and the TA-GVHD expressed under these circumstances may be expected to occur regardless of the host's immune status because the failure to eliminate donor-derived T lymphocytes is based on the genetics of the HLA system rather than on variables that contribute to immune competence per se.

In both immunocompetent and immunodeficient hosts, TA-GVHD is characterized by inexorable proliferation of donor T lymphocytes and rapid elimination of all circulating host cellular blood elements; an elegant demonstration of this immunologic basis for the disease was provided by Ito et al.[6] Furthermore, in one patient with chronic myelogenous leukemia who received a T-cell-depleted histocompatible marrow allograft, both graft rejection and GVHD developed, and a variety of tests confirmed that cells in the peripheral blood and bone marrow were not derived from either the donor or the recipient.[11] These cells were thought to represent a population of proliferating transfused cells that were alloreactive against both donor and host.

Lee et al.[12] applied a quantitative allele-specific polymerase chain reaction (PCR) to follow the fate of donor leukocytes after transfusion into humans and dogs. Their preliminary results demonstrate rapid clearance of cells on the first day followed by a transient 1 to 2 log expansion after 4 to 6 days, presumably reflecting delayed clonal expansion of selected cells. The characteristics of the proliferating leukocytes, the mechanism for their subsequent elimination, and the role of HLA antigens in this process are all unknown, but such studies are central to the understanding of TA-GVHD. The minimal number of donor lymphocytes required to mediate TA-GVHD is unclear; Von Fliedner et al.[5] surmised that transfusion of at least 10^7 lymphocytes/kg was

necessary, although the disease has been reported with transfusion of as few as 10^4 lymphocytes/kg.[13]

HISTORICAL PERSPECTIVE AND RISK GROUPS

In 1955, Shimoda[14] reported on the first Japanese case of "post-operative erythroderma," now considered to be the same disease as TA-GVHD. The syndrome was later described after transfusion in immunodeficient children in 1965.[15] Over the next 15 years, 38 cases of TA-GVHD were described in patients with severe combined immunodeficiency and Wiskott-Aldrich syndromes; in newborns with erythroblastosis fetalis; and in patients with hematologic malignancies, including Hodgkin's disease and non-Hodgkin's lymphoma, acute lymphoblastic and myelocytic leukemia, and chronic lymphocytic leukemia.[5] Although its true incidence remains unknown, TA-GVHD was estimated to occur in 0.1 to 1.0 percent of patients with hematologic malignancies or lymphoproliferative diseases, and all patients with the above diagnoses were believed to be at risk for TA-GVHD. The risk of developing TA-GVHD was also identified in patients with neuroblastoma and those who received intrauterine or exchange transfusions for hemolytic disease of the newborn.[16] In a 1987 review of 27 reported cases of TA-GVHD in patients with both hematologic malignancies and solid tumors (neuroblastoma, rhabdomyosarcoma, and glioblastoma), Kessinger et al.[17] noted that all affected patients had received cytotoxic chemotherapy and 13 had received prior radiation therapy. Cases of TA-GVHD have been documented in patients with Hodgkin's disease who were treated with either chemotherapy alone[18] or with a combination of chemotherapy and ionizing radiation.

TA-GVHD continues to be reported, albeit rarely, in patients with malignancies. It was originally recognized in patients with solid tumors who received intensive therapy for neuroblastoma.[19,20] Four of 34 patients with solid tumors (lung and germ cell cancer) who were treated with high doses of chemotherapy and autologous marrow infusions and subsequently received transfusions of nonirradiated blood cells also had TA-GVHD.[21] Case reports documenting TA-GVHD in patients with cervical, renal, esophageal, lung, bladder, and prostate carcinomas who did not receive aggressive chemotherapy indicate that a broader spectrum of patients with solid tumors may be at risk.[10,15,22–24] Cases of TA-GVHD have also been documented in premature infants who received unirradiated blood products in the setting of hyaline membrane disease or suspected sepsis and respiratory distress syndrome;[25,26] these patients did not have congenital immunodeficiency syndromes or erythroblastosis fetalis.

It is interesting that there have been no reported cases of TA-GVHD in patients with acquired immunodeficiency syndrome (AIDS). Perhaps some of the signs and symptoms (rashes, pancytopenia, and liver function abnormalities) presently attributed to infections, drug reactions, and other coexisting medical conditions in patients with AIDS are related to TA-GVHD. Alternatively, qualitative aspects of the nature of the immune deficit in AIDS may not predispose patients to the development of TA-GVHD. In addition, the disease has only rarely been reported in patients receiving immunosuppressive medications.

Solid organ transplant recipients might be expected to have a high incidence of TA-GVHD because they receive aggressive immunosuppressive treatment and are frequently transfused. Indeed, a number of patients have had GVHD develop after solid organ transplantation, particularly after liver transplantation.[2,27–34] However, in all but one of the cases in which the source of transplanted foreign cells was identified, their origin was the transplanted organ rather than the transfused blood products. The single exception occurred in a renal transplant recipient in whom life-threatening TA-GVHD developed after transfusion of whole blood in association with the transplant.[34]

Finally, TA-GVHD has been reported in individuals without obvious immunodeficiencies. In 1986, the syndrome was described after blood transfusion to an immunocompetent Japanese patient who had undergone surgery for an aortic aneurysm.[3] A survey of 340 Japanese hospitals documented "postoperative erythroderma," identical to TA-GVHD, in 96 of the 63,257 patients who underwent cardiac surgery, with a mortality rate of 90 percent.[35] Cases of TA-GVHD after cardiac surgery were subsequently reported from the United States and Israel.[36,37] More recently, fatal GVHD has been reported in a number of HLA-heterozygous transfusion recipients who shared a haplotype with related or unrelated HLA-homozygous donors (one-way HLA match).[10,38,39] Clinical settings in which TA-GVHD has been reported in immunocompetent hosts include pregnancy; cardiac, vascular, orthopaedic, and abdominal surgeries; cholecystectomy; α thalassemia; rheumatoid arthritis; trauma; and short-course glucocorticoid therapy.[39–45]

The groups of patients at risk for acquiring TA-GVHD are summarized in Table 42-1. It appears that many, but not all, conditions or treatments that compromise immunity predispose patients to the development of TA-GVHD. At the same time, immunocompetent individuals are not necessarily protected, particularly in the event of a one-way HLA match. The lack of uniform GVHD after transfusion of unirradiated blood components to patients who are known to be immunodeficient, coupled with the development of this syndrome in patients without in vitro immune dysfunction, suggests that the risk

Table 42-1. Risk Groups for Transfusion-Associated Graft-Versus-Host Disease

Patient groups at significant risk
    Bone marrow transplant recipients
    Congenital immunodeficiency syndromes
    Intrauterine transfusions
    Transfusions from blood relatives
    Premature newborns
    Neonates receiving exchange transfusion
    Patients receiving HLA-matched platelet transfusions
    Patients with Hodgkin's disease
Patient groups in which occasional case reports suggest some increased relative risk
    Hematologic malignancies other than Hodgkin's disease
        Acute leukemia
        Non-Hodgkin's lymphoma
    Solid organ transplant recipients
    Solid tumors treated with chemotherapy or radiation therapy
        Neuroblastoma
        Glioblastoma
        Rhabdomyosarcoma
        Immunoblastic sarcoma
No defined increased risk compared with the general population
    Full-term neonates
    Patients with acquired immunodeficiency syndrome
    Patients receiving immunosuppressive medications

factors predisposing to TA-GVHD are only partially defined. Blood transfusion itself may be immunosuppressive,[46] and the argument can be made that almost every patient who requires transfusion of a blood product is potentially immunocompromised in some way that could facilitate the development of TA-GVHD. The low incidence of TA-GVHD in presumably immunocompetent patients may result from under-recognition of the syndrome, as discussed above, but more likely reflects effective defense against it in individuals with truly intact immune function.

EPIDEMIOLOGY

All of the available epidemiologic data on TA-GVHD are based on reports of single or very small groups of patients. A prospective study on the development of this disease has never been undertaken and would, in fact, be very difficult to perform. Estimates of the incidence and identification of patient groups at risk are therefore subject to all the limitations of retrospective data; perhaps foremost among these are the under-reporting of cases and the absence of definitive diagnostic studies in many instances. At least two factors may contribute to the under-reporting of cases of TA-GVHD. First, the diagnosis may not be considered, and, second, it may be difficult or impossible to establish with certainty. Thus, although more than 200 cases of presumed TA-GVHD have been reported or referenced in the Japanese and English language literature, definitive diagnostic tests have been performed in only a handful of cases. Lists of published case reports and small series have been compiled in several review articles.[39,47,48] The overall reported mortality rate is approximately 90 percent, although rare survivors have been documented.[42,49]

CLINICAL MANIFESTATIONS

The clinical manifestations of TA-GVHD are similar to those of GVHD in other settings and include fever, rash, watery or bloody diarrhea, elevated liver enzymes, and hyperbilirubinemia. In addition, bone marrow failure, which manifests as pancytopenia, is a characteristic feature of the terminal phase of the disease and distinguishes it from GVHD that occurs after bone marrow or organ transplantation. The rash usually begins as an erythematous maculopapular eruption centrally, spreads to the extremities, and may progress to generalized erythroderma and bullous formation in severe cases. Similarly, diarrhea may be severe, and elevation of liver function test results can be extreme, reflecting extensive hepatocellular damage. Additional manifestations may include anorexia, nausea, and vomiting. Clinical and histopathologic features of the rash are shown in Figure 42-1 and the typical time course of findings and laboratory abnormalities in Figure 42-2.

Most cases of TA-GVHD are rapidly fatal. The time from onset of symptoms to death can be less than 1 week and rarely exceeds 3 weeks. Patients usually die of complications of bone marrow failure, primarily infection.

Because there are no pathognomonic features of GVHD, this syndrome is sometimes difficult to distinguish from viral infections or drug reactions. This assumes particular clinical importance in the transfusion-related disease, in which the index of suspicion for this diagnosis may be low and a patient who has required blood product support may harbor significant comorbidity. Nonetheless, characteristic changes are demonstrable on skin biopsy, including degeneration of the epidermal basal cell layer with vacuolization; dermal-epithelial layer separation and bullae formation; mononuclear cell migration into, and infiltration of, the upper dermis; hyperkeratosis; and degenerative dyskeratosis (Fig. 1B).[50,51] Liver biopsies reveal degeneration and eosinophilic necrosis of the small bile ducts with intense periportal inflammation and mononuclear (lymphocytic) infiltration.[52] Bone marrow aspirates reveal lymphocytic infiltration, pancytopenia, and possibly fibrosis.

DIAGNOSIS

Although the clinical syndrome associated with TA-GVHD is dramatic and frequently fatal, the differential diagnosis is broad. Myriad factors can result in the development of fevers, rashes, and liver function abnormalities. Certainly, other etiologic factors such as infection and drug reaction are more commonly encountered in clinical practice and more likely to be investigated. Although histologic findings in the skin and gastrointestinal tract may suggest the diag-

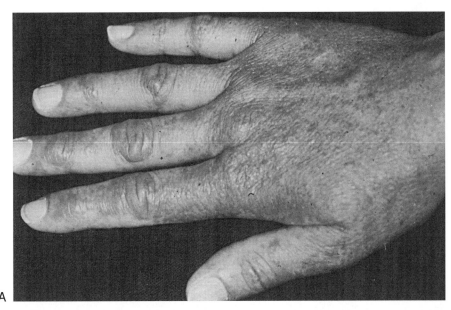

A

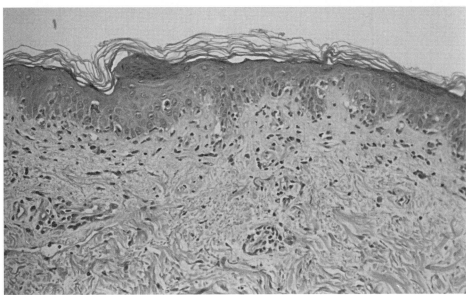

B

Fig. 42-1. **(A)** Typical rash seen in patients with TA-GVHD. (Courtesy of Richard Johnson, M.D.) **(B)** Typical skin biopsy appearance in patients with TA-GVHD. For details of each, see text.

nosis of TA-GVHD, they are not pathognomonic. The most conclusive evidence for the diagnosis of TA-GVHD rests on the demonstration of donor-derived lymphocytes in the circulation of a patient with characteristic clinical findings. This requires either careful HLA typing or some other technique that

reliably distinguishes between host and donor cells.[53–56] However, because the disease involves rapid elimination of circulating host blood cells, samples adequate for HLA typing frequently are not available. Some workers have circumvented this problem by using PCR-based methods for HLA typ-

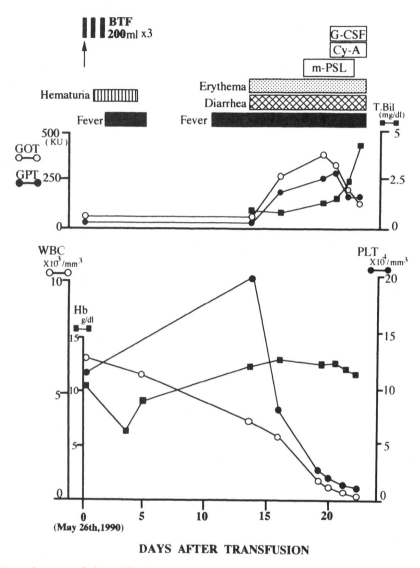

Fig. 42-2. Typical course of clinical findings and laboratory abnormalities in patients with TA-GVHD. Days after the implicated blood transfusion (arrow) are indicated on the x-axis. BTF, blood transfusion; M-PSL, methyl-prednisolone; T. BIL, total bilirubin; WBC, white blood cells; PLT, platelets; HB, hemoglobin; GOT, glutamic-oxaloacetic transaminase; GPT, glutamic-pyruvic transminase. *Abbreviations:* G-CSF, granulocyte colony stimulating factor; Cy-A, Cyclosporine A. (From Kobayashi et al.,[45] with permission.)

ing[24,53,54] or by deducing the patient's HLA type from those of surviving first-degree relatives.[10] Cytogenetic methods have been used in the event that donor and recipient have been of different gender or when the disease has followed transfusion of granulocytes donated by individuals with Philadelphia chromosome-positive chronic myeloid leukemia.[23] Increasingly sophisticated techniques for confirming the diagnosis of TA-GVHD have included the detection of polymorphisms for restriction fragment lengths and human microsatellite markers.[39,55] Even so, all too often the diagnosis is made postmortem.

Table 42-2. Methods Used to Diagnose or Document Transfusion-Associated Graft-Versus-Host Disease

Conventional HLA typing

Deduction of patient's HLA type from those of family members

DNA-based HLA typing using the polymerase chain reaction

Cytogenetic methods

Restriction fragment length polymorphisms

Polymorphism of human microsatellite markers

Identification of donor T cells by above techniques in skin biopsy samples

Table 42-3. Blood Products Implicated in Transfusion-Associated Graft-Versus-Host Disease

Whole blood, fresh or stored

Packed red blood cells

Platelet concentrates

Leukocytes
   From normal donors
   From donors with chronic myeloid leukemia

Liquid plasma

Methods that have been used to document TA-GVHD are summarized in Table 42-2.

The demonstration of donor-derived lympho-hematopoietic cells in a transfusion recipient is not diagnostic of TA-GVHD per se. As mentioned previously, preliminary data by Lee et al.[12] indicated that donor leukocytes can be detected in the recipient's circulation by sensitive recombinant DNA techniques 4 to 6 days after transfusion. Further studies are necessary to determine the frequency, extent, and significance of these findings. In addition, cells of donor origin may populate the blood and tissues of liver transplant recipients, resulting in a state of chimerism. This is not associated with GVHD, but, instead, donor-derived cells may induce tolerance to graft antigens.[57–62] Also, mixed hematopoietic chimerism has frequently been reported after ABMT, not necessarily in association with GVHD.[63–65] Indeed, some studies suggest that the development of mixed chimerism may induce transplantation tolerance,[66] and the incidence of acute GVHD after ABMT may be lower in patients with mixed chimerism than in patients with complete chimerism.[64,65]

BLOOD PRODUCTS IMPLICATED IN TA-GVHD

This syndrome has developed after exchange and intrauterine transfusions and after transfusion of whole blood, plasma, red blood cells, and platelets. Leukocytes harvested from normal donors and from donors with chronic myelocytic leukemia have also been transfused into patients with hematologic malignancies and have been implicated in TA-GVHD.

To date, transfusions of fresh frozen plasma, frozen deglycerolized red blood cells, and clotting factor concentrates have not been implicated as causes of TA-GVHD. This information is summarized in Table 42-3.

The risk of developing TA-GVHD appears to be related to the presence of functional contaminating T lymphocytes rather than to any specific blood product. Transfusions of red cells or platelets account for most cases, reflecting the higher frequency of transfusion of these components relative to other cellular blood products. Many affected patients received transfusions of freshly donated (i.e., not stored) cellular blood products. Because fresh blood contains larger numbers of viable (and presumably competent) lymphocytes than blood that has been stored for a period before transfusion,[56] the use of unstored blood surfaced as a major risk factor for the development of TA-GVHD in univariate analysis.[39] In view of this, the practice of transfusing freshly donated unirradiated blood is strongly discouraged, even in Japan, where this was, until recently, a common clinical practice. However, it appears that lymphocytes that survive the storage process can mediate TA-GVHD in some patients because cases of TA-GVHD have occurred after transfusion of blood products that have been stored for variable times.[43,56]

Cases of TA-GVHD after transfusions of cellular blood products that had been irradiated or depleted of leukocytes by filtration are discussed below.

TA-GVHD IN IMMUNOCOMPETENT PATIENTS

Initial reports of TA-GVHD were limited to patients with either demonstrated or presumed immunodeficiency, which led to the belief that this was a prerequisite for the development of the disease.[5] Indeed, immunodeficient patients constitute the largest group at risk for TA-GVHD within the United States. Since 1986, however, the syndrome has been reported among apparently immunocompetent individuals from Japan, Israel, Great Britain, Australia, and the United States.[3,10,37,42,43] The clinical course and outcome in immunocompetent patients does not appear to be any different from those in immunocompromised hosts. A one-way HLA match, or significant sharing of HLA antigens between donor and recipient, may account for many of the cases of TA-GVHD in immunocompetent patients and may be a contributing factor in at least some of the cases in immunocompromised patients. Based on the likelihood of a one-way HLA match, certain groups are intrinsically at risk for the development of TA-GVHD, that is, patients who receive blood products donated by close relatives and individuals from a population with limited genetic heterogeneity who receive blood products donated by other individuals within the same population.

Related-donor transfusions account for about one-half of the cases of TA-GVHD reported in presumed immunocompetent patients.[39] Kanter[67] used a mathematic model to derive the risk of transfusion of blood from an HLA-homozygous donor to related HLA-heterozygous recipients who share that haplotype. Parents and children presented the greatest risk; surprisingly, second-degree related donors as a group presented a slightly greater risk than siblings. Most importantly, in this analysis, there was no sharp cutoff of risk among the various classes of related donors. In a retrospective analysis of published cases of TA-GVHD in patients who received chemotherapy for hematologic or solid neoplasms, Charpentier et al.[68] noted that 7 of 26 patients had received blood components donated by parents, children, or siblings and that a one-way HLA match was verified in 3 of these 7 cases. These data indicate that HLA relatedness or haploidentity may account for a significant proportion of cases of TA-GVHD, even in immunocompromised patients. They underscore the notion that a one-way HLA match presents a risk for the development of TA-GVHD independent of the host's immune status.

Most reported cases of TA-GVHD that occurred in patients who were presumed to be immunocom-

petent and who were transfused with blood products donated by an unrelated individual have been reported from Japan, where the population is relatively homogeneous. The application of mathematic models to population data on HLA haplotypes in various countries has yielded estimates for the probability of transfusion of blood from HLA homozygotes to heterozygotes with a shared haplotype. Takahashi et al.[69] estimated the probability as 1 in 312 in Japan, 1 in 1,024 in European whites, and 1 in 797 in North American whites. Ohto et al.[70] calculated the risk of HLA homozygosity of a donor for a haplotype shared by an unrelated Japanese patient as 1 in 874, with the relative risk of such an occurrence in Canadian, German, and U.S. whites being 1.9, 3.5, and 8.2, respectively. Interestingly, six of the eight Japanese cases of TA-GVHD in recipients of transfusions from unrelated donors involved the most common HLA haplotype in that country's population, HLA-A2Bw52C____,[38] and two other cases involved an HLA haplotype that is represented in 5.8 percent of the Japanese population.

These estimates, which suggest an approximately two- to fourfold difference between the frequency of HLA homozygosity of the donor for a haplotype shared by a patient in Japan and the frequency in whites, do not seem entirely to explain the strikingly higher incidence of TA-GVHD in immunocompetent patients in Japan. Thus, it appears that other factors also contribute to the frequency of TA-GVHD in Japan, particularly the common use of fresh blood, that is, blood used within 96 hours of collection (often used "immediately"). A combination of predisposing factors is likely to be present in many cases. A one-way HLA match may be critical, but it may not be sufficient to cause TA-GVHD unless it is combined with other factors, such as some degree of immune deficiency and/or the use of fresh blood.[39]

TREATMENT

Results on the treatment of TA-GVHD have been uniformly dismal, accounting for the high mortality rate associated with the disease. Attempted immunosuppressive therapies have included glucocorticoids, antithymocyte globulin, cyclosporine, cyclophosphamide, and anti-T-cell monoclonal antibodies.[10,17,20,39,71–74] Although some of these agents have been successful in the treatment of post-BMT GVHD, by and large, they have been ineffective for TA-GVHD. Resistance to treatment appears to reflect the pathophysiologic conditions rather than the common delays in diagnosis because patients whose conditions are diagnosed early in the course of the disease fare no better than those diagnosed later.

Rare responses to some of the commonly used agents have been reported.[43,49] However, it is difficult to extract meaningful guidelines for clinical practice from these anecdotal experiences. Because the disease has an immune basis, clinicians may consider a therapeutic trial of glucocorticoids despite the low likelihood of efficacy. TA-GVHD is a serious and increasingly frequent disease that demands a search for effective treatment.

γ IRRADIATION OF CELLULAR BLOOD COMPONENTS FOR PREVENTION OF TA-GVHD

Because attempts at treatment of TA-GVHD have been unsuccessful, the primary emphasis has been on prevention. Prevention of GVHD by γ irradiation of blood was first described in mice[75] and in humans 2 years later.[76,77] As little as 500 cGy of γ irradiation can abrogate the response of lymphocytes to allogeneic cells in a mixed lymphocyte culture, and 1,500 cGy can reduce the response to mitogen-induced stimulation by 90 percent.[78,79] Button et al.[80] examined the function of blood components after irradiation doses of 500 to 20,000 cGy and demonstrated that doses up to 5,000 cGy decreased mitogen stimulation by 98.5 percent without compromising the function of cells other than lymphocytes; specifically, red blood cells that were transfused without further storage after irradiation had no change in survival; granulocytes had normal in vitro bacterial killing capacity, chemotactic mobility, and superoxide production; and transfused irradiated platelets produced the expected increases in platelet counts and controlled hemostasis in thrombocytopenic patients. However, doses of 5,000 cGy decreased the yield of platelets post transfusion by one-third. Limiting dilution experiments suggest that the frequency of irradiated lymphocytes able to respond to mitogen is reduced by 5 to 6 $\log_{10}$ by irradiation at 1,500 to 2,000 cGy compared with nonirradiated controls,[11]

but a small percentage of lymphocytes do survive irradiation at these doses. The reactivity of T cells in mixed lymphocyte cultures and limiting dilution assays presumably serve as the best predictors for development of GVHD, and studies utilizing such assays indicate that doses of 2,500 to 3,000 cGy may be required for the complete inactivation of T cells in transfused cellular blood products.[81,82] The American Association of Blood Banks (AABB) *Standards for Blood Banks and Transfusion Services* indicates that, when irradiated blood products are indicated, blood and cellular components should be irradiated with a minimum of 2,500 cGy.[83] Ninety-seven percent of AABB institutions surveyed in 1989 utilized doses of 1,500 to 3,500 cGy.[84] The issue of quality control and standards for radiation treatment has merited some attention[85] and led to the recommendations by the Food and Drug Administration that validation studies be performed annually and after mechanical repairs. Also, the use of indicator devices, which signal exposure of the blood product container to radiation, is encouraged.

Several studies address the potential adverse consequences of irradiation followed by storage of blood products. Ramirez et al.[86] irradiated red cell concentrates at 3,000 cGy and noted a threefold elevation in potassium levels relative to controls. Rivet et al.[87] confirmed that potassium levels increase with length of storage in both irradiated and nonirradiated red cell concentrates, that the length of storage before irradiation does not significantly affect the potassium level, and that manual washing and reconstitution with fresh frozen plasma was effective in reducing the potassium levels of all red cell concentrates. The total infusion load of potassium appears to be clinically insignificant in adults[88] but may be substantial in neonates.[89–91] This has led to the recommendation that blood required for intrauterine, neonatal, or pediatric transfusion not be stored after irradiation[86] or that irradiated red cell concentrates used for neonatal transfusions be washed manually to reduce potassium levels.[87]

This issue has been thoughtfully reviewed by Strauss[92] who pointed out that the plasma level of K^+ of red cells irradiated and stored for up to 14 days before transfusion does not pose a risk to most neonatal patients who require small-volume transfusions given slowly. Even if the K^+ level is as high as

68 mM after storage, a 1-kg neonatal patient given 10 ml of sedimented red cells (hematocrit 80 percent) receives a total dose of only 0.136 mmol of K^+. The 24-hour maintenance requirement for K^+ of a 1-kg neonatal patient is about 1 mmol or 0.093 mmol/hr. Accordingly, routinely washing of irradiated red cells to remove excessive K^+ seems unwarranted. Obviously, good medical practice may dictate the need for washing irradiated red cells before transfusion to selected, problem patients (e.g., those to whom large volumes of red cells will be given during exchange transfusions or extracorporeal circulation, neonatal patients already being treated for documented hyperkalemia, and patients with pronounced renal failure).

Most recent studies have documented decreases in adenosine triphosphate, increases in potassium, and increases in plasma hemoglobin after irradiation of red cells (3,000 to 3,500 cGy) and storage for 42 days.[93,94] Red cell survival has been reported to be decreased after transfusion of stored irradiated (68 percent survival) vs. stored nonirradiated red cells (78 percent survival).[94] In contrast, studies to date suggest that γ irradiation of platelets with 2,000 to 3,000 cGy and subsequent storage for 5 days does not adversely affect in vitro platelet function or in vivo post-transfusion recovery and survival.[95,96]

Although γ irradiation remains the best proven method for abrogating the risk of TA-GVHD, it should be noted that at least three cases of GVHD after transfusion of irradiated blood components have been reported.[97,98] One occurred after transfusion of red cells and platelets treated with 1,500 cGy into a 10-year-old girl receiving chemotherapy for acute myelocytic leukemia, which had recurred after BMT.[97] The other two cases occurred after irradiation of blood products with 2,000 cGy.[11,98]

CURRENT PRACTICES AND GUIDELINES FOR THE PREVENTION OF TA-GVHD

Two attempts have been made to survey blood component irradiation practices. Greenbaum[48] surveyed 100 physicians selected at random from the membership directories of professional societies. Among 66 responders from 56 institutions, 30, 10, and 40.5 percent indicated that they provided irradiated blood products to all patients, potential or post-BMT

patients, and selected patients, respectively. Blood component irradiation practice has also been examined in a survey of 2,250 blood centers, hospital blood banks, or transfusion services that are institutional members of the AABB;[84] 12.3 percent of the institutions had on-site facilities for the irradiation of blood components. Of 9.4 million components transfused in 1989, 10.1 percent were irradiated, and 44 cases of TA-GVHD were identified. There was marked variability in blood component irradiation practice, even among groups in whom the risk of TA-GVHD is well defined. For example, 12, 19, and 32 percent of institutions did not provide irradiated components to recipients of ABMT, patients receiving autologous BMT, and those with congenital immunodeficiencies, respectively. Irradiated blood components were provided by 51.4, 34, 32, and 20 percent of institutions to patients with leukemias, Hodgkin's disease, non-Hodgkin's lymphoma, and solid tumors, respectively, and 24.5 percent provided irradiated blood products to patients with AIDS.

The AABB has delineated patient groups currently believed to be at risk for TA-GVHD and who should therefore receive only irradiated cellular blood components. The *Standards for Blood Banks and Transfusion Services* indicates that these patient categories are fetuses receiving intrauterine transfusions, selected immunoincompetent or immunocompromised recipients, recipients of donor units known to be from a blood relative, and recipients who have undergone bone marrow transplantation.[83] The major difficulty in complying with these standards is the problem in defining the "selected" immunoincompetent or immunocompromised recipients. Table 42-1 lists our assessment of patient groups at various relative risks for the development of TA-GVHD. This classification is based on clinical judgment and an analysis of the frequency of reported cases but is necessarily somewhat arbitrary and imprecise.

Directed donations from family members increase the likelihood of TA-GVHD because such donors have a higher probability than unrelated donors of sharing HLA antigens with recipients.[67] Irradiation of blood components from directed donations from relatives should be utilized to avoid this complication, and the AABB has broadened its original recommendation, now indicating that cellular blood components donated by a blood relative should be irradiated with at least 2,500 cGy before transfusion.[83]

In alloimmunized patients refractory to standard platelet transfusion therapy, the provision of HLA-matched platelets has been demonstrated to result in improved platelet count increments.[99] However, the provision of HLA-matched platelets increases the probability of transfusing a cellular blood product with a one-way HLA-match. Zeger et al.[100] indicated that 12 percent of HLA-matched plateletpheresis products were most likely homozygous for HLA-A and -B antigens, and 32 percent of these were transfused to a patient who shared one HLA-A and -B haplotype with the donor. Grishaber et al.[101] reported that 15 of 65 patients (23 percent) who received HLA-matched platelets received at least one transfusion from a donor who provided a one-way HLA match. Benson et al.[102] reported a case of fatal TA-GVHD associated with transfusions of HLA-matched, HLA-homozygous platelets from an unrelated donor. On the basis of these data, a number of investigators have suggested that it is prudent to irradiate HLA-matched platelet products.[39,100–102]

The cases of TA-GVHD reported after cardiac surgery in both Israel and Japan occurred after transfusion of fresh whole blood, presumably used for its purported improved hemostatic effects.[35,37] Indeed, in a review of TA-GVHD in immunocompetent patients, 33 of 39 patients had been transfused with "fresh" blood (less than 96 hours old).[39] Although a prospective randomized study provided no support for the use of fresh blood in adult patients undergoing coronary bypass surgery,[103] fresh blood did offer some advantage in children younger than 2 years old who underwent complex cardiac surgery, presumably because of improved platelet function.[104] However, there is no reason to alter storage time between donation and transfusion of blood components in an attempt to avoid TA-GVHD. Irradiation of blood products administered to the appropriate risk groups is a more reasonable course of action.

The relatively low frequency of TA-GVHD in immunocompetent patients who receive blood donated by unrelated donors has thus far precluded the broad application of γ irradiation to all transfused cellular blood products. Issues relating to cost, the logistics of irradiation in emergency and small clinic settings, and the exceedingly low risk of TA-GVHD have also been raised.[105]

FUTURE DIRECTIONS

There are two potential alternatives to γ irradiation for the prevention of TA-GVHD, but both are presently unproved. The first involves depletion of lymphocytes from blood products before transfusion. Reductions occur in both the incidence and severity of GVHD post-ABMT when T cells are eliminated from the donor marrow by a variety of techniques before grafting.[106,107] Most currently utilized ex vivo methods are capable of removing more than 90 percent of T cells from donor marrow, with approximately 10^7 residual marrow T lymphocytes.[108–111] Although it may not be either possible or practical to treat blood components in a similar fashion, techniques are presently available for the reduction of leukocytes from red cells, such as elimination of the buffy coat after centrifugation, direct or inverted dilution-centrifugation, washing, cotton or cellulose acetate filtration, and freezing.[112] Leukocytes can be removed from platelets by centrifugation and cotton or acetate filtration.[113–116] These techniques all deplete 2 to 3 $\log_{10}$ of leukocytes so that treated products would contain a residual of about 10^6 to 10^7 leukocytes. These efforts have evolved for the avoidance of leukocyte-related transfusion reactions or alloimmunization and are under investigation for viral depletion. However, because the number and precise T-cell populations required to mediate TA-GVHD remain undefined, it is unknown whether depletion of leukocytes with these currently available techniques would decrease the risk of TA-GVHD. It is known that frozen deglycerolized blood contains less than 2 percent residual lymphocytes with intact proliferative ability,[112] confirming that some immunocompetent T cells are present and suggesting that leukocyte reduction techniques may not constitute effective prophylaxis against TA-GVHD. Indeed, at least three cases of TA-GVHD have been reported after transfusion of leukocyte-reduced (filtered) red cells.[117–119] If leukocyte reduction can be shown to prevent TA-GVHD effectively, the cost-effectiveness of transfusions could be improved by allowing filtration to accomplish more than one objective.

Second, a canine model has been used to demonstrate that ultraviolet (UV) rather than γ irradiation of transfused leukocytes can abrogate GVHD in recipient animals.[120] Four dogs who received unirradiated leukocytes, two of three dogs given leukocytes irradiated with 20 mJ/cm^2 of UV light (200 to 300 nm), and none of three dogs transfused with leukocytes irradiated to 1,000 mJ/cm^2 developed GVHD. Preliminary studies in humans utilized UV irradiation of blood components to minimize alloimmunization.[121] Future studies will determine whether UV light can avoid either alloimmunization or TA-GVHD in transfusion recipients without adverse effects on in vitro function or in vivo recovery of treated red cells and platelets.

Finally, van der Mast et al.[122] raised the provocative suggestion that host T cells may exert protective effects against the development of TA-GVHD, at least in immunocompetent patients. It remains to be seen whether such an effect can ever be harnessed therapeutically. Meanwhile, the practical emphasis remains on γ irradiation, which has been shown to be effective not only in vitro in preventing lymphocyte reactivity but appears also to have initiated a decrease in the incidence of TA-GVHD.[123]

REFERENCES

1. Ferrara JL, Deeg HJ: Graft versus host disease. N Engl J Med 324:667, 1991
2. Burdick JF, Vogelsang GB, Smith WJ et al: Severe graft-versus-host disease in a liver transplant recipient. N Engl J Med 318:689, 1988
3. Hathaway WE, Fulginiti VA, Pierce CW et al: Graft versus host reaction following a single blood transfusion. JAMA 201:139, 1967
4. Dinsmore RE, Straus DJ, Pollack MS et al: Fatal graft-versus-host disease following blood transfusion in Hodgkin's disease documented by HLA typing. Blood 55:831, 1980
5. Von Fliedner V, Higby DJ, Kim U: Graft versus host reaction following blood transfusion. Am J Med 72:951, 1982
6. Ito K, Yoshida H, Yanagibashi K et al: Change of HLA phenotype in postoperative erythroderma (letter). Lancet 2:413, 1988
7. Sakakibara T, Juji T: Post-transfusion graft-versus-host disease after open heart surgery (letter). Lancet 2:1099, 1986
8. Sakakibara T, Ida T, Mannouji E et al: Post-transfusion graft-versus-host disease following open heart surgery: report of six cases. J Cardiovasc Surg (Torino) 30:687, 1989
9. Billingham RE: The biology of graft-versus-host reactions. Harvey Lect 62:21, 1967
10. Shivdasani RA, Haluska FG, Dock NL et al: Graft-versus-host disease associated with transfusion of blood from unrelated HLA-homozygous donors. N Engl J Med 328:766, 1993
11. Drobyski W, Thibodeau S, Truitt RL et al: Third party mediated graft rejection and graft-versus-host disease after T cell depleted bone marrow transplantation, as demonstrated by hypervariable DNA probes and HLA-DR polymorphism. Blood 74:2285, 1989
12. Lee TH, Donegan E, Slichter S, Busch MP: In vivo proliferation of donor leukocytes following allogeneic transfusions of immunocompetent recipients, abstracted. Transfusion, suppl. 33:51S, 1993
13. Rubinstein A, Radl J, Cottier H et al: Unusual combined immunodeficiency syndrome exhibiting kappa-IgD paraproteinemia, residual gut immunity and graft-versus-host reaction after plasma infusion. Acta Paediatr Scand 62:365, 1973
14. Shimoda T: The case report of post-operative erythroderma. Geka 17:487, 1955
15. Hathaway WE, Githens JH, Blackburn WR et al: Aplastic anemia, histiocytosis, and erythroderma in immunologically deficient children. N Engl J Med 273:953, 1965
16. Weiden P: Graft-vs-host disease following transfusion. Arch Intern Med 144:1557, 1984
17. Kessinger A, Armitage JO, Klassen LW et al: Graft versus host disease following transfusion of normal blood products to patients with malignancies. J Surg Oncol 36:206, 1987
18. Ekert H, Waters KD, Smith PJ et al: Treatment with MOPP or ChlVPP chemotherapy only for all stages of childhood Hodgkin's disease. J Clin Oncol 6:1845, 1988
19. Woods WG, Lubin BH: Fatal graft-versus-host disease following a blood transfusion in a child with neuroblastoma. Pediatrics 67:217, 1981
20. Kennedy JS, Ricketts RR: Fatal graft versus host disease in a child with neuroblastoma following a blood transfusion. J Pediatr Surg 21:1108, 1986
21. Postmus PE, Mulder NH, Elema JD: Graft versus host disease after transfusion of non-irradiated blood cells in patients having received autologous bone marrow. Eur J Cancer 24:889, 1988
22. Capon SM, DePond WD, Tynan DB et al: Transfusion-associated graft-versus-host disease in an immu-

nocompetent patient. Ann Intern Med 114:1025, 1991

23. Matsushita M, Shibata Y, Fuse K et al: Sex chromatin analysis of lymphocytes invading host organs in transfusion-associated graft-versus-host disease. Virchows Arch B Cell Pathol 55:237, 1988

24. Saito M, Takamatsu H, Nakao S et al: Transfusion-associated graft-versus-host disease after surgery for bladder cancer (letter). Blood 82:326, 1993

25. Sanders M, Graeber J, Zehnbauer B et al: Post transplant graft-versus-host disease in a premature infant without known risk factors, abstracted. Blood, suppl. 1, 72:384a, 1988

26. Berger RS, Dixon SL: Fulminant transfusion-associated graft-versus-host disease in a premature infant. J Am Acad Dermatol 20:945, 1989

27. Deierhoi MH, Sollinger HW, Bozdech MJ, Belzer FO: Lethal graft-versus-host disease in a recipient of a pancreas-spleen transplant. Transplantation 41:544, 1986

28. Collins RH, Jr, Cooper B, Nikaein A et al: Graft-versus-host disease in a liver transplant recipient. Ann Intern Med 116:391, 1992

29. Marubayashi S, Matsuzaka C, Takeda A et al: Fatal generalized acute graft-versus-host disease in a liver transplant recipient. Transplantation 50:709, 1990

30. Grant D, Garcia B, Wall W et al: Graft-versus-host disease after clinical small bowel/liver transplantation. Transplant Proc 22:2464, 1990

31. Jamieson NV, Joysey V, Friend PJ et al: Graft-versus-host disease in solid organ transplantation. Transplant Int 4:67, 1991

32. Roberts JP, Ascher NL, Lake J et al: Graft vs. host disease after liver transplantation in humans: a report of four cases. Hepatology 14:274, 1991

33. Corry RJ, Ngheim DD, Schulak JA et al: Surgical treatment of diabetic nephropathy with simultaneous pancreatic duodenal and renal transplantation. Surg Gynecol Obstet 162:547, 1986

34. Andersen CB, Ladefoged SD, Taaning E: Transfusion-associated graft-versus-graft and potential graft-versus-host disease in a renal allotransplanted patient. Hum Pathol 23:831, 1992

35. Juji T, Takahashi K, Shibata Y et al: Post-transfusion graft-versus-host disease in immunocompetent patients after cardiac surgery in Japan (letter). N Engl J Med 321:56, 1989

36. Arsura EL, Bertelle A, Minkowitz S et al: Transfusion-associated graft-versus-host disease in a presumed immunocompetent patient. Arch Intern Med 148:1941, 1988

37. Thaler M, Shamiss A, Orgad S et al: The role of blood from HLA-homozygous donors in fatal transfusion-associated graft-versus-host disease after open heart surgery. N Engl J Med 321:25, 1989

38. Otsuka S, Kunieda K, Kitamura F et al: The critical role of blood from HLA-homozygous donors in fatal transfusion-associated graft-versus-host disease in immunocompetent patients. Transfusion 31:260, 1991

39. Petz LD, Calhoun L, Yam P et al: Transfusion-associated graft-versus-host disease in immunocompetent patients. Report of a fatal case associated with transfusion of blood from a second-degree relative, and a survey of predisposing factors. Transfusion 33:742, 1993

40. Otsuka S, Kunieda K, Hirose M et al: Fatal erythroderma (suspected graft-versus-host disease) after cholecystectomy. Transfusion 29:544, 1989

41. Sheehan T, McLaren KM, Brettle R, Parker AC: Transfusion-induced graft versus host disease in pregnancy. Clin Lab Haematol 9:205, 1987

42. Prince M, Pedersen JS, Szer J et al: Transfusion associated graft-versus-host disease after cardiac surgery: response to antithymocyte globulin and corticosteroid therapy. Aust N Z J Med 21:43, 1991

43. O'Connor NTJ, Mackintosh P: Transfusion associated graft versus host disease in an immunocompetent patient. J Clin Pathol 45:621, 1992

44. Bell C: Fatal transfusion-associated graft-versus-host disease caused by blood from an unrelated donor in an immunocompetent patient (letter). Transfusion 33:785, 1993

45. Kobayashi H, Kitano K, Kishi E et al: Transfusion-associated graft-versus-host disease in an immunocompetent patient following accidental injury. Am J Hematol 43:51, 1993

46. Perkins HA: Transfusion-induced immunologic unresponsiveness. Transfusion Med Rev 2:196, 1988

47. Anderson KC, Weinstein HJ: Transfusion-associated graft-versus-host disease. N Engl J Med 323:315, 1990

48. Greenbaum BH: Transfusion associated graft versus host disease: historical perspectives, incidence, and current use of irradiated blood products. J Clin Oncol 9:1889, 1991

49. Cohen D, Weinstein H, Mihm M, Yankee R: Nonfatal graft-versus-host disease occurring after transfusion with leukocytes and platelets obtained from normal donors. Blood 53:1053, 1979

50. DeDobbeleer GD, Ledoux-Corbusier MH, Achten GA: Graft versus host reaction. An ultrastructural study. Arch Dermatol 111:1597, 1975

51. Sale GE, Lerner KG, Barker EA et al: The skin biopsy

in the diagnosis of acute graft versus host disease in man. Am J Pathol 89:621, 1977

52. Sale GE, Storb R, Kolb H: Histopathology of hepatic acute graft versus host disease in the dog. Transplantation 26:102, 1978

53. Kunstmann E, Bocker T, Roewer L et al: Diagnosis of transfusion-associated graft-versus-host disease by genetic fingerprinting and polymerase chain reaction. Transfusion 32:766, 1992

54. Hayakawa S, Chishima F, Sakata H et al: A rapid molecular diagnosis of posttransfusion graft-versus-host disease by polymerase chain reaction. Transfusion 33:413, 1993

55. Wang L, Juji T, Tokunaga K et al: Polymorphic microsatellite markers for the diagnosis of graft-versus-host disease. N Engl J Med 330:398, 1994

56. Suzuki K, Akiyama H, Takamoto S et al: Transfusion-associated graft-versus-host disease in a presumably immunocompetent patient after transfusion of stored packed red cells. Transfusion 32:358, 1992

57. Starzl TE, Demetris AJ, Murase N et al: Cell migration, chimerism, and graft acceptance. Lancet 1:1579, 1992

58. Starzl TE, Demetris AJ, Trucco M: Chimerism after liver transplantation for type IV glycogen storage disease and type 1 Gaucher's disease. N Engl J Med 328:745, 1993

59. Starzl TE, Demetris AJ, Trucco M et al: Cell migration and chimerism after whole-organ transplantation: the basis of graft acceptance. Hepatology 17:1127, 1993

60. Steinman RM, Inaba K, Austyn JM: Donor-derived chimerism in recipients of organ transplants. Hepatology 17:1153, 1993

61. Schlitt HJ, Kanehiro H, Raddatz G et al: Persistence of donor lymphocytes in liver allograft recipients. Transplantation 56:1001, 1993

62. Nagler JA, Ilan Y, Amniel A, Tur-Kaspa R: Systemic chimerism in sex-mismatched liver transplant recipients detected by fluorescence in situ hybridization. Transplantation 57:1458, 1994

63. Petz LD, Yam P, Wallace RB et al: Mixed hematopoietic chimerism following bone marrow transplantation for hematologic malignancies. Blood 70:1331, 1987

64. Hill RS, Petersen FB, Storb R et al: Mixed hematologic chimerism after allogeneic marrow transplantation for severe aplastic anemia is associated with a higher risk of graft rejection and a lessened incidence of acute graft-versus-host disease. Blood 67:811, 1986

65. Bertheas MF, Lafage M, Levy P: Influence of mixed chimerism on the results of allogeneic bone marrow transplantation for leukemia. Blood 78:3103, 1991

66. Ildstad ST, Sachs DH: Reconstitution with syngeneic plus allogeneic or xenogeneic bone marrow leads to specific acceptance of allografts or xenografts. Nature 307:168, 1984

67. Kanter MH: Transfusion-associated graft-versus-host disease: do transfusions from second-degree relatives pose a greater risk than those from first-degree relatives? Transfusion 32:323, 1992

68. Charpentier F, Bracq C, Bonin P et al: HLA-matched blood products and post-transfusion graft-versus-host disease (letter). Transfusion 30:850, 1990

69. Takahashi K, Juji T, Miyazaki H: Post-transfusion graft-versus-host disease occurring in non-immunosuppressed patients in Japan. Transfusion Sci 12:281, 1991

70. Ohto H, Yasuda H, Noguchi M, Abe R: Risk of transfusion-associated graft-versus-host disease as a result of directed donations from relatives (letter). Transfusion 32:691, 1992

71. Sanders M, Graeber J: Post-transfusion graft-versus-host disease in infancy. J Pediatr 117:159, 1990

72. Burns LJ, Westburg MW, Burns CP et al: Acute graft versus host disease resulting from normal donor blood transfusion. Acta Haematol 71:270, 1984

73. Schmidmeier W, Feil W, Gebhart W et al: Fatal graft versus host reaction following granulocyte transfusions. Blut 45:115, 1982

74. Strobel S, Morgan G, Simmonds AH et al: Fatal graft-versus-host disease after platelet transfusions in a child with purine nucleoside phosphorylase deficiency. Eur J Pediatr 148:312, 1989

75. Goodman JW, Congdon CC: The killing effect of blood-bone marrow mixtures given to irradiated mice. Radiat Res 12:439, 1960

76. Cole LJ, Garver RM: Abrogation by injected mouse blood of the protective effect of foreign bone marrow in lethally x-irradiated mice. Nature 184:1815, 1959

77. Thomas ED, Herman EC, Jr, Greenough WB III et al: Irradiation and marrow infusion in leukemia. Arch Intern Med 107:829, 1961

78. Sprent J, Anderson RE, Miller JFAP: Radiosensitivity of T and B lymphocytes. II. Effect of radiation on response of T cells to alloantigens. Eur J Immunol 4:204, 1974

79. Valerius NH, Johansen KS, Nielson OS et al: Effect of in vitro x-irradiation on lymphocyte and granulocyte function. Scand J Hematol 27:9, 1981

80. Button LN, DeWolf WC, Newburger PE et al: The effects of irradiation on blood components. Transfusion 21:419, 1981

81. Rosen NR, Weidner JG, Boldt HD, Rosen DS: Prevention of transfusion-associated graft-versus-host disease: selection of an adequate dose of gamma radiation. Transfusion 33:125, 1993

82. Pelszynski MM, Moroff G, Luban NLC et al: Effect of γ irradiation of red blood cell units on T-cell inactivation as assessed by limiting dilution analysis: implications for preventing transfusion-associated graft-versus-host disease. Blood 83:1683, 1994

83. Widmann FK (ed): Standards for Blood Banks and Transfusion Services. 15th Ed. American Association of Blood Banks, Bethesda, MD, 1993

84. Anderson KC, Goodnough LT, Sayers M et al: Variation in blood component irradiation practice: implications for prevention of transfusion-associated graft-versus-host disease. Blood 77:2096, 1991

85. Leitman SF: Dose, dosimetry, and quality improvement of irradiated blood components (editorial). Transfusion 33:447, 1993

86. Ramirez AM, Woodfield DG, Scott R, McLachlan J: High potassium levels in stored irradiated blood (letter). Transfusion 27:444, 1987

87. Rivet C, Baxter A, Rock G: Potassium levels in irradiated blood (letter). Transfusion 29:185, 1989

88. Ferguson DJ: Potassium levels in irradiated blood (letter). Transfusion 29:749, 1989

89. Rock G, Shear JM: Potassium levels in irradiated blood (letter). Transfusion 29:749, 1989

90. Bernard DR, Chapman RG, Simmons MA et al: Blood for use in exchange transfusions in the newborn. Transfusion 20:401, 1980

91. Hall TL, Barnes A, Miller JR et al: Neonatal mortality following transfusion of red cells with high plasma potassium levels. Transfusion 33:606, 1993

92. Strauss RG: Routinely washing irradiated red cells before transfusion seems unwarranted. Transfusion 30:675, 1990

93. Hillyer CD, Tiegerman KO, Berkman EM: Evaluation of the red cell storage lesion after irradiation in filtered packed red cell units. Transfusion 31:497, 1991

94. Davey RJ, McCoy NC, Yu M et al: The effect of prestorage irradiation on posttransfusion red cell survival. Transfusion 32:525, 1992

95. Rock G, Adams GA, Labow RS: The effects of irradiation on platelet function. Transfusion 28:451, 1988

96. Read EJ, Kodis G, Carter CS, Leitman SF: Viability of platelets following storage in the irradiated state. Transfusion 28:446, 1988

97. Lowenthal RM, Challis DR, Griffiths AE: Transfusion-associated graft-versus-host disease: report of an occurrence following the administration of irradiated blood. Transfusion 33:524, 1993

98. Sproul AM, Chalmers EA, Mills KI et al: Third party mediated graft rejection despite irradiation of blood products. Br J Haematol 80:251, 1992

99. Yankee RA, Grumet FC, Rogentine GN: Platelet transfusion therapy: the selection of compatible platelet donors for refractory patients by lymphocyte HLA typing. N Engl J Med 281:1208, 1969

100. Zeger G, Vengelen-Tyler V, McGrath C: The possibility of graft vs host disease in recipients of HLA matched plateletpheresis products, abstracted. p. 120. In Book of Abstracts, Joint Congress of ISBT and AABB, Los Angeles, CA, Nov 10-15, 1990

101. Grishaber JE, Birney SM, Strauss RG: Potential for transfusion-associated graft-versus-host disease due to apheresis platelets matched for HLA class I antigens. Transfusion 33:910, 1993

102. Benson K, Marks AR, Marshall J, Goldstein JD: Fatal graft-versus-host disease associated with HLA-matched, HLA-homozygous platelet transfusions from unrelated donors. Transfusion 34:432, 1994

103. Wasser MN, Houblers JG, D'Amaro J et al: The effect of fresh versus stored blood on post-operative bleeding after coronary bypass surgery: a prospective randomized study. Br J Haematol 72:81, 1989

104. Manno CS, Hedberg KW, Kim HC et al: Comparison of the hemostatic effects of fresh whole blood, stored whole blood, and components after open heart surgery in children. Blood 77:930, 1991

105. Lind SE: Has the case for irradiating blood products been made? Am J Med 78:543, 1985

106. Sprent J, Von Boehmer H, Nabholz M: Association of immunity and tolerance to host H-2 determinants in irradiated F1 hybrid mice reconstituted with bone marrow cells from one parental strain. J Exp Med 142:321, 1975

107. Korngold R, Sprent J: T cell subsets and graft-versus-host disease. Transplantation 44:335, 1987

108. Filipovich AH, Vallera DA, Youle RJ et al: Graft-versus-host disease prevention in allogeneic bone marrow transplantation from histocompatible siblings: a pilot study using immunotoxins for T cell depletion of donor bone marrow. Transplantation 44:62, 1987

109. Anderson KC, Nadler LM, Takvorian T et al: Monoclonal antibodies: their use in bone marrow transplantation. p. 137. In Brown E (ed): Progress in Hematology. Grune & Stratton, Orlando, 1981

110. Reisner Y, Kapoor N, Kirkpatrick D et al: Transplantation for acute leukaemia with HLA-A and B nonidentical parental marrow cells fractionated with soy-

bean agglutinin and sheep red blood cells. Lancet 2: 327, 1981

111. de Witte T, Hoogengout J, de Pauw B et al: Depletion of donor lymphocytes by counterflow centrifugation successfully prevents acute graft-versus-host disease in matched allogeneic marrow transplantation. Blood 5:1302, 1988

112. Crowley JP, Skrabut EM, Valeri CR: Immunocompetent lymphocytes in previously frozen washed red cells. Vox Sang 26:513, 1974

113. Schiffer CA, Dutcher JP, Aisner J et al: A randomized trial of leukocyte depleted platelet transfusion to modify alloimmunization in patients with leukemia. Blood 62:815, 1983

114. Eernisse JG, Brand A: Prevention of platelet refractoriness due to HLA antibodies by administration of leucocyte-poor blood components. Exp Hematol 9: 77, 1981

115. Murphy MF, Metcalfe P, Thomas H et al: Use of leukocyte-poor blood components and HLA matched platelet donors to prevent HLA alloimmunization. Br J Haematol 62:529, 1986

116. Sniecinski I, O'Donnell MR, Nowicki B, Hill LR: Prevention of refractoriness and HLA-alloimmunization using filtered blood products. Blood 71:1402, 1988

117. Akahoshi M, Takanashi M, Masuda M et al: A case of transfusion-associated graft-versus-host disease not prevented by white cell-reduction filters. Transfusion 32:169, 1992

118. Heim MU, Munker R, Sauer H et al: Graft-versus-Host Krankheit (GVH) mit letalem Ausgang nach der Gabe von gefilterten Erythrozytenkonzentraten (EK), abstracted. Infusionstherapie, suppl. 18:8, 1991

119. Hayashi H, Nishiuchi T, Tamura H, Takeda K: Transfusion-associated graft-versus-host disease caused by leukocyte-filtered stored blood. Anesthesiology 79:1419, 1993

120. Deeg HJ, Graham TC, Gerhard Miller L et al: Prevention of transfusion-induced graft-versus-host disease in dogs by ultraviolet irradiation. Blood 74: 2592, 1989

121. Brand A, Class FHJ, van Rood JJ: UV-irradiated platelets: ready to use? Transfusion 29:377, 1989

122. van der Mast BJ, Hornstra N, Ruigrok MB et al: Transfusion-associated graft-versus-host disease in immunocompetent patients: a self-protective mechanism. Lancet 343:753, 1994

123. Hato T, Yasukawa M, Takeuchi N: Decrease in transfusion-associated graft-versus-host disease. Transfusion 34:457, 1994

Chapter 43

Plasma and Plasma Derivatives

Scott N. Swisher and Lawrence D. Petz

In this chapter, we review indications for the use of fresh frozen plasma (FFP) and the current status of solvent-detergent-treated plasma (see Chs. 8, 18, 25, 27, 30, and 35 for more specific details on coagulation factor replacement therapy). We next review albumin products and plasma substitutes (i.e., gelatins and dextrans). (Oxygen-carrying blood substitutes are reviewed in Ch. 44).

PLASMA

Plasma as a Volume Expander

During World War II, large amounts of lyophilized human plasma were produced and used as a blood volume expander in the acute treatment of battle injuries. It was soon recognized that this practice resulted in the transmission of hepatitis, then called "homologous serum hepatitis." Fatalities occurred, but the benefit in that situation was thought to outweigh the risks. This situation fueled the intensive efforts in the laboratories of Cohn and colleagues that led to plasma fractionation by cold ethanol precipitation, a process that still survives despite technical and scientific advances that could supplant it. The main objective, development of a stabilized albumin preparation that would withstand viral inactivation by heat, was achieved, however.

Today, albumin, other colloid solutions, and crystalloid solutions are readily available for use as vol-ume expanders. Nevertheless, liquid plasma products that can transmit infectious agents are often used inappropriately for this purpose.

FRESH FROZEN PLASMA

FFP is plasma that is separated from the red blood cells and platelets of whole blood donations and placed at $-18°C$ or below within 8 hours after collection.[1] Single-donor plasma units may also substitute. FFP contains the labile and stable components of the coagulation, fibrinolytic, and complement systems; the proteins that maintain oncotic pressure and modulate immunity; and other proteins that have diverse activities. In addition, fats, carbohydrates, and minerals are present in concentrations similar to those in circulation.[2] In recent decades, the use of FFP has increased 10-fold in the United States, and Devine et al.[3] estimate that 1.8 million units were transfused in the United States in 1990.

Unfortunately, studies of the use of FFP show that it is often misused.[4,5] This is largely due to the misconceptions regarding its hemostatic effectiveness and inadequate knowledge of the situations in which its use is appropriate.[4]

Indications

Indications for the use of FFP have been reviewed by a National Institutes of Health Consensus Conference,[2] by a task force of the College of American

Table 43-1. Indications and Contraindications for the Use of Fresh Frozen Plasma

Indications
 Replacement of isolated coagulation factor deficiencies
 Reversal of warfarin effect
 Vitamin K deficiency
 Liver disease
 Massive transfusion
 Thrombotic thrombocytopenic purpura
 Acute disseminated intravascular coagulation
 Cl esterase inhibitor deficiency
Situations in which Fresh Frozen Plasma has been used without justification
 As volume expander in hypovolemia
 Nutritional support
 Protein-losing states
 Immunodeficiency states
 Reconstitution of whole blood

Pathologists,[1] and by the British Committee for Standards in Haematology.[4] FFP is indicated for some isolated coagulation protein deficiencies; for patients with multiple coagulation defects such as with warfarin therapy, vitamin K deficiency, or liver disease; for some patients who require massive transfusion; in conjunction with therapeutic plasma exchange for thrombotic thrombocytopenic purpura (TTP); for some patients with disseminated intravascular coagulation (DIC); and for patients with acute symptoms associated with C1 esterase deficiency. Its use in most other cases should be discouraged (Table 43-1).

Replacement of Isolated Coagulation Factor Deficiencies

More specific factor concentrates are becoming available for clinical use, and FFP is only required when specific or combined factor concentrates are unavailable. The dose depends on the specific factor being replaced, as both the half-life and plasma concentration required for hemostasis vary for individual factors.

Replacement therapy for factors II and X can be accomplished with a concentrate of combined factors II, IX, and X, and this is recommended rather than FFP. Cryoprecipitate, which contains fibrinogen, fibronectin, and factor VIII, should be used as the replacement therapy in patients with a deficiency of fibrinogen (factor I).[4]

A deficiency of von Willebrand factor should not be corrected with FFP because alternative therapy is available, especially desmopressin acetate and some intermediate-purity factor VIII concentrates.[4]

When specific component therapy is not available or not appropriate, FFP is efficacious for bleeding or prophylactically for surgery or an invasive procedure for patients with congenital deficiency of factors II, V, VII, IX, X, XI, or XIII.[1,2]

Therapy is not considered necessary unless (1) the prothrombin time (PT) is greater than 1.5 times the midpoint of the normal range (usually more than 18 seconds), (2) the activated partial thromboplastin time (aPTT) is greater than 1.5 times the top of the normal range (usually more than 55 to 60 seconds), and (3) a coagulation factor assay finding is less than 25 percent activity.[1]

Requirements for FFP vary with the specific factor being replaced. For example, hemostatic levels of factor IX in a patient with severe deficiency are difficult to achieve with FFP alone, whereas patients with severe factor X deficiency require factor levels of about 10 percent to achieve hemostasis and are easily treated with FFP.[2] For most disorders, a recommended starting dose is 15 ml/kg.[6] (If platelets are also being transfused, it must be remembered that for every 5 to 6 units of platelets or 1 plateletpheresis unit, the patient is receiving a volume equivalent of 1 unit of FFP; therefore, smaller doses of FFP may be needed.)

After completion of the initial infusion, if the PT is greater than 18 seconds or the aPTT is greater than 60 seconds, more FFP may be needed. To determine the need for repeating FFP transfusions, the half-lives of the coagulation factors must be considered. Because factor VII has a much shorter half-life than the other factors (5 to 6 hours), the PT may become prolonged sooner than the aPTT after plasma transfusion. Therefore, if the PT is not determined within 1 to 2 hours after transfusion, the aPTT is a better indicator of the initial efficacy of treatment.[1] The patient's clinical bleeding must also be continuously assessed.

Other Coagulation Factor Deficiencies

FFP may be used to treat patients with a deficiency of antithrombin III (when a concentrate is not available), heparin cofactor II, protein C, or protein S.[1]

Reversal of Warfarin Effect

Patients who are anticoagulated with warfarin are deficient in the functional vitamin K-dependent coagulation factors II, VII, IX, and X and proteins C and S. These functional deficiencies can be reversed by the administration of vitamin K. However, 4 to 6 hours must be allowed for adequate clinical response in the average patient so that, for anticoagulated patients who are actively bleeding or who require emergency surgery, FFP (about 1 l for an adult) can be used to achieve immediate hemostasis.[2]

Vitamin K Deficiency

Hemorrhagic disease of the newborn, and conditions that may impair vitamin K absorption, such as biliary duct obstruction, are associated with a coagulation abnormality similar to that described with oral anticoagulant therapy. If bleeding results, a regimen similar to that for reversal of warfarin effect should be used.[4]

Liver Disease

A variety of abnormalities of coagulation are seen in patients with liver disease (see Chs. 18 and 35). Bleeding seldom occurs as a result of a hemostatic defect alone but usually has a precipitating cause such as surgery. FFP is indicated if the patient is bleeding or if an invasive procedure is planned. However, because of the large volumes of FFP required by patients who already have an expanded plasma volume as a result of ascites and edema and the short biologic half-life of some of the coagulation factors, complete correction of coagulation test abnormalities may not be possible. There is little information regarding the levels of coagulation test abnormalities that are safe for patients with liver disease before invasive procedures. A PT of 1.6 to 1.8 times the control value is probably realistic.[4]

Massive Transfusion

Use of FFP in massive blood transfusion, which may be defined as the replacement of the patient's total blood volume with stored blood in less than 24 hours, appears to have increased in frequency, possibly due in part to the relative unavailability of whole blood.[2] Pathologic hemorrhage in the massively transfused patient is caused more frequently by

thrombocytopenia than be depletion of coagulation factors. The prophylactic administration of FFP according to a set formula that depends on the amount of stored blood transfused usually results in unnecessary transfusion because such formulae overestimate the probability of coagulation factor deficiencies.[7-9] Moreover, when coagulation factor replacement is necessary, usually in association with a consumptive disorder, these formulae generally provide inadequate replacement therapy. Thus, prophylactic component supplementation according to a set formula is both unnecessary and insufficient.[7] To prevent the indiscriminate use of blood components in patients receiving massive transfusion, early laboratory assessment is needed to determine the precise nature of any disorders of coagulation which may be present (see Chs. 18, 25, and 35).

Thrombotic Thrombocytopenic Purpura

FFP is the accepted form of treatment for TTP, generally in conjunction with plasma exchange (see Ch. 46).

Disseminated Intravascular Coagulation

DIC, which can be associated with shock, trauma, and sepsis, results in variable deficiencies of factors V and VIII, fibrinogen, and platelets because of activation of the coagulation and fibrinolytic systems. The spectrum of presentation is wide, ranging from a decompensated state of hemostasis, with abnormalities of coagulation demonstrable only in the laboratory, to a fulminant form with major bleeding and thrombotic complications.

The treatment of all patients must first be directed at the cause of the DIC. There is no evidence that any supportive or replacement therapy is beneficial unless it is possible to correct the underlying condition.

Replacement therapy is indicated in acute DIC when there is hemorrhage and abnormality of coagulation. The infusion of FFP, cryoprecipitate, and platelet concentrates forms the basis of initial therapy. The response should be closely monitored by repeated laboratory tests and clinical assessment and further replacement judged by both (see Ch. 18).

C1 Esterase Inhibitor Deficiency

FFP is indicated as short-term prophylactic therapy before surgery to prevent laryngeal edema in patients with hereditary angioedema (congenital C1 esterase inhibitor deficiency).[10–12] This is particularly important for patients scheduled for dental surgery or who are expected to require endotracheal intubation. The transfusion of 2 units of FFP to an adult patient causes a modest increase in the level of the C1 inhibitor, which is sufficient to prevent attacks of hereditary angioedema. Levels return to the previous subnormal values in 1 to 4 days.[10]

Life-threatening acute attacks of laryngeal edema have also been treated successfully with infusions of FFP,[13] although FFP contains both the C1 inhibitor and components of complement so that it is theoretically possible that the sudden availability of these components may transiently exacerbate the attack.[14,15]

C1 esterase deficiency may also occur rarely as an acquired disorder associated with lymphoproliferative diseases.[16] The therapy of acquired C1 esterase inhibitor deficiency has not been subjected to controlled studies, but it is reasonable to anticipate a similar usefulness of FFP.[17]

A concentrate of C1 inhibitor has been produced (C1-Inactivator, HS, Behring, Marburg, Germany) and, if available, may be preferable to FFP because it avoids the risk of infectious disease transmission and does not cause the sudden replenishment of components of complement.[18]

Special Pediatric Indications

FFP has been suggested as being useful in infants with secondary immunodeficiency associated with severe protein-losing enteropathy and in whom total parenteral nutrition is ineffectual.[2] However, other workers do not consider FFP efficacious in this setting.[4]

In pediatric patients with severe sepsis, including sepsis in the newborn, therapy with FFP and cryoprecipitate has been advocated for the provision of clotting factors, complement, fibronectin, and protease inhibitors, which may be deficient in these infants. However, no evidence confirming the efficacy of this use of FFP is yet available.[4]

Cardiopulmonary Bypass Surgery

Most adult patients undergoing cardiopulmonary bypass surgery do not have significant coagulation abnormalities. In most studies, nonsurgical bleeding has been attributed to platelet dysfunction rather than to a deficiency of plasma coagulation factors. FFP should only be used in those patients in whom bleeding is associated with proven abnormalities of coagulation other than residual heparin effect. Such patients have usually been massively transfused and may have had consumptive coagulopathy develop.

Unwarranted Situations for Use

Hypovolemia

There is no place for FFP as a volume expander for the management of hypovolemia because safer alternative therapies exist, including crystalloids, synthetic colloids, and human albumin solutions.[1,2,4] It is discouraging to note that some estimates have suggested that almost 50 percent of the FFP used in the United States is transfused as a volume expander.[5]

Nutritional Support and Protein-Losing States

There is no justification for the administration of FFP for nutritional purposes, for chronic cases of cirrhosis with ascites and nephrosis, or for chronic thoracic duct drainage.[4]

Treatment of Immunodeficiency States

In the past, FFP has been used as a source of immunoglobulins in the treatment of inherited immunodeficiency states. Purified intravenous immunoglobulin is now available and has replaced the need for FFP in these patients (see Ch. 45).

Reconstitution of Whole Blood

A particularly objectionable use of FFP is its addition to units of separated red cells, in effect, to reconstitute a unit of whole blood. This has the undesirable consequence of exposing the recipient to two donors rather than to one. The same effect is achieved by the serial administration of 1 unit of red cells followed by 1 unit of FFP. This practice could be acceptable, when logistically necessary, if the separated plasma could be returned to the red cells of the same donor or if these two components could be coadministered. If the two components are not physically separated, the plasma cannot be frozen. If the plasma is separated, the product management program and the transfusion procedure must guarantee that both components from the same donor are reunited. This creates a difficult management problem and an obvious potential for errors. It is much more reasonable to maintain, distribute, and use an inventory of whole blood where needed.

SOLVENT-DETERGENT-TREATED PLASMA

Concern about transfusion-transmitted diseases, especially acute since the appearance of the human immunodeficiency virus (HIV), has driven a growing number of measures aimed at improving the safety of transfusion therapy. One such approach is the application of the solvent-detergent method of inactivation of lipid-enveloped viruses to FFP.[19] The resulting product, frozen plasma, solvent/detergent treated (FP S/DT), has been extensively evaluated both in the US and Europe. This product has been used clinically in Europe but, as of late 1994, has not been approved by the Food and Drug Administration (FDA) for use in the United States; approval is expected in 1995.[20,21] The product will be provided largely in the frozen state, although it can be lyophilized for special needs such as military and emergency use or for distribution in areas where frozen refrigeration is not available. Lyophilization adds greatly to the cost and imposes some loss of activity. The product will be distributed as ABO-specific subproducts.

FP S/DT is essentially the same as FFP as a replacement for those hemostatic factors for which a concentrated product is not available.[22] It also appears to be equivalently effective in the treatment of TTP by exchange transfusion.[23] It can be used as a diluent for resuspension of platelets when this is indicated with maintenance of platelet function and viability.[24]

The solvent-detergent process does not inactivate viruses without a lipid envelope. Two such agents are of concern in transfusion medicine: hepatitis A and parvovirus B19. There is evidence of transmission of these agents by infusion of hemostatic factor concentrates, although overt disease is rare. This may be due to the presence of antibody against these agents in the original plasma pool. Because the FP S/DT is prepared from pools of donor plasma, the possibility of occasional contamination of a pool by an asymptomatic but viremic donor is present. Here, the coinfusion of antibody against these agents that is present in donors' plasma may also reduce the risk

of transmission of infection. This caveat will certainly be reflected in the required labeling when the product is released for distribution.[25]

Cost-Effectiveness

Reducing viral transmission is an important goal of transfusion medicine, and the FP S/DT treatment process offers this prospect for about 2 million units of plasma transfused annually in the United States. However, because of the current remarkable safety of the blood supply, FP S/DT provides relatively small health benefits at high societal cost.

AuBuchon and Birkmeyer[26] studied the public health and economic implications of FP S/DT. They used a decision analysis model to assess transfusion-related outcomes in hypothetic cohorts of plasma recipients. In-hospital mortality rates and other characteristics were determined in 61 patients who received plasma transfusions at a medium-sized tertiary care center to provide data for the model. Other parameters were obtained from the medical literature.

Compared with untreated plasma, 1 unit of FP S/DT produces a net benefit of 35 minutes in quality-adjusted life expectancy at a cost of about $19. Extrapolated to an estimated 2.2 million plasma units transfused annually in the United States, FP S/DT would save 147 quality-adjusted life-years at a cost of $42.5 million. In sensitivity analysis, the net benefit of FP S/DT was negated by the existence of even a minute risk of nonenveloped virus infection. It was the opinion of the authors that the relatively high costs and small benefits of reducing enveloped virus infection risks with FP S/DT do not appear to justify widespread implementation of this new technology. The use of FP S/DT does not compare favorably with many common therapeutic medical interventions as a public health investment.

Transfusion medicine specialists are, therefore, caught between two strong, competing pressures. Concern about HIV transmission and other risks of transfusion continues to drive the blood banking system toward developing increased safety at any cost. On the other hand, recognition that health care resources are necessarily limited, means that physicians are being urged (forced) to control costs. If FP S/DT is approved by the FDA, health care providers and payers will have to consider these difficult trade-offs when deciding about broad implementation of this new technology. Similar considerations concerning the cost-effectiveness of measures designed to increase the safety of transfusion apply to predeposit autologous donation (see Ch. 11).

This cost-to-benefit analysis of FP S/DT is given here as an example of the kind of evaluation that many new products, drugs, devices, tests, and procedures will face in the near future when further changes in the funding of health care are instituted. It will be important for the transfusion medicine community to take a proactive role in this regard, rather than to respond after possibly inappropriate decisions are made by others.

HUMAN SERUM ALBUMIN PRODUCTS

Human serum albumin products are by far the most commonly used plasma volume expanders in use in the United States and Canada. These products are "artificial" in that they are produced from human plasma by a manufacturing process referred to as fractionation. The alternative to fractionated human serum albumin—unfractionated whole human plasma—is much less useful because the product (1) contains isoagglutinins; (2) contains proteins such as fibrinogen, which may be unwanted; and (3) most importantly, cannot be heat sterilized. Pooled, lyophilized human plasma used during World War II resulted in a seriously high incidence of hepatitis before albumin became available. Albumin products have great logistic advantages. They are stable under reasonable storage conditions and can be concentrated to 25 percent solutions for shipment to areas where diluent can be prepared locally. Thus, these products had great appeal to the military medical services and to civil defense and disaster management authorities for treatment of war casualties and civilian disaster victims. As albumin products became available, interest in the artificial colloids of nonhuman origin promptly waned. Clinical use diminished rapidly as did further research and development in the field in the United States.

Growth in the use of albumin was essentially controlled only by the available supply. Although albumin was first introduced as a plasma volume expander, a wide variety of other uses were soon proposed. Many of these uses were justified on strictly empiric

grounds (i.e., if the patient's serum albumin level was low, it could frequently be raised by albumin infusions). Data indicating that this therapy had a beneficial effect on the clinical outcome of the treated patients were frequently lacking. Many early studies of the efficacy of albumin were poorly designed and inadequately executed or analyzed when viewed from the standpoint of modern standards. Indeed, it is only recently that the community of clinical investigators fully realized the difficulties and sources of error inherent in studying a problem of efficacy of this sort. The primary problem is the inherent great variability in the treated patient population, which makes it almost impossible to obtain comparable groups of treated and control patients or groups treated in two different ways. Thus, it is not surprising that much of the available information about the efficacy of albumin therapy in a wide variety of circumstances remains inconclusive.

Military medical research has been of great value in studies of the problems of trauma and shock. These patient populations are more homogeneous, and their management can be standardized more readily in spite of the vicissitudes of doing such studies in a theater of war. The subjects of military medical research are primarily young men in excellent physical condition. Although this provides some degree of limitation on the translation of wartime experience to civilian practice involving children, female patients, elderly patients, and those otherwise ill, the general principles clarified by these studies are nonetheless transferable and have been found to be of real value in civilian practice of traumatology and major surgery. One can only admire investigators who have contributed this knowledge under such demanding conditions.[27–29]

As supplies of albumin increased, its marketers promoted uses for which there was little or no supporting evidence of a benefit. These uncritical uses have led to a number of efforts to define appropriate and inappropriate uses of these products.[30–33] Several of these studies were motivated by issues of supply, sources of commercially obtained plasma, and costs.[30] The major effort in this regard was made by the Division of Blood Diseases and Resources, National Heart and Lung Institute of the National Institutes of Health. In February 1975, they sponsored a conference on the scientific basis of the clinical uses of albumin. The proceedings of this conference have been published and provide a valuable document in this area.[34] In early 1977, Tullis,[35,36] who summarized the conference, published two articles on the physiology and use of albumin that were based largely on the results of the 1975 conference. These provided the first scientifically based comprehensive guidelines to the appropriate use of albumin materials. In the time since they were published, it has become clear that these guidelines, believed to be overly restrictive by some when first published, are actually fairly liberal.

Characteristics and Physiology

Human albumin is a highly soluble, symmetric, slightly heterogeneous protein that weighs about 67,000 D (584 amino acid residues) with 17 internal disulfide bridges. It carries a high net negative charge of -19. The high negative charge results in albumin's binding of a large number of compounds, including drugs. Albumin contains a large amount of aspartic and glutamic acids and is relatively deficient in leucine and tryptophan, particularly the latter. It is synthesized in the liver, normally at from one-third to one-half the maximal rate, which is thought to be controlled largely by the oncotic pressure of the interstitial fluid. The synthesis of albumin is rapid, but hepatic reserves of albumin are small.[37]

Albumin is responsible for 80 percent of the colloid oncotic pressure (COP) of the plasma, normally about 27 mmHg; reduction of COP to about 20 mmHg, corresponding to a total serum protein of about 5.2 g/dl, has been regarded as a "critical value," leading to an excessively expanded interstitial volume (about $+50$ percent).

Albumin is a dynamic protein. Total body stores approximate 300 g in a 70-kg adult, of which 60 to 65 percent is extravascular in skin, muscle, and gut primarily.[34,35] These pools have been regarded as "reserves," but it is more probable that the albumin here is part of a complex regulatory process of fluid exchange involving hydrostatic and osmotic forces. The various extravascular pools equilibrate with intravascular albumin at various rates but generally rapidly. About 15 g of albumin (4 to 5 percent) is metabolized and synthesized daily in the normal steady state. Small amounts are normally lost in the gut. A wide variety of factors influence both the synthesis and degradation of albumin. Albumin production is decreased by malnutrition, hormonal influences, and a wide range of diseases, particularly chronic liver disease. Refeeding results in the onset of albumin synthesis in minutes in the presence of adequate hepatic function.[38]

Available Products

Three manufactured albumin products are available in the United States: human serum albumin 5 percent solution; human serum albumin 25 percent solution; and plasma protein fraction (PPF). The latter contains at least 83 percent albumin as a 5 percent electrolyte solution, with the remainder of the protein made up of α- and β-globulins and traces of many other plasma proteins. Twenty-five percent human serum albumin is usually diluted to 5 percent in electrolyte solution before infusing.

PPF yields somewhat more useful protein per liter of starting plasma in the fractionating process. The nonalbumin proteins are probably quickly removed from the circulation because of heat denaturation. All these products are freed of hepatitis and other viruses by heating after chemical stabilization of the protein with the additives caprylate and/or acetyltryptophanate. Variable amounts of albumin dimers and oligomers result from the fractionation process and storage. The functional significance of these and their in vivo persistence is unknown. Shelf life depends on storage temperature; 3 years is permitted at below 37°C and 5 years at 2 to 10°C. After the expiration of storage life, albumin can be "reworked," although this practice was largely confined to military and civil defense stockpiles of albumin. Albumin is no longer stockpiled in large amounts in the United States for these purposes.

Newer Methods of Fractionation of Plasma Proteins

All of the albumin products manufactured in the United States and Canada are produced by variations of the basic Cohn process, which was developed by the late E. J. Cohn et al.[39] during World War II. This process also yielded fibrinogen and γ-globulin. Fibrinogen has been removed from the market because of its high risk of transmitting hepatitis. The Cohn process, now almost 50 years old, is based on differential precipitation of proteins by varying concentrations of alcohol and pH in the cold. Its great advantage lies in its proven safety. Albumin products withstand virus inactivation by heat. The Cohn fractionation process efficiently inactivates HIV; as a result, there has never been a documented transmission of HIV from any preparation of intravenous immune globulin.[40] Unfortunately, the hepatitis C virus is more resistant, and its transmission has been reported rarely after intravenous immune globulin administration (see Ch. 45).

A number of new methods of plasma protein fractionation that use a variety of physicochemical principles have been developed.[41-44] Several of these, particularly column chromatographic separation techniques, have the potential for isolating a number of presently unavailable plasma proteins of possible therapeutic value. Examples of such proteins are C1 esterase inhibitor, α_1-antitrypsin, fibronectin, β_2-macroglobulin, proteins C and S, metal- and enzyme-binding proteins, transport proteins, and many others. Presumably, these new methods would yield albumin products at least as good as or better than present products. Production of these proteins will be facilitated by the development of improved methods of in vitro sterilization of plasma derivatives. The solvent-detergent method now in use is one such technology.

Unfortunately, commercial development of many of these products is financially not feasible at the present time.[44] Pilot-scale quantities of the proteins are needed to investigate their usefulness. The course of such clinical investigations is prolonged, made very difficult because of present restrictions on investigation in human subjects, and extremely costly. By the time regulatory approval could be obtained, the investment, even in a potentially very useful and marketable product is so high as to be practically unrecoverable in a reasonable period.

Rational Use

The administration of albumin in the clinical setting continues to be controversial. Availability and cost concerns have forced many hospitals to review their guidelines for albumin administration. However, the lack of transmission of hepatitis virus and HIV has made albumin solutions appealing relative to blood products.[33]

Blood Volume Expansion

This is the primary indication for the administration of albumin, although authorities on the management of trauma and shock differ as to its value. Several studies comparing albumin with crystalloid solutions have been published subsequent to the National Institutes of Health Workshop on Albumin held in 1975.[34] These studies were summarized by Erstad et al.[33]

Albumin titrated to achieve a predetermined albumin concentration of COP has not been shown to provide benefits beyond those obtained with crystalloid solutions alone when used for intravascular expansion. In addition, crystalloids have been as effective as albumin when the dose of albumin was titrated according to either an empiric formula or hemodynamic stabilization in most patients undergoing surgery. However, albumin may be useful in the elderly population who requires volume expansion because these patients may not tolerate the large volume of crystalloid solutions often needed for resuscitation.

Paracentesis

Albumin has been shown to be beneficial in preventing acute complications such as hyponatremia and renal impairment associated with paracentesis. Studies are needed to compare the less expensive saline solutions with albumin for the acute stabilization of problems associated with paracentesis. The only randomized trial in patients with cirrhosis not undergoing paracentesis found no benefits from the addition of albumin administration to diet and diuretic therapy.[33]

Nephrotic Syndrome

Albumin may be useful in combination with diuretic therapy for patients with edema secondary to the nephrotic syndrome when diuretics alone have failed. A randomized trial with furosemide titrated to effect or adverse reactions, compared with a combined albumin and furosemide regimen, should be performed. Such a study should include patients with complications related to their edema.[33]

Thermal Injuries

Despite a number of resuscitation formulae that are recommended for patients with thermal injuries, only one randomized trial conducted in humans has compared a crystalloid with a crystalloid and albumin combination. That study found that albumin given within the first 24 hours postburn may increase the lung water level during the following week compared with crystalloid solutions. Comparative studies using albumin and crystalloids after the first 24 hours postburn should be performed because this is when advocates of colloids often use them.[33]

Total Parenteral Nutrition

One study found decreased complications but not length of stay when albumin was given in conjunction with total parenteral nutrition. A second trial using albumin in patients receiving total parenteral nutrition did not find benefits associated with supplemental albumin administration. A trend toward increased complications, length of hospital stay, and days of ventilatory therapy dependence was found in patients receiving albumin in the second trial.[33]

Therapeutic Plasma Exchange

FFP, albumin, or other plasma derivatives such as PPF can be used to provide the colloid necessary to replace the patient's plasma. The optimal replacement fluid varies, depending on the indication for the procedure. For example, for TTP, plasma is the replacement fluid of choice, but, for most other procedures, albumin or PPF has been the colloid used because of the risk of infectious disease transmission by plasma.[33]

Other Uses of Albumin

Albumin has been recommended alone or in conjunction with other therapeutic modalities for a number of uses, including patients with cerebral ischemia, renal transplantation, and liver resections without definitive evidence of efficacy.[33]

Misuses

Malnutrition

The use of albumin to treat malnutrition is inefficient and expensive and may defer proper measures to restore caloric and amino acid intake. Albumin is of absolutely no value in "toning up the system," a use once proposed to one of us. Only about 45 percent of infused albumin as a total protein source en-

ters the body protein pool of protein-depleted isocaloric patients.[45]

Situations of Chronic Albumin Loss

Chronic albumin loss, such as in chronic nephrosis and cirrhosis of the liver, are not improved by long-term albumin administration.

Adverse Effects

Albumin products are inherently surprisingly safe. Only a few significant adverse effects are reported in the literature. Some of these are due to technical accidents during manufacture. Probably more frequent are adverse effects caused by inappropriate or incorrect administration.[35]

Bacterial Contamination

Rarely, a lot of an albumin product has been found to be contaminated with bacteria, particularly with Pseudomonas spp. These lots produced febrile reactions, transient bacteremia, shock, and possible sepsis in the recipient.[46] Human serum albumin 25 percent is a good culture medium for a number of organisms. Not only does it support growth, but it appears to stabilize certain organisms and preserve viability.[47]

It is important to note that the heating step in the manufacture of albumin products, at 60°C for 10 hours, is done to inactivate hepatitis and other viruses, not to ensure bacterial sterility, which would require autoclaving.[48] Albumin cannot withstand these temperatures. Extreme care in preventing contamination during manufacture and filtration before bottling are required to prevent contamination. All lots released by the FDA are tested for contamination and pyrogenicity. In spite of these precautions, bacterial contamination can occur and should be considered in any patient who has an episode of fever, particularly with shaking chills, during or shortly after albumin administration. It is important that samples of the administered material and other vials of the same lot be preserved for investigation. Both the manufacturer and the FDA should be notified of such reactions.

Pyrogenic Reactions

Reactions characterized by chills and fever constitute about 75 percent of all reported reactions. It is difficult to be sure that the cause of these reactions, in fact, was due to albumin administration or that they were truly pyrogenic in nature. The fact that only a single patient may be reported as reacting to a single lot of albumin suggests that most such reactions are of other origin. These reactions are rarely severe, but, if they are suspected to be related to albumin product administration, they should be reported to the manufacturer for appropriate investigation.

Hepatitis and Human Immunodeficiency Viruses

When properly heated and protected from subsequent contamination, human serum albumin and PPF are unable to transmit hepatitis.[49] Nevertheless, an outbreak of hepatitis traceable to PPF prepared by one manufacturer occurred in 1973.[50] It is probable that a defect in the heating process accounted for this episode, but this was never proved. It is interesting that serum albumin products prepared simultaneously by this manufacturer from similar source plasma were not infective. The requirement to screen for hepatitis B surface antigen (HB$_s$Ag) and anti-HIV and eliminate those plasma specimens that are positive has resulted in a sharp decline in the amount of HB$_s$Ag detectable in albumin products. This may contribute to the safety of the product, and it also reduces the amount of passively transferred HB$_s$Ag given to recipients, which may cause diagnostic confusion.

Fortunately, the Cohn fractionation process efficiently inactivates HIV,[51] and we are not aware of any reported instances of transmission of HIV by transfusion of albumin products.

Hypotension

It has been known for some time that the rapid administration of PPF is frequently associated with transient hypotension. Rarely, lots of human serum albumin had been thought to evoke a similar reaction. This topic was investigated in great detail after an episode in which somewhat more severe hypotension was found to follow the administration of PPF prepared by one manufacturer in 1977. Although this reaction was thought to be due to the presence of bradykinin in trace amounts, these investigations demonstrated that prekallikrein activator (PKA), which is present in PPF and in a few lots of human serum albumin, was responsible. The PKA activates the production of bradykinin from the recipient's

own kinin system. This problem has been resolved by changes in the manufacturing process that result in the inactivation of PKA.[52]

Other Reactions

A number of other reactions have been reported in relation to the administration of albumin products. Of these, urticaria is the most believable. Many such reports may involve coincidences that do not involve a cause-and-effect relationship.

Risks Caused by Improper Administration

Excessive administration of albumin should be avoided. If the concentration of albumin is raised artificially above about 5.5 g/dl in the plasma, a hyperoncotic state is induced that, in the absence of available extracellular fluid, results in increased albumin catabolism and decreased hepatic synthesis. If there is excessive extracellular fluid, excessive albumin administration will result in a rise in intravascular volume and possible pulmonary edema. The same effect can occur if excessive amounts of albumin and crystalloid are given simultaneously. These adverse reactions are more frequent and severe in patients with intrinsic heart disease who have lowered cardiac functional reserves. Both the rate of administration and amount given are important. Pulmonary edema can occur in both the clinical context of treatment of hypovolemia with rapid fluid and albumin administration and in the more leisurely paced treatment of other hypoalbuminemic states. Careful, frequent evaluation of the patient, with preliminary calculation of the replacement need in both amount and rate will minimize these adverse reactions.

ARTIFICIAL BLOOD SUBSTITUTES

Blood substitutes are of two general types: (1) those designed to provide colloid osmotic activity to maintain or expand the plasma volume and (2) those able to transport oxygen. The latter are reviewed in detail in Chapter 44.

A number of nonmetabolizable artificial plasma substitutes have been investigated. Table 43-2 summarizes the characteristics of the principal candidate materials currently used as artificial plasma expanders. Because there is relatively little use of any of

Table 43-2. Characteristics of Principal Plasma Substitute Colloids[a]

Material	Solution Concentrations (%)	Source Material	Chemical Structure	M_n[b]	Excretion Route	Intravascular Persistence	Comments
Gelatins							
Oxypolygelatin (OPG)	5–6	Hydrolysis of animal collagen	Protein Condensed with glyoxal and oxidized with H_2O_2	23,300	All largely renal excretion; some proteolytic metabolism	About as for MFG	Gelatins are now largely prepared by European firms and marketed in Europe
Modified fluid gelatin (MFG)	3–4		Degraded and coupled with polycarboxylic acid anhydrides	22,600		50% of volume persists 4 to 5 hr postinfusion	OPG may be most antigenic in humans
Urea-linked gelatin (ULG)	3–4 (all with electrolytes)		Cross-linked with di-isocyanate (urea bridges)	24,500	75% excreted 1 wk	About as for MFG	MFG most widely used at present
Dextrans							
D70 "high molecular weight"	6	Bacterial synthesis by *Leukonostoc mesenteroides* from sucrose substrate	Complex Carbohydrate Polymers of D-glucopyranose linked (1–6); partial acid hydrolysis with fractionation by molecular size	35,000–40,000	Largely renal excretion; some metabolism to CO_2	Longer than gelatins, 50% of volume persist 8 hr postinfusion	Used primarily for plasma volume expansion, M_w,[b] nominal 70,000
D40, "low molecular weight"	10 (both with electrolytes)			25,000	55% excreted in urine, in 4 hr	Shorter than D70	Also used for "flow promotion" in capillary bed and antithrombotic prophylaxis. M_w,[b] nominal 40,000
Starch							
Hydroxyethyl starch (HES) (hetastarch)	6 (with electrolyte)	Waxy maize starch (amylopectin)	Complex Carbohydrate Highly branched glucose polymer; hydroxyethylation with ethylene oxide to slow rate of enzymatic hydrolysis in vivo	See the text	Renal excretion and metabolism ?Other routes of excretion	HES 25/75 about same as albumin	Several preparations with variable intrinsic viscosity and degree of hydroxyethylation HES 25/75 resembles D70 HES 16/43 resembles D40 (see the text)

Abbreviations: M_n, number average molecular weight; M_w, weight average molecular weight.

[a] There is a great deal of variation in figures reported for molecular weight, excretion rate, and intravascular persistence. Some of this is explained by methodologic differences and experimental variability. Reported differences in concentration suggest that a number of different formulations have been studied from time to time and that the formulation of even a trade name product may also have changed periodically. Thus, the characteristics of these materials given above should not be regarded as specific for any product. Rather, they are general descriptions of preparations that have been in clinical use. (Data from Prince et al.,[53] Consensus Development Panel, National Institutes of Health,[2] Gruber,[54] and Jamieson and Greenwalt.[55]

[b] M_w > M_n for polydisperse colloid.

these materials for this purpose in the United States at present, they will not be discussed in great detail in this text. Clearly, none have advantages over human albumin products from the practical point of view.

Gelatins

Gelatin was the first of the artificial colloids used to treat shock during World War I.[56] It was not until the modern era of investigation of shock in humans after World War II that interest in these materials redeveloped. Three derivative products of gelatin, listed in Table 43-2, were developed between 1951 and 1962.[57–60] Problems associated with gelatin at the lower temperatures that were characteristic of early preparations resulted in decreased interest in gelatin products in the United States. They were rejected by the U.S. Military for this reason. At present, the low-temperature fluidity of modern gelatin preparations is satisfactory, but they have been used and further developed mostly in Europe.[61,62]

Like all other artificial colloids used as plasma expanders, gelatins are polydisperse, that is, variable in molecular size and configuration. This is in contrast to albumin, which is essentially homogeneous (monodisperse), except for the presence of variable, usually small amounts of dimer and oligomers that are found in the usual clinical preparations of this protein. The variability in molecular weight and molecular configuration of a polydisperse colloid affect its intravascular persistence and pattern of elimination and its viscosity and oncotic effect. A simple description of all of these physicochemical characteristics is not possible. The number average molecular weight is somewhat more informative for purposes of comparing colloids than is weight average molecular weight (Mw). Other notations, such as those used to describe preparations of hydroxyethyl starch (HES), which are discussed in more detail later in this chapter, use intrinsic viscosity measurements as one of the descriptors.

Although their use has been largely abandoned in the United States, gelatin preparations, particularly modified fluid gelatin (MFG), have been widely used in Europe. They are of intermediate effectiveness in plasma volume expansion, that is, superior to electrolyte solutions but less effective in this respect than are long-persisting artificial colloids such as dextran (D70). That gelatins have found a clinical role in

Europe was attested to by the report of Nahas et al.[62] in 1978 who showed that more than 2.2 million units of 500 ml each were given to about 1 million patients in France during the period from 1973 to 1976. In 1976, fluid gelatins constituted 58.7 percent of all artificial plasma expanders used in France where the use of electrolyte solutions alone for volume expansion is not widely practiced.

Undesirable Effects

There is little question that modern preparations of gelatin are effective plasma volume expanders. However, they are alleged to share two problems common to all artificial colloids: (1) alteration of the hemostatic mechanism[63,64] and (2) transient effects on renal tubular function.[62] The effect of colloids on hemostasis is discussed in more detail in connection with the use of dextrans. Neither of these effects seems to be clinically significant in the French experience.[50] Lundsgaard-Hansen and Tschirren[61] cite evidence that gelatins have neither of these undesirable characteristics, other opinions notwithstanding.[61]

Most artificial colloids also have at least some antigenic potential in humans. The incidence of significant reactions of the anaphylactic type to gelatin products appears to be comparable to that of other artificial colloids. Wide ranges of reaction frequencies are reported for all such colloids, from 2.5 in 10,000 units to 1 in 300,000 units for dextran. Nahas et al.[62] estimate the frequency of such reactions to gelatin to be in the range of 1 in 40,000 to 1 in 100,000 units. In many instances, the immunologic basis of such reactions is doubtful or unproved. The risk of anaphylaxis is thus not great, and very large volumes of MFG—15 to 20 L—have been given without event to numbers of patients. Nevertheless, concerns about safety appear to be the principal factor mitigating against the wider use of gelatin and other artificial colloid materials in the United States at present.

Dextran

Experimental evaluations of dextrans as a plasma volume expander in humans began in 1944.[65] A clinical product, D70, was introduced for this purpose in 1947; in 1961, so-called low-molecular-weight dextran, D40, was available for use in situations characterized by low perfusion of the capillary bed.[66] These materials largely displaced interest in gelatin products in the United States where they became the principal artificial colloids in clinical use over the next decade. It has been estimated that more than 60 million units of dextran have been used, primarily for volume expansion, since its introduction.[67]

Volume Expansion Effects

Dextrans appeared to be preferable to gelatin because they do not gel at lowered temperatures and were thus better adapted for military and emergency use. D70 has a powerful volume expansion effect, at least as great or greater than albumin, and a relatively long intravascular persistence.[68] Only 30 to 40 percent of D70 is excreted in the urine during the first 12 hours after infusion.[69] There is a substantial body of physiologic research documenting its efficacy in this respect. Investigations that compare its efficacy with that of other colloids such as albumin on outcomes in patients so treated are lacking in the early literature. Indeed, this controversy regarding the relative efficacy of colloids of all types and crystalloids in the management of patients still persists.

Low-molecular-weight dextran, D40, has a higher oncotic effect per gram of infused material than does D70. Because about 63 percent of the molecules of D40 are below 50,000 Mw, the approximate renal excretion threshold size, this colloid has a much shorter intravascular persistence. Arturson and Wallenius[69] showed that 60 to 70 percent of an infused dose was excreted in the urine over a period of 12 hours, with about 50 percent lost in 5 hours. In spite of its relatively short intravascular persistence, D40 appears to produce satisfactory temporary plasma volume support.

Capillary Flow Promotion

Greater investigative interest in D40 was based on the proposal that this colloid improved perfusion of the capillary bed in the clinical setting of trauma, shock, or sepsis. Much interest in the problem of intravascular red cell aggregation and capillary perfusion was generated by the work of Kniseley et al.[70] in 1945 and Kniseley[71] in 1951. As a result of observations that indicated red cell disaggregation by the administration of the smaller-sized range of dextran molecules in experimental shock, Gelin and Ingel-

man[66] suggested the use of a specially prepared low-molecular-weight dextran for this purpose in 1961. Because D70 preparations contain a significant proportion of molecules in this small size range, similar effects on capillary circulation were also found for this preparation. Interest in the use of D70 for volume expansion gradually waned as concern about its adverse effect on hemostasis grew.

Antithrombotic Effects

The possible role of dextran in the prevention of thrombosis may be related to the red cell-disaggregating effect of dextran and/or to its still poorly understood interference with blood coagulation and hemostasis. Thoren[67] was among the principal advocates of this use of dextran as a measure to reduce the incidence of postoperative deep vein thrombosis and pulmonary embolism. He assembled the evidence supporting this use of D70. He reported the combined results of 11 studies, largely European, in which 1,722 patients were given D70 prophylactically, with 6 fatal cases of pulmonary embolism resulting, as opposed to 1,801 untreated controls with 36 such fatalities, all verified at autopsy ($P < 0.001$). Similar data for D40 were also found. Thoren also summarized the information regarding the possible mechanism of this effect, which still remains obscure. Other European authors also reviewed this topic and reached similar conclusions.[53,72,73] In spite of this opinion, dextran is not presently used to any great extent for this purpose in the United States.

Undesirable Effects

Immunologic Effects

Disadvantages of dextran as an artificial plasma colloid include anaphylactoid reactions of variable severity similar to those found with all other colloid solutions. As discussed in relation to gelatin solutions, various reports give widely different incidence figures for these reactions. Mild reactions include rashes, fever, tachycardia, hypotension, or respiratory symptoms and may occur in about 5 percent or more of patients, according to Thompson.[74] Other authors report incidence figures two to three orders of magnitude lower.[66,74] One can only conclude that the true incidence of these reactions is uncertain, but it probably is less than 1 percent because the bulk of the reports cluster around low-incidence figures. One source of confusion in the literature is the fact that some reports are based on reactions encountered per 100 infusions; others report the percentage of patients given infusions who react unfavorably.

By contrast, it is generally agreed that the incidence of severe reactions, including the few that are lethal, is very low; on the basis of a number of estimates, it appears to be in the range of 8 per 100,000 infusions.[66,73–76] In contrast with the infrequency of severe anaphylactoid reactions, preformed dextran-reactive hemagglutinating antibodies are found frequently; such antibodies have been demonstrated in more than two-thirds of the patients in one study. Some of these dextran-reactive hemagglutinating antibodies may be the result of exposure to other natural complex carbohydrate immunogens by other routes.[67] They do not appear to be involved in anaphylactic reactions.[77] High-molecular-weight dextrans are immunogenic as demonstrated by Kabat et al[78], but clinical materials are not immunogenic as a rule.[78–81] Thus, it is not clear what component of a dextran solution may be responsible for the clinically observed reactions. A bacterial by-product of the biosynthesis process might be responsible. It is also noteworthy that reaction rates of similar magnitude are reported for human plasma and plasma derivatives.

Viscosity-Related Effects

Dextrans have high intrinsic viscosity. Their concentration in the urine may become very high after the administration of D40 because of elevation of urine viscosity. This produces diuresis and a type of transient tubular obstruction and change in renal function, particularly when renal perfusion is reduced.[74] This may be associated with transient oliguria and decreased renal function. As Thoren[67] and others[69] have pointed out, this phenomenon, easily demonstrable in dogs, is more difficult to evaluate in clinical practice because dextran D40 is frequently given in the presence of other factors that may cause or contribute to renal failure. It is generally agreed that dextrans by themselves do not cause significant renal damage.

Hemostatic Defects Caused by Dextran and Other Artificial Colloids

Concern about the effect of dextrans on the hemostatic mechanism was initiated by the report of Carbone et al.[82] in 1954. They observed an increase in bleeding time in about 5 percent of otherwise normal subjects given dextran. Many studies since that time have confirmed and amplified this observation.[64] Several of these reports involved clinically significant hemostatic defects secondary to dextran administration.[83,84] By 1958, it had been shown that nearly one-half of patients given 1 L or more of clinical dextran showed increased bleeding time and that daily administration or administration of larger volumes resulted in abnormalities of bleeding in virtually all patients. Coexistent thrombocytopenia aggravates the bleeding tendency, as does simultaneous administration of dicumarol or aspirin.[85–87] Other artificial colloids have similar but less marked effects. The problem may be most severe, and thus most significant, in severely traumatized patients.

The mechanism of bleeding from dextran administration has been investigated extensively. The subject was reviewed by Alexander et al.[63] and Alexander[64], who have also made important contributions to this work. Although the mechanism of increased bleeding after dextran administration is still incompletely understood, these authors argued that it is comparable to an induced form of von Willebrand's disease. This is based on the demonstration of defects in platelet function, factor VIII, and von Willebrand factor activities and capillary changes, all of which resemble those seen in von Willebrand's disease. This may be caused by slow macromolecular precipitation of fibrinogen (factor I), fibrin monomer, and factor VIII, including von Willebrand factor, and by direct effects on platelet and endothelial surfaces. Hemodilution of coagulant proteins does not account for the effects.[64] These mechanisms may also account for the antithrombogenic effects of dextrans, although this remains unproved.

Concern over induction of abnormal bleeding undoubtedly was the principal factor that caused the decline in clinical use of dextran in the United States. Increased availability of human albumin products certainly has contributed to the declining usage. The bleeding tendency was rarely found to be severe with limited administration of dextran, and its use in significant quantities as a plasma volume expander continued in other countries, even though increased availability of albumin has also decreased the use of dextran there.

Hydroxyethyl Starch

This family of substances is the most recently introduced artificial intravascular colloid.[88] One of the principal advantages of HES is that its molecular size and rate of elimination can be relatively precisely controlled. A further advantage lies in its enzymatic degradability by α-amylases, which are widespread in tissues; this results in only small amounts of long-term storage of the compound. Enzymatic hydrolysis of the starch, normally fairly rapid, is decreased by hydroxyethylation with ethylene oxide in alkaline solutions. The degree of hydroxyethylation can be controlled over a wide range of molecular substitution ratios. For a given molecular weight, HES compounds are much less filterable through the glomerulus or capillaries than are dextrans because of their "dense" molecular configuration.[74]

These polydisperse colloids are described in terms of their intrinsic viscosity (i.e., the limiting viscosity of a polymer in a solution as the concentration is extrapolated to zero). The molecular substitution ratio of hydroxyethyl groups is the second pertinent description. Thus, hetastarch, which has been used clinically in the United States, is described as HES-25/75; the intrinsic viscosity is 25 ml/g, and the ratio of hydroxyethyl groups to anhydroglucose units is 0.75. Other colloids include HES-16/43 and HES-90/50. The effects of HES-25/75 resemble those of D70, and HES-16/43 behaves much as D40 does.[74]

Volume Expansion Effects

HES-25/75 is an effective plasma volume expander with a somewhat longer intravascular persistence than the comparable dextran. The administration of a single unit of HES-25/75 resulted in the excretion of 39 percent of the dose in the urine in 24 hours compared with 45 percent of D70.[89,90] The incidence of anaphylactoid reactions and abnormalities of hemostasis may be somewhat lower than is the case with other artificial colloids. Significant tissue injury secondary to transient storage in the reticulo-

endothelial system or uptake by renal tubular cells has not been observed or demonstrated physiologically. HES appears to be nonantigenic in humans,[91-93] and it does not appear to have an antithrombogenic effect.

Use in Leukapheresis

One of the more important uses of HES has been in the collection of donor granulocytes by continuous-flow or cyclic machine centrifugation. In this application, it acts to increase red cell sedimentation and speed centrifugal separation. Many leukapheresis donors have been so treated without untoward reactions. The large amounts given to some of these repeated donors constitutes substantial evidence of its safety. Although an ideal system of donor granulocyte procurement or therapeutic leukapheresis would involve no modification of the donor, the use of HES for this purpose appears to be acceptably safe.

The clinical utility of HES compounds has not yet been fully explored. Extensive clinical use under a wide variety of conditions will be required to determine their ultimate utility and place in transfusion practice. When these materials have been fully developed, HES may well prove to be the colloid of choice for most purposes if any of the artificial colloids again attain widespread use as plasma volume expanders.

REFERENCES

1. Development Task Force of the College of American Pathologists: Practice parameters for the use of fresh-frozen plasma, cryoprecipitate, and platelets. Fresh-frozen plasma, cryoprecipitate, and platelet administration practice guidelines. JAMA 271:777, 1994
2. NIH Consensus Conference: Fresh-frozen plasma. Indications and risks. JAMA 253:551, 1985
3. Devine P, Linden JV, Hoffstadter LK et al: Blood donor-, apheresis-, and transfusion-related activities: results of the 1991 American Association of Blood Banks Institutional Membership Questionnaire. Transfusion 33:779, 1993
4. Contreras M, Ala FA, Greaves M et al: Guidelines for the use of fresh frozen plasma. British Committee for Standards in Haematology, Working Party of the Blood Transfusion Task Force. Transfusion Med 2:57, 1992

5. Cash J: Fresh frozen plasma: is it farewell? Vox Sang 67:121, 1994

6. Stehling L, Luban NL, Anderson KC et al: Guidelines for blood utilization review. Transfusion 34:438, 1994

7. Ciavarella D, Reed RL, Counts RB et al: Clotting factor levels and the risk of diffuse microvascular bleeding in the massively transfused patient. Br J Haematol 67: 365, 1987

8. Mannucci PM, Federici AB, Sirchia G: Hemostasis testing during massive blood replacement. A study of 172 cases. Vox Sang 42:113, 1982

9. Counts RB, Haisch C, Simon TL et al: Hemostasis in massively transfused trauma patients. Ann Surg 190: 91, 1979

10. Frank MM, Gelfand JA, Atkinson JP: Hereditary angioedema: the clinical syndrome and its management. Ann Intern Med 84:580, 1976

11. Jaffe CJ, Atkinson JP, Gelfand JA, Frank MM: Hereditary angioedema: the use of fresh frozen plasma for prophylaxis in patients undergoing oral surgery. J Allergy Clin Immunol 55:386, 1975

12. Wall RT, Frank M, Hahn M: A review of 25 patients with hereditary angioedema requiring surgery (see comments). Anesthesiology 71:309, 1989

13. Pickering RJ, Good RA, Kelly JR, Gewurz H: Replacement therapy in hereditary angioedema. Successful treatment of two patients with fresh frozen plasma. Lancet 1:326, 1969

14. Rosen FS, Austen KF: The "neurotic edema" (hereditary angioedema) (Review). N Engl J Med 280:1356, 1969

15. Donaldson VH: Therapy of "the neurotic edema." N Engl J Med 286:835, 1972

16. Geha RS, Quinti I, Austen KF et al: Acquired C1-inhibitor deficiency associated with antiidiotypic antibody to monoclonal immunoglobulins. N Engl J Med 312: 534, 1985

17. Gelfand JA, Boss GR, Conley CL et al: Acquired C1 esterase inhibitor deficiency and angioedema: a review. Medicine (Baltimore) 58:321, 1979

18. Sim TC, Grant JA: Hereditary angioedema: its diagnostic and management perspectives (see comments) (Review). Am J Med 88:656, 1990

19. Horowitz B, Bonomo R, Prince AM et al: Solvent/detergent-treated plasma: a virus-inactivated substitute for fresh frozen plasma. Blood 79:826, 1992

20. Solheim BG, Svenning DL, Mohr B et al: The use of Octaplas in patients undergoing open heart surgery. p. 253. In Muller-Berghaus G et al (eds): DIC: Pathogenesis, Diagnosis, and Therapy of Disseminated Intravascular Fibrin Formation. Elsevier, Amsterdam, 1993

21. Inbal A, Epstein O, Blickstein D et al: Evaluation of solvent/detergent treated plasma in the management of patients with hereditary and acquired coagulation disorders. Blood Coagul Fibrinolysis 4:599, 1993

22. Piquet Y, Janvier G, Selosse P et al: Virus inactivation of fresh frozen plasma by a solvent detergent procedure: biological results. Vox Sang 63:251, 1992

23. Pehta J, Horowitz M, S/D Plasma Study Group: Clinical studies of solvent detergent-treated plasma. Proceedings of the FDA/NHLBI Workshop on Solvent/Detergent Virus Inactivation, Bethesda, March 23, 1994

24. Tocci LJ, Napychank PA, Cable RG, Snyder EL: The effect of solvent/detergent-treated plasma on stored platelet concentrates. Transfusion 33:145, 1993

25. Horowitz B: Viral safety and biochemical characterization of solvent-detergent plasma. Proceedings of the FDA/NHLBI Workshop on Solvent/Detergent Virus Inactivation, Bethesda, March 23, 1994

26. AuBuchon JP, Birkmeyer JD: Safety and cost-effectiveness of solvent-detergent--treated plasma. In search of zero-risk blood supply. JAMA 272:1210, 1994

27. Beecher HK, Burnett CH, Shapiro SL et al: The Physiologic Effects of Wounds. Medical Department of the US Army; Surgery in WW II. Office of the Surgeon General, Department of the Army, Washington, DC, 1952

28. Simmons RL, Heisterkamp CA, Doty DB: Post-resuscitative blood volumes in combat casualties. Surg Gynecol Obstet 128:1193, 1969

29. Collins JA, Simmons RL, James PM et al: Acid-base status of seriously wounded combat casualties. I. Before treatment. Ann Surg 171:595, 1970

30. Sgouris JT, Dorsey HW: Survey of the use of plasma expanders in the United States. p. 137. In Sgouris JT, René A (eds): Proceedings of the Workshop on Albumin, 1975. Publication no. (NIH) 76-925. National Heart and Lung Institute, National Institutes of Health, Department of Health, Education and Welfare, Bethesda, 1976

31. Lundh B: The consumption of albumin at the University Hospital, Lund, Sweden. p. 239. In Sgouris JT, Rene A (eds): Proceedings of the Workshop on Albumin, 1975. Publication no. (NIH) 76-925. National Heart and Lung Institute, National Institutes of Health, Department of Health, Education and Welfare, Bethesda, 1976

32. Swisher SN (ed): Report of Panel 6 on Safety and Efficacy of Blood and Blood Derivatives. Bureau of Biologics, Food and Drug Administration. The Federal Register, 1980

33. Erstad BL, Gales B, Rappaport WD: The use of albumin in clinical practice. Arch Intern Med 151:901, 1991

34. Sgouris JT, Rene A (eds): Proceedings of the Workshop on Albumin, 1975. Publication no. (NIH) 76-925. National Heart and Lung Institute, National Institutes of Health, Department of Health, Education and Welfare, Bethesda, 1976

35. Tullis JL: Albumin. 1. Background and use. JAMA 237:335, 1977

36. Tunis JL: Albumin. 2. Guidelines for clinical use. JAMA 237:460, 1977

37. Urban J, Inglis AS, Edwards K: Chemical evidence for the difference between albumins from microsomes and serum and a possible precursor product relationship. Biochem Biophys Res Commun 61:444, 1974

38. Rothschild MA, Oratz M, Mongelli J: Effects of a short-term fast on albumin synthesis: studies in vivo, in the perfused liver, and on amino acid incorporation by hepatic microsomes. J Clin Invest 47:2591, 1968

39. Cohn EJ, Oncley JL, Strong LE et al: A system for the separation into fractions of the protein and lipoprotein components of biological tissues and fluids. J Am Chem Soc 68:459, 1946

40. Schiff RI: Transmission of viral infections through intravenous immune globulin. N Engl J Med 331:1649, 1994

41. Polson A, Potgieter GM, Largier JF et al: The fractionation of protein mixtures by linear polymers of high molecular weight. Biochim Biophys Acta 82:463, 1964

42. Watt JG: Automatically controlled continuous recovery of plasma protein fractions for clinical use. A preliminary report. Vox Sang 18:42, 1970

43. Condie RM, Hull BL, Howard RJ et al: Treatment of life-threatening infections in renal transplant recipients with high dose IV human IgG. Transplant Proc 11:66, 1979

44. Sandberg HE: Proceedings of the International Workshop on Technology for Protein Separation and Improvement of Blood Plasma Fractionation. Publication no. (NIH) 78-1422. National Institutes of Health, U. S. Department of Health, Education and Welfare, Washington, DC, 1978

45. Waterhouse C, Bassett SH, Holler J: Metabolic studies on protein depleted patients receiving a large part of their nitrogen intake from human serum albumin administered intravenously. J Clin Invest 28:245, 1949

46. Steere AC: Adverse reactions to albumin caused by bacterial contamination. p. 278. In Sgouris JT, René A (eds): Proceedings of the Workshop on Albumin, 1975. Publication no. (NIH) 76-925. National Heart and Lung Institute, National Institutes of Health, Department of Health, Education and Welfare, Bethesda, 1976

47. Hochstein HD, Seligmann EB: Microbial contamination in albumin. p. 284. In Sgouris JT, René A (eds): 4D. Proceedings of the Workshop on Albumin, 1975. Publication no. (NIH) 76-925. National Heart and Lung Institute, National Institutes of Health, Department of Health, Education and Welfare, Bethesda, 1976

48. Barker LF: Albumin products and the Bureau of Biologics. p. 22. In Sgouris JT, René A (eds): Proceedings of the Workshop on Albumin, 1975. Publication no. (NIH) 76-925. National Heart and Lung Institute, National Institutes of Health, Department of Health, Education and Welfare, Bethesda, 1976

49. Hoofnagle JH, Barker LF: Hepatitis B virus and albumin products. p. 305. In Sgouris JT, René A (eds): Proceedings of the Workshop on Albumin, 1975. Publication no. (NIH) 76-925. National Heart and Lung Institute, National Institutes of Health, Department of Health, Education and Welfare, Bethesda, 1976

50. Pattison CP, Klein CA, Leger RT et al: Field studies of type B hepatitis associated with transfusion of plasma protein fraction. p. 315. In Sgouris JT, René A (eds): Proceedings of the Workshop on Albumin, 1975. Publication no. (NIH) 76-925. National Heart and Lung Institute, National Institutes of Health, Department of Health, Education and Welfare, Bethesda, 1976

51. Wells MA, Wittek AE, Epstein JS et al: Inactivation and partition of T-cell lymphotrophic virus, type III, during ethanol fractionation of plasma. Transfusion 26:210, 1986

52. Alving BM, Hojima Y, Pisano JJ et al: Hypotension associated with prekallikrein activator (Hageman-factor fragments) in plasma protein fraction. N Engl J Med 299:66, 1978

53. Prince AM, Horowitz B, Horowitz MS, Zang E: The development of virus free labile blood derivatives—a review. Eur J Epidemiol 3:103, 1987

54. Gruber UF: Blood Replacement. Springer-Verlag, Berlin, 1969

55. Jamieson GA, Greenwalt TJ: Blood substitutes and plasma expanders. Prog Clin Biol Res 19:1, 1978

56. Hogan JJ: Intravenous use of colloidal (gelatin) solutions in shock. JAMA 64:721, 1915

57. Campbell DH, Koepfli JB, Pauling L et al: The preparation and properties of a modified gelatin (oxypolygelatin) as an oncotic substitute for serum albumin. Tex Rep Biol Med 9:235, 1951

58. Tourtelotte D, Williams HE: Acylated gelatins and their preparations. U.S. Patent No. 2:817:19D8

59. Tourtelotte D, Williams HE: Chemical modifications of gelatin for use as plasma volume expander. p. 246. In Stainsby G (ed): Recent Advances in Gelatin and Glue Research. Pergamon Press, London, 1957

60. Schmidt-Thome J, Mager A, Schone HH: Zur Chemie einer neuen Plasmaexpanders. Arzneimittelforschung 12:378, 1962

61. Lundsgaard-Hansen P, Tschirren B: Modified fluid gelatin as a plasma substitute. Prog Clin Biol Res 19:227, 1978

62. Nahas GG, Vourch G, Tannieres ML: The current use in France of modified fluid gelatins as plasma expanders. Prog Clin Biol Res 19:259, 1978

63. Alexander B, Odake K, Lawler D, Swanger M: Coagulation, hemostasis, and plasma expanders: a quarter century enigma. Fed Proc 34:1429, 1975

64. Alexander B: Effects of plasma expanders on coagulation and hemostasis: dextran, hydroxyethyl starch, and other macromolecules revisited. Prog Clin Biol Res 19:293, 1978

65. Gronwall A, Ingelman B: Untersuchunger uber Dextran und sein Verhalten be parenteraler Zufuhr. Acta Physiol Scand 7:97, 1944

66. Gelin L-E, Ingelman B: Rheomacrodex—a new dextran solution for rheological treatment of impaired capillary flow. Acta Chir Scand 122:294, 1961

67. Thoren L: Dextran as a plasma volume substitute. Prog Clin Biol Res 19:265, 1978

68. Arturson G, Wallenius G: The intravascular persistence of dextran of different molecular sizes in normal humans. Scand J Clin Lab Invest 16:76, 1964

69. Arturson G, Wallenius G: The renal clearance of dextran of different molecular sizes in normal humans. Scand J Clin Lab Invest 16:81, 1964

70. Kniseley MH, Eliot TS, Bloch EH: Sludged blood in traumatic shock. I. Microscopic observations on the precipitation and agglutination of blood flowing through the vessels in crushed tissues. Arch Surg 51:221, 1945

71. Kniseley NH: An annotated bibliography on sludged blood. Postgrad Med 10:15, 1951

72. Steinmann E, Duckert F, Gruber UF: Wert von Dextran 70 zur thromboembolie Prophylaxe in der Allgemeinen. Chirurgie, Orthopadie, Urologie, und Gynakologie, abstracted in English. Schweiz Med Wochenschr 105: 1637, 1975

73. Verstraete M: The prevention of postoperative deep vein thrombosis and pulmonary embolism with low dose subcutaneous heparin and dextran. Surg Gynecol Obstet 143:981, 1976

74. Thompson WL, Jr: Hydroxyethyl starch. Prog Clin Biol Res 19:283, 1978

75. Lundsgaard-Hansen P, Bucher U, Tschirren B et al: Red cells and gelatin as the core of a unified program for the national procurement of blood components and derivatives. Prediction, performance and impact on supply of albumin and factor VIII. Vox Sang 34: 261, 1978

76. Ring J, Messmer K: Incidence and severity of anaphylactoid reactions to colloid volume substitutes. Lancet 1:466, 1977

77. Hedin H, Richter W, Ring J: Dextran-induced anaphylactoid reactions in man: role of dextran reactive antibodies. Int Arch Allergy Appl Immunol 52:145, 1976

78. Kabat EA, Berg D: Dextran—an antigen in man. J Immunol 70:514, 1953

79. Allen PZ, Kabat EA: Persistence of circulating antibodies in human subjects immunized with dextran, levan, and blood group substances. J Immunol 80:495, 1958

80. Kabat EA, Turino GM, Tarrow AB, Maurer PH: Studies on the immunochemical basis of allergic reactions to dextran in man. J Clin Invest 36:1160, 1957

81. Kabat EA, Bezer AE: The effect of variations in molecular weight on the antigenicity of dextran in man. Arch Biochem 78:306, 1958

82. Carbone JV, Furth FW, Scott R, Crosby WH: A hemostatic defect associated with dextran infusion. Proc Soc Exp Biol Med 85:101, 1954

83. Bronwell AW, Artz CP, Sako Y: Evaluation of blood loss from a standardized wound after dextran. Surg Forum 5:809, 1954

84. Horvath SM, Hamilton LH, Spurr GB et al: Plasma expanders and bleeding time. J Appl Physiol 7:614, 1955

85. Adelson E, Crosby WH, Roeder W: Further studies of a hemostatic defect caused by intravenous dextran. J Lab Clin Med 45:441, 1955

86. Adelson E: Bleeding time prolongation after dextran infusion. Bibl Haematol 7:275, 1958

87. Brodman RF, Sarg M, Veith FJ, Spaet T: Dextran 40-induced coagulopathy confused with von Willebrand's disease. Arch Surg 112:321, 1977

88. Munsch CM, MacIntyre E, Machin SJ et al: Hydroxyethyl starch: an alternative to plasma for postoperative volume expansion after cardiac surgery. Br J Surg 75: 675, 1988

89. Metcalf W, Darzan EL, Hehre EL et al: Clinical physiological characterization of a new dextran. Surg Gynecol Obstet 115:199, 1962

90. Metcalf W, Papadopoulas A, Tufaro R, Barth A: A clinical physiologic study of hydroxyethyl starch. Surg Gynecol Obstet 131:255, 1970

91. Salvaggio J, Kayman H, Leskowitz S: Immunologic responses of atopic and normal individuals to aerosolized dextran. J Allergy 38:31, 1966

92. Brickman RD, Murray GF, Thompson WL, Ballinger WF: The antigenicity of hydroxyethyl starch in humans. JAMA 198:1277, 1966

93. Maurer PH, Berardinelli B: Immunologic studies with hydroxyethyl starch (HES), a proposed plasma expander. Transfusion 8:265, 1968

Chapter 44

Blood Substitutes

Richard K. Spence

The search for a clinically useful blood substitute has been underway for almost as long as blood transfusion has been practical. Early experiments with a hemoglobin solution injected into dogs, conducted by Nauyn in the 1860s, set the stage for subsequent work in the twentieth century by numerous investigators.[1,2] Hamlin's[3] advocacy in 1874 of milk as a blood substitute presaged later investigations of casein derivatives and starchs.[4] These initial experiments were prompted by both scientific curiosity and the recognition that blood transfusion was a technically demanding specialty that was not readily available to the practicing physician. Since World War II, the search has been driven primarily by the desire to have an effective alternative to blood that can be stockpiled for use during wartime or large-scale civilian disasters. The last 10 years have witnessed significant progress in the development of the two major classes of substitutes that carry oxygen directly: hemoglobin solutions and perfluorocarbon (PFC) emulsions. With this advance has come an increased recognition of the toxicities and inherent limitations of these products, which has led to a gradual redefinition of their potential clinical uses. This chapter focuses on recent developments in these two classes of substitutes as they might apply to the field of transfusion medicine in the future.

None of the products under development have entered clinical practice to any significant extent, and only one product, a PFC compound, Fluosol (Green Cross, Osaka, Japan), has gained regulatory approval for limited use. This chapter has been included to provide a summary of this field of investigation because of widespread interest in the topic. Research and development in this area continues as of this writing, and much new and important information may be expected in subsequent years.

HEMOGLOBIN-BASED SUBSTITUTES

The earliest experiments with this class of substitutes used stroma-free hemoglobin (SFH) derived from outdated blood. SFH is prepared by lysing red cells in hypotonic media (e.g., distilled water) followed by removal of stroma by a variety of methods, including centrifugation, filtration, and chemical extraction (Figure 44-1).[5] The advantages of these solutions over blood are found primarily in their suitability for prolonged shelf storage and their lack of antigenicity (i.e., no need for crossmatching).[6–8] Amberson et al.'s[2] review of their and others' work with SFH up to the 1940s struck a discouraging note with their description of studies as a "quest" rather than a "conquest." Their reasons for concern were based on the knowledge that SFH had limited usefulness because of its high oxygen affinity, elevated oncotic pressures, rapid intravascular clearance, toxicity, and technical difficulties in preparation. Subsequent

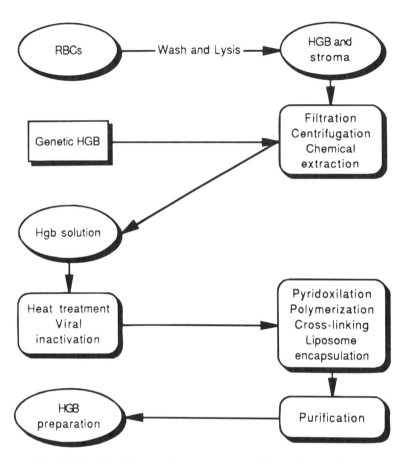

Fig. 44-1. Possible steps for preparation of hemoglobin solution.

work in this field has been directed at solving these problems (Table 44-1).

Oxygen Affinity

Organic phosphates, primarily 2,3-diphosphoglyceric acid (2,3-DPG) and adenosine triphosphate, interact with hemoglobin to produce a lower oxygen affinity (i.e., the O_2 tension at which oxygen is released from the red cell to the tissues) (Fig 44-2).[9] Free hemoglobin is devoid of these compounds, leading to a high oxygen affinity, which results in a lower than normal P_{50} of 12 to 14 mmHg (normal = 26.5 mmHg).[5,10] This, in turn, may lead to potentially deleterious decreases in mixed venous oxygen tension at the tissue level after infusions of hemoglobin solutions. Gould et al.[11] showed lower mixed venous oxygen tensions in primates

that were transfused with pyridoxalated hemoglobin compared with control, hemodiluted animals. MacDonald and Winslow[12] demonstrated that a hemoglobin solution with a normal P_{50} was superior to one with a higher oxygen affinity in preserving contractility and function in a rabbit heart preparation.

Oxygen transport characteristics of free hemoglobin preparations can be improved in a number of ways. Benesh and Benesh[13] increased the P_{50} by binding the artificial organic phosphate, pyridoxal 5′-phosphate (PLP) to free hemoglobin. Moss et al.[10] subsequently produced a similar pyridoxalated and polymerized SFH with a P_{50} of 20 to 22 mmHg. Dellacherie and Vigneron[14] took a somewhat different approach by designing new polymers from dextran and polycarboxylates, which mimic 2,3-DPG. By co-

Table 44-1. Modification of Hemoglobin

To improve oxygen-transport capabilities
    Pyridoxalation with phosphates (e.g., pyridoxal 5′-phosphate)
    Polymerization with various substances (e.g., o-raffinose, dextran, or polycarboxylates)
    Encapsulation with phosphates
    Crosslinking (e.g., diaspirin)
    Bovine hemoglobin
    Genetically engineered hemoglobin
To improve intravascular retention
    Polymerization and crosslinking (e.g., glutaraldehyde or polyethylene glycol)
    Conjugation
    Liposome encapsulation
    Genetic engineering
To reduce toxicity
    Polymerization (e.g., glutaraldehyde)
    Liposome encapsulation
    Treatment with nitric oxide inhibitors

valently fixing these polymers onto oxyhemoglobin, P_{50} values higher than native hemoglobin were attained.[15] Hsia et al.[16] reported on initial success with an o-raffinose polymerized human hemoglobin.

Organic phosphates such as 2,3-DPG and PLP can be encapsulated in liposome-hemoglobin products.[17–20] These preparations closely mimic the red cell in terms of oxygen dynamics, but problems may exist with both membrane stability and hydrolysis of the phosphate compounds. Stabilization of the hemoglobin tetramer by crosslinking α chains with the diaspirin reagent 3,5-dibromosalicyl-bis-fumarate increases P_{50} to 30 to 35 mmHg.[21,22] Creating multiple links produces more stable hemoglobins.[23,24] Acylation of the lysine residue 82 of the β chain by reacting hemoglobin with mono-(3,5-dibromosalicyl) fumarate produces a solution with low oxygen affinity and the potential advantages of both improved resistance to oxidative damage caused by hydrogen peroxide and retention of oxygen-carrying capacity at low temperatures.[25,26] Reaction of deoxyhemoglobin with mellitic dianhydride produces a compound with decreased oxygen affinity.[27]

Decreased oxygen affinity and normalization of P_{50} can be attained by using nonhuman or genetically engineered hemoglobins. Bovine hemoglobin in its natural state has a P_{50} of approximately 30 mmHg.[28] Feola et al.[29] developed a polymerized bovine product with a P_{50} of 18 to 22 mmHg. Bucci et al.[30] applied crosslinking technology and polyaspirin reactions to both human and bovine hemoglobins to produce formulations with P_{50} values ranging from 10 to 50 mmHg. Hemoglobins synthesized in *Escherichia coli* have oxygen affinities much lower than that of native hemoglobin.[31,32]

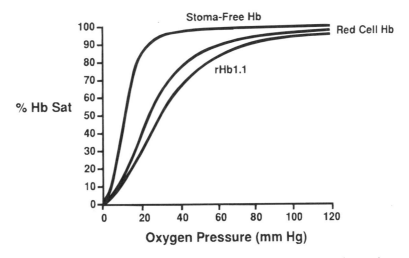

Fig. 44-2. Oxygen dissociation curves for hemoglobin solutions. rHB 1.1, recombinant hemoglobin (Somatogen, Boulder, CO). (From Shoemaker,[149] with permission.)

Oncotic Pressure

Initial formulations of SFH with normal hemoglobin concentrations (i.e., 14 g/dl) were hyperoncotic.[33] Moss et al.[10] solved this problem by polymerization with glutaraldehyde, which increased the molecular size of the product while decreasing the overall number of molecules present in solution. Their formulation, Poly SFH-P, has a normal oncotic pressure of approximately 22 mmHg. Unfortunately, polymerization is not always uniform and may produce a variety of large and small forms.[5] A preponderance of large polymers can lead to unacceptable increases in viscosity.[34,35] This tendency may be corrected by the use of "designer" polymers.[15,36] Liposome encapsulation can produce artificial red cells with acceptable osmotic properties.[19,20,37]

Intravascular Retention

Unmodified SFH dissociates from the tetrameric form into low molecular weight dimers and monomers that are readily filtered by the kidney, resulting in an intravascular half-life of approximately 4 hours.[5,38,39] Such a short half-life places severe limitations on the clinical usefulness of SFH. Fortunately, modifications undertaken to improve oxygen affinity characteristics also lead to decreased renal elimination and increased intravascular retention. Glutaraldehyde treatment of hemoglobin, either human or bovine, can yield solutions with a range of polymers and a half-life of 24 to 48 hours.[28,29,40-42] In a trial of polymerized hemoglobin in chimpanzees undergoing partial exchange transfusion of hemoglobin solution for whole blood (mean exchange = 56.7 ± 7.1 percent), the mean intravascular half-life was 14.6 ± 3.2 hours.[43] Intravascular retention appears to be directly proportional to the number of large polymers in solution. Bleeker et al.[44] found a plasma half-life of 12 to 26 hours for large polymers compared with a 4-hour half-life for 64-kD monomers. Keipert et al.[45] found similar results with a variety of polymerized and crosslinked hemoglobins. The half-life of o- hemoglobin varies from 4 hours for monomeric fragments to up to 15 hours for nanomers.[16]

Crosslinking of free hemoglobin prolongs the intravascular half-life. Coupling of the β chains of hemoglobin produces a solution with an expected half-life of 8 hours in humans.[15,25,34] Crosslinking, like polymerization, produces high-molecular-weight species. It is no surprise that plasma retention is dependent on the number of crosslinked tetramers in these preparations.[46] Liposome encapsulation can also prolong the plasma half-life. Rudolph et al.[47] and Phillips et al.[48] measured circulation half-lives of just over 10 and 20 hours in the mouse and rabbit, respectively, with a liposome-encapsulated hemoglobin. Finally, hemoglobin can be genetically engineered to create fused subunits that resist dissociation into dimers, increasing the half-life to approximately 8 hours.[32]

Modifications that produce prolonged intravascular retention are not without a price. Higher-molecular-weight polymers and liposomes are removed initially from the circulation by the reticuloendothelial cell system (RES) and stored in the liver and spleen.[49-51] The potential for overloading the RES, even for a short time, will most likely limit the absolute amount of these solutions that can be infused at a given time.[52]

Toxicity

Toxicity remains the main barrier to the rapid advancement of hemoglobin solutions into the clinical arena. Unmodified SFH decreases the glomerular filtration rate, leading to renal damage (Table 44-2).[2,5,38,53] This may be caused by excessive glomerular filtration of hemoglobin dimers and tubular obstruction. However, evidence that large amounts of free hemoglobin produced either during cardiac bypass or by improperly thawing blood can be filtered by the kidneys without apparent damage brings this mechanism into question.[54] Polymerized hemoglobin reportedly does not traverse the renal tubule; therefore, its renal toxicity should be negligible.[10,45] However, as noted above, polymerization reactions

Table 44-2. Toxicities of Hemoglobin Solutions

Unmodified hemoglobin
    Renal tubular obstruction
    Decreased glomerular filtration rate
Modified hemoglobin
Vasoconstriction
Contaminants/endotoxins
    Complement activation
    Free radical production

produce a wide variety of forms, some of which can damage the kidney. Takahashi et al.[35] reported transient renal tubular vacuole formation after multiple injections of a polymerized hemoglobin solution.

Endotoxin contaminants, residual cellular stroma, and lipid fragments generated during production of hemoglobin solutions are known mediators of toxicity.[5,53] Several investigators have shown that even small amounts of these substances can cause significant side effects, including vasoconstriction, complement activation, and generation of free radicals.[55–61] Because modifications of SFH do not prevent these problems, production of a highly purified product is essential, as is some uniformity in testing standards.[62–69] Hemoglobin solutions do not appear to be immunogenic when given intravenously and have no appreciable effect on coagulation parameters.[70–73]

Recently, attention has been focused on nitric oxide as the agent responsible for the vasoconstriction produced by hemoglobin solutions. Nitric oxide, an endothelial cell-derived relaxing factor, induces vasodilation and reduces blood pressure by stimulating the release of cyclic guanosine monophosphate in smooth muscle.[74] Several investigators showed that small amounts of free or modified hemoglobin solutions can produce hypertension.[59,75–77] The role of nitric oxide in producing this phenomenon has been demonstrated by studies using either nitric oxide synthase inhibitors or stimulators.[77,78] Katsuyama et al.[76] used N^G-nitro-L-arginine methyl ester to inhibit nitric oxide synthase and L-arginine, a precursor of nitric oxide, in a rat model of hemodilution with diaspirin-crosslinked hemoglobin (DCLHb). The former agent prevented the occurrence of DCLHb-mediated hypertension; the latter reversed the effect. In the dog model of Rooney et al.,[78] using hemodilution with a hemoglobin solution and nitroprusside infusions in supranormal doses led to a modest decrease in the SFH-induced hypertension, implicating nitric oxide as the mediator. Encapsulation of hemoglobin in the liposome may eliminate some of the hypertensive effect by reducing direct contact of hemoglobin with the endothelial cell.[79,80]

Clinical Uses

A large number of animal studies have investigated the potential role of hemoglobin solutions in transfu-

Table 44-3. Potential Clinical Uses of Hemoglobin Substitutes

Treatment of hemorrhagic shock
Battlefield resuscitation
Organ preservation
Cardioplegia
Adjunct to preoperative autologous donation
Short-term blood substitute (e.g., sickle crisis)
Iron loading

sion medicine (Table 44-3). Hemoglobin solutions can sustain life during hemodilution to low hematocrits in a variety of animals, ranging from the rat to the primate.[10,43,60,78–81] The outcome in hemorrhagic shock is comparable to that seen after resuscitation with shed blood and is better than that observed with both crystalloid and colloid solutions.[53,76,77,82–88] Hemoglobin solutions have also been used successfully in animal models to preserve isolated organs,[89–91] as a cardioplegic agent,[92] and as an adjunct to preoperative autologous blood donation.[93] One must be careful not to extrapolate from these data to the human clinical setting because of the wide variety of preparations used and the lack of uniformity in study design. At best, this work can only be used as an indication of the *potential* for clinical use of hemoglobin solutions.

Very little exists in the literature regarding human studies of hemoglobin solutions. Feola et al.[94] tested a 10 percent bovine hemoglobin solution in nine anemic children with sickle cell disease with no comparable controls. Patients infused with an average 25 percent of blood volume reported improvement in clinical symptoms and no obvious adverse effects. The solution produced an erythropoietic response with elevations in reticulocyte counts, probably from the iron load.

Initial phase I safety trials of several hemoglobin products were halted by the Food and Drug Administration after reports of a high incidence of adverse effects.[54] Moss et al.[95] reported a mild "allergic reaction" in one patient during infusion of a polymerized hemoglobin. Hypertension was a common finding in many patients. In 1992, Winslow[96] reported that 26 of 52 patients who had received hemoglobin solutions had had a hypertensive reaction.

Modifications to the solutions allowed testing to resume. Somatogen reported successful administration of recombinant hemoglobin to 70 patients without significant adverse effects.[97] At least three products—polyhemoglobin, DCLHb, and recombinant hemoglobin—were in clinical efficacy trials as of mid-1994 in trauma patients.[98–100]

At the time of this writing, the clinical future of hemoglobin solutions is unknown. Multiple products exist, including polymerized, pyridoxalated, crosslinked, genetically engineered, recombinant, and liposome-encapsulated hemoglobins, all with different effects and reactions. Problems with preparation of large quantities of purified, residue, and endotoxin-free solutions remain to be solved.[101] Dosage levels thus far are limited, with the maximal amount of product transfused safely to date being the equivalent of 1 unit of red cells.[100] Toxicity persists as a problem, to the point that some investigators have suggested that the untoward effect of nitric oxide-induced hypertension may require concurrent treatment if hemoglobin solutions are to be used successfully.

PERFLUOROCARBONS

PFCs represent the second class of oxygen-carrying red cell substitutes. PFCs are chemically inert compounds consisting of fluorine-substituted hydrocarbons. Unlike hemoglobin, PFCs do not chemically interact with oxygen but dissolve it and other gases in accordance with Henry's law.[102] This relationship is linear (i.e., the amount of oxygen dissolved in a PFC is directly related to the partial pressure of oxygen [PO_2]); it does not follow a hemoglobin-like dissociation curve (Fig. 44-3). Typical oxygen solubility for a PFC is 40 to 50 volumes percent.[103] PFCs provide their main benefit by increasing the oxygen solubility of the plasma compartment.[104] Unlike oxygen that is chemically bound to hemoglobin in the red cell, this dissolved oxygen is not subject to the effects of temperature, pH, 2,3-DPG, and so forth. In addition, PFCs appear to facilitate the transfer of oxygen from the red cell to tissues.[54]

Because they are insoluble in water, PFCs must be emulsified for intravenous use. This was first accomplished by Sloviter[105] using albumin and subsequently by Geyer et al.[106] using Pluronic F-68 (Wyan-

dotte Chemicals, St. Louis, MO), a mixture of short chain polymers. PFCs were first considered as potential blood substitutes in the 1960s by Clark and Gollan,[107] who demonstrated their ability to dissolve enough oxygen to allow survival of PFC-liquid-breathing mice. Subsequently, varying combinations of PFCs were tested in a search for a balance between oxygen-carrying ability and tissue retention, eventually resulting in production and testing of Fluosol-DA 20 percent (Green Cross, Osaka, Japan).[108] This first commercially available PFC used Pluronic F-68 as an emulsifier. Concerns over complement activation caused by Pluronic F-68 eventually led to its reduction and partial replacement by egg yolk phospholipids.[109,110]

Fluosol contained two PFCs, perfluorodecalin (FDC) and perfluorotrypropylamine (FTPA), each with markedly different tissue half-lives. FDC was the primary component and oxygen carrier, with FTPA serving primarily to provide stability.[5,111] The emulsion was approximately 11 percent PFC by volume with a 70:30 ratio of FDC to FTPA, for a total weight/volume of 14 percent FDC and 6 percent FTPA. The particle size was 0.2 μm or less, although uniformity of size was uncertain. Stability required that the emulsion be stored in a frozen state and reconstituted just before it was to be used. Its effective intravascular half-life was no more than 3 to 6 hours, primarily because of the rapid clearance of FDC.[54] A significant drawback was the prolonged tissue retention of FTPA, which persisted for months after infusion in the experimental animal.[112]

Fluosol arrived on the U.S. clinical scene in the early 1980s, accompanied by much fanfare. The excitement produced by the promise of a readily available artificial blood substitute for the treatment of anemic patients was fueled in part by the recent acknowledgment that the world's blood supply was infected by the virus responsible for acquired immunodeficiency syndrome. PFCs were ideal candidates as a substitute because they carried oxygen efficiently and in large quantities, were not biologically active, and did not have the problems and encumbrances associated with allogeneic blood transfusion—or so it was thought. The desire to have such a substitute moved Fluosol into clinical trials rapidly.

Unlike hemoglobin solutions, PFCs have an extensive clinical history. Ohyanagi and Saitoh[108] re-

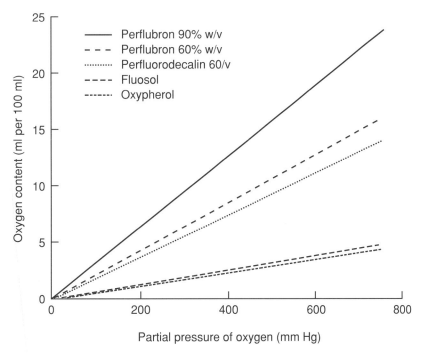

Fig. 44-3. Theoretic relationships between oxygen content and PO_2 for a number of PFC emulsions. (From Faithfull,[145] with permission.)

ported that, as of 1986, more than 400 patients had been treated in Japan with Fluosol. These patients were all Jehovah's Witnesses who had had recent bleeding. After an initial test dose of 0.5 ml, they all received an infusion of 30 ml/kg of Fluosol. PFC and plasma phase oxygen contents increased, although overall oxygen content did not change. Hemodynamic properties remained stable, and no adverse reactions were noted.

Three reports of clinical trials of Fluosol performed in the United States have been published along with a few reports of individual cases. Tremper et al.[113] described the initial U.S. experience in 1982 with 13 patients. Six had been treated as part of a humanitarian protocol, with no data collection. His article summarized the results of the seven remaining severely anemic patients (hemoglobin range = 1.9 to 7.5 g/dl) who had been entered into a trial designed to evaluate the clinical safety of Fluosol and to determine the product's effect on both oxygen transport and hemodynamic variables. Two of the seven patients reacted to an initial test dose, one with

vague symptoms and the other with a "noticeable clinical reaction." The authors also noted transient decreases in white blood cell counts in three patients. These adverse effects were thought to be due to complement activation, and premedication with steroids was suggested as a possible preventive treatment. The arterial oxygen content was significantly increased in these patients by 0.8 volume percent, and oxygen consumption also increased. The cardiac index was also noted to decrease from an elevated mean level of 5.3 ± 1.6 L/min/M^2 of body surface area. All patients were reported to have had an objective improvement.

These investigators subsequently reported on the use of Fluosol in six bleeding Jehovah's Witnesses.[114] It is unclear whether these patients were included in the initial report. None of these patients had adverse reactions to the test dose, but one became hypotensive when the infusion volume and rate were increased. Five of six had a transient decrease in white cell count. Moreover, in three patients, syndromes developed, consisting of fever, leukocytosis, and infiltrates on chest roentgenogram. It was impossible to determine whether Fluosol was responsible for these changes. All patients showed a small increase in calculated arterial oxygen content while breathing 100 percent oxygen after the infusion was complete. This was a significant change compared with the increase noted with oxygen alone before infusion. Five of the six also had increases in oxygen consumption, but the importance of this change in terms of overall oxygen dynamics and outcome was not determined. The authors primarily emphasized both the nature and the severity of the adverse reactions encountered in this small group.

Karn et al.[115] reported their experience with two patients who had received Fluosol after massive postpartum hemorrhage. Both had hemoglobin concentrations of 3 g/dl or lower. Arterial PO_2 rose after Fluosol infusion in both patients, and both heart rate and cardiac index decreased. However, the effect was transient.

Perhaps the most significant report, at least in terms of its effect on the future of Fluosol as a blood substitute, appeared in 1986. Gould et al.[116] reported on their experience in using Fluosol in a small number of patients with hemoglobin concentrations below 3 g/dl. The need for additional oxygen had been demonstrated by the patients' failure to respond to 100 percent oxygen breathing with a change in oxygen extraction ratio. Although Fluosol had a measurable effect in increasing both oxygen delivery and consumption, the authors concluded that the emulsion was of no benefit as a blood substitute in the anemic patient, in part because of the lack of any improvement in patient survival. Other investigators took issue with this conclusion, pointing out that Fluosol had improved oxygenation and that this group of patients was probably beyond salvage, even if they had received red cell transfusions.[117,118]

The randomized clinical trial of Fluosol in the treatment of severe anemia was stopped in the mid-1980s; the results found in the accumulated group of approximately 70 patients were never published. Our report of 46 patients involved in this study appeared in 1990.[119] All patients were Jehovah's Witnesses who refused blood transfusion and were severely anemic (mean hemoglobin = 4.6 g/dl) after acute blood loss. A total of 30 ml/kg of Fluosol was infused after a test dose of 0.5 ml, which produced no reaction. Fluosol successfully increased dissolved or plasma oxygen content 12 hours after infusion but not overall oxygen content compared with the control group. In addition, a significant change from baseline values was noted in the treated patients. None of the patients had adverse reactions to either the test dose or the infusion, but several had been pretreated with corticosteroids. Moreover, the infusion protocol was not continued in four other patients who had reactions to the test dose characterized by chest pain and transient elevations in pulmonary pressure. Fluosol's beneficial effect persisted for up to 12 hours postinfusion but had no apparent effect on survival.

Unfortunately, Fluosol did not live up to its clinical expectation as a blood substitute. Its failure to improve survival in the anemic Jehovah's Witnesses was considered proof of lack of efficacy, preventing its approval for clinical use.[54] Lack of clinical efficacy was thought to be a result of poor understanding of Fluosol's limitations in emulsion design and concentration plus an inappropriate study design, rather than an inherent defect in PFCs. All of the clinical studies had demonstrated in one form or another that PFCs could increase dissolved oxygen content during 100 percent oxygen breathing in the clinical setting. Safety issues remained a concern in spite of reformulation of Fluosol to include egg yolk phospholipid emulsion and less Pluronic F-68.[120–122] As the first chapter in the use of PFCs as blood substitutes came to an end, the challenges confronting investigators were to maximize the oxygen-carrying potential of PFCs, to minimize side effects, and, most importantly, to develop appropriate clinical uses for PFCs.

Second-Generation Perfluorocarbons

Reiss and LeBlanc[102] summarized the desirable characteristics of a PFC intended for intravascular use as a blood substitute. These include (1) large oxygen-dissolving capacity, (2) fast excretion (i.e., lack of long-term tissue retention), (3) absence of clinically significant side effects, (4) good definition and purity, and (5) large-scale industrial availability. They identified three PFCs—FDC, perfluorooctyl bromide (PFOB), and bis(perfluorobutyl)ethylene (Therox, Dupont, Wilmington, DE) as the best can-

Table 44-4. First-Generation Versus Second-Generation Fluorocarbon Emulsions: The Progress

Better defined, pure fluorocarbons

Improved knowledge of fluorocarbons and fluorocarbon emulsions ex vivo and in vivo

Faster excretion

Better accepted surfactants (Pluronic → egg yolk phospholipids)

Higher O_2 carrying capacity (linear fluorocarbons, fluid concentrated emulsions)

Prolonged shelf stability

Ready for use and user friendly

Clinical evaluation in progress (hemodilution, cancer, blood pool imaging, and lymph node imaging)

Limited side effects (+ prophylaxis)

Higher versatility/adaptation

I.V. persistence: no progress

(From Reiss and LeBlanc,[102] with permission.)

didates to meet these criteria (Table 44-4). PFOB, known in its emulsion as Oxygent (Alliance Pharmaceuticals, San Diego, CA) is Reiss's[123] choice as the best candidate because of its stability and high excretion rate. Most of the current work done with PFC emulsions has been performed with Oxygent, although other products are under investigation.[124–126]

The choice of a PFC for clinical use requires balancing oxygen-transport capabilities with both intravascular half-life and tissue retention. Factors that determine oxygen-carrying capacity include the choice of PFC and both the concentration and particle size of the emulsion. Linear PFCs (e.g., PFOB) dissolve oxygen better than cyclic ones (e.g., FDC).[127] Oxygen solubility is inversely proportional to molecular weight and directly proportional to the number of fluorine atoms in the chemical. Ninety percent weight/volume emulsions of PFOB have been developed that can contain four times the amount of oxygen contained in an equal volume of a first-generation PFC.[128] Expressed in other terms, PFOB emulsions could deliver equivalent amounts of oxygen with smaller volumes. The emulsion concentration can be varied, depending on the intended use. Small-droplet-size emulsions favor oxygen-carrying capacity.

Because PFCs are chemically inert, they are not metabolized. Droplets are removed rapidly from the circulation by the RES and are stored primarily in the liver and spleen for subsequent exhalation through the lungs (Fig. 44-4). Intravascular persistence of PFCs is limited by the action of the RES, which removes most of the chemical within 4 to 12 hours. Smaller particles are cleared more slowly than larger ones, but there is a limit to how much droplet size can be decreased and still maintain an effective emulsion. Increasing either concentrations or doses in hopes of prolonging the half-life merely leads to increased tissue deposition and potential damage.[129,130] Unfortunately, little is known at this time about the long-term effects of PFC retention. This concern limited the amount of Fluosol that was given to patients in the anemia trials to a one-time dose of 30 ml/kg. As a result, the emulsion's effect was short-lived. Lessons learned from liposome technology may be applicable to PFCs to produce steric, hydrophilic barriers that minimize droplet removal.[131]

Side effects seen with second-generation PFCs can be divided into acute and late occurrences, based on animal and clinical experience with PFOB (Table 44-5). Acute, transient effects may include facial flushing and back pain; fever and flu-like symptoms may occur 1 to 4 hours postinfusion.[132,133] These symptoms were reported in awake patients receiving PFOB as an imaging agent. In a study of anesthetized surgical patients, acute reactions were not seen,

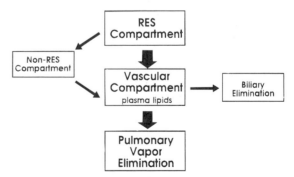

▶ Major elimination as pulmonary vapor

Fig. 44-4. Pharmacokinetic properties of distribution and elimination of Oxygent PFC emulsion. (Courtesy of N. S. Faithfull, M.D.)

Table 44-5. Side Effects/Toxicities of Perfluorocarbons

Perfluorocarbon (dose and drug related)
Facial flushing
Fever
Flu-like symptoms
Thrombocytopenia
Pulmonary gas trapping
Organ retention in liver and spleen
Surfactant/endotoxin
Complement activation
Free radical production

but some patients had minimal temperature elevations of 1°F.[134] These side effects appear to be caused by the normal clearance of PFC droplets by the RES. Opsonization and phagocytosis of droplets lead to the activation of macrophages and release of both prostaglandins and cytokines by the arachadonic acid pathway.[132] It may be possible to block these effects with the use of cyclo-oxygenase inhibitors such as nonsteroidal anti-inflammatory drugs. Unlike first-generation Fluosol, PFOB preparations do not activate complement because they do not contain Pluronic F-68.[109,110]

Inhibition of platelet aggregation has been reported with 90 percent weight/volume PFOB emulsions in an in vivo porcine model and an in vitro human setting.[135] Inhibition was dose dependent and decreased when doses were changed to 1.0 ml/kg or less. Preliminary data from our studies of similar doses of PFOB in anesthetized humans undergoing surgery shows measurable but clinically insignificant decreases in platelet counts; no counts were below 80,000/μl. These decreases occurred 2 to 4 days postinfusion, often after the patient had been discharged from the hospital. No clinical, adverse effects were seen, and counts returned to the normal range within 7 days. This decrease is thought to be caused by an interaction between the platelet's surface and the emulsion, leading to removal of senescent platelets by the RES.

Pulmonary hyperinflation has been reported after infusion of PFOB emulsions in some animal species.[128,132,136] PFOB bubbles formed by vaporization from the circulation into the alveoli of the lung may trap atmospheric gases, causing alveolar expansion and increased pulmonary residual volume. No histo-

logic changes have been observed with this phenomenon.[128] It is both species specific, occurring primarily in rabbits, pigs, and monkeys, and PFC specific. Hyperinflation occurs more often with first-generation, decalin-containing PFC emulsions (e.g., Fluosol) than with second-generation emulsions. There is no evidence that this phenomenon occurs in humans.

Because PFCs are stored temporarily in the liver, it is appropriate to determine whether any hepatotoxicity results. Both first- and second-generation PFCs cause temporary histologic changes in the liver in animals, causing enlargement and histiocytosis, or the appearance of vacuolated macrophages.[103,129–132,137] Hepatic enzymes may be activated, particularly cytochrome P450, leading to changes in the metabolism of various drugs.[137–139] Animal studies show prolongation of this effect with barbiturates and alterations in metabolism and persistence of drugs as diverse as lidocaine and tamoxifen.[139–141] Most of these changes were seen with Fluosol or similar emulsions and may be attributable in part to the effect of the Pluronic F-68 emulsifier. It remains to be seen whether PFOB has a similar effect. Both Zarif et al.[142] and Pelura et al.[143] experimented with a variety of surfactants and emulsifiers in an attempt to improve both stability and biocompatibility. Both the purity and the completeness of the emulsification process have an effect on biocompatibility, stressing once again the need for superior quality control in manufacturing.

Information on both animal and human use of second-generation PFC emulsions is limited (Table 44-6). Goodin et al.[124] demonstrated the ability of a proprietary 40 percent volume/volume PFC emulsion to restore tissue oxygenation and improve survival after experimental hemorrhagic shock. Other investigators have focused on demonstrating the oxygen-transport capabilities of PFOB in the hemodiluted state. Cain et al.[144] isovolemically hemodiluted dogs under air-breathing conditions to hematocrit levels of 25 percent followed by infusions of 6 ml/kg of PFOB emulsion. The animals were then bled until they reached a critical level of oxygen delivery, as determined by whole body, gut, and hindlimb oxygen-extraction ratios. Their results showed no significant differences between control and air-breathing PFOB-treated animals, suggesting that the dog was

Table 44-6. Potential Clinical Uses of Perfluorocarbon
Substitutes

Adjunct to hemodilution
Adjunct to autologous blood donation
Temporary blood substitute
Organ preservation
Myocardial protection during angioplasty
Reduction of acute myocardial ischemia
Treatment of acute cerebral ischemia
Battlefield resuscitation
Oxygen sensitizers during radiotherapy
Oxygen sensitizers during chemotherapy
Liquid ventilation
X-ray visualization
Carbon monoxide therapy
Treatment of gas embolism

able to maintain sufficient delivery and diffusion of oxygen to tissues during controlled hemodilution. However, the authors suggested that PFOB emulsions may play a role in those states in which oxygen diffusion is abnormal and oxygen consumption becomes supply dependent (e.g., sepsis).

Subsequent experiments in a similar canine model hemodiluted to hematocrit levels of approximately 10 percent have been reported by Keipert et al.[104] An infusion of 3.3 ml/kg of PFOB emulsion supplied 30 percent of oxygen-delivery needs and led to a significant increase in mixed venous oxygen tension (PvO_2), suggesting that oxygenation at the tissue level was improved by the emulsion. From these data, Faithfull[145] created an elegant computer model that demonstrates the potential benefit of this elevation in PvO_2 in the clinical setting of hemodilution in the surgical patient (Fig. 44-5). Assume a transfusion threshold of 7 g/dl of hemoglobin in a theoretic surgical patient who has donated 3 units of autologous blood and is bleeding at a rate of 1 L/hr. Once the trigger is reached, the patient can be transfused with autologous blood to maintain safe oxygen delivery, defined as a PvO_2 of 45 mmHg. If the patient is given a 1.35 g/kg of PFC infusion (Oxygent) instead, PvO_2 will be raised to 55 mmHg, providing a considerable margin of safety during further blood loss. Transfusion can be avoided until PvO_2 decreases, which represents a further blood

loss of approximately 2,800 ml. The transfused patient would have used 3 units of blood to maintain acceptable oxygen delivery and would now require allogeneic blood. In contrast, the Oxygent-treated patient would have 3 units of autologous blood remaining (Fig. 44-6). This scenario points out the potential benefit of the PFOB emulsion as an adjunct to hemodilution and avoidance of allogeneic transfusion.

This computer simulation was compared with a canine model of surgical hemodilution.[146] Splenectomized beagles were hemodiluted to hemoglobin levels of 7 g/dl with Ringer's lactate. After treatment with either 0.9 g/kg of PFC (Oxygent) or an equivalent volume of 6 percent hydroxyethyl starch, the dogs were bled in 1-g/dl decrements while cardiopulmonary parameters were followed. Oxygent-treated animals had significantly higher PvO_2, mean arterial pressure, cardiac output, and oxygen delivery than controls during profound hemodilution to 4 g/dl of hemoglobin. A pilot study of seven surgical patients gave similar findings, demonstrating maintenance of PvO_2 values of 55 to 60 mmHg at 30 minutes after a single dose of 0.9 g/kg of PFC (Oxygent) in spite of surgical bleeding and decrease in hemoglobin from 8.3 to 5.9 g/dl.[147] A multicenter, phase II evaluation of Oxygent in this setting is currently underway.

As can be seen from this review, most of the available information about this class of blood substitutes is preclinical in nature. A definitive evaluation of their impact on transfusion medicine is far in the future. What can we say about their potential utility in patient care? Short half-life, prolonged tissue retention, and potential toxicity will most likely place limitations on their usage. Given these constraints, the focus has shifted from the unrealistic goal of completely replacing red blood cells to one of using these products as complementary oxygen transport vehicles. Temporary use during stabilization when blood is not available (e.g., prehospital or battlefield resuscitation from hemorrhagic shock or intraoperative infusion as an adjunct to normovolemic hemodilution) can provide additional oxygen and possibly a margin of safety not obtainable from standard crystalloid and colloid solutions.

The military services certainly have a continuing interest in further development of these products

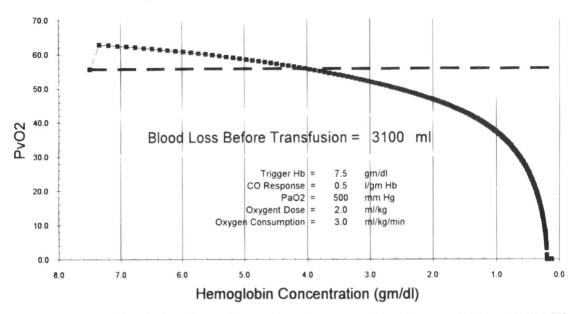

Fig. 44-5. Potential benefit of an infusion of PFC emulsion, Oxygent, in a hemodilution model. (From Faithfull,[145] with permission.)

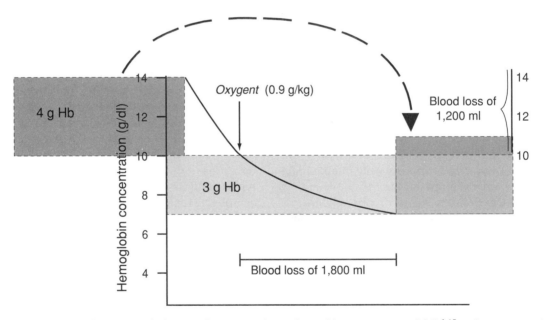

Fig. 44-6. Blood savings with the use of Oxygent during hemodilution. (From Faithfull,[145] with permission.)

and will probably continue their support of this work. Transfusion requirements that appear in parts of the world where the threat of human immunodeficiency virus (HIV) infection of the blood supply is unacceptably high and where safe blood products are not available on short notice is another major potential use. Other potential uses may develop when and if licensed products become widely available, as has been the case with many other products in the past.

Several other issues will be faced in further development of these transfusion materials. One of the principal motivations for their development in the past has been the problem of HIV infection, which is transmissible by transfusion. However, current donor qualification practices have reduced this risk to a negligible point. Public appreciation of this fact lags far behind, however. If the problem of short intravascular persistence is not solved, the use of an oxygen-carrying blood substitute in many instances will only defer not eliminate the need for transfusion with a red cell product. Thus, these materials will function more as an adjunct to prevailing transfusion practices.

Issues of cost, cost relative to benefit, and the availability of starting materials for the preparation of hemoglobin-based products will all have to be evaluated in a health care system that is undergoing major economic and political change. The regulatory process for biologic materials imposed by the Food and Drug Administration is increasingly demanding, costly, and time consuming.[148] All new biologic products face similar problems. These factors lead inevitably to the conclusion that these products will not be available to meet practical transfusion needs any time soon. The problems in the field and the newly available information about them still remains a topic of great theoretic and practical interest.

REFERENCES

1. Nauyn B: Untersuchungen uber bluterinnungen lebenden thiere und ihre Folgen. Arch Pathol Pharmakol 1:1, 1873
2. Amberson WR, Jacobs JE, Hisey A et al: Hemoglobin-saline solutions as transfusion media. p. 156. In Mudd S, Thalhimer W (eds): Blood Substitutes and Blood Transfusion. Charles C Thomas, Springfield, 1942
3. Hamlin AC: Transfusion, 1874. Presented at the Maine Medical Association, June 1874
4. Madden SC, Zeldis LJ, Hengerer AD et al: Casein digests parenterally utilized to form blood plasma protein. p. 201. In Mudd S, Thalhimer W (eds): Blood Substitutes and Blood Transfusion. Charles C Thomas, Springfield, 1942
5. Faithfull NS: Artificial oxygen carrying blood substitutes. Adv Exp Med Biol 317:55, 1992
6. Greenburg AG, Ginsburg K, Peskin GW: Preservation of stroma-free hemoglobin solution. Surg Forum 29:5, 1977
7. De Venuto F: Stability of crystalline hemoglobin solution during extended storage. J Clin Lab Med 92:976, 1978
8. Cochin A, Das Gupta TK, De Woskin R et al: Immunogenic properties of stroma vs stroma-free hemoglobin solution, Surg Forum 24:19, 1972
9. Benesh R, Benesh RE: Intracellular organic phosphates as regulators of oxygen release by hemoglobin. Nature 221:618, 1969
10. Moss GS, Gould SA, Sehgal LB et al: Polyhemoglobin and fluorocarbon as blood substitutes. Biomater Artif Cells Artif Org 15:333, 1981
11. Gould SA, Rosen A, Sehgal L et al: The effect of altered hemoglobin-oxygen affinity on oxygen transport by hemoglobin solution. J Surg Res 28:246, 1980
12. MacDonald VW, Winslow RM: Oxygen delivery and myocardial function in rabbit hearts perfused with cell-free hemoglobin. J Appl Physiol 72:476, 1992
13. Benesh RE, Benesh RE: The effect of organic phosphates from the human erythrocyte on the allosteric properties of hemoglobin. Biochem Biophys Res Commun 26:162, 1967
14. Dellacherie E, Vigneron C: Hemoglobin-based artificial blood: new polymeric derivatives of hemoglobin with low oxygen affinity. Int J Artif Organs 14:28, 1991
15. Prouchayret F, Dellacherie E: Low oxygen affinity derivatives of human hemoglobin by fixation of polycarboxylic dextran to the oxyform. Bioploymers 33:1903, 1993
16. Hsia JC, Song DL, Er SS et al: Pharmacokinetic studies in the rat on a o-raffinose polymerized human hemoglobin. Biomater Artif Cells Immobil Biotechnol 20:587, 1992
17. Farmer MC, Rudolph AS, Vandergriff KD et al: Liposome-encapsulated hemoglobin: oxygen binding properties and respiratory function. Biomater Artif Cells Artif Cells Artif Organs 16:289, 1988
18. Cliff RO, Ligler F, Goins B et al: Liposome encapsulated hemoglobin: long-term storage stability and in

vivo characterization. Biomater Artif Cells Immobil Biotechnol 20:619, 1992

19. Usuba A, Motoki R, Suzuki K et al: Study of the effect of the newly developed artificial blood Neo Red Cells (NRC) on hemodynamics and blood gas transport in canine hemorrhagic shock. Biomater Artif Cells Immobil Biotechnol 20:531, 1992

20. Takeoka S, Hasegawa E, Nishide H et al: Oxygen-transport and solution properties of polylipid/Hb vesicles (ARC). Biomater Artif Cells Immobil Biotechnol 20:399, 1992

21. Chatterjee R, Welty EV, Walder RY et al: Isolation and characterization of a new hemoglobin derivative cross-linked between the alpha chains (lysine 99 alpha$_1$ to lysine 99 alpha$_2$). J Biol Chem 261:9929, 1986

22. Winslow RM: Advances in Blood Substitute Research. Alan R Liss, New York, 1989

23. Olsen KW, Zhang QY, Huang H et al: Stabilities and properties of multilinked hemoglobins. Biomater Artif Cells Immobil Biotechnol 20:283, 1992

24. Kluger R, Wodzinska J, Jones RT et al: Three-point cross-linking: potential red cell substitutes from the reaction of trimesoyl tris(methyl phosphate) with hemoglobin. Biochemistry 31:7551, 1992

25. Osawa Y, Darbyshire JF, Meyer CA et al: Differential susceptibilities of the prosthetic heme of hemoglobin-based red cell substitutes. Implications in the design of safer agents. Biochem Pharmacol 46:2299, 1993

26. Alayash AI, Fratantoni JC: Effects of hypothermic conditions on the oxygen carrying capacity of cross-linked hemoglobins. Biomater Artif Cells Immobil Biotechnol 20:259, 1992

27. Currell DL, Chow R, Yimenu T: The functional properties of hemoglobin modified with mellitic dianhydride: possible applications as a blood substitute. Biomater Artif Cells Immobil Biotechnol 21:153, 1993

28. Sheffield CL, Spates GE, DeLoach JR: Hypoosmotic dialysis and ultrafiltration technique for preparation of mammalian hemoglobins: a comparison of three species. Biomater Artif Cells Artif Organs 16:887, 1988–9

29. Feola M, Gonzalez H, Canizaro PC et al: Development of a bovine stroma-free hemoglobin as a blood substitute. Surg Gynecol Obstet 157:399, 1983

30. Bucci E, Fronticelli C, Razynska A et al: Hemoglobin tetramers stabilized with polyaspirins. Biomater Artif Cells Immobil Biotechnol 20:243, 1992

31. Baudin V, Pagnier J, Lacaze N et al: Allosteric properties of haemoglobin beta 41 (C7) Phe→Tyr: a stable, low-oxygen affinity variant synthesized in *Escherichia coli*. Biochim Biophys Acta 1159:223, 1992

32. Looker D, Abbott-Brown D, Cozart O et al: A human recombinant haemoglobin designed for use as a blood substitute. Nature 356:258, 1992

33. Kaplan HR, Murthy VS: Hemoglobin solution: a potential oxygen transporting plasma volume expander. Fed Proc 34:1461, 1975

34. Bakker JC, Berbers GA, Bleeker WK et al: Preparation and characterization of crosslinked and polymerized hemoglobin solutions. Biomater Artif Cells Immobil Biotechnol 20:233, 1992

35. Takahashi T, Iwasaki K, Malchesky PS et al: Renal effects of multiple infusion of pyridoxalated-hemoglobin-polyoxyethylene conjugate (PHP) solution in dogs. Artif Organs 17:153, 1993

36. Potzschke H, Barnikol WK: A new type of artificial oxygen carrier: soluble hyperpolymeric haemoglobin with negligible oncotic pressure—production of thermally stable hyperpolymers from human blood with glutaraldehyde as cross-linker. Biomater Artif Cells Immobil Biotechnol 20:287, 1992

37. Zheng S, Zheng Y, Beissinger RL et al: Liposome-encapsulated hemoglobin processing methods. Biomater Artif Cells Immobil Biotechnol 20:355, 1992

38. Savitsky JP, Doczi J, Black J et al: A clinical safety trial of stroma-free hemoglobin. Clin Pharmacol Ther 23:73, 1978

39. Bonhard K: Acute oxygen supply by infusion of hemoglobin solutions. Fed Proc 34:1466, 1975

40. Sehgal LR, Gould SA, Rosen AR et al: Polymerized pyridoxalated hemoglobin: a red cell substitute with normal O$_2$ capacity. Surgery 95:433, 1984

41. DeVenuto F, Zegna A: Preparation and evaluation of pyridoxalated polymerized human hemoglobin. J Surg Res 34:205, 1983

42. Keipert PE, Chang TMS: Preparation and in vitro characteristics of a blood substitute based on pyridoxalated polyhemoglobin. Appl Biochem Biotech 10:133, 1984

43. Lenz G, Junger H, Schneider M et al: Elimination of pyridoxalated polyhemoglobin after partial exchange transfusion in chimpanzees. Biomater Artif Cells Immobil Biotechnol 19:699, 1991

44. Bleeker WK, Berbers GA, den Boer PJ et al: Effect of polymerization on clearance and degradation of free hemoglobin. Biomater Artif Cells Immobil Biotechnol 20:747, 1992

45. Keipert PE, Gomez CL, Ganzales A et al: The role of the kidneys in the excretion of chemically modified hemoglobins. Biomater Artif Cells Immobil Biotechnol 20:737, 1992

46. Manning LR, Morgan S, Beavis RC et al: Preparation, properties, and plasma retention of human hemoglo-

bin derivatives: comparison of uncrosslinked carboxymethylated hemoglobin with crosslinked tetrameric hemoglobin. Proc Natl Acad Sci U S A 88:3329, 1991

47. Rudolph AS, Cliff RO, Klipper R et al: Circulation persistence and biodistribution of lyophilized liposome-encapsulated hemoglobin: an oxygen carrying resuscitative fluid. Crit Care Med 22:142, 1994

48. Phillips WT, Rudolph AS, Goins B et al: Biodistribution studies of liposome encapsulated hemoglobin (LEH) studied with a newly developed 99m-technetium liposome label. Biomater Artif Cells Immobil Biotechnol 20:757, 1992

49. Kim HW, Clancy T, Chen F et al: Hepatic reticuloendothelial function following resuscitation with hemoglobin solutions. Biomater Artif Cells Immobil Biotechnol 20:789, 1992

50. Anderson PJ, Ning J, Biro GP: Clearance of differentially labeled infused hemoglobin and polymerized hemoglobin from dog plasma and accumulation in urine and selected tissues. Biomater Artif Cells Immobil Biotechnol 20:781, 1992

51. Beach MC, Morley J, Spirdya L et al: Effects of liposome encapsulated hemoglobin on the reticuloendothelial cell system. Biomater Artif Cells Immobil Biotechnol 20:771, 1992

52. Kim HW, Chen F, Greenburg AG: A double (exchange transfusion-carbon clearance) model for testing post-resuscitation reticuloendothelial function. Biomater Artif Cells Immobil Biotechnol 20:777, 1992

53. Ning J, Peterson LM, Anderson PJ et al: Systemic hemodynamic and renal effects of unmodified SFHS in dogs. Biomater Artif Cells Immobil Biotechnol 20:723, 1992

54. Zuck TF, Reiss JG: Current status of injectable oxygen carriers. p. 295. In Hindmarsh JT, Goldberg DM (eds): Clinical Reviews in Clinical Laboratory Sciences. CRC Press, Boca Raton, FL, 1994

55. Lieberthal W, LaRaia J, Valeri CR: Role of thromboxane in mediating the intrarenal vasoconstriction induced by unmodified strom free hemoglobin in the isolated perfused rat kidney. Biomater Artif Cells Immobil Biotechnol 20:663, 1992

56. Feola M, Simoni J, Tran R et al: Nephrotoxicity of hemoglobin solutions. Biomater Artif Cells Artif Organs 18:233, 1990

57. Biessels PT, Hak JB, Bleeker WK et al: Effects of modified hemoglobin solutions on the isolated rabbit heart. Biomater Artif Cells Immobil Biotechnol 20:693, 1992

58. Gotoh K, Morioka T, Nishi K: Effects of pyridoxalated hemoglobin polyoxyethylene conjugate (PHP)

and stroma free hemoglobin (SFH) on pulmonary vascular responsiveness to various vasoactive substances in isolated perfused rat lungs. Biomater Artif Cells Immobil Biotechnol 20:721, 1992

59. Matsumura H, Araki H, Morioka T et al: Pyridoxalated hemoglobin polyoxyethylene conjugate (PHP) on the endothelium-dependent relaxation in rat mesenteric arterioles. Biomater Artif Cells Immobil Biotechnol 20:679, 1992

60. Feola M, Simoni J, Dobke M et al: Complement activation and the toxicity of stroma-free hemoglobin solutions in primates. Circ Shock 25:275, 1988

61. Alayash AI, Fratantoni JC, Bonaventura C et al: Consequences of chemical modifications on the free radical reactions of human hemoglobin. Arch Biochem Biophys 298:114, 1992

62. Biessels PT, Berbers GA, Broeders GC et al: Detection of erythrocyte membrane components in hemoglobin-based blood substitutes. Clin Chim Acta 212:113, 1992

63. Greenburg G, Kim HW: Evaluating new red cell substitutes: a critical analysis of toxicity models. Biomater Artif Cells Immobil Biotechnol 20:575, 1992

64. Tani T, Chang TM, Kodama M et al: Endotoxin removed from hemoglobin solution using polymyxin-B immobilized fibre (PMX-F) followed by a new turbidometric endotoxin assay. Biomater Artif Cells Immobil Biotechnol 20:457, 1992

65. Marshall T, Weltzer J, Hai T et al: Trace element analyses of diaspirin cross-linked hemoglobin solutions. Biomater Artif Cells Immobil Biotechnol 20:453, 1992

66. Nakai K, Abe H, Matsuda N et al: Development of analytical methods to evaluate SFH. Biomater Artif Cells Immobil Biotechnol 20:447, 1992

67. Menu P, Faivre B, Labrude P et al: Possible importance of chromatographic purification position in a blood substitute elaboration process. Biomater Artif Cells Immobil Biotechnol 20:443, 1992

68. Sekiguchi S: Studies on the quality control of stroma-free hemoglobin. Biomater Artif Cells Immobil Biotechnol 20:407, 1992

69. Feola M, Simoni J, Canizaro PC: Quality control of hemoglobin solutions. I. The purity of hemoglobin before modification. Science 253:32, 1991

70. Chang TM, Lister C, Nishiya A et al: Immunological effects of hemoglobin, encapsulated hemoglobin, polyhemoglobin and conjugated hemoglobin using different immunization schedules. Biomater Artif Cells Immobil Biotechnol 20:611, 1992

71. Estep TN, Gonder J, Bornstein I et al: Immunogenicity of diaspirin cross-linked human hemoglobin solu-

tions. Biomater Artif Cells Immobil Biotechnol 20: 603, 1992

72. Kim HW, Stubdal H, Greenburg AG: Coagulation dynamics after hemodilution with polyhemoglobin. Surg Gynecol Obstet 175:219, 1992

73. Reiss RF, Caballero R, Hess J: Effects of X-linked hemoglobin on in-vitro platelet function. Biomater Artif Cells Immobil Biotechnol 20:651, 1992

74. Moncada S, Palmer RMJ, Higgs EA: Nitric oxide: physiology, pathophysiology, and pharmacology. Pharmacol Rev 43:109, 1991

75. Alayash AI, Fratantoni JC, Bonaventura C et al: Nitric oxide binding to human ferrihemoglobins cross-linked between alpha or β subunits. Arch Biochem Biophys 303:332, 1993

76. Katsuyama SS, Cole DJ, Drummond JC et al: Nitric oxide mediates the hypertensive response to a modified hemoglobin solution (DCLHb) in rats. Artif Cells Blood Substit Immobil Biotechnol 22:1, 1994

77. Hess JR, MacDonald VW, Brinkley WW: Systemic and pulmonary hypertension after resuscitation with cell-free hemoglobin. J Appl Physiol 74:1769, 1993

78. Rooney MW, Hirsch LJ, Aasen MK et al: Lack of increased cardiac output during hemoglobin hemodilution can be reversed with sodium nitroprusside. Biomater Artif Cells Immobil Biotechnol 20:689, 1992

79. Rabinovici R, Rudolph AS, Ligler FS et al: Biological responses to exchange transfusion with liposome-encapsulated hemoglobin. Circ Shock 37:124, 1992

80. Nakai K, Matsuda N, Amano M et al: Acellular and cellular hemoglobin solutions as vasoconstrictive factor. Artif Cells Blood Substit Immobil Biotechnol 22:559, 1994

81. Lenz G, Junger H, van den Ende R et al: Hemodynamic effects after partial exchange transfusion with pyridoxalated polyhemoglobin in chimpanzees. Biomater Artif Cells Immobil Biotechnol 19:709, 1991

82. Usuba A, Motoki R, Suzuki K et al: Study of the effect of newly developed artificial blood Neo Red Cells (NRC) on hemodynamics and blood gas transport in canine hemorrhagic shock. Biomater Artif Cells Immobil Biotechnol 20:531, 1992

83. Chang TM, Varma R: Effect of single replacement of one of Ringer lactate, hypertonic saline/dextran, 7 g% albumin, stroma-free hemoglobin, o-raffinose polyhemoglobin or whole blood on the long term survival of unanesthetized rats with lethal hemorrhagic shock after acute 67% blood loss. Biomater Artif Cells Immobil Biotechnol 20:503, 1992

84. Hess JR, MacDonald VW, Winslow RM: Dehydration and shock: an animal model of hemorrhage and re-suscitation of battlefield injury. Biomater Artif Cells Immobil Biotechnol 20:499, 1992

85. Malcolm D, Kissinger D, Garrioch M: Diaspirin cross-linked hemoglobin solution as a resuscitative fluid following severe hemorrhage in the rat. Biomater Artif Cells Immobil Biotechnol 20:495, 1992

86. Schultz SC, Hamilton IN, Jr, Malcolm DS: Use of base deficit to compare resuscitation with lactated Ringer's solution, Haemaccel, whole blood, and diaspirin cross-linked hemoglobin following hemorrhage in rats. J Trauma 35:6, 1993

87. Hodakowski GT, Svizzero T, Jacobs EE, Jr et al: Acute effects of massive transfusion of a bovine hemoglobin blood substitute in a canine model of hemorrhagic shock. Eur J Cardiothorac Surg 6:649, 1992

88. Bosman RJ, Minten J, Lu HR et al: Free polymerized hemoglobin versus hydroxyethyl starch in resuscitation of hypovolemic dogs. Anesth Analg 75:811, 1992

89. Liu H, Agishi T, Kawai T et al: Evaluation of a pyridoxalated hemoglobin polyoxyetheylene conjugate solution as a perfusate for small intestine preservation. Biomater Artif Cells Immobil Biotechnol 20: 557, 1992

90. Horiuchi T, Ohta Y, Hashimoto K et al: Machine perfusion of isolated kidney at 37 degrees C using pyridoxalated hemoglobin polyoxyetheylene (PHP) solution, UW solution and its combination. Biomater Artif Cells Immobil Biotechnol 20:549, 1992

91. Agishi T, Sonda K, Nakajima I et al: Modified hemoglobin solution as possible perfusate relevant to organ transplantation. Biomater Artif Cells Immobil Biotechnol 20:539, 1992

92. Schistek R, Pohla G, Samhaber E et al: Artificial blood and extracorporeal circulation (ECC). Biomater Artif Cells Immobil Biotechnol 20:731, 1992

93. Stanetz PJ, Lee R, Page R et al: Hemoglobin blood substitutes in extended preoperative autologous blood donation: an experimental study. Surgery 115: 246, 1994

94. Feola M, Simoni J, Angelillo R et al: Clinical trial of a hemoglobin based blood substitute in patients with sickle cell anemia. Surg Gynecol Obstet 174:379, 1992

95. Moss GS, Gould SA, Rosen AL et al: Results of the first clinical trial with a polymerized hemoglobin solution, abstracted. Biomater Artif Cells Artif Organs 17:633, 1989

96. Winslow RW: Hemoglobin-Based Red Cell Substitutes. Johns Hopkins University Press, Baltimore, 1992

97. Clinical testing of recombinant hemoglobin to begin, Blood Weekly, August 9, 1993, p. 3

98. Baxter to test blood substitute in the US. Blood Weekly, August 9, 1993, p. 3

99. Safety study of recombinant hemoglobin advances. Blood Weekly, October 4, 1993, p. 13

100. Blood substitute moves into trauma trials. Blood Weekly, October 25, 1993, p. 10

101. Chapman KW, Snell SM, Jesse RG et al: Pilot scale production of pyrogen-free human hemoglobin for research. Biomater Artif Cells Immobil Biotechnol 20:415, 1992

102. Reiss JG, LeBlanc M: Solubility and transport phenomena in perfluorochemicals relevant to blood substitution and other medical applications. Pure Appl Chem 54:2383, 1982

103. Lowe KC: Synthetic oxygen transport fluids based on perfluorochemicals: applications in medicine and biology. Vox Sang 60:129, 1991

104. Keipert PE, Faithfull NS, Bradley JAD et al: Oxygen delivery augmentation by low-dose perfluorochemical emulsion during profound normovolemic hemodilution. p. 197. In Vampel P, Zander R, Bruley DF (eds): Oxygen Transport to Tissue XV. Plenum, New York, 1994

105. Sloviter HA: Perfusion of the brain and other isolated organs with dispersed perfluoro compounds. p. 28. In Blood Substitutes and Plasma Expanders. Alan R Liss, New York, 1978

106. Geyer RP, Monroe RG, Taylor K: Survival of rats totally perfused with a fluorocarbon-detergent preparation. p. 85. In Norman JC (ed): Organ Perfusion and Preservation. Appleton-Century Crofts, East Norwalk, CT, 1968

107. Clark LC, Jr, Gollan F: Survival of mammals breathing organic liquids equilibrated with oxygen at atmospheric pressure. Science 152:1755, 1966

108. Ohyanagi H, Saitoh Y: Development and clinical application of perfluorochemical artificial blood. Int J Artif Organs 9:363, 1986

109. Hammerschmidt DE, Vercellotti GM: Limitation of complement activation by perfluorocarbon emulsions: superiority of lecithin-emulsified preparations. p. 431. In Chang TM, Geyer RP (eds): Blood Substitutes. Marcel Dekker, New York, 1989

110. Hong F, Shastri KA, Logue GL et al: Complement activation by artificial blood substitute Fluosol: in vitro and in vivo studies. Transfusion 31:642, 1991

111. Biro GP: Perfluorocarbon-based red blood cell substitutes. Transfusion Med Rev 7:84, 1993

112. Yokoyama K, Yamanouchi K, Ohyanagi H et al: Fate of perfluorocarbons in animals after intravenous injection of hemodilution with their emulsions. Chem Pharm Bull (Tokyo) 26:956, 1978

113. Tremper KK, Friedman AE, Levine EM et al: The preoperative treatment of severely anemic patients with a perfluorochemical oxygen-transport fluid. Fluosol-DA. N Engl J Med 307:277, 1982

114. Waxman K, Tremper KK, Cullen BF et al: Perfluorocarbon infusion in bleeding patients refusing blood transfusions. Arch Surg 119:721, 1984

115. Karn KE, Ogburn PL, Jr, Julian T et al: Use of a whole blood substitute, Fluosol-DA 20%, after massive postpartum hemorrhage. Obstet Gynecol 65:127, 1985

116. Gould SA, Rosen AL, Sehgal LR et al: Fluosol-DA as a red cell substitute in acute anemia. N Engl J Med 314:1653, 1986

117. Spence RK: Fluosol-DA as a red cell substitute in acute anemia (correspondence). N Engl J Med 315:1677, 1987

118. Reiss JG: Fluorocarbon-based in vivo oxygen transport and delivery systems. Vox Sang 61:225, 1991

119. Spence RK, McCoy S, Costabile J et al: Fluosol DA-20 in the treatment of severe anemia: randomized controlled study of 46 patients. Crit Care Med 18:1227, 1990

120. Ingram DA, Forman MB, Murray JJ: Phagocytic activation of human neutrophils by the detergent component of Fluosol. Am J Pathol 140:1081, 1992

121. Kent KM, Cleman MW, Cowley MJ et al: Reduction of myocardial ischemia during percutaneous transluminal coronary angioplasty with oxygenated Fluosol. Am J Cardiol 66:279, 1990

122. Flain SF: Pharmacokinetics and side effects of perfluorocarbon-based blood substitutes. Biomater Artif Cells Immobil Biotechnol 22:1043, 1994

123. Reiss JG: Overview of progress in the fluorocarbon approach to in vivo oxygen delivery. p. 24. In Chang TM (ed): Blood Substitutes and Oxygen Carriers. Marcel Dekker, New York, 1993

124. Goodin TH, Grossbard EB, Kaufman RJ et al: A perfluorochemical emulsion for prehospital resuscitation of experimental hemorrhagic shock: a prospective, randomized, controlled study. Crit Care Med 22:680, 1994

125. Thoolen MJMC, Rasbach DE, Shaw JH et al: Preservation of regional and global left ventricular function by intracoronary infusion with oxygenated fluorocarbon emulsion Therox in dogs. Biomater Artif Cells Immobil Biotechnol 21:53, 1993

126. Meinert H, Fackler R, Knoblich A et al: On the perfluorocarbon emulsions of second generation. Biomater Artif Cells Immobil Biotechnol 20:95, 1992

127. Reiss JG, Le Blanc M: Preparation of perfluorochemical emulsions for biomedical use: principles, materials and methods. p. 94. In Lowe KC (ed): Blood Substitutes: Preparation, Physiology and Medical Applications. Ellis Horwood, Chichester, 1988

128. Reiss JG: The design and development of improved fluorocarbon-based products for use in medicine and biology. Artif Cells Blood Substit Immobil Biotechnol 22:215, 1994

129. Bentley PK, Johnson OL, Washington C et al: Lymphoid tissue responses to concentrated perfluorochemical emulsions in rats. Biomater Artif Cells Immobil Biotechnol 20:1033, 1992

130. Lowe KC, Bentley PK: Retention of perfluorochemicals in rat liver and spleen. Biomater Artif Cells Immobil Biotechnol 20:1029, 1992

131. Woodle MC, Lasic DD: Sterically stabilized liposomes. Biochim Biophys Acta 1113:171, 1992

132. Flaim SF, Hazard DR, Hogan J et al: Characterization and mechanism of side-effects of Oxygent HT (highly concentrated fluorocarbon emulsion) in swine. Biomater Artif Cells Immobil Biotechnol 19:383, 1991

133. Bruneton JN, Falewee MN, Francois E et al: Preliminary clinical results using perfluorocetylbromide (PFOB) for CT imaging of the liver, spleen and vessels. Radiology 170:179, 1989

134. Cernaianiu AC, Spence RK, DelRossi AD et al: A safety study of the perfluorochemical emulsion, Oxygent, in anesthetized surgical patients, abstracted. Anesthesiology 81:A397, 1994

135. Smith DJ, Lane TA: Effect of a high concentration perfluorocarbon emulsion on platelet function. Biomater Artif Cells Immobil Biotechnol 20:1045, 1992

136. Clark LC, Hoffman RE, Davis SL: Response of the rabbit lung as a criterion of safety for fluorocarbon breathing and blood substitutes. Biomater Artif Cells Immobil Biotechnol 20:1085, 1992

137. Adrianov NV, Achakov AI, Zigler M: Induction of cytochrome P-450 by perfluorodecalin in mouse liver microsomes. Bull Exp Biol Med (USSR) 108:164, 1989

138. Lowe KC, Armstrong FH: Biocompatibility studies with perfluorochemical oxygen carriers. Biomater Artif Cells Immobil Biotechnol 20:993, 1992

139. Armstrong FH, Lowe KC: Effects of emulsified perfluorochemicals on liver cytochrome P-450 in rats. Compar Biochem Physiol 94C:345, 1989

140. Shah IG, Parsons DL: Human albumin binding of tamoxifen in the presence of a perfluorochemical erythrocyte substitute. J Pharm Pharmacol 43:790, 1991

141. Hoke JF, Ravis WR: Effect of a perfluorochemical erythrocyte substitute on the in vitro metabolism of lidocaine using rat liver slices. Res Commun Chem Pathol Pharmacol 73:333, 1991

142. Zarif L, Reiss JG, Pucci B et al: Biocompatibility of alkyl and perfluoralkyl surfactants derived from THAM. Biomater Artif Cells Immobil Biotechnol 21:597, 1993

143. Pelura TJ, Johnson CS, Tarara TE et al: Stabilization of Perflubron emulsions with egg yolk phospholipid. Biomater Artif Cells Immobil Biotechnol 20:845, 1992

144. Cain SM, Curtis SE, Bradley WE: Facilitation of oxygen transfer by Perflubron in hemodiluted dogs. Adv Exp Med Biol 317:479, 1992

145. Faithfull NS: Mechanisms and efficacy of fluorochemical oxygen transport and delivery. Biomater Artif Cells Immobil Biotechnol 22:181, 1994

146. Cernaianu AC, Spence RK, Vasilidze T et al: Improvement in circulatory and oxygenation status with Perflubron (Oxygent HT) in a canine model of surgical hemodilution. Artif Cells Blood Substit Immobil Biotechnol 81:A313, 1994

147. Wahr JA, Trouwborst A, Spence RK et al: A pilot study of the efficacy of an oxygen carrying emulsion, Oxygent HT, in patients undergoing surgical blood loss, abstracted. Anesthesiology (in press)

148. Fratantoni JC: Points to consider on efficacy evaluation of hemoglobin- and perfluorocarbon-based oxygen carriers. Transfusion 34:712, 1994

149. Shoemaker SA, Gerber MJ, Evans GL et al: Initial clinical experience in the rationally designed, genetically engineered recombinant human hemoglobin. Artif Cells Blood Substit Immobil Biotechnol 22:457, 1994

Chapter 45

Immunoglobulin Therapy

Roger H. Kobayashi and E. Richard Stiehm

Immunoglobulin therapy (passive immunization) is the administration of antibody from an immune subject to a nonimmune subject to provide temporary protection against a microbial agent, toxin, poison, or cell. Passive immunity (unlike active immunity, in which antigen is administered) is usually used when a subject is exposed to an infectious disease in which active immunization is either unavailable or has not been given before exposure (e.g., tetanus or rabies). Immunoglobulin therapy is also used in certain disorders associated with toxins (e.g., diphtheria), in certain bites (e.g., snake or spider), and as a specific (e.g., Rho[D] immunoglobulin) or as a nonspecific (e.g., antithymocyte globulin) immunosuppressive. Large doses of human intravenous immunoglobulin (IVIG) are also used as replacement therapy in antibody deficiencies and as an anti-inflammatory and immunomodulatory agent in a variety of autoimmune disorders.

Five types of preparations are used in immunoglobulin therapy (1) standard human immune serum globulin (ISG) for general use, given intramuscularly or subcutaneously; (2) standard human IVIG; (3) special high-titered human immune globulins with a known antibody content for specific diseases; (4) animal antisera and antitoxins; and (5) other miscellaneous therapeutic antibodies, including monoclonal antibodies and antibody fragments. These are listed in Table 45-1.

Passive immunization for an infectious disease is not always effective; the duration of action is short and variable (1 to 6 weeks); and undesirable side reactions may occur, particularly if the immunoglobulin is of nonhuman origin. The special high-titered human immunoglobulins are identical to ISG (or in the case of cytomegalovirus [CMV]-IVIG, to IVIG) except they are obtained from immunized or convalescing donors, and their antibody titer is assayed. They are valuable in several disorders in which ISG or IVIG are of little or no value.

In addition to the preparations listed in Table 45-1, several new immunoglobulin products are under development and may enter the therapeutic cornucopia by the time this chapter reaches the reader's eye. These include respiratory syncytial virus IVIG (RSV-IVIG),* hepatitis B IVIG, and Pseudomonas IVIG.

ANIMAL SERUMS AND ANTITOXINS

These are derived from the serum of immunized animals, usually horses (equine antiserum). Because these serums are foreign proteins, there is a significant risk to their use. Thus, they should be administered only when specifically indicated, after sensitivity tests, and by a physician prepared to deal with a hypersensitivity reaction.

A careful history must be taken before an animal

---

* Licensed as RespiGam in January, 1996 by the U.S. FDA for the prevention of serious lower respiratory tract infections caused by RSV in children under 24 months of age with bronchopulmonary dysplasia or a history of premature birth (≤35 weeks' gestation). It is given monthly during the respiratory virus season.

Table 45-1. Antibody Preparations Available for Passive Immunity

Product	Abbreviations or Brand Names	Principal Use
Standard human immune serum globulins	γ Globulin	
Intravenous immune globulin	IVIG, IGIV	Treatment of antibody deficiency, immune thrombocytopenia purpura, Kawasaki disease, other inflammatory diseases
Intramuscular immune globulin	ISG	Treatment of antibody deficiency, prevention of measles, hepatitis, etc.
Special human immune serum globulins[a]		
Hepatitis B immune globulin	HBIG	Prevention of hepatitis B
Varicella-zoster immune globulin	VZIG	Modification or prevention of chicken pox
Rabies immune globulin	RIG	Prevention of rabies
Tetanus immune globulin	TIG	Prevention or treatment of tetanus
Vaccinia immune globulin[b]	VIG	Prevention or treatment of smallpox, vaccinia
Western equine encephalitis immune globulin[b]	WEE-IG	Prevention, after laboratory accident with WEE virus
Rho(D) immune globulin	Rho-GAM	Prevention of Rh hemolytic disease
Cytomegalovirus immune globulin intravenous	CMV-IVIG	Prevention and treatment of cytomegalovirus infections
Animal serums and globulins		
Tetanus antitoxin (equine)	TAT	Prevention or treatment (when TIG unavailable)
Diphtheria antitoxin[b] (equine)		Prevention or treatment of diphtheria
Rabies immune serum (equine)		Prevention (when RIG unavailable)
Botulism antiserum (equine)		Treatment of botulism
Latrodectus mactans antivenin (equine)		Treatment of black widow spider bites
Crotalidae polyvalent antivenin (equine)		Treatment of most snake bites
Micrurus fulvius antivenin (equine)		Treatment of coral snake bites
Digoxin immune Fab fragments (ovine)	Digibind	Digoxin or digitoxin overdose
Anti-CD3 monoclonal antibody (murine)	Muromonab-CD3 OKT3	Immunosuppression
Lymphocyte immune globulin, antithymocyte globulin (equine)	ATG, Atgam	Immunosuppression

[a] All but CMV-IVIG are for intramuscular or subcutaneous use.
[b] Available through the Centers for Disease Control and Prevention (Atlanta, GA), telephone number (404)639-3670.

serum is injected. Inquiry must be made about asthma, hay fever, urticaria, and previous injections of animal serums. Patients with a history of asthma, allergic rhinitis, or other allergic symptoms on exposure to horses may be dangerously sensitive to the corresponding serum and should receive it only with the utmost caution.

Sensitivity Tests for Animal Serum

A scratch test or an eye test, followed by an intradermal skin test, must be performed before any injection of animal serum, whether or not the patient has had the serum previously. A scratch test is performed by applying a drop of 1:100 dilution in saline of the serum to the site of a superficial scratch and observing it for 30 minutes. A positive reaction consists of erythema or wheal formation.

An eye test is performed by instilling a drop of 1:10 saline dilution of serum in one eye and a drop of saline in the other eye to serve as a control. A positive reaction consists of lacrimation and conjunctivitis appearing in 10 to 30 minutes in the eye used for testing. If the scratch or eye test is negative, an intradermal test is performed by injecting 0.1 ml of a 1:100 saline dilution. The reaction is read after 10 to 30 minutes and is positive if a wheal appears. In persons with a history of allergy, the intradermal dose is reduced to 0.05 ml of a 1:1,000 dilution.

Although intradermal skin tests have resulted in fatalities, eye and scratch tests have not. Therefore, a skin test should never be performed (nor a serum injected) unless a syringe containing 1 ml of 1:1,000 epinephrine is within immediate reach.

Skin and eye tests can indicate the probability of sensitivity. However, a negative skin or eye test result is not an absolute guarantee of absence of sensitivity. Therefore, either a specific history of allergy or a positive skin or eye test result with horse serum is sufficient reason for special caution. A positive history of sensitivity to horse dander is an indication of the need for extreme caution.

Administration of Animal Serum

If the history and sensitivity tests are negative, the indicated dose of serum may be given intramuscularly. Intravenous injection may be indicated if a high concentration of circulating antibody is required rapidly, as in severe tetanus or diphtheria.

In such instances, a preliminary dose of 0.5 ml of serum should be diluted in 10 ml of either physiologic saline or 5 percent glucose solution. This preparation should be given over 5 minutes, and the patient should be watched for 30 minutes for reactions. If no reaction occurs, the remainder of the serum, diluted 1:20, may be given at a rate not to exceed 1 ml/min.

If the skin test result is positive or there is a general history of allergy in a person for whom the need for serum is unquestioned (and epinephrine is at hand), 1 ml of 1:10 dilution of the serum in physiologic saline may be administered subcutaneously and the patient observed for another 0.5 hour. If there still is no reaction, proceed as indicated in the previous paragraph.

If a reaction occurs, a procedure commonly called "desensitization" is undertaken, but it is dangerous to assume that any significant desensitization occurs. It is more likely that this procedure merely results in establishing the tolerance level of the patient. A satisfactory procedure is available.[1]

Hypersensitivity Reactions to Animal Serum

Hypersensitivity reactions to animal serum may be of four general types: (1) anaphylactic reactions, consisting of urticaria, dyspnea, cyanosis, shock, and unconsciousness occurring seconds to minutes after an injection; (2) acute febrile reactions, consisting of moderate or severe hyperpyrexia within 2 hours after an injection; (3) serum sickness reactions, consisting of urticaria, arthritis, adenopathy, and fever occurring hours to days after an injection, depending on the dose and the presence or degree of prior sensitization (serum sickness occurs within hours or a few days after the second injection and within 7 to 12 days after the first injection); and (4) delayed reactions of varying nature, including peripheral neuritis (serum neuritis).

Use of Diphtheria Antitoxin

An example of the use of an animal serum is in the management of diphtheria. The damaging effects of diphtheria are in large part due to the toxin elaborated during the disease, which damages the central nervous system, kidneys, and other organs. Thus, optimal treatment requires both antibiotic and antitoxin therapy.

Antitoxin of animal origin remains the mainstay of treatment, as it was in the era before antibiotic therapy. Diphtheria was the first illness in which antiserum was used as standard therapy; proof of its efficacy was established by Fibiger[2] in 1898 when he showed that 5 of 204 patients given horse antitoxin died, whereas 14 of 201 not given antiserum died.

Equine diphtheria antitoxin is indicated in all suspected or proven cases of diphtheria. Before its administration, it is necessary to perform skin or conjunctival tests for sensitivity, as outlined above. The amount of antitoxin given depends on the location and the extensiveness of the diphtheritic membrane, the degree of systemic toxicity, and the duration of illness. In severe and late cases, intravenous use is indicated; in mild forms, intramuscular administration suffices. In all cases, diphtheria antitoxin should be given promptly rather than delayed while waiting for bacterial confirmation of the diagnosis. Further details of treatment are available elsewhere.[3]

Other Animal Serums

For rabies and tetanus prophylaxis, both human and equine preparations are available. Animal antisera is also available for several other illnesses, poisons, and bites (Table 45-1). Details of their use can be found elsewhere.[1,3]

HUMAN IMMUNE SERUM GLOBULIN

ISG for general use (administered intramuscularly or subcutaneously) has been available since 1945 and is primarily used for replacement therapy in antibody immunodeficiencies and for hepatitis A and measles prophylaxis. It can also be used for hepatitis B, varicella, rubella, and poliovirus prophylaxis.

Pharmacology

ISG is prepared from pooled human serum by Cohn's alcohol fractionation procedure (thus deriving its alternative name of Cohn fraction II). In this procedure, most other serum proteins and live viruses (e.g., hepatitis B virus [HBV] and human immunodeficiency virus [HIV]) are removed, thus providing a sterile product for intramuscular injection. ISG is reconstituted as a sterile 16.5 percent solution (165 mg/ml) with thimerosal as a preservative.* It contains a wide spectrum of antibodies to viral and bacterial antigens.

ISG is 95 percent IgG, but trace quantities of IgM and IgA and other serum proteins are present. The IgM and IgA are therapeutically insignificant because of their rapid half-lives (less than 7 days) and their low concentrations in ISG, which contains all IgG subclasses and allotypes.

ISG is for intramuscular or subcutaneous use; intravenous use is contraindicated. It aggregates in vitro to form complexes, which are strongly anticomplementary. These aggregates are probably responsible for the occasional systemic reactions to ISG. The incidence of these reactions is increased if the recipient has received ISG in the past. Small intradermal injections of ISG are of no value.

Use in Immunodeficiency

The usual dose of ISG for antibody immunodeficiency is 100 mg/kg/month, about equivalent to 0.7 ml/kg/month of the 16.5 percent solution. A double or triple dose is given at the onset of therapy, by repeating the 0.7 ml/kg dose on successive days. The maximal dose should not exceed 20 or 30 ml/week or 5 ml at any one site.

The maximal increase of the serum IgG level after

a standard ISG injection varies from patient to patient and from dose to dose because of different rates of absorption, local proteolysis at the injection site, and distribution within the tissues. An intramuscular injection of 100 mg/kg of ISG usually raises the IgG serum level by 100 to 125 mg/dl after 2 to 4 days.[4] Thus, a recent ISG injection usually does not obscure the diagnosis of hypogammaglobulinemia.

Adverse Effects

Although ISG is one of the safest biologics available, rare anaphylactic reactions have been reported, particularly in patients who required repeat injections.[5,6] The British Medical Research Council Working Party[6] noted such reactions in 33 of 175 patients (19 percent) treated over a 10-year period. In all, there were 85 reactions to about 40,000 injections. In eight patients, the injections were stopped owing to these adverse effects, and one death was recorded. The symptoms include anxiety, nausea, vomiting, malaise, flushing, facial swelling, cyanosis, and loss of consciousness. Immediate treatment with epinephrine and antihistamines is indicated.

Individuals who experience such reactions should be evaluated before a repeat injection. Skin testing using several lots of ISG should be done.[4,5] A skin test result that is positive for an old but not a new lot of ISG may indicate a particular idiosyncratic reaction to a particular unit. Under these circumstances, incremental doses of ISG from a new lot are recommended. In other patients, IgE antibodies to IgG develop, resulting in positive immediate skin test results.[7] In others, no cause of the reactions can be found. Some of these patients tolerate repeated small doses of ISG, particularly if they are premedicated with aspirin, diphenhydramine, or corticosteroids. Finally, a few patients have had IgG or IgE antibodies develop to the IgA present in minute quantities in the ISG; these anti-IgA antibodies can be detected by serologic means in several laboratories. IVIG with low IgA content or IgA-deficient plasma can be used under these circumstances.

Patients with antibodies to IgA may have a reaction to ISG or IVIG as a result of the trace quantities of IgA in these products.[8] However, some patients with combined IgA and IgG$_2$ deficiency with anti-IgA antibodies tolerate treatment with IVIG, particularly an IVIG with low levels of IgA.[9]

---

* In the United States; in many other countries, ISG is preservative-free.

Administration of exogenous immunoglobulin may inhibit the endogenous synthesis of immunoglobulin. Premature infants given ISG monthly in the first year of life had lower IgG levels at 1 year than albumin-treated controls.[10]

Immunoglobulin injections or infusions may also inhibit antibody responses to vaccine antigens, particularly measles. Siber et al.[11] recommend an interval of 3 months between immunoglobulin therapy and vaccination after immunoglobulin doses less than 40 mg/kg, 6 months for doses of 40 to 80 mg/kg, 8 months for doses of 80 to 400 mg/kg, and 12 months for large doses of 1 to 2 g/kg. Late side effects to ISG are uncommon; in a few patients, fibrosis of the buttocks or localized subcutaneous atrophy develops at the site of repeated injections. Repeat injections of ISG may result in high levels of mercury as a result of the thimerosal preservative. Although mercury toxicity (acrodynia) developed in one patient as a result of such therapy,[12] most patients remain asymptomatic.

Slow Subcutaneous Infusions

As an alternative to intramuscular injections or IVIG, ISG can be given to immunodeficient patients by slow (1 to 2 ml/kg/hr) subcutaneous injections.[13,14] These injections are self-administered into the abdominal wall with the use of a battery-operated pump (Auto syringe). They are well tolerated and enable the patient to maintain high serum levels of IgG. In some countries, for some patients, where the cost of IVIG is prohibitive, subcutaneous ISG infusions are used regularly. We have utilized this method successfully in individuals with anaphylactic reactions to intramuscular ISG or IVIG.[15]

Measles

Studies by Stokes et al.[16] and Ordman et al.[17] in 1944 established that (1) large doses (0.05 ml/kg) of ISG given immediately after exposure could prevent measles, (2) lesser doses (0.01 ml/kg) given immediately after exposure could modify measles, and (3) large doses (0.05 ml/kg) given in the early stages of clinical illness could lessen the severity of measles. ISG is still used in the prevention and modification of measles in unimmunized children.

In nonvaccinated normal infants and children exposed to measles, a preventive dose of ISG (0.25 ml/kg intramuscularly) should be given as soon as possible after exposure. Twelve or more weeks later, measles vaccine should be given for permanent immunity. Alternatively, an attenuating dose of ISG can be given at a lower dose (0.05 ml/kg). In normal infants 6 to 15 months of age with a high risk of exposure to measles (e.g., an infant traveling to a country where there is endemic measles), 0.25 ml/kg of ISG can be given at 3-month intervals to prevent measles. Measles vaccination before 15 months of age may not be effective and can lead to a partial state of tolerance to subsequent vaccine.[18]

High-risk children exposed to measles (those with leukemia, lymphoma, generalized malignancy, immunodeficiency, or who are taking immunosuppressive drugs) should be given a larger dose (0.5 ml/kg, maximum 15 ml). Immunodeficient children receiving regular doses of ISG or IVIG do not require additional ISG on measles exposure.

Hepatitis A

The widest use of ISG is in the prevention of hepatitis A. Its efficacy has been demonstrated repeatedly since the 1945 studies of Stokes and Neefe[19] in which an epidemic was aborted in a children's summer camp, of Havens and Paul[20] who controlled an institutional epidemic, and of Gellis et al.[21] who prevented hepatitis A in the Mediterranean theater of operations at the close of World War II. There is no other effective means of prophylaxis for close family contacts (although scrupulous cleanliness may interrupt the intestinal-oral circuit of transmission when contacts are not using the same hygienic facilities).

ISG is efficacious in hepatitis A if given any time during the incubation period up until 6 days before the onset of disease. The protection persists for a period of 6 to 8 weeks. Stokes et al.[22] noted that a single small dose of ISG (0.02 ml/kg) provided a degree of protection for up to 9 months for individuals residing at an institution in which hepatitis A was endemic.

The effectiveness of ISG in hepatitis A prophylaxis varies from 80 to 95 percent, depending on how soon it is administered after exposure and the severity of the exposure.[23] ISG suppresses the clinical manifestations of the disease. Anicteric hepatitis is not prevented, however, and the ratio of anicteric hepatitis to icteric hepatitis may be as high as 12:1.[24]

The development of antibody tests for hepatitis A provides a way to determine the (1) immunity of subjects, (2) presence of inapparent infection, (3) titer of hepatitis A virus in lots of ISG, and (4) validity of the passive-active immunity concepts.[23–25]

Most lots of ISG have antibodies to hepatitis A virus by a competitive-inhibition radioimmunoassay (RIA). Titers greater than 1:100 are protective. There is some evidence that more recent lots of ISG contain more antibodies to hepatitis A virus than lots obtained earlier.[26]

Individual Exposure

Individuals, either adults or children, with a known intimate exposure to hepatitis A such as a household or child care contact should be given a single dose of 0.02 ml/kg of ISG. This includes newborns of mothers with hepatitis. Serologic testing for hepatitis A positivity is unnecessary and may delay administration of ISG. The use of ISG more than 2 weeks after exposure is not indicated.

ISG is usually unnecessary for children exposed to hepatitis A at day school. However, ISG prophylaxis is recommended for children exposed at a boarding school or in a school for retarded children, where the opportunities for fecal-oral route transmission are increased. Hospitalized children exposed to another child with hepatitis A on the hospital ward need not be given ISG.

Institutional Outbreaks

Institutional hepatitis A outbreaks, such as in a boarding school, day care center, facility for the mentally retarded, or prison, require aggressive action. Other cohorts, employees, and adult members of households with infants who wear diapers and who attend these facilities should be treated immediately with 0.02 mg/kg of ISG. If recognition of the initial case is delayed 3 or more weeks or if it appears that spread is occurring to other cohorts, staff, or household contacts, all personnel (staff and children) should be given ISG. If an outbreak of hepatitis A is traced to food handlers, ISG should be given to their close contacts and other restaurant employees.[27]

Foreign Travel

Ordinary tourist travel does not require ISG prophylaxis. However, individuals going to developing countries should receive 0.02 ml/kg of ISG if they intend to stay less than 3 months. If longer stays are anticipated, testing for immunity to hepatitis A virus is advisable. Nonimmune individuals should receive 0.06 ml/kg of ISG, repeated every 4 to 5 months. Some recommend stopping after one or two supplemental injections with the hope that active immunization has ensued. It seems relatively innocuous to continue the ISG until there is serologic evidence that active immunity has been established. Most individuals who reside permanently (longer than 2 years) in endemic areas do not maintain their ISG injections.

Primate Exposure

Certain subhuman primates such as chimpanzees may carry hepatitis A virus. Animal handlers should observe scrupulous hygiene and be tested for hepatitis A virus antibody. If they are found to be susceptible, prophylaxis with ISG, 0.06 ml/kg every 5 months, is advisable.

Needle Exposure

ISG is indicated for individuals accidentally inoculated with blood or serum from a patient with hepatitis A. The recommended dose is 0.02 ml/kg of ISG. Pregnancy is not a contraindication of ISG.

Newborn Infants of Infected Mothers

Unless the mother is jaundiced at the time of delivery, no special care of the infant is necessary, such as ISG administration or recommendations against breast feeding. If the mother is jaundiced, the infant can be given 0.02 ml/kg of ISG; efficacy is not established.

SPECIAL HIGH-TITERED IMMUNE SERUM GLOBULINS

Several special human immune globulins are available; these are identical to ISG except they have high titers to an infectious agent or the Rh antigen. They are listed in Table 45-1.

Hepatitis B Immune Globulin

Soon after the identification of hepatitis B surface antigen (HB$_s$Ag) and its antibody (anti-HB$_s$Ag), it became evident that measurement of the antibody content of ISG would permit selection of lots (or donors) with high titers of anti-HB$_s$Ag; such selection results in lots with anti-HB$_s$Ag titers of at least 1: 100,000 by RIA. This product (HBIG) has been licensed since 1978 for prevention of HBV infection.[28,29] Alternatively, large doses of ISG can be used.[3]

HBIG is recommended after parenteral or mucous membrane (oral, sexual, or ophthalmic) contact with individuals with HBV infection or with HB$_s$Ag-positive materials (e.g., blood or plasma) and for neonates born to HB$_s$Ag-positive mothers. It is available in 1- and 5-ml vials.

Exposure to Blood Products Containing Hepatitis B Surface Antigen

There are no prospective studies testing the efficacy of a combination of HBIG and HBV vaccine in preventing HBV infection after accidental exposure. This includes exposure by the percutaneous, ocular, and mucous membrane routes and by human bites that penetrate the skin. Because health care workers at risk for such accidents are HBV vaccine candidates and because the combination HBIG and HBV vaccine is more effective than HBIG alone in perinatal exposure, this combination is also recommended after accidental exposure.

If the blood or secretions come from an individual known to be HB$_s$Ag positive or if the status of the exposure donor is unknown, immediate prophylaxis is indicated. A single dose of HBIG (0.06 ml/kg or 5 ml for adults) should be given as soon as possible, preferably within 24 hours of exposure. HBV vaccine should be given simultaneously at a different site and repeated after 1 and 6 months.

After massive exposure (e.g., a blood transfusion), much larger doses of HBIG are probably indicated. If HBIG is unavailable, ISG may be given at an equivalent or double dose (0.12 ml/kg or 10 ml for adults).

If an individual has received at least two doses of HBV vaccine before accidental exposure, HBIG is unnecessary if serologic tests show adequate anti-HB$_s$Ag titers (greater than 10 international units/ml by RIA). If HBV vaccine is not given, two doses of HBIG should be used, the second given 1 month after the first.

Perinatal Exposure of Infants

If the mother is HB$_s$Ag and hepatitis B antigen positive, 85 percent of her offspring will become infected and will become chronic carriers, some of whom will develop chronic hepatitis, cirrhosis, or hepatic cancer. If the mother is HB$_s$Ag positive only, the risk of her offspring becoming carriers is considerably less but still significant. Accordingly, these infants are also candidates for prophylaxis.

For optimal passive-active immunity, HBIG is given (0.5 ml), and HBV vaccination is begun simultaneously and repeated at 1 and 6 months. This combination is only about 90 percent effective in preventing the carrier state because intrauterine infection is not prevented.

HBIG effectiveness is markedly diminished if administration is delayed beyond 48 hours. Nevertheless, if the mother is found to be HB$_s$Ag positive at birth, HBIG and HBV vaccine should be given to her infant even if there has been a significant delay. The infant should be tested for HB$_s$Ag and anti-HB$_s$Ag at 12 to 15 months to determine the success of the HBIG and HBV vaccine regimen. If HB$_s$Ag is present, the infant probably is a carrier; if HB$_s$Ag is absent and anti-HB$_s$Ag is present, the child has been successfully immunized. HBIG administration at birth should not interfere with polio or diphtheria-pertussis-tetanus vaccines starting at 2 months of age.

Sexual Exposure to Hepatitis B or a Hepatitis B Carrier

Sexual exposure to an individual who has or who has HBV infection develop is an indication for HBIG (0.06 ml/kg, 5-ml maximum). This should be effective for about 14 days after the exposure. If the contact's HB$_s$Ag status is not known, it should be determined; if the contact is HB$_s$Ag positive, HBIG should be given. If sexual contact continues and if the contact remains HB$_s$Ag positive for more than 3 months, a second HBIG dose is recommended.

HBIG should also be given if sexual contact with a HB$_s$Ag-positive individual is anticipated. Contacts who remain HB$_s$Ag positive are probably carriers, and HBV vaccine should be given to their regular sexual partners.

For sexual exposures among homosexual men, HBIG is given, and HBV vaccine should be given simultaneously; indeed, HBV vaccine is recommended for all susceptible sexually active homosexual men. Additional doses of HBIG are unnecessary if HBV vaccine is given.

Possible Exposures

After possible exposures (percutaneous, ingestion, or sexual) to an unidentified person or body fluid in which the HB$_s$Ag status is unknown, a decision to treat with HBIG (or ISG) must be made individually, based on the likelihood that the source is HB$_s$Ag positive and the seriousness of the exposure.

Ideally, the source should be tested for HB$_s$Ag positivity; if the results are available within 7 days, ISG (0.06 ml/kg) can be given immediately, followed by HBIG at 7 days (0.06 ml/kg, 5-ml maximum) and again at 1 month if the source is HB$_s$Ag positive. When the source cannot be tested or when the source is likely to be HB$_s$Ag positive, HBIG is given immediately and again at 1 month.

If the exposed individual is a high-risk patient (e.g., immunodeficient, immunosuppressed, institutionalized, Down syndrome, Asian, or undergoing hemodialysis) or is in a unit for which past environmental control measures have been ineffective, prophylaxis should be given. The staff of such units (e.g., mental institutions or hemodialysis units) with considerable patient contact are also candidates for prophylaxis.

HBIG or ISG is not indicated on a routine basis after blood transfusions. A school or hospital exposure is not an indication for HBIG or ISG.

Use of Immune Serum Globulin Instead of Hepatitis B Immune Globulin

Lots of ISG must have an anti-HB$_s$Ag of 1:100 by RIA; this titer may be protective but is considerably less than the anti-HB$_s$Ag content of HBIG (at least 1:100,000). ISG can no longer be recommended as an alternative to HBIG.

Rabies, Rabies Immune Globulin, and Hyperimmune Rabies Serum

Rabies is the ideal disease for passive immunization because the exact moment, the exact source, and the exact location of exposure are known. Furthermore, the long incubation period and the fact that the virus remains localized to the wound for several days enhance the effectiveness of passive immunization.

Optimal treatment for rabies exposure requires both active and passive immunization. Before 1971, the available antiserum was of equine origin. Since then, human rabies immune globulin (RIG) has also been available in the United States and many other countries and is preferred because of the lessened risk of serum reactions.

RIG (or rabies antiserum) is recommended in nonimmunized individuals for all bites by animals in which rabies cannot be ruled out and for nonbite exposure to animals proved or suspected of being rabid.[30] Such treatment should be given as early as possible after exposure but should be used regardless of the interval between exposure and treatment. One-half of the RIG (or rabies antiserum) should be injected locally at the wound site and the rest given intramuscularly. Vaccine should then be given at a different site with a different needle and syringe.

RIG (or antiserum) should not be administered after rabies exposure (1) if the person has had adequate pre- or postexposure prophylaxis with rabies vaccine or (2) has known a protective antirabies titer after another vaccine regimen. These persons are given two doses of rabies vaccine only, on the day of exposure and on day 3.

When both preparations are available, human RIG is preferred because of the decreased risk of serum reactions. If RIG is unavailable, equine rabies antiserum should be used. If an individual is known to be allergic to horse serum, RIG must be used or a schedule of desensitization employed.

RIG is not used simultaneously when rabies vaccine is given prophylactically to unexposed high-risk individuals.

RIG and rabies antiserum are of no value in the treatment of established rabies infection.

Tetanus Immune Globulin and Tetanus Antitoxin

Antitoxin in the treatment of tetanus was introduced in medicine by Behring and Kitasato in 1890; large doses (50 to 100 ml) of serum from horses immunized with tetanus toxin were used.[31] The mechanism of action of tetanus antitoxin (TAT) is to neutralize the toxin before its arrival in the nervous system by way of the circulation. It can also neutralize toxin locally and prevent its systemic absorption. Thus, TAT should be given at the site of toxin production (e.g., at the site of a wound) and intravenously (in severe cases) or intramuscularly, with the latter being reserved for less severe cases.

Rubbo and Suri[32] and Rubinstein[33] showed that human tetanus immune globulin (TIG) given intramuscularly (5 to 10 units/kg) provides adequate circulating antitoxin levels and is maintained in the circulation for a considerably longer time than is equine TAT.

TIG can be given along with tetanus toxoid (10 Lf units) for passive-active immunization. A dose of 250 units of TIG given intramuscularly at a site different from that of the toxoid does not interfere with the active antibody response.[34]

Prophylaxis

If a nonimmunized individual sustains a serious injury or a bite, 250 to 500 units of TIG should be given intramuscularly. The larger dose should be used if there is an extensive wound or delay in treatment. Alum-precipitated toxoid to initiate active immunity is given at a different site, using a separate syringe. If TIG is unavailable, 3,000 to 5,000 units of TAT (bovine or equine) are given (after screening and testing the patient for serum sensitivity).

Treatment

In addition to antibiotics and wound management, TIG in doses of 500 to 3,000 units should be given, part infiltrated near the wound and the rest given intramuscularly.

If TIG is unavailable, equine TAT should be given in a single dose of 50,000 to 100,000 units with 20,000 units given intravenously (after appropriate testing for sensitivity). In severe cases, up to 50,000 units of TAT should be given intravenously. Intrathecal TIG or TAT is usually unnecessary and is not recommended. On recovery, primary immunization should be undertaken.

Varicella-Zoster Immune Globulin

Ross[35] in 1962 gave 242 children ISG in doses of 0.1 to 0.6 ml/lb within 3 days of exposure to chickenpox; 209 similarly exposed, uninjected children were used as controls. The attack rate was the same (97 percent) in both groups, which indicated that ISG

does not prevent varicella under these conditions. However, with doses of ISG above 0.2 ml/kg, the severity of the disease was reduced, as indicated by a decreased number of pox and lessened temperature.

The value of large ISG doses in decreasing the incidence and severity of varicella led to the trial of high-titered plasma or γ globulin preparations to prevent varicella. These preparations include zoster immune globulin and zoster immune plasma from convalescing patients with herpes zoster and varicella-zoster immune globulin (VZIG) prepared from high-titered normal adults. Several studies have established that VZIG is useful in modifying the severity of chickenpox (varicella) in immunocompromised hosts but will not reliably prevent its occurrence.

For normal children exposed to varicella, standard ISG can be expected to modify the disease and VZIG to prevent it.[36] However, because varicella is a mild disease in most children, prophylaxis is usually not indicated. In high-risk immunocompromised children and in normal and high-risk adults, the decision to administer VZIG or ISG is based on the likelihood of susceptibility, the nature of the exposure, and the risk of developing varicella. VZIG is expensive ($220 for 125 units or $1,100 for an adult who weighs more than 40 kg), and the modified infection that ensues may or may not lead to lifelong immunity and may or may not decrease the risk of developing herpes zoster later in life.

Determination of Susceptibility

This is usually based on historic information elicited by an experienced interviewer. Varicella-zoster virus antibody tests to determine varicella susceptibility are not widely available and are often unreliable. Complement fixation, fluorescent antibody, enzyme-linked immunosorbent assay, and neutralizing antibody tests are available, but they may give negative results despite immunity. When the results are positive, they may not indicate immunity, particularly in neonates and immunocompromised subjects.

With the exception of bone marrow transplant recipients, healthy and immunocompromised individuals who by history have had prior varicella infection are considered immune. Healthy adults and children 15 years of age and older with a negative or uncertain history are generally considered immune; however, those who are immunocompromised are considered susceptible. Approximately 85 to 95 percent of adults and children 15 years of age and older with a negative or uncertain history of prior varicella are immune, particularly those who are older siblings in large families and those whose children have had varicella. Children who are younger than 15 years of age and do not have a history of varicella are considered susceptible unless proved otherwise using a sensitive serologic assay; however, the results of these assays must be interpreted cautiously in immunocompromised children. Children or adults who have received bone marrow transplants should be considered susceptible to varicella regardless of prior history of the disease in the donor or recipient. Bone marrow transplant recipients with varicella or herpes zoster after transplantation can subsequently be considered immune.

Normal Children

As noted, prophylaxis for most normal children is not indicated. However, special circumstances (e.g., future travel, surgery, or risk of exposure of an immunocompromised sibling) may require its use; the dose is identical to that for immunocompromised children.

Immunocompromised Children

The principal use of VZIG is after exposure to herpes zoster or chickenpox in susceptible immunocompromised children. This includes children with primary immunodeficiency or neoplastic diseases and those receiving immunosuppressive therapy, including corticosteroids. VZIG may only modify varicella rather than prevent it. Although children who have neoplastic disease or are receiving immunosuppressive therapy and who have a definitive history of varicella are considered immune, patients with primary antibody or cellular immunodeficiency or children receiving bone marrow transplants should be considered to be susceptible regardless of prior history.

Newborns

VZIG is recommended for a newborn whose mother develops varicella within 5 days before or 48 hours after delivery, regardless of whether the mother received VZIG. Varicella infection is life threatening in these newborns, and VZIG may be expected to modify but not prevent the disease. VZIG is probably unnecessary for term newborns whose mothers develop varicella more than 5 days before delivery, inasmuch as they will receive some transplacental immunity and will be protected from severe disease.

Postnatal exposure to varicella infection does not represent a threat to normal infants, particularly if the mother has had varicella, because transplacental antibodies modify or protect the infant. In all exposed infants younger than 28 weeks old or who weigh less than 1,000 g, VZIG is recommended because transplacental passage of IgG is significantly lessened and the infant's cellular immune system is immature.

In larger premature infants who are exposed by a contact other than the mother, VZIG is recommended for those whose mothers do not report a history of varicella infection.

Immunocompromised Adults

Exposed immunocompromised adults who are believed susceptible should receive VZIG. Many (most) are probably immune, but in this high-risk situation, prophylaxis is justified.

Normal Adults

Adults are more susceptible to severe varicella than are children; the death rate from varicella in adults is 50 per 100,000 compared with 2 per 100,000 in children, and the complication rate is increased 9- to 25-fold. Accordingly, some exposed adults, depending on their health and the need to avoid or modify varicella, are candidates for VZIG. Although the cost of VZIG is substantial, under certain circumstances, the benefits clearly outweigh this expense.

Pregnant Women

Exposed pregnant women should be considered the same as other exposed adults. There is no evidence that VZIG given during pregnancy will prevent intrauterine, congenital, or neonatal varicella. It is unlikely that VZIG given to a pregnant woman with varicella within 5 days of delivery will result in sufficient transplacental passage to modify or prevent varicella in her infant. Accordingly, the infant should be given VZIG regardless of whether the mother has received VZIG prenatally.

Hospital Personnel Exposures

Recommendations for exposed hospital personnel and ward management of exposure problems are available.[1]

Dosage

VZIG should be given as soon as possible after exposure but probably is effective if given within 4 or 5 days after exposure. VZIG is not valuable in the treatment of varicella or herpes zoster. VZIG probably confers protection for 3 weeks. Antibody determinations before and 2 months after administration may help to determine the immune status of the individual and whether subclinical or modified infection has resulted.

VZIG is supplied in vials of 125 units (about 1.25 ml). The recommended dose is 125 units/10 kg, up to a maximum of 625 units (five vials). The minimal dose is 125 units. The approximate cost is $220/vial!

INTRAVENOUS IMMUNOGLOBULIN

IVIG is further treated human ISG that has been rendered free of complexes and thus safe for intravenous infusion. This product can be given rapidly in large quantities for antibody deficiencies[37] and several autoimmune and inflammatory disorders.[38,39] Several methods to treat Cohn fraction II have been used to eliminate high-molecular-weight complexes; these include treatment with proteolytic enzymes, ultracentrifugation, reduction of sulfhydryl bonds followed by alkylation, and incubation at low pH. Although these additional procedures increase its production cost, IVIG has several advantages over intramuscular ISG, including (1) larger quantities of IgG can be given; (2) high levels of serum IgG can be achieved rapidly; (3) painful, intramuscular injections are avoided; (4) tissue pooling or proteolysis is avoided; and (5) self-administration is possible.[3]

The first IVIG produced in the United States in 1981 was Gamimune (Cutter Laboratories, Berkeley, CA), a reduced and alkylated 5 percent solution containing 10 percent maltose (Table 45-2). The second IVIG produced was prepared by acidification and treatment with pepsin; the lyophilized powder could be reconstituted as a 3, 6, or 12 percent solution (Sandoglobulin, Sandoz Pharmaceuticals, East Hanover, NJ). Since then, several other IVIGs have been introduced by different manufacturers (Table 45-2). Some are 5 to 10 percent solutions; others are lyophilized powders that are reconstituted as 3 to 12 percent solutions.

Although these products vary slightly,[40] they are generally therapeutically equivalent and are usually selected on the basis of cost and convenience. There are minor IgA and IgG subclass differences.[41,42] Antibody titers may also vary from lot to lot and among different IVIGs.[42] Products low in IgA content such as Gammagard or Polygam (American Red Cross, Washington, DC) are used to minimize reactions in patients with hypogammaglobulinemia and concurrent IgA deficiency or when anti-IgA antibodies are present in the recipient. Very sensitive patients may not tolerate any IVIG. Premixed liquids have the advantage of convenience because the reconstitution step is not required; however, they must be kept refrigerated.

All currently available IVIG products have adequate serum half-lives (15 to 25 days), a wide spectrum of antibody activity, and minimal anticomplementary activity, and they are free of bacterial and viral contamination. Hepatitis C has been transmitted through certain experimental IVIG lots[43] and in some European preparations.[44-47] In the report by Bjoro et al.,[47] immunocompromised patients had a severe and rapidly progressive course of hepatitis C infection, and the responses to interferon were poor.

Until the report of an outbreak of hepatitis C published in 1994,[48] there had never been a report in the United States of hepatitis associated with any commercially available IVIG preparation. As of October 1994, there were reports of 137 suspected cases, 88 of which were confirmed.[49] Fifty-one of the 88 patients (58 percent) had primary immunodeficiencies, and 63 percent eventually became symptomatic. The Gammagard involved in the outbreak has been replaced with Gammagard-S/D, the manufacture of which includes treatment with a solvent and a detergent to inactivate hepatitis C virus and other membrane-enveloped viruses. Manufacturers of other preparations have also incorporated procedures to inactivate hepatitis C virus and most other viruses. Each of the various methods seems effective,

Table 45-2. Intravenous Immunoglobulin Preparations Available in the United States

Name of Preparation, Year Released, and Manufacturer	Isolation Method	Product from (Stabilizers)	pH	IgA Content	Comments
Sandoglobulin (1984) Sandoz Pharmaceuticals, E. Hanover, NJ	Acid and pepsin	Lyophilized. Reconstituted as 3, 6, and 12% solution. Available in 1-, 3-, and 6-g bottles (5% sucrose)	6.6	VH	Reaction rates may be somewhat higher than other IVIG products. Storage: Room temperature.
Gammagard (1986), -S/D (1995) Baxter HealthCare Co., Hyland Division, Glendale, CA	PEG and ultrafiltration -SD ion-exchange and ultrafiltration	Lyophilized. Reconstituted as a 5% solution. 0.5-, 2.5-, and 10-g bottles (glycine, albumin, and 2% glucose). SD reconstituted as 5% solution. 2.5-, 5-, and 10-g bottles.	6.8	L	A number of hepatitis C cases reported. Withdrawn from the market in 1994. Recommended for patients with absent IgA. A detergent, S/D treated form available in 1995. Storage: Room temperature.
Gamimune-N (1986–5%) (1992–10%) Cutter Laboratories, Berkeley, CA	Acid and diafiltration	Liquid. Reconstituted as a 5% or 10% solution. Available in 0.5-, 2.5-, 5-, and 12.5-g bottles (10% maltose)	4.25	H	Low rate of side effects. Storage: Refrigerated.
Iveegam (1988) Immuno-US, Rochester, MI	Trypsin and PEG	Lyophilized. Reconstituted as 5% solution. Available in 0.5-, 1-, 2.5-, and 5-bottles (5% glucose)	6.8	VL	First used in Kawasaki Syndrome trials. No longer available in the United States. Storage: Refrigerated.
Venoglobulin-I (1988) Alpha Therap. Corp., Los Angeles, CA	PEG-DEAE-sephadex fractionation	Lyophilized. Reconstituted as 5% solution. Available in 0.5-, 2.5-, 5-, and 10-g bottles (albumin 2% mannitol)	6.8	L	Storage: Room temperature.
Polygam (1988), S/D (1995) America Red Cross, Washington, D.C.	PEG and ultrafiltration	Lyophilized. Reconstituted as 5% solution. Available in 2.5-, 5-, and 10-g bottles (glycine, albumin, and 2% glucose)	6.8	L	Manufactured for the American Red Cross by Baxter Pharmaceuticals from volunteer donors. No cases of hepatitis C reported, however, removed from the market in 1994 along with Gammagard.[a] Reintroduced 1995 as Polygam S/D Storage: Room temperature.
Gammar-IV (1989) Armour Pharmaceuticals, Chicago, IL	Low-ionic-strength ethanol fractionation	Lyophilized. Reconstituted as 5% solution. Available in 1-, 2.5-, and 5-g bottles (albumin and 5% sucrose)	7.0	L	Storage: Room temperature.
CytoGam (1991) Med Immune, Inc., Gaithersburg, MD	Polyethylene glycol (PEG) and ultrafiltration	Lyophilized. Reconstituted as 5% solution. Available in 2.5-g bottles (5% sucrose and albumin)	NA	NA	Enriched for CMV antibodies. Manufactured by the Massachusetts Public Health Biologic Laboratories for Med Immune, Inc. Storage: Room temperature.
Venoglobulin-S (1992) Alpha Therapeutics, Los Angeles, CA	PEG and DEAE-Sephadex fractionation followed by solvent detergent treatment	Liquid. Reconstituted as 5% solution. Available in 2.5-, 5-, and 10-g bottles (5% D-sorbitol)	5.2	L	Storage: Room temperature.

Abbreviations: VL, very low; L, low; H, high; VH, very high; PEG, polyethylene glycol; DEAE, diethylaminoethyl
[a] (From Centers for Disease Control.[48])

but none can guarantee the total absence of infectious virus.

However, no cases of HIV transmission have ever been reported with IVIG administration.[49–51]

Administration

IVIG administration requires venous access, sometimes a problem in small children. It also requires close monitoring during the infusion. Adverse reactions to IVIG tend to occur more frequently and are more severe than with ISG injections. Between 2 and 10 percent of IVIG infusions may be associated with adverse reactions; typically, these include headaches, nausea and vomiting, flushing, chills, myalgia, arthralgia, and abdominal pain. Occasionally, chest tightness, hives, and anaphylactoid reactions can occur. Very rarely, severe life-threatening anaphylactic reactions can occur. Late but very rare side reactions include aseptic meningitis,[52] renal insufficiency,[53] and hemolytic anemia.[54] Thus, IVIG infusions should be supervised by individuals with the experience, skill, and knowledge to handle these reactions. Nurses, parents, or others who perform home infusions must be taught to recognize and treat adverse reactions.

IVIG is contraindicated in patients who have had an anaphylactic reaction to IVIG or other blood products. IVIG is given with great caution in those patients who have hypogammaglobulinemia with IgA deficiency and/or anti-IgA antibodies.[55]

Typically, an IVIG infusion requires 1 to 4 hours to administer. The initial rate is 0.01 ml/kg/min, and this can be doubled at 20- to 30-minute intervals if there are no side effects to a maximal rate of 0.08 ml/kg/min. Adverse effects tend to be associated with rapid infusion rates in patients with concurrent acute infections, in previously untreated patients, or when significant time between infusions has transpired (greater than 6-week intervals). Immediate minor reactions can be avoided or diminished by slowing the infusion rate. Patients who experience minor side effects such as headaches, shaking chills, nausea and vomiting, or myalgia/arthralgia can be pretreated with aspirin, diphenhydramine, or hydrocortisone (1 hour before infusion). Occasionally, switching to a different product (generally one available as a solution) may alleviate the reactions.

A few investigators have given high concentrations (9 and 12 percent solutions) infused rapidly over a period of 20 to 40 minutes; this rapid rate can be tolerated by some patients.[56] However, this should not be done except by experienced personnel equipped to manage adverse reactions. In responsible, older patients who receive infusions without adverse effects, infusion by home self-administration can be accomplished at great cost savings.[57–59] However, in most cases, IVIG infusions are performed in the clinic setting or by home infusion teams.

Primary Immunodeficiencies

IVIG is indicated in patients with profound antibody deficiency (quantitative and qualitative), in patients with combined immunodeficiencies, and in those with secondary immunodeficiency with significant antibody abnormalities (Table 45-3). For patients with agammaglobulinemia or hypogammaglobulinemia, regular infusions of IVIG can keep them free

Table 45-3. Some Immunodeficiencies in Which Human Intravenous Immunoglobulin May be Beneficial

Antibody deficiencies
    X-linked agammaglobulinemia
    Common variable immunodeficiency
    Immunodeficiency with hyper-IgM
    Transient hypogammaglobulinemia of infancy (sometimes)
    IgG subclass deficiency IgA deficiency (sometimes)
    Antibody deficiency with normal immunoglobulins
Combined deficiencies
    Severe combined immunodeficiencies (all types)
    Wiskott-Aldrich syndrome
    Ataxia-telangiectasia
    Short-limbed dwarfism
    X-linked lymphoproliferative syndrome
Secondary immunodeficiencies
    Malignancies with antibody deficiencies; multiple myeloma, chronic lymphocytic leukemia, other cancers
    Protein-losing enteropathy with hypogammaglobulinemia
    Nephrotic syndrome with hypogammaglobulinemia
    Pediatric acquired immunodeficiency syndrome
    Intensive care patients: trauma, surgery, or shock
    Post-transplantation period
    Burns
    Prematurity

from infections for long periods of time or lessen the severity and frequency of chronic infections. Patients with X-linked agammaglobulinemia, common variable immunodeficiency, and the hyper-IgM syndrome clearly benefit from replacement therapy. In disorders characterized by combined antibody and cellular defects and in those with secondary immunodeficiencies, IVIG serves as an important ancillary treatment but does not correct the associated T-cell defect or underlying secondary immunodeficiency.

Given at comparable doses (100 mg/kg/month) IVIG has been shown to be as effective as ISG in antibody immunodeficiency.[60] Other studies that used IVIG at larger doses (150 to 200 mg/kg/every 3 to 4 weeks) demonstrated therapeutic superiority over ISG.[61–64] Subsequent studies have suggested that patients who received high IVIG doses (500 mg/kg/month) had fewer sinopulmonary infections than those who received conventional doses (150 mg/kg/month).[64] When patients have chronic lung disease or continued infection despite usual doses of IVIG, higher doses (400 to 600 mg/kg/month) may result in improved pulmonary function and fewer infections.[65]

These large doses of IVIG are not warranted in patients who do well on conventional doses because of the increased costs. Our practice is to administer between 300 and 400 mg/kg/month of IVIG to keep the serum IgG trough level above 500 mg/dl (near-normal levels) or 300 mg/dl above the pretreatment level. Some patients with severe disease do not respond to higher doses or more frequent infusions because of permanent tissue damage or deep-seated chronic infection.

IVIG is also used in patients with recurrent infections with antibody deficiency and normal or near-normal immunoglobulin levels. Rarely, IVIG is indicated in infants with transient hypogammaglobulinemia with persistent infection that is nonresponsive to antibiotics. IVIG has also been used in patients with IgG subclass deficiencies, but controlled studies demonstrating efficacy are lacking.[66–68]

A syndrome of polymyositis and/or chronic encephalopathy caused by persistent viral infection of the central nervous system in patients with agammaglobulinemia has been treated successfully with very high doses of IVIG.[69,70] However, there have been patients who did not respond.[71]

Secondary Immunodeficiencies

Some patients with secondary immunodeficiencies have low immunoglobulin levels, poor response to antigenic challenge, and low levels of natural antibodies. This may be the result of loss of immunoglobulin, loss of immune cells, or the toxic effect of therapy or infection on the immune system. Table 45-3 includes those diseases and conditions in which secondary immune deficiency can occur. Laboratory criteria that support the use of IVIG include (1) significant hypogammaglobulinemia (serum IgG less than 200 mg/dl or total immunoglobulin level [IgG + IgM + IgA] less than 400 mg/dl), (2) absent or low natural antibody levels, (3) absent or poor response to antigenic challenge (e.g., tetanus or pneumococcal vaccines), and (4) lack of an antibody response to the infecting organisms.

Hematologic-Oncologic Diseases

Antibody deficiencies can occur with multiple myeloma, chronic lymphocytic leukemia, lymphomas, and advanced cancer. A large, double-blind multicenter study concluded that the prophylactic infusion of 400 mg/kg of IVIG every 3 weeks reduced the incidence of bacterial infections in patients with chronic lymphocytic leukemia,[72] although serious concerns have been raised about the cost-effectiveness of IVIG in this setting.[73,74] The treatment group had fewer infections with *Streptococcus pneumoniae* and *Haemophilus influenzae*, but there was no difference in incidence of infection from other gram-negative bacteria, fungi, or viruses. In an earlier crossover study, IVIG was also shown to reduce the incidence of infections in patients with multiple myeloma.[75]

Premature Infants

All premature infants have very low serum levels of IgG, IgM, and IgA. In addition, they have decreased complement levels and diminished T cell and natural killer cell function. These combine to make the premature infant highly susceptible to severe, disseminated viral and bacterial infections. Early, preliminary studies of the routine use of IVIG in prematures to prevent infection appeared promising, but subsequent controlled studies did not show efficacy.[76,77] Thus, IVIG is not recommended for routine prophylaxis of infection in low-birth-weight infants.[78]

Severely Ill Patients: Burns, Trauma, Surgery, or Shock

Patients with extensive burns may experience secondary hypogammaglobulinemia from protein loss. Gram-negative sepsis is the leading cause of death in these patients. IVIG has been used in burn patients,[79] but proof of efficacy is lacking. Similarly, severely injured patients or those recovering from surgery also have an increased rate of infection, but IVIG administration has not decreased this rate.[80,81] To combat gram-negative sepsis, IVIG with antiendotoxin activity has been used, but the results were disappointing; trials with monoclonal antibody preparations are also underway, but the results are inconclusive.[82]

Nephrotic Syndrome and Protein-Losing Enteropathies

In patients with severe protein loss, hypogammaglobulinemia can result. Treatment with IVIG is indicated in those individuals with profound hypogammaglobulinemia (IgG less than 200 mg/dl) and recurrent infections.

Post-Transplantation

Conditioning regimens to eliminate host hematopoietic and immunologic defense systems during bone marrow transplantation procedures leave the patient extremely susceptible to infection.[83] Complications from viral infections, particularly CMV, may occur.

The use of IVIG to prevent opportunistic infections, particularly sepsis, pneumonia, or gastrointestinal infections, has met with limited success,[84–86] with the exception of preventing complications from CMV infection (discussed in the next section). Nevertheless, one report demonstrated some benefit from infusions of IVIG in a controlled trial on 382 bone marrow recipients.[87] The patients received 500 mg/kg/dose of IVIG weekly for 90 days and then monthly for 1 year, with a resultant decrease in the number of infections, the number of platelet transfusions, and the incidence of graft-versus-host disease. A more recent review from the same group of investigators concluded that IVIG was beneficial in reducing the rate of septicemia, interstitial pneumonia, fatal CMV disease, acute graft-versus-host disease, and transplant-related death in adult recipients of related marrow transplants.[88] Its use has been recommended for allogenic marrow transplant recipients[39,89] but not for autologous transplantation.[90,91]

Viral Infections

Cytomegalovirus Infection

IVIG or enriched IVIG (CMV-IVIG) has proven benefit in treating symptomatic CMV infection in transplantation patients[92] and preventing infection in CMV-negative recipients. In combination with ganciclovir, IVIG may be more efficacious than either alone in treating established CMV infections in bone marrow transplantation recipients.[93,94]

Other studies, although limited in number, have shown some benefit of IVIG in preventing CMV infection in CMV-negative kidney[95–97] and liver transplant recipients.[98,99] The optimal dose and dose scheduling regimens for CMV-IVIG are yet to be established, but it will likely be high and frequent and, thus, expensive. Furthermore, the successful use of ganciclovir in prevention may lessen the need for IVIG in CMV infection.

Other Herpesviruses

IVIG has been used in chronic Epstein-Barr (EBV) infection[100] and in patients with X-linked lymphoproliferative syndrome to prevent EBV infection. However, controlled studies are lacking and a recent report described an initially seronegative college student with this syndrome who died from overwhelming EBV infection while receiving monthly IVIG prophylaxis.[101]

IVIG can also be used prophylactically in immunodeficient patients on exposure to varicella-zoster infection if VZIG is unavailable.[102] Comparable levels of antivaricella antibody titers can be achieved with either.

Human Immunodeficiency Virus Infections

The rationale for the use of IVIG in HIV-infected patients includes their increased susceptibility to common bacterial infections (particularly children)[103,104] and the increased incidence of HIV-induced immune thrombocytopenic purpura (ITP). A large National Institutes of Child Health and Human Development double-blind placebo-controlled study confirmed that IVIG was effective in preventing infections in HIV-infected children with

CD4 counts greater than 200/mm³.[105] Infections were less frequent, and more patients were infection-free longer in the treatment group than in the placebo group; however, there was no difference in survival between the two groups. In a continuation of this study, the placebo group was allowed to cross-over to receive IVIG, with a subsequent drop in the rate of serious infections and hospitalizations.[106]

In HIV-associated ITP, IVIG has been shown to be effective in adults[107,108] and possibly in children.[109]

IVIG is less effective in preventing infection if the HIV-infected children receive continuous trimetho-prom-sulfamethoxazole prophylaxis for *Pneumocystis carinii* pneumonia.[110] Hyperimmune HIV-IVIG is under study to prevent maternal-fetal HIV transmission and to modify progression in advanced HIV infection.

Parvovirus Infections

Parvovirus B19 can cause transient aplastic anemia in normal individuals and chronic aplastic anemia in immunodeficient or severely immunosuppressed patients. High-dose IVIG can cure B19 infection with reversal of the anemia.[111,113]

Respiratory Syncytial Viral Infections

RSV causes considerable morbidity in very young children; premature infants; and children with pre-existing pulmonary, cardiac, or immune disease. Pilot studies using IVIG indicated possible benefit with attenuation of disease severity.[114,115] A large multicenter study that used RSV-IVIG in high-risk infants (bronchopulmonary dysplasia, congenital heart disease, or prematurity) was conducted comparing high-dose (750 mg/kg/month) versus low-dose (150 mg/kg/month) versus no treatment. The high-dose group experienced fewer lower respiratory tract infections, fewer hospitalizations, fewer hospital days, fewer days in the neonatal intensive care unit, and less use of the antiviral drug ribavirin than the other regimens.[116]

Other Respiratory Viruses

IVIG contains antibodies against numerous respiratory viruses, including adenovirus, influenza, and parainfluenza viruses. Although IVIG has been used to prevent or treat these respiratory infections, proof of efficacy is lacking. Lack of standardized or high-titered products make it difficult to evaluate the effectiveness of treatment. Furthermore, as in other viral infections, IVIG is unlikely to eradicate entrenched infections.

Bacterial Infections

Passive immunity for bacterial infections or toxins has been used for nearly a century. In the preantibiotic era, antiserum was used for whooping cough and bacterial meningitis (*H. influenzae* and *Neisseria meningitides*). Antitoxin is still necessary in infections in which toxins are produced (e.g., diphtheria and tetanus). Effective vaccines and antibiotics have diminished the need for passive immunity; however, there are certain clinical situations in which IVIG or hyperimmune IVIG may be useful. These include toxic shock syndrome,[117] gram-negative sepsis, and Pseudomonas infections; however, improved products and controlled studies are required. IVIG has also been used in the pulmonary infections of cystic fibrosis with transient benefit.[118]

Autoimmune and Inflammatory Diseases

High-dose IVIG has immunosuppressive and anti-inflammatory effects that make it a valuable agent in the treatment of several autoimmune or inflammatory disorders (Table 45-4). High-dose IVIG (1 to 2 g/kg/dose) inhibits antibody synthesis (possibly by a direct effect on proliferating B cells), combines directly with autoimmune antibodies (because it contains anti-idiotypic antibodies[119]), blocks the uptake of antibody-coated cells in the spleen and liver (Fc receptor blockade of antibody-dependent cellular cytotoxicity), and downregulates immune activation with inhibition of inflammatory cytokine release.[38] The latter may be associated with specific neutralization of superantigens associated with toxins or bacteria.[120]

The best documented uses of high-dose IVIG as an immunoregulator are in the treatment of Kawasaki disease and ITP. In other disorders, the reports of efficacy are based on smaller studies or case reports (Table 45-4).

Kawasaki Disease

Kawasaki disease is an acute, inflammatory febrile childhood disorder of unknown cause.[121] Generalized vasculitis is common, but coronary artery ob-

Table 45-4. Other (Noninfectious) Uses of Human Intravenous Immunoglobulin

Proven benefit[a]
   Kawasaki syndrome
   Immune thrombocytopenic purpura
   Guillain-Barré syndrome
   Dermatomyositis
Probable benefit[b]
   Neonatal isoimmune or autoimmune thrombocytopenic purpura
   Postinfectious thrombocytopenic purpura
   Immune neutropenia (including neonatal)
   Autoimmune hemolytic anemia
   Chronic inflammatory myelinating polyneuropathy
   Myasthenia gravis
Possible benefit[c]
   Anticardiolipin antibody syndrome
   Toxic shock syndrome
   Coagulopathy with factor VIII inhibitor
   Bullous pemphigoid
   Churg-Strauss vasculitis
Unproven benefit[d]
   Intractable seizures
   Steroid-dependent asthma
   Eczema
   Juvenile rheumatoid arthritis
   Lupus erythematosus
   Recurrent abortion
   Hemolytic-uremic syndrome

[a] Controlled studies demonstrate efficacy
[b] Several case reports or uncontrolled series are convincing.
[c] Preliminary studies are encouraging but incomplete.
[d] Prelinary studies are limited or equivocal.

struction or aneurysm can cause long-term morbidity and, on occasion, death. The major goal of therapy is to reduce the rate of coronary artery disease. IVIG was initially shown to reduce coronary artery complications and to shorten the febrile period.[122,123] A large U.S. multicenter study compared aspirin alone with high-dose IVIG (400 mg/kg/day for 4 days) plus aspirin.[124] The IVIG-aspirin combination was superior to aspirin alone in preventing coronary artery abnormalities. A subsequent controlled study showed that a single 2-g/kg dose of IVIG was superior to four daily 400-mg/kg doses (both groups received aspirin) in reducing the rate of coronary artery disease.[125] Thus, current optimal treatment includes a single high dose of IVIG (1 to 2 g/kg) together with aspirin.

Immune Thrombocytopenic Purpura

ITP is an autoimmune disease caused by an antibody directed against platelet antigens, leading to platelet destruction in the spleen. Imbach et al.[126] first described the response of thrombocytopenia to IVIG in patients with Wiskott-Aldrich syndrome. Subsequently, a number of studies confirmed the efficacy of IVIG in acute and chronic ITP, ITP associated with pregnancy, and neonatal alloimmune thrombocytopenia.[127–131] Currently, IVIG is approved for the treatment of acute and chronic ITP with standard doses of 400 mg/kg/day for 5 days; however, higher doses over 1 to 2 days are just as effective[130,131] and, because of convenience and expense, are preferred.

Guillain-Barré Syndrome

IVIG is effective in the treatment of Guillain-Barré syndrome, possibly by interfering with antineuronal antibodies.[132,133] A large Dutch study compared plasmapheresis (n = 73) with IVIG (n = 74) in moderate to severely affected patients.[134] Improvement was seen in both treatment groups, but those treated with IVIG responded faster and had greater improvement. IVIG is much easier to use and less expensive than plasmapheresis; therefore, if the efficacy is comparable, IVIG is indicated.

Dermatomyositis

Dermatomyositis is an autoimmune, inflammatory disease of muscles, small blood vessels, and skin. IVIG has been used with some benefit in dermatomyositis.[135–137] A recent, small double-blind placebo-controlled study involving 15 patients (ages 18 to 55 years) with treatment-resistant disease concluded that IVIG was safe and effective in treating dermatomyositis.[138] Patients were randomized to receive IVIG (n = 8; 2,000 mg/kg/month) or placebo (n = 7) for 3 months. All patients in the treatment group had significant improvement compared with none in the placebo group. The patients were given the option of crossing over; a total of 12 patients received IVIG, and 9 had major improvement, 2 had mild improvement, and 1 had no improvement. Further studies involving larger number of patients and longer observation periods are indicated.

Diseases in Which Intravenous Immune Globulin May Be Valuable

Neurologic Diseases

IVIG has been used in a number of inflammatory neurologic diseases. It has been of considerable value in myasthenia gravis.[139,140] IVIG has also been successful in many patients with chronic inflammatory demyelinating polyneuropathy.[141,142] A few children with intractable seizures and IgG subclass deficiencies have received benefit from IVIG.[143,144] IVIG has also been used in chronic fatigue syndrome,[145,146] multiple sclerosis,[147] Sydenham's chorea,[148] and other neurologic disorders.[38]

Hematologic Diseases

IVIG has also been used in autoimmune neutropenia in adults[149] and children[150] and autoimmune hemolytic anemia[151,] based on the success of IVIG in ITP. Patients with hemophilia and antifactor VIII antibodies may benefit from large doses of IVIG.[152] Two children with severe combined immunodeficiency and adenosine deaminase deficiency had an antibody develop to exogenously administered polyethylene glycol-bovine adenosine deaminase and were successfully treated with large doses of IVIG together with prednisone therapy.[153]

Collagen Vascular Diseases

High-dose IVIG has been used in systemic lupus erythematosus[154] and juvenile rheumatoid arthritis[155,156] with mixed results. One report suggested benefit in a patient with polymyositis.[157] IVIG was used in a patient with Churg-Strauss syndrome (pulmonary vasculitis) with anecdotal benefit.[158] Patients with bullous pemphigoid, a skin disease characterized by antiepidermal antibodies, had improvement of their illness with high-dose IVIG.[159] IVIG has been used in women with recurrent spontaneous abortions,[160-162] although a therapeutic effect could not be verified in a randomized, double-blind, multicenter trial in comparison with 5 percent human albumin, which was used as a placebo.[163]

Allergic Diseases

Several studies have suggested the efficacy of high-dose IVIG in patients with asthma and subtle antibody deficiency[164] and in steroid-dependent asthmatic pa-

tients without antibody defect.[165] In one patient with severe intractable atopic dermatitis, high-dose IVIG infusions led to significant clinical improvement and a marked decrease in serum IgE levels.[166]

SPECIAL ANTIBODY PREPARATIONS FOR NONINFECTIOUS USE

Rho (D) Immune Globulin

Anti D immune globulin (Rho-Gam, Ortho, Raritan, NJ) is a high-titer human antirhesus immune serum globulin used in the prevention of Rh hemolytic disease of newborns. It is given by intramuscular injection to Rh-negative mothers after delivery of an Rh-positive infant or after miscarriage or abortion. It should also be used after inadvertent transfusion of an Rh-negative individual with Rh-positive blood.

Experimental lots of anti-D intravenous immune globulin have been used successfully in the treatment of ITP in Rh-positive individuals.[167,168] Salama and Mueller-Eckhardt[168] proposed that the anti-D coats red cells, which in turn causes reticuloendothelial blockage, similar to the effect of high-dose IVIG in this disorder.

Immunosuppressive Antibodies

Two antibodies—one a mouse monoclonal antibody directed against human CD3 T lymphocytes (Muromonab, Ortho Biotech, Raritan, NJ) and another, antithymocyte globulin (Atgam, Upjohn, Kalamazoo, MI), a polyclonal equine preparation—are used for immunosuppression, particularly for transplant procedures.

Antivenins

Three equine antivenins are available for bites by black widow spiders, coral snakes, and other poisonous snakes (Table 45-1).

Digoxin Antibody

An ovine (sheep) antibody fragment (Fab portion of IgG) binds to digoxin and digitoxin (Digibind, Burroughs Wellcome, Research Triangle Park, NC) and is valuable in the treatment of digitalis toxicity or overdose by accidental ingestion. Fragmentation of the antibody results in rapid catabolism; after its intravenous infusion, it combines with the drug and removes it rapidly from the serum.

USE OF IMMUNE GLOBULINS BY UNUSUAL ROUTES

Administration of immune globulin orally to provide antimicrobial activity in the gastrointestinal tract mimics the action of antibody-rich colostrum and breast milk. In humans, little or no ingested immune globulin is absorbed intact into the systemic circulation.[169] Some oral immune globulin traverses the entire gastrointestinal tract undigested, particularly in premature infants.[170] Oral immune globulin may neutralize microorganisms, inhibit their colonization, and prevent their attachment to the gastrointestinal mucosa.

Barnes et al.[171] fed human γ globulin for 7 days or a placebo to premature infants in a nursery in which rotavirus was endemic. Rotavirus-associated diarrhea developed in 6 of 11 babies given placebo and in 1 of 14 given oral γ globulin. Losonsky et al.[172] used oral human immune globulin successfully to interrupt the excretion of rotavirus in immunodeficient patients chronically infected with rotavirus.

Eibl et al.[173] were able to prevent necrotizing enterocolitis in all 90 infants given oral immune globulin rich in serum IgA. There were 6 cases among 91 control infants. Bovine colostrom has been used successfully to treat Cryptosporidium diarrhea in HIV infection.[174] Oral human immune globulin has also been used in the period after bone marrow transplantation to prevent viral gastroenteritis[175] and in nonspecific diarrhea in immunodeficient subjects.[176]

Human immunoglobulin has been used intrathecally in the treatment of viral encephalomyelitis in antibody deficiency[177] and as respiratory aerosol in the treatment of RSV infection.[178]

FUTURE DIRECTIONS IN IMMUNOGLOBULIN THERAPY

Several high-titer human immune globulins are being tested for clinical efficacy, including group B streptococcal IVIG (for premature infants), a bacterial polysaccharide immune globulin (for high-risk infants), a Pseudomonas IVIG (for burn patients),

and an HIV IVIG (for HIV treatment and prevention). Other therapeutic immune globulins under investigation include an *Escherichia coli* endotoxin antibody (for shock or surgery), an antimalarial antibody, and an anti-RSV immune globulin for RSV infection. Intravenous preparations of HIBG are being developed for the prevention of HBV infection after liver transplantation.

The use of other monoclonal antibodies, both human and murine, to treat specific infections will be forthcoming. These monoclonal antibodies may be used alone or added to polyvalent IVIG to increase the titer to a specific microorganism.

The use of monoclonal antibodies to neutralize cells, bind to cytokines or receptors, and detoxify certain drugs will also be forthcoming. Monoclonal anti-idiotypic antibodies may also be used to suppress autoimmune disease or inhibit a specific harmful autoantibody.

The use of monoclonal antibodies directed to specific tumor cells or organs to deliver radioisotopes or chemotherapeutic agents is feasible. Such antibodies can also be used diagnostically for tumor cell or infection localization.

Chimeric antibodies that contain the antigen-reactive site of a mouse monoclonal antibody attached to the constant regions of a human antibody can be made; these "humanized" monoclonals have a longer half-life and better complement-fixation ability than the intact mouse monoclonal antibody. A final advance is to use engineered antibodies by genetically recombining the L chain and H chain gene from different antibody clones for maximal binding activity.[179]

REFERENCES

1. American Academy of Pediatrics: Active and passive immunization. p. 7. In Peter G (ed): 1994 Red Book: Report of the Committee on Infectious Diseases. 23rd Ed. American Academy of Pediatrics, Elk Grove Village, 1994
2. Fibiger J: Om serum Behandling af Difteri. Hospitalstidende 6:337, 1898
3. Stiehm ER: Passive immunization. p. 2261. In Feigen RD, Cherry JD (eds): Textbook of Pediatric Infectious Diseases. 3rd Ed. WB Saunders, Philadelphia, 1992
4. Stiehm ER: Immunodeficiency disorders: general considerations. p. 157. In Stiehm ER (ed): Immuno-

logic Disorder in Infants and Children. 3rd Ed. WB Saunders, Philadelphia, 1989

5. Ellis EF, Henney CS: Adverse reactions following administration of human gammaglobulin. J Allergy 43: 45, 1969

6. Medical Research Council Working Party: Hypogammaglobulinemia in the United Kingdom. Lancet 1: 163, 1969

7. Burks AW, Sampson HA, Buckley RH: Anaphylactic reactions after gamma globulin administration in patients with hypogammaglobulinemia. N Engl J Med 314:560, 1986

8. Vyas GN, Perkins HA, Yaug YM, Basantanix GK: Healthy blood donors with selective absence of immunoglobulin A: prevention of anaphylactic transfusion reactions caused by antibodies to IgA. J Lab Clin Med 85:838, 1975

9. Björkander J, Hammarstrom L, Smith CIE et al: Immunoglobulin prophylaxis in patients with antibody deficiency syndromes and anti-IgA antibodies. J Clin Immunol 7:8, 1987

10. Amer J, Ott E, Ibbott FA et al: The effect of monthly gamma globulin administration on morbidity and mortality from infection in premature infants during the first year of life. Pediatrics 32:4, 1963

11. Siber GR, Werner BG, Halse NA et al: Interference of immune globulin with measles and rubella immunization. J Pediatr 122:204, 1993

12. Matheson DS, Clarkson TW, Gelfand EW: Mercury toxicity (acrodynia) induced by long-term injection of gamma globulin. J Pediatr 97:153, 1980

13. Gardulf A, Hammarstrom L, Smith CIE: Home treatment of hypogammaglobulinaemia with subcutaneous gammaglobulin by rapid infusion. Lancet 338: 162, 1991

14. Berger M, Cupps TR, Fauci A: Immunoglobulin replacement therapy by slow subcutaneous infusion. Ann Intern Med 93:55, 1980

15. Welch MJ, Stiehm ER: Slow subcutaneous immunoglobulin therapy in a patient with reactions to intramuscular immunoglobulin. J Clin Immunol 3:285, 1983

16. Stokes J, Jr, Maris EP, Gellis SS: Chemical, clinical and immunological studies on the products of human plasma fractionation. XI. The use of concentrated normal human serum in the prophylaxis and treatment of measles. J Clin Invest 23:531, 1944

17. Ordman CS, Jennings CG, Jr, Janeway CA: Chemical clinical and immunological studies on the products of human plasma fractionation. XII. The use of concentrated normal human serum gamma globulin (human immune serum globulin) in the prevention and attenuation of measles. J Clin Invest 23:541, 1944

18. Black FL, Berman LL, Libel M et al: Inadequate immunity to measles in children vaccinated at an early age: effect of revaccination. Bull World Health Organ 62:315, 1984

19. Stokes J, Jr, Neefe JR: The prevention and attenuation of infectious hepatitis by gamma globulin. JAMA 127:144, 1945

20. Havens WP, Jr, Paul JR: Prevention of infectious hepatitis with gamma globulin. JAMA 129:270, 1945

21. Gellis SS, Stokes J, Jr, Brother GM et al: The use of human immune serum globulin (gamma globulin) in infectious (epidemic) hepatitis in the Mediterranean theater of operations. I. Studies on prophylaxis in two epidemics of infectious hepatitis. JAMA 128: 1062, 1945

22. Stokes J, Jr, Farquhar JA, Drake ME et al: Infectious hepatitis: length of protection of immune serum globulin (gamma globulin) during epidemics. JAMA 147:714, 1951

23. Ward R, Krugman S: Etiology, epidemiology and prevention of viral hepatitis. Prog Med Virol 4:87, 1962

24. Krugman S, Ward R, Giles JP et al: Infectious hepatitis: studies on the effectiveness of gamma globulin and on the incidence of inapparent infection. JAMA 174:823, 1960

25. Ward R, Krugman S, Giles JP et al: Infectious hepatitis. Studies of its natural history and prevention. N Engl J Med 258:407, 1958

26. Smallwood LA, Tabor E, Finlayson JS et al: Antibodies in hepatitis A virus in immune serum globulin. J Med Virol 7:21, 1981

27. Carl M, Francis DP, Maynard JE: Food-borne hepatitis A: recommendations for control. J Infect Dis 148: 1133, 1983

28. Centers for Disease Control: Postexposure prophylaxis of hepatitis B. MMWR Morb Mortal Wkly Rep 33:285, 1984

29. Centers for Disease Control: Recommendations for protection against viral hepatitis. MMWR Morb Mortal Wkly Rep 34:313, 1985

30. Centers for Disease Control: Rabies prevention United States 1984: recommendations of the Immunization Practices Advisory Committee. MMWR Morb Mortal Wkly Rep 33:393, 1984

31. Patel JC, Mehta BC, Nanavati BH et al: Role of serum therapy in tetanus. Lancet 1:740, 1963

32. Rubbo SD, Suri JC: Passive immunization against tetanus with human immune globulin. BMJ 2:79, 1962

33. Rubinstein HM: Studies on human tetanus antitoxin. Am J Hyg 76:276, 1962

34. McComb JA, Dwyer RC: Passive-active immunization with tetanus immune globulin (human). N Engl J Med 268:857, 1963

35. Ross AH: Modification of chickenpox in family contacts by administration of gamma globulin. N Engl J Med 267:369, 1962

36. Brunell PA, Gershon AA: Passive immunization against varicella-zoster infections. J Infect Dis 127:415, 1973

37. Buckley RH, Schiff RI: The use of intravenous immune globulin in immunodeficiency diseases. N Engl J Med 325:110, 1991

38. Dwyer JM: Manipulating the immune system with immune globulin. N Engl J Med 326:107, 1992

39. Keller T, McGrath K, Newland A et al: Indications for use of intravenous immunoglobulin. Recommendations of the Australasian Society of Blood Transfusion consensus symposium. Med J Aust 159:204, 1993

40. Skavaril F, Gardi A: Differences among available immunoglobulin preparations for intravenous use. Pediatr Infect Dis, suppl. 7:43, 1988

41. Apfelzweig R, Piszkiewicz D, Hooper JA: Immunoglobulin A concentrations in commercial immune globulins. J Clin Immunol 7:46, 1987

42. Chehimi H, Peppard J, Immanuel D: Selection of an intravenous immunoglobulin for immunoprophylaxis of cytomegalovirus infections: an *in vitro* comparison of currently available and previously effective immune globulins. Bone Marrow Transplant 2:395, 1987

43. Ochs HD, Fischer SH, Virant FS et al: Non-A non-B hepatitis and intravenous immunoglobulin. Lancet 1:404, 1985

44. Bjorkander J, Cunningham-Rundles C, Ludon P: Intravenous immunoglobulin prophylaxis causing liver damage in 16 of 77 patients with hypogammaglobulinemia or IgG subclass deficiency. Am J Med 84:107, 1988

45. Lehner PJ, Webster AD: Hepatitis C from immunoglobulin infusion. BMJ 306:1541, 1993

46. Williams PE, Yap PL, Gillon J et al: Transmission of non-A non-B hepatitis by pH4 treated intravenous immunoglobulin. Vox Sang 57:15, 1989

47. Bjoro K, Froland SS, Yun Z et al: Hepatitis C infection in patients with primary hypogammaglobulinemia after treatment with contaminated immune globulin. N Engl J Med 331:1607, 1994

48. Centers for Disease Control: Outbreak of hepatitis C associated with intravenous immunoglobulin administration—United States, October 1993–June 1994. MMWR Morb Mortal Wkly Rep 43:505, 1994

49. Schiff RI: Transmission of viral infections through intravenous immune globulin. N Engl J Med 331:1649, 1994

50. Imbach P, Perret B, Babington R et al: Safety of intravenous immunoglobulin preparations. Vox Sang 61:1, 1991

51. Henin Y, Marechal V, Barre F et al: Inactivation and partition of HIV during Kistler and Nitschmann fractionation of human blood plasma. Vox Sang 54:78, 1988

52. Kato E, Shindo S, Eto Y et al: Administration of immune globulin associated with aseptic meningitis. JAMA 259:3267, 1988

53. Rault R, Piraino B, Johnston JR et al: Pulmonary and renal toxicity of intravenous immunoglobulin. Clin Nephrol 36:83, 1991

54. Brox AG, Courmoyer D, Sternbach M et al: Hemolytic anemia following intravenous immunoglobulin administration. Am J Med 82:633, 1987

55. Cunningham-Rundles C, Bjorkander J, Hanson LA: Therapeutic use of an IgA depleted intravenous immunoglobulin patient. p. 87. In Morell A, Nydegger UE (eds): Clinical Use of Intravenous Immunoglobulin. Academic Press, London, 1986

56. Schiff RI, Sedlak D, Buckley RH: Rapid infusion of Sandoglobulin in patients with primary humoral immunodeficiency. J Allergy Clin Immunol 88:61, 1991

57. Ashida ER, Saxon A: Home intravenous immunoglobulin infusion by self-infusion. J Clin Immunol 6:306, 1986

58. Sorensen RU, Kallick MD, Berger M: Home treatment of antibody deficiency syndromes with intravenous immunoglobulin. J Allergy Clin Immunol 80:810, 1987

59. Kobayashi RH, Kobayashi AD, Lee N et al: Home self-administration of intravenous immunoglobulin in children. Pediatrics 85:705, 1990

60. Ammann AJ, Ashman RF, Buckley RH et al: Use of intravenous immunoglobulin in antibody deficiency: results of a multi-center controlled trial. Clin Immunol Immunopathol 22:60, 1982

61. Cunningham-Rundles C, Siegal FP, Smithwick EM et al: Efficacy of intravenous immunoglobulin in primary humoral immunodeficiency. Ann Intern Med 101:435, 1984

62. Nolte NT, Pirofsky B, Gerritz GA et al: Intravenous immunoglobulin therapy for antibody deficiency. Clin Exp Immunol 36:237, 1979

63. Pirofsky B, Anderson CJ, Bardana EJ: Therapeutic and detrimental effects of intravenous immunoglobulin therapy. p. 15. In Alving BM, Finlayson JS (eds): Immunoglobulins: Characteristics and Uses of Intra-

venous Preparations. DHHS publication no. FDA 80-9005. Food and Drug Administration, Bethesda, 1980

64. Montanaro A, Pirofsky B: Prolonged intervals of high dose IVIG in patients with primary immune deficiency states. Am J Med, suppl. 3A, 76:67, 1984

65. Roifman CM, Livison H, Gelfand EW: High dose vs low dose intravenous immunoglobulin in hypogammaglobulinemia and chronic lung disease. Lancet 1:1075, 1987

66. Bjorkander J, Bengtsson U, Oxelius VA et al: Symptoms and efficacy of intravenous immunoglobulin prophylaxis in patients with low serum levels of IgG subclasses. J Allergy Clin Immunol 77:124, 1986

67. Silk H, Geha RS: Intravenous immunoglobulin prophylaxis in children with IgG subclass 2 deficiency. J Allergy Clin Immunol 79:188, 1987

68. Knudson AP: Patients with IgG subclass and/or selective antibody deficiency to polysaccharide antigens: initiation of a controlled clinical trial of intravenous immunoglobulin. J Allergy Clin Immunol 84:640, 1989

69. Meese PJ, Ochs HD, Wedgwood RJ: Successful treatment of echovirus meningoencephalitis and myositis-fasciitis with intravenous immune globulin therapy in a patient with X-linked agammaglobulinemia. N Engl J Med 304:1278, 1981

70. Erlandsson K, Schwart T, Dwyer JM: Successful reversal of echovirus encephalitis in X-linked hypogammaglobulinemia by intraventricular administration of immunoglobulin. N Engl J Med 312:351, 1985

71. Crennan JM, Van Scoy RE, McKenna CH et al: Echovirus polymyositis in patients with hypogammaglobulinemia: failure of high dose intravenous gammaglobulin therapy and review of the literature. Am J Med 81:35, 1986

72. Cooperative Group for the Study of Immune Globulin in Chronic Lymphocytic Leukemia: Intravenous immunoglobulin for the prevention of infection in chronic lymphocytic leukemia—a randomized, controlled trial. N Engl J Med 319:902, 1988

73. Weeks JC, Tierney MR, Weinstein MC: Cost-effectiveness of prophylactic intravenous immune globulin in chronic lymphocytic leukemia. N Engl J Med 325:81, 1991

74. Weeks JC, Tierney MR, Weinstein MC: Prophylactic immune globulin in chronic lymphocytic leukemia (correspondence). N Engl J Med 326:139, 1992

75. Schedel I: Application of immune globulin preparations in multiple myeloma. p. 123. In Morrell A, Nydegger UE (eds): Clinical Use of Intravenous Immunoglobulins. Academic Press, New York, 1986

76. Magny JF, Bremard-Oury C, Brault D et al: Intravenous immunoglobulin therapy for prevention of infection in high-risk premature infants: report of a multi-center, double-blind study. Pediatrics 88:437, 1991

77. Fanaroff AA, Korones SB, Wright LL et al: A controlled trial of intravenous immune globulin to reduce nosocomial infections in very low-birth-weight infants. N Engl J Med 330:1107, 1994

78. NIH Consensus Development Statement: Intravenous Immunoglobulin: Prevention and Treatment of Disease. May 21-23, 1990. Vol. 8. National Institutes of Health, Bethesda, 1990

79. Shirani KZ, Vaughan GN, McManus AT et al: Replacement of therapy with modified immune globulin G in burn patients: preliminary kinetics studies. Am J Med 76:175, 1984

80. Glinz W, Grob PV, Nydegger UE et al: Polyvalent immunoglobulin for the prophylaxis of bacterial infections in patients following multiple trauma. Intensive Care Med 11:288, 1985

81. DeSimone C, Delogu, Corbetta G: Intravenous immunoglobulins in association with antibiotics. A therapeutic trial in septic intensive care unit patients. Crit Care Med 16:23, 1988

82. Suffredini AF: Current prospects for the treatment of clinical sepsis. Crit Care Med 22:S12, 1994

83. Tutscha PJ: Diminishing morbidity and mortality of bone marrow transplantation. Vox Sang, Suppl. 2, 51:87, 1986

84. Sullivan KM: Intravenous immune globulin in recipients of a marrow transplant. J Allergy Clin Immunol 84:632, 1989

85. Sullivan KM: Immunoglobulin therapy in bone marrow transplantation. Am J Med, suppl. 4A, 83:34, 1987

86. Graham-Pole J, Camitta B, Casper J et al: Intravenous immunoglobulin may lessen all forms of infection in patients receiving allogeneic bone marrow transplantation for acute lymphoblastic leukemia: a Pediatric Oncology Group study. Bone Marrow Transplant 3:559, 1988

87. Sullivan KM, Kopecky KJ, Jocom J et al: Immunomodulatory and antimicrobial efficacy of intravenous immunoglobulin in bone marrow transplantation. N Engl J Med 323:705, 1990

88. Siadak MF, Kopecky K, Sullivan KM: Reduction in transplant-related complications in patients given intravenous immune globulin after allogeneic marrow transplantation. Clin Exp Immunol, suppl. 1, 97:53, 1994

89. Rowe JM, Ciobanu N, Ascensao J et al: Recommended guidelines for the management of autolo-

gous and allogeneic bone marrow transplantation. Ann Intern Med 120:143, 1994

90. Wolff SN, Fay JW, Herzig RH et al: High-dose weekly intravenous immunoglobulin to prevent infections in patients undergoing autologous bone marrow transplantation or severe myelosuppressive therapy. A study of the American Bone Marrow Transplant Group. Ann Intern Med 118:937, 1993

91. Guglielmo BJ, Wong-Beringer A, Linker CA: Immune globulin therapy in allogeneic bone marrow transplant: a critical review. Bone Marrow Transplant 13:499, 1994

92. Winston DJ: Intravenous immunoglobulins as therapeutic agents: use in viral infections. Ann Intern Med 107:371, 1987

93. Winston DJ, Ho WG, Chaplin RE: Ganciclovir and intravenous immunoglobulin in bone marrow transplantation. p. 337. In Champlin RE, Gale RP (eds): New Strategies in Bone Marrow Transplantation. Wiley-Liss, New York, 1991

94. Emmanuel D, Cunningham I, Jules-Elysee K et al: Cytomegalovirus pneumonia after bone marrow transplantation successfully treated with the combination of ganciclovir and high-dose intravenous immune globulin. Ann Intern Med 109:777, 1988

95. Snydman DR, Werner BG, Heinze-Lacey B et al: Use of cytomegalovirus immune globulin to prevent cytomegalovirus disease in renal transplant recipients. N Engl J Med 317:1049, 1987

96. Snydman DR: Cytomegalovirus immunoglobulins in the prevention and treatment of cytomegalovirus disease. Rev Infect Dis, suppl. 7, 12:839, 1990

97. Steinmueller DR, Graneto D, Swift C et al: Use of intravenous immunoglobulin prophylaxis for primary cytomegalovirus infection post living-related-donor renal transplantation. Transplant Proc 21:2069, 1989

98. Cofer JB, Morris CA, Sutker WL et al: The effect of prophylactic immune globulin on cytomegalovirus infection and liver transplants. p. 229. In Imbach P (ed): Immunotherapy With IVIG. Academic Press, London, 1991

99. Bell R, Shei A, McDonald JA et al: The role of CMV immune prophylaxis in patients at risk for primary CMV infection following orthoptic liver transplantation. Transplant Proc 21:3781, 1989

100. Tobi M, Strauss SE: Chronic Epstein-Barr virus disease: a workshop held by the National Institute of Allergy and Infectious Diseases. Ann Intern Med 103:951, 1985

101. Okano M, Pirruccello SJ, Grierson HL et al: Immunovirological studies of fatal infectious mononucleo-sis in a patient with X-linked lymphoproliferative syndrome treated with intravenous immunoglobulin and interferon-α. Clin Immunol Immunopathol 54:410, 1990

102. Paryani SG, Arvin AM, Koropchak CM et al: Comparison of varicella-zoster antibody titers in patients given intravenous immune serum globulin or varicella-zoster immune globulin. J Pediatr 105:200, 1984

103. Bernstein LJ, Krieger BZ, Novic B et al: Bacterial infections in acquired immunodeficiency syndrome of children. Pediatr Infect Dis 4:472, 1985

104. Ochs HD: Intravenous immunoglobulin in the treatment and prevention of acute infections in pediatric acquired immunodeficiency syndrome patients. Pediatr Infect Dis 6:509, 1987

105. NICHD Intravenous Immunoglobulin Study Group: Intravenous immune globulin for the prevention of bacterial infections in children with symptomatic human immunodeficiency virus infection. N Engl J Med 325:73, 1991

106. Mofenson LM, Moye J, Korelitz J et al: Cross-over of placebo patients to intravenous immunoglobulin confirms efficacy for prophylaxis of bacterial infections and reduction of hospitalization in human immunodeficiency virus infected children. Pediatr Infect Dis J 13:477, 1994

107. Pollach AN, Janinis J, Green D: Successful intravenous immunoglobulin therapy for human immunodeficiency virus-associated thrombocytopenia. Arch Intern Med 148:695, 1988

108. Bussel JB, Himi JS: Isolated thrombocytopenia in patients infected with HIV: treatment with intravenous gammaglobulin. Am J Hematol 28:79, 1988

109. Kurtzberg J, Friedman HS, Kinney PR et al: Management of human immunodeficiency virus-associated thrombocytopenia with intravenous gammaglobulin. Am J Pediatr Hematol Oncol 9:299, 1987

110. Spector SA, Gelber RD, McGrath N et al: A controlled trial of intravenous gamma globulin for prevention of serious bacterial infections in children with advanced human immunodeficiency virus infection receiving zidovudine. N Engl J Med 331:1181, 1994

111. Koch WC, Massey G, Russel CE et al: Manifestations and treatment of human parvovirus B19 infection in immunocompromised patients. J Pediatr 116:355, 1990

112. Kurtzman G, Frickhofen N, Kimball J et al: Pure red cell aplasia of 10 years duration due to persistent parvovirus B19 infection and its cure with immunoglobulin treatment. N Engl J Med 321:519, 1989

113. Tang ML, Kemp AS, Moaven LD: Parvovirus B19-associated red blood cell aplasia in combined immu-

nodeficiency with normal immunoglobulins. Pediatr Infect Dis J 13:539, 1994

114. Hemming VG, Rodriguez W, Kim HW et al: Intravenous immunoglobulin treatment of respiratory syncytial virus infections in infants and young children. Antimicrob Agents Chemother 31:1882, 1987

115. Groothuis JR, Levin MJ, Rodriguez W et al: Use of intravenous gammaglobulin to passively immunize high risk children against respiratory syncytial virus: safety and pharmacogenetics. Antimicrob Agents Chemother 35:1469, 1991

116. Groothuis JR, Simoes EA, Levin MJ et al: Prophylactic administration of respiratory syncytial virus immune globulin to high-risk infants and young children. N Engl J Med 329:1524, 1993

117. Barry W, Hudgins L, Donta T et al: Intravenous immunoglobulin therapy for streptococcal toxic shock syndrome. JAMA 267:315, 1992

118. Winnie GB, Cowan RG, Wade NA: Intravenous immune globulin treatment of pulmonary exacerbations in cystic fibrosis. J Pediatr 114:309, 1989

119. Silvestris F, Cafforio P, Dammacco F: Pathogenic anti-DNA idiotype-reactive IgG in intravenous immunoglobulin preparations. Clin Exp Immunol 97:19, 1994

120. Takei S, Arora YK, Walker SM: Intravenous immunoglobulin contains specific antibodies inhibitory to activation of T cells by staphylococcal toxin superantigens. J Clin Invest 91:602, 1993

121. Leung DY, Burns J, Newberger J et al: Reversal of immunoregulatory abnormalities in Kawasaki syndrome by intravenous gammaglobulin. J Clin Invest 79:468, 1987

122. Furusho K, Nakano H, Shinomya K et al: High-dose intravenous immunoglobulins for Kawasaki disease. Lancet 2:1055, 1984

123. Furusho K, Kamiya T, Nakano H et al: Japanese gammaglobulin trials for Kawasaki disease. p. 425. In Shulman ST (eds): Progress in Clinical and Biologic Research. Kawasaki Disease. Vol. 250. Alan R Liss, New York, 1987

124. Newburger JW, Takahashi M, Burns JC et al: The treatment of Kawasaki syndrome with intravenous gammaglobulin. N Engl J Med 315:341, 1986

125. Newburger JW, Takahashi M, Beiser AS et al: A single intravenous infusion of gammaglobulin as compared with 4 infusions in the treatment of acute Kawasaki syndrome. N Engl J Med 324:1633, 1991

126. Imbach T, D'Apuzzo V, Hirt A: High-dose intravenous gammaglobulin for idiopathic thrombocytopenic purpura in childhood. Lancet 1:1228, 1981

127. Bussel JB, Pham LC, Aledort L et al: Maintenance treatment of adults with chronic refractory immune thrombocytopenic purpura using repeated intravenous infusions of gammaglobulin. Blood 72:121, 1988

128. Bussel JB, Berkowitz R, McFarland J et al: Antenatal treatment of neonatal alloimmune thrombocytopenia. N Engl J Med 319:1374, 1988

129. Hollenberg JP, Subak LL, Ferry JJ et al: Cost effectiveness of splenectomy vs intravenous gammaglobulin in the treatment of chronic immune thrombocytopenic purpura in childhood. J Pediatr 112:530, 1988

130. Rosthoj S, Steffensen GK, Glud TK: Simplified immunoglobulin treatment of idiopathic thrombocytopenic purpura. Acta Paediatr Scand 76:631, 1987

131. Bussel JB, Pham LC: Intravenous treatment with gammaglobulin in adults with immune thrombocytopenic purpura; review of the literature. Vox Sang 52:206, 1987

132. Vermeulen M, VanDerMeche FG, Steelman JD et al: Plasma and gammaglobulin infusion in chronic inflammatory polyneuropathy. J Neurol Sci 70:317, 1985

133. Kleyweg RP, VanDerMeche FG, Meulstee J: Treatment of Guillain-Barré syndrome with high-dose gammaglobulin. Neurology 38:1639, 1988

134. VanDerMeche FG, Schmitz PI: A randomized trial comparing intravenous immunoglobulin and plasma exchange in Guillain-Barré syndrome. N Engl J Med 326:1123, 1992

135. Roifman CM, Schaffer FN, Wachsmuth SE et al: Reversal of chronic polymyositis following intravenous immune globulin therapy. JAMA 258:513, 1987

136. Lang BA, Laxer RM, Murphy G et al: Treatment of dermatomyositis with intravenous immunoglobulin. Am J Med 91:169, 1991

137. Cherin P, Herson S, Wechsler B et al: Efficacy of intravenous gammaglobulin therapy in chronic refractory polymyositis and dermatomyositis: an open study with 20 adult patients. Am J Med 91:162, 1991

138. Dalakas MC, Illa I, Dambrosia JM et al: A controlled trial of high-dose intravenous immune globulin infusions as treatment for dermatomyositis. N Engl J Med 329:1993, 1993

139. Arsura E: Experience with intravenous immunoglobulin in myasthenia gravis. Clin Immunol Immunopathol 53:S170, 1989

140. Liblau R, Gajdos PH, Bustarret FA et al: Intravenous gamma-globulin in myasthenia gravis: interaction with anti-acetylcholine receptor autoantibodies. J Clin Immunol 11:128, 1991

141. VanDerMeche FG, Vermeulen N, Busch HF: Chronic inflammatory demyelinating polyneuropathy: conduction failure before and during immunoglobulin of plasma therapy. Brain 112:1553, 1989

142. Faed JM, Day B, Pollock M et al: High-dose intravenous human immunoglobulin in chronic inflammatory demyelinating polyneuropathy. Neurology 39: 422, 1989

143. Arizumi N, Babba K, Shiira H et al: High-dose gammaglobulin for intractable childhood epilepsy. Lancet 2:162, 1983

144. Schwartz SA, Gordon KE, Johnston MV et al: Use of intravenous immunoglobulin in the treatment of seizure disorders. J Allergy Clin Immunol 84:603, 1989

145. Lloyd A, Hickie I, Wakefield D et al: A double-blind placebo controlled trial of intravenous immunoglobulin therapy in patients with chronic fatigue syndrome. Am J Med 89:561, 1990

146. Peterson PK, Shepard J, Macres M et al: A controlled trial of intravenous immunoglobulin G in chronic fatigue syndrome. Am J Med 89:554, 1990

147. Achiron A, Pras E, Gilad R et al: Open controlled therapeutic trial of intravenous immune globulin in relapsing-remitting multiple sclerosis. Arch Neurol 49:1233, 1992

148. Swedo SE, Leonard HL, Schapiro MB et al: Sydenham's chorea: physical and psychological symptoms of St. Vitus dance. Pediatrics 91:706, 1993

149. Pollack S, Cunningham-Rundles C, Smithwick EM et al: High-dose intravenous immunoglobulin for autoimmune neutropenia (letter). N Engl J Med 307:253, 1982

150. Bussel JB, Lalezari P, Hilgartner M et al: Reversal of neutropenia with intravenous gammaglobulin in autoimmune neutropenia of infancy. Blood 62:398, 1983

151. MacIntyre EA, Linch DC, Macey MG et al: Successful response to intravenous immunoglobulin in autoimmune hemolytic anaemia. Br J Haematol 60:387, 1985

152. Gianella-Gorradori A, Hirt A, Luthy A et al: Hemophilia due to factor VIII inhibitors in a patient suffering from an autoimmune disease. Treatment with intravenous immunoglobulin. Blood 48:403, 1984

153. Chaffee S, Mary A, Stiehm ER et al: IgG antibody response to polyethylene glycol-modified adenosine deaminase (PEG-ADA) in patients with adenosine deaminase deficiency. J Clin Invest 89:1643, 1992

154. Jordan SC: Intravenous gammaglobulin therapy in systemic lupus erythematosus and immune complex disease. Clin Immunol Immunopathol, suppl., 53: 164, 1989

155. Silverman ED, Laxer RN, Greenwald M et al: Intrave-

nous immunoglobulin therapy and systemic juvenile rheumatoid arthritis. Arthritis Rheum 33:1015, 1990

156. Ballow M, Parke A: The uses of intravenous immunoglobulin in collagen vascular disorders. J Allergy Clin Immunol 84:608, 1989

157. Roifman CM, Schaffer FM, Wachsmuth SE et al: Reversal of chronic polymyositis following intravenous immune serum globulin therapy. JAMA 258:513, 1987

158. Hamilos DL, Christensen J: Treatment of Churg-Strauss syndrome with high dose intravenous immunoglobulin. J Allergy Clin Immunol 88:823, 1991

159. Godard W, Roujeau JC, Guillot B et al: Bullous pemphigoid and intravenous gamma globulin (letter). Ann Intern Med 103:964, 1985

160. Park A, Maier D, Wilson D: Intravenous gammaglobulin, anti-phospholipid antibodies and pregnancy. Ann Intern Med 110:495, 1989

161. Carreras LO, Perez G, Vega HR: Lupus anti-coagulant and recurrent fetal loss: successful treatment with gammaglobulin. Lancet 11:393, 1988

162. Coulam C, Peters A, MacIntyre J et al: The use of IVIG for the treatment of recurrent spontaneous abortion. p. 394. In Imbach P (ed): Immunotherapy With Intravenous Immunoglobulins. Academic Press, London, 1991

163. Heine O, Mueller-Eckhardt G: Intravenous immune globulin in recurrent abortion. Clin Exp Immunol, suppl. 1, 97:39, 1994

164. Page R, Masur BD, Friday G et al: Asthma in selective immunoglobulin subclass deficiency: improvement of asthma after immunoglobulin replacement therapy. J Pediatr 112:127, 1988

165. Masur BD, Gelfand EW: An open-label study of high-dose IVIG in severe childhood asthma. J Allergy Clin Immunol 87:976, 1991

166. Greenberg BK, Kobayashi RH, Katz RN et al: The use of intravenous immunoglobulin in a patient with severe atopic dermatitis. J Allergy Clin Immunol 85: 206A, 1990

167. Bussel JB, Graziano JN, Kimberly RP et al: Intravenous anti-D treatment of immune thrombocytopenic purpura: analysis of efficacy, toxicity, and mechanism of effect. Blood 77:1884, 1991

168. Salama A, Mueller-Eckhardt C: Use of Rh antibodies in the treatment of autoimmune thrombocytopenia. Transfusion Med Rev 6:17, 1992

169. Ammann AJ, Stiehm ER: Immune globulin levels in colostrum and breast milk, and serum from formula- and breast-fed newborns. Proc Soc Exp Biol Med 122: 1098, 1966

170. Blum PM, Phelps DL, Ank BJ et al: Survival of oral

human immune serum globulin in the gastrointestinal tract of low birth weight infants. Pediatr Res 15: 1256, 1981

171. Barnes NL, Doyle LW, Hewson PH et al: A randomized trial of oral gammaglobulin in low-birth-weight infants infected with rotavirus. Lancet 1:1371, 1982

172. Losonsky GA, Johnson J, Winkelstein JA et al: Oral administration of human serum immunoglobulin in immunodeficient patients with viral gastroenteritis: a pharmacokinetic and functional analysis. J Clin Invest 76:2362, 1985

173. Eibl MM, Wolf HM, Furnkranz H et al: Prevention of necrotizing enterocolitis in low-birth-weight infants by IgA-IgG feeding. N Engl J Med 319:1, 1988

174. Borowitz SM, Saulsbury FT: Treatment of chronic cryptosporidial infection with orally administered human serum immune globulin. J Pediatr 119:593, 1991

175. Copelon EA, Tutschka PJ: Immunoglobulin in bone marrow transplantation. p. 117. In Morell A, Nydegger UE (eds): Clinical Use of Intravenous Immunoglobulins. Academic Press, New York, 1986

176. Melamed I, Griffiths AM, Roifman CM: Benefit of oral immune globulin therapy in patients with immunodeficiency and chronic diarrhea. J Pediatr 3:486, 1991

177. Erlendsson K, Swartz T, Dwyer JM: Successful reversal of echovirus encephalitis in X-linked hypogammaglobulinemia by intraventricular administration of immunoglobulin. N Engl J Med 312:351, 1985

178. Rimensberger PC, Schaad UB: Clinical experience with aerosolized immunoglobulin treatment of respiratory syncytial virus infection in infants. Pediat Infect Dis J 13:328, 1994

179. Barbas CF III, Hu D, Dunlop N et al: In vitro evolution of a neutralizing human antibody to human immunodeficiency virus type I to enhance affinity and broaden strain cross-reactivity. Proc Natl Acad Sci U S A 91:3809, 1994

Chapter 46

Therapeutic Hemapheresis

Harvey G. Klein

Therapeutic hemapheresis traces its roots to the therapeutic bloodletting described in ancient teachings and to the Greek medical theory of humors. The term *apheresis,* coined at the beginning of the century from a Greek verb meaning to take away or withdraw, describes the removal of one component of blood and the return of the remaining components to the donor.[1] Although the concept of apheresis applied originally to removal of plasma (plasmapheresis) or cells (plateletpheresis or leukapheresis) by centrifugal or filtration technology, apheresis is now used more widely to refer also to such extracorporeal manipulation of blood as the removal of plasma components by column adsorption and even to exposure of blood in an extracorporeal circuit to ultraviolet light (photopheresis), in which no blood component is actually removed from the patient. Like therapeutic bleeding, which the ancients used to purify the blood, hemapheresis has assumed an almost spiritual appeal to physician and patient alike. Advocates occasionally forget that the effectiveness of the procedure should be judged not by the volume of blood processed or by the number of cells or amount of solute removed but by objective measures of patient improvement.

PRINCIPLES OF APHERESIS

The principal objective of apheresis is efficient removal of some circulating blood component, either cells or some plasma constituent. For most disorders,

the treatment goal is to deplete the circulating cell or substance directly responsible for the disease process. Apheresis can also mobilize cells and plasma components from tissue depots. For example, peripheral lymphocytes may be mobilized from the spleen and lymph nodes of some patients with chronic lymphocytic leukemia, and low-density lipoproteins (LDL) can be removed from tissue stores in patients with familial hyperlipoproteinemia. Apheresis may have other, more subtle effects. Lymphocyte depletion may modify immune responsiveness in some disease states, possibly by disturbing the control mechanisms of cellular immune regulation.[2] Plasmapheresis enhances splenic clearance of immune complexes in certain autoimmune disorders.[3]

Current automated apheresis instruments use microprocessor technology to draw and anticoagulate blood, separate components either by centrifugation or by filtration, collect the desired component, and recombine the remaining components for return to the patient. The equipment has disposable plastic software in the blood path and uses anticoagulants that contain citrate or combinations of citrate and heparin that do not result in clinical anticoagulation. Most instruments function well at blood flow rates of 30 to 80 ml/min and can operate from peripheral venous access or from a variety of multilumen central venous catheters.[4]

Several mathematical models formulated for different clinical conditions describe the kinetics of apheresis.[5-7] Removal of most blood components follows a logarithmic model described by the following equation: $C/C_0 = e^{-x}$ where C_0 is the initial concentration of the component, C is the concentration at a point in time after the procedure has begun, and x is the number of blood or plasma volumes exchanged. This model assumes that the component removed is neither synthesized nor degraded substantially during the procedure, remains within the intravascular compartment, and mixes instantaneously and completely with any plasma replacement solution. When the goal of plasmapheresis is to supply a deficient substance, for example plasma factors in the treatment of thrombotic thrombocytopenic purpura (TTP), replacement follows logarithmic kinetics similar to those developed for solute removal. One and one-half to 2 volumes, the usual definition of a therapeutic procedure, reduces an intravascular substance by about 60 percent. Processing larger volumes results in little additional gain.

Specific cell removal with centrifugal automated cell separators depends on the number of cells available, the volume of blood processed, the efficiency of the particular instrument, and the separation characteristics of the different cells.[8] Most commercially available instruments remove platelets and lymphocytes extremely efficiently. Granulocytes and monocytes cannot be cleanly separated from other cells by standard centrifugal apheresis equipment. Optimal harvesting of these cells requires special techniques such as pretreating the patient with corticosteroids or cytokines and adding sedimenting agents to enhance cell separation.

Because the ideal method for treating disorders mediated by abnormal plasma components is to remove the offending substance selectively, a variety of on-line filtration and column adsorption techniques have been introduced or proposed. Filtration instruments use the sieving properties of a wide variety of membranes to separate cells from plasma and to isolate specific plasma solutes. Filtration therapy has successfully removed LDL from patients with familial hypercholesterolemia.[9] Cascade filtration uses two or more filters in tandem (Fig. 46-1). Although the principle of cascade filtration is differential filtration based on membranes of different pore size, the filtration kinetics are complex.[10] Filtration in-

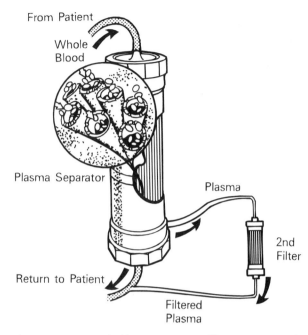

Fig. 46-1 Cascade filtration. Primary filter separates cells from plasma. A second-stage filter is designed to retain plasma solutes by specific molecular weight.

struments are generally smaller than centrifugal blood cell separators, have a smaller extracorporeal volume, and produce plasma free of cells and cell fragments.

A further technical refinement involves pairing an absorption column with a filter to remove a specific plasma component from the separated plasma. Ligands bound to a column matrix may be relatively nonspecific chemical sorbents such as charcoal or heparin or specific ligands such as monoclonal antibodies and recombinant protein antigens. The two most successful clinical columns use staphylococcal protein A and dextran sulfate cellulose. Staphylococcal protein A has high affinity for the Fc portion of IgG_1, IgG_2, and IgG_4 and for immune complexes that contain these IgG subtypes. The dextran sulfate cellulose columns selectively remove LDL and are effective in managing patients with homozygous hyperlipoproteinemia (Fig. 46-2).

A procedure related to hemapheresis, although not strictly a removal technique, has been termed photopheresis.[11] This is an automated extracorporeal photochemotherapeutic treatment that involves

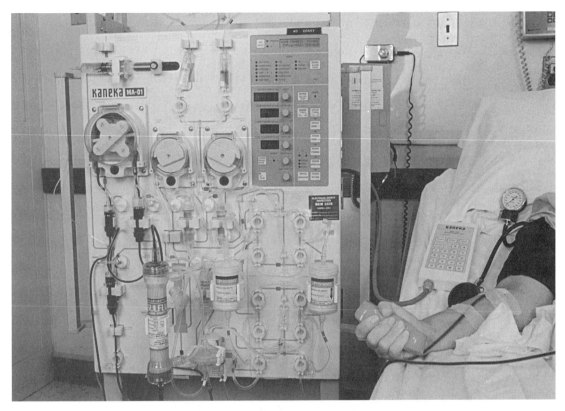

Fig. 46-2 Two-stage therapeutic plasmapheresis. Plasma is separated from cells by filtration and then passed through parallel adsorption columns to remove LDL from a patient with homozygous familial hyperlipoproteinemia.

oral administration of a light-sensitizing agent, 8-methoxy-psoralen, followed by leukapheresis and ex vivo ultraviolet A irradiation of leukocytes. The treated cells are reinfused. Photopheresis has induced remissions in patients with Sézary syndrome and is being investigated as a treatment for scleroderma and organ graft rejection.[12] The mechanism of action of photopheresis is unknown.

THERAPEUTIC CYTAPHERESIS

Common indications for therapeutic cell removal are listed in Table 46-1.

Red Cell Exchange

Red cell exchange (erythrocytapheresis) is used most often to manage or prevent the acute vaso-occlusive complications of sickle cell disease. Mechanical cell separators offer the advantages of speed and ease compared with manual exchange transfusion and avoid the potential risks from rapid alterations in blood volume and whole blood viscosity that result from simple transfusion.[13] Exchange transfusion should improve tissue oxygenation and prevent microvascular sickling by diluting the patient's abnormal red cells with normal cells, thus simultaneously correcting anemia and favorably altering whole blood viscosity and rheology.[14] No clinical data support a single optimal level of hemoglobin A. However, as few as 30 percent of transfused cells markedly decrease blood viscosity, and at mixtures of 50 percent and greater, resistance to membrane filterability approaches normal.[15,16] Achieving such levels requires one red cell volume exchange, about 4 to 6 units, in an adult with a hematocrit of about 25 percent. Although 50 percent hemoglobin A is a frequently quoted target level of exchange transfusion,

Table 46-1. Common Indications for Therapeutic Cytapheresis

Red cell exchange
    Sickle cell disease
        Acute vaso-occlusive complications
        Prophylaxis for recurrent stroke
        Frequent, severe pain crises
    Malaria with hyperparasitemia
Leukapheresis
    Leukemia with hyperleukocytosis syndrome
    Rheumatoid arthritis
Plateletpheresis
    Symptomatic thrombocythemia

some patients remain symptomatic when maintained at levels of 80 percent and above. Such failures may be due in part to pre-existing irreversible ischemic organ damage.

Clinical indications for exchange transfusion remain controversial. Simple transfusion has improved renal concentrating ability and splenic function in young sickle cell patients; exchange transfusion has improved exercise tolerance and reversed the periodic oscillations in cutaneous blood flow noted in this disease.[17–20] Such observations have encouraged the use of exchange transfusion for acute complications of sickle cell disease such as acute chest syndrome, priapism, severe painful crises, retinal artery occlusion, and intrahepatic cholestasis. Exchange transfusion for patients with sickle cell disease has also been used for prophylaxis during pregnancy, before surgery, or for patients who have suffered a stroke.[21] However, a multicenter randomized trial of transfusion during pregnancy reported that transfusion sufficient to reduce the incidence of painful crises did not reduce other maternal morbidity or perinatal mortality rates, which suggests that the effects of transfusion on the pathophysiology of sickle cell disease may be more complex than originally thought.[22] Prophylactic exchange transfusion before elective surgery is currently under study in a randomized, prospective trial.

Exchange transfusion, although relatively safe and convenient, carries all of the complications of red cell transfusion. Patients are exposed to a large number of donors and are at substantial risk for contracting hepatitis and other blood-borne infections. As many as one-third of all patients have alloanti-

bodies develop, and life-threatening delayed hemolytic transfusion reactions have been reported.[23,24] Unexplained neurologic complications, including subarachnoid hemorrhage, have also been seen in association with erythrocytapheresis, although neither the cause nor the pathophysiology of these events has been demonstrated definitively.[25] Despite the removal of cells during exchange, patients remain in positive iron balance, although iron accumulation is slow, and chelation is rarely required to prevent transfusional hemosiderosis.[26] Most centers avoid inducing nonhemolytic transfusion reactions by using washed or filtered red cells and perform extended red cell phenotyping to avoid alloimmunization to clinically important red cell antigens.

Other indications for red cell exchange are rare. The procedure has been used for patients with overwhelming red cell parasitic infections such as severe and complicated malaria and babesiosis.[27,28] In these situations, red cell exchange decreases the concentration of circulating parasites and may help sustain life until conventional therapy and natural immunity take effect. Automated red cell removal with volume replacement, isovolemic hemodilution, can be performed rapidly and safely in polycythemic subjects.[29] This maneuver should be reserved for polycythemic patients with an urgent clinical indication to lower the hematocrit, for example, evolving thrombotic stroke, for which standard single-unit manual phlebotomy might be inadvisably slow.

Leukapheresis

Therapeutic leukapheresis has been used most successfully to help manage patients with acute or chronic leukemia and extremely high white blood cell numbers, so-called hyperleukocytic leukemias.[30,31] When the fractional volume of leukocytes (leukocrit) exceeds 20 percent, blood viscosity increases, and leukocytes can interfere with pulmonary and cerebral blood flow and compete with tissue for oxygen in the microcirculation.[32] A single leukapheresis procedure generally reduces the white blood cell count by 20 to 50 percent. Ordinarily, leukapheresis is indicated when the blast count exceeds $100,000/\mu l$ or when rapidly rising blast counts exceed $50,000/\mu l$ (leukocrit greater than 10 percent), especially when evidence of central nervous system or pulmonary symptoms appears.[33] The effects of a single leukapheresis are transient, and chemotherapy should be instituted when the decision to perform leukapheresis is made. Although repeated leukapheresis has adequately reduced the white cell count in a series of patients with chronic myelocytic leukemia, improved patient survival has not been demonstrated.[34] Chronic leukapheresis can provide acceptable control of the peripheral white cell count in clinical situations such as pregnancy, when cytotoxic agents may best be avoided. Cytoreduction alone does not appear to alter the course of chronic myelocytic leukemia.

Cytoreduction for managing other leukemic processes has limited usefulness. Some studies of patients with chronic lymphocytic leukemia suggested short-term clinical benefit, but long-term support of patients in whom disease is refractory to chemotherapy does not appear to prolong life.[35] Transient responses to leukapheresis used alone or in combination with low-dose chemotherapy have been reported in a variety of lymphoproliferative disorders. However, most patients quickly have relapses and do not respond to further leukapheresis therapy.[36–39]

Therapeutic lymphocyte depletion has been used to modify patient immune responsiveness. Removal of large numbers of lymphocytes over a period of a few weeks can suppress peripheral lymphocyte counts in patients with rheumatoid arthritis for as long as 1 year and alter laboratory measurements of immune responsiveness to a variety of stimulants.[40] Selected patients experience a modest but significant reduction in disease activity; however, the subset of patients who may derive substantial benefit from this therapy is difficult to identify.[41,42] Lymphocyte removal by apheresis has also been used to treat patients with multiple sclerosis, to enhance allograft survival, and to reverse graft rejection, but evidence of clinical efficacy in these situations is unconvincing.

Plateletpheresis

Therapeutic plateletpheresis is generally reserved for patients with myeloproliferative disorders and hemorrhage or thrombosis associated with an increased number of circulating platelets. Because thrombocytosis from other causes such as iron deficiency rarely results in thrombosis, other factors, such as a clone of functionally abnormal cells, may cause the symptoms attributed to elevated platelets in myeloproliferative disorders. Many centers undertake plateletpheresis when the patient's peripheral platelet count exceeds $10^6/\mu l$, although no consistent relationship between the level of platelet elevation and the occurrence of symptoms has been found.[43,44] Unfortunately, no generally accepted assay of platelet dysfunction predicts patients at increased risk.

When therapeutic plateletpheresis is indicated, generally in symptomatic patients, a single procedure can lower the platelet count by 30 to 50 percent. Attempts to maintain thrombocythemic patients at normal platelet counts by cytapheresis alone have not been successful; more practical long-term therapy, such as chemotherapy, should be instituted concurrently with the cytapheresis program. Because most patients with thrombocytosis, even those with myeloproliferative disorders, do not have symptoms, prophylactic plateletpheresis seems unwarranted, regardless of the platelet count.[45]

THERAPEUTIC PLASMAPHERESIS

Plasmapheresis has been used empirically to treat hundreds of different disorders. Common clinical indications for therapeutic plasmapheresis are outlined in Table 46-2. A committee appointed by the American Society of Apheresis reviewed the experience with therapeutic hemapheresis and offered guidelines for clinical practice. Disorders that have been treated with therapeutic hemapheresis were placed into four categories as follows.

Category I: Therapeutic hemapheresis is standard and acceptable

Category II: Therapeutic hemapheresis is generally accepted

Category III: Reported evidence is insufficient to establish the efficacy of therapeutic hemapheresis and/or a favorable benefit-to-risk ratio has not been clearly documented

Category IV: Available controlled trials have shown lack of therapeutic efficacy for therapeutic hemapheresis. Category I and II disorders are listed in Table 46-2.

Table 46-2. Disorders Designated as Category I or Category II as a Provisional Guide for Selecting Therapeutic Hemapheresis as a Management Option

Disorders	Category
Autoimmune	
Human immunodeficiency virus related syndromes	
Polyneuropathy	I
Hyperviscosity	I
Thrombotic thrombocytopenic purpura	I
Immune thrombocytopenia	II
Bullous pemphigoid	II
Pemphigus vulgaris	II
Raynaud's disease	II
Systemic lupus erythematosus	II
Systemic vasculitis	II
Hematology and Oncology	
Thrombotic thrombocytopenic purpura	I
Hemolytic uremic syndrome	II
ABO-incompatible marrow transplant	I
Myeloma and paraproteinemias	II
Cryoglobulinemia	I
Erythrocytosis, polycythemia vera	I
Leukocytosis and thrombocytosis	I
Post-transfusion purpura	I
Sickle cell disease complications (erythrocyte exchange)	I
Coagulation factor inhibitors	II
Cutaneous lymphoma (photopheresis)	I
Metabolic	
Refsum's disease	I
Familial hypercholesterolemia	II
Poisoning	II
Neurology	
Acute Guillain-Barré syndrome	I
Chronic inflammatory demyelinating polyneuropathy	I
Eaton-Lambert myasthenic syndrome	I
Myasthenia gravis	I
Paraproteinemic peripheral neuropathy	II
Renal	
Goodpasture syndrome	I
Rapidly progressive nephritis (without anti-GBM)	II

Some of the disorders placed into categories III or IV are progressive systemic sclerosis (III), rheumatoid arthritis (III), psoriasis (IV), autoimmune hemolytic anemia (III), hemolytic disease of the newborn (III), immune thrombocytopenia (III), platelet refractoriness (III), multiple sclerosis (III), amyotrophic lateral sclerosis (IV), and renal allograft rejection (IV).

Comprehensive reviews that describe the rationale for using plasmapheresis in a wide variety of disease states can be found elsewhere.[46,47] Some of the least controversial indications for plasmapheresis are supported by small series of uncontrolled cases that rely on objective clinical or laboratory measurements of patient improvement. Such studies support the use of plasmapheresis for treating the hyperviscosity syndrome resulting from paraproteinemia, for cryoglobulinemia, and for poisoning with albumin-bound toxins.[48–52] In the case of paraproteinemic hyperviscosity syndrome, symptoms of hyperviscosity correlate well with measurements of serum viscosity and respond promptly to plasmapheresis.[53] Hyperviscosity may be managed for years with repeated plasmapheresis; however, plasmapheresis does not alter the underlying course of the disease. Patients with cold agglutinin disease and cryoglobulinemia usually respond transiently and incompletely; however, cytotoxic therapy is usually necessary for long-term control of symptoms, and plasmapheresis is not of major importance in managing these disorders.

Metabolic Disorders

Evidence that both the cutaneous and vascular lesions of familial hypercholesterolemia regress as LDL levels are controlled by plasmapheresis has encouraged the use of plasmapheresis and several related extracorporeal procedures for patients with homozygous disease and for poorly controlled heterozygous patients.[52–55] Although the ideal plasma LDL level is controversial, the frequency of apheresis necessary to achieve a target value can be predicted.[56] By extension, plasmapheresis is used for other inherited metabolic disorders such as Refsum disease.[54–57] The frequency of exchange depends primarily on total body burden, rate of synthesis, and plasma concentration of the compound to be removed. Column technology designed to remove the specific toxic metabolite in different metabolic disorders has the advantages of preserving beneficial plasma solutes, such as high-density lipoproteins, and obviating the need for replacement solutions.

Immune Disorders

Plasmapheresis appears to have at least a temporary adjunctive role in managing some disorders characterized by circulating autoantibodies. Early success was reported in patients with Goodpasture syndrome, a disease characterized by a specific pathogenic autoantibody (anti-GBM) directed against the renal glomerular and pulmonary alveolar basement membrane.[58,59] The anti-GBM titer correlates with disease activity, and a declining titer during therapy predicts recovery of renal function. Success in rapidly progressive glomerular nephritis without demonstrable autoantibodies has also been observed. Plasmapheresis has enjoyed similar success in other disorders associated with specific autoantibodies, including myasthenia gravis (antiacetylcholine receptor), pemphigus, and Eaton-Lambert syndrome; however, long-term remissions without concurrent drug therapy are not ordinarily expected.[60-62] In still other immune-mediated disorders, such as immune thrombocytopenic purpura (ITP), post-transfusion purpura, and immune inhibitors to coagulation proteins, plasmapheresis may be helpful during a catastrophic event, but continued benefit in chronic disorders is generally not achieved.[63-67]

Controlled clinical trials of plasmapheresis were effective in at least two of the polyradiculoneuropathies.[68,69] In acute Guillain-Barré syndrome (GBS), a rapidly evolving neuropathy associated with antibodies to peripheral nerve myelin and circulating immune complexes, plasmapheresis has significant clinical benefit, especially when instituted early.[69,70] Infusion of intravenous immunoglobulin (IVIG) was equally effective, however.[71] The choice between therapeutic plasmapheresis and IVIG, for GBS or for other immune-mediated disorders such as ITP, will depend on such factors as ready availability, cost, and safety for a specific patient.

Although therapeutic plasma exchange has been used in a variety of other "immune" disorders, such as systemic lupus erythematosus, Raynaud's disease, and rheumatoid vasculitis, its efficacy remains unproved. The only two controlled trials of plasmapheresis in lupus nephritis did not demonstrate efficacy.[72,73] Lymphoplasmapheresis and lymphocytapheresis have resulted in temporary and modest improvement in patients with refractory rheumatoid arthritis.[74,75] Plasmapheresis appears to be less effective.[76] For these disorders, therapeutic apheresis should be reserved at best for circumstances in which a vital organ or life itself is endangered.

Controversy surrounds the practice of combining cytotoxic drug therapy with plasmapheresis to prevent rapid resynthesis of antibody, so-called antibody rebound. Although the rebound phenomenon is well established in animal models, investigational studies in healthy volunteers suggest that antibody rebound is not common.[77] Controlled trials of plasmapheresis therapy in lupus nephritis and polymyositis have been criticized for not including a plasmapheresis-with-immunosuppression treatment arm.[73,78] Because many uncontrolled treatment protocols use immunosuppressive drugs and plasmapheresis concurrently, an apparent favorable trial outcome may result from the independent effects of the different treatments, from some synergistic effect, or from neither.

The role of therapeutic apheresis in the treatment of multiple sclerosis remains controversial despite trials in patients with both acute relapsing and chronic progressive disease.[79-82] These studies are difficult to compare because different treatment protocols, schedules of apheresis, length of treatment, and patient groups were involved. Plasmapheresis appears most likely to benefit patients in the following circumstances: (1) in acute relapsing multiple sclerosis, when corticosteroid therapy is ineffective, especially when the attack is severe; (2) when conventional therapy is contraindicated; and (3) when chronic disease progresses despite optimal use of conventional therapy. In chronic progressive disease, exchanges may have to be repeated for 15 to 20 weeks.

Thrombotic Thrombocytopenic Purpura

The success of therapeutic apheresis procedures seldom depends on the composition of the replacement solution that is used. The single exception seems to be TTP. Numerous reports support the use of fresh frozen plasma or cryoprecipitate-poor plasma as a specific therapeutic replacement fluid, possibly to replace a labile inhibitor of platelet aggregation.[83,84] For TTP, plasmapheresis is the treatment of choice and should be initiated as soon as possible after diagnosis. Frequent clinical assessment and monitoring of renal function, platelet count, and serum lactate dehydrogenase level are necessary to guide therapy. Although TTP is thought to be a relatively rare disorder, plasma exchange is clearly lifesaving therapy in many patients who have not responded to conventional treatment. The incidence of this disorder of still unknown cause may be increasing or at least more frequently recognized. In some instances, plasma exchange can be regarded as a true emergency in the patient with rapid onset of severe symptoms.

Replacement Fluids

Because less than 50 ml of volume is removed during most cytapheresis procedures, no replacement beyond the anticoagulant and saline priming solution is required. With therapeutic plasmapheresis, the primary function of the replacement solution is to maintain intravascular volume, and replacement with 5 percent albumin or with combinations of albumin and crystalloid solution suffices.[85] Additional features deemed desirable for a replacement fluid include restoration of important plasma proteins, maintenance of colloid osmotic pressure, maintenance of electrolyte balance, and preservation of trace elements lost during a prolonged course of plasmapheresis procedures. In moderately well-nourished subjects, homeostatic mechanisms normally obviate the need for precise plasma replacement. Other patients should receive solutions prepared specifically to meet their individual requirements. Routine supplementation with calcium, potassium, or immunoglobulins is unnecessary.

Complications of Apheresis

When performed by experienced personnel, automated apheresis is a minimal risk procedure. The current generation of blood cell separators is reliable and equipped with sensitive detection and alarm systems to alert the operator to potential problems. Nevertheless, at least 59 deaths have been associated with these therapeutic procedures, an estimated mortality rate of 3 in 10,000 procedures. However, most deaths are related to cardiac and respiratory

causes in patients who are critically ill before apheresis.[86] National incidence figures for Canada in 1985 indicate that 12 percent of 5,235 therapeutic procedures and 40 percent of the 627 patients had treatment side effects. Most of these were of little clinical significance, and no treatment-related deaths occurred.[87]

Complications of apheresis are associated with vascular access, hemodynamic alterations, mechanical problems related to instrumentation, depletion of cellular and plasma components, reactions to replacement solutions (including anticoagulants, improper additives, and bacterial contaminants), and allergic reactions. If citrate-induced hypocalcemia, vasovagal reactions, clotting of fistulae and catheters, and urticaria are included, about 10 percent of procedures have medical complications (Table 46-3). Hemodynamic complications are readily prevented by careful fluid replacement calculations and familiarity with the extracorporeal volume requirements of the different blood cell separators. Vascular access problems occur primarily with multilumen catheters designed for long-term access. The most common problems are catheter occlusion, vessel thrombosis, infection, and vessel perforation.[88] The frequency and severity are determined by the nature and location of the catheter. Various soft, flexible catheters are available for therapeutic apheresis, and various procedures to maintain catheter patency and

Table 46-3. Complications of Therapeutic Apheresis

Citrate effect	Acral or circumoral paresthesias
Citrate toxicity	Nausea, vomiting, tetany, arrhythmias
Vasovagal reactions	Bradycardia, hypotension, seizures
Volume alteration	Hypotension, tachycardia, hypertension, pulmonary edema
Vascular access	Hematoma, phlebitis, neuropathy
Anaphylaxis	Related to infusion, ethylene oxide, angiotensin-converting enzyme inhibitors
Sepsis	Related to infusion
Loss of blood components	Anemia (10–20% decrease) Thrombocytopenia (30% decrease) Hypofibrinogenemia (50% decrease)

decrease local thrombosis have been used.[89] Clot aspiration and local instillation and thrombolytic agents are often effective when catheter occlusion occurs during a procedure.

Some depletion of plasma electrolytes, plasma proteins, platelets, and lymphocytes is expected and usually clinically unimportant. Electrolytes and small molecules are not removed efficiently by plasmapheresis. Although small fluctuations in calcium and potassium levels can result in important clinical consequences, changes during apheresis are ordinarily minimal and transient. High concentrations of citrate in patients with renal and hepatic dysfunction may require intravenous calcium replacement for symptomatic hypocalcemia. Many plasma proteins are removed efficiently by plasmapheresis, but clinical problems such as bleeding or immunosuppression are rare.[90] A decrease in hemoglobin of 10 to 20 percent and in platelet count of about 30 percent result from a combination of dilution and cell loss. Clinical problems related to chronic protein, platelet, and leukocyte loss have been sought for years, but even long-term serial apheresis seems exceptionally safe.[91,92]

The most severe allergic complications are related to sensitivity to plasma proteins and occur when plasma is used as the replacement solution. Most of these reactions are mild and transient, but fatal anaphylaxis has occurred. Anaphylactoid reactions to ethylene oxide, an agent used in sterilization of the plastic disposables, are well documented; severe reactions have not been reported.[93] Of more concern are the anaphylactic reactions reported in patients receiving angiotensin-converting enzyme inhibitor medications while undergoing different apheresis procedures.[94] Such medications should be discontinued at least 24 hours before apheresis.

Because plasma carries most of the infectious risks of whole blood, including hepatitis and human immunodeficiency virus, 5 percent albumin in saline is the most commonly used replacement solution. If fever and hypotension develop during a procedure, bacterial contamination of the replacement solution should be considered. Concern that plasmapheresis somehow predisposes patients with glomerulonephritis to an increased risk of bacterial infection appears to be unfounded.[95]

REFERENCES

1. Abel JJ, Rowntree LG, Turner BB: Plasma removal with return of corpuscles (plasmapheresis). J Pharmacol Exp Ther 5:625, 1914
2. Wright DG, Karsh J, Fauci AS et al: Lymphocyte depletion and immunosuppression with repeated leukapheresis by continuous flow centrifugation. Blood 58: 451, 1981
3. Lockwood SM, Worlledge S, Nicholas A et al: Reversal of impaired splenic function in patients with nephritis or vasculitis by plasma exchange. N Engl J Med 300: 524, 1979
4. Hodgson WJB, Mercan S: Hemapheresis listening post. Optimal venous access. Transfusion Sci 12:274, 1991
5. Weiner AS, Wexler IB: The use of heparin when performing exchange blood transfusions in newborn infants. J Lab Clin Med 31:1016, 1946
6. Collins JA: Problems associated with the massive transfusion of stored blood. Surgery 75:274, 1974
7. McCullough J, Chopek M: Therapeutic plasma exchange. Lab Med 12:745, 1981
8. Hester JP, Kellogg RM, Mulzet AP et al: Principles of blood separation and component extraction in a disposable continuous-flow single-stage channel. Blood 54:254, 1978
9. Leitman SF, Smith JW, Gregg RE: Homozygous hypercholesterolemia: selective removal of low density lipoproteins by secondary membrane filtration. Transfusion 29:341, 1989
10. Lysaght MJ, Samtleben W, Schmidt B, Gurland HJ: Closed-loop plasmapheresis. In MacPherson JL, Kasprisin DO (eds): Therapeutic Hemapheresis. Vol. 1. CRC Press, Boca Raton, 1985
11. Rook AH, Cohen JH, Lessin SR, Vowels BR: Therapeutic applications of photopheresis. Dermatol Clin 11:339, 1993
12. Rook AH, Freundlich B, Jegasothy BV et al: Treatment of systemic sclerosis with extracorporeal photochemotherapy. Arch Dermatol 128:337, 1992
13. Wayne AS, Kevy SW, Nathan DG: Transfusion management of sickle cell disease. Blood 81:1109, 1993
14. Schmalzer EA, Lee JO, Brown AK et al: Viscosity of mixtures of a sickle cell and normal red cells at varying hematocrit levels: implications for transfusion. Transfusion 27:228, 1987
15. Anderson R, Cassell M, Mullinax GL et al: Effect of normal cells on viscosity of sickle-cell blood: in vitro studies and report of six years experience with a prophylactic program of "partial exchange transfusion." Arch Intern Med 111:286, 1963

16. Lessin LS, Kurantsin-Mills J, Klug PP et al: Determination of rheologically optimal mixture of AA and SS erythrocytes for transfusion. Prog Clin Biol Res 20: 123, 1978

17. Keitel HG, Thompson D, Itano HA: Hyposthenuria in sickle cell anemia: a reversible renal defect. J Clin Invest 35:998, 1956

18. Pearson HA, Cornelius EA, Schwartz AD et al: Transfusion-reversible functional asplenia in young children with sickle-cell anemia. N Engl J Med 283:334, 1970

19. Miller DM, Winslow RM, Klein HG et al: Improved exercise performance after exchange transfusion in subjects with sickle cell anemia. Blood 56:1127, 1980

20. Rodgers GP, Schechter AN, Noguchi CT et al: Periodic microcirculatory flow in patients with sickle cell disease. N Engl J Med 311:1534, 1984

21. Klein HG: Transfusion support of hemoglobinopathies. p. 198. In Cash J (ed): Progress in Transfusion Medicine. Vol. 3. Churchill Livingstone, Edinburgh, 1987

22. Koshy M, Burd L, Wallace D et al: Prophylactic red-cell transfusions in pregnant patients with sickle cell disease. N Engl J Med 319:1447, 1988

23. Coles SM, Klein HG, Holland PV: Alloimmunization in two multitransfused patient populations. Transfusion 21:462, 1981

24. Diamond WJ, Brown FL, Bitterman P et al: Delayed hemolytic transfusion reactions presenting as sickle cell crisis. Ann Intern Med 93:231, 1980

25. Rackoff WR, Ohene-Frempong K, Month S et al: Neurologic events after partial exchange transfusion for priapism in sickle cell disease. J Pediatr 120:882, 1992

26. Kim HC, Dugan NP, Silber JH et al: Erythrocytapheresis therapy to reduce iron overload in chronically transfused patients with sickle cell disease. Blood 83: 1136, 1994

27. Miller KD, Greenberg AE, Campbell CC: Treatment of severe malaria in the United States with a continuous infusion of quinidine gluconate and exchange transfusion. N Engl J Med 321:65, 1989

28. Jacoby JA, Hunt JV, Kosinski KS et al: Treatment of transfusion-transmitted babesiosis by exchange transfusion. N Engl J Med 303:1098, 1980

29. Winslow RM, Monge CC, Brown EG et al: The effect of hemodilution on O_2 transport in high altitude polycythemia. J Appl Physiol 59:1495, 1985

30. Freireich EJ, Thomas LB, Frei E III et al: A distinctive type of intracerebral hemorrhage associated with "blastic crisis" in patients with leukemia. Cancer 13: 146, 1960

31. Lester TJ, Johnson JW, Cuttner J: Pulmonary leukostasis as the single worst prognostic factor in patients with acute myelocytic leukemia and hyperleukocytosis. Am J Med 79:43, 1985

32. Lichtman MA, Rowe JM: Hyperleukocytic leukemias: rheological, clinical, and therapeutic considerations. Blood 60:279, 1982

33. Cuttner J, Holland JF, Norton L et al: Therapeutic leukapheresis in acute myelocytic leukemia. Med Pediatr Oncol 11:76, 1983

34. Hester JP, McCredie KB, Freirich EJ: Response to chronic leukapheresis procedures and survival of chronic myelogenous leukemia patients. Transfusion 22:305, 1982

35. Lowenthal RM, Buskard NA, Goldman JM et al: Intensive leukapheresis as an initial therapy for chronic granulocytic leukemia. Blood 46:835, 1975

36. Goldfinger D, Capostagno V, Lowe C et al: Use of long-term leukapheresis in the treatment of chronic lymphocytic leukemia. Transfusion 20:450, 1980

37. Cooper IA, Ding JC, Adams PB: Intensive leukapheresis in the management of cytopenias in patients with chronic lymphocytic leukemia (CLL) and lymphocytic lymphoma. Am J Hematol 6:387, 1979

38. Fay JW, Moore JO, Logue GL et al: Leukapheresis therapy of leukemic reticuloendotheliosis (hairy cell leukemia). Blood 54:747, 1979

39. Golomb HM, Kraut EH, Oviatt DL et al: Absence of prolonged benefit of initial leukapheresis therapy for hairy cell leukemia. Am J Hematol 14:49, 1983

40. Wright DG, Karsh J, Fauci AS et al: Lymphocyte depletion and immunosuppression with repeated leukapheresis by continuous flow centrifugation. Blood 58: 451, 1981

41. Karsh J, Klippel JH, Plotz PH et al: Lymphapheresis in rheumatoid arthritis: a randomized trial. Arthritis Rheum 24:867, 1981

42. Wallace DJ, Goldfinger D, Lowe C et al: A double-blind controlled study of lymphoplasmapheresis versus sham apheresis in rheumatoid arthritis. N Engl J Med 306:1406, 1982

43. Chievitz E, Thiede T: Complications and causes of death in polycythemia vera. Acta Med Scand 172:51, 1962

44. Dawson AA, Ogston D: The influence of the platelet count on the incidence of thrombotic and hemorrhagic complications in polycythemia vera. Postgrad Med J 46:76, 1970

45. Kessler CM, Klein HG, Havlik RJ: Uncontrolled thrombocythemia in myeloproliferative disorders. Br J Haematol 50:157, 1982

46. Leitman SF, Ciavarella D, Kucera E et al: Guidelines for Therapeutic Hemapheresis. American Association of Blood Banks, Bethesda, 1992

47. Strauss RG, Ciavarella D, Gilcher R et al: Clinical applications of therapeutic apheresis: report of the Clinical Applications Committee. J Clin Apheresis 8:4, 1993

48. Solomon A, Fahey JL: Plasmapheresis therapy in macroglobulinemia. Ann Intern Med 58:799, 1963

49. Taft EG, Propp RP, Sullivan SA: Plasma exchange for cold agglutinin hemolytic anemia. Transfusion 17:173, 1977

50. Silberstein LE, Berkman EM: Plasma exchange in autoimmune hemolytic anemia. J Clin Apheresis 1:238, 1983

51. Geltner D, Kohn RW, Gorevic PD et al: The effect of combination chemotherapy (steroids, immunosuppressives and plasmapheresis) on 5 mixed cryoglobulinemia patients with renal, neurologic and vascular involvement. Arthritis Rheum 24:1121, 1981

52. Miller J, Sanders E, Webb D: Plasmapheresis for paraquat poisoning. Lancet 1:875, 1978

53. Beck JR, Quinn BM, Meier FA, Rawnsley HM: Hyperviscosity syndrome in paraproteinemia: managed by plasma exchange; monitored by serum tests. Transfusion 22:51, 1982

54. King ME, Breslow JL, Lees RS: Plasma-exchange therapy of homozygous familial hypercholesterolemia. N Engl J Med 302:1457, 1979

55. Gordon BR, Kelsey SF, Bilheimer DW et al: Treatment of refractory familial hypercholesterolemia by low-density lipoprotein apheresis using an automated dextran sulfate cellulose adsorption system. The Liposorber Study Group. Am J Cardiol 70:1010, 1992

56. Jacob BG, Richter WO, Schwandt P et al: Therapy of severe hypercholesterolemia by low-density lipoprotein apheresis with immunoadsorption: effects of the addition of 3-hydroxy-3-methylglutaryl coenzyme A reductase inhibitors to therapy. Clin Invest 71:908, 1993

57. Gibberd FB, Billimoria JD, Page NGR, Retsas S: Heredopathia atactica polyneuritiformis (Refsum's disease) treated by diet and plasma-exchange. Lancet 1:575, 1979

58. Lockwood CM, Boulton-Jones JM, Jowenthal RM et al: Recovery from Goodpasture's syndrome after immunosuppressive treatment and plasmapheresis. BMJ 2:252, 1975

59. Johnson JP, Whitman W, Briggs WA et al: Plasmapheresis and immunosuppressive agents in antibasement membrane antibody-induced Goodpasture's syndrome. Am J Med 64:354, 1978

60. Rodnitzky RL, Bosch EP: Chronic long-interval plasma exchange in myasthenia gravis. Arch Neurol 41:715, 1984

61. Kornfield P, Ambinder EP, Mittag T et al: Plasmapheresis in generalized refractory myasthenia gravis. Arch Neurol 38:478, 1972

62. Roujeau JC, Kalis B, Lauret P et al: Plasma exchange in corticosteroid-resistant pemphigus. Br J Dermatol 106:103, 1982

63. Pintado T, Taswell HF, Bowie EJW: Treatment of life-threatening hemorrhage due to acquired factor VIII inhibitor. Blood 46:535, 1975

64. Nilsson I, Jonsson S, Sundquist S et al: A procedure for removing high titer antibodies by extracorporeal protein-A-Sepharose adsorption in hemophilia substitution therapy and surgery in a patient with hemophilia B antibodies. Blood 58:38, 1981

65. Marder VJ, Nusbacher J, Anderson FW: One-year follow-up of plasma exchange therapy in 14 patients with idiopathic thrombocytopenic purpura. Transfusion 21:291, 1981

66. Cimo PL, Aster RH: Post-transfusion purpura: successful treatment by exchange transfusion. N Engl J Med 287:290, 1972

67. Snyder HW, Cochran SK, Balint JP et al: Experience with protein A-immunoadsorption in treatment resistant immune thrombocytopenic purpura. Blood 79:2237, 1992

68. Dyck PJ, Daube J, O'Brien P et al: Plasma exchange in chronic inflammatory demyelinating polyradiculoneuropathy. N Engl J Med 314:461, 1986

69. The Guillain-Barré Study Group. Plasmapheresis and acute Guillain-Barré syndrome. Neurology 35:1096, 1985

70. French Cooperative Group on Plasma Exchange in Guillain-Barré Syndrome: Efficiency of plasma exchange in Guillain-Barré syndrome: role of replacement fluid. Ann Neurol 22:753, 1987

71. van der Meche FGA, Schmitz PIM, The Dutch Guillain-Barré Study Group: A randomized trial comparing intravenous immune globulin and plasma exchange in Guillain-Barré syndrome. N Engl J Med 326:1123, 1992

72. Huston DP, White MJ, Mattioli C et al: A controlled trial of plasmapheresis and cyclophosphamide therapy of lupus nephritis. Arthritis Rheum 26:S33, 1983

73. Lachin JM, Lan SP: Termination of a clinical trial with no treatment group difference: the Lupus Nephritis Study Group. Control Clin Trials 13:62, 1992

74. Wallace DJ, Goldfinger D, Lowe C et al: A double blind, controlled study of lymphoplasmapheresis versus sham pheresis in rheumatoid arthritis. N Engl J Med 306:1406, 1982

75. Karsh J, Klippel JH, Plotz PH et al: Lymphapheresis in rheumatoid arthritis. Arthritis Rheum 24:867, 1981

76. Dwosh IL, Giles AR, Ford PM et al: Plasmapheresis therapy in rheumatoid arthritis: a controlled double-blind study. N Engl J Med 308:1124, 1983

77. Derksen RHWM, Schuurman HJ, Gmelig Meyling FHJ et al: Rebound and overshoot after plasma exchange in humans. J Lab Clin Med 104:35, 1984

78. Miller FW, Leitman SF, Cronin ME et al: Controlled trial of plasma exchange and leukapheresis in polymyositis and dermatomyositis. N Engl J Med 326:1380, 1992

79. Hauser SL, Dawson DM, Lehrich JR et al: Intensive immunosuppressive therapy in progressive multiple sclerosis: a randomized three-arm study of high-dose intravenous cyclophosphamide, plasma exchange and ACTH. N Engl J Med 308:173, 1983

80. Khatri BO, McQuillen MP, Harrington GJ et al: Chronic progressive multiple sclerosis: double-blind controlled study of plasmapheresis in patients taking immunosuppressive drugs. Neurology 35:312, 1985

81. Weiner HL, Dau PC, Khatri BO et al: Double-blind study of true vs. sham plasma exchange in patients treated with immunosuppression for acute attacks of multiple sclerosis. Neurology 39:1143, 1989

82. The Canadian Cooperative Multiple Sclerosis Study Group: The Canadian cooperative trial of cyclophosphamide and plasma exchange in progressive multiple sclerosis. Lancet 337:441, 1991

83. Rock GA, Shumak KH, Buskard NA et al: Comparison of plasma exchange and plasma infusion in the treatment of thrombotic thrombocytopenic purpura. N Engl J Med 325:393, 1991

84. Bell WR, Braine HG, Ness PM, Kickler TS: Improved survival in thrombotic thrombocytopenic purpura-hemolytic uremic syndrome. N Engl J Med 325:398, 1991

85. Lasky LC, Finnerty EP, Genis L, Polesky HF: Protein and colloid osmotic pressure changes with albumin and/or saline replacement during plasma exchange. Transfusion 24:256, 1984

86. Huestis DW: Complications of therapeutic apheresis. p. 179. In Valbonesi M, Pineda AA, Biggs JC (eds): Therapeutic Hemapheresis. Wichtig Editore, Milan, 1986

87. Sutton DMC, Nair RC, Rock G, The Canadian Apheresis Study Group: Complications of plasma exchange. Transfusion 29:124, 1989

88. Jacobs MB, Yeager M: Thrombotic and infectious complications of Hickman-Broviac catheters. Ann Intern Med 144:1597, 1984

89. Haire WD, Edney JA, Landmark JD, Kessinger A: Thrombotic complications of subclavian apheresis catheters in cancer patients: prevention with heparin infusion. J Clin Apheresis 5:188, 1990

90. Klein HG: Effect of plasma exchange on plasma constituents: choice of replacement solutions and kinetics of exchange. p. 3. In McPherson JL, Kasprisin DO (eds): Therapeutic Hemapheresis. Vol. 2. CRC Press, Boca Raton, 1985

91. Wasi S, Santowski T, Murray SA et al: The Canadian Red Cross Plasmapheresis Donor Safety Program: changes in plasma proteins after long-term plasmapheresis. Vox Sang 60:82, 1991

92. Heal JM, Horan PK, Schmitt TC et al: Long-term follow-up of donors cytapheresed more than 50 times. Vox Sang 45:14, 1983

93. Leitman SF, Boltansky H, Alter HJ et al: Allergic reactions in healthy plateletpheresis donors caused by sensitization to ethylene oxide gas. N Engl J Med 315:1192, 1986

94. Owen HG, Brecher ME: Atypical reactions associated with ACE inhibitors and apheresis. Transfusion 34:891, 1994

95. Pohl MA, Lan S-P, Berl T et al: Plasmapheresis does not increase the risk of infection in immunosuppressed patients with severe lupus nephritis. Ann Intern Med 114:924, 1991

Chapter 47

Biologic Response Modifiers—Hematopoietic Growth Factors

Margot S. Kruskall

Biologic response modifiers, or cytokines, are biologically active glycoproteins secreted by a variety of cells that influence the biologic behavior of cells.[1] More than 35 have been described; they fall into six broad classes, including interferons, interleukins (IL), tumor necrosis factors, transforming growth factors, miscellaneous growth factors such as monocyte chemoattractant factor, and colony-stimulating factors. The last group, including granulocyte-macrophage colony-stimulating factor (GM-CSF), granulocyte colony-stimulating factor (G-CSF), erythropoietin, and the recently discovered thrombopoietin, have the most immediate potential effect on transfusion practices and are the subject of this chapter.

The first evidence of the existence of a hematopoietic cytokine (erythropoietin) appeared at the turn of the century; granulocyte factors were identified in the 1960s.[2] Identification and purification of these factors from urine allowed amino acid sequencing, from which complementary DNA probes identified the genes.

The pluripotent stem cell has the potential to differentiate along a number of different pathways, as shown in Figure 47-1. Although this differentiation appears to be stochastic (random), biologic response modifiers affect stem cells by enhancing proliferation and by preventing apoptosis (cell death).[3] Biologic response modifiers have activity at multiple points in differentiation. Some, such as erythropoietin, are relatively lineage specific and affect predominantly one cell line (erythroid); however, most cytokines have been shown to have biologic effects on multiple cell lines.[4] Of concern is the potential for growth factors to stimulate neoplastic cell growth; in vitro stimulation by G-CSF and GM-CSF of small cell lung cancer and colon cancer have been demonstrated. Synergy between cytokines (e.g., GM-CSF and IL-3) may be necessary for optimal proliferation of marrow precursors.[5]

Receptors for hematopoietic cytokines and other growth factors are responsible for translating the binding of a cytokine into an intracellular message, which induces growth and development. Many receptors share common features and appear to be part of a superfamily; for example, receptors for IL-2, IL-3, IL-4, IL-7, GM-CSF, G-CSF, erythropoietin, and the hormone prolactin all share amino acid structures common to cell surface adhesive molecules and are important to cytokine binding.[4,6]

ERYTHROPOIETIN

The hematopoietic growth factor erythropoietin is a glycoprotein (molecular weight 30,400) that regulates the feedback between tissue oxygenation, through a renal oxygen sensor, and red cell mass, through erythroid progenitors.[7] Erythropoietin is

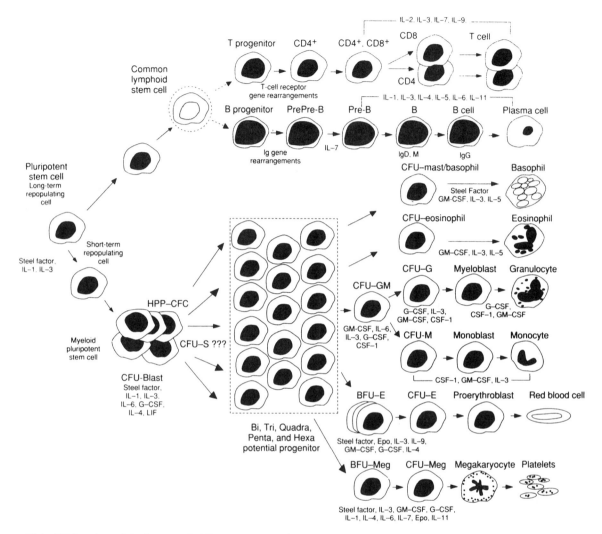

Fig. 47-1. A model of stem cell differentiation. Biologic response modifiers exert their effects at many points. CFU, colony-forming unit; CFU-S, colony-forming unit-spleen; CFU-GM, colony-forming unit-granulocyte-macrophage; CFU-M, colony-forming unit-macrophage; BFU-E, burst-forming unit-erythroid; CFU-E, colony-forming unit-erythroid; BFU-Meg, burst-forming unit-megakaryocyte; CFU-Meg, colony-forming unit-megakaryocyte. (From Quesenberry,[4] with permission.)

the only growth factor identified to date that works like a hormone in that its deficiency results in anemia.[8] In the normal individual, a serum erythropoietin level between 5 and 25 milliunits/ml is adequate for replacement of cells lost through senescence and maintenance of a normal red cell mass (25 to 30 ml/kg).[7,8] The concentration of erythropoietin may rise by 1,000-fold in anemia.[7]

Although produced in both the liver and kidney in utero, erythropoietin production comes largely from the kidneys by the time of birth and in adults.[9] Renal peritubular interstitial cells produce erythropoietin and probably also contain the renal oxygen sensor, a heme protein, which is thought to undergo a conformational change in the presence of oxygen.[10] The rate of production of erythropoietin is

Table 47-1. Approved Indications for Recombinant Human Erythropoietin

Anemia of chronic renal failure

Anemia in zidouvidine-treated, human immunodeficiency virus-infected patients

Anemia in patients with cancer who are undergoing chemotherapy

dictated by the extent of renal hypoxia. Renal oxygen tension is correlated with hemoglobin concentration, pulmonary function, cardiac output, and blood flow to the kidneys.[7]

Erythropoietin works on erythroid-committed stem cells (blast-forming unit-erythroid [BFU-E] and colony-forming unit-erythroid [CFU-E]) to prevent premature cell death (apoptosis)[11] and possibly also to enhance red cell proliferation.[12] Cells responsive to erythropoietin have erythropoietin-specific receptors that can bind with the hormone at high affinity.[13]

Erythropoietin was discovered in 1950 by Reissmann,[14] who used a parabiotic rat model to demonstrate the presence of a humoral factor that stimulated erythropoiesis. The cytokine was purified from the urine of patients with aplastic anemia in 1977.[15] A recombinant product, produced in tissue culture from Chinese hamster ovarian cells, was first made available for clinical use in 1985.[16] The recombinant protein has an identical amino acid structure to the native protein and only subtle differences in glycosylation; as a result, antierythropoietin antibodies do not develop in treated subjects.[17]

The first clinical trials with recombinant erythropoietin, for the anemia associated with renal failure, were reported in 1987.[18] A testimony to the success of these and later studies is published data showing that more than 0.5 million patients had been treated with erythropoietin as of the end of 1992.[19] At present, the use of the cytokine is approved in the United States for three indications (Table 47-1), and many others are under active investigation.

Anemia of Chronic Renal Failure

Although many factors contribute to the anemia of renal failure, erythropoietin deficiency is clearly the most important. As many as 25 percent of patients who require chronic hemodialysis are transfusion dependent because their diseased kidneys are unable to produce adequate levels of erythropoietin, and therefore these individuals cannot maintain red cell production (Fig. 47-2).[20,21] In the first phase I and II studies of recombinant erythropoietin in patients with renal failure, doses of 50 units/kg or more raised hematocrits and eliminated transfusion requirements in all patients.[18] In a follow-up multicenter phase III trial, 97.4 percent of 333 anemic patients with renal failure were able to achieve hematocrits of at least 35 percent within 18 weeks of starting recombinant erythropoietin therapy.[22] From this, it has been estimated that the use of recombinant erythropoietin in transfusion-dependent patients with end-stage renal disease could eliminate

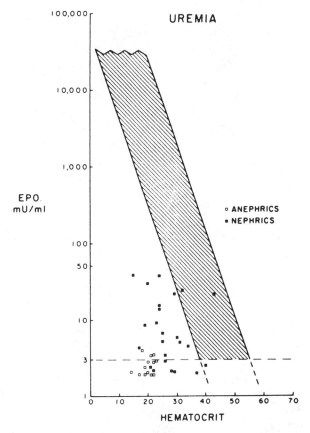

Fig. 47-2. Relationship between hematocrit and plasma erythropoietin concentrations in patients with chronic renal failure. The range of serum concentrations of erythropoietin in patients with anemia uncomplicated by either renal failure or inflammation is shown in the cross-hatched area. (From Erslev et al.,[21] with permission.)

500,000 transfusions annually or 3 percent of red cell use in the United States.[20] Furthermore, despite concerns that predialysis patients with renal failure have (dialyzable) inhibitors of erythropoiesis, which could blunt the effect of recombinant erythropoietin, the cytokine has also been successfully utilized in this population to increase hematocrits.[23]

The dosage of recombinant erythropoietin to attain target hematocrits varies among patients, in part because of factors that interfere with the erythropoietic response (including iron, folate, or vitamin B_{12} deficiency; inflammatory states; and aluminum overload) and also according to the route of administration (subcutaneous versus intravenous).[24] In one recent analysis of recombinant erythropoietin use in renal failure, the authors found that, to maintain a hematocrit of 30 percent, maintenance doses of recombinant erythropoietin averaged 122 units/kg/week when administered by the intravenous route and 88 units/kg/week when administered subcutaneously.[25] Others substantiated a 25 to 50 percent reduction in dose of recombinant erythropoietin when the subcutaneous route was substituted.[26] The improved effectiveness of subcutaneous recombinant erythropoietin is related to its pharmacokinetic properties, which result in a longer sustained plasma concentration than intermittent intravenous bolus doses.[27]

Serious side effects are not seen with recombinant erythropoietin. Exacerbation of hypertension in 25 to 35 percent of recipients and seizures in another 5 percent have been reported, usually in association with rapid increases in red cell mass.[22] Falls in serum ferritin levels and transferrin saturation are common, although they are not always low enough to meet laboratory definitions of iron deficiency. Nonetheless, the response to recombinant erythropoietin often dwindles; this "functional iron deficiency" can be corrected by iron supplementation.[28] Recombinant erythropoietin administration does not increase the risk of vascular access thrombosis and also does not significantly impair dialysis efficacy despite the increased hematocrit.[22]

Anemia in Zidouvidine-Treated Patients With Human Immunodeficiency Virus Infections

Most patients with acquired immunodeficiency syndrome (AIDS) are anemic, and most require transfusion. Impaired erythropoiesis occurs as a result of viral infection of marrow precursors and lower than appropriate erythropoietin levels for the degree of anemia. In addition, antiviral agents (in particular, zidovudine) cause bone marrow suppression. Although the pathophysiology of the anemia, and other cytopenias, is incompletely understood, administration of a variety of cytokines has been shown to stimulate hematopoiesis.[29] In a randomized controlled trial in which recombinant erythropoietin was administered to patients with AIDS being treated with zidovudine, the number of patients requiring transfusions fell by nearly 50 percent in the recombinant erythropoietin treatment arm.[30] The drug appeared most beneficial to patients with comparatively low serum erythropoietin levels (500 milliunits/ml or less).[31]

Anemia in Patients With Cancer Who Are Receiving Chemotherapy

The anemia associated with malignant disease may have any of a number of causes, including blood loss from the tumor site, nutritional deficiencies (iron or folate), marrow infiltration, hemolysis, and the effects of chemotherapy and radiation treatments. However, most commonly, the anemia resembles the anemia of chronic disease, in that patients have reticulocytopenia, low serum iron levels, marrow erythroid hypoplasia, increased iron stores, and inappropriately low erythropoietin levels for the degree of anemia,[32] which become still worse during periods of chemotherapy.[33] Recombinant erythropoietin has been studied in more than 500 patients with cancer, both during and without chemotherapy, in more than 20 different studies.[34] Approximately one-half of treated patients (range 32 to 85 percent) responded to doses of drug between 100 and 150 units/kg subcutaneously three times a week with increases in hematocrit of 6 percent or more.[35–37] The factors that affect the patient's response to erythropoietin are not understood; patients with high serum ferritin (more than 400 ng/ml) and high serum erythropoietin levels (more than 100 milliunits/ml) after 2 weeks of therapy are unlikely to respond to longer courses of therapy.[36]

Anemia Associated With Multiple Myeloma

Anemia is a common complication of multiple myeloma. However, its cause is uncertain; marrow replacement with tumor frequently causes pancytopenia, but some patients have selective anemia, and other factors that suppress erythropoiesis may be involved. In a study of patients with advanced myeloma and hemoglobin levels less than 11 g/dl, subcutaneous erythropoietin administered three times a week resulted in 11 of 13 patients increasing their hemoglobin levels by at least 2 g/dl within 2 months.[38] The authors found a correlation between pretreatment erythropoietin level and eventual response similar to that seen in human immunodeficiency virus infected patients, and proposed that responders had relative deficiencies in erythropoietin.

Anemia of Prematurity

Anemia is a common problem in the low-birth-weight premature infant, which develops between 4 and 12 weeks of age, and is characterized by reticulocytopenia despite adequate erythroid progenitor cells and inappropriately low erythropoietin levels.[39,40] The problem is aggravated by frequent blood sampling for laboratory tests. A significant proportion of these infants (30 percent of infants small than 1,300 g and nearly 100 percent of infants who weighed less than 1,000 g) are treated with blood transfusions.[41] A number of recent studies looked at the role of recombinant erythropoietin in preventing transfusions in preterm infants.[42–46] The largest study to date, with 241 subjects randomized to receive either recombinant erythropoietin (250 units subcutaneously three times a week) or no treatment beginning on days 3 to 5 of life, reported fewer patients transfused and less blood used in the recombinant erythropoietin treatment arm.[47] However, recombinant erythropoietin was least effective in infants who weighed less than 1,200 g, the group most likely to be transfused. Similarly, in a study that included infants with complications such as respiratory distress who required artificial respiration, transfusion requirements were not reduced.[42]

Even as these investigations are being carried out, the use of transfusions in neonates has been decreasing in hospitals independent of the use of erythropoietin, probably as a result of improvements in respiratory care and more conservative transfusion indications.[41] Furthermore, the administration of erythropoietin to all very low-birth-weight infants would be more costly than the use of transfusions for currently accepted indications.[48] At the present time, therefore, the use of recombinant erythropoietin to correct the anemia of prematurity is of uncertain value and awaits larger, controlled studies (see Ch. 28.)

Myelodysplastic Syndromes

Myelodysplastic syndromes (MDS) are clonal disorders of stem cells that result in quantitative and qualitative abnormalities in red cells, white cells, and platelets. Anemia is an early and prominent feature, and many patients become transfusion dependent. The cause of the anemia is multifactorial, and in vitro response of erythroid progenitors to erythropoietin is poor.[49] However, some investigators predicted that recombinant erythropoietin could stimulate residual normal marrow precursors, direct differentiation of the abnormal clone, or reverse the erythropoietic inhibitory effects of cytokines such as IL-1.[50] For these reasons, more than 300 patients with MDS have been treated with high doses of recombinant erythropoietin (in some studies, up to 12,000 units/kg three times a week).[50,51] Overall, only 20 to 25 percent of patients responded, usually those with serum erythropoietin levels less than 500 units/L and minimal transfusion requirements.[51–54] Combinations of recombinant erythropoietin and other cytokines, such as G-CSF, are also under investigation,[55] although initial results are not encouraging.[56]

Postoperative Anemia

Some investigators have suggested that postoperative endogenous erythropoietin levels may be suboptimal for the degree of anemia engendered by surgical blood loss, perhaps because many other factors besides blood oxygen content affect the concentration of erythropoietin.[57–59] In an animal model of acute isovolemic anemia after laparotomy, the daily administration of recombinant erythropoietin accelerated the appearance of reticulocytes and halved the time to return to baseline hematocrit (9.9 versus 17.4 days).[60] In humans, daily subcutaneous administration of recombinant erythropoietin (300 units/kg) for 10 days before surgery and 4 days postoperatively resulted in substantially increased reticulocyte counts and hematocrits (Fig. 47-3) and fewer postoperative transfusions. The largest effect was in patients with baseline hemoglobin levels less than 13.5

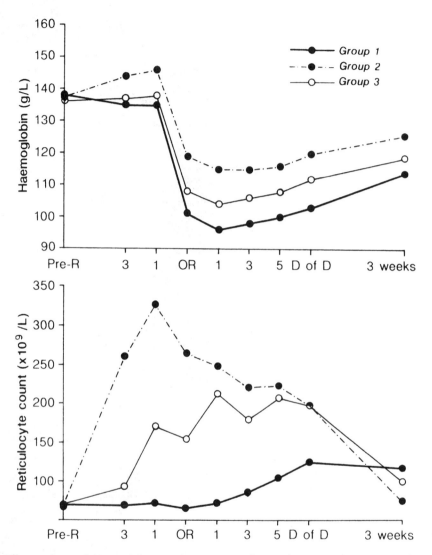

Fig. 47-3. Effect on hemoglobin and the reticulocyte count of recombinant erythropoietin administered in the perioperative period. Patients in group I received a placebo for 14 days, beginning 11 days before surgery; patients in group II received recombinant erythropoietin for 14 days; and patients in group III received placebo for 5 days, followed by erythropoietin for 9 days. (From the Canadian Orthopedic Perioperative Erythropoietin Study Group,[61] with permission.)

g/dl; the likelihood of transfusion was reduced from 74 percent in the placebo group to 33 percent.[61]

Anemia in Jehovah's Witnesses

Jehovah's Witnesses do not allow the use of blood transfusions in their care; this religious tenet is based on a literal interpretation of instructions in the bible forbidding the eating of blood (see Ch. 27).[62] The care of such patients in the setting of surgery and hemorrhage poses great challenges. In addition to other blood-conservation measures, such as minimizing iatrogenic blood loss, supplementation with hematinics and oxygen, extreme hemodilution during surgery, and autotransfusion with an uninterrupted circuit during surgery,[63] a number of groups have reported the use of recombinant erythropoietin to stimulate erythropoiesis, either in advance of elective surgery or after hemorrhage.[64] All current formulations of recombinant erythropoietin include small amounts of human albumin as a stabilizing agent; however, most Jehovah's Witnesses will accept this serum component as part of the drug.[62] Recombinant erythropoietin has been used to avoid transfusions in these patients during and after a variety of surgical procedures, including cardiac surgery,[65,66] renal transplantation,[67] and neurosurgery,[68,69] and in the settings of burns[70] and after childbirth.[71]

Recombinant Human Erythropoietin and Autologous Blood Donation

Autologous blood donations are limited by the shelf life of liquid blood at 1 to 6°C and the speed with which the donor regenerates red cells after phlebotomy.[72] Although mild anemia develops quickly after donations, the rate of red cell regeneration is slowed by low serum erythropoietin levels.[73,74] For this reason, the utility of administering recombinant erythropoietin to nonanemic subjects to improve autologous blood collections has been studied in both animals and humans. Most studies readily demonstrate that recombinant erythropoietin enhances erythropoiesis; fewer have translated this into useful clinical results.

In baboons, the intravenous administration of recombinant erythropoietin over a 5-week period allowed a 35 percent increase in autologous blood collections and a more rapid appearance of reticulocytes.[75] In humans, case reports have suggested that the cytokine may be valuable in enhancing erythropoiesis in special circumstances, such as in patients with the anemia of chronic disease and multiple red cell alloantibodies.[76,77] In larger studies, the results have been more controversial. In a randomized controlled trial of intravenous recombinant erythropoietin before orthopaedic surgery, 23 erythropoietin recipients were able to donate 5.4 units (of a total of 6 units possible) of autologous blood over 3 weeks versus 4.1 units by control subjects.[78] Because recombinant erythropoietin recipients had less anemia throughout the donation period, the difference in the volume of red cells donated was even greater (911 ml versus 568 ml).[79] However, the use of allogeneic blood, which was lim-

ited in the placebo group (2 of 24 patients) was not affected by recombinant erythropoietin administration (1 of 23 patients).[78] Other studies have drawn similar conclusions: although the administration of recombinant erythropoietin enhances erythropoiesis, control populations of autologous donors also increase red cell production in response to anemia, often in sufficient magnitude to allow adequate collection of autologous blood for their procedures.[80–82] In a few reports, especially involving procedures with large transfusion requirements, more salutary effects on transfusion use were found.[83,84] In one multicenter trial of erythropoietin use in 205 patients undergoing open heart surgery in Japan, the proportion of patients with moderate perioperative blood losses (15 to 50 ml/kg) who used homologous blood transfusions was reduced from 40 percent (in control subjects) to 21 percent (in patients given intravenous recombinant erythropoietin and allowed to donate 3 units of autologous blood before surgery).[83]

Trials with recombinant human erythropoietin have been more successful in facilitating donations by patients with mild anemias. Mercuriali et al.[85] found that a twice-weekly regimen of intravenous recombinant erythropoietin (either 300 or 600 units/kg) increased the reticulocyte count and the mean number of units of blood donated. Furthermore, the use of allogeneic blood decreased from a mean of 1.2 ± 1.4 units in placebo patients to 0.4 ± 0.8 units in recombinant erythropoietin-treated patients; and 75 to 84 percent of recombinant erythropoietin-treated patients, but only 50 percent of placebo control patients, avoided allogeneic transfusions.

However, both the modest results and the expense of the drug (approximately $0.01 per unit) have kept recombinant erythropoietin from being widely used to enhance autologous donations in the United States. Attempts to maximize the efficacy of the cytokine have focused on the route of administration. As in dialysis patients, subcutaneous, rather than intravenous, administration appears to increase the efficacy of recombinant erythropoietin here.[86] Furthermore, iron deficiency can blunt the response to recombinant erythropoietin. However, adequate baseline iron stores plus dietary and even supplemental oral iron administration are often not sufficient to prevent a state of functional iron defi-

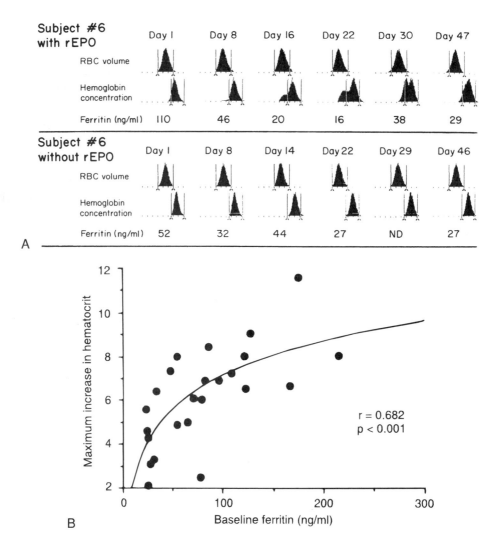

Fig. 47-4. Qualitative and quantitative effects of functional iron deficiency occurring during administration of recombinant erythropoietin. **(A)** This subject was given either daily recombinant erythropoietin (200 units/kg/day subcutaneously) and oral iron for the first 21 days (top) or oral iron alone (bottom) while twice-weekly donations of blood (450 ml) were made. Despite normal baseline iron stores, markedly underhemoglobinized cells appeared by day 8 during erythropoietin administration. (From Brugnara et al.,[87] with permission.) **(B)** In 24 healthy men with normal iron stores given recombinant erythropoietin (total dose 1,200 units/kg over 10 days), the maximal increase in hematocrit was directly correlated with the serum ferritin level. (From Rutherford et al.,[88] with permission.)

ciency.[28] In autologous donors, this results in both underhemoglobinized red cells (Fig. 47-4A)[87] and a blunted response to recombinant erythropoietin (Fig. 47-4B).[88,89] Optimal response to recombinant erythropoietin may therefore require the use of parenteral iron. In the Mercuriali et al. study,[85] the ad-

ministration of intravenous iron saccharate improved red cell regeneration in all treatment arms, including a placebo group. Further studies of these variables are needed before recombinant erythropoietin can be considered an accepted strategy for the collection of autologous blood.

Miscellaneous Indications

Most patients with the anemia associated with rheumatoid arthritis respond, albeit slowly, to recombinant erythropoietin.[90] Recombinant erythropoietin has been used to ameliorate hypotension in patients with autonomic neuropathy who are also anemic and who are symptomatic despite the use of mineralocorticoids.[91] The hormone has also been effective in eliminating the transfusion requirement of a patient with an artificial heart valve and hemolysis caused by a paravalvular leak.[92] In a handful of cases, recombinant erythropoietin has been effective in restoring erythropoiesis in pure red cell aplasia, even though baseline serum erythropoietin levels were already elevated.[93]

GRANULOCYTE AND GRANULOCYTE-MACROPHAGE COLONY-STIMULATING FACTORS

Four cytokines are currently known to stimulate myeloid cell proliferation and differentiation: G-CSF, GM-CSF, macrophage colony-stimulating factor, and IL-3.[94] Only two, G-CSF and GM-CSF, are commercially produced and in use in clinical trials. The primary indication for these cytokines is the supplementary augmentation of endogenous cytokines; in contrast to erythropoietin, absolute deficiency states of these myeloid cytokines have not been identified.[94]

The complementary DNA sequence for GM-CSF was cloned in 1984[95,96] and G-CSF 2 years later.[97] GM-CSF is a 127-amino acid glycosylated polypeptide located on human chromosome 5q21-32.[98] G-CSF, on chromosome 17, consists of 174 amino acids, also glycosylated.[99] G-CSF and GM-CSF have numerous effects on hematopoietic (and nonhematopoietic) cells and share many of these actions. Both cytokines cause transient leukopenia within 1 hour of injection, followed by an increase in peripheral blood neutrophils over the following days. G-CSF increases the neutrophil count to a greater extent than GM-CSF does.[94] Peripheral blood progenitors cells of all hematopoietic lineages are increased, as is bone marrow cellularity.[2,94] Each cytokine also has distinct actions, both because of their own characteristics and the secondary cytokine production that

Table 47-2. Approved Indications for Granulocyte and Granulocyte-Macrophage Colony-Stimulating Factors

Acceleration of myeloid recovery during autologous bone marrow transplantation for lymphoma (granulocyte-macrophage colony-stimulating factor)

Treatment of neutropenia in patients with nonmyeloid malignancies who are undergoing chemotherapy (granulocyte colony-stimulating factor)

they stimulate; for example, GM-CSF also stimulates the growth of nonhematopoietic cells (such as endothelial cells); enhances functions of neutrophils, monocytes, and macrophages such as phagocytosis and antigen presentation; recruits production of other cytokines; enhances antigen presentation by mononuclear cells; and augments antibody-mediated cell and tumor cytotoxicity.[2]

Both G-CSF and GM-CSF are associated with side effects. The most common complication of G-CSF administration is bone pain, typically a mild and transient ache, seen in up to 20 percent of patients.[100] Reactions to GM-CSF are more frequent and sometimes more severe. Minor complications include fever, myalgias, bone pain, anorexia, flushing, skin eruptions, and local inflammation at the site of injection.[101] GM-CSF is a potent stimulator of endothelial cells, and this effect may be related to a capillary leak syndrome seen in association with the use of this cytokine.[4]

These cytokines are used to reduce the period and depth of neutropenia after chemotherapy. Although only two indications have been approved by the Food and Drug Administration (Table 47-2), many others are under active investigation by many groups.

Acceleration of Myeloid Recovery During Autologous Bone Marrow Transplantation for Lymphoma

GM-CSF administered after high-dose intensive chemotherapy and autologous bone marrow transplantation hastens the recovery of neutrophils and platelets.[102,103] The administration of this cytokine appears to be cost-effective in this setting; in one randomized, controlled study of autologous bone marrow transplantation in patients with Hodgkin's disease, the median hospital charge was reduced from $62,500 to $39,800 because hospital stays and the use of blood products were reduced.[104]

Treatment of Neutropenia in Patients With Nonmyeloid Malignancies Undergoing Chemotherapy

G-CSF has been used in a number of studies to increase the neutrophil count after chemotherapy (Fig. 47-5).[100,105] GM-CSF has also been studied[106] but is used less often because it frequently causes fever, a troubling and diagnostically confusing side effect in patients who are neutropenic.[101]

Marrow Graft Failure

GM-CSF can increase neutrophil and monocyte counts during the second and third week after the marrow transplant and results in fewer cases of pneumonia and other bacterial infections.[107,108] In situations in which the transplanted marrow (either autologous or allogeneic) did not engraft and second

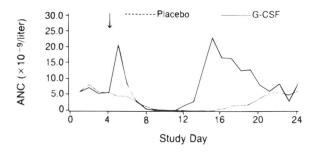

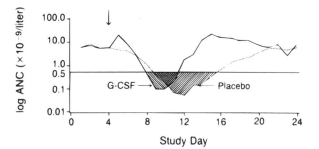

Fig. 47-5. Effect of G-CSF administered after chemotherapy. Daily G-CSF or placebo was administered beginning (arrow) 1 day after the end of chemotherapy. Median absolute neutrophil counts are shown with a linear scale (top) or logarithmic scale (bottom). The period of neutropenia (granulocyte count less than $0.5 \times 10^9/mm^3$) is shown in the hatched areas. (From Crawford et al.,[100] with permission.)

marrow transplants were not feasible or considered unlikely to work, the use of GM-CSF in one study resulted in neutrophil counts greater than $500/mm^3$ in most patients and an improved survival rate compared with historical controls.[109]

Treatment of Congenital Neutropenias

G-CSF has been used to treat patients with congenital and idiopathic neutropenias. Although baseline serum levels of the endogenous cytokine are typically elevated in these patients, supplementation with the recombinant hormone led to increased numbers of neutrophils and resolution in many cases of chronic infections.[110]

The treatment of aplastic anemia has been less satisfactory; although the neutrophil count can be increased transiently with G-CSF, patients with severe hypoplasia do not respond.[111] Furthermore, the authors of one trial reported that, in three children treated with G-CSF, myelodysplasia developed which, in two, progressed to acute myelomonocytic leukemia.[112]

Treatment of Neutropenia in Acquired Immunodeficiency Syndrome

Administration of either G-CSF or GM-CSF has been shown to increase neutrophil counts in patients with AIDS and leukopenia.[113,114] Increases in p24 antigen during treatment with GM-CSF have been documented; further studies are needed to evaluate the benefits versus the possible adverse effects on the underlying viral infection associated with the use of these cytokines.

Treatment of Acute Myeloid Leukemia and Myelodysplastic Syndromes

Colony-stimulating factors have been shown to hasten the recovery of granulocytes after intensive chemotherapy for leukemia and to reduce the incidence of bacterial infections.[115] Leukemic myeloid cells bear receptors for colony-stimulating factors; therefore, the use of G-CSF and GM-CSF to treat neutropenia could also enhance growth of leukemia.[116] Studies to date have not documented any apparent adverse effect regarding remission induction or duration, although further studies are needed to verify this.

G-CSF and GM-CSF have each been used in the

treatment of MDS; each has resulted in increased neutrophil counts in most patients and, in some patients, improvement also in the hematocrits.[117,118] However, the progression to leukemia that occurs with these syndromes was unaffected; therefore, it is unlikely that these cytokines will affect survival.

Collection of Peripheral Blood Stem Cells

Peripheral blood myeloid progenitors, normally found in only very small numbers in the circulation, increase 5- to 20-fold after recovery from chemotherapy-induced nadirs;[119] this effect is further magnified by the postchemotherapy administration of GM-CSF.[120] Autologous peripheral blood stem cells have now been used to augment autologous bone marrow in a large number of reports of patients being treated with myeloablative regimens for lymphoma and breast cancer.[121] This subject is covered in more detail in Chapter 48.

Collection of White Cells From Donors

Transfusions of granulocytes were first attempted 30 years ago to treat bacterial infections in the setting of neutropenia. Successful results were directly related to the volume of cells collected by apheresis techniques. Some of the best results occurred with collections from donors with chronic myelogenous leukemia, who could donate 10-fold more white cells than normal donors.[122] Although regimens were developed to treat healthy donors with steroids to demarginate neutrophils and sedimenting agents such as hydroxyethyl starch were added to the centrifugation bowl to improve the efficiency of white cell separation, many transfusion failures occurred, often in association with suboptimal collections (less than 1 to 2 $\times$ 10^{10} cells).[123]

Treatment of healthy donors with G-CSF to increase circulating white cell levels has recently reported by a number of groups. In Switzerland, a single subcutaneous injection of G-CSF (300 μg) 12 to 16 hours before leukapheresis resulted in a mean of 4.4 $\times$ 10^{10} granulocytes collected or two to four times the current minimum for an adequate collection.[124] In the United States, daily administration of a weight-related dose of G-CSF (5 μg/kg/day) resulted in a similar increase in the number of granulocytes collected (4.2 $\times$ 10^{10}).[125] Another U.S. group reported that G-CSF-stimulated collections resulted in extended post-transfusion survival of the infused granulocytes (half-life of 24 hours versus the normal intravascular half-life of 6 hours); the author postulated that this might be due to the collection of less mature, and therefore longer-lived, myeloid progenitors.[122] None of the donors in any of the studies suffered ill effects from the cytokine injections. Granulocyte transfusions are administered very infrequently at present; in many situations, broad-spectrum antibiotics appear to be adequate. Whether the enhanced collections facilitated by G-CSF will revive their use is unclear.

THROMBOPOIETIN

For more than 40 years, researchers have hypothesized that humoral factors ("thrombopoietin" and megakaryocyte colony-stimulating factor) must exist that specifically control the proliferation and maturation of megakaryocytes and the production of platelets. This hypothesis stemmed from experiments using plasma from thrombocytopenic animals or humans, injections of which reproducibly increased the peripheral platelet count of animals, and which also enhanced proliferation of megakaryocyte precursors when added to in vitro cultures.[126] Although many cytokines have been shown to have modest effects on the platelet count, including IL-1, IL-3, IL-6, IL-11, GM-CSF, and c-Kit ligand, the increase in count is slow to occur, and many unwanted effects on other cells are the price paid; thus, none of these factors fit the definition of a lineage-specific thrombopoietin.[127–131]

Recently, three groups independently identified the genes for both a human and murine cytokine that has the characteristics of thrombopoietin.[132–135] This long-awaited finding was based on studies in 1990 of a proto-oncogene (*MPL*) encoded by a murine leukemia retrovirus. The gene has substantial homology to other hematopoietic growth factor receptor genes.[136] *MPL* antisense oligonucleotides were subsequently shown to inhibit megakaryocyte colony formation, with no effect on erythroid or growth in vitro, suggesting that the MPL ligand could be thrombopoietin.[137] Although each research group used different techniques to identify thrombopoietin (e.g., affinity purification of thrombocytopenic pig plasma using a MPL column, generation

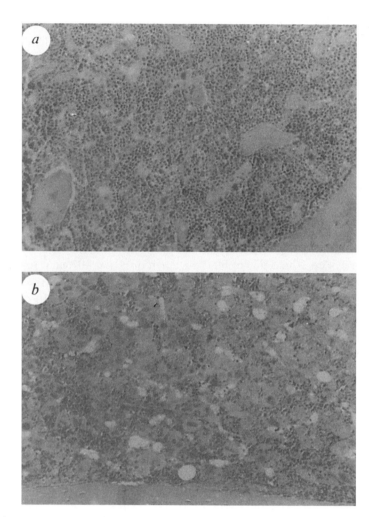

Fig. 47-6. Histologic examination of the marrow of mice given either thrombopoietin or placebo. After daily injections of either placebo or purified thrombopoietin, platelet counts, but not hematocrits or white counts, rose in the cytokine-treated group. Femoral sections from a control mouse (a) and a thrombopoietin-treated mouse (b) are shown. (From Kaushansky et al.,[133] with permission.)

of complementary DNA, and production of recombinant hormone[135] versus screening of mutant cell clones that expressed MPL to look for autonomous expression of the MPL ligand[132,133]), the resulting protein was the same: a polypeptide with two domains and substantial homology to erythropoietin at the N-terminal domain. Injection of this protein into mice resulted greater than in a fourfold increase in the platelet count at day 7 and substantial increases in marrow and spleen megakaryocytes (Fig. 47-6).[133] The in vitro effects of thrombocytopenic

serum (which contains this protein) on both megakaryocyte proliferation and differentiation can be blocked by absorption of the sera with MPL receptor, which suggests that thrombopoietin itself may be a, or the sole, megakaryocyte colony-stimulating factor.[134]

The impending availability of recombinant human thrombopoietin is likely to have a substantial impact on the care of patients with chemotherapy-induced thrombocytopenia and with some congenital and acquired thrombocytopenic states. In addition, if recombinant thrombopoietin is without significant side effects, it is conceivable that it could be used in normal donors (both allogeneic and autologous) to enhance apheresis platelet collections.[130]

REFERENCES

1. Blajchman MA: Cytokines in transfusion medicine. Transfusion 33:1, 1993
2. Neumanitis J: Granulocyte-macrophage colony-stimulating factor: a review from preclinical development to clinical application. Transfusion 33:70, 1993
3. Ogawa M: Differentiation and proliferation of hematopoietic stem cells. Blood 81:2844, 1993
4. Quesenberry PJ: Biomodulation of chemotherapy-induced myelosuppression. Semin Oncol 19:8, 1992
5. Metcalf D: Hematopoietic regulators: redundancy or subtlety? Blood 82:3515, 1993
6. Bazan JF: Structural design and molecular evolution of a cytokine receptor superfamily. Proc Natl Acad Sci U S A 87:6934, 1990
7. Erslev AJ: The therapeutic role of recombinant erythropoietin in anemic patients with intact endogenous production of erythropoietin. Semin Oncol 19:14, 1992
8. Spivak JL: The application of recombinant erythropoietin in anemic patients with cancer. Semin Oncol 19:25, 1992
9. Zanjani ED, Ascensao JL, McGlave PB et al: Studies on the liver to kidney switch of erythropoietin production. J Clin Invest 67:1183, 1981
10. Spivak JL: Recombinant erythropoietin. Annu Rev Med 44:243, 1993
11. Koury MJ, Bondurant MC: The molecular mechanism of erythropoietin action. Eur J Biochem 210:649, 1924
12. Spivak JL, Pham T, Isaacs M, Hankins WD: Erythropoietin is both a mitogen and a survival factor. Blood 77:1228, 1991
13. Dong YJ, Goldwasser E: Evidence for an accessory component that increases the affinity of the erythropoietin receptor. Exp Hematol 21:483, 1993
14. Reismann KR: Studies on the mechanisms of erythropoietic stimulation in parabiotic rats during hypoxia. Blood 5:372, 1950
15. Miyake T, Kung CK-H, Goldwasser E: Purification of human erythropoietin. J Biol Chem 252:5558, 1977
16. Adamson JW, Spivak JL: Physiologic basis for the pharmacologic use of recombinant human erythropoietin in surgery and cancer treatment. Surgery 115:7, 1994
17. Erslev AJ: Erythropoietin. N Engl J Med 324:1339, 1991
18. Eschbach JW, Egrie JC, Downing MR et al: Correction of the anemia of end-stage renal disease with recombinant human erythropoietin: results of a combined phase I and II clinical trial. N Engl J Med 316:73, 1987
19. Adamson JW: Introduction. Semin Oncol 19:1, 1992
20. Adamson JW: Cytokine biology: implications for transfusion medicine. Cancer 67:2708, 1991
21. Erslev AJ, Caro J, Miller O, Silver R: Plasma erythropoietin in health and disease. Ann Clin Lab Sci 10:250, 1980
22. Eschbach JW, Abdulhadi MH, Browne JK et al: Recombinant human erythropoietin in anemic patients with end-stage renal disease: results of a phase III-multicenter clinical trial. Ann Intern Med 111:992, 1989
23. Lim VS, DeGowin RL, Zavala D et al: Recombinant human erythropoietin treatment in pre-dialysis patients: a double-blind placebo-controlled trial. Ann Intern Med 110:108, 1989
24. Humphries JE: Anemia of renal failure: use of erythropoietin. Med Clin North Am 76:711, 1992
25. Levin NW, Lazarus JM, Nissenson AR: Maximizing patient benefits with epoetin alfa therapy: National Cooperative rHu Erythropoietin Study in Patients with Chronic Renal Failure—an interim report. Am J Kidney Dis, suppl. 1, 22:3, 1993
26. Besarab A: Optimizing epoetin therapy in end-stage renal disease: the case for subcutaneous administration. Am J Kidney Dis, suppl. 1 22:13, 1993
27. McMahon FG, Vargas R, Ryan M et al: Pharmacokinetics and effects of recombinant human erythropoietin after intravenous and subcutaneous injections in healthy volunteers. Blood 76:1718, 1990
28. Macdougall IC, Cavill I, Hulme B et al: Detection of functional iron deficiency during erythropoietin treatment: a new approach. BMJ 304:225, 1992
29. Groopman JE, Feder D: Hematopoietic growth factors in AIDS. Semin Oncol 19:408, 1992
30. Fischl M, Galpin JE, Levine JD et al: Recombinant human erythropoietin for patients with AIDS treated with zidovudine. N Engl J Med 322:1488, 1990
31. Henry DH, Beall GN, Benson CA et al: Recombinant human erythropoietin in the treatment of anemia associated with human immunodeficiency virus (HIV) infection and zidovudine therapy. Ann Intern Med 117:739, 1992
32. Lee GR: The anemia of chronic disease. Semin Hematol 20:61, 1983
33. Miller CB, Jones RJ, Piantadosi S et al: Decreased

erythropoietin response in patients with the anemia of cancer. N Engl J Med 322:1689, 1990

34. Spivak JL: Recombinant human erythropoietin and the anemia of cancer. Blood 84:997, 1994

35. Henry DH, Abels RI: Recombinant erythropoietin in the treatment of cancer and chemotherapy-induced anemia: results of double-blind and open-label follow-up studies. Semin Oncol, suppl. 3, 21:21, 1994

36. Ludwig H, Fritz E, Leitgeb et al: Prediction of response to erythropoietin treatment in chronic anemia of cancer. Blood 84:1056, 1994

37. Cascinu S, Fedeli A, Del Ferro E et al: Recombinant human erythropoietin treatment in cisplatin-associated anemia: a randomized double-blind trial with placebo. J Clin Oncol 12:1058, 1994

38. Ludwig H, Fritz E, Kotzmann H et al: Erythropoietin treatment of anemia associated with multiple myeloma. N Engl J Med 322:1693, 1990

39. Gallagher PG, Ehrenkranz RA: Erythropoietin therapy for anemia of prematurity. Clin Perinatol 20:169, 1993

40. Shannon KM, Naylor GS, Torkildson JC et al: Circulating erythropoietin progenitors in the anemia of prematurity. N Engl J Med 317:728, 1987

41. Strauss RG: Erythropoietin and neonatal anemia. N Engl J Med 330:1227, 1994

42. Soubasi V, Kremenopoulos G, Diamandi E et al: In which neonates does early recombinant human erythropoietin treatment prevent anemia of prematurity? Results of a randomized, controlled study. Pediatr Res 34:675, 1993

43. Messer J, Haddad J, Donato L et al: Early treatment of premature infants with recombinant human erythropoietin. Pediatrics 92:519, 1993

44. Ohls RK, Christensen RD: Recombinant erythropoietin compared with erythrocyte transfusion in the treatment of anemia of prematurity. J Pediatr 119:781, 1991

45. Meyer MP, Meyer JH, Commerford A et al: Recombinant human erythropoietin in the treatment of the anemia of prematurity: results of a double-blind, placebo-controlled study. Pediatrics 93:918, 1994

46. Shannon KM, Mentzer WC, Abels RI et al: Enhancement of erythropoiesis by recombinant human erythropoietin in low birth weight infants: a pilot study. J Pediatr 120:586, 1992

47. Maier RF, Obladen M, Scigalla P et al: The effect of epoetin beta (recombinant human erythropoietin) on the need for transfusion in very-low-birth-weight infants. N Engl J Med 330:1173, 1994

48. Shireman TI, Hilsenrath PE, Strauss RG et al: Recombinant human erythropoietin vs. transfusions in the treatment of anemia of prematurity. Arch Pediatr Adolesc Med 148:582, 1994

49. Merchav S, Nielson OJ, Rosenbaum H et al: In vitro studies of erythropoietin-dependent regulation of erythropoiesis in myelodysplastic syndromes. Leukemia 4:771, 1990

50. Mittleman M: Recombinant erythropoietin in myelodysplastic syndromes: whom to treat and how? More questions than answers. Acta Haematol 90:53, 1993

51. Stein RS, Abels RI, Krantz SB: Pharmacologic doses of recombinant human erythropoetin in the treatment of myelodysplastic syndromes. Blood 78:1658, 1991

52. Bowen T, Culligan D, Beguin Y et al: Estimation of effective and total erythropoiesis in myelodysplasia using serum transferrin receptor and erythropoietin concentrations, with automated reticulocyte parameters. Leukemia 8:151, 1994

53. Stenke L, Wallvik J, Celsing F, Hast R: Prediction of response to treatment with human recombinant erythropoietin in myelodysplastic syndromes. Leukemia 7:1324, 1993

54. Bowen D, Culligan D, Jacobs A: The treatment of anaemia in the myelodysplastic syndromes with recombinant human erythropoietin. Br J Haematol 77:419, 1991

55. Schuster M: Will cytokines alter the treatment of myelodysplastic syndrome? Am J Med Sci 305:72, 1993

56. Imamura M, Kobayashi M, Kobayashi S et al: Failure of combination therapy with recombinant granulocyte colony-stimulating factor and erythropoietin in myelodysplastic syndromes. Ann Hematol 68:163, 1994

57. Levine EA, Rosen AL, Sehgal LR et al: Erythropoietin deficiency after coronary artery bypass procedures. Ann Throac Surg 51:764, 1991

58. Clemens J, Spivak JL: Serum immunoreactive erythropoietin during the perioperative period. Surgery 115:510, 1994

59. Lorentz A, Eckhardt K-U, Osswald PM, Kruse C: Perioperative plasma erythropoietin levels in hip arthroplasty. Ann Hematol 68:117, 1994

60. Levine EA, Rosen AL, Sehgal LR et al: Treatment of acute postoperative anemia with recombinant human erythropoietin. J Trauma 29:1134, 1989

61. Canadian Orthopedic Perioperative Erythropoietin Study Group: Effectiveness of perioperative recombinant human erythropoietin in elective hip replacement. Lancet 341:1227, 1993

62. Dixon JL: Jehovah's Witnesses: the surgical/ethical challenge. JAMA 246:2471, 1981

63. Spence RK, Alexander JB, DelRossi AJ et al: Transfu-

sion guidelines for cardiovascular surgery: lessons learned from operations in Jehovah's Witnesses. J Vasc Surg 16:825, 1992

64. Mann MC, Votto J, Kambe J, McNamee MJ: Management of the severely anemic patient who refuses transfusion: lessons learned during the care of a Jehovah's Witness. Ann Intern Med 117:1042, 1992

65. Gaudiani VA, Mason HDW: Preoperative erythropoietin in Jehovah's Witnesses who require cardiac procedures. Ann Thorac Surg 51:823, 1991

66. Fullerton DA, Campbell DN, Whitman GJR: Use of human recombinant erythropoietin to correct severe preoperative anemia. Ann Thorac Surg 51:825, 1991

67. Akingbola OA, Custer JR, Bunchman TE, Sedman AB: Management of severe anemia without transfusion in a pediatric Jehovah's Witness patient. Crit Care Med 22:524, 1994

68. Schiff SJ, Weinstein SL: Use of recombinant human erythropoietin to avoid blood transfusion in a Jehovah's Witness requiring hemispherectomy. J Neurosurg 79:600, 1993

69. Kantrowitz AB, Spallone A, Taylor W et al: Erythropoietin-augmented isovolemic hemodilution in skull-base surgery. J Neurosurg 80:740, 1994

70. Boshkov LV, Tredget EE, Janowska-Wieczorek A: Recombinant human erythropoietin for a Jehovah's Witness with the anemia of thermal energy. Am J Hematol 37:53, 1991

71. Koenig HM, Levine EA, Resnick DJ, Meyer WJ: Use of recombinant human erythropoietin in a Jehovah's Witness. J Clin Anesth 5:244, 1993

72. Goodnough LT, Wasman J, Corlucci K, Chernosky A: Limitations to donating adequate autologous blood prior to elective orthopedic surgery. Arch Surg 124: 494, 1989

73. Kickler TS, Spivak JL: Effect of repeated whole blood donations on serum immunoreactive erythropoietin levels in autologous donors. JAMA 260:65, 1988

74. Lorentz A, Hendrissek A, Eckhardt KU et al: Serial immunoreactive erythropoietin levels in autologous blood donors. Transfusion 31:650, 1991

75. Levine EA, Rosen AL, Gould SA et al: Recombinant human erythropoietin and autologous blood donation. Surgery 104:365, 1988

76. Graf H, Watzinger U, Ludvik B et al: Recombinant human erythropoietin as adjuvant treatment for autologous blood donation. BMJ 300:1627, 1990

77. Thompson FL, Powers JS, Graber SE, Krantz SB: Use of recombinant human erythropoietin to enhance autologous blood donation in a patient with multiple red cell allo-antibodies and the anemia of chronic disease. Am J Med 90:398, 1991

78. Goodnough LT, Rudnick S, Price TH et al: Increased preoperative collection of autologous blood with recombinant human erythropoietin: a controlled trial. N Engl J Med 321:1163, 1989

79. Goodnough LT, Price TH, Rudnick S, Soegiarso RW: Preoperative red cell production in patients undergoing aggressive autologous blood phlebotomy with and without erythropoietin therapy. Transfusion 32: 441, 1992

80. Tasaki T, Ohto H, Hashimoto C et al: Recombinant human erythropoietin for autologous blood donation: effects on perioperative red-blood-cell and serum erythropoietin production. Lancet 339:773, 1992

81. Beris P, Mermillod B, Levy G: Recombinant human erythropoietin as adjuvant treatment for autologous blood donation: a prospective study. Vox Sang 65: 212, 1993

82. Goodnough LT, Price TH, Friedman KD et al: A phase III trial of recombinant human erythropoietin therapy in nonanemic orthopedic patients subjected to aggressive removal of blood for autologous use: dose, response, toxicity, and efficacy. Transfusion 34: 66, 1994

83. Kyo S, Ozmoto R, Hirashima K et al: Effect of human recombinant erythropoietin on reduction of homologous blood transfusion in open-heart surgery: a Japanese multicenter study. Circulation, suppl. 2, 86:II-413, 1992

84. Kajikawa M, Nonami T, Kurokawa T et al: Autologous blood transfusion for hepatectomy in patients with cirrhosis and hepatocellular carcinoma: use of recombinant human erythropoietin. Surgery 115: 727, 1994

85. Mercuriali F, Zanella A, Barosi G et al: Use of erythropoietin to increase the volume of autologous blood donated by orthopedic patients. Transfusion 33:55, 1993

86. Hiyashi J, Kumon K, Takanashi S et al: Subcutaneous administration of recombinant human erythropoietin before cardiac surgery: a double-blind, multicenter trial in Japan. Transfusion 34:142, 1994

87. Brugnara C, Chambers LA, Malynn E et al: Red blood cell regeneration induced by subcutaneous recombinant erythropoietin: iron-deficient erythropoiesis in iron-replete subjects. Blood 81:956, 1993

88. Rutherford CJ, Schneider TJ, Dempsey H et al: Efficacy of different dosing regimens for recombinant human erythropoietin in a simulated perisurgical setting: the importance of iron availability in optimizing response. Am J Med 96:139, 1994

89. Biesma DH, van de Wiel A, Beguin Y et al: Erythro-

poietic activity and iron metabolism in autologous blood donors during recombinant human erythropoietin therapy. Eur J Clin Invest 24:426, 1994

90. Pincus T, Olsen NJ, Russell IJ et al: Multicenter study of recombinant human erythropoietin in correction of anemia in rheumatoid arthritis. Am J Med 89:161, 1990

91. Hoeldtke RD, Streeten DHP: Treatment of orthostatic hypotension with erythropoietin. N Engl J Med 329:611, 1993

92. Kornowski R, Schwartz D, Jaffe A et al: Erythropoietin therapy obviates the need for recurrent transfusions in a patient with severe hemolysis due to prosthetic valves. Chest 102:315, 1992

93. Zeigler ZR, Rosenfeld CS, Shadduck RK: Resolution of transfusion dependence by recombinant human erythropoietin (rHuEPO) in acquired pure red cell aplasia (PRCA) associated with myeloid metaplasia. Br J Haematol 83:28, 1993

94. Lieschke GJ, Burgess AW: Granulocyte colony-stimulating factor and granulocyte-macrophage colony-stimulating factor (first of two parts). N Engl J Med 327:28, 1992

95. Gough NM, Gough J, Metcalf D et al: Molecular cloning of cDNA encoding a murine haematopoietic growth regulator, granulocyte-macrophage colony stimulating factor. Nature 309:763, 1984

96. Wong GG, Witek JS, Temple PA et al: Human GM-CSF: molecular cloning of the complementary DNA and purification of the natural and recombinant proteins. Science 228:810, 1985

97. Souza LM, Boone TC, Gabrilove J et al: Recombinant human granulocyte colony-stimulating factor: effects on normal and leukemic myeloid cells. Science 232:61, 1986

98. Huebner K, Isobe M, Croce CM et al: The human gene encoding GM-CSF is at 5q21-q32, the chromosome region deleted in the 5q-anomaly. Science 230:1282, 1985

99. Zsebo K, Cohen AM, Murdock DC et al: Recombinant human granulocyte colony stimulating factor: molecular and biological characterization. Immunobiology 172:175, 1986

100. Crawford J, Ozer H, Stoller R et al: Reduction by granulocyte colony-stimulating factor of fever and neutropenia induced by chemotherapy in patients with small-cell lung cancer. N Engl J Med 325:164, 1991

101. Peters WP, Shogan J, Shpall EJ et al: Recombinant human granulocyte-macrophage colony-stimulating factor produces fever. Lancet 1:950, 1988

102. Neumanitis J, Rabinowe SN, Singer JW et al: Recombinant granulocyte-macrophage colony-stimulating factor after autologous bone marrow transplantation for lymphoid cancer. N Engl J Med 324:1773, 1991

103. Neumanitis J, Singer JW, Buckner CD et al: Use of recombinant human granulocyte-macrophage colony-stimulating factor in autologous marrow transplantation for lymphoid malignancies. Blood 72:834, 1988

104. Gulati SC, Bennett CL: Granulocyte-macrophage colony-stimulating factor (GM-CSF) as adjunct therapy in relapsed Hodgkin disease. Ann Intern Med 116:177, 1992

105. Gabrilove JL, Jakubowski A, Scher H et al: Effect of granulocyte colony-stimulating factor on neutropenia and associated morbidity due to chemotherapy for transitional-cell carcinoma of the urothelium. N Engl J Med 318:1414, 1988

106. Antman KS, Griffin JD, Elias A et al: Effect of recombinant human granulocyte-macrophage colony-stimulating factor on chemotherapy-induced myelosuppression. N Engl J Med 319:593, 1988

107. De Witte T, Gratwohl A, Van Der Lely N et al: Recombinant human granulocyte-macrophage colony-stimulating factor accelerates neutrophil and monocyte recovery after allogeneic T-cell-depleted bone marrow transplantation. Blood 79:1359, 1992

108. Brandt SJ, Peters WP, Atwater SK et al: Effect of recombinant human granulocyte-macrophage colony-stimulating factor on hematopoietic reconstitution after high-dose chemotherapy and autologous bone marrow transplantation. N Engl J Med 318:869, 1988

109. Neumanitis J, Singer JW, Buckner CD et al: Use of recombinant human granulocyte-macrophage colony-stimulating factor in graft failure after bone marrow transplantation. Blood 76:245, 1990

110. Bonilla MA, Gillio AP, Ruggeiro M et al: Effects of recombinant human granulocyte colony-stimulating factor on neutropenia in patients with congenital agranulocytosis. N Engl J Med 320:1574, 1989

111. Kojima S, Fukuda M, Miyajima Y et al: Treatment of aplastic anemia in children with recombinant human granulocyte colony-stimulating factor. Blood 77:937, 1991

112. Kojima S, Tsuchida M, Matsuyama T: Myelodysplasia and leukemia after treatment of aplastic anemia with G-CSF. N Engl J Med 326:1294, 1992

113. Miles SA, Mitsuyasu RT, Moreno J et al: Combined therapy with recombinant granulocyte colony-stimulating factor and erythropoietin decreases hematologic toxicity from zidovudine. Blood 77:2109, 1991

114. Groopman JE, Mitsuyasu RT, DeLeo MJ et al: Effect of recombinant human granulocyte-macrophage col-

ony-stimulating factor on myelopoiesis in the acquired immunodeficiency syndrome. N Engl J Med 317:593, 1987

115. Ohno R, Tomonaga M, Kobayashi T et al: Effect of granulocyte colony-stimulating factor after intensive induction therapy in relapsed or refractory acute leukemia. N Engl J Med 323:871, 1990

116. Buchner T, Hiddeman W, Koenigsman M et al: Recombinant human granulocyte-macrophage colony-stimulating factor after chemotherapy in patients with acute myeloid leukemia at higher age or after relapse. Blood 78:1190, 1991

117. Negrin RS, Haeuber DH, Nagler A et al: Maintenance treatment of patients with myelodysplastic syndromes using recombinant human granulocyte colony-stimulating factor. Blood 76:36, 1990

118. Vadhan-Raj S, Keating M, LeMaistre A et al: Effects of recombinant human granulocyte-macrophage colony-stimulating factor in patients with myelodysplastic syndromes. N Engl J Med 317:1545, 1987

119. Stiff PJ, Murgo AJ, DeRisi MF, Clarkson B: Quantification of the peripheral blood colony forming unit-culture rise following chemotherapy: could leukocytapheresis replace bone marrow for autologous transplantation? Transfusion 23:500, 1983

120. Siena S, Bregni M, Brando B et al: Circulation of CD34+ hematopoietic stem cells in the peripheral blood of high-dose cyclophosphamide-treated patients: enhancement by intravenous recombinant human granulocyte-macrophage colony-stimulating factor. Blood 74:1905, 1989

121. Elias AD, Ayash L, Anderson KC et al: Mobilization of peripheral blood progenitor cells by chemotherapy and granulocyte-macrophage colony-stimulating factor for hematologic support after high-dose intensification for breast cancer. Blood 79:3036, 1992

122. Freireich EJ: White cell transfusion born again. Leukemia Lymphoma, suppl. 2, 11:161, 1994

123. Strauss RG: Therapeutic granulocyte transfusions in 1993. Blood 81:1675, 1993

124. Caspar CB, Seger RA, Burger J, Gmur J: Effective stimulation of donors for granulocyte transfusions with recombinant methionyl granulocyte colony-stimulating factor. Blood 81:2866, 1993

125. Bensinger WI, Price TH, Dale DC et al: The effects of daily recombinant human granulocyte colony-stimulating factor administration on normal granulo-cyte donors undergoing leukapheresis. Blood 81:1883, 1993

126. McDonald TP: Thrombopoietin: its biology, clinical aspects, and possibilities. Am J Pediatr Hematol Oncol 14:8, 1992

127. Du XX, Neben T, Goldman S, Williams DA: Effects of recombinant human interleukin-11 on hematopoietic reconstitution in transplant mice: acceleration of recovery of peripheral blood neutrophils and platelets. Blood 81:27, 1993

128. Weber J, Yang JC, Topalian SL et al: Phase I trial of subcutaneous interleukin-6 in patients with advanced malignancies. J Clin Oncol 11:499, 1993

129. D'Hondt V, Weynants P, Humblet Y et al: Dose-dependent interleukin-3 stimulation of thrombopoiesis and neutropoiesis in patients with small-cell lung carcinoma before and following chemotherapy: a placebo-controlled randomized phase Ib study. J Clin Oncol 11:2063, 1993

130. Gordon MS, Hoffman R: Growth factors affecting human thrombocytopoiesis: potential agents for the treatment of thrombocytopenia. Blood 80:302, 1992

131. Robinson BE, McGrath HE, Quesenberry PJ: Recombinant murine granulocyte-macrophage colony-stimulating factor has megakaryocyte colony-stimulating activity and augments megakaryocyte colony stimulation by interleukin 3. J Clin Invest 79:1648, 1987

132. Lok S, Kaushansky K, Holly RD et al: Cloning and expression of murine thrombopoietin cDNA and stimulation of platelet production in vivo. Nature 369:565, 1994

133. Kaushansky K, Lok S, Holly RD et al: Promotion of megakaryocyte progenitor expansion and differentiation by the c-mpl ligand thrombopoietin. Nature 369:568, 1994

134. Wendling F, Maraskovsky E, Debill N et al: c-Mpl ligand is a humor regulator of megakaryocytopoiesis. Nature 369:571, 1994

135. de Sauvage FJ, Hass PE, Spencer SD et al: Stimulation of megakaryocytopoiesis and thrombopoiesis by the c-mpl ligand. Nature 369:533, 1994

136. Souyri M, Vigon I, Penciolelli J-F et al: A putative truncated cytokine receptor gene transduced by the myeloproliferative leukemia virus immortalizes hematopoietic progenitors. Cell 63:1137, 1990

137. Methia N, Louache F, Vainchenker W, Wendling F: Oligodeoxynucleotides antisense to the proto-oncogene c-mpl specifically inhibit in vitro megakaryocytopoiesis. Blood 82:1935, 1993

Chapter 48

Peripheral Stem Cell Transplantation

Anne Kessinger

HISTORY AND BACKGROUND

Autologous bone marrow transplantation (ABMT) has been used with increasing frequency since the late 1970s to restore marrow function that was damaged by the administration of high-dose myelotoxic radiation therapy and/or chemotherapy.[1] After the discovery was made that hematopoietic precursors, apparently similar to precursors in the bone marrow, are normally and routinely present in the circulation,[2] an interest in the ability of these peripheral stem cells (PSC) to sustain marrow function after transplantation was stimulated. A number of animal models were developed to test the feasibility of autologous and allogeneic PSC transplants.[3,4]

In 1977, after the initial preclinical trials were successful, a large clinical trial began involving patients with chronic myelogenous leukemia (CML). The patients had PSC collected and stored during the chronic phase of the disease. Under usual circumstances, the number of hematopoietic progenitors in the circulation is meager; this cell population is normally much less prevalent in peripheral blood than in bone marrow. Patients with CML, however, have greatly increased numbers of circulating progenitors, and the increase is accounted for by an accumulation of leukemic PSC. Therefore, most collected progenitor cells in this early study contained the disease. When the CML in these patients transformed to an accelerated phase, high-dose therapy

was administered followed by a PSC autotransplant. This attempt to convert the disease back to the chronic phase by destroying the accelerated phase disease and replacing it with hematopoietic cells containing the chronic phase was successful in most patients so treated.[5] Unfortunately, the second chronic phase was short lived and provided essentially no advantage to the patient, but the study did demonstrate that leukemic hematopoietic progenitor cells collected from blood could restore (leukemic) marrow function when autografted.

In 1979 and 1980, two failed attempts at successful syngeneic PSC transplantation were reported along with the caution that nonleukemic PSC transplantation may not be able to restore marrow function.[6,7] In retrospect, the failures were most likely a result of technique (too few cells transfused over a prolonged period of time) and not the inability of hematopoietic PSC to restore marrow function. Publications regarding clinical PSC transplantation eventually resurfaced in 1985[8] in 1986, six independent investigators reported successful PSC transplantations.[9–14] From that time, the number of reports in the literature regarding PSC transplantation seem to have increased at an exponential rate.

The term "PSC transplant" has been the subject of criticism in recent times mainly because the definition of a stem cell has changed over the years. Very early publications referred to those hematopoietic cells that required additional mitotic activity to achieve terminal differentiation as *committed stem cells* or simply *stem cells* and referred to those cells that were able to provide continuous and sustained marrow function as *uncommitted stem cells*.[15,16] As older studies have given way to new ones, facilitated especially by hematopoietic growth factor research, the term "progenitor" has replaced "committed stem cell," and the "uncommitted stem cell" is now called the "pluripotent" or "totipotent stem cell." Stem cell now is sometimes assumed to mean pluripotent stem cell, and all other hematopoietic precursors are called progenitors. Because an assay to identify the pluripotent stem cell is not yet available, some investigators have argued that, because the only currently identifiable hematopoietic precursor cells in autologous blood cells transplanted to restore iatrogenically damaged marrow function are progenitors, such transplants should be called peripheral blood progenitor cell transplants. The term "autologous PSC transplant" is used here because this nomenclature is prevalent in the literature, with the understanding that progenitor cells are included in the transplant product. The possibility that pluripotent stem cells do circulate in human blood seems likely, however.

HARVESTING FOR AUTOLOGOUS TRANSPLANTATION

The number of circulating progenitors in humans varies but normally is considerably less that the number present in bone marrow.[5] Although a sufficient number of marrow cells for autografting a 70-kg individual is contained in a marrow harvest product of approximately 742 ml,[17] a similarly sized person with a blood volume of 4.5 L and unperturbed or "steady-state" bone marrow function must undergo apheresis of about 14 blood volumes to collect enough cells for a PSC transplant.[18] As a result of the number of cells available, PSC for autografting are usually collected with a series of apheresis procedures. The operating manuals for all apheresis devices currently on the market include descriptions of the procedure(s) to be used for PSC collections. In general, the machine is programmed to collect low-density mononuclear cells or lymphocytes.

Usually, a central venous catheter is used to gain venous access for apheresis collections. When possible, central venous catheters that can also be used later during high-dose therapy and PSC transplantation are chosen to keep the number of catheter insertion and removal procedures at a minimum. To provide adequate access for apheresis, a catheter specially designed for apheresis is optimal because these catheters have the larger lumens and thicker walls that permit the necessary high flow rates.[19]

Patients who are undergoing repetitive autologous PSC collections are subject to the side effects of frequent apheresis procedures, which include anemia, thrombocytopenia, and the symptoms of hypovolemia and hypocalcemia. Because these collections are from patients and not normal donors, the susceptibility to and the severity of these side effects may be accentuated, depending on the individual circumstances involved.

MOBILIZATION

If the numbers of progenitors that normally circulate could be increased above steady state or baseline during the collection process, apheresis procedures would harvest the PSC autograft product more efficiently. Circulating PSC numbers have been reported to vary normally; for example, more colony forming units-granulocyte-macrophage (CFU-GM) and colony forming units-granulocyte, erythrocyte, monocyte, megakaryocyte (CFU-GEMM) are present in the circulation during the afternoon than in the morning.[20,21] Certain clinically impractical manipulations have been noted to result in large increases of circulating progenitors, including endotoxin administration,[22] epinephrine administration,[23] and exercise.[24] Two clinically applicable methods used to mobilize progenitors into the circulation have also been described: myelotoxic chemotherapy administration[25] and administration of certain hematopoietic growth factors.[26,27] Almost certainly, mechanisms responsible for the increase in numbers of progenitors (mobilization) differ according to the stimulus applied. Exercise can produce mobilization in less than 1 minute, although the effect persists for only a few minutes more even when the exercise is continued,[24] which perhaps can be explained as a result of demargination. Growth factor administration causes detectable mobilization in 3 or 4 days, and the effect apparently persists as long as the administration continues,[18] although the maximal effect may be limited to a few days. Growth factors might conceivably produce a mobilization effect by altering the adhesion molecules of progenitor cells. Approximately 2 weeks after myelosuppressive chemotherapy administration, mobilization effects become measurable[28] and may be the result of endogenous cytokine production.

Concerns have arisen regarding the specific progenitors that respond to mobilization attempts. Do only very committed progenitors mobilize? Is mobilization accomplished at the expense of the most primitive progenitors or even the pluripotent stem cell?[29] As assays for more and more primitive progenitors become available, studies suggest that all categories of progenitors respond to mobilization efforts, although the degree of response is not necessarily equivalent for each progenitor subtype.[30]

Mobilization After Myelosuppressive Chemotherapy

Chemotherapy-induced mobilization was the first technique used clinically to increase the number of circulating progenitors during harvesting. Myelosuppressive agents given either singly[28] or in combination[31] result in peripheral cytopenia that reaches a nadir about 2 weeks after administration. When recovery from cytopenia begins, the number of progenitors in the circulation increases, and apheresis is instituted. The time to begin the collections has been variously defined as the first day of a spontaneous rise in platelet numbers,[28] the day the recovering total white blood count reaches a target number,[32] the day the percentage of monocytes in the recovering white blood cell population reaches a certain number,[33] and the day the recovering granulocytes reach a specific number.[34] More recently, flow cytometric assays to detect circulating cells that express the CD34 differentiation antigen (a hematopoietic progenitor cell marker) have been utilized to determine the precise onset of the mobilization effect.[35] The duration of a chemotherapy-induced mobilization effect is variable, but typically is 5 days, with a range of 1 to 8 days.[28]

These characteristics of chemotherapy-induced mobilization are responsible for some of the clinical liabilities of this mobilization technique. Neutropenic fever has been described in patients as they reach the nadir of myelosuppression. Nearly one-third of patients who received chemotherapy for mobilization were reported to require hospitalization, mostly for neutropenic fever.[36] Sepsis and, rarely,

death have been reported after chemotherapy for mobilization.[28] If patients experience neutropenic fever at the time apheresis is scheduled to begin, concern arises about the possibility of collecting a bacterially contaminated product. In addition, the entire mobilization process is time consuming because the mobilization effect does not begin until approximately 2 weeks after the chemotherapy is administered.

One especially troubling feature of chemotherapy-induced mobilization is that some patients do not respond to the mobilizing attempt. Those who seem most at risk for failure are patients who have already received considerable amounts of antineoplastic therapy for their underlying disease before becoming eligible for PSC collection.[37] The amount of prior therapy necessary to impede successful chemotherapy-induced mobilization is difficult to quantify, but patients who have had more than six cycles of combination chemotherapy or have received radiation therapy to more than 20 percent of their bone marrow have been reported to respond poorly to mobilization attempts. The bone marrow in patients with metastatic malignant cells detected there on routine biopsy also does not routinely mobilize well with chemotherapy.[28]

When mobilization attempts are successful, the number of apheresis procedures necessary to collect a PSC autograft product can be markedly reduced. As many as 21 apheresis procedures have been reported to be necessary to collect a nonmobilized product,[38] although successful chemotherapy-induced mobilization often permits collections with three procedures.[28] Minimizing the number of apheresis procedures is useful, but successful mobilization provides an even greater clinical benefit than collection efficiency. The speed of hematopoietic recovery after autotransplantation of well-mobilized cells is accelerated by 1 week or more when compared with recovery after ABMT or nonmobilized PSC transplant.[39] Earlier hematopoietic recovery can result in earlier dismissal from the hospital and fewer infections, blood product transfusions, and days of fever.

Mobilization After Cytokine Administration

In 1988, administration of granulocyte-macrophage colony-stimulating factor[40] and granulocyte colony-stimulating factor (G-CSF)[27] were reported to mobilize hematopoietic progenitors into the circulation. Initial concern about using growth factors to facilitate stem cell collections revolved around the possibility that growth factors would encourage stem cells down differentiation pathways, would not increase the number of noncommitted stem cells in the circulation, and would result in an apheresis product devoid of cells that could support sustained hematopoietic recovery. Therefore, early studies added growth factor-mobilized PSC to autologous marrow harvests at the time of autografting in an effort to promote rapid hematopoietic recovery with the peripheral cells while providing sufficient pluripotent stem cells with the marrow to ensure sustained function.[41] Growth factor administration after chemotherapy provided the most prodigious mobilizing effect except for patients who had already been treated with myelosuppressive therapy (radiation therapy or chemotherapy). PSC were not mobilized in these patients when growth factor was administered after chemotherapy.[37]

In 1990, a series of five patients treated with high-dose therapy and growth factor-mobilized PSCT were reported to have experienced sustained recovery of hematopoietic function.[42] This important observation provided a starting point for studies of PSC transplant using cells mobilized only with growth factor(s). Growth factor mobilization eliminates some of the liabilities of chemotherapy-induced mobilization: neutropenia is avoided completely, the mobilization effect appears in 3 or 4 days after initiation of growth factor administration, and the mobilization effect can be extended with continued growth factor administration. However, growth factor administration can result in confounding side effects, including fever, bone pain, and fluid retention. A recent report described successful mobilization using a single cytokine for patients who had received considerable prior treatment. The mobilized cells were collected with fewer apheresis procedures, and the mobilized autografts resulted in earlier hematopoietic recovery compared with nonmobilized PSC transplants.[18]

The appearance of malignant cells in the circulation associated with the administration of mobilizing doses of G-CSF has been recently reported in a patient with progressive multiple myeloma.[43] This same report described two additional patients with myeloma who received G-CSF for mobilization without the subsequent appearance of circulating myeloma cells. The status of their disease at the time of G-CSF administration (i.e., progressive or in remission) was not described. The possibility exists that growth factors alone should not be used for patients with certain diseases that are progressing at the time of PSC collection. Additional studies are required to confirm or refute this potential concern.

Mobilization After Chemotherapy and Cytokine Administration

The use of cytokine or growth factor alone for mobilization typically results in a less vigorous response than the combination of cytotoxic chemotherapy plus growth factor.[37,40] Cytokine therapy is usually begun a few days after the myelosuppressive chemotherapy is given and continues until the collections are complete. The maximal mobilization effect is generally noted about 2 weeks after the chemotherapy is administered.[37] Collection of sufficient numbers of peripheral stem cells mobilized with growth factor and myelosuppressive chemotherapy to serve as a successful autograft in pretreated patients with lymphoma has occurred with a single apheresis procedure.[44]

A recent report suggested that chemotherapy plus cytokine-induced mobilization sometimes results in the appearance of, or an increase in the number of, measurable circulating malignant cells.[45] This effect was noted for patients with breast and lung cancer. The malignant cell detection assays used were not designed to determine the potential of the mobilized tumor cells to establish malignancies should they be reinfused at the time of autografting. Such studies are currently underway, however.

QUALITY ASSURANCE

Two general issues of quality assurance arise when considering a PSC autograft product: (1) the suitability of the product for transplantation and (2) the caliber of the laboratory practices involved during collection, processing, and infusion of the cells. The responsibility for these assurances varies from one transplant center to another, but the processing laboratory is always responsible for the quality assurance of the processing, cryopreservation, and storage procedures. The progenitor assay laboratory, if separate from the processing laboratory, maintains the quality of the assays. The director(s) of the laboratory(ies) can advise and assist the responsible physician caring for the patient as a final decision is made regarding the suitability of the product for transplant.

PSC should be collected, processed, and cryopreserved according to protocols defined in each facility's procedure manual. A system should be in place to track the individual responsible for each step of the collection, processing, cryopreservation, and infusion of each PSC product. General laboratory quality assurance is an integral component of the assurance process, including documentation of continued competence and proficiency testing of both the medical technologists involved in processing and of the medical personnel who collect the cells with apheresis techniques. Currently, there are few (if any) externally available proficiency testing programs applicable to PSC collection, processing, and/or infusion. Therefore, each transplant program needs to develop its own set of internal proficiency testing procedures.

The definition of an adequate collection is made by each transplant center because no universally accepted definition exists. The usual surrogate markers for a suitable collection include mononuclear cell (only for nonmobilized PSC), CD34+ cell, and/or CFU-GM content. The definition of an adequate collection is made in part by determining the numbers of these surrogate markers in the transplanted product, which are associated with satisfactory engraftment at the particular transplant center under consideration. Approximate or "ballpark" values at many institutions are 6 to 8 $\times$ 10^8 mononuclear cells/kg for nonmobilized cells,[38] 2.5 to 50 $\times$ 10^4 CFU-GM/kg for mobilized cells,[46,47] and 1 to 5 $\times$ 10^6 CD34+ cells/kg for mobilized cells.[48,49] The number of CD34+ cells necessary for a suitable collection is unique to each transplant center because flow cytometric analysis of these cells is not standardized and varies considerably.

The efficiency of mononuclear cell collection by the particular apheresis device used and the platelet, but especially the red cell content of each apheresis product, should be monitored to ensure product consistency. The laboratory should also monitor

problems associated with infusion of the cells and maintain data regarding hematopoietic recovery after transplant. The markers used to determine suitability of the autograft should be reviewed periodically to ensure that they correlate with hematopoietic recovery, realizing that correlations may vary with the characteristics of the patients treated, the particular mobilization technique used, and/or the high-dose therapeutic regimen utilized.

The American Association of Blood Banks' standards for processing PSC products include bacterial and fungal cultures for each product just before cryopreservation.[50] This quality assurance procedure, designed to monitor sterile collection and processing techniques and reagents, currently is not performed on every collection product at all hematopoietic stem cell processing laboratories but seems especially important for collections from febrile patients and for cells undergoing unusual processing, for example, purging or CD34+ cell selection.

The physician who is directing the care of the patient should supply the laboratory with an order or a "prescription" for the appropriate processing and cryopreservation technique to be used if more than one is available. After processing, the product should be labeled with appropriate donor and intended recipient identification, date of collection, a designation as a PSC collection (rather than bone marrow), and, when appropriate, an indication that the product is contained in more than one storage bag. The label should also indicate the approximate volume, the name of the facility, the temperature of storage, and, where appropriate, the expiration date. Instructions to the infusionist should accompany the component. The characteristics of each processed product (e.g., mononuclear cell count, differential count, progenitor cell content, microbial culture results, cell viability, and so forth) should be provided for inclusion in the patient's medical record. A record of the cooling curve during cryopreservation should be maintained in the laboratory. The precise location of the product in the storage freezer must also be maintained by the laboratory.

Each center should develop and follow a protocol for infusion of the cells. In most centers, these protocols have been adapted from protocols for infusion of cryopreserved autologous marrow. Generally, intravenous hydration is provided along with diphen-hydramine hydrochloride and meperidine hydro-chloride before infusion to prevent or decrease the toxicities that can occur during infusion of the cells. These toxicities include hemoglobinuria, nausea, fever, chills, vomiting, abdominal cramping, diar-rhea, and headache, among others.[51] The cells are checked out from the laboratory while frozen, with the usual documentation procedure ensuring that the recipient's identification code corresponds to the identification code of the product bags. One bag is thawed in a water bath at the bedside, and the con-tents are then administered intravenously. Adverse reactions, if they occur, are recorded, and the next bag is not thawed until the patient is well enough to receive the infusion. Cells should be thawed for as short of a period as possible before infusion. Leuko-depletion filters should not be used, and of course the product should not be treated with γ irradiation before infusion.

CRYOPRESERVATION AND STORAGE

Two methods of cryopreservation and storage have been used clinically to maintain the long-term viabil-ity of harvested PSC (Table 48-1). One method uses 10 percent, by volume, dimethyl sulfoxide (DMSO) as the cryoprotectant, controlled-rate cooling, and storage in a liquid nitrogen freezer. This technique, adapted with little change from that used for bone marrow cryopreservation, is the traditional method.[52] The second procedure, also borrowed from the bone marrow cryopreservation laboratory, uses 5 percent DMSO and 6 percent hydroxyethyl

Table 48-1. Cryopreservation of Peripheral Stem Cells

	Method 1	Method 2
Media	Tissue culture media	Albumin, dextrose
Cryoprotectant	10% DMSO	5% DMSO 6% Hydroxyethyl starch
Cooling	Controlled rate	Direct
Storage	−196°C	−80°C

Abbreviation: DMSO, dimethyl sulfoxide.

starch as the cryoprotectant and does not call for controlled-rate freezing. Rather, the cells are placed directly in a −80°C, or colder, freezer and stored there until needed.[53] Although the number of CFU-GM colonies recovered from cells processed with each of these two techniques is equivalent,[54] no ran-domized study of differences in the clinical effective-ness of cells processed with each of the methods is available. Suggestions have been made that cells not stored in liquid nitrogen freezers be used within 4 months of processing.[55]

ALLOGENEIC TRANSPLANTATION

In the past, two concerns curbed the enthusiasm of investigators who contemplated clinical allogeneic PSC transplantation. The first concern was that the presence of the pluripotent stem cell in the human circulation has never been documented because no assay for that cell exists. The fact that autologous PSC transplantation after potentially marrow-lethal total body radiation has been associated with full and sustained recovery of hematopoiesis[56] does not prove that a pluripotent hematopoietic stem cell was transplanted because autochthonous marrow recov-ery cannot be discounted as the source of sustained hematopoiesis for these patients. Total body irradia-tion does not always result in permanent marrow ablation, and markers to distinguish progeny from transplanted autologous PSC versus recovering mar-row were not available. If pluripotent stem cells were not returned to patients who had received truly mar-row-lethal therapy, marrow aplasia would be the ulti-mate consequence. The second concern was for the development of severe graft-versus-host disease. This illness, mediated by T lymphocytes, was feared to be a larger problem with allogeneic PSC trans-plantation because considerably more T lympho-cytes are present in a PSC collection than in a mar-row harvest.[57]

In 1989, an allogeneic PSC transplant was re-ported, using cell collections that were partially T cell depleted before transplantation.[58] Nonmobi-lized PSC were transplanted because mobilization with cytotoxic chemotherapy could not be consid-ered in a normal donor and hematopoietic growth factors were not yet routinely available. After transplantation, the cells that reappeared in the peripheral blood of the patient were found to be exclusively of donor origin. Acute graft-versus-host disease developed but was mild, confined to the skin, and responded completely to steroid therapy. Unfortunately, the patient died of a systemic fungal infection 1 month after transplantation. Obviously, the survival of the patient was not long enough to determine whether sustained donor engraftment resulted. Sustained engraftment of donor origin would prove that pluripotent stem cells had been collected from the bloodstream of the donor and were successfully transplanted.

In 1993, five syngeneic PSC transplants for four patients were reported using cells that had been mobilized with G-CSF.[59] The only immediate toxicity from G-CSF administration experienced by the normal donors was bone pain. The patients experienced timely hematopoietic recovery, which was sustained to a maximal follow-up interval of 214 days. However, like autologous PSC transplantation, this experience cannot answer the question as to whether the pluripotent stem cell is present in the human circulation.

Two apparently successful allogeneic PSC transplants using cells mobilized with G-CSF were reported in 1993.[60,61] One followed two allogeneic bone marrow transplants from the same donor, neither of which restored hematopoiesis in a timely fashion.[61] An active cytomegalovirus infection was believed to be the cause of marrow failure. The PSC were infused 91 days after the initial bone marrow transplant and immediately after a course of ganciclovir. Initial marrow recovery was noted 11 days later. Follow-up 260 days after the procedure revealed continued trilineage marrow function of donor origin. Mild to moderately acute graft-versus-host disease, confined to the skin, responded well to therapy. The patient subsequently had mild chronic graft-versus-host disease develop, again confined to the skin. The continuing marrow function cannot be absolutely attributed to the allogeneic PSC transplant, however, because cells introduced with the prior allogeneic bone marrow transplants (BMT) could have been the source of the sustained engraftment.

The second reported allogeneic PSC transplant did not follow a failed BMT but constituted the only transplant for this patient.[60] Recovery of granulocyte and platelet counts was not accelerated when compared with usual recovery rates after BMT, but no graft-versus-host disease was encountered. Follow-up at the time of the report was only 58 days; therefore, the permanence of the restored marrow function had not been determined.

These experiences with nonautologous PSC transplant suggest that allogeneic PSC transplant may be a satisfactory alternative to allogeneic BMT. Whether mobilization of donor cells before collection is necessary and, if so, what the ideal mobilization technique will be in this situation awaits further studies. However, if allogeneic PSC transplantation proves to be reliable, one can imagine how blood is likely to become the preferred source of hematopoietic allographs.

PRESENT AND FUTURE ROLE

Currently, PSC transplantation is used routinely for patients eligible for high-dose therapy who have marrow that, for some reason, is not suitable for autografting. PSC transplantation is also used in some instances when faster hematopoietic recovery than might be expected after ABMT is anticipated. The long-term progression-free survival of patients who receive a PSC transplant after high-dose therapy seems to be at least as good as that observed after ABMT.[62] There is some preliminary evidence that, for some diseases, specifically the intermediate-grade non-Hodgkin lymphomas, patients may have an advantage in disease-free survival after PSC transplant compared with ABMT.[63] Confirmation of the findings of this retrospective study will require randomized prospective studies, which are ongoing, but proposed explanations for better tumor control after PSC transplantation (Table 48-2) have been explored with resultant supportive preliminary data.

Patients might expect to experience a better disease-free survival after high-dose therapy and PSC transplantation rather than ABMT if occult clonal tumor cells in autologous stem cell collections, which can restore disease when infused with the autograft product, are less frequent in PSC collections than in marrow harvest products. This situation is likely to

Table 48-2. Potential Advantages of Peripheral Stem Cell Transplantation Other Than Hematopoietic Recovery

Fewer tumor cells capable of re-establishing disease may be present in a PSC collection than in a bone marrow harvest.

A PSC collection contains more lymphocytes than a bone marrow harvest. These and other accessory cells provide minimal direct antitumor activity, which could be augmented with further manipulation.

Immune reconstitution after high-dose therapy is different after PSC transplantation than after ABMT. Faster recovery of more effective immune activity may provide elimination of minimal residual disease.

Abbreviations: PSC, peripheral stem cell; ABMT, autologous bone marrow transplantation.

be specific to the malignancy being treated; for diseases such as non-Hodgkin's lymphoma and breast cancer, however, occult malignant cells capable of growth have been encountered less frequently in PSC collections than in bone marrow.[64,65]

Minimal residual disease in the patient after high-dose therapy is postulated to be responsible for some tumor relapses observed after transplantation.[66] The baseline cytotoxicity of mononuclear cells in PSC collections measured with chromium release assays has been reported to be approximately 8 percent.[67] This degree of cytotoxicity seems unlikely to have more than a slight effect on minimal residual disease in the patient at the time of transplantation or on any occult tumor cells contained in the PSC collection product. However, this cytotoxic activity can be increased 10-fold with cytokine incubation.[68] In the future, cytokine incubation of the nonhematopoietic cells in the graft product might provide a meaningful therapeutic effect to the transplanted cells.

Faster recovery of CD3+ cells (T cells) after PSC transplantation than after ABMT has been reported.[69] Immune reconstitution after PSC transplantation has been reported to result in an immune status that was functionally superior to that seen in the patient at the time of diagnosis of a malignant disease and before the transplant.[70] Immune reconstitution after high-dose therapy has been reported to develop differently after ABMT than after PSC

transplantation.[71] These differences, at least in part, are suspected to be due to the larger numbers of lymphocytes contained in a PSC collection compared with bone marrow.[72] If immune surveillance were restored more quickly and completely, minimal residual disease remaining after high-dose therapy might be more susceptible to immune-mediated eradication.

The known and anticipated qualities of PSC transplantation suggest the role of this procedure will continue to expand. One can speculate that in the not-too-distant future, PSC transplantation, both autologous and allogeneic, will become the preferred means with which to restore iatrogenically damaged or destroyed bone marrow.

ALLOGENEIC CORD BLOOD TRANSPLANTATION

The blood that remains in the umbilical cord and placenta at the time of birth contains an immense number of hematopoietic precursors.[73] These cord blood cells, which are never referred to as PSC, can also restore hematopoietic function when transplanted.[74] Cord blood has theoretic advantages over bone marrow as a source of hematopoietic stem cells for allografting because the accessory cells in cord blood are more immunologically naive and may result in less graft-versus-host disease. If cord blood, which is routinely discarded after birth, were HLA typed and banked instead, a larger proportion of patients in search of a source of hematopoietic stem cells for allografting might be served.[75] The first recipient of a cord blood transplant has been followed more than 5 years and has demonstrated sustained hematopoiesis of donor origin.

Cord blood transplantation techniques are new, and a number of issues are not yet resolved.[76] Thus far, the only recipients of cord blood allografts have been children because the total number of hematopoietic cells in a cord blood harvest is smaller than that number traditionally believed to be required for successful transplantation to an adult. Hematopoietic recovery after cord blood transplants has been slower than the speed of recovery after allogeneic bone marrow transplantation.[75] Nonetheless, the future of cord blood transplantation seems bright. If the cord blood of each infant could be banked in a cost-effective manner and if hematopoietic stem cell transplantation continues to be a valuable therapeutic tool, the next century might find that cord blood is the source of all hematopoietic stem cell grafts, autologous and allogeneic.

REFERENCES

1. Keating A: Autologous bone marrow transplantation. p. 162. In Armitage JO, Antman KH (eds): High-Dose Cancer Therapy Pharmacology, Hematopoietins, Stem Cells. Williams & Wilkins, Baltimore, 1992
2. McCredie KB, Hersh EM, Freireich EJ: Cells capable of colony formation in the peripheral blood of man. Science 171:387, 1971
3. Cavins JA, Scheer SC, Thomas ED, Ferrebee JW: The recovery of lethally irradiated dogs given infusions of autologous leukocytes preserved at −80° C. Blood 23:38, 1964
4. Storb R, Graham TC, Epstein RB et al: Demonstration of hemopoietic stem cells in the peripheral blood of baboons by cross circulation. Blood 50:537, 1977
5. McCarthy DM, Goldman JM: Transfusion of circulating stem cells. Crit Rev Clin Lab Sci 20:1, 1984
6. Hershko C, Gale RP, Ho WG et al: Cure of aplastic anaemia in paroxysmal nocturnal haemoglobinuria by marrow transfusion from identical twin: failure of peripheral-leukocyte transfusion to correct marrow aplasia. Lancet 1:945, 1979
7. Abrams RA, Glaubiger D, Appelbaum FR et al: Result of attempted hematopoietic reconstitution using isologous, peripheral blood mononuclear cells: a case report. Blood 56:516, 1980
8. Juttner CA, To LB, Haylock DN et al: Circulating autologous stem cells collected in very early remission from acute non-lymphoblastic leukaemia produce prompt but incomplete haemopoietic reconstitution after high dose melphalan or supralethal chemoradiotherapy. Br J Haematol 61:739, 1985
9. Castaigne S, Calvo F, Doulay L et al: Successful haematopoietic reconstitution using autologous peripheral blood mononucleated cells in a patient with acute promyelocytic leukaemia. Br J Haematol 62:209, 1986
10. Reiffers J, Bernard P, David B et al: Successful autologous transplantation with peripheral blood hemopoietic cells in a patient with acute leukemia. Exp Hematol 14:312, 1986
11. Korbling M, Dorken B, Ho AD et al: Autologous transplantation of blood-derived hemopoietic stem cells after myeloablative therapy in a patient with Burkitt's lymphoma. Blood 67:529, 1986
12. Tilly H, Bastit D, Lucet JC et al: Haemopoietic reconstitution after autologous peripheral blood stem cell transplantation in acute leukemia. Lancet 2:154, 1986
13. Bell AJ, Figes A, Oscier DG, Hamblin TJ: Peripheral blood stem cell autografting. Lancet 1:1027, 1986
14. Kessinger A, Armitage JO, Landmark JD, Weisenburger DD: Reconstitution of human hematopoietic function with autologous cryopreserved circulating stem cells. Exp Hematol 14:192, 1986
15. Fliedner TM, Calvo W, Korbling M et al: Hematopoietic stem cells in blood: characteristics and potentials. p. 193. In Golde DW (ed): Hematopoietic Cell Differentiation. Academic Press, New York, 1978
16. Gidali J, Feher I, Antal S: Some properties of the circulating hemopoietic stem cells. Blood 43:573, 1974
17. Jin NR, Hill RS, Petersen FB et al: Marrow harvesting for autologous marrow transplantation. Exp Hematol 13:879, 1985
18. Bishop MR, Anderson JR, Jackson JD et al: High-dose therapy and peripheral blood progenitor cell transplantation: effects of recombinant human granulocyte-macrophage colony-stimulating factor on the autograft. Blood 83:610, 1994
19. Haire WD: Hickman line management. p. 419. In Armitage JO, Antman KH (eds): High-Dose Cancer Therapy Pharmacology, Hematopoietins, Stem Cells. Williams & Wilkins, Baltimore, 1992
20. Verma DS, Fisher R, Spitzer G et al: Diurnal changes in circulating myeloid progenitor cells in man. Am J Hematol 9:185, 1980
21. Lasky LC, Ascensao J, McCullough J, Zanjani ED: Steroid modulation of naturally occurring diurnal variation in circulating pluripotential haemotopoietic cells (CFU-GEMM). Br J Haematol 55:615, 1983
22. Cline MJ, Golde DW: Mobilization of haematopoietic stem cells (CFU-C) into the peripheral blood of man by endotoxin. Exp Hematol 5:1977, 1977
23. Morra L, Ponassi A, Caristo G et al: Comparison between diurnal changes and changes induced by hydrocortisone and epinephrine in circulating human hemopoietic progenitor cells (CFU-GM) in man. Biomed Pharmacother 38:167, 1984
24. Barrett AJ, Longhurst P, Sneath P et al: Mobilisation of CFU-C by exercise and ACTH induced stress in man. Exp Hematol 6:590, 1978
25. To LB, Haylock DN, Kimber RJ, Juttner CA: High levels of circulating haemopoietic stem cells in very early remission from acute nonlymphoblastic leukaemia and their collection and cryopreservation. Br J Haematol 58:399, 1984
26. Socinski MA, Cannistra AS, Elias A et al: Granulocyte-

macrophage colony stimulating factor expands the circulating haemopoietic progenitor cell compartment in man. Lancet 1:1194, 1988

27. Duhrsen U, Villeval JL, Boyd J et al: Effects of recombinant human granulocyte colony-stimulating factor on hematopoietic progenitor cells in cancer patients. Blood 72:2074, 1988

28. To LB, Shepperd KM, Haylock DN et al: Single high doses of cyclophosphamide enable the collection of high numbers of hemopoietic stem cells from the peripheral blood. Exp Hematol 18:442, 1990

29. Tavassoli M: Expansion of blood stem cell pool or mobilization of its marrow counterpart? Exp Hematol 21:1205, 1993

30. Bender JG, Lum L, Unverzagt KI et al: Correlation of colony-forming cells, long-term culture initiating cells and CD34+ cells in apheresis products from patients mobilized for peripheral blood progenitors with different regimens. Bone Marrow Transplant 13:479, 1994

31. To LB, Haylock DN, Thorp D et al: The optimization of collection of peripheral blood stem cells for autotransplantation in acute myeloid leukaemia. Bone Marrow Transplant 4:41, 1989

32. Pettengell R, Testa NG, Swindell R et al: Transplantation potential of hematopoietic cells released into the circulation during routine chemotherapy for non-Hodgkin's lymphoma. Blood 82:2239, 1993

33. Ventura GJ, Barlogie B, Hester JP et al: High dose cyclophosphamide, BCNU and VP-16 with autologous blood stem cell support for refractory myeloma. Bone Marrow Transplant 5:265, 1990

34. Kotasek D, Shepherd KM, Sage RE et al: Factors affecting blood stem cell collections following high-dose cyclophosphamide mobilization in lymphoma, myeloma and solid tumors. Bone Marrow Transplant 9:11, 1992

35. Siena S, Bregni M, Brando B et al: Flow cytometry for clinical estimation of circulating hematopoietic progenitors for autologous transplantation in cancer patients. Blood 77:400, 1991

36. Schwartzberg LS, Birch R, Hazelton B et al: Peripheral blood stem cell mobilization by chemotherapy with and without recombinant human granulocyte colony-stimulating factor. J Hematother 1:317, 1992

37. Brugger W, Bross K, Frisch J et al: Mobilization of peripheral blood progenitor cells by sequential administration of interleukin-3 and granulocyte-macrophage colony-stimulating factor following polychemotherapy with etoposide, ifosfamide and cisplatin. Blood 79:1193, 1992

38. Kessinger A, Bierman PJ, Vose JM, Armitage JO:

High-dose cyclophosphamide, carmustine, and etoposide followed by autologous peripheral stem cell transplantation for patients with relapsed Hodgkin's disease. Blood 77:2322, 1991

39. Kessinger A: Reestablishing hematopoiesis after dose-intensive therapy with peripheral stem cells. p. 182. In Armitage JO, Antman KH (eds): High-Dose Cancer Therapy Pharmacology, Hematopoietins, Stem Cells. Williams & Wilkins, Baltimore, 1992

40. Socinski MA, Cannistra SA, Elias A et al: Granulocyte-macrophage colony stimulating factor expands the circulating haemopoietic progenitor cell compartment in man. Lancet 1:1194, 1988

41. Gianni AM, Bregni M, Siena S et al: Rapid and complete hemopoietic reconstitution following combined transplantation of autologous blood and bone marrow cells. A changing role for high dose chemo-radiotherapy? Hematol Oncol 7:139, 1989

42. Haas R, Ho AD, Bredthauer U et al: Successful autologous transplantation of blood stem cells mobilized with recombinant human granulocyte-macrophage colony-stimulating factor. Exp Hematol 18:94, 1990

43. Vora AJ, Toh CH, Peel J, Greaves M: Use of granulocyte colony-stimulating factor (G-CSF) for mobilizing peripheral blood stem cells: risk of mobilizing clonal myeloma cells in patients with bone marrow infiltration. Br J Haematol 86:180, 1994

44. Pettengell GR, Morgenstern GR, Woll PJ et al: Peripheral blood progenitor transplantation in lymphoma and leukemia using a single apheresis. Blood 82:3770, 1993

45. Brugger W, Bross KJ, Glatt M et al: Mobilization of tumor cells and hematopoietic progenitor cells into peripheral blood of patients with solid tumors. Blood 83:636, 1994

46. Takaue Y, Watanabe T, Abe T et al: Experience with peripheral blood stem cell collection for autografts in children with active cancer. Bone Marrow Transplant 10:241, 1992

47. To LB, Dyson PG, Branford AL et al: Peripheral blood stem cells collected in very early remission produce rapid and sustained autologous haemopoietic reconstitution in acute nonlymphoblastic leukaemia. Bone Marrow Transplant 2:103, 1987

48. Handgretinger R, Klingebiel TH, Baden B et al: Stem cell mobilization, collection and transplantation in patients with pediatric tumors. Cancer Res Ther Control 3:43, 1992

49. Hohaus S, Goldschmidt H, Ehrhardt R, Haas R: Successful autografting following myeloablative conditioning therapy with blood stem cells mobilized by

chemotherapy plus rhG-CSF. Exp Hematol 21:508, 1993

50. Widmann FK (ed): Standards for Blood Banks and Transfusion Services. 15th Ed. American Association of Blood Banks, Bethesda, 1993

51. Kessinger A, Schmit-Pokorny K, Smith D, Armitage J: Cryopreservation and infusion of autologous peripheral blood stem cells. Bone Marrow Transplant, suppl. 1, 5:25, 1990

52. Law P, Meryman H: Cryopreservation of human bone marrow grafts. p. 332. In Gee AP (ed): Bone Marrow Processing and Purging: A Practical Guide. CRC Press, Boca Raton, 1991

53. Stiff PJ: Simplified bone marrow cryopreservation using dimethyl sulfoxide and hydroxyethyl starch as cryoprotectants. p. 341. In Gee AP (ed): Bone Marrow Processing and Purging: A Practical Guide. CRC Press, Boca Raton, 1991

54. Jackson J, Kloster T, Welniak L et al: Peripheral blood-derived stem cells can be successfully cryopreserved without using controlled-rate freezing. p. 367. In Worthington-White DA, Gee AP, Gross S (eds): Advances in Bone Marrow Purging and Processing. Wiley-Liss, New York, 1992

55. Stiff PJ, Koester AR, Weidner MK et al: Autologous bone marrow transplantation using unfractionated cells cryopreserved in dimethylsulfoxide and hydroxyethyl starch without controlled-rate freezing. Blood 70:974, 1987

56. Kessinger A, Vose JM, Bierman PJ, Armitage JO: High-dose therapy and autologous peripheral stem cell transplantation for patients with bone marrow metastases and relapsed lymphoma: an alternative to bone marrow purging. Exp Hematol 19:1013, 1991

57. Dooley DC, Law P, Alsop P: A new density-gradient for the separation of large quantities of rosette-positive and rosette-negative cells. Exp Hematol 15:296, 1987

58. Kessinger A, Smith DM, Strandjord SE et al: Allogeneic transplantation of blood-derived, T cell-depleted hemopoietic stem cells after myeloablative treatment in a patient with acute lymphoblastic leukemia. Bone Marrow Transplant 4:643, 1989

59. Weaver CH, Buckner CD, Longin K et al: Syngeneic transplantation with peripheral blood mononuclear cells collected after the administration of recombinant human granulocyte colony-stimulating factor. Blood 82:1981, 1993

60. Russell NH, Hunter A, Rogers S et al: Peripheral blood stem cells as an alternative to marrow for allogeneic transplantation. Lancet 341:1482, 1993

61. Dreger P, Suttorp M, Haferlach T et al: Allogeneic granulocyte colony-stimulating factor-mobilized peripheral blood progenitor cells for treatment of engraftment failure after bone marrow transplantation. Blood 81:1404, 1993

62. Kessinger A: Utilization of peripheral blood stem cells in autotransplantation. Hematol Oncol Clin North Am 7:535, 1993

63. Vose JM, Anderson JR, Kessinger A et al: High-dose chemotherapy and autologous hematopoietic stem cell transplantation for aggressive non-Hodgkin's lymphoma. J Clin Oncol 11:1846, 1993

64. Sharp JG, Kessinger A, Armitage JO et al: Clinical significance of occult tumor cell contamination of hematopoietic harvests in non-Hodgkin's lymphoma and Hodgkin's disease. p. 123. In Zander AR, Barlogie B (eds): Autologous Bone Marrow Transplantation for Hodgkin's Disease, Non-Hodgkin's Lymphoma and Multiple Myeloma. Springer-Verlag, Berlin, 1993

65. Ross AA, Cooper BW, Lazarus HM et al: Detection and viability of tumor cells in peripheral blood stem cell collections from breast cancer patients using immunocytochemical and clonogenic assay techniques. Blood 82:2605, 1993

66. Sharp JG, Kessinger A: Minimal residual disease and blood stem cell transplants. p. 75. In Gale RP, Juttner CA, Henon P (eds): Blood Stem Cell Transplants. Cambridge University Press, Cambridge, 1994

67. Verbik DJ, Jackson JD, Pirruccello SJ et al: Characterization of GM-CSF mobilized human peripheral stem cell harvests obtained from consecutive collections. Blood 82:654a, 1993

68. Verbik DJ, Jackson JD, Pirruccello SJ et al: Augmentation of cytotoxicity of peripheral blood stem cells after in vitro activation with cytokines. Blood 80:433a, 1992

69. Roberts MM, To LB, Gillis D et al: Immune reconstitution following peripheral blood stem cell transplantation, autologous bone marrow transplantation and allogeneic bone marrow transplantation. Bone Marrow Transplant 12:469, 1993

70. Scambia G, Panici PB, Pierelli L et al: Immunological reconstitution after high-dose chemotherapy and autologous blood stem cell transplantation for advanced ovarian cancer. Eur J Cancer 29A:1518, 1993

71. Gordy C, Perry G, Thomas M et al: Immune function and phenotype of peripheral blood and bone marrow stem cell products and peripheral blood reconstitution. J Cell Biochem 18B:100, 1994

72. Weaver CH, Longin K, Buckner CD, Bensinger W: Lymphocyte content in peripheral blood mononu-

clear cells collected after the administration of recombinant human granulocyte colony-stimulating factor. Bone Marrow Transplant 13:411, 1994

73. Broxmeyer HE, Douglas GW, Hangoc G et al: Human umbilical cord blood as a source of transplantable hematopoietic stem/progenitor cells. Proc Natl Acad Sci USA 86:3828, 1989

74. Gluckman E, Broxmeyer HE, Auerbach AD et al: Hematopoietic reconstitution in a patient with Fanconi's anemia by means of umbilical-cord blood from an HLA-identical sibling. N Engl J Med 321:1174, 1989

75. Wagner JE, Broxmeyer HE, Byrd RL et al: Transplantation of umbilical cord blood after myeloablative therapy: analysis of engraftment. Blood 79:1874, 1992

76. Nicol AJ, Hows JM, Bradley BA: Cord Blood transplantation: a practical option? Br J Haematol 87:1, 1994

Chapter 49

Adoptive Immunotherapy

Janice P. Dutcher

Although the humoral component of the immune system has been studied and utilized clinically for years, by both passive and active immunization, the cellular component of the immune system has only recently begun to be utilized for clinical benefit. Cell-mediated immunity functions as both a broad defense and as a specific antigen-driven immune response. Lymphocytes are the effector cells that recognize specific antigens, and they can generate a cellular immune response, utilizing cytokines such as interleukin-2 (IL-2) and γ interferon as mediators of subsequent cellular activation. Like humoral immunity, the cellular response can be highly specific, responding to distinct antigens or portions thereof called epitopes, and effector cells can also have immunologic memory (see Glossary 49-1 for definitions of terms).

Cellular immunity involves the activation of cells that secrete cytokines and activated cytolytic cells that function as effector cells with the capacity to kill targets.[1-3] Cellular immunity is important clinically in a number of ways, including being the major source of the antimicrobial response to agents such as tuberculosis and viruses. Cellular immunity also mediates autoimmune diseases and graft-versus-host disease, and there appears to be endogenous and inducible cellular activity against tumors.[3] Deficiencies in cellular and humoral immunity can lead to immunodeficiency syndromes of varying severity.

Acquired immunodeficiency syndrome (AIDS) represents the most obvious clinical example of the loss of cellular immunity.

Adoptive immunotherapy is the transfer of active immunity, in particular, cellular immunity, either directed against a specific immunogen or broad-based cellular immune activation. This concept is analogous to administration of a specific hyperimmune globulin versus broad-spectrum γ globulin. Clinical studies of adoptive cellular immunotherapy utilize activated autologous immune cells, such as lymphokine-activated killer (LAK) or cytolytic T cells.[4-6] The relationship of immune cell activation to major histocompatibility complex (MHC) identification and the possibility of graft-versus-host reaction makes an allogeneic approach to adoptive immunotherapy much more difficult than in a serologic immune response. Ongoing clinical trials evaluating the efficacy of adoptive immunotherapy are being done primarily as antitumor therapy but also in immunodeficiency diseases.

COMPONENTS OF THE CELLULAR IMMUNE RESPONSE

Lymphocytes represent the major component of the cellular immune response, with T cells functioning as the mediators of cell-mediated immunity. All mature T cells carry the antigen, CD3, and subsets carry

CD4 (helper cells) or CD8 (suppressor/cytotoxic cells) antigens.[1,2] These antigen molecules have several functions, including binding to MHC molecules and serving as cell-cell adhesion molecules. Cytolytic T cells (CD3+, CD8+) can kill tumors in experimental animal systems.[3]

Natural killer (NK) cells are also a component of the cellular immune system and are a subset of lymphocytes found in blood and lymphoid tissues, especially the spleen.[4] NK cells are also identified as large granular lymphocytes and represent a primitive cytotoxic lymphocyte that lacks the specific T-cell receptor for antigen recognition. Phenotypically, they are characterized as CD3−,CD16+ or CD3−, CD56+. NK cells have the ability to kill certain tumor cells and normal cells infected with virus. They are also mediators of antibody-dependent cell-mediated cytotoxicity.

LAK cells are NK cells that have been activated by the cytokine IL-2 and exhibit enhanced and broad antitumor cytotoxicity.[5–7] LAK cells have been generated in the human clinical protocols of adoptive immunotherapy.

The term tumor-infiltrating lymphocytes (TIL) describes the lymphoid cells that are noted histologically to infiltrate tumors.[8] These cells are believed to generate a local antitumor immune response, although there continues to be some debate.[8–12] The characteristics of these cells are different in different tumor types. Some have the antigenic characteristics of T cells, but others have the features of NK cells. Studies are ongoing to adapt these cells to adoptive immunotherapy.

The mechanism for activation of killer cells appears to be by cytokine exposure. Peripheral blood lymphocytes cultured in vitro with IL-2 develop the capacity of becoming LAK cells.[5] Similarly, TILs cultured in vitro for a longer period of time with IL-2 develop enhanced antitumor activation. After such activation, in vitro studies of cytotoxicity using chromium-51 release assays demonstrate killing of more than 95 percent of tumor cells.

Systemic administration of IL-2 to patients produces in vivo activation of killer cells from peripheral blood lymphocytes, which also demonstrate LAK-type killing capability.[13,14] Although there may be enhanced activation through ex vivo lymphocyte culture with IL-2, there is clearly antitumor activity generated in vivo by systemic administration of IL-2. These activated cells can be detected by studying their cytotoxicity against tumor cells; in some cases, persistence of "in vivo cytotoxicity" can be demonstrated long after IL-2 has been administered.

ROLE OF INTERLEUKIN-2

IL-2 is a cytokine produced by T lymphocytes, normally in small quantities, and was initially identified as a substance called T-cell growth factor. It is an essential requirement for the sustained growth of normal lymphocytes in vitro. IL-2 is not usually measurable in normal serum and appears to act locally in lymphoid tissue in both autocrine and paracrine fashion to maintain T-cell function. Through in vitro study of its role in the immune system, it is now clear that not only does IL-2 maintain lymphocyte growth and function but it is a mediator of lymphocyte activation and proliferation. When administered in supraphysiologic doses to animals, it can restore previously suppressed cellular immunologic function. It has also been shown in animal studies that IL-2 exposure can lead to the generation of large quantities of activated killer cells.[5]

IL-2 appears to be the primary activation cytokine for both cytolytic T cells and for the development of LAK antitumor activity.[5,9] This is somewhat surprising because antimicrobial NK cell activity is frequently associated with interferon. However, it has been amply demonstrated that, in the case of LAK activation, the cytokine mediator is IL-2.[16] Nevertheless, the expression of other cytokines is noted in the generalized killer cell antitumor response, including γ interferon, IL-1, and tumor necrosis factor (TNF).[17] Animal and human studies have demonstrated that the administration of IL-2 systemically can generate in vivo killer cell activity and also primes lymphoid cells in vivo for further activation when exposed to IL-2 in vitro.[18–20]

IL-2 can also be administered locally into lymph nodes to generate local activation of cellular immunity. This led to studies of injection of IL-2 directly into lymph nodes that were draining tumors with the hypothesis that this approach would stimulate antigen-stimulated cellular immunity.[21,22]

INITIAL CLINICAL TRIALS

A large body of animal work suggested the potential value of adoptive immunotherapy as a mechanism to control tumors. Initial experimental studies utilized mice injected with tumor cells that predictably had metastatic tumor nodules develop. When these animals were then treated with IL-2 with or without IL-2-activated syngeneic splenic lymphocytes, the growth of tumor nodules could be reduced or eradicated. Animals with immunogenic tumors often responded to IL-2 alone, but animals with nonimmunogenic tumors required infusions of both IL-2 plus activated killer cells to achieve tumor reduction.[13,18,19] Therefore, this approach entered human clinical investigation.

The initial human studies, in patients with metastatic renal cell cancer and melanoma, were designed to mimic the animal studies. Human tumors are believed to be analogous to the nonimmunogenic tumors of animals, despite the often observed host "immune response" described in the above two tumor types. The clinical trials began with infusions of IL-2 systemically to activate cellular immunity in vivo. IL-2 was given in a variety of doses and schedules, often exposing the patient to maximally tolerated toxicity.[23] These toxicities include hypotension-requiring pressors, tachypnea, pulmonary infiltrates, oliguria, and arrhythmias. They are managed by withholding doses of IL-2 until improvement; once the drug is removed, they resolve very quickly. There have been no long-term sequelae, although, in early studies, patients did have cardiac ischemia and myocardial infarctions and even died.

More recently, however, the incidence of serious complications has diminished. This is a result of both greater experience on the part of a number of treating physicians and a number of changes in the treatment protocol. The most significant change in terms of preventing cardiac toxicity is the requirement for prescreening for cardiopulmonary disease and eliminating patients with occult coronary artery disease, who may not tolerate moderate hypotension and tachycardia, from high-dose IL-2 therapy. Such patients may tolerate lower dose regimens. In addition, the elimination of ex vivo-activated LAK cells from the regimen has markedly reduced the acute pulmonary toxicity that resulted directly from the infusion of these cells with accumulation in the pulmonary capillary bed. Although IL-2 itself may induce a capillary leak in the pulmonary vasculature, this effect is considerably more manageable and rarely leads to life-threatening toxicity. Thus, the current approach to high-dose IL-2 is considerably safer than that used in earlier reports.

Within 48 hours of completing the IL-2 therapy, patients routinely had a marked peripheral blood lymphocytosis develop with white blood cell counts in the 20,000 range and the lymphocyte count being greater than 50 percent. During this "rebound" lymphocytosis, patients underwent lympocytopheresis to remove preactivated lymphocytes, which were then placed in large-volume tissue culture systems and exposed to additional IL-2. This process yielded a high volume of LAK cells with broad antitumor cytotoxicity, which routinely demonstrated killing against more than 95 percent of targets in chromium-51 release cytotoxicity assays.[24] When these cells reached maximal activation, they were reinfused into the patients with additional IL-2. The cells generated during this process were subjected to intense scrutiny, and there was initial debate as to the origin of the "killer" cell. However, the consensus appears to be that this process primarily develops an NK-derived LAK cell with broad antitumor cytotoxicity and, to a lesser degree, cytotoxic T cells.[13,15,20]

Other types of culture techniques generated cells known as adherent LAK cells, which seemed to expand faster than nonadherent cells and grew in slightly different culture conditions.[25] The cytotoxic activity appeared to be similar, although animal studies suggested enhanced activity. In addition, others have attempted to generate specific killer cells by activating cells derived from the lymph nodes that drain the area of the tumor.

Surprisingly, these initial studies yielded some dramatic clinical responses, in patients with metastatic, chemotherapy-refractory diseases such as melanoma and renal cell cancer. In these two diseases, approximately 20 percent of patients demonstrated greater than 50 percent shrinkage of total tumor volume, and some (5 percent) patients had complete eradication of metastatic cancer.[26-32] The median survival of complete responders has not been reached at 5 to 8 years of follow-up, and 75 to 80

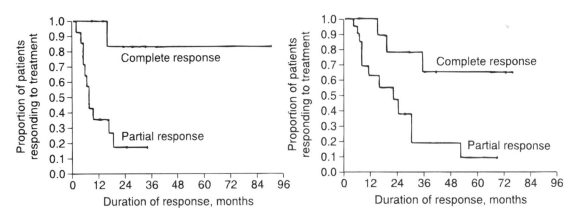

Fig. 49-1 The duration of complete and partial responses in patients with metastatic melanoma (left) and metastatic renal cell cancer (right) treated with high-dose bolus IL-2, as assessed in June 1993. (From Rosenberg et al.,[32] with permission.)

percent of complete responders continue disease-free at more than 8 years since initial treatment (Fig. 49-1 and 49-2 and Table 49-1). Figures 49-1 and 49-2 present long-term follow-up data from studies of IL-2 therapy alone, completed at the National Cancer Institute.[32] Attempts to identify particular pa-

tient characteristics of responders have not yet been successful enough to make therapeutic recommendations (Table 49-2).

Once activity was demonstrated, clarification of the mechanism and role of the therapeutic components was initiated. The role of ex vivo activation of

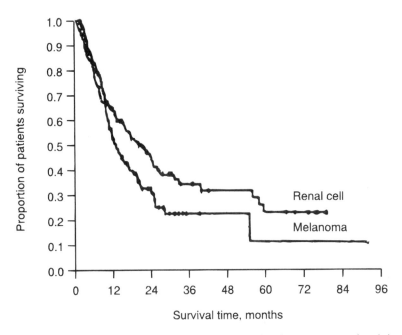

Fig. 49-2 Survival of patients with metastatic melanoma and renal cell cancer treated with high-dose bolus IL-2, as assessed in June 1993. (From Rosenberg et al.,[32] with permission.)

Table 49-1. Summary of Results of Interleukin-2 Therapy in Patients With Renal Cell Cancer and Melanoma

Regimen	Response Rate	Complete Response Rate	Duration
High-dose IL-2			
+ LAK cells	15–25%	4–6%	Up to 8+ yrs
alone	15–25%	4–6%	Up to 7+ yrs
Moderate-dose IL-2			
Continuous infusion	15–25%	4–6%	Up to 2+ yrs
Subcutaneous	15–25%	3–5%	Up to 2+ yrs
High-dose IL-2 + TIL	25–50% of those cultured Represents 50% of those entered (50% of 50% = 25%)		NA[a]

Abbreviations: NA, not available; IL-2, interleukin-2; TIL, tumor-infiltrating lymphocytes.

[a] Note: Partial responders to high-dose IL-2 have a median duration of response of 20+ months and often respond to retreatment. Data are not yet available for this in lower dose regimens. The median response duration of complete responders to high-dose regimens has not yet been reached. An additional 25% of treated patients remain stable for 1–3+ years.

LAK cells was debated. Subsequently, data from the initial National Cancer Institute and a multicenter comparative trial suggested that there was no difference in response rate between patients treated with IL-2 with or without ex vivo activated LAK cells.[33,34] The question of response duration has not yet been addressed. However, as a result of the lack of response difference and because of the increased cost, labor and greater toxicity with the addition of ex vivo-activated LAK cells, it is now recommended that this approach utilize simply IL-2 alone, relying on in vivo LAK activation for the cellular antitumor response. IL-2 is currently the approved treatment for metastatic renal cell cancer.

Much work is yet to be done to determine the optimal dose and schedule for this agent and the potential for its activity in other diseases. Immunologic activation occurs in all patients, and the data to date do not allow us to predict responders to this therapeutic approach based on cellular immune parameters. The relative role of the various cellular components continues to be debated.

TECHNOLOGY OF LAK AND TIL PRODUCTION

The intensity of effort to develop technology to generate large quantities of activated lymphocytes has had some very positive spinoffs. Initially, LAK cell production was a manual operation that was both costly and labor intensive. Each leukapheresis collection of peripheral blood lymphocytes required liters of tissue culture medium, culturing at a concentration of 1.5 to 3.0×10^9 cells/L of medium with the addition of IL-2.[24,35] The manual process, repeated for each leukapheresis, required 0.5 day of technician time. Rather quickly, automated cellular processing was attempted, borrowing from work done in processing marrow for transplantation. Several technical protocols arose for the preparation of LAK cells for culture and for harvesting them after the 72-hour IL-2 culture period. Some utilized the apheresis equipment itself; others used blood cell washers to process the leukapheresis product.[36,37] The latter system was particularly helpful in concentrating the large volumes of culture material utilized

Table 49-2. Clinical Features of Renal Cell Cancer and Melanoma Associated With Response to Adoptive Immunotherapy

Site of disease: Lymph node, lung, soft tissue
Performance status: 0 ≫ 1
Factors evaluated and *not* correlating with response:
  Size of tumor
  Prior nephrectomy
  Number of lymphokine-activated killer cells generated
  HLA-DR expression on tumor
  Phenotype of killer cells
  Types of cytokines released
  Level of in vitro cytotoxicity

in LAK generation and in providing a volume reduction of the cell product to be infused. Even with the automated systems, there were open steps, and each collection and processing required microbiologic verification of sterility before administration (Gram stain was used for screening, but all were subsequently cultured). All serial collections were also tested for generation of cytotoxic activity.

More recently, in the development of technology for the production of TIL cells, which requires considerably longer culture times, small, continuous-flow cell culture generators have been developed.[38,39] These maintain the lymphocytes in a closed system while renewed culture material continuously flows through to provide nourishment and a source of IL-2. Modified versions of these are also being studied to attempt to generate highly specific lymphocyte cultures (i.e., CD8+ cells only).[40] These systems are important for cell culture in gene therapy studies, and some are currently also being re-adapted to use in long-term bone marrow culture and stem cell generation.

CELULLAR SPECIFICITY

Although encouraged by the initial success and activity of IL-2 plus LAK cells as an antitumor approach, there was concern that the LAK cell was too primitive and nonspecific for optimal tumor kill. Therefore, great interest has remained in isolating and utilizing a more specific killer cell. However, the exact characteristics of such a cell are yet to be defined. Some studies indicate that the TILs noted in some immunoresponsive tumors represent this type of specific cell; they are immunized to the tumor by direct contact. A great deal of effort has been expended to characterize these cells and their activity and to develop techniques to study them clinically.[10,11,40–42]

Therefore, the next generation of antitumor studies in adoptive immunotherapy moved to the production and study of TIL cells. Of interest is that TILs from melanomas are almost exclusively cytotoxic T cells but only demonstrate their cytotoxicity after ex vivo culture with IL-2.[9] TILs from head and neck cancer appear to have the immunologic phenotype of LAK cells rather than T cells.[13] TILs from renal cell cancers bear properties of NK cells, and some studies suggest that they are deficient in in

vitro studies in autologous antitumor activity.[11] Studies are ongoing to determine whether these cells can be revitalized with ex vivo culture with IL-2. Other studies have shown that a small percentage of the TILs recovered have enhanced antitumor activity, and work is ongoing to develop methods to expand this specific population of TIL.[40]

Clinical trials utilizing TILs began with the extraction of these cells from tumors and long-term ex vivo culture with IL-2 plus tumor cells to expand, immunize, and activate such cells. Clinical results of studies of TIL infusions in conjunction with IL-2 yielded apparently higher response rates among patients who were treated; among all patients entered, however, the overall response rate was no different than with IL-2 plus LAK cells.[43–45] There was a 50 percent fall off for patients whose TIL cells did not grow ex vivo. Thus, the current assessment is that TIL plus IL-2 studies are equivalent to LAK plus IL-2 studies, which are equivalent to IL-2 alone (Table 49-1).[33,34,43–45]

The interest in developing and characterizing TIL continues, however, with the goal of using these highly specific cells as messengers of additional anti-tumor agents. Studies of radiolabeled TIL have demonstrated localization to tumor and survival of the cells in vivo.[46]

ONGOING INVESTIGATIONAL STUDIES

The use of specific immunologic cells as vehicles for antitumor agents is under active investigation. Areas being developed include attachment of monoclonal antibodies, which add to the specificity; attachment of toxins or radioisotopes; and insertion of genes that encode for antitumor cytokines, which are then expressed at the site of the tumor. In the latter, called gene therapy, the cell is transfected with a gene for an antitumor cytokine, which then travels to the tumor by way of the immunized lymphocyte. Expression of the gene is then a local phenomenon, with the goal of producing high concentrations of the antitumor cytokine at the site of the tumor and not systemically, yielding a highly specific and localized immune response. Preliminary studies have been accomplished to demonstrate the safety of using the viral vector to insert the gene, and now studies are ongoing using marker genes.[47] Ongoing studies to insert the gene for TNF into TIL and study the antitumor response have begun at the Surgery Branch of the National Cancer Institute (Rosenberg SA, personal communication). Studies that are proposed will insert the TNF gene into preimmunized TIL or peripheral blood lymphocytes and monitor the trafficking of these cells to the tumor with the potential for a local antitumor response. Other groups are pursuing this approach with other transfected genes, including the gene for IL-2.

Interestingly, the development of gene therapy has led adoptive immunotherapy full circle. The initial goal of the generation of long-term lymphocyte culture with IL-2 was to provide a source of immune cells for immune reconstitution, in clinical situations such as AIDS. Early studies were unsuccessful because they preceded effective antiviral therapy and the lymphocytes were killed by the virus. Now this approach is being revisited in conjunction with more effective antiviral therapy.

Similarly, with gene therapy and the ability to transfect lymphocytes with genes safely, an example of immune reconstitution has already been achieved, in children with immunodeficiency due to the absence of the gene for adenine deaminase (ADA).[48] Two children have had their immunodeficiency successfully reconstituted by production of autologous lymphocytes transfected with the ADA gene, which then has produced the missing enzyme.

The ability to generate such cells in culture now provides a tool and a modality for further innovative studies. Ongoing investigational studies will utilize these technologies. Therefore, the technology to produce, grow safely, and expand both peripheral blood lymphocytes and TILS will need to become more standardized and automated. Some of the "cell generators" (in vitro system for long-term culture of lymphocytes or stem cells) have clearly begun to be developed with this in mind.

Other investigative approaches with the goal of utilizing the cellular immune system have directed their approach to identification of the putative "tumor-specific" antigen, planning to utilize the epitope to induce specifically an enhanced cellular and serologic immune response. One such series of investigations is identifying unusual proteins in the mucin secreted by certain adeocarcinomas. Immune responses to these have shown MHC-restricted and unrestricted recognition of mucin by T cells. Such T cells can then be isolated from regional lymph nodes and expanded in vitro.[49]

Another approach is the use of bispecific monoclonal antibodies, which bind to the tumor and to the immunologically active cell and thus help mediate cellular cytotoxicity. Ring et al.[50] developed one such molecule, which binds to the Fc fragment on the surface of T cells and also binds to ERBB2, a cell surface receptor found only on tumor cells that is encoded by an oncogene. The hypothesis is that one can bind the antibody with specificity for certain tumors that carry this receptor to T cells, and this will then direct cytotoxic T cells to the tumor. Phase I clinical trials are ongoing.

Both of the trials discussed above involve ex vivo manipulation of autologous lymphocytes. One aim is to isolate immunized regional lymphocytes and reinfuse them when they have enhanced activation, and the other is to manipulate the lymphocytes to bind to the bispecific antibody. To investigate the promise of these innovative ideas fully, the studies will rely on the technology developed in the processing of TIL and LAK cells. Thus, the ideas for enhancing and studying cellular immunity rely on the ability to obtain, grow, and study the cells themselves.

FUTURE DIRECTIONS

Adoptive immunotherapy, the transfer of ex vivo-activated cellular immunity, by expanding cells involved in the antitumor immune response, has allowed us to study the potential efficacy of this approach. The goals for future studies, therefore, to harness the cellular immune response, include attempts to enhance specificity and efficacy while reducing toxicity. The appropriate way to utilize this system, including the cytokines and the activated cells, clinically, is still the subject of much discussion and clinical investigation. Adoptive immunotherapy approaches are changing and evolving weekly, which requires rapid changes in technology and laboratory expertise. Although some approaches have not been as successful as hoped, the reproducible demonstration of antitumor response and enhanced survival should encourage research in this difficult area to continue. Similarly, the rapid development of gene therapy technology will likely lead to applications in therapy of other diseases in addition to cancer, including immunodeficiencies and inborn errors. Offshoots of this technology are likely to lead to progress in our understanding of the immune system and its role in cancer, AIDS, and autoimmune diseases. Our development of research in cellular immunity has opened a vast area of both investigation and technology. This continues to be a highly productive endeavor scientifically, and the clinical results will follow.

REFERENCES

1. Bierer BE, Sleckman BP, Ratnofsky SE, Burakoff SJ: The biologic roles of CD2, CD4 and CD8 in T-cell activation. Annu Rev Immunol 7:579, 1989

2. Parnes JR: Molecular biology and function of CD4 and CD8. Adv Immunol 44:265, 1989

3. Kupfer A, Singer SJ: Cell biology of cytotoxic and helper T-cell functions. Annu Rev Immunol 7:309, 1989

4. Trinchier G: Biology of natural killer cells. Adv Immunol 47:187, 1989

5. Grimm EA, Mazumder A, Zhang HZ, Rosenberg SA: The lymphokine activated killer cell phenomenon: lysis of NK resistant fresh solid tumor cells by IL-2 activated autologous human peripheral blood lymphocytes. J Exp Med 155:1823, 1982

6. Grimm EA, Ramsey KM, Mazumder A et al: Lymphokine-activated killer cell phenomenon: II. The precursor phenotype is serologically distinct from peripheral T lymphocytes, memory CTL, and NK cells. J Exp Med 157:884, 1983

7. Yang JC, Mule JJ, Rosenberg SA: Characterization of the murine lymphokine-activated killer precursor and effector cell. Surg Forum 36:408, 1985

8. Yron I, Wood TA, Spiess P, Rosenberg SA: In vitro growth of murine T cells: V. The isolation and growth of lymphoid cells infiltrating syngeneic solid tumors. J Immunol 125:238, 1980

9. Itoh K, Tilden AB, Balch CM: Interleukin 2 activation of cytotoxic T-lymphocytes infiltrating into human metastatic melanomas. Cancer Res 46:3011, 1986

10. Itoh K, Hayakawa K, von Eschenbach AC, Morita T: Natural killer cells in human renal cancer. p. 95. In Klein EA, Bukowski RM, Finke JH (eds): Renal Cell Carcinoma. Marcel Dekker, New York, 1993

11. Finke JH, Rayman P, Edinger M et al: Characterization of tumor-infiltrating lymphocyte lines derived from renal cell carcinoma. p. 115. In Klein EA, Bukow-

ski RM, Finke JH (eds): Renal Cell Cancinoma. Marcel Dekker, New York, 1993

12. Heo DS, Whiteside TL, Johnson JT et al: Long-term interleukin-2-dependent growth and cytotoxic activity of tumor-infiltrating lymphocytes from human squamous cell carcinomas of the head and neck. Cancer Res 47:6353, 1987

13. Ettinghausen SE, Lipford EH, Mule JJ, Rosenberg SA: Systemic administration of recombinant interleukin-2 stimulates in vivo lymphoid cell proliferation in tissues. J Immunol 135:1488, 1985

14. Walewski J, Paietta E, Dutcher JP, Wiernik PH: Evaluation of natural killer and lymphokine-activated killer (LAK) cell activity in vivo in patients treated with high dose interleukin-2 and adoptive transfer of autologous LAK cells. J Cancer Res Clin Oncol 115:170, 1989

15. Grimm EA, Robb RJ, Roth JA et al: Lymphokine-activated killer cell phenomenon: III. Evidence that IL-2 is sufficient for direct activation of peripheral blood lymphocytes into lymphokine-activated killer cells. J Exp Med 158:1356, 1983

16. Damle NK, Doyle LV: Interleukin-2 activated human killer lymphocytes: lack of involvement of interferon in the development of IL2-activated killer cells. Br J Cancer 40:519, 1987

17. Gemlo BT, Palladino MA, Jaffe HS et al: Circulating cytokines in patients with metastatic cancer treated with recombinant interleukin-2 and lymphokine-activated killer cells. Cancer Res 48:5864, 1988

18. Mule JJ, Shu S, Schwarz SL, Rosenberg SA: Adoptive immunotherapy of established pulmonary metastases with LAK cells and recombinant interleukin-2. Science 225:1487, 1984

19. Mule JJ, Shu S, Rosenberg SA: The anti-tumor efficacy of lymphokine-activated killer cells and recombinant interleukin-2 in vivo. J Immunol 135:646, 1985

20. Ettinghausen SE, Lipford EH, Mule JJ, Rosenberg SA: Recombinant interleukin-2 stimulates in vivo proliferation of adoptively transferred lymphokine activated killer (LAK) cells. J Immunol 135:3623, 1985

21. Forni G, Cavallo GP, Giovarelli M et al: Tumor immunotherapy by local injection of IL-2 and non-reactive lymphocytes. Experimental and clinical results. Prog Exp Tumor Res 32:187, 1988

22. Vlock DR, Snyder C, Johnson J et al: Phase Ib trial of the effect of peritumoral and intranodal injections of interleukin-2 in patients with advanced squamous cell carcinoma of the head and neck: an Eastern Cooperative Oncology Group trial. J Immunother 15:134, 1994

23. Margolin K, Rayner AA, Hawkins M et al: Toxicity of

interleukin-2 and lymphokine-activated killer (LAK) cell therapy. J Clin Oncol 7:486, 1989

24. Boldt DH, Mills BJ, Gemlo BT et al: Laboratory correlates of adoptive immunotherapy with recombinant interleukin-2 and lymphokine-activated killer cells in humans. Cancer Res 48:4409, 1988

25. Melder RJ, Whiteside TL, Vujanovic NL et al: A new approach to generating antitumor effectors for adoptive immunotherapy using human adherent lymphokine-activated killer cells. Cancer Res 48:3461, 1988

26. Rosenberg SA, Lotze MT, Muul LM et al: A progress report on the treatment of 157 patients with advanced cancer using lymphokine activated killer cells and interleukin-2 or high dose interleukin-2 alone. N Engl J Med 316:889, 1987

27. West WH, Tauer KW, Yannelli JR et al: Constant infusion recombinant interleukin-2 in adoptive immunotherapy of advanced cancer. N Engl J Med 316:898, 1987

28. Fisher RI, Coltman CA, Doroshow JH et al: Phase II clinical trial of interleukin II plus lymphokine activated killer cells in metastatic renal cancer. Ann Intern Med 108:518, 1988

29. Dutcher JP, Creekmore S, Weiss GR et al: A phase II study of high dose interleukin-2 and lymphokine activated killer cells in patients with metastatic malignant melanoma. J Clin Oncol 7:477, 1989

30. Schoof DD, Gramolini BA, Davidson DL et al: Adoptive immunotherapy of human cancer using low-dose recombinant interleukin 2 and lymphokine-activated killer cells. Cancer Res 48:5007, 1988

31. Weiss GR, Margolin KA, Aronson FR et al: A randomized phase II trial of continuous infusion interleukin-2 or bolus injection interleukin-2 plus lymphokine-activated killer cells for advanced renal cell carcinoma. J Clin Oncol 10:275, 1992

32. Rosenberg SA, Yang JC, Topalian SL et al: Treatment of 283 consecutive patients with metastatic melanoma or renal cell cancer using high-dose bolus interleukin-2. JAMA 271:907, 1994

33. McCabe MS, Stablein D, Hawkins MJ: The modified group C experience—phase III randomized trials of IL-2 vs IL-2/LAK in advanced renal cell carcinoma and advanced melanoma. Proc Am Soc Clin Oncol 10:213, 1991

34. Rosenberg SA, Lotze MT, Yang JC et al: Prospective randomized trial of high-dose interleukin-2 alone or in conjunction with lymphokine-activated killer cells for the treatment of patients with advanced cancer. J Natl Cancer Inst 85:622, 1993

35. Muul LM, Director EP, Hyatt CL, Rosenberg SA: Large scale production of human lymphokine activated killer cells for use in adoptive immunotherapy. J Immunol Methods 88:265, 1986

36. Aebersold P, Carter CS, Hyatt C et al: A simplified automated procedure for generation of human lymphokine-activated killer cells for use in clinical trials. J Immunol Methods 112:1, 1988

37. McMannis J, Paietta E, Mills B et al: Automated procedure for bulk culture of human lymphokine activated killer (LAK) cells. FASEB J 2:688, 1988

38. Alter BJ, Ochoa AC, Gruenberg ML et al: The growth of cells with LAK activity in an automated tissue culture system (Acusyst P). p. 301. In Truitt RL, Gale RP, Bortin MM (eds): Progress in Clinical and Biological Research. Alan R Liss, New York, 1987

39. Tanji M, Tanaka T, Taguchi T: The culture of LAK cells with hollow-fiber bioreactor. Biotherapy (Tokyo) 2:361, 1988

40. Figlin R, Pierce W, deKernion J et al: The biology and clinical activity of CD8+ tumor infiltrating lymphocytes in patients with metastatic renal cell carcinoma. Proc Am Soc Clin Oncol 12:288, 1993

41. Topalian SL, Muul LM, Solomon D et al: Expansion of human tumor infiltrating lymphocytes for use in immunotherapy trials. J Immunol Methods 102:127, 1987

42. Whiteside TL, Heo S, Adler A et al: Expansion of tumor-infiltrating lymphocytes from human solid tumors in interleukin-2. Fed Proc 46:1341, 1987

43. Rosenberg SA, Packard BS, Aebersold PM et al: Use of tumor-infiltrating lymphocytes and interleukin-2 in the immunotherapy of patients with metastatic melanoma: a preliminary report. N Engl J Med 319:1676, 1988

44. Topalian SL, Solomon D, Avis FP et al: Immunotherapy of patients with advanced cancer using tumor-infiltrating lymphocytes and recombinant interleukin-2: a pilot study. J Clin Oncol 6:839, 1988

45. Rosenberg SA, Schwarz SL, Spiess PJ: Combination immunotherapy for cancer: synergistic antitumor interactions of interleukin-2, alfa interferon and tumor-infiltrating lymphocytes. J Natl Cancer Inst 80:1393, 1988

46. Fisher B, Packard BS, Read EJ et al: Tumor localization of adoptively transferred indium-111 labeled tumor-infiltrating lymphocytes in patients with metastatic melanoma. J Clin Oncol 7:250, 1989

47. Culver K, Cornetta K, Morgan R et al: Lymphocytes as cellular vehicles for gene therapy in mouse and man. Proc Natl Acad Sci U S A 88:3155, 1991

48. Blaese RM, Culver KW, Chang L et al: Treatment of severe combined immunodeficiency (SCID) due to adenine deaminase deficiency with CD34+ selected autologous peripheral blood cells transduced with a human ADA gene. Hum Gene Ther 4:521, 1993

49. Gendler SJ, Burchell JM, Duhig T et al: Cloning of a partial cDNA encoding differentiation and tumor-associated mucin glycoproteins expressed by human mammary epithelium. Proc Natl Acad Sci U S A 84: 6060, 1987

50. Ring DB, Shi T, Hsieh MA ST et al: Targeted lysis of human breast cancer cells by human effector cells armed with bispecific antibody 2B1 (anti-c-erbB-2/anti-Fc G receptor III). In Ceriani R (ed): Proceedings of the International Workshop on Monoclonal Antibodies and Breast Cancer. San Francisco 11/5–6/90. Plenum, New York, 1991

Appendix 49-1
Glossary

T cell T lymphocyte without subset definition

CD4+ T cell Helper T cell

CD8+ T cell Suppressor/cytotoxic T cell

NK cell Natural killer cell: primitive cellular surveillance; less MHC restriction than T cells

LAK cell Lymphokine-activated killer cell: an activated derivative cell of the natural killer cell lineage

A-LAK cells Adherent LAK cells: adhere to in vitro culture plates; may have differential activity compared with LAK

TIL Tumor-infiltrating lymphocyte: histologically observed to be infiltrating tumors; may be T cell; may be NK cell

IL-2 Interleukin-2: T-cell growth factor produced by T lymphocytes; allows growth of lymphoid cells in vitro; expands T cell, NK cell, LAK cell, and TIL cell populations in vitro

γIFN "Immune interferon": cytokine produced by macrophages during IL-2 therapy; synergistic with IL-2 in antitumor studies; approved for therapy of combined immunodeficiency syndrome

TNF Tumor necrosis factor: cytokine produced by natural killer cells during IL-2 therapy; mediator of hypotension in sepsis and IL-2 therapy; has direct antitumor activity when administered in animals

MHC Major histocompatibility complex: the protein structure on the surface of cells that provides specificity for immune recognition of the cell.

Chapter 50

Gene Therapy

John A. Zaia and Priscilla Yam

DEFINITIONS AND SCOPE OF GENE THERAPY

The hematology community is familiar with successful attempts to cure selected acquired or inborn genetic abnormalities by the use of bone marrow transplantation (BMT) intended to provide donor cells for correction of a specific chemical or cellular defect. Thus, for the past two decades, BMT has been used to treat diseases ranging from Philadelphia chromosome-positive leukemias, thalassemia, and sickle cell disease to rarer conditions such as combined immune deficiency disorders, storage diseases, white cell disorders, and osteoporosis.[1] In the broader sense of the word, this is therapy directed at genetic diseases, but it is not considered *gene therapy*. Gene therapy is defined as the introduction of new genetic material into a cell for the purposes of correcting a specific disease. This also needs to be distinguished from *somatic cell therapy*, which is the introduction of ex vivo processed cells, not genetically manipulated, for the treatment of a specific disease. This is not just a semantic distinction because the regulatory aspects of patient treatment make a clear distinction between gene and somatic cell therapy.

Gene therapy was originally thought to be a potential method for correction of inborn errors of metabolism or of primary immune deficiencies such as those noted in Table 50-1. Until 1990, gene therapy seemed to be merely an intellectual pursuit that might have promise at some unknown future time. However, with the rapid development of gene transfer methodology in the mid-1980s, and particularly with the demonstration of safety of retrovirus-based gene transfer in animals, it became possible to introduce these new therapeutic approaches effectively into the clinic.[2-7] The dawn of the era of gene therapy technically began with the use of genetic marking of lymphocytes used in somatic cell therapy in cancer treatment.[8,9] A marker gene is one that encodes an enzyme or other protein that can be detected by either functional or antigenic detection methods and is used for tracking the genetically altered cell (see section on marker studies). The first therapeutic use of gene therapy followed soon after this with the successful introduction of the adenosine deaminase (ADA) gene into two children with severe combined immunodeficiency (SCID).[10,11] These pioneering clinical applications of gene therapy have unleashed a relative abundance of research protocols designed either to study the effects of various forms of somatic cell therapy using genetic markers or to investigate the safety of treating other inborn genetic abnormalities, cancer, or acquired abnormalities such as acquired immunodeficiency syndrome (AIDS).

The advent of gene therapy brings with it a new technology and discipline which promises to trans-

Table 50-1. Candidate Diseases for Gene Therapy

Defective Gene	Disease
Inborn errors of metabolism	
Arginosuccinate synthetase	Citrullinemia
αL-Fucosidase	Fucosidosis
Glucocerebrosidase	Gaucher's disease
β-Glucuronidase	Mucopolysaccharidosis type VII
αL-Iduronidase	Mucopolysaccharidosis type I
Ornithine transcarbamylase	Hyperammonemia
Sphingomyelinase	Niemann-Pick disease
Phenylalanine hydroxylase	Phenylketonuria
Other single-gene mutations	
α₁-Antitrypsin	Emphysema
Cystic fibrosis transmembrane regulator	Cystic fibrosis
Low-density lipoprotein receptor	Familial hypercholesterolemia
Dystrophin	Muscular dystrophy
Immunohematologic disease	
Adenosine deaminase	Severe combined immunodeficiency
CD-18	Leukocyte adhesion deficiency
Factor IX	Hemophilia B
Factor VIII	Hemophilia A
β-Globin	Sick cell anemia, thalassemia
Purine nucleoside phosphorylase	Severe combined immunodeficiency

form certain aspects of medical practice.[12] This will have a particularly significant effect on the blood bank community because cell collection, cryopreservation, and quality control will undoubtedly become the responsibility of this group. It is for this reason that persons involved with this area of medicine should become active participants in this developing field. Thus, this chapter is designed to review the current status of gene therapy and to encourage those with blood banking experience to explore this new field.

METHODS OF GENE TRANSFER

Virus Vectors

The agent used for genetic transfer to and alteration of a cell is called a *vector,* and, just as in nature, the vectors used for gene transfer have been viruses, which can package and target genetic material to cells. Although it is possible to use direct transfer of DNA into mammalian cells, a process called *transfection,* in general, DNA is transferred by a viral infection, a process called *transduction.* Viruses not only efficiently package and stabilize DNA, but they also facilitate targeting to specific cells or organs for which the virus is tropic. Thus, a variety of viruses have been used in the initial attempts at gene transfer, and vector selection has been based on the efficiency of DNA integration into the host genome and on the tropism of the vector for the target tissue. Viruses, of course, have constitutive genes that facilitate virus replication and spread, and this can produce disease. The goal of vector development is to eliminate the pathogenic elements of a virus genome by making a recombinant virus that cannot replicate. To accomplish this, artificial virus packaging systems are used that can produce infectious virions, containing the gene of interest and other genes necessary for DNA integration but lacking genes that are necessary for replication. Such recombinant viruses are referred to as *replication incompetent.*[13] With this in mind, recombinant vectors have been made from a variety of native viruses (Table 50-2). At the present

Table 50-2. Gene Transfer Vectors

Recombinant viruses
Murine RV
Other retroviruses (e.g., HIV-1 and Harvey RV)
Adenovirus
Adenoassociated virus
Herpesvirus (e.g., HSV and VSV)
Poliovirus
Vaccinia virus
Synthetic vector
Liposomes-DNA complex
Polylysine-antibody DNA complex
Protein receptor-DNA complex
Accelerated particle-DNA
Plasmid-DNA

Abbreviations: RV, retrovirus; HIV-1, human immunodeficiency virus type 1; HS, herpes simplex virus; VZV, varicella-zoster virus.

time, three viral vectors have been approved for human gene therapy: Moloney murine leukemia virus, adenovirus, and adenoassociated virus (AAV).

Retrovirus-Based Vectors

Retroviruses are a family of enveloped, double-stranded RNA viruses that utilize virion-associated reverse transcriptase to make DNA copies of the virus genome and then integrate this into the host genome.[14] Retrovirus infections in various animal species are associated with a variety of hematologic diseases ranging from leukemia/lymphoma to anemia to immunodeficiency. Despite this, retroviruses were considered to be potentially ideal vectors for gene therapy because of their ability to integrate into a host genome permanently and produce stable transduction of cells.[15]

Retroviral gene integration occurs presumably as a relatively random event. It is possible that such integration can disturb normal cell function and might even lead to disruption of important control mechanisms that regulate cell replication. Thus, retroviral integration can lead to oncogenic change in cells, and this is the major concern regarding the safety of exogenous gene introduction by retroviruses.[6,16] There is also the possibility that the original *gag/pol/env* functions of the virion can recombine with the portion of the retrovirus that contains the packaging element and produce replication competent retrovirus (RCR).[16] It has been shown that, when RCR is present in a vector used to transduce hematopoietic cells in nonhuman primates, subsequent lymphoma can result.[17,18] This process is thought to develop only when there is a chronic retroviremia and eventual random integration and disruption of genetic control at sites that are linked to cell growth. Thus, the regulatory agencies involved in ensuring the safety of retroviral vectors are most concerned with a demonstration that clinical grade vectors lack RCR.[6] It should be realized, however, that primate studies suggest that both high-grade RCR exposure and immunosuppression are necessary for development of retrovirus-induced neoplasm.[18,19] Based on these animal studies, it is estimated that a severely immunosuppressed person would need to be exposed to 2×10^7 focus-forming units (ffu) of RCR, and this is well within the detection range for quality

control (QC) determinations for vector production lots.[19,20] If we assume that RCR exposure is less than that detectible by such QC tests (1 RCR ffu/ml), then the degree of risk for new cancer development has been estimated to be 0.0000003, a risk substantially less than the risk of nearly 10 percent associated with severe immunosuppression itself.[21] It is important to realize that this vector was not developed for human use without a vast amount of safety testing. Improved methods have now appeared to ensure the safety and efficacy of transduction using retrovirus-based vectors.[22,23]

The process of retroviral vector production is shown in Figure 50-1.[24–26] A helper virus genome is modified by altering the packaging signal (ψ), which permits the introduction into a tissue culture cell of the *gag*, *pol*, and *env* portions of the retroviral genome.[22,27–30] This cell now lacks the critical packaging signal for putting viral elements together into the form of infectious virions. The gene of interest is then introduced into a modified retrovirus-based DNA plasmid that contains the normal packaging signal but lacks the other critical elements necessary for virus replication.[24,29] The resultant producer cell is able to package the new gene into virions, but, without *gag*, *pol*, and *env*, these virions cannot undergo subsequent replication. Nevertheless, these replication-incompetent retroviruses are infectious and can transduce cells and cause integration of the transmitted gene.[24]

Successful retroviral cell transduction requires entry of the recombinant retrovirus into the target cell, which is a receptor-mediated event.[15] It is possible that the efficiency of retroviral transduction in certain cells is limited by the absence of such a putative receptor. In addition, successful integration requires that the cells are replicating. This has serious implications for transduction of primitive stem cells, especially hematopoietic cells necessary for successful marrow transplantation. The use of growth factors for the induction of such replication can induce differentiation of uncommitted stem cells, potentially resulting in limited transduction of marrow elements. Despite these concerns, Brenner et al.[31,32] showed that retroviral transduction of marrow cells, administered to humans, can engraft and result in marker genes becoming present in multiple hemato-

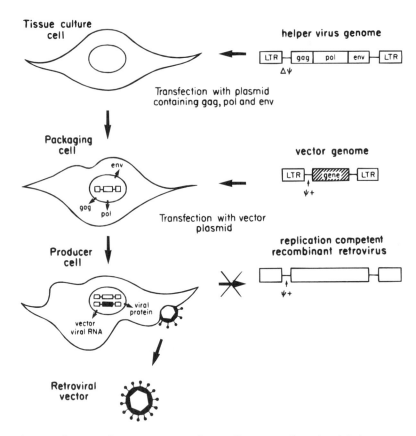

Fig. 50-1. Production of retroviral vectors. Tissue culture cells are transfected with helper virus DNA containing an altered packaging signal ($\Delta\Psi$), and the resulting packaging cell line expresses retroviral proteins (gag, pol, and env) but no infectious virus. This is then transfected with retroviral DNA containing the transgene and a wild-type packaging signal ($\Psi+$), and the resulting producer cells make infectious virions, which, because they lack gag, pol, and env, are replication incompetent.

poietic cell lines (see section on Therapeutic Gene Therapy Studies).

Pseudotype Retroviruses

Viruses have the ability to exchange coat proteins, and a virus with the genetic element of one virus and the envelope of another is called a *pseudotype virus.* The limited tropism of one virus can thus be overcome by exchanging a surface protein of another virus. Vesicular stomatitis viral G-protein has been expressed in cells that, when used as producer cells for retrovirus vectors, can generate pseudotyped recombinant retrovirus vectors.[33] These viruses are now being evaluated for their ability to improve the efficiency and cellular transduction range of retroviral vectors.

Adenoassociated Viruses

AAV are relatively small DNA viruses that are ubiquitous in nature.[34,35] They are replication incompetent and require a helper virus such as adenovirus or herpesviruses to contribute essential factors for AAV replication.[36] Virtually all persons become infected with AAV in childhood, and there are no known pathologic effects of this virus.[34] In addition, AAV is a very stable virus and can resist heating at 56°C for 18 hours. More importantly, these viruses can infect a wide variety of human cells and have been shown to integrate into nondividing cells,[37] including hematopoietic stem cells.[38,39] In addition, after wild AAV infection, DNA integration is site specific, with integration occurring in a small region of human chromosome 19.[40] It is not yet known whether recombinant AAV vectors will share this same property for site-specific integration, but, if they do, the absence of random integration should lessen any potential for oncogenic changes in transduced cells.

The production of recombinant AAV vectors is somewhat different than that for retroviral vectors.[35,41] As shown in Figure 50-2, two plasmid vectors, a helper AAV, which contains the genetic coding sequences for AAV *rep* and *cap* proteins, and the vector plasmid, which contains the AAV inverted terminal repeat sequences, are cotransfected into the 293 cell line. These cells are then infected with either adenovirus or with herpes simplex virus type 1 (HSV-1) to facilitate AAV replication. Subsequently, a crude cell lysate is collected that contains the recombinant vector-DNA packaged as a recombinant AAV and contaminating helper virus. This mixture of virions is then heated to inactivate the helper virus, and then the more stable AAV is separated on a cesium chloride gradient. This vector is then used to transduce cells, as shown, which can be tested for transgene activity. There is no stable packaging cell line for AAV, and the scale-up for production of sufficient quantities of AAV vector necessary for clinical gene therapy requires transfection of large numbers of tissue culture plates followed by separation of contaminating adenovirus or HSV-1. Despite these problems, a clinical protocol for the treatment of persons with cystic fibrosis (CF) using a recombinant AAV vector, containing the gene for CF regulatory protein, has been approved for human use.[42]

Adenovirus-Based Vectors

Adenoviruses are large, double-stranded DNA viruses that can efficiently infect nondividing cells and are produced in high titer.[43,44] Adenovirus virions are relatively stable and can be purified and concentrated using cesium chloride similar to the method used for AAV, as shown in Figure 50-2. Adenovirus infects cells by receptor-mediated endocytosis, and the viral DNA migrates to the nucleus after disruption of the endosome, where it remains as an extrachromosomal form in the nucleus. Although integra-

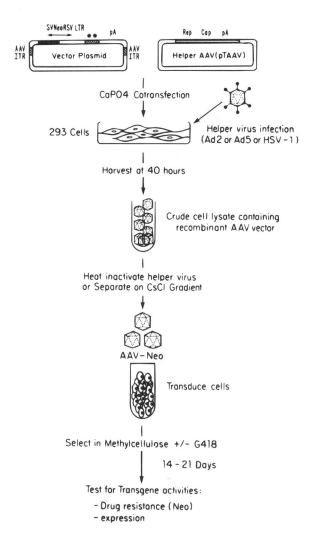

Fig. 50-2. Production of AAV vectors. The vector plasmid DNA, containing the AAV inverted terminal repeat (ITR) sequences plus the transgene (**) under the control of a Rous sarcoma virus (RSV) promoter and adjacent to the neomycin (Neo) resistance gene under the control of a simian virus 40 (SV40) promoter is transfected into 293 cells. At the same time, an AAV plasmid containing the *rep* and *cap* gene of AAV is transfected into these cells. A helper virus infection with either adenovirus 2 or 5 (Ad2 or Ad5) or with herpes simplex virus type 1 (HSV-1) activate the AAV replication. The helper virus is inactivated with heat, and the AAV vector is separated on a cesium chloride (CsCl) gradient. Target cells are then infected with AAV vector, and transduced cells are selected for Neo-resistance in medium containing G418 antibiotic.

tion of viral DNA is possible at high multiplicities of infection, it is inefficient, and it remains to be determined whether or not adenovirus transduction will produce long-term stable transformation. Nevertheless, there is reason to want transient expression of certain genes, and adenovirus is well suited for this propose. It appears to be particularly suited for gene therapy of the respiratory tract, and an adenovirus-based vector is approved for use in gene therapy of CF.[43]

Nonviral Transfer Methods

Viruses have not been the only vectors proposed for use in gene therapy. Nonviral methods for DNA transfer have included the use of liposomes,[45–48] of DNA-protein complexes, and of direct injection of free DNA.[49] Because these methods avoid the regulatory problems associated with recombinant viral vector production, they have been the focus of rapid application to the clinical setting. The first direct therapeutic injection of DNA for gene therapy was performed using liposomes containing DNA for HLA-B7 antigen.[48] By complexing DNA with adenovirus protein with or without transferrin[50–53] or with ligands for cellular receptors,[54–56] enhanced DNA transfer has been demonstrated. In addition, DNA transfer can be accomplished by physical means such as electroporation[57] or by complexing the DNA to particles with mass and accelerating them into cells either in vitro or in vivo. This latter method has already been approved for gene therapy of AIDS and will be compared with retroviral-based methods.[58]

REGULATORY ISSUES

General Considerations

The regulation of gene therapy by governmental bodies is given the highest priority because of the novelty of this activity and because the work involves manipulation of the human genome.[59] In addition to review by the Food and Drug Administration (FDA) and by comparable bodies in other countries, specific scientific and ethical review committees have been established in most countries of Western Europe and Japan. In the United States, the review process for gene therapy research protocols is described in Fig-

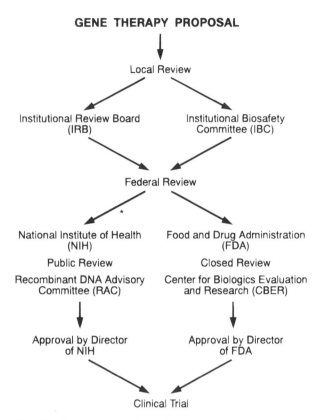

Fig. 50-3. Review and regulation of gene therapy protocols. * The RAC is revising its procedures for review of certain protocols that do not involve novel strategies or untested vectors.

ure 50-3. Gene therapy is restricted to somatic cell manipulation, and any procedure that involves germline alteration or that could produce spread of the genetic vector to germ tissue is not permitted.[60,61] The initial review of all protocols is the responsibility of the research institution at which the work will be performed. This consists of review by the local institutional biosafety committee and by the institutional review board for human subject research. After this, the protocol is reviewed at the national level by the Recombinant DNA Advisory Committee (RAC), a panel that makes recommendations to the Director of the National Institutes of Health, who has final authority over the approval of the proposal. After approval by the RAC, clinical protocols are regulated as Investigational New Drug exemptions by the FDA before human subject trials may begin.

Recombinant DNA Advisory Committee

The RAC of the National Institutes of Health oversees all gene therapy protocols funded by federal sources. It serves to provide a peer review of scientific and ethical evaluation of proposed studies. This is the only public forum at which gene therapy research and development is reviewed. The increasing activity of the RAC is shown in Figure 50-4. Since 1990, there has been a steady increase in the number of protocols reviewed. The marker studies related to cancer protocols formed a major portion of all gene therapy studies in the early years, but, since 1992, there is increasing application of gene therapy to treatment-related projects.

The RAC reviews the scientific aspects of a gene therapy project, the proposed method, and the ethical aspects of the work. This involves a series of important questions, which, when answered, create a detailed justification of the proposal. For example, as outlined in Table 50-3, there are several questions that focus on the specific pathologic process that is the target of genetic manipulation and on whether existing treatment already exists for this disease. Gene therapy research is currently restricted to applications for which there is no adequate alternative therapeutic approach. The questions address which vector will be

Table 50-3. Questions to Consider in Gene Therapy

Is there a specific pathological process that can be corrected by genetic manipulation?

Is there an adequate alternative therapy?

Is there an accessible target cell population for gene therapy?

What is the vector for DNA delivery and can the candidate gene by delivered to these cells?

After such delivery, is gene expression stable, and is it adequate for effect?

Has the test of concept been proved in a laboratory or an animal model?

What are the ethical concerns regarding this method of gene therapy?

used for delivery of the gene of interest, whether the gene can be delivered to the target cell population, and whether there is stable expression without obvious side effects. This requires documentation of the complete sequence of the vector; review of open reading frames, which could be the basis of recombination with other viruses, leading to replication-competent viruses; and demonstration of safety in laboratory animals. In addition, it is important to show that a "test of concept" exists, which might indicate that the disease process could be influenced by the genetic manipula-

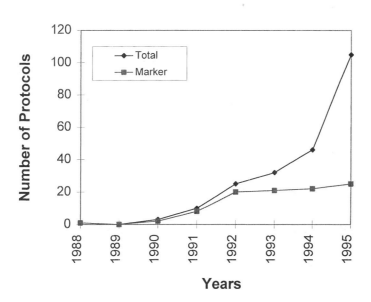

Fig. 50-4. RAC approval of gene therapy protocols. Time course of total number of approved protocols and marker gene protocols are presented here.

tion. Finally, there are the ethical concerns regarding risks taken by the subjects participating in this research, the correct explanation of such risks in the informed consent, and the potential benefits.

Food and Drug Administration Regulation

In the United States, the FDA has authority over all production and safety testing of biologics, and gene therapy vectors fall into this category of medicinals.[62] The Center for Biologics Evaluation and Research (CBER) oversees this activity. FDA publishes a review outline called "Points to Consider," which, although not an official guideline, addresses all relevant issues regarding safety, production, and potential for efficacy.[63] In addition to the consideration of issues relating to gene therapy, there are several other "Points to Consider" documents that involve such related topics as production and testing of new drugs and biologics produced by recombinant DNA technology; collection, processing, and testing of mononuclear leukocytes in somatic cell therapy; and characterization of cell lines used to produce biologics. (These materials can be obtained free of charge by writing to the Division of Congressional and Public Affairs, CBER, Food and Drug Administration, 1401 Rockville Pike, Rockville, Maryland 20852.)

Preparation and Purification of Vectors

Safety testing of products used in clinical trials that involve human subjects focuses on the correct characterization of the cell preparations used. Producer cells used for vector production must be shown to be free of microbiologic contamination, including the absence of replication-competent viruses. In addition, a master cell bank must be established that defines cytogenetic and other evidence of cell derivation and from which the working producer cell banks are derived. These lines must be maintained with laboratory procedures that meet Good Laboratory Practice guidelines.[63]

Clinical Cell Transduction Laboratory

The clinical facility used for transduction, amplification, and preparation of human material used for gene therapy must be guided by the regulations currently considered for somatic cell therapy ("Points to Consider in Human Somatic Cell Therapy and

Gene Therapy," CBER, FDA, 1991). In the immediate future, regulations for the use of blood products in gene therapy will be formulated, but, at the time of this printing, these have not yet been developed.

CURRENT STATUS OF GENE THERAPY PROTOCOLS

As noted in the section on the Definitions and Scope of Gene Therapy, there are two types of gene therapy protocols: marker studies and therapeutic studies. Marker studies utilize a transferred gene (termed a *transgene*) product for determination of cell trafficking patterns or for demonstration of ontologic potential of transduced stem cells. Therapeutic studies to date are usually phase I protocols that focus on safety rather than efficacy. However, because a biologic effect can be observed, as with the ADA transgene experiment, there is a phase II component to many of these studies. Representative initial marker and therapeutic research protocols will be illustrated below.

Marker Studies

The value of marker studies is exemplified by the work of Brenner et al.[32] in tracing the origin of relapse after marrow transplantation for acute leukemia. In this study, the neomycin-resistance (NEO^R) transgene was inserted into a fraction of marrow cells before autologous BMT to determine whether the processed marrow itself contributed to relapse or relapse derived only from residual host disease. Clearly, this is a question of major importance because, if the marked cells are the source of relapsed leukemia, then this would have a profound influence on the need to purge marrow more effectively before BMT. Alternatively, if no marker appeared in the relapsed leukemia, then it could be inferred that the source of relapse was residual disease in the host, and better ablative therapies would be indicated.

In this experiment, bone marrow was harvested for autologous BMT for the treatment of acute myelogenous leukemia (AML) in remission, and approximately one-third of this marrow was exposed to a retroviral vector that contained the marker gene NEO^R. Children with AML in remission were treated with ablative therapy that consisted of busulfan and cyclophosphamide, and the gene-marked marrow was reinfused 14 days after harvesting and transduction. Two patients subsequently had relapses; in both patients, the populations of leukemic cells were positive for the marker gene, as measured by the polymerase chain reaction. To confirm that the marker was actually in leukemic cells, purified blast cells were cultured in methylcellulose with and without G418 (an analogue to neomycin) to determine whether any malignant cells expressed NEO[R]. Approximately 2 to 3 percent of these blast cells were G418 resistant. Concomitant analysis of these NEO[R]-resistant clones from one patient confirmed the presence of the tumor marker *AML1/ETO*, which results from an 8:12 chromosome translocation. This was the first demonstration that relapse derives in part from cells present in autologous marrow at the time of transplantation, and this has obvious significance for further improvement in this method of treatment.[32]

Gene-marking studies have also been used to determine whether there is long-term hematopoiesis after autologous BMT.[31] This experiment utilized the same marker technique of NEO[R] transduction of autologous marrow cells and asked the question whether long-term progeny are derived from these transplanted cells. Twenty patients were studied during autologous BMT for either AML or neuroblastoma. The transduction of approximately one-third of the marrow cells resulted in an efficiency of 6.5 percent transfer of the marker gene for patients with AML and 4 percent for the patients with neuroblastoma. The laboratory manipulation of the marrow specimens had no adverse effect on the time of engraftment with the median time to recovery of the absolute neutrophil count to 500/μl of 35 and 27 days for AML and neuroblastoma populations, respectively, with the time to reach 2×10^4 platelets/μl of 36 and 27 days, respectively. NEO[R] was detected in marrow mononuclear cells in 14 of 18 patients at 1 month, and the presence of the marker in hematopoietic progenitor cells was confirmed by cloning in methylcellulose for 15 of 18 patients. NEO[R] progenitor cells persisted for 6 months in eight of nine patients and for 1 year for all five patients studied. NEO[R] was present in erythroid, myeloid, myelocytic, and multilineage progenitors at some time postengraftment. The marker gene was also present after more than 1 year in peripheral blood mononuclear cells, including T cells, B cells, and neutrophils. Thus, hematopoietic progenitor

cells can be transduced with a retrovirus vector, and the progeny of these cells survive for at least 1 year after transplantation.[31] This information provides a justification for exploring the use of therapeutic transgenes in the setting of BMT.

Therapeutic Gene Therapy Studies

The first gene therapy with therapeutic intent was the transfer of the ADA gene into CD4 + T cells from two children with SCID.[10,11] The analysis of "Points to Consider" for this project illustrates the way in which a candidate proposal for genetic treatment of a disease should be assessed.[64] The pathogenesis of SCID is well understood, and one variant of SCID is due to lack of a functional ADA, which is harmful to T cells.[65] ADA catalyzes the deamination of deoxyadenosine to deoxyinosine, and an absence of ADA permits the accumulation of deoxyadenosine to levels that are toxic to T cells. As a consequence, these children have a cellular immune defect and are at risk of having life-threatening infections. The available treatment for this potentially fatal disease is polyethylene glycol-ADA, but this is an orphan drug that is very expensive and not completely effective.[66] Thus, from the standpoint of therapeutic need, ADA deficiency represented a life-threatening disease for which there was no curative treatment and for which existing therapy was unsatisfactory.

The gene for ADA had been cloned, and its size was suitable for insertion into a retroviral vector.[67] In addition, only T cells need be transduced to cure the disease, and this target population is readily accessible. Furthermore, only 5 to 10 percent of normal ADA protein is needed to maintain a functional immune system.[68] Finally, in vitro laboratory evidence indicates that the enzymatic defect could be corrected by retrovirus-mediated transduction.[10,67] Thus, ADA deficiency appeared to have all the elements necessary for the ideal situation for which gene therapy could be attempted.

The clinical ADA protocol involved the isolation of T cells, which were then stimulated to divide in culture using monoclonal antibody to the T cell receptor (OKT-3) and interleukin-2 (IL-2), and transduced with retrovirus vector that contained the ADA transgene and NEO[R].[64] The cells were subsequently expanded to several billion and then transfused into the patient. The results to date have shown that, first, lymphocytes isolated from an immunodeficient subject can be cultivated, transduced with a gene for ADA using a retroviral vector, selected with NEO^R, and safely administered to a patient with SCID. Second, the two children enrolled in the study demonstrated an increase in lymphocyte counts to normal levels, with the presence of the ADA transgene being found months after administration. During this period, the genetically altered lymphocytes were administered on multiple occasions. Whether there is a requirement for continued intermittent infusions of treated T cells is not known. Third, both patients had improved in vivo immunologic function, as shown by positive skin tests and by improved quality of life with fewer infections.

A revised protocol, which has been used to treat three neonates with prenatally diagnosed SCID, investigated the use of transduced CD34-positive cells to test whether hematopoietic stem cells can be transduced with this retroviral vector and engrafted into an unconditioned autologous donor.[69]

APPLICATION OF GENE THERAPY TO TREATMENT OF CANCER

Rationale

Although the initial considerations regarding gene therapy focused on its use in the treatment of inborn genetic diseases, the most prominent use of gene therapy to date has been in the field of cancer. This is because the insertion of new genetic information has multiple potential applications for cancer therapy, ranging from the correction of genetic abnormalities related to the causes of oncogenic transformation to enhancement of immunity against cancer, introduction of toxins that could inhibit neoplastic growth, and protection of the patient with cancer from the side effects of chemotherapy. As shown in Table 50-4, gene therapy has been applied to the treatment of patients with cancer in four general areas. The first is the use of marker genes to determine the biologic effects of somatic cell therapy.[70] The second is the enhancement of immunologic antitumor mechanisms by the induction of cytokine expression in tumor-infiltrating lymphocytes or onto autologous cancer cells[8,9] or the expression of a foreign major histocompatibility complex antigen on

Table 50-4. Gene Therapy for Cancer

Immunologic approaches
    Cytokine expression in tumor-infiltrating lymphocytes
    Cytokine expression in autologous cancer cells
    Foreign major histocompatibility complex antigen expression in cancer cells
Antitumor treatment
    Expression of potential toxins, thymidine kinase, CD16
    Expression of antioncogene, antisense, ribozymes
Enhanced chemotherapy
    Protection from chemotherapy (e.g., *MDR1* and *MGM*)

the tumor with the intent of promoting an immune recognition of the tumor.[48] A third area in which gene therapy has been applied to cancer is the direct expression of toxins that are normally not present in the tumor but, if present, could serve to mediate an antitumor effect. Such candidate genetic treatments include the use of antisense RNA, ribozyme, herpes simplex virus thymidine kinase, or CD16 protein. The fourth area of application of gene therapy to cancer is the attempt to protect patients from the side effects of chemotherapy using genes such as the multidrug-resistance gene (*MDR1*), which are designed to protect the marrow from toxicity and permit more effective use of chemotherapy.

Marking Studies in Patients With Cancer

The first approved gene therapy protocol in the United States was for marking tumor-infiltrating lymphocytes in patients with advanced cancer. This protocol received RAC approval on October 3, 1988 and National Institutes of Health approval on March 2, 1989. Subsequent to this, marker studies were proposed for a variety of studies relating to trafficking of anticancer lymphocytes and hematopoiesis.[70,71] Two of these, the studies of the origin of relapsed leukemia after bone marrow transplantation and of long-term hematopoeisis after BMT, are described in the section on Marker Studies above.

Immunologic Approaches to Gene Therapy of Cancer

As noted above, attempts are currently in progress to support immune-based methods of cancer treatment using cytokine or growth factor expression either in tumor-infiltrating lymphocytes[72,73] or in autologous cancer cells.[74] The cytokines include tumor necrosis factor, IL-2, IL-4, IL-7, IL-12, and granulocyte-macrophage colony-stimulating factor gm-CSF. In addition, introduction of a foreign HLA-B7 antigen has been completed in an initial series of patients.[48] In this study, the expression of HLA-B7 was transferred directly to melanoma nodules in an attempt to induce immune-mediated tumor rejection.

Use of Direct Gene Therapy-Based Antitumor Treatment for Enhanced Chemotherapy

Because new growth factors can result from the production of new genes after chromosomal translocation with subsequent neoplasm, it has been proposed that antitumor RNA might be useful for control of selected tumors. Thus, for example, in chronic myelogenous leukemia, in which the *BCR-ABL* translocation results in a new protein, which explains, in part, the growth of the leukemia, it is proposed to use either antisense or ribozyme for inhibition of this protein synthesis.[75] This method may have particular utility for the purging of tumor cells from marrow in the process of autologous BMT.

One of the most exciting and rapidly moving areas of solid tumor treatment is the introduction of an HSV-1 thymidine kinase gene, which is nontoxic to cells except in the present of ganciclovir or acyclovir. The enzyme phosphorylates ganciclovir and acyclovir to a toxic form, resulting in cell death.[76–78] Because retroviruses require dividing cells for efficient integration, the rationale for the treatment of a brain tumor is to place retrovirus-based vector-producing cells at the site of a brain tumor by stereotactic injection and then allow the dividing tumor cells to be transduced by the thymidine kinase vector. The nondividing normal adjacent brain should be protected from retroviral thymidine kinase transduction and therefore will not be killed by the ganciclovir treatment. Studies in mice have demonstrated the test of concept for this novel method of treating central nervous system tumors.[76] At present, a protocol is actively enrolling patients for direct inoculation of producer cells into central nervous system tumors for subsequent treatment with ganciclovir.

Use of Gene Therapy for Enhanced Chemotherapy

The *MDR1* gene has been isolated from tumors that are resistant to multiple forms of chemotherapy.[79]

It has been suggested that introduction of this gene into marrow progenitor cells may spare the marrow of toxic effects of chemotherapy. The test of concept for this proposal has been demonstrated in a murine model.[80,81] At present, attempts are focusing on introduction of the *MDR1* gene into hematopoietic cells to determine whether this will permit more intensive chemotherapy to be used for advanced solid tumors.[82,83]

GENE THERAPY OF CLASSIC GENETIC DISEASES

As shown in Figure 50-4, an increasing number of gene therapy protocols for treatment-related studies have been approved. These include such diseases as ADA deficiency, as described before, familial hypercholesterolemia;[84–86] CF;[87] and glucocerebrosidase deficiency (Gaucher's disease);[88–90] although the bulk of studies remain focused on cancer.

Treatment of Cystic Fibrosis With Gene Therapy

CF is the most common lethal autosomal recessive disease in the United States and has an estimated incidence of 1 in 2,000.[91,92] The basic defect in CF is an abnormality of cyclic adenosine monophosphate (cAMP)-regulated chloride secretion by epithelial cells, which causes dysfunction of exocrine glands, primarily in the bronchial tree and intestinal tract.[92,93] The failure of chloride secretion by these cells produces dehydration of glandular secretions, which become too viscid to flow freely. CF then presents as obstructive pulmonary disease with infection, as gastrointestinal malabsorption and small bowel obstruction, as biliary cirrhosis, and as vas deferens obstruction with azoospermia. CF is inherited as an autosomal recessive disease, and the gene is located on the long arm of chromosome 7.[94] The human cystic fibrosis transmembrane regulator (*CFTR*) gene encodes a polypeptide of 1,480 amino acids with distinct structure-containing transmembrane segments. This protein is membrane bound and is responsible for hydrolysis of adenosine triphosphate. It has been shown that gene transfer of the full-length complementary DNA for *CFTR* confers cAMP-dependent chloride channel activity that will correct the chloride transport defect characteristic of cells derived from patients with CF.[95,96] The most common mutation that produces CF is a deletion of phenylalanine at position 508 of the CFTR protein.[97,98] Although this defect accounts for 70 percent of CF cases, there are other multiple distinct genetic alterations that have been found in *CFTR*, which was cloned in 1989 and subsequently cloned into vectors derived from retroviruses and from the respiratory viruses, adenovirus and AAV, and has corrected the metabolic CF defect in respiratory epithelium.[99] Initial protocols are attempting to demonstrate the safety of transduction of the *CFTR* transgene using either adenovirus-based[43] or AAV-based vectors.[42,100]

APPLICATION OF GENE THERAPY TO AIDS

Rationale

Although one might think that the complexity of virologic, immunologic, and biologic events that occur in the pathogenesis of AIDS would make this disease an unlikely target for gene therapy, AIDS is actually a prime candidate for application of gene therapy studies.[101] The reason for this is that the molecular biologic aspects of human immunodeficiency virus type 1 (HIV-1) gene regulation are well understood, and HIV infection presents an opportunity to treat a viral infection for which there is inadequate therapy (Table 50-5). The transactivational protein, tat, and the messenger RNA regulatory protein, rev, provide targets for the introduction of competitive transdominant mutations. The introduction of a modified protein that would compete with the

Table 50-5. Gene Therapy of Acquired Immunodeficiency Syndrome

Immunologic restoration
    Adoptive immunotherapy
    Universal CD8+ T cells
    Vaccination with genetic vectors
Transdominant negative mutant proteins
    Antirev
    Antitat
    Antigag
    Antienv
Signal decoy-based inhibition
    TAR
    Rev-responsive element
Antisense and ribozyme

parent protein for biologic sites of action has been termed *intracellular immunization*.[102] In addition to regulatory proteins, structural proteins such as gag and env have been used as targets for these transdominant negative mutants. In addition, the RNA regulatory sites, tat activation response element (TAR), and the rev-responsive element (RRE) can be introduced and expressed in a cell, and these serve as decoys that competitively inhibit the interaction of the regulatory proteins with viral RNA. Other RNA-based mechanisms for inhibition of HIV include antisense and ribozyme (see section on Inhibition Using Antisense or Ribozyme below). Thus, there are protein-, RNA-, and immune-based methods of gene therapy for AIDS.

Intracellular Immunization

Inhibition Using Transdominant Negative Mutant Proteins

Transdominant negative proteins are mutant proteins that have phenotypes that compete with the parent protein for sites of activity and produce inhibition.[103] HIV-1 inhibition has been shown in vitro using transdominant negative rev,[104] tat,[105,106] env,[107] and gag.[108]

The rev mutation, termed *revM10*, has been developed for clinical application.[109] The rev protein consists of 116 amino acids and can be divided into an N-terminal half, which contains an arginine-rich region necessary for nuclear localization of the rev protein,[110] and a C-terminal half, which contains midportion domain residues 78 and 79 that are essential for transactivation. Approximately 15 different rev mutants have been reported to have transdominant negative activity; however, most studies have focused on the *revM10* mutant, which has a missense substitution at residues 78 and 79 of this C-terminal peptide.[111] Cells transduced with and stably expressing *revM10* and challenged with cloned isolates of HIV-1 demonstrated inhibited virus replication.[104,112]

The mechanism of action of the transdominant negative rev mutants is thought to be due to a combination of the transdominant rev with wild-type rev to form an inactive multimer complex or to compete directly with wild-type rev in binding to the RRE target. Recent studies suggest that rev forms multimers at the RRE site,[111] and this multimer complex binds to RRE and alters the normal interaction of rev with cellular factors necessary for transport of the RNA from the nucleus.

RNA Decoys

The RNA sites of protein binding that are important in the regulation of HIV-1 gene transcription and processing can be used to compete with viral RNA sites and inhibit HIV replication. TAR, a cis-acting target for tat binding, located within the long terminal repeat (LTR) of the virus at positions -17 to $+80$, is essential for tat activation of the LTR. TAR decoy sequences were expressed in HIV-1-susceptible cells with a Moloney murine virus vector, which contains the coding sequence for a transfer RNA-TAR decoy in its 3′ LTR. When the sequence was incorporated into the target cell, the transfer RNA-TAR template was duplicated and subsequently expressed from both proviral LTR sites. The resultant transduced cells were challenged with HIV-1 and were found to inhibit virus replication by 99 percent.[113] Subsequently, it was shown that concatemers of TAR could inhibit HIV-1 LTR-based functions, and tandem sequences could be expressed in cells and limit the replication of HIV-1.[106,114]

The RRE is a cis-acting sequence that is important in viral replication and is located within a highly structured sequence of RNA present in the coding region for the *env* gene. Interaction of rev with RRE results in the cytoplasmic accumulation of large, unspliced, or singly spliced transcripts that serve both as retroviral genome and as templates for essential viral structural elements. This rev-RRE interaction is crucial in the viral life cycle and permits a switch from small highly spliced messenger RNA to the large RNA necessary for viral encapsidation. The overexpression of RRE decoy sequences has been shown to limit rev binding to wild-type RRE[115] and to inhibit HIV-1 replication.[116] However, inhibition of HIV-1 by RRE decoys has not yielded results as favorable as those found using TAR decoys that were expressed under similar systems.

Inhibition Using Antisense or Ribozyme

Antisense is DNA or RNA that is complementary to messenger RNA transcripts. Antisense compounds are currently being used in clinical research studies to introduce DNA into cells and inhibit gene processing, but this is not considered a form of gene therapy

unless expression of antisense messenger RNA occurs in targeted cells. Various antisense sequences have been designed that bind to messenger RNA transcripts that encode HIV-1 proteins and to untranslated regions of HIV-1, including the LTR and the primer binding site. Effective targets reported to date include TAR;[117] the 5′ LTR-gag region[118,119]; the coding exons of tat and rev[117]; and the initiation codons of tat, rev, vpu, and env.[120] Many of these targets, such as the 5′ end, the primer binding site, all initiation codons, and all splice sites were compared in a study that tested 20 binding sites on HIV-1 transcripts.[121] Antisense sequences complementary to any of the 20 sites showed antiviral activity, but the most active inhibition was seen with sequences complementary to the 5′ untranslated end, the polyadenylation signal, the region adjacent to the primer binding site, and splice acceptor sites. In all the antiviral studies that used these sequences, cells transfected or transduced with genes that encoded for antisense sequences showed variable resistance to HIV-1.[112,118–120] The highest inhibition was reported for a sequence targeting both a stretch in the 5′ untranslated LTR sequence, including TAR, and a portion of the 3′ end, including a part of the polyadenlytion signal.[117] Transduced CD4-positive cells, challenged with HIV-1, demonstrated inhibition of virus replication by 98 percent for up to 20 days.

Ribozymes are RNA sequences that have the ability to cleave RNA,[122] and there are two ribozyme motifs that have been identified and classified as a "hammerhead"[123] or as "hairpin" structure.[124] Although the ribozymes found in nature react by way of a cis-acting mechanism, in which the required sequences are located on one strand of RNA, it has been possible to create ribozymes that will form by trans configuration, in which the required sequences are on two separate strands.[125,126] Hammerhead ribozymes were the first to be shown to cleave HIV-1 RNA and to inhibit HIV replication in vitro.[127] More recently, transduction of cells with ribozymes targeted to the 5′ LTR[128] or to tat[129] inhibit HIV-1 in vitro. Ribozymes targeted to as many as 10 different sites on the envelope glycoprotein (GP120) have been shown to inhibit HIV-1 in vitro.[130] Both tat and the tat/rev common exon have been targeted, and it has been shown that dual ribozyme expression can effectively inhibit HIV-1 infection in vitro.[131]

The hairpin ribozyme has also been successfully used to inhibit HIV-1 replication. These hairpin ribozymes have been targeted to the viral messenger RNA coding for tat[132] and to the messenger RNA sequences of the 5′ HIV-1 LTR[133] and have shown reduced virus production in transduced T cells. Hairpin ribozymes have been approved for clinical use and are entering trials.[134]

Inhibition Using Modified Lysosomal Degradation

Because CD4 is a receptor for HIV-1 GP120, attempts have been made to utilize intracellular expression of CD4 to interrupt normal viral envelope production. The soluble CD4 coding sequence was modified to contain an amino acid sequence that retains soluble proteins in the lumen of the endoplasmic reticulum and prevents the secretion of the protein.[135] Cells that express this modified CD4 could not secrete HIV-1 GP120 after transfection with a plasmid coding for GP120. These cells also did not form syncytia, which suggests that the endoplasmic reticulum retention of GP120 prevented surface expression of this protein. A more direct approach to enhanced degradation of GP120 has been to modify CD4 to contain a lysosomal targeting domain. Transformed cells that express this protein inhibit the expression of HIV-1 after infection. This inhibition was due to transport of GP160 to lysosomes by the SCD4-fusion molecules.

Current Gene Therapy Protocols

Immunotherapy Using CD8 Lymphocytes

The first gene therapy protocol approved for use in patients with AIDS was developed by Greenberg and Riddell.[136] The goal of this protocol is to clone CD8 cells with cytotoxic T-lymphocyte (CTL) function specific for HIV-1, to mark these cells with a retroviral vector, and to transfer them adoptively to a patient with AIDS. These cells will be derived from a person undergoing allogeneic BMT for AIDS-related lymphoma, and the study will evaluate the safety, stability, and antiviral effect of these adoptively transferred CTL clones in vivo.

In addition, a DNA-based vaccine to HIV-1 envelope glycoprotein gp160 has been approved by the RAC as a therapeutic vaccine.[137] This protocol was originally intended to utilize autologous fibroblasts transduced with a retroviral vector-containing gp160. Because of the recent awareness that direct injection of DNA can result in transgene expression and immune response, this protocol has been expanded to include direct DNA injection.

Rev Transdominant Mutant Therapy

The first protocol to utilize a method of intracellular immunization for treatment of AIDS was developed by Nabel et al.[109] This proposal will evaluate the use of *revM10* or an inactive *revM10* in CD4 cells from HIV-1-infected persons. The CD4 cells will be transduced with either *revM10* or control vector, selected in tissue culture, and then infused into the patient. The mode of transduction will compare retrovirus-mediated transduction to particle-mediated cell transduction. The initial clinical patients treated in this way have received cells transduced by an accelerated particle-mediated method of cell transduction, and the results are still pending.

Ribozyme Gene Therapy

The first clinical trial to evaluate the safety and effects of ribozymes for the treatment of AIDS was developed by Leavitt et al.[134] The goals of this phase 1 trial are to determine the safety of infusing autologous CD4 cells that have been transduced ex vivo with a retroviral vector that contains a hairpin ribozyme targeted to the HIV-1 LTR and to compare the survival of ribozyme-transduced cells and control cells transduced with a similar vector that contains no ribozyme sequence.

FUTURE APPLICATIONS OF GENE THERAPY

This has been a review of representative applications of gene therapy to medical problems. It is anticipated that demonstration of the safety and efficiency of newer methods of DNA transfer will have application to a wide range of common situations from immunizations[138] to management of coronary artery restenosis[139] and improvement of outcome from hip and knee prosthetic surgery.[140] It is anticipated that the Human Genome Project will have considerable influence on gene therapy applications.[141] Although the complexity of in vitro cell transduction creates a problem for efficient application of gene therapy to medicine, the recent use of direct DNA injection suggests that less complex approaches to the application of gene therapy will be possible in the future. This could allow use of gene therapy in many situations in which a protein-based approach is rational but not yet feasible because of problems of drug design, manufacture, or delivery. Such diseases include not only the rare problems such as antitrypsin deficiency[142] and hemophilia[143] but also extend to kidney stones[144] and atherosclerosis.[145] Gene therapy promises to influence the practice of medicine significantly in the future, and it is clear from the rapid progress since 1990 that this future is with us now.

REFERENCES

1. Forman SJ, Blume KB, Thomas ED: Bone Marrow Transplantation. Blackwell Scientific Publications, Boston, 1994

2. Cournoyer D, Scarpa M, Jones SN et al: Gene therapy: a new approach for the treatment of genetic disorders. Clin Pharmacol Ther 47:1, 1990

3. Badman DG, Schechter AN: NIDDK symposium on the impact of molecular genetics on the treatment of genetic diseases. Hum Gene Ther 4:635, 1993

4. Blaese RM, Culver KW: Prospects for gene therapy of human disease. Allergy Immunopathol 19:25, 1991

5. Anderson WF: Human gene therapy. Science 256: 808, 1992

6. Cornetta K, Morgan RA, Anderson WF: Safety issues related to retroviral-mediated gene transfer in humans. Hum Gene Ther 2:5, 1991

7. Beutler E, Sorge J: Gene transfer in the treatment of hematologic disease. Exp Hematol 18:857, 1990

8. Rosenberg SA, Aebersold P, Cornetta K et al: Gene transfer into humans—immunotherapy of patients with advanced melanoma, using tumor-infiltrating lymphocytes modified by retroviral gene transduction (see comments). N Engl J Med 323:570, 1990

9. Rosenberg SA: Immunotherapy and gene therapy of cancer. Cancer Res, Suppl. 18, 51:5074s, 1991

10. Culver KW, Osborne WR, Miller AD et al: Correction of ADA deficiency in human T lymphocytes using retroviral-mediated gene transfer. Transplant Proc 23:170, 1991

11. Culver KW, Blaese RM: Gene therapy for adenosine deaminase deficient and malignant solid tumors. p. 256. In Wolff JA (ed): Gene Therapeutics. Birkhauser, Boston, 1994

12. Morgan RA, Anderson WF: Human gene therapy. Annu Rev Biochem 62:191, 1993

13. Armentano D, Yu SF, Kantoff PW et al: Effect of internal viral sequences on the utility of retroviral vectors. J Virol 61:1647, 1987

14. Cullen BR: Mechanism of action of regulatory proteins encoded by complex retroviruses. Microbiol Rev 56:375, 1992

15. Miller AD: Progress toward human gene therapy. Blood 76:271, 1990

16. Temin HM: Safety considerations in somatic gene therapy of human disease with retrovirus vectors. Hum Gene Ther 1:111, 1990

17. Donahue RE, Kessler SW, Bodine D et al: Helper virus induced T cell lymphoma in nonhuman primates after retroviral mediated gene transfer. J Exp Med 176:1125, 1992

18. Anderson WF: Editorial: what about those monkeys that got T-cell lymphoma? Hum Gene Ther 4:1, 1993

19. Anderson WF, McGarrity GJ, Moen RC: Report to the NIH Recombinant DNA Advisory Committee on murine replication-competent retrovirus (RCR) assays. Hum Gene Ther 4:311, 1993

20. Gunter KC, Khan AS, Noguchi PD: The safety of retroviral vectors. Hum Gene Ther 4:643, 1993

21. Anderson WF: Editorial: was it just stupid or are we poor educators. Hum Gene Ther 5:791, 1994

22. Miller AD, Rosman GJ: Improved retroviral vectors for gene transfer and expression. Biotechniques 7: 980, 1989

23. Kotani H, Newton PB III, Zhang S et al: Improved methods of retroviral vector transduction and production for gene therapy. Hum Gene Ther 5:19, 1994

24. Mulligan RC: The basic science of gene therapy. Science 260:926, 1993

25. Eglitis MA, Kantoff PW, Gilboa E, Anderson WF: Gene expression in mice after high efficiency retroviral-mediated gene transfer. Science 230:1395, 1985

26. Eglitis MA, Anderson WF: Retroviral vectors for introduction of genes into mammalian cells. Biotechniques. 6:608, 1988

27. Adam MA, Miller AD: Identification of a signal in a murine retrovirus that is sufficient for packaging of nonretroviral RNA into virions. J Virol 62:3802, 1988

28. Bender MA, Palmer TD, Gelinas RE, Miller AD: Evidence that the packaging signal of Moloney murine leukemia virus extends into the gag region. J Virol 61:1639, 1987

29. Linial ML, Miller AD: Retroviral RNA packaging: se-

quence requirements and implications. Curr Top Microbiol Immunol 157:125, 1990

30. Miller AD, Buttimore C: Redesign of retrovirus packaging cell lines to avoid recombination leading to helper virus production. Mol Cell Biol 6:2895, 1986

31. Brenner MK, Rill DR, Holladay MS et al: Gene marking to determine whether autologous marrow infusion restores long-term haemopoiesis in cancer patients. Lancet 342:1134, 1993

32. Brenner MK, Rill DR, Moen RC et al: Gene-marking to trace origin of relapse after autologous bone-marrow transplantation. Lancet 341:85, 1993

33. Burns JC, Friedmann T, Driever W et al: Vesicular stomatitis virus G glycoprotein pseudotyped retroviral vectors: concentration to very high titer and efficient gene transfer into mammalian and non-mammalian cells. Proc Natl Acad Sci U S A 90:8033, 1993

34. Muzyczka N: In vitro replication of adeno-associated virus DNA. Virology 2:281, 1991

35. Muzyczka N: Use of adeno-associated virus as a general transduction vector for mammalian cells. Curr Top Microbiol Immunol 158:97, 1992

36. Kotin RM: Prospects for the use of adeno-associated virus as a vector for human gene therapy. Hum Gene Ther 5:793, 1994

37. Podsakoff G, Wong KK, Jr, Chatterjee S: Gene transfer into non-dividing cells by AAV vectors. J Virol 68:5656, 1994

38. Zhou SZ, Cooper S, Kang LY et al: Adeno-associated virus-mediated high efficiency gene transfer into immature and mature subsets of hematopoietic progenitor cells in human umbilical cord blood. J Exp Med 179:1867, 1994

39. Goodman S, Xiao X, Donahue RE et al: Recombinant adeno-associated virus-mediated gene transfer into hematopoietic progenitor cells. Blood 84:1492, 1994

40. Kotin RM, Siniscalco M, Samulski RJ et al: Site-specific integration by adeno-associated virus. Proc Natl Acad Sci U S A 87:2211, 1990

41. Hamada K, Akagi T, Okano A et al: A new method of gene transfer into hematopoietic progenitors using liquid culture with interleukin-3 and interleukin-6. J Immunol Methods 141:177, 1991

42. Flotte TR, Afione SA, Conrad C et al: Stable in vivo expression of the cystic fibrosis transmembrane conductance regulator with an adeno-associated virus vector. Proc Natl Acad Sci U S A 90:10613, 1993

43. Rosenfeld MA, Siegfried W, Yoshimura K et al: Adenovirus-mediated transfer of a recombinant alpha 1-antitrypsin gene to the lung epithelium in vivo. Science 252:431, 1991

44. Rosenfeld MA, Yoshimura K, Trapnell BC et al: In vivo transfer of the human cystic fibrosis transmembrane conductance regulator gene to the airway epithelium. Cell 68:143, 1992

45. Stewart MJ, Plautz GE, Del Buono L et al: Gene transfer in vivo with DNA-liposome complexes: safety and acute toxicity in mice. Hum Gene Ther 3:267, 1992

46. Mannino RJ, Gould-Fogerite S: Liposome mediated gene transfer. Biotechniques 6:682, 1988

47. Felgner PL, Rhodes G: Gene therapeutics. Nature 349:351, 1991

48. Nabel GJ, Nabel EG, Yang Z-Y et al: Direct gene therapy transfer with DNA-liposome complexes in melanoma: expression, biologic activity, and lack of toxicity in humans. Proc Natl Acad Sci U S A 90:11307, 1993

49. Wolff JA, Malone RW, Wiliams P et al: Direct gene transfer into mouse muscle in vivo. Science 247:1465, 1990

50. Wagner E, Zenke M, Cotten M et al: Transferrin-polycation conjugates as carriers for DNA uptake into cells. Proc Natl Acad Sci U S A 87:3410, 1990

51. Wagner E, Cotten M, Foisner R, Birnstiel ML: Transferrin-polycation-DNA complexes: the effect of polycations on the structure of the complex and DNA delivery to cells. Proc Natl Acad Sci U S A 88:4255, 1991

52. Curiel DT, Agarwal S, Wagner E, Cotten M: Adenovirus enhancement of transferrin-polylysine-mediated gene delivery. Proc Natl Acad Sci U S A 88:8850, 1991

53. Cotten M, L'angle-Rouault F, Kirlappo H et al: Transferrin-polycation-mediated introduction of DNA into human leukemic cells: stimulation by agents that affect the survival of transfected DNA or modulate transferrin receptor levels. Proc Natl Acad Sci U S A 87:4033, 1990

54. Wu CH, Wilson JM, Wu GY: Targeting genes: delivery and persistent expression of a foreign gene driven by mammalian regulatory elements in vivo. J Biol Chem 264:16985, 1989

55. Wu GY, Wilson JM, Shalaby F et al: Receptor-mediated gene delivery in vivo. Partial correction of genetic analbuminiemia in Nagase rats. J Biol Chem 266:14338, 1991

56. Wu GY, Wu CH: Delivery systems for gene therapy. Biotherapy 3:87, 1991

57. Keating A, Toneguzzo F: Gene transfer by electroporation: a model of gene therapy. Prog Clin Biol Res 333:491, 1990

58. Gupta S, Lee CD, Vemuru RP, Bhargava KK: [111]Indium labeling of hepatocytes for analysis of short-

term biodistribution of transplanted cells. Hepatology 19:750, 1994

59. Epstein SL: Regulatory concerns in human gene therapy. Hum Gene Ther 2:243, 1991

60. Danks DM: Germ-line gene therapy—no place in treatment of genetic disease. Hum Gene Ther 5:151, 1994

61. Davis BD: Limits to genetic intervention in humans: somatic and germline. Ciba Found Symp 149:81, 1990

62. Kessler DA, Siegel JP, Noguchi PD et al: Regulation of somatic-cell therapy and gene therapy by the Food and Drug Administration. N Engl J Med 329:1169, 1993

63. Points to consider in human somatic cell therapy and gene therapy. Hum Gene Ther 2:251, 1991

64. Anderson WF, Blaese RM, Culver K: Treatment of severe combined immunodeficiency disease (SCID) due to adenosine deaminase (ADA) deficiency with autologous lymphocytes transduced with a human ADA gene. Hum Gene Ther 1:331, 1990

65. Hirschhorn R: Adenosine deaminase deficiency. Immunodefic Rev 2:175, 1990

66. Fischer A: Primary immunodeficiencies: molecular aspects and treatment. Bone Marrow Transplant 1:39, 1992

67. Kantoff PW, Kohn DB, Mitsuya H et al: Correction of adenosine deaminase deficiency in cultured human T and B cells by retrovirus-mediated gene transfer. Proc Natl Acad Sci U S A 83:6563, 1986

68. Parkman R, Gelfand EW: Severe combined immunodeficiency disease, adenosine deaminase deficiency and gene therapy. Curr Opin Immunol 3:547, 1991

69. Cournoyer D, Scarpa M, Mitani K et al: Gene transfer of adenosine deaminase into primitive human hematopoietic progenitor cells. Hum Gene Ther 2:203, 1991

70. Rill DR, Moen RC, Buschle M et al: An approach for the analysis of relapse and marrow reconstitution after autologous marrow transplantation using retrovirus-mediated gene transfer. Blood 79:2694, 1992

71. Dunbar CE, Nienhuis AW, Stewart FM et al: Amendment to clinical research projects. Genetic marking with retroviral vectors to study the feasibility of stem cell gene transfer and the biology of hemopoietic reconstitution after autologous transplantation in multiple myeloma, chronic myelogenous leukemia, or metastatic breast cancer. Hum Gene Ther 4:205, 1993

72. Culver K, Cornetta K, Morgan R et al: Lymphocytes as cellular vehicles for gene therapy in mouse and man. Proc Natl Acad Sci U S A 88:3155, 1991

73. Kasid A, Morecki S, Aebersold P et al: Human gene transfer: characterization of human tumor-infiltrating lymphocytes as vehicles for retroviral-mediated gene transfer in man. Proc Natl Acad Sci U S A 87:473, 1990

74. Schmidt-Wolf IGH, Huhn D, Neubauer A, Wittig B: Clinical protocol: interleukin-7 gene transfer in patients with metastatic colon carcinoma, renal cell carcinoma, melanoma, or with lymphoma. Hum Gene Ther 5:1161, 1994

75. Nadkarni KS, Datar RH, Rao SG: Antisense RNA therapy for CML—an hypothesis. Med Hypotheses 35:307, 1991

76. Culver KW, Ram Z, Wallbridge S et al: In vivo gene transfer with retroviral vector-producer cells for treatment of experimental brain tumors. Science 256:1550, 1992

77. Barba D, Hardin J, Sadelain M, Gage FH: Development of anti-tumor immunity following thymidine kinase-mediated killing of experimental brain tumors. Proc Natl Acad Sci U S A 91:4348, 1994

78. Moolten FL, Wells JM: Curability of tumors bearing herpes thymidine kinase genes transferred by retroviral vectors. J Natl Cancer Inst 82:297, 1990

79. Germann UA, Chin KV, Pastan I, Gottesman MM: Retroviral transfer of a chimeric multidrug resistance-adenosine deaminase gene. FASEB J 4:1501, 1990

80. Podda S, Ward M, Himelstein A et al: Transfer and expression of the human multiple drug resistance gene into live mice. Proc Natl Acad Sci U S A 89:9676, 1992

81. Sorrentino BP, Brandt SJ, Bodine D et al: Selection of drug-resistant bone marrow cells in vivo after retroviral transfer of human MDR1. Science 257:99, 1992

82. Ward M, Richardson C, Pioli P et al: Bank. Transfer and expression of the human multiple drug resistance gene in human CD34+ cells. Blood 84:1408, 1994

83. Hesdorffer C, Antman K, Bank A et al: Clinical protocol: human MDR gene transfer in patients with advanced cancer. Hum Gene Ther 5:1151, 1994

84. Grossman M, Raper SE, Kozarsky K et al: Successful ex vivo gene therapy directed to liver in a patient with familial hypercholesterolemia. Nature 6:335, 1994

85. Dichek DA, Bratthauer GL, Beg ZH et al: A genetic therapy for familial hypercholesterolemia. Trans Assoc Am Physicians 103:73, 1990

86. Chowdhury JR, Grossman M, Gupta S et al: Long-term improvement of hypercholesterolemia after ex

vivo gene therapy in LDLR-deficient rabbits. Science 254:1802, 1991

87. Welsh MJ, Smith AE: Cystic fibrosis gene therapy using an adenovirus vector—in vivo safety and efficacy in nasal epithelium. Hum Gene Ther 5:209, 1994

88. Weinthal J, Nolta JA, Yu XJ et al: Expression of human glucocerebrosidase following retroviral vector-mediated transduction of murine hematopoietic stem cells. Bone Marrow Transplant 8:403, 1991

89. Xu L, Stahl SK, Dave HP et al: Correction of the enzyme deficiency in hematopoietic cells of Gaucher patients using a clinically acceptable retroviral supernatant transduction protocol. Exp Hematol 22:223, 1994

90. Kohn DB, Nolta JA, Weinthal J et al: Toward gene therapy for Gaucher disease. Hum Gene Ther 2:101, 1991

91. Boat TF, Welsh MJ, Beaudet AL: Cystic fibrosis. p. 2649. In Scriver CR, Beaudet AL, Sly WS, Valle D (eds): The Metabolic Basis of Inherited Disease. McGraw-Hill, New York, 1989

92. Wood RE, Boat TF, Doershuk CF: Cystic fibrosis. Am Rev Respir Dis 113:833, 1976

93. Porteous DJ, Dorin JR: Cystic fibrosis. 3. Cloning the cystic fibrosis gene: implications for diagnosis and treatment. Thorax 46:46, 1991

94. Rommens JM, Iannuzzi MC, Kerem BS et al: Identification of the cystic fibrosis gene: chromosome walking and jumping. Science 245:1059, 1989

95. Drumm ML, Pope HA, Cliff WH et al: Correction of the cystic fibrosis defect in vitro by retrovirus-mediated gene transfer. Cell 62:1227, 1990

96. Rich DP, Anderson MP, Gregory RJ et al: Expression of cystic fibrosis transmembrane conductance regulator corrects defective chloride channel regulation in cystic fibrosis airway epithelial cells. Nature 347:358, 1990

97. Kerem BS, Rommens JM, Buchanan JA et al: Identification of the cystic fibrosis gene: genetic analysis. Science 245:1073, 1989

98. Riordan JR, Rommens JM, Kerem BS et al: Identification of the cystic fibrosis gene: cloning and characterization of complementary DNA. Science 245:1066, 1989

99. Olsen JC, Gohnson LG, Stutts MJ et al: Correction of the apical membrane chloride permeability defect in polarized cystic fibrosis airway epithelia following retroviral-mediated gene transfer. Hum Gene Ther 3:253, 1992

100. Flotte TR, Afione SA, Solow R et al: Expression of the cystic fibrosis transmembrane conductance regulator

from a novel adeno-associated virus promoter. J Biol Chem 268:3781, 1993

101. Dropulic B, Jeang K-T: Gene therapy for human immunodeficiency virus infection: genetic antiviral strategies and targets for intervention. Hum Gene Ther 5:927, 1994

102. Baltimore D: Intracellular immunization. Nature 335:395, 1988

103. Herskowitz I: Functional inactivation of genes by dominant negative mutations. Nature 329:219, 1987

104. Malim MH, Freimuth WW, Liu J et al: Stable expression of transdominant rev protein in human T cells inhibits human immunodeficiency virus replication. J Exp Med 176:1197, 1992

105. Balboni PG, Bozzini R, Zocchini S et al: Inhibition of human immunodeficiency virus reactivation from latency by a tat transdominant negative mutant. J Med Virol 41:289, 1993

106. Lisziewicz J, Sun D, Smythe G et al: Inhibition of human immunodeficiency virus type 1 replication by regulated expression of a polymeric tat activation response RNA decoy as a strategy for gene therapy in AIDS. Proc Natl Acad Sci U S A 90:8000, 1993

107. Freed EO, Delwart EL, Buchschacher GL, Jr, Panganiban AT: A mutation in the human immunodeficiency virus type 1 transmembrane glycoprotein gp41 dominantly interferes with fusion and infectivity. Proc Natl Acad Sci U S A 89:70, 1992

108. Trono D, Feinberg MB, Baltimore D: HIV-1 gag mutants can dominantly interfere with the replication of the wild-type virus. Cell 59:113, 1989

109. Nabel GJ, Fox BA, Post L et al: A molecular genetic intervention for AIDS—effects of a transdominant negative form of rev. Hum Gene Ther 5:79, 1994

110. Malim MH, McCarn DF, Tiley LS, Cullen BR: Mutational definition of the human immunodeficiency virus type 1 rev activation domain. J Virol 65:4248, 1991

111. Malim MH, Bohnlein S, Hauber J, Cullen BR: Functional dissection of the HIV-1 rev trans-activator-derivation of a trans-dominant repressor of rev function. Cell 58:205, 1989

112. Bahner I, Zhow C, Yu X-J et al: Comparison of transdominant inhibitory mutant human immunodeficiency virus type 1 genes expressed by retroviral vectors in human T lymphcytes. J Virol 67:3199, 1993

113. Sullenger BA, Gallardo HF, Ungers GE, Gilboa E: Analysis of trans-acting response decoy RNA-mediated inhibition of human immunodeficiency virus type 1 transactivation. J Virol 65:6811, 1991

114. Sullenger BA, Gallardo HF, Ungers GE, Gilboa E: Overexpression of TAR sequences renders cells resis-

tant to human immunodeficiency virus replication. Cell 63:601, 1990

115. Graham GJ, Maio JJ: RNA transcripts of the human immunodeficiency virus transactivation response element can inhibit action of the viral transactivator. Proc Natl Acad Sci U S A 87:5817, 1990

116. Lee TC, Sullenger BA, Gallardo HF et al: Overexpression of RRE-derived sequences inhibits HIV-1 replication in CEM cells. New Biologist 4:66, 1992

117. Chatterjee S, Johnson PR, Wong KK, Jr: Dual-target inhibition of HIV-1 in vitro by means of an adeno-associated virus antisense vector. Science 258:1485, 1992

118. Joshi S, Van Brunschot A, Asad S et al: Inhibition of human immunodeficiency virus type 1 multiplication by antisense and sense RNA Expression. J Virol 65:5524, 1991

119. Sczakiel G, Pawlita M: Inhibition of human immunodeficiency virus type 1 replication in human T cells stably expressing antisense RNA. J Virol 65:468, 1991

120. Rhodes A, James W: Inhibition of human immunodeficiency virus replication in cell culture by endogenously synthesized antisense RNA. J Gen Virol 71:1965, 1990

121. Goodchild J, Agrawal S, Civeira MP et al: Inhibition of human immunodeficiency virus replication by antisense oligodeoxynucleotides. Proc Natl Acad Sci U S A 85:5507, 1988

122. Cech TR, Bass BL: Biological catalysis by RNA. Annu Rev Biochem 55:599, 1986

123. Odai O, Kodama H, Hiroaki H et al: Synthesis and NMR study of ribooligonucleotides forming a hammerhead-type RNA enzyme system. Nucleic Acids Res 18:5955, 1990

124. Hampel A, Tritz R, Hicks M, Cruz P: "Hairpin" catalytic RNA model: evidence for helices and sequence requirement for substrate RNA. Nucleic Acids Res 18:299, 1990

125. Koizumi M, Iwai S, Ohtsuka E: Cleavage of specific sites of RNA by designed ribozymes. FEBS Lett 239:285, 1988

126. Jeffries AC, Symons RH: A catalytic 13-mer ribozyme. Nucleic Acids Res 17:1371, 1989

127. Sarver N, Cantin EM, Chang PS et al: Ribozymes as potential anti-HIV-1 therapeutic agents. Science 247:1222, 1990

128. Weerasinghe M, Liem SE, Asad S et al: Resistance to human immunodeficiency virus type 1 (HIV-1) infection in human lymphocyte-derived cell lines conferred by using retroviral vectors expressing an HIV-1 RNA-specific ribozyme. J Virol 65:5531, 1991

129. Lo KMS, Biasolo MA, Dehni G et al: Inhibition of replication of HIV-1 by retroviral vectors expressing tat-antisense and anti-tat ribozyme RNA. Virology 190:176, 1992

130. Chen C-J, Banerjea AC, Harmison GG et al: Multitarget-ribozyme directed to cleave at up to nine highly conserved HIV-1 env RNA regions inhibits HIV-1 replication—potential effectiveness against most presently sequenced HIV-1 isolates. Nucleic Acids Res 20:4581, 1992

131. Zhou C, Bahner IC, Larson GP et al: Inhibition of HIV-1 in human T-lymphocytes by retrovirally transduced anti-tat and rev hammerhead ribozymes. Gene 149:33, 1994

132. Ojwang JO, Hampel AP, Looney DJ et al: Inhibition of human immunodeficiency virus type 1 expression by a hairpin ribozyme. Proc Natl Acad Sci U S A 89:10802, 1992

133. Yu M, Ojwang J, Yamada O et al: Hairpin ribozyme inhibits expression of diverse strains of human immunodeficiency virus type 1. Proc Natl Acad Sci U S A 90:6340, 1993

134. Leavitt MC, Yu M, Yamada O et al: Transfer of an anti-HIV-1 ribozyme gene into primary human lymphocytes. Hum Gene Ther 5:1115, 1994

135. Lin X, Dashti A, Schinazi RF, Tang J: Intracellular diversion of glycoprotein gp160 of human immunodeficiency virus to lysosomes as a strategy of AIDS gene therapy. FASEB J 7:1070, 1993

136. Greenberg P, Riddell S: Clinical protocol: adoptive immunotherapy for AIDS. Hum Gene Ther 3:319, 1992

137. Laube LS, Burrascano M, DeJesus CE et al: Cytotoxic T lymphocyte and antibody responses generated in rhesus monkeys immunized with retroviral vector-transduced fibroblasts expressing human immunodeficiency virus type-1 IIIB env/rev proteins. Hum Gene Ther 5:853, 1994

138. Ulmer JB, Donnelly JJ, Parker SE et al: Heterologous protection against influenza by injection of DNA encoding a viral protein. Science 259:1745, 1993

139. Nabel EG, Plautz G, Nabel GJ: Site-specific gene expression in vivo by direct gene transfer into the arterial wall. Science 249:1285, 1990

140. Bonadio J, Jepson KJ, Mansoura MK et al: A murine skeletal adaptation that significantly increases cortical bone mechanical properties: implications for human skeletal fragility. J Clin Invest 92:1697, 1993

141. Green ED, Waterston RH: The human genome project. Prospects and implications for clinical medicine. JAMA 266:1966, 1991

142. Gilardi P, Courtney M, Pavirani A, Perricaudet M: Expression of human alpha 1-antitrypsin using a re-

combinant adenovirus vector. FEBS Lett 267:60, 1990

143. Kay MA, Landen CN, Rothenberg SR et al: In vivo hepatic gene therapy—complete albeit transient correction of factor IX deficiency in hemophilia B dogs. Proc Natl Acad Sci U S A 91:2353, 1994

144. Lung HY, Cornelius JB, Peck AB: Cloning and expression of the oxalyl-CoA decarboxylase gene from the bacterium, *Oxalobacter formigenes*: prospects for gene therapy to control Ca-oxalate kidney stone formation. Am J Kidney Dis 17:381, 1991

145. Wilson JM, Chowdhury JR: Prospects for gene therapy of familial hypercholesterolemia. Mol Biol Med 7:223, 1990

Index

Note: Page numbers followed by f indicate figures; those followed by t indicate tables.

A

AABB. *See* American Association of Blood Banks (AABB).
Abdominal aortic aneurysms, blood saving strategies for, 529
ABO blood group system, 77–78
  ABH-soluble substances, 78
  antibodies, 79–81
    differential absorption technique and, 482
    in pregnancy, 80
  antibody typing
    in autoimmune hemolytic anemia, 474–475, 474t
    for autologous component therapy, 311
    historical aspects of, 200
    for pediatric transfusion, 328
    procedure for, 201
  antigens, 78
    biosynthesis of, 76–77, 77f
    disease associations of, 83–84
    minor incompatibilities and, 769
    precursors of, 81–82, 82t
  biochemistry, 81–82, 82t
  clinical significance, 83–84
  compatibility
    for component therapy, 320, 320t
    for granulocyte transfusion, 425–426
    for liver transplantation, 794–795
    matched platelets, for platelet transfusion refractoriness, 388
    for platelet transfusions, 378–379
  conversion, by surface antigen removal, 223

discovery, 24, 71
genetics, 81
incompatibility, 83
  in bone marrow transplantation, plasma exchange for, 743
  delayed hemolytic transfusion reactions and, 922, 923f
  hemolysis from, 397–399, 523–524, 575
  with pregnancy, 41
  transfusion reactions and, 510, 523–524, 575
phenotypes, 81–83
secretors, 76, 78, 84, 88
subgroups, 78–79, 79t, 80t
Abruptio placentae, 583
Abscesses, granulocyte transfusions for, 418
Accreditation Association for Ambulatory Health Care, 296
Accutane (isotretinoin), 261
Acid-citrate-dextrose (ACD), 28
Acidosis, in shock, 566
Acquired immunodeficiency syndrome (AIDS), 351. *See also* Human immunodeficiency virus (HIV).
  anemia, in zidouvidine-treated patients, 1026
  cytomegalovirus infection risk and, 879
  Epstein-Barr virus infection and, 886
  gene therapy for, 1076–1078, 1076t
  graft-versus-host disease and, 933
  granulocyte transfusions for, 421
  health care delivery and, 296

progression
  in heavily transfused patients, 60
  from HIV-I infection, 828
  risk perception, 813
  transfusion-related transmission
    community education programs and, 250
    exclusion of donor groups/sites and, 247–248
    risk of, 827, 827f
Activated clotting time, for heparin therapy monitoring, 735
Activated partial thromboplastin time (aPTT), in von Willebrand's disease, 598
Acute chest syndrome, erythrocytopheresis for, 746–747, 747f
Acute lymphoblastic leukemia (ALL), 705
  platelet transfusions, 709
    alloimmunization and, 721, 721t
Acute nonlymphoblastic leukemia (ANLL)
  bleeding risk, 361–362
  platelet transfusions, 710
    alloimmunization and, 721, 721t
Acute RNA tumor viruses, 824–825
Acute T-cell leukemia (ATL), HTLV-I and, 835
Acyclovir, 884
Additive solutions, for red blood cell concentrates, 571
Adenoassociated virus vectors, 1068–1069, 1069f
Adenosine triphosphate (ATP), 308, 576